1 MONT
FREE
READING

at

www.ForgottenBooks.com

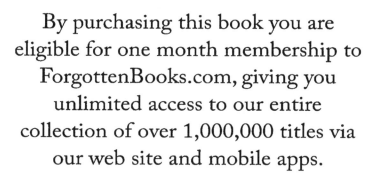

By purchasing this book you are eligible for one month membership to ForgottenBooks.com, giving you unlimited access to our entire collection of over 1,000,000 titles via our web site and mobile apps.

To claim your free month visit:

www.forgottenbooks.com/free1374921

* Offer is valid for 45 days from date of purchase. Terms and conditions apply.

1,000,000 Books

are available to read at

ISBN 978-1-397-31319-5
PIBN 11374921

THE

JOHNS HOPKINS HOSPITAL

BULLETIN

VOLUME XVII

BALTIMORE
THE JOHNS HOPKINS PRESS
1906

The Friedenwald Company
BALTIMORE, MD., U. S. A.

BULLETIN

OF

THE JOHNS HOPKINS HOSPITAL

Entered as Second-Class Matter at the Baltimore, Maryland, Postoffice.

Vol. XVII.—No. 178.]   BALTIMORE, JANUARY, 1906.   [Price, 25 Cents.

CONTENTS.

DR. GARTH: THE KIT-KAT POET.*

(1661-1718.)

BY HARVEY CUSHING, M. D.

IN the reign of Queen Anne, a pasty-cook, one Christopher or Kit for short, 'immortal made by his pyes,' kept a tavern near Temple Bar at the Sign of the Cat and Fiddle. Here was wont to gather a group of the most distinguished men of the time, the patriots that saved Britain, according to the opinion of one who in the succeeding generation bore the name of not the least illustrious of them; leaders of the fashionable world, noblemen, poets, statesmen, soldiers; all fine gentlemen, all earnest Whigs, firmly sworn to support the Protestant succession in the house of Hanover. Of this famous club there were first and last some forty-eight members, including the great Marlborough, Robert Walpole, Godolphin, and Halifax, Addison and Steele, Kneller the artist, and Vanbrugh the builder of Blenheim, Jacob Tonson the famous book-seller—Pope's left leg'd Jacob—and many more

besides the subject of this sketch, the popular, the generous, the companionable Garth.

Mary Pierrepont, the daughter of Lord Kingston, one of the noblemen who helped to make up this distinguished coterie, was during her childhood an object of her father's special pride and fondness, and the following incident which in later years she loved to recall has been thus related by her granddaughter. "One day at a meeting to choose toasts for the year, a whim seized him to nominate her, then not eight years old,[1] a candidate, alleging that she was far prettier than

---

* Read at a Meeting of the Johns Hopkins Hospital Historical Club, December 12, 1904.

[1] Lady Mary, according to recent authority (Firth, DICT. OF NAT. BIOG.), was born in May, 1689, and the Kit-Kat Club, as such, was supposedly not founded until 1703, so that unless the Club held meetings, as is quite possible, before the designation of Kit-Kats was given them, she was not the child she feigned to have been. There is much confusion in regard to dates of many events of these times, especially in regard to such hearsay ones.

The Friedenwald Company
BALTIMORE, MD., U. S. A.

BULLETIN

OF

THE JOHNS HOPKINS HOSPITAL

Entered as Second-Class Matter at the Baltimore, Maryland, Postoffice.

Vol. XVII.—No. 178.]   BALTIMORE, JANUARY, 1906.   [Price, 25 Cents.

CONTENTS.

DR. GARTH: THE KIT-KAT POET.*

(1661-1718.)

By Harvey Cushing, M. D.

In the reign of Queen Anne, a pasty-cook, one Christopher or Kit for short, 'immortal made by his pyes,' kept a tavern near Temple Bar at the Sign of the Cat and Fiddle. Here was wont to gather a group of the most distinguished men of the time, the patriots that saved Britain, according to the opinion of one who in the succeeding generation bore the name of not the least illustrious of them; leaders of the fashionable world, noblemen, poets, statesmen, soldiers; all fine gentlemen, all earnest Whigs, firmly sworn to support the Protestant succession in the house of Hanover. Of this famous club there were first and last some forty-eight members, including the great Marlborough, Robert Walpole, Godolphin, and Halifax, Addison and Steele, Kneller the artist, and Vanbrugh the builder of Blenheim, Jacob Tonson the famous book-seller—Pope's left leg'd Jacob—and many more

besides the subject of this sketch, the popular, the generous, the companionable Garth.

Mary Pierrepont, the daughter of Lord Kingston, one of the noblemen who helped to make up this distinguished coterie, was during her childhood an object of her father's special pride and fondness, and the following incident which in later years she loved to recall has been thus related by her granddaughter. "One day at a meeting to choose toasts for the year, a whim seized him to nominate her, then not eight years old,[1] a candidate, alleging that she was far prettier than

* Read at a Meeting of the Johns Hopkins Hospital Historical Club, December 12, 1904.

[1] Lady Mary, according to recent authority (Firth, Dict. of Nat. Biog.), was born in May, 1689, and the Kit-Kat Club, as such, was supposedly not founded until 1703, so that unless the Club held meetings, as is quite possible, before the designation of Kit-Kats was given them, she was not the child she feigned to have been. There is much confusion in regard to dates of many events of these times, especially in regard to such hearsay ones.

any lady on the list. The other members demurred because the rules of the club forbade them to elect a beauty whom they had never seen. 'Then you shall see her,' cried he; and in the gaiety of the moment sent orders home to have her finely dressed, and brought to him at the tavern; where she was received with acclamations, her claim unanimously allowed, her health drunk by every one present, and her name engraved in due form on a drinking glass. The company consisting of some of the most eminent men in England, she went from the lap of one poet or patriot or statesman to the arms of another, was feasted with sweet-meats, overwhelmed with caresses, and," Lady Louisa Stewart adds with a touch of irony, "what perhaps already pleased her better than either, heard her wit and beauty loudly extolled on every side. Pleasure, she said, was too poor a word to express her sensations; they amounted to ecstasy; never again throughout her whole future life, did she pass so happy a day."

It is pleasing to think that Samuel Garth, the single medical member of the club, may have participated in this scene, and that the child toast, whom he, unlike some others, continned to admire throughout his life, was passed to him in turn for a greeting. Little could he then have thought that her name, both in medicine and letters, would almost outshine and outlive his own: for the child heroine of this episode was none other than the Lady Mary Wortley Montague whose gallant struggle against the popular prejudice and professional jealousy of the times, in her effort to introduce the practice of "ingrafting" against the small-pox, must ever make her an object of interest to medical men.

One may perchance be the more readily excused for plunging into an incident almost in Garth's middle life, inasmuch as there are no details of

> How the dim speck of entity began
> T'extend its recent form, and stretch to man;
> *The Dispensary,* CANTO I.

and but scant ones of the time intervening until he became the popular and well known figure in the metropolis. He was born of a good family in Yorkshire,[1] probably in 1661; was at school in the village of Ingleton, a neighborhood of most romantic scenery; a student at Peterhouse, the eldest of the Cambridge Colleges, where he matriculated July 6, 1676, received his B. A. in 1679, and five years later a Master's degree in arts. These are the bare facts which carry us through the first twenty-five years of Garth's life without further illumination from contemporary writings. What induced him to take up Physick for his life's work seems not to be known, unless it was the direct influence of his college,[2] and the

[1] The eldest son of Wm. Garth of Bowland Forest in the West Riding (DICT. OF NAT. BIOG.).

[2] "Among the colleges at least one (Peterhouse) had in past times a laudable custom of urging her fellows to determine themselves in the line of some faculty—going on 'the Law line,' or that of Physic, or of Divinity." Wordsworth's SCHOLAE ACADEMICAE; Some account of the studies at the English Universities in the eighteenth century. Cambridge, 1877.

promise for the better in medicine of Sydenham's and Locke's recent and great reforms. The colleges, however, at the time, had only theoretical instruction in preparation for practice, and it was the custom for those very few students, who like Garth took their degree in arts before entering upon their professional studies, to look elsewhere for opportunities to gain practical knowledge. With this object in 1687 he repaired to Leyden, then approaching the zenith of its medical fame; and there Garth may possibly have touched elbows in his classes with the young Dutchman who was destined to become the greatest clinician of his time, and whose name made that of his university famous to the ends of the earth. Four years later (July 7, 1691) Garth received from his alma mater the degree of M.D., and repairing to the metropolis he was promptly admitted (June 26, 1693) a Fellow of the College of Physicians.

He must early have distinguished himself, for in the following year he is said to have delivered the Gulstonian Lecture, choosing *De Respiratione* as his text. Although a request was made that he should do so, Garth never published this discourse, and consequently we have lost the only one of his strictly medical writings of which knowledge has come down to us.

A further and still greater compliment was paid the young physician three years later, in 1697, when he was asked to deliver the annual oration in Latin before the College on St. Luke's Day—better known to us as the Harveian Oration.[3]

ORATIO LAUDATORIA
IN AEDIBUS
COLLEGII REGALIS MED. LOND.
17MO DIE SEPTEMBRIS
HABITA
A. SAM GARTH
COLL. REG. MED. LOND. SOC.
LONDINI
MDCXCVII.

The public tribute that Garth on this occasion paid to William III, as well as the tirade, at the close of the oration, against the professional quackery of the times, proved doubly influential in his career; the tribute, an open demonstration of his political affiliations, bringing him later on his Knighthood; the tirade, immediately, as it made him the acknowledged champion of the College of Physicians in a famous quarrel: for thus he was led to write the poem on which alone his position among the English poets rests. But to explain this I must retrace my steps.

THE DISPENSARIAN QUARREL.

A CERTAIN lack of sympathy seems always to have existed between those privileged to prescribe, and those who are restricted by law to the dispensation alone of drugs; and at the time of which we are writing a combination of circumstances had fanned latent animosity into a public

[3] An original paper copy of this oration will be found in the Surgeon-General's Library in Washington.

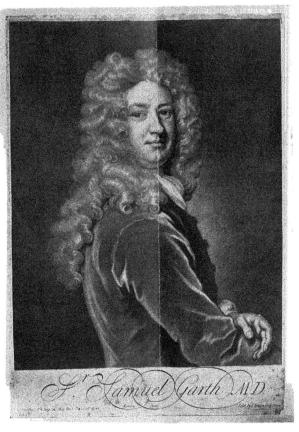

any lady on the list.. The other members demurred because the rules of the club forbade them to elect a beauty whom they had never seen. 'Then you shall see her,' cried he; and in the gaiety of the moment sent orders home to have her finely dressed, and brought to him at the tavern; where she was received with acclamations, her claim unanimously allowed, her health drunk by every one present, and her name engraved in due form on a drinking glass. The company consisting of some of the most eminent men in England, she went from the lap of one poet or patriot or statesman to the arms of another, was feasted with sweet-meats, overwhelmed with caresses, and,' Lady Louisa Stewart adds with a touch of irony, " what perhaps already pleased her better than either, heard her wit and beauty loudly extolled on every side. Pleasure, she said, was too poor a word to express her sensations; they amounted to ecstasy; never again throughout her whole future life, did she pass so happy a day."

It is pleasing to think that Samuel Garth, the single medical member of the club, may have participated in this scene, and that the child toast, whom he, unlike some others, continned to admire throughout his life, was passed to him in turn for a greeting. Little could he then have thought that her name, both in medicine and letters, would almost outshine and outlive his own: for the child heroine of this episode was none other than the Lady Mary Wortley Montague whose gallant struggle against the popular prejudice and professional jealousy of the times, in her effort to introduce the practice of " ingrafting " against the small-pox, must ever make her an object of interest to medical men.

One may perchance be the more readily excused for plunging into an incident almost in Garth's middle life, inasmuch as there are no details of

> How the dim speck of entity began
> T'extend its recent form, and stretch to man;
> *The Dispensary*, CANTO I.

and but scant ones of the time intervening until he became the popular and well known figure in the metropolis. He was born of a good family in Yorkshire,' probably in 1661; was at school in the village of Ingleton, a neighborhood of most romantic scenery; a student at Peterhouse, the eldest of the Cambridge Colleges, where he matriculated July 6, 1676, received his B. A. in 1679, and five years later a Master's degree in arts. These are the bare facts which carry us through the first twenty-five years of Garth's life without further illumination from contemporary writings. What induced him to take up Physick for his life's work seems not to be known, unless it was the direct influence of his college,' and the

---

' The eldest son of Wm. Garth of Bowland Forest in the West Riding (DICT. OF NAT. BIOG.).

' " Among the colleges at least one (Peterhouse) had in past times a laudable custom of urging her fellows to determine themselves in the line of some faculty—going on 'the Law line,' or that of Physic, or of Divinity." Wordsworth's SCHOLAE ACADEMICAE; Some account of the studies at the English Universities in the eighteenth century. Cambridge, 1877.

promise for the better in medicine of Sydenham's and Locke's recent and great reforms. The colleges, however, at the time, had only theoretical instruction in preparation for practice, and it was the custom for those very few students, who like Garth took their degree in arts before entering upon their professional studies, to look elsewhere for opportunities to gain practical knowledge. With this object in 1687 he repaired to Leyden, then approaching the zenith of its medical fame; and there Garth may possibly have touched elbows in his classes with the young Dutchman who was destined to become the greatest clinician of his time, and whose name made that of his university famous to the ends of the earth. Four years later (July 7, 1691) Garth received from his alma mater the degree of M.D., and repairing to the metropolis he was promptly admitted (June 26, 1693) a Fellow of the College of Physicians.

He must early have distinguished himself, for in the following year he is said to have delivered the Gulstonian Lecture, choosing *De Respiratione* as his text. Although a request was made that he should do so, Garth never published this discourse, and consequently we have lost the only one of his strictly medical writings of which knowledge has come down to us.

A further and still greater compliment was paid the young physician three years later, in 1697, when he was asked to deliver the annual oration in Latin before the College on St. Luke's Day—better known to us as the Harveian Oration.'

ORATIO LAUDATORIA
IN AEDIBUS
COLLEGII REGALIS MED. LOND.
17MO DIE SEPTEMBRIS
HABITA
A. SAM GARTH
COLL. REG. MED. LOND. SOC.
LONDINI
MDCXCVII.

The public tribute that Garth on this occasion paid to William III, as well as the tirade, at the close of the oration, against the professional quackery of the times, proved doubly influential in his career; the tribute, an open demonstration of his political affiliations, bringing him later on his Knighthood; the tirade, immediately, as it made him the acknowledged champion of the College of Physicians in a famous quarrel: for thus he was led to write the poem on which alone his position among the English poets rests. But to explain this I must retrace my steps:

THE DISPENSARIAN QUARREL.

A CERTAIN lack of sympathy seems always to have existed between those privileged to prescribe, and those who are restricted by law to the dispensation alone of drugs; and at the time of which we are writing a combination of circumstances had fanned latent animosity into a public

---

'. An original paper copy of this oration will be found in the Surgeon-General's Library in Washington.

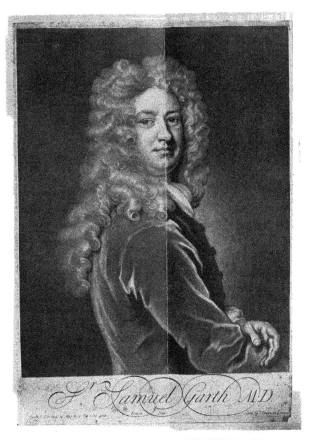

Sr Samuel Garth M.D

FROM JACOB TONSON'S MEZZOTINT REPRODUCTIONS OF KNELLER'S PORTRAITS OF THE KIT-KAT CLUB MEMBERS.

broil. The apothecaries, for the most part, were uneducated men and at a somewhat earlier period their relation to the community was so loosely controlled that even the grocers and pepperers were privileged to dispense drugs and the fact that they were legalized, under certain circumstances, to perform phlebotomy sufficed to bring them intimately into contact with the people as patients. By a charter, granted early in the reign of James I, they had been made "Freemen of the Mystery of Grocers and Apothecaries of the City of London," but soon such remonstrance was raised on all sides against their incompetence and such scandal over the adulteration of their commodities that in 1617, owing to the intervention of one of the few distinguished members of their fraternity, Gideon de Laune, the apothecaries were separated by charter from their former associates, the grocers. The new grant placed them under the control of the College of Physicians and to this body was given the power of inspecting their wares and regulating their actions. This restraint was far from agreeable; its consequences were inevitable. The medical therapy of the time was based almost entirely on empiricism and the vendors of drugs found therefore that it was a simple matter to compete with the qualified practitioners. They encroached more and more on the physician's province; some of them indeed amassing large fortunes thereby.

> So modern 'Pothecaries taught the art
> By Doctors bills to play the Doctor's part
> Bold in the practice of mistaken rules
> Prescribe, apply, and call their masters fools.
> *Essay on Criticism.*

Thus Pope, some years later, described the situation as analogous in a measure to that occupied by the critics who had come to turn their own arms against the poets from whom they had first learned to write. It has been said by Jeaffreson that the doctors of the day knew so little that the apothecaries found little difficulty in knowing as much and there need be little wonder at the story that has come down to us of one of Radcliffe's patients who left him preferring to be treated by a well known apothecary. Thus it was not long before the apothecaries grew away from the restraint legally imposed upon them and regardless of the College began to prescribe widely on their own responsibility. Were they threatened with punishment, they retaliated by refusing to call in consultation the physician who had censured them; an action that in many cases might have completely ruined his practice. The dependence that many placed on these consultations, even at a later date, is illustrated by the story of Mead, who in the morning at Batson's coffee-house, in the evening at Tom's, used to receive apothecaries and charge only half-guinea fees for prescriptions written without seeing the patient. The situation was a most entangled one. The apothecaries defended themselves on the ground that they would prescribe and care for the poor who could not afford to pay the physician's fees in addition to the expense of the drugs; possibly a just claim were our beliefs in their charitable pretenses not shaken by a knowledge of what were their actual practices.

In 1687 the first effort to counteract these abuses was made by the College. An edict was unanimously passed by that body (July 28, 1687), requiring all the fellows, candidates and licentiates to give gratuitous advice to their neighboring poor; but the solution of the difficulty was not so simple. It was in the first place, as at the present day, difficult to designate those who were to be considered "poor," and the practice not only led to abuses but was further frustrated by the inordinately high price immediately put upon all drugs by the apothecaries. As the patients had not the wherewithal to get them filled, prescriptions were thrown to the winds. Under the shadow of benevolence, too, there is said to have lurked animosity toward the apothecaries; a spirit which of itself, if we are to believe the slander, would certainly have been fatal to the successful carrying out of the edict. With the

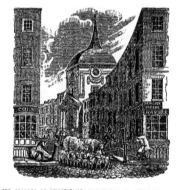

OLD COLLEGE OF PHYSICIANS, WARWICK LANE, NEAR NEWGATE.

From a print in the THE GOLD HEADED CANE.*

> Not far from that most celebrated Place
> Where angry Justice shews her awful face;
>   * * * * *
> There stands a Dome, Majestick to the Sight,
>   * * * * *
> A golden Globe placed high with artful Skill,
> Seems to the distant Light, a gilded Pill:
> *The Dispensary.*

view, however, of rendering it more effectual, it was determined by a vote in the following year (August 13, 1688), to accommodate the laboratory of the College to the purpose of preparing medicines; the contributors toward the expense were themselves to manage the charity. Such a philanthropy properly controlled would have effectually done away with the

---

* Especially in Munk's edition there is a full account of the various homes and places of meeting of the College from its establishment in 1518.

abuses of indiscriminate dispensing of drugs, had the apothe-caries submitted to it. Not so. They claimed that it was a money-making scheme on the part of the physicians who aimed thereby merely to undersell them. They even succeeded in raising an opposition in the very College itself [a] among those who at heart and for selfish reasons favored the old system; so that Dispensarians found themselves arrayed against Anti-Dispensarians and the design failed of being carried into execution.

At this juncture, with the College in an embroiled state, Garth, fresh from the university, appeared at the metropolis; he was early admitted a fellow and allied himself unhesitat-ingly with the Dispensarian party. Courageously, too, since for a youth on foot with little more than his diploma in his pocket to take a stand openly against ' affluent tradesmen,' rolling by in their carriages,' as Jeaffreson puts it, who might absolutely injure his prospects, must have required the cour-age of conviction.

In 1694, the College again succeeded in issuing an order demanding from all members strict obedience to the edict of 1688; and in the following year [b] this new order was presented to the city authorities in the hope of gaining their support; a hope unfortunately defeated. Not discouraged, the physicians of the Dispensarian party actually raised a subscription (December 22, 1696), from among those favoring the charity, each subscribing ten pounds, the money to be " expended in preparing and delivering medicines to the poor at their intrinsic value." To disarm the insinuations of their oppo-nents and to show that the undertaking had the sanction of a College act, the names of all the subscribers, fifty-one in number, were appended to a printed sheet which was widely distributed.[c] Thus for a time, there was an actual distribu-tion to the needy of drugs at cost price, and though the experiment was perhaps poorly conducted, its philanthropic intent was genuine enough; as Garth says, it was managed with an integrity and disinterest suitable to so charitable a

---

[a] Perhaps made the more easy as one of the members, Francis Bernard had formerly been an apothecary; but owing to distin-guished services had been elevated to the post of assistant physi-cian to St. Bartholomew's and also elected to the College in 1687. He was an able and very scholarly man and, remaining loyal to his former guild, must have been a formidable opponent to the Dispensarian party. He is the ' Horoscope' of Garth's poem.

[b] A Short Account of the Proceedings of the College of Physi-cians, London, in Relation to the Sick Poor, 1697. See, also, The Copy of an Instrument Subscribed by the President, Censors, Most of the Elects, Senior Fellows, Candidates, etc., of the Col-lege of Physicians in Relation to the Sick Poor.

[c] Among the names occur those of Sir Thos. Millington, who with Boyle, Wrenn, Willis and others had helped found the Royal Society, and who was then president of the College; of Sir Hans Sloane, a later President of the College, who subse-quently served in that capacity for sixteen years, and who founded the British Museum; of Edward Browne, scholar and traveller, el-dest son of the author of the *Religio Medici*; Robert Brady, the historian and friend of Sydenham; Charles Goodall, also a later president; Sir Edward Hulse and many others.

design, though the effort sufficed only to make the long stand-ing disagreement " break out to fury and excess." The usual form of warfare—a paper warfare, emanating from Grub Street—arose. There are many references to the controversy, even in the more stable writings of the time, and it is apparent that most of the men of education outside the profession upheld the cause of the Dispensarians. Among them was Dryden, as shown by the following lines inscribed to a relative, who ' blessed led a country life.'

> The tree of knowledge, once in Eden placed,
> Was easy found, but was forbid the taste;
> O, had our grandsire walked without his wife,
> He first had sought the better plant of life!
> Now both are lost: yet wandering in the dark,
> Physicians for the tree have found the bark;
> They, laboring for relief of human kind,
> With sharpened sight some remedies may find;
> The apothecary-train is wholly blind.
> From files a random recipe they take,
> And many deaths of one prescription make.
> Garth, generous as his Muse, prescribes and gives;
> The shopman sells and by destruction lives;
> Ungrateful tribe! who, like the viper's brood,
> From Medicine issuing, suck their mother's blood!   .
> Let these obey and let the learned prescribe,
> That men may die without a double bribe;
> . Let them, but under their superiors, kill,
> When doctors first have signed the bloody bill:
> He 'scapes the best, who, nature to repair,
> Draws physic from the fields in draughts of vital air.[d]

Garth, seemingly, first became an active belligerent in this warfare from the vantage ground of his Harveian Oration, when, as above mentioned, he took the opportunity of " public-ally ridiculing the multifarious classes of quacks, with spirit and not without humor." [e] Though by nature averse to any violent partisanship, his keen mind, ready wit and facile pen must have made him a formidable champion for any cause which he felt himself called upon to support. " In those old days," says Lady Louisa Stewart, " people's brains being more active than their fingers, ballads swarmed as abundantly as caricatures are swarming at present, and were struck off almost as hastily, whenever humor or malice and scurrility formed a theme to fasten upon." One of Garth's chance shafts was winged at this time against another rhyming physician, Sir Richard Blackmore, who, Saintsbury says, has been made

---

[d] John Dryden. To my Honored Kinsman, John Driden, of Chesterton. vs. 96-116. Garth well proved his generosity in Dryden's case, as a later incident will show.

[e] There is some difference of opinion as to the literary merit of this oration. Johnson quotes the single paragraph with which he was familiar and adds sarcastically, " this was cer-tainly thought fine by the author, etc.," but inasmuch as Garth's life was one of the hurried parts of the Biographical Series, Johnson doubtless made no effort to read his writings even were they accessible to him. Chalmers (Bioo. Dict. 1814) says of this speech, " which being soon after published, left it doubtful whether the poet or the orator was most to be admired."

immortal by his satirists" and seems to have been heartily abominated by all for his pomposity and 'amiable faith in himself.' Garth, ordinarily charitable enough, especially toward his professional brethren and political party, could not overlook Blackmore's anti-Dispensarian attitude and to ridicule him composed the following lines,—"To the Merry Poetaster at Sadler's Hall in Cheapside."

> Unwieldy pedant, let thy aukward muse
> With censures praise, with flatteries abuse.
> To lash, and not be felt, in thee's an art;
> Thou ne'er mad'st any but thy school-boys, smart.
> Then be advis'd and scribble not again;
> Thou'rt fashion'd for a flail, and not a pen.
> If B——l's immortal wit thou would'st descry,
> Pretend 'tis he that writ thy poetry.
> Thy feeble satire ne'er can do him wrong;
> Thy poems and thy patients live not long.

Poor as they are, there is nothing seriously objectionable in the ridicule of these lines and they suffice merely to illustrate the form of these poetical duels. The bad taste in twitting Blackmore with his early life as a school-master is nothing to the vulgarity, even more in accord with the times, which made physical infirmities a favorite object of satire. Dr. Garth, happily may not be accused of this offence.

"The Dispensary."

G ARTH, however, was capable of better things than the writing of doggerel verses. There appeared in 1699, in broadside paper form after the fashion of the times, an anonymous poem in six cantos called The Dispensary, in which the history of the attempt to establish gratuitous dispensation of drugs was put into rhyme. The poem had an immediate and unexpected success; was soon after printed in book form; went through two other editions before the year was out; and was so widely read during the next two decades, when its characters and subject matter were still of public interest, that ten authorized and some pirated editions were issued. There were several factors which must have contributed to its success: first among them, the rapidly spreading popularity of the author, whose touch must immediately have been recognized; the unusual form of versification, also, for Garth was among the first to show the influence which Boileau, the great French versifier, was to have on English poetry; possibly, too, the curiosity that must have been aroused by the fact that so many public characters figured in the poem either under fictitious names or with their actual ones feebly masked

by hyphenating the consonants." In his preface to the second edition, the author states his main purpose in writing the poem, for "finding the Animosities amongst the Members of the College of Physicians encreasing daily (not withstanding the frequent Exhortations of our Worthy President to the contrary) I was persuaded to attempt something of this nature, and to endeavor to Rally some of our disaffected Members into a sense of their Duty, who have hitherto most obstinately oppos'd all manner of Union; and have continu'd so unreasonably refractory, etc.," much such a purpose as an editorial in the Times or Lancet might have served today.

The poem, mock heroic in kind, opens with a description of the College "Rais'd for Use as Noble as its Frame," but in which the God of Sloth had made his lair; disturbed out of his lethargy by the enterprize attending the building of the Dispensary, the slumbering God sends his Phantom to summon Envy "to blast their Hopes and baffle their Designs."

In Canto II, Envy, the famish'd Fiend, rejoicing at the task, assumes the form of one Colon (Mr. Lee, Warden of Apothecaries Hall) and appears before Horoscope (Dr. Bernard) in his apothecary shop, where "Mummies lay most reverently stale" etc., and where Horoscope was found environed by a crowd of gullible people, promising them future Health for present Fees. Into his breast the Fury breathed a storm of envy against the Dispensarian movement and left it there like a Brood of Maggots to develop.

Horoscope, in Canto III, through his coadjutor, 'officious Squirt,' calls for a meeting of the Apothecaries at their Hall in Blackfriars; meanwhile he invokes to their aid the Harpy, Disease, "Begot by Sloth, maintain'd by Luxury," through a burnt offering of drugs and old prescriptions. Ill omen attends this sacrifice. The apothecaries meet; one advocates friendly advances to the Faculty; another, a bold fight at Honor's call; another, Askaris, more slyly urged a consultation with their friends the disaffected members of the Faculty, "who Int'rest prudently to Oaths prefer." The assemblage was scattered by an explosion in the laboratory of Apothecaries Hall.

Canto IV. At a tavern near Drury Lane, frequented by the apothecaries and where "want of Elbow-room's supply'd in Wine," the company again gather, together with some unprincipled members of the College whom they propose to use as their unwilling accomplices as "Boys hatch Game-Eggs under Birds o' Prey." There an altercation takes place between those advising caution and those clamoring for war.

" In the Spectator (No. 567, July 14, 1714) Addison ascribes this particular style of writing, so common in Anne's time, to Thomas Brown—the 'I do not love thee Dr. Fell' Thomas Brown—saying, "Some of our authors indeed, when they would be more satirical than ordinary, omit only the vowels of a great man's name, and fall most unmercifully upon all the consonants. This way of writing was first of all introduced by T—m B—wn of facetious memory."

This same Brown, in a broad-side—"Physic lies a Bleeding"—published in the heat of the Dispensarian quarrel, had himself a fling at the apothecaries!

Physic lies a Bleeding: or, The Apothecary turned Doctor. A Comedy acted almost every Day in most Apothecaries Shops in London. And more especially to be seen, by Those who are willing to be cheated, the First of April, every year. Absolutely necessary for all Persons that are Sick (or) may be Sick. (Quot. from Juvenal) by Tho. Brown. Dedicated to that worthy and ingenious Gentleman Dr. J. B. 4to, 1697.

" For example, one of Thomas Moore's epigrams runs:

> 'Twas in his carriage the sublime
> Sir Richard Blackmore used to rhyme,
> And if the wits don't do him wrong,
> 'Twixt death and epics passed his time
> Scribbling and killing all day long.

It ends in Horoscope being wafted away to the Fortunate Isles to consult the Goddess there. In oracular fashion she tells him that "Wars must insue, the Fates will have it so."

> "Dread Fates shall follow, and Disasters great,
> Pills charge on Pills, and Bolus Bolus meet:
> Both sides shall conquer and yet Both shall fall;
> The Mortar now, and then the Urinal."

CANTO V. Mirmillo, one of the traitorous physicians, begins to feel alarm for his safety in this alliance and is on the point of withdrawing when the Fury, *Discord*, appearing before him frightens him into joining the fray. The apothecary legions meet, the contestants in all manner of armament. Thus, Querpo

> "A Pestle for his Truncheon, led the Van
> And his high Helmet was a Close-Stool pan."

Rumor brought the news of the intended attack to Warwick Hall where preparations are hurriedly made to receive the assault. In mock heroic fashion the clash takes place with caustics, emetics, cathartics, syringes and what not, as weapons, while "Pestles peal a martial Symphony."

CANTO VI. In the midst of the battle the Goddess of *Health* appears, calls "enough" and bids Machaon (Millington, President of the College) send a messenger to the Elysian Fields to consult the immortal Harvey as to the best method of terminating their woes. Carus (Garth) is chosen for this mission and, Dante fashion, with *Hygeia* as his guide, he visits the lower regions. There, together with all sorts of wondrous subterranean phenomena, he sees old Chaos, an awkward Lump of shapeless Anarchy, with dull Night, his melancholy Consort; pale Fear and dark Distress; parch'd Eye'd Febris; bloated Hydrops; meagre Phthisis; Lepra the loathsome; as well as other Sights that go to "make up the frightful Horror o' the Place." They are at last ferried across the Styx and in the delightful Plain, "where the glad Manes of the Bless'd remain" the Shade of Harvey is found. The Venerable Sage addresses himself to *Hygeia* on the dissentions of the Faculty

> "Where sick'ning Art now hangs her Head,
> And once a Science, is become a Trade."

He finally turns to her companion, Carus, with the admonition, that by attending to Science more, and to Lucre less, and by letting Nassau's (that is King William's or England's) health be their chief aim, the College could once more become restored to the position it held under Willis and Wharton, Bates and Glisson.

A storm of unfriendly criticism was aroused by the first appearance of the poem. The design was bad. The execution was poor. The best part of the poem was in imitation of Boileau's *Lutrin* [12]—and much more besides. Garth, however,

[12] Nicolas Boileau, or M. Despréaux as he was usually called in the memoirs of the time, was one of the favorite writers of the day and his poetry exercised great influence, not only over French, but also over later English verse. *Lutrin* was possibly his best poem. There is an interesting allusion to him and to the Sir Richard Blackmore referred to above, in Lord Hervey's letters. He writes to Lady Mary Wortley Montague, Oct. 28, 1728, "Boileau can write a *Lutrin* what one can read with pleasure a thousand times, and Blackmore cannot write upon the *Creation* anything that one shall not yawn ten times over, before one has read it once."

At the hands of his own countrymen Boileau did not escape animadversions or at least until Voltaire's *mot*, "Don't say harm of Nicolas, it brings ill-luck," passed into a proverb.

in the preface written for the later editions, gracefully disarms all of these animadversions of his critics. He was proud of the imputation of imitating Boileau and points out the very lines in which he had done so; he defends his scheme on classical authority and modestly said, "However, I shall not be much concerned not to be thought excellent in an amusement I have very little practiced hitherto, nor perhaps ever shall again."

A dedicatory letter addressed to the gifted Sir Anthony Henley,[13] appropriately introduces these later editions, for Henley, judging from Garth's words must openly have expressed his approval of the poem when it first appeared. "Your approbation of this poem, is the only exception to the opinion the world has of your judgment, etc."

As was the custom, too, the poem in its later editions, is prefaced by commendatory verses by friendly hands.[14] And Garth, referring to those that might feel the sting of his satire, says "If I am hard upon anyone, it is my reader: but some worthy gentlemen, as remarkable for their humanity as their extraordinary parts, have taken care to make him amends for it, by prefixing something of their own."

Of the literary merit displayed in *The Dispensary*, liberally though it was applauded at the time, diverse opinions have been given by later critics. All of them, however, are unanimous in according to it an important position through the influence that it exercised upon the poetical style which continued into the following century.[15] Garth seems, as it were,

[13] Henley is noted for having been 'fed with soft dedications' by authors to whom he had been generous. He was one of the foremost wits and was a quasi friend of Swift in so far as the Dean could occasionally get a dinner out of him. "He has not seen me for some time in the Coffee-house, and asking after me, desired Lord Herbert to tell me I was a beast forever, after the order of Melchisedec. Did you ever read the Scripture? It is only changing the word priest to beast." *Journal to Stella.*

[14] Among them were the Earl of Orrery (C. Boyle) and C. Codrington. It was Boyle whose struggle with Bentley, the Oxford scholar, over some manuscripts led to Swift's "Battle of the Books." He was a member of Swift's 'The Club.' Codrington, a soldier, born in the Barbadoes, friend of the poets, left a large library to Christ Church. He says of Garth:

> "Thou hast no faults, or I no faults can spy,
> Thou art all beauty, or all blindness I."

[15] Oliver Goldsmith (*The Beauties of English Poetry*, 1767) commends highly Canto VI. It is interesting to note that in 1767 he was unable to find a first edition. He says ' the praises' bestowed on this poem are more than have been given to any other; but our approbation at present is cooler, for it owed part of its fame to party."

Johnson, in the Lives, characteristically says of Garth, " his poetry has been praised at least equally to its merit," and of *The Dispensary*, " no passages fall below mediocrity, and a few rise much above it." He continues in a more commendatory strain; " the composition can seldom be charged with inaccuracy or negligence. The author never slumbers in self indulgence; his full vigor is always exerted, scarcely a line is left unfinished; nor is it easy to find an expression used by constraint or a thought imperfectly expressed."

Henry Hallam (*Introduction to the Literature of Europe*, 1837-

to have introduced Boileau to Alexander Pope and Pope's praise of the poem, it will be remembered, was unstinted. In *The Dunciad* appear these lines,

> Be thine, my stationer, this magic gift;
> Cook shall be Prior, and Concanen, Swift;
> So shall each hostile name become our own,
> And we too boast our Garth and Addison.

and in the foot-notes,—Pope's own,—it is said, "nothing is more remarkable than our author's love of praising good writings. . . . It must have been particularly agreeable to him to celebrate Dr. Garth, both as his constant friend and as his predecessor in this kind of satire."

Equally unanimous is the opinion of the later critics, that this once celebrated poem after fifty years of celebrity has ceased to excite common interest. To the medical profession, however, if not to the community in general, it must always remain of historic import, commemorating as it does the first attempt to establish those out-patient rooms for the dispensation of medicines, which since have become such a universal charity. And whatever may be the actual merits of the poem, Garth, seemingly with no particular literary ambition, nevertheless with this single effort placed himself forever high in the ranks of the English Poets. There are other physicians who have courted the Muses and who, unlike Garth, have become renowned more as poets than physicians. Horace Walpole, as a rule none too lenient in matters of literary criticism, in one of his letters, while most flatteringly commending some poetry of Dr. Darwin's, continues, " Is it not extraordinary, dear Sir, that two of our very best poets, Garth and Darwin, should have been physicians? I believe they have left all the lawyers wrangling at the turnpike of Parnassus . . . ." [18]

THE DRYDEN EPISODE.

A FEW months after Garth had so abruptly stepped into his place in the ranks of English poets, there died the man who had succeeded Ben Jonson in the post of literary dictator and who was to be followed after a fashion

by Addison, Pope and the great lexicographer in turn. From John Dryden, Garth had borrowed the form of couplet which he had so improved, and from him Garth, the physician, ' generous as his Muse,' had received the immortal tribute of praise in verse. It is pouring old wine into new bottles to attempt anew the relation of a story, of which so many versions have come down to us that it is now difficult to tell wherein lies the truth." Authentic, however, seem these facts. John Dryden died in the house still standing on Gerrod Street in narrow and neglected circumstances on the Mayday of 1700, at three o'clock of a Wednesday morning. His body lay in state, twelve days later at no less curious a place than the Hall of the College of Physicians, where on Monday, May the 13th, Garth pronounced his funeral oration and with many others, ' fifty carriages of friends and fifty more besides,' attended the body to Westminster where it was interred between the graves of Chaucer and Cowley in the Poets' Corner.

Garth is generally considered to have rescued Dryden's body from a supposedly ignominious burial, but whatever part he may actually have played in the matter, certain it is that he obtained permission from the Board of Censors to allow the funeral exercises to be held at the College." Invitations, specimens of which are still extant,[19] were issued to attend the ceremony at this place.

That there is any truth in the wild story of the vexatious events that happened at his funeral, as told in Johnson's Lives and elsewhere, there is no trustworthy evidence. Misstatements, long passing as genuine,[20] were founded on a jocular letter by Farquhar, the comic dramatist, addressed to ' his Dear Madam,' and a poem [21] by Tom Brown, and were revived thirty years later for a monetary consideration, seemingly, by the unfortunate Mrs. Thomas (' Corinna '), then a prisoner for debt. The sources are equally unreliable. Farquhar, indeed, begins the very letter [22] in which his infamous burlesque appears, with,—" I was so fuddled, that I hardly remember whether I writ or not."—certainly an indifferent authority. According to Johnson, who, it must be confessed, accepted the story somewhat unwillingly, a private interment was to have been held at the expense of Lord Halifax—the Mæcenas of Garth's day. So on the Saturday following his death, the funeral procession with a ' velvet hearse ' was about

---

1839) says, " Garth, as has been observed, is a link of transition between the style and turn of poetry under Charles and William, and that we find in Addison, Prior, Tickell and Pope during the Reign of Anne."

George Saintsbury (*English Poets*, 1880, Vol. III, p. 13) comments, " Garth is mainly interesting at the present day because he was the first writer who took the couplet, as Dryden had fashioned it, from Dryden's hands, and displayed it in the form it maintained throughout the Eighteenth Century. In some respects it may be said that no advance in this particular mode was ever made on The Dispensary. * * * Except for its versification, which not only long preceded Pope, but also anticipated Addison's happiest efforts by some years, The Dispensary is not now an interesting poem."

[18] The Letters of Horace Walpole. Cunningham's Ed'n. 1877, Vol. IX, p. 372. Letter to Thos. Barrett Esq. May 14, 1792. Cunningham's note on this passage says " We had two better poets physicians, Akenside and Armstrong; but this Walpole would not have admitted."

[17] Arbuthnot, in The Gold Headed Cane, tells the story as commonly related, in an imaginary conversation at Mead's.

[18] Annals of the College of Physicians; May 3, 1700.

[19] They must be very rare. There is no example preserved among the archives of the Royal College of Physicians; none in the British Museum. A copy recently came under the hammer at Sotheby's among some Dryden manuscripts and was secured by Mr. Harold Peirce of Philadelphia, to whom I am greatly indebted for the accompanying photograph.

[20] Until refuted by Malone (*Miscellaneous Prose Works of John Dryden*, 1800, pp., 355-382). Sir Walter Scott (*Life of John Dryden*) also accepted the tale as a romance and gives references for those who wish to consult them.

[21] A Description of Mr. D——n's Funeral.

[22] The Works of Mr. George Farquhar. Edn. IX. Lond., 1760. Vol. I, p. 73.

to leave Dryden's door, when Lord Jeaffries with some rakish companions, happening by, interrupted the proceedings on learning whose private burial it was, promising a large sum for a public funeral and a monument in the Abbey. Reluctantly the company was persuaded to disperse while the body was sent to an undertaker's. On the morrow, Jeaffries excused his action as part of a drunken frolic. Lord Halifax also, naturally disgruntled, refused to concern himself further with the matter after once having had the Abbey lighted and prepared. The chagrin of the family may be imagined. Their circumstances were such as to make it impossible for them to bear the expense of a funeral; and this is the less to be wondered at when one considers what formidable functions they were at this time. At this embarrassing juncture, Garth, as Johnson says, "withal a man of generosity and great humanity sent for the corpse to the College of Physicians in Warwick Lane and proposed a funeral by public subscription to which he himself set a noble example." Though the improbability of much of this story was pointed out years later by Malone, the fact of Dryden's actual interment on the second of May at

St. Anne's in Soho has only recently come to light by the chance discovery of an entry to that effect in the parish register.[22] The circumstances of the disinterment, of the embalming at Russel's and of the transfer to the College continue to be obscured by uncertainties and the finale of this marvellous structure of fable as Johnson relates it, is too absurd to credit;[23] that Garth delivered his oration with much good nature from the top of a beer barrel the head of which fell in during the course of the proceedings; that confusion and ribald disorder reigned during the ceremony, at the College, at the Abbey, and on the march thither. For all of this we are probably indebted to the fanciful imaginings of the befuddled Farquhar. It is perhaps worthy of note that Garth's share alone of the proceedings did not suffer burlesque from his

SIR,

YOU are defired to Accompany the Corps of Mr. John Dryden, from the College of Phyficians in Warwick-Lane, to Weftminfter Abby; on Monday the 13th of this Inftant May, 1700. at Four of the Clock in the Afternoon exactly, it being refolved to be moving by Five a Clock. And be pleafed to bring this Ticket with you.

Dated April 20th

CARD OF INVITATION, ISSUED BY GARTH FROM THE COLLEGE OF PHYSICIANS, TO ATTEND DRYDEN'S FUNERAL.

---

[22] A Burial Mystery. Soho Monthly Paper. June, 1904, p. 143. Also, The Athenaeum of July 30, 1904.

[23] Those who wish to peruse this memorable romance will find it in Dryden's Works, Vol. XVIII, p. 200. It was first published in Wilson's Life of Congreve, 1730. Mr. Malone has pointed out the falsity of the tale in almost all its parts. Independently of

pen for he said,—" The oration indeed was great and ingenious, worthy the subject and like the author; whose prescriptions can restore the living and his pen embalm the dead."

There is one feature of the ceremony, as related by Thomas Hearne,[*] that deserves passing mention, indicating as it does a side of Garth's character of which more will be said anon. " Mr. John Dryden, the great poet, was buried in Westminster Abbey among the old poets in May, 1700, being carried from the College of Physicians, where an oration was pronounced by the famous Dr. Garth, in which he did not mention one word of Jesus Christ, but made an oration as an apostrophe to the great god Apollo, to influence the minds of the auditors with a wise, but, without doubt, poetical understanding, and, as a conclusion, instead of a psalm of David, repeated the 30th ode of the third book of Horace's odes beginning " Exegi monumentum, etc." He made a great many blunders in the pronunciation." Hearne is not the only one who has thus commented on Garth's apparent irreligion; but why should he have been expected to deliver a sermon under those unusual circumstances? That the proceedings were dignified cannot be doubted and Garth's selection of the Ode to Melpomene, which was sung to music, was certainly a fitting and beautiful one.

> " I have reared a monument, my own,
> More durable than brass.
> Yea, kingly pyramids of stone
> In height it does surpass."

It is almost prophetic of the fact that the spot where Dryden was interred long remained undistinguished by mark of any kind. Not until thirty years later did the Duke of Buckingham place a tablet there inscribed simply with Dryden's name.[*]

ANNE'S REIGN AND THE KIT-KAT CLUB.

ALMOST coincident with Dryden's death and the birth of a new century, Anne came to the throne and with her reign began what has been called the Augustan era in England. There are, as Goldwin Smith has pointed out,

the extreme improbability of the whole story, it is clear from Ward's account, written at the time, that Lord Jeaffries who, it is pretended, interrupted the funeral, did, on the contrary, largely contribute in helping Garth subsequently to bring it about.

In a letter from Doctor, afterward Bishop Tanner, dated May 6th, 1700, quoted by Malone, there appears the following paragraph: " Mr. Dryden died a Papist if at all a Christian. Mr. Montague had given orders to bury him; but some Lords (my Lord Dorset, Jeaffries, et al.) thinking it would not be splendid enough, ordered him to be carried to Russel's; there he was embalmed; and now lies in state at the Physician's College and is to be buried with Chaucer, Cowley, etc., at Westminster Abbey, on Monday next." MSS. Ballard in Bibl. Bodl. Vol. VI, p. 29.

[*] *Reliquiae Hearnianae*, Edn. Bliss, 1726. Vol. II, p. 267.

[*] In his preface to the translation of Ovid's Metamorphoses (1717) Garth says of Dryden, " The man, that could make kings immortal, and raise triumphal arches to heroes, now wants a poor square foot of stone, to show where the ashes of one of the greatest poets, that ever was upon earth, are deposited."

certain grounds that substantiate the comparison. Peace, at home at all events, for Marlborough's operations leading up to Blenheim constituted largely a war of the allies and happily a victorious one; poetry and literature in the persons of Pope, Swift, Addison, Steele and DeFoe; the restoration of classical learning under Bentley's scholarship; and statesmen who almost with uniformity were patrons of letters. But underneath there was much vulgarity, ignorance and excess. Even in literature, good breeding as evidenced by such as Addison and Garth, was rare and barely sufficed to safeguard even them against the coarse demands of the popular taste. The Queen, when she felt so disposed, resumed the practice of touching for the evil. Marauders after nightfall, calling themselves Mohawks, terrorized the citizens by their depredations, and animosities, resultant to party feeling, seem to have been almost equally disturbing to the peace.

The period, too, at least for the fine gentlemen, was one of the tavern and coffee-house, where in lieu of the daily press the news of the day and the gossip of yesterday were washed down, often with so many bottles that the resultant conviviality commonly saw the day become the morrow. Thus ductile people like poor Dick Steele were led to send late messengers with lanterns to their Dear Prues, begging them to go to bed and promising to come home " within a pint of wine,"—a bibulous way of recording the hours.

Many hearsay incidents of these coffee-house festivities have come down to us, some of them hardly acceptable to modern ears. Of Garth there are numerous anecdotes, indicative for the most part of his readiness and wit. He was sitting one day in the coffee room of the Cocoa Tree Tavern,. near his home in St. James Street, conversing with two persons of quality, when the poet Rowe, a vain fellow, fond of being noticed, entered the door. He sat in a box nearly opposite to Garth, looking frequently around in the hope of catching his eye. Not succeeding in this, he desired the waiter to ask the Doctor for the loan of his snuffbox, which he knew to be a rare one, set with diamonds and the gift of royalty. After taking a pinch and returning it without Garth's deigning to notice him, he sent again for it, and soon again. Finally Garth, who knew him well and saw through his purpose from the beginning, took out his pencil and wrote on the lid the two Greek characters,—P —, Fie! Rowe! The mortified poet ceased his persecutions.

It was a coffee-house custom for every one to pay his share of the entertainment, to contribute his club, as it was expressed,[*] and it was not long before this term, coupled with some appropriate adjective, became commonly used in designation of one or another coterie of friends. Gastronomy was at first the chief reason for a club's existence. " Our modern

[*] Thus Swift writes to Stella, Oct. 13, 1710, " The fine fellows are always inviting him (young Harrison, the poet) to the tavern and make him pay his club. Henley (that is Anthony Henley, to whom Garth dedicated The Dispensary) is a great crony of his: they are often at the tavern at six or seven shillings reckoning, and he always makes the poor lad pay his full share."

celebrated clubs" Addison says, " are founded on eating and drinking, which are points wherein most men agree." Somewhat later Dr. Johnson gave his properly indefinite definition of " An assembly of good fellows meeting under certain conditions." The number of these organizations multiplied enormously; many of them, in addition to mere conviviality, fostered objects of a more lofty nature, as literature and the fine arts. A few of them ultimately developed into powerful political machines and of these there are two that continue to be of considerable historical interest; one of them made up largely of active Whig members; the other, the October Club, comprising those desirous of the Stewart succession, the active members of the Tory party.

Garth's Harveian Oration, with its reference to William III, had early been the straw to show the direction of his political tendencies, and though never a violent partisan at a time when political partisanship meant intolerance, his culture, wit and elegance doubtless made him a companion eagerly sought for by the clique forming the famous Kit-Kat Club, in which, as Macaulay says, were gathered all the various talents and accomplishments which then gave lustre to the Whig party.

The early beginnings of this society, its purpose and the source from which its name was derived are all shrouded in some obscurity. It seems probable, however, that Jacob Tonson, the celebrated book-seller, one of the dwellers in ' Little Britain,' was its prime mover; some have said that for selfish reasons he gathered the young and budding wits of his own party, at his own expense to the mutton-pie feasts, hoping through this association with them to obtain the refusal of their youthful publications. Tonson seems to have been no more deserving of affection than other publishers of his time, so bitterly stung by the ' Wasp of Twickenham ' in the Dunciad, especially if we are to judge from the stories of his relations with Dryden, a triplet from whose pen portrays him, physically at least, in no very favorable light.[29] He had acquired wealth partly, it is said, by a lucky stroke in the Mississippi Scheme, partly, also, through success in his trade; for during the Whig administration he was stationer, binder,

book-seller and printer to the Crown. After the change in government in 1710, it was largely through his influence that the club held together and out of its peaceable origin grew into an organization that exerted a powerful influence in political affairs. It was no longer at a tavern but at his country home in Barn Elms, Surrey, that the meetings ultimately became held,—

" One night in seven at this convenient seat
Indulgent Bocaj (Jacob) did the Muses treat."[30]

and it was to decorate their convivium that Godfrey Kneller painted the celebrated portraits " of the members, exerting himself, it is said, as he seldom did at other times.

As described by Steele in the Tatler, the custom of making toasts of the fashionable beauties of the time was peculiar to and originated with the society out of which the Kit-Kat Club was formed and the scene with which this sketch opened was an instance of the annual election. The ' toasts ' were formally determined by balloting and when elected they reigned, says the Tatler, indisputably, like the Doge in Venice. One finds mentioned in many a paragraph or letter the names of those who were thus forever celebrated by the attention of that illustrious gathering. When the ' toasts ' for the year had been chosen it was customary for their names to be scratched with a diamond on a drinking glass and, ballads being the fashion of the day, rhymes were often added as well. Garth semes to have had an especial facility for turning out these jingles and many of the verses have been attributed to his fancy; one illustration, however, will suffice to show what

---

[28] According to Ward, in a curious old book,—"The Secret History of Clubs"—the name took its origin from Christopher or ' Kit,' whose tavern, the first place of meeting, was at the Sign of the Cat and Fiddle; later on the Club moved with him from his original humble surroundings, to the Fountain Tavern in the Strand.

" The Kit-Cat Club came to be so-called from one Christopher Catting (a pudding pye-man) with whose puddings and conversation the first founders of the society were well pleased." Reliquiae Hearnianae. Edn., Bliss, I, 74.

In the Spectator, No. 9, Addison, who, being a member, should have known, says,—"The Kit-Cat itself is said to have taken its original from a mutton-pye." Thus the pies were called kit-cats long before the club was so named.

" The fact is, that on account of its excellence it was called a Kit-Cat as we now say a Sandwitch." Malone.

[29] With leering looks, bull-faced, and freckled fair,
With two left legs and Judas colour'd hair,
And frowsy pores, that taint the ambient air.

---

[30] Sir Richard Blackmore. The Kit-Cats. A Poem. London H. Hills, 1708.

[31] These portraits in Horace Walpole's opinion, (Anecdotes of Painting, Vol. II, p., 204.) possess great sameness and no imagination. " See but a head, it interests you—uncover the rest of the canvas, you wonder faces so expressive could be employed so insipidly." Faint praise indeed; others have not so damned them.

Inasmuch as the room in which these portraits were to be hung was quite low, the usual half-length (thirty guinea) size could not be used, so that Kneller had to content himself—except in the case of his own portrait which was half-length—with the head and one hand. Thus it was that this particular size and arrangement became known as a ' Kit-Kat portrait.' They measured 28 by 36 inches. While they were at Barn Elms mezzotint engravings were made of the entire series and were published in 1723 by Tonson (cf. Frontispiece). They were republished in 1795 by J. Faber and were reproduced in 1821 in a volume entitled " Memoirs of the Celebrated Persons comprising the Kit-Cat Club,"—a volume not to be commended for its accuracy of facts. The collection of portraits is said to have been kept intact by Tonson's descendants and is now at Bayfordbury in Herts. A portrait, supposed however to be Kneller's original Kit-Kat portrait, was presented in 1763 by Dr. Chauncey to the College of Physicians and now hangs in the Censor's Room at the left hand just as you enter the door. It is certainly a very good picture, though possibly a copy. It looks the opposite way from the mezzotint which was possibly reversed by the engraver. In the national Portrait Gallery there is another portrait supposedly by Kneller—a head alone.

doggerel rhymes they were. The stanza is dedicated to Lady Hyde,—Prior's Kitty, beautiful and young,—and runs,

> The God of wine grows jealous of his art;
> He only fires the head, but Hyde the heart.
> The Queen of love looks on and smiles to see
> A nymph more mighty than a deity.

No one would have lamented more than Garth the perpetuation of such vapid lines as these and on a later occasion he excused them as having been spontaneously struck off to meet post-prandial demands. They led nevertheless to his being designated as the Kit-Kat poet. The whole custom suffered ridicule at the hands of Pope or Arbuthnot, one of whom wrote,

> Whence deathless Kit-Cat took its name,
> Few critics can unriddle;
> Some say from pastry-cook it came,
> And some from Cat and Fiddle.
>
> From no trim beaux its name it boasts,
> Gray statesmen or green wits;
> But from this pell-mell pack of toasts,
> Of old "Cats" and young "Kits."

There are many stories, oft told, of Garth and his friends at these meetings. Some of them are neither credible nor creditable. One night while lounging over his wine he was jokingly rebuked by Steele for neglecting his patients. "Nay, nay, Dick," said he, pulling out his consulting list, " it is no urgent matter after all, for nine of them have such bad constitutions that not all the physicians in the world could save them; and the other six have such good constitutions that all the physicians in the world could not kill them."

After some twenty years of life, together with the thinning which death made in the Club's ranks, the gatherings themselves died away. In 1725 Vanbrugh wrote to Tonson, " You may believe, when I tell you, you were often talked of, both during the journey and at home; and our former Kit-Cat days were remembered with pleasure. We were one night reckoning who were left, and both Lord Carlisle and Cobham expressed a great desire of having one meeting next winter if you came to town; not as a club, but as old friends that have been of a club, and the best club that ever met."

GARTH THE PHYSICIAN AND FRIEND.

> Whenever Garth shall raise his sprightly song,
> Sense flows in easie numbers from his tongue;
> Great Phoebus in his learned son we see
> Alike in Physic as in Poetry.
>
> JOHN GAY.   Poems 1714. To Bernard Lintot.

Few indeed have been the disciples of Aesculapius who have climbed 'the severe ascent of high Parnassus' and at the same time been faithful to their vocation. Too often has this divided allegiance meant the unqualified sacrifice of Physic upon the shrine of the Corycian nymphs: for the public has ever been shy of the physician who allows his mind to soar above the level of most practical and mundane things, and a genius so inclined, has, in reciprocation, not uncommonly failed of success in his profession from an equal shyness of the public. As indicated by Gay's lines, such a fate

was not meted out to Garth, for he continued throughout life to be for the members of the Whig party what his equally talented contemporary—the author of John Bull—was for the Tories; the fashionable and honored medical consultant. " Never," says Leigh Hunt, " were two better men sent to console the ailments of two witty parties, or show them what a nothing party is, compared with the humanity remaining under the quarrels of both." Their intolerance of one another was said to have been such that a Whig invalid seemed to think it impossible that he could derive any benefit from the advice of a Tory physician and upon the same principle a Tory patient industriously avoided calling on a Whig practitioner. Garth, however, much like Addison in his charitableness and tolerance, seems to have stood aloof from petty professional jealousies and political rivalries and though zealous for and constant to his party, yet he was very far from having the narrow and malicious spirit, so characteristic of the times, and which led, often enough, to hatred of those holding opposite political beliefs. Even Dr. Johnson acknowledges that Garth imparted his kindness equally among those who were and those who were not supposed to favor his principles. But even had he shared in these rivalries, the change in government that followed Anne's death in 1714, with Swift's fall and the reinstation of the Whigs, would have placed him on the top wave of political preference.[20]

With the inauguration of the Hanoverian dynasty, Garth was made the King's Physician in Ordinary, Physician General to the Army, and in the same year was knighted with the hero of Blenheim's sword, so the story runs; presumably the famous diamond-hilted sword, which in after years Marlborough's widow, the celebrated Sarah, plead for in Chancery lest she should live to see her profligate grandchild, who had succeeded to the title, squander for cash the jewels with which it was adorned.[21]

---

[20] Radcliffe, it will be remembered, died a few months after Anne (Nov. 1, 1714), having been unable or unwilling to answer the call to her bedside; frightened to death, 'twas said, by the threats of the Tories, who blamed him for not keeping her alive. " You know your doctor (Radcliffe) is gone the way of all his patients, and was hard put to it how to dispose of an estate miserably unwieldy and splendidly unuseful to him. " I consider myself as a poor passenger; and that the earth is not to be forsaken for the rocks removed from me." (Pope to Martha Blount.) When Garth learned what disposition Radcliffe had made of his property, he said that for him to establish a library was as inappropriate as for a eunuch to found a seraglio.

Arbuthnot had been Physician in Ordinary to the Queen—she had always been a Tory at heart—and the change in government removed him, too, permanently from the political horizon. In Swift's correspondence (Unpublished Letters of Dean Swift. Birkbeck Hill. 1899) there is a letter from Arbuthnot on " the terrible shock " which the Queen's death had given him. " I consider myself as a poor passenger; and that the earth is not to be forsaken nor the rocks removed from me." Reason enough for Arbuthnot's downfall has been given by ' the immortal Tit-mouse ' in the description of the part he played in the conspiracy to place the young pretender on the throne—he who preferred Beatrice to the crown.

[21] " That sword," said she, " that sword, my Lord would have car-

These honors, according to Chalmers, were no more than the just rewards of his medical merit though there need be no doubt that they were influenced by his known political affiliations. His social position, his oratorical and poetical success, coupled with the philanthropic spirit that led up to the latter, possibly, too, the part played in the Dryden incident, as well as his natural ability and popularity, all combined to lead him rapidly into an extensive and profitable practice. Cibber says, " He had the happiness of an early acquaintance with some of the most powerful, wisest, and wittiest men of the age in which he lived. He attached himself to a party, which at last obtained the ascendant, and he was equally successful in his fortune as his friends. Persons in these circumstances are seldom praised, or censured with moderation." In 1702, Garth became a Censor of the College, practising always, 'tis said, ' in strict regard to the honor and interest of the faculty; never stooping to prostitute the dignity of his profession through mean and sordid views of self interest by courting even the most popular and wealthy apothecaries '—a stand which contrasts badly with the story of Mead, the succeeding luminary in the medical sky, and his half guinea prescriptions. In strong contrast also to Mead's predecessor in possession of the Gold Headed Cane, does Garth stand out as one who endeared himself to his patients as well as to his friends by his politeness, accomplishments and consideration. He was one who knew that the

> Same nerves are fashion'd to sustain
> The greatest pleasure and the greatest pain.
> *The Dispensary.* CANTO I.

In contemporary writings there are many references to his professional skill and reputation. Lady Mary Wortley Montague writes in 1714 to her husband, " But I should be very glad if you saw Dr. Garth if you would ask his opinion concerning the use of cold baths for young children," and again, " I hope the child is better than he was but I wish you would let Dr. Garth know—he has a bigness in his joints, but not much; his ankles seem chiefly to have a weakness. I should be very glad of his advice upon it and whether he approves rubbing them with spirits, which I am told is good for him." In the collected works of the notorious Mr. Thomas Brown appears the following epistle addressed :

TO DOCTOR GARTH:
    Whether your letter or your prescription has made me well, I protest I cannot tell; but this much I can say, That as the one was the most nauseous thing I ever knew, so the the other was the most entertaining. I would gladly ascribe my cure to the last; and if so, your practice will become so universal you must keep a secretary as well as an apothecary.
    The observations I have made are these: that your prescription staid not long with me, but your letter has, especially that part of it where you told me I was not altogether out of your memory; you'll find me much altered in everything when you see me, but in my esteem for yourself: I that was as lank as a *crane* when I left you at *London*, am now as

ried to the Gates of Paris. Am I to live to see the diamonds picked off one by one and lodged at the pawn-brokers?" *Introductory Anecdotes.* Stewart.

plump as an *ortolan*. I have left off my false calves, and had yesterday a great belly laid to me. A facetious widow, who is my confident in this affair, says you ought to father the child; for he that lends a man a sword is in some part accessory to the mischief is done with it; however, I'll forgive you the inconvenience you've put me to. I believe you were not aware you were giving life to two people. Pray let me have a consolatory letter from you upon this new calamity; for nothing can be so welcome, excepting rain in this sandy country where we live. The widow saith, she resolves to be sick on purpose to be acquainted with you; but I'll tell her she'll relish your prescriptions better in full health, and if at this distance you can do her no service, pray prescribe her

Your humble Servant.

And so the Churchills, and Lady Hervey—beautiful Molly Lepel—the Walpoles and others among those, who, through their letters, are still well known to us, despite the gap of almost two hundred years, often make mention of Garth the Aesculapian as well as of Garth the companion. But intimate as he seems to have been with those who were socially and politically among the great, his benevolence and true professional kindliness toward the needy seems in no way to have suffered. His reputation for charitableness, as one learns from many sources, was well deserved. " No physician knew his art more nor his trade less."

Poor Dick Steele never forgot his own indebtedness to Garth. He dedicated his play, *The Lover,* to him, saying, " The pitiful artifices which empyrics are guilty of, to drain cash out of valetudinarians, are the abhorrence of your generous mind; and it is as common with Garth to supply indigent patients with money for food, as to receive it from wealthy ones for physic." And, hardly in accord with the story of the consultation list related above, Steele says farther on, " This tenderness interrupts the satisfaction of conversation, to which you are so happily turned; but we forgive you that our mirth is often insipid to you, while you sit absent to what passes amongst us, from your care of such as languish in sickness. We are sensible that their distresses, instead of being removed by company, return more strongly to your imagination, by comparison of their condition with the jollities of health. But I forget I am writing a dedication   *   *   *   ."

The best of all of Steele's tributes to his friend and physician I cannot help quoting still more at length. The genuine and warm-hearted gratitude which it displays as well as the gracefully indirect method in which this has been expressed make it an acknowledgment of services such as even the most deserving rarely receive. In the *Tatler,* No. 78, Saturday, October 8, 1709, Isaac Bickerstaff records that he has received the following letter :

" Sir,
    I am just recovered out of a languishing sickness by the care of Hippocrates, who visited me throughout my whole illness, and was so far from taking any fee, that he inquired into my circumstances, and would have relieved me also that way, but I did not want it. I know no method of thanking him, but recommending it to you to celebrate so great humanity in the manner you think fit, and to do it with the spirit and sentiments of a man

National Bank.

£27

Samuel Garth

ORder is taken this 27 Day of Febry 1715 by Vertue and in Pursuance of an Act lately paſſed in Parliament, (Entituled, An Act for Granting an Aid to His Majeſty, by a Land-Tax in Great Britain, for the Service of the Year 1716.) That you deliver and pay of ſuch His Majeſty's Treaſure as remains in your Charge, ariſing by Vertue of the ſaid Act, unto Samuel Garth

or his Aſſigns, the Sum of Two hundred pound &c

in Repayment of the like Sum by him lent upon Credit of the ſaid Act, and paid into the Receipt of His Majeſty's Exchequer the ſaid given Day of Febry 1715 as by a Talley bearing Date the ſame Day appears; together with Intereſt for the ſame, after the Rate of Six Pounds per Cent per Annum, at the End of every Three Months, from the Date of the ſaid Talley, until the Repayment of the Principal. And theſe, together with — or his Aſſigns Acquittance, ſhall be your Diſcharge herein.......

in Repayment of Loan on — Diſcharged 4 Act —
June 1716.

This document, which is reproduced chiefly for the sake of showing Garth's signature as it was incised two years before his death, is interesting as well from the indication it gives of an income sufficient to let him respond generously to Walpole's call for a national loan to meet the government expenditure connected with the Rising of 1715.

Dr. Stone has called my attention to a paragraph in Dowell's History of Taxation in England, Vol. II, p.30, where it is stated that 'the expedient incurred in the summons of the attempt of the Pretender rendered necessary the grant of a 4s. land tax for 1716.' It is evident that the Garth loaned the Government on February 26th, 1715, the sum of £200, and was given as security the special tax (the high 4s. Act), of which security this document is the certificate. On March 7, 1716, the loan was repaid and the Signature attached.

It will be remembered that the Calendar-Amendment Act, establishing January 1st as the beginning of each year (instead of Lady-Day, March 25) was not adopted until 1752, so that the dates on this document refer to the julian or old style calendar.

just relieved from grief, misery and pain, to joy, satisfaction and ease; in which you will represent the grateful sense of your obedient servant,

I. B."

" I think the writer of this letter has put the matter in as good a dress as I can for him; yet I cannot but add my applause to what this distressed man has said. There is not a more useful man in the commonwealth than a good physician, and, by consequence, no worthier a person than he that uses his skill with generosity even to persons of condition, and compassion to those who are in want: which is the behavior of Hippocrates, who shows as much liberality in his practice, as he does wit in his conversation, and skill in his profession. A wealthy doctor, who can help a poor man, and will not without a fee, has less sense of humanity than a poor ruffian who kills a rich man to supply his necessities. It is something monstrous to consider a man of a liberal education tearing at the bowels of a poor family, by taking for a visit what would keep them a week. Hippocrates needs not the comparison of such extorsion to set off his generosity, but I mention his generosity to add shame to such extorsion."

Many years later when writing of Garth in his *Lives of the Poets*, Johnson, as will be remembered, was led for similar reasons and in like vein, to pay the medical profession one of the most appreciated bits of praise it has ever received. "Whether what Temple says be true, that physicians have had more learning than the other faculties, I will not stay to enquire; but I believe every man has found in physicians great liberality and dignity of sentiment, very prompt effusion of beneficence and willingness to exert a lucrative art, where there is no hope of lucre." [34]

CHARACTER AND PRIVATE LIFE.

I T is regrettable that we have so little information, beyond that conveyed by anecdote, of Garth's private life; regrettable too that much of what we know serves merely to indicate the character of the day rather than of the individual. The customs, the fashions, the morals were not our own and our judgment upon them must be given with a light hand. There are some things held up against him—notably irreligion and libertinism—which only the coarseness of the times enables us to excuse as being less bad in him than in the company he kept. Garth's own reflection upon Ovid's writings, we may,

[34] It is interesting to note that Boswell quoted this paragraph in the letters to Cullen, Munro and Hope of the Edinburgh School, when he appealed to them for advice in Johnson's last illness. To which letter and " its venerable object, all of them paid the most polite attention " as would have been expected even without the quotation.

Through the many illnesses of his life as well as in this last one, had Johnson been considerably cared for by many distinguished medical men. " A few days after his departure, Dr. Brocklesby and Mr. Cruikshank who with great assiduity and humanity (and I must add generosity for neither they, nor Dr. Heberden nor Warren, nor Dr. Butler would accept any fees) had attended him, signified a wish that his body might be opened." G. Birkbeck Hill; *Johnsonian Miscellanies.* 1897. Vol. II, p. 136.)

however, appropriately turn upon his own character. He says, " It must be granted that when there appears an infinite variety of inimitable excellences, it would be too harsh and disingenuous to be severe on such faults, as have escap'd rather thro' want of leisure, and opportunity to correct, than thro' the erroneous turn of a deprav'd judgment."

During his early life in London, Garth is said to have resided in humble quarters in the Haymarket—according to the Rate Books of St. Martin's-in-the-Fields, ' on the East side six doors from the top.' It was in a garret of this same street that Addison lived when he wrote *The Campaign,* the poem that started his political fortune rolling, and it is quite probable that both of them were among the distinguished company present at the laying of the corner stone of the Queen's Theatre—now the Haymarket Opera House—designed by their friend Vanbrugh. Another bystander was the much abused laureate Colley Cibber, who subsequently wrote, " of this theatre I saw the first stone laid on which was inscribed THE LITTLE WHIG in honor of a lady of extraordinary beauty, then the celebrated Toast and Pride of that party." This was Lady Sunderland, Marlborough's second daughter, and it was to her and Vanbrugh that Garth referred in the line, " By beauty founded and by wit designed," which occurs in his Prologue, subsequently read at the formal opening of this famous Opera House." [35]

In the same year—1705—Garth removed to more fashionable quarters, to St. James in fact, where he resided near his friends the Churchills, whose particular favor and esteem he always enjoyed. Here he was married to Martha, the daughter of Sir Henry Beaufoy, and here, so far as is known, he continued to dwell until later in life a country home at Harrow-on-the-Hill was taken by him for Lady Garth and Martha, his only daughter.

Though his professional labors must have kept him much in town, his affection for ' The Hill ' where many delightful social hours were passed with his friends, was such that he determined it should be his final resting place and a vault was prepared in the church for the purpose. [36]

The visitations between neighboring country houses, then as now, were many and Garth's companionship, whether as guest or entertainer, must have been eagerly courted. " On the morrow I am engaged to go to Harrow-on-the-Hill with company," writes Pope in a note to Kneller, and in return we find Garth at the Twickenham Grotto, whence Pope sends

[35] The Haymarket Opera House opened April 9, 1705, with a performance of Dryden's ' Indian Emperor.'
[36] In Hay's *Religio Philosophi* the circumstances of Garth's ordering a vault for himself and his wife in Harrow Church is spoken of as the result of some accidental whim. His will is dated 20th May 1717; and his property including Edgecott in Bucks he bequeaths to his daughter, Martha Beaufoy Boyle (Cunningham). This will was made shortly after the death (May 1st, 1717) of Lady Garth, he being himself in ill health at the time. The daughter had become the wife of Col. William Boyle, son of the Hon. Col. Henry Boyle, uncle of the last Earl of Burlington of that name.

word to Lady Mary Wortley Montague (October, 1717), who is still in Constantinople and still an object of Pope's fickle admiration,—"Dr. Garth makes epigrams in prose when he speaks of you." It is perhaps but another evidence of that desirable quality for which Garth was so distinguished—his good nature—that his friendships endured so long. It is a quality to which so many allusions are made and with such a

known for this character. that an epistle so directed would find its way to you without your name: and I believe nobody but yourself would deliver such a superscription to any other person."

The adulation of soft dedications of the 18th century must of course be taken into account in this eulogy, though there need be little doubt of the genuineness of Steele's feeling; but

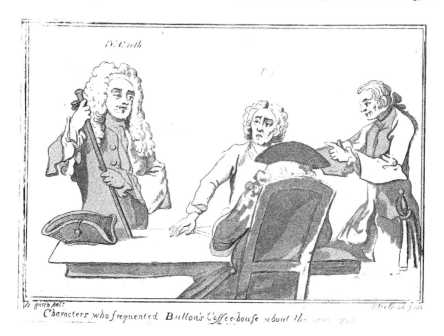

Characters who frequented Button's Coffee-house about th—

unanimity of opinion that one would weary of it were it not for the realization that two hundred years ago the designation had a widely different meaning from that into which it has now become corrupted—with a suggestion of complaisance and the mental inactivity that accompany ready adjustment to the moods of others. and that too often belong to a wearisome though amiable personality. Of all his contemporaries not even Addison seems to have been so universally liked. In Steele's dedication, from which I have already so freely borrowed. he says, "As soon as I thought of making the *Lover* a present to one of my friends, I resolved without distracting my choice to send it to the BEST NATURED MAN. You are so universally

there were others notoriously of less kindly instincts who had the same regard for Garth. Eminent among them was "he, who hardly drank tea without a stratagem." Garth's friendship with Pope began when the latter was a mere boy and although Arbuthnot and Swift may at one time have been his closer intimates, nevertheless cordial relations with Garth were continued with a constancy which the younger man rarely exhibited. The ease with which Pope's animosities were aroused on seemingly the most trivial grounds makes it all the more creditable that Garth remained among the few who first or last suffered in no way from the stings of the poet's satire. His 'Pastorals' were written by the stripling minstrel of Binfield when only sixteen and the second of them—Summer—was dedicated to Garth."

So later, in his 'Epistle to Arbuthnot,' he refers to Garth's early encouragement of his work in the lines—

> "But why then publish? Granville the polite
> And knowing Walsh, would tell me I could write;
> Well natured Garth, inflamed with earthly praise;
> And Congreve lov'd, and Swift endur'd by lays."

Good reason indeed had he to feel gratitude toward this patron of his youth, if we are to credit—as we should, for it comes through the Rev. Jos. Spence from Pope's own lips—the story of how Garth with Addison and Congreve brought him before Lord Halifax for a reading of the first sections of his translation of the Iliad, how his Lordship criticised several passages, requesting that they be altered and how Garth, who took Pope home in his chariot, laughed at his embarrassment and told him to leave them as they were, but to thank his Lordship and then go and read them again to him after a few months, which he did to the gratification of Lord Halifax who cried out, "Ay now, Mr. Pope, they are perfectly right! Nothing can be better."

During their town life they were found together at Button's Coffee House, where they were immortalized by Hogarth's pencil,[38] and they continued to fraternize after Pope left the dear, damn'd distracting town to pass the remainder of 'that long illness, his life,' at Twickenham. And there Garth, no longer needed as literary patron, probably did more to encourage the poet's feeble body than his verse. Indeed the tables were so turned, that Pope became the advocate of his friend's Muse, announcing to Richardson "that there was hardly an alteration in *The Dispensary* of the innumerable ones through every edition that was not for the better; and that he took Garth to be one of the few truly judicious authors." For Garth did not live up to his threat of writing no more. The most pretentious as well as the last work in which he engaged was the editing of a beautiful great folio of Ovid's Metamorphoses.[39] Of this Wharton says, "About this time it became fashionable among the wits at ' Button's,' the mob of gentlemen that wrote with ease, to translate Ovid. Their united performances were published in form by Garth, with a preface written in a flowery and lively style, but full of strange opinions." And soon after its appearance Pope wrote to Curyll, August 6, 1717.—" Dr. Garth has published

---

[37] Of this, Wharton says, "It is unfortunate that this second pastoral, the worst of the four, should be inscribed to the best of all Pope's four friends to whom they were addressed "—to Sir Wm. Trumbull, Garth, Mr. Wycherley and Mrs. Tempest.

[38] I do not know, in this sketch, who can be the third person who stands by the table at the artist's right. Another similar sketch, also attributed to Hogarth, is reproduced in B. W. Richardson's *Disciples of Aesculapius*. In this one a figure, undoubtedly Arbuthnot, appears sitting between Garth and Pope. "You may know Arbuthnot because he can only sit," says Swift, in the *Journal to Stella.*

[39] Published by J. Tonson in 15 books, 1717.

a translation of Ovid's Metamorphoses by several hands with a preface and a dedication in a new fashion, Folio, price 20s. I advise you to borrow it." Between *The Dispensary*, his first, and this, Garth's last literary venture, there appeared several minor poems, one of which must needs be mentioned, as an incident arising from it seems to show how well the author deserved his epithet of good nature. In 1710 when the Government changed hands, Garth wrote a short poem of kindly address dedicated to Lord Godolphin on the reverse of his political fortunes. In the Tory paper, the *Examiner*, No. 6, this poem was attacked by Prior, not only for its sense but for its versification and with all the outrage of party virulence. Garth had poise enough not to retaliate, but his satisfaction must have been great at the appearance of an unanswerable defence made for him by Addison, who concluded by observing that " the same person who has endeavored to prove that he who wrote *The Dispensary* was no poet, will very suddenly undertake to show that he who gained the battle of Blenheim was no general."

With like restraint Garth had not deigned to reply to the accusation of an earlier time that *The Dispensary* was really the product of another's pen, a slander, raised by the envy of authorship, that would now be forgotten were it not for Pope's lines:

> With him most authors steal their works, or buy;
> Garth did not write his own Dispensary.
> *Essay on Criticism.*

It was the lack of just such good nature that led to the sorry breach between Addison and Pope, which arose out of the jealousies engendered by Pope's and Tickell's translations of the Iliad. We find the fat, cringing Gay adding fuel to the fire in a letter addressed to Pope, July 8, 1715:—

> " I have just set down Sir Samuel Garth at the Opera. He bids me tell you that everybody is pleased with your translation but a few at Button's; and that Sir Richard Steele told him that Mr. Addison said Tickell's translation was the best that was ever in any language. He treated me with extreme civility, and out of kindness gave me a squeeze by the forefinger. I am informed that at Button's your character is made very free with as to morals etc., and one Mr. A(ddison) says that your translation and Tickell's are both very well done, but the latter has more of Homer. I am etc."

The extreme civility Garth doubtless gave to all, but his companion deserved it little more than the squeeze by the forefinger.

GARTH'S RELIGION, ILLNESS AND DEATH.

IT must have seemed odd to all who have interested themselves in Garth's life that, considering the scant notes which are accessible, there is so much said on the subject of his religion or irreligion. It naturally brings to mind the sorry publicity thrust 150 years later upon the beliefs of another agnostic, to whom might also be applied the sentiment in Pope's oft repeated statement that " if ever there was a good Christian without knowing himself to be so it was Dr.

Garth." * His presumed hostility to every form of Christian faith seems to have been due partly to the irregularity of the exercises at Dryden's funeral, over which he presided, as well as to an early epitaph on St. Evremond, accredited to him and intended for Westminster Abbey, in which he commended him for his indifference to all religion. It does not seem to have been Garth's practice, however, to parade his personal beliefs or disbeliefs, for the tale has come down to us that being one day questioned by Addison upon his religious creed, he replied that he was of the religion of wise men, and being asked to explain himself further, he added that wise men kept their own secrets. Whatever may have been these secrets, his friends knew that, as his days became numbered, doubt and uncertainties arose in his mind and as he neared the end Addison made a futile effort to console him with the hope of a life hereafter, but was turned off with the reply that the doctrines of Christianity were incomprehensible. If, however, we are to believe the story which came from Mr. Blount, the father of Pope's Martha, to Pope, and through him to be recorded among the first of Spence's anecdotes, he repented this attitude on his deathbed. " It was usual for him to say: ' That if there was any such thing as religion 'twas among the Roman Catholics.' Probably from the efficacy we give the sacraments. He died a Papist; as I was assured by Mr. Blount, who carried the Father to him in his last hours." He did not take any care of himself in his last illness; and had talked for three or four years as though tired of life; in short, I believe he was willing to go."

Indeed, not only did he take no care of himself in his last illness, but he actually essayed to have his end hurried, if we are to place further credence on the hearsay anecdotes of the time. I cannot do better than quote again from Spence, who says:

When Dr. Garth had been for a good while in a bad state of health, he sent one day for a physician with whom he was particularly intimate and conjured him by their friendship and by everything that was most sacred (if there was anything more sacred), to tell him sincerely whether he thought he should ever be able to get rid of his illness or not. His friend, thus conjured, told him that he thought that he might struggle on with it perhaps for some years, but that he much feared that he would never get the better of it entirely. Dr. Garth thanked him for dealing so fairly with him, turned

* The same expression Pope put in verse when, shortly before Garth's death, he wrote his farewell to London " Dear, damn'd distracting town, farewell."

> " Farewell Arbuthnot's railing
> On every learned sot
> And Garth the best good Christian he,
> Although he knew it not."

Here in the same stanza Pope links his two distinguished medical friends—Tory and Whig.

* On which Johnson observes that " a mind wearied with perpetual doubt willingly seeks repose in the bosom of an infallible Church."

the discourse to other things and talked very cheerfully all the rest of the time he staid with him. As soon as he was gone, he called for his servant, said he was a good deal out of order and would go to bed; he then sent him for a surgeon to bleed him. Soon after he sent for a second surgeon, by a different servant, and was bled in the other arm. He then said he wanted rest, and when everybody had quitted the room, he took off the bandages and lay down with the design of bleeding to death. His loss of blood made him faint away, and that stopped the bleeding; he afterwards sunk into a sound sleep, slept all the night, waked in the morning without his usual pains, and said if it would continue so he would be content to live on.

It was perhaps this acknowledged attempt to speed the end of his sufferings, coupled with the playful remark accredited to him that he was glad he was dying, for he was weary of having his shoes pulled on and off, which led " ill tongues and worse hearts," as Pope said, " to brand even his last moments as wrongfully as they did his life with irreligion." Can we not commiserate him? A physician who held not the layman's fear of death; wifeless, for Lady Garth had been buried at Harrow the year before; not having the solace brought by religious faith; and doomed to linger on with a painful illness. It was a Baconian saying that man fears not being dead, but only the stroke of death; but to Garth and many others of his kind, necessarily familiar with death, not even the event is fearful—Garth's " friendly stroke."

> To die is landing on some silent shore
> Where billows never beat, nor tempests roar,
> Ere well we feel the friendly stroke, 'tis o'er.
> *The Dispensary.*

Memorable are the words of William Hunter to Dr. Combe. " If I had strength enough to hold a pen, I would write how easy and pleasant a thing it is to die."

Beautiful as the view still remains, the pointed spire of St. Mary's of Harrow-on-the-Hill no longer looks out, as in Garth's day, on unbroken woodland and country side, but on the smoke and roofs of approaching London, apart from whose strife and turmoil he had hoped forever to rest. Forgotten and half hidden by some modern furnishings, in the corner of the chancel one may find a large gray flag stone, on which a part at least of this simple inscription may still be read:

IN THIS VAULT LIES YE BODY
OF YE LADY GARTH LATE WIFE
OF SAMUEL GARTH, KT.
WHO DYED YE 1 OF MAY,
IN YE YEAR 1717.

SIR SAMUEL GARTH
OBIIT JAN. THE 18, 1718.

THE RELATIONSHIP OF THE STATE TO THE TUBERCULOSIS QUESTION.[1]

By John P. C. Foster, M. D.,

New Haven, Conn.

It is unnecessary for me to waste a moment of your time in picturing the havoc wrought by tuberculosis. The story is an old one, and to many of us has a personal bearing. Nor will I attempt to establish the claim that it is the duty of the state to assume the responsibility for the eradication of such a scourge. The health of every community is the measure of its well-being. After centuries of singular indifference the general public is gradually awakening to a proper conception of disease, and of the great economic importance of intelligent and systematic measures to control it. The old teaching that led to the belief that sickness was punishment for sin was accepted by the world with marvelous complacency. Even to-day there is a considerable following of the old teaching, and modern research as it discloses the true origin of one disease after another is regarded as the machination of the devil. Ignorance, prejudice, and heartless greed have ever been ready to block all efforts to control the spread of contagious disease. In contending with such unreasonable influences the task of the workers for sanitary reform has been filled with difficulty and discouragement. Experience has at last made apparent to even the most sceptical the advantages secured to every community by organized effort to control the acute contagious diseases.

With tuberculosis the conditions are not so satisfactory. It is only within a few years that the methods of transmission in this disease have been fully understood. Its development is so subtle that the danger is not so apparent as to arouse public solicitude. The acute character of a yellow fever epidemic appeals directly to the public imagination and justifies any action to secure relief. The insidious development of a more destructive disease, that slowly tortures its victims to death, creates so slight an impression upon the imagination that efforts to control it are not properly appreciated. Men are sceptical as to the curability of tuberculosis, and object to sanitary regulations that do not show immediate results. This scepticism must ultimately yield to the efforts of those who are interested in the tuberculosis question. The time, I believe, is near when state control will be accepted without question. What will be the duty of the state when that happy day shall dawn?

The essentials of success are: First, measures to arrest the development of the disease; and second, the systematic care of all sufferers who may in any way be dependent upon the public for their support.

Measures to control the development of tuberculosis include:

Scientific supervision of all water and milk supplies.

Rational tenement house legislation.

Registration of all cases of tuberculosis in every community.

Control of indiscriminate expectoration.

Intelligent efforts to educate the public as to proper sanitary precautions.

Each of these measures is worthy of careful consideration and has enlisted the sympathy and earnest efforts of philanthropists and sanitary reformers the world over. Time will allow but a brief consideration of them to-night.

Water and Milk Supply.—So much has been said about the public water and milk supply that discussion may seem unnecessary. It may be that the public are already sufficiently aroused upon the water question, but there is yet much to be done to secure suitable milk. Nothing bears more powerfully upon the tuberculosis question than the proper control of the milk supply. Humanity is more dependent upon milk and more widely exposed to disease through its contamination than through any other product. The healthy are infected through its use, and poor sufferers from tuberculosis use it freely as the cheapest and most nutritious food at their command, when in fact it may be the cause of their undoing. In no direction is the responsibility of the state greater, and yet there is a carelessness or indifference that is to be explained chiefly by an unwillingness to antagonize the farmers. Politics and sanitation are poor bedfellows.

It is true that attempts have been made to exterminate tuberculosis in the cow, and many valuable cattle affected with the disease have been destroyed by law. This is well as far as it goes, but intelligent legislation would accomplish much more if it was directed to the preservation of the health of the cattle and to guarding them against the development of tuberculosis especially. The occasional examination of herds and the extermination of tuberculous cattle is right. The municipal examination of milk and the enforcement of a required standard is right. The duty of the state goes farther. All farms should be subjected to regular inspection. No farmer should be allowed to sell milk without a license. Any farmer discovered housing his cattle improperly should be deprived of his license until he has corrected the evil.

Examination into the cattle barns about the country to-day would reveal a condition of filth and neglect that is little suspected by those who are not familiar with the subject. Some time ago I was inspecting a farm with reference to purchasing it for sanatorium work. The place was one of rare natural

[1] Read before the Laennec Society at the Johns Hopkins Hospital, Thursday evening, November 23, 1905.

beauty, and the tenant, I was informed, had used it for years as a milk farm to supply a milk route which he owned in a neighboring city. I saw no evidence of any herd as I walked over the place. Finally, while inspecting the main barn, I noticed a hole in the floor in which a ladder led down into utter darkness. I started to descend upon a tour of investigation, when a voice from below called to me to be cautious and step upon a stone when I reached the bottom of the ladder or I would sink in. I found the stone, and after my eyes became accustomed to the darkness the forms of poor unfortunate cattle began to be evident. The farmer was wading among them in rubber boots. I was told that the cows were never let out, because when housed they gave more milk. From this sink hole of filth milk was carried every day to hundreds of innocent customers, among them unquestionably victims of tuberculosis who were hoping to regain their health by the liberal use of the very milk that had caused their disease. I was told in response to my remonstrance that I would find pretty much the same condition all about the country. I cannot believe this to be true, but I am confident that there is a widespread disregard of all sanitary rules that the state should correct. It can be corrected at small cost, and at no cost to the farmer, if the work is undertaken in the proper spirit.

I am not contending that the state should take measures to enforce fancy dairy development. Farms where cows are washed and curried and where the milkers are forced to wear slippers and refrain from profanity lest they disturb the peace of mind of the cow and induce serious changes in the quality of the milk are all very well, but they are luxuries for the rich who can pay and will pay fifteen to twenty cents a quart for milk. It is the milk of the poor man that I would protect, and there is no possible reason why it cannot be clean and wholesome if the state meets the requirements of the case firmly and intelligently.

Tenement House Regulation.—Of even greater importance is the regulation by law of all tenement house construction. That the crowded tenement is the most prolific breeding spot for tuberculosis has been so clearly demonstrated and the knowledge of the fact has been so widely disseminated, that further delay in legislation to arrest this monstrous evil is criminal. No intelligent and honest man, be he layman or physician, contradicts the statement that impure air and overcrowding are the chief factors in developing disease. The charts showing the results of the efforts that have been made by the health authorities of New York City to control the tenement evil offer a picture that must appeal to every honest man. Is it not marvelous that, with the facts staring us in the face and universally recognized, we should find in this field of reform the bitterest and most powerful opposition? The united tenement house owners, caring for naught but interest upon their investment, are ready to furnish money and personal effort to check legislation. In the field of politics they are a power through the support that they receive, singularly enough, from their victims. The well-to-do, busy with their own affairs, take little interest in the poor, and ignorantly suppose

that the cleaning up of the tenement abuses has no bearing upon their own well-being. This is a fatal error. We cannot live in any community without sharing to some degree its dangers. The yellow fever may lie concealed in some low Italian tenement while those who are long to fall under its power live in the fancied security of wealth. Tuberculosis is wider spread, more difficult to control, more fatal. The elimination of the tenement house infection works for the welfare of the whole community, and should receive the support of the most selfish as well as of those who feel interested to improve the condition of the poor. The state should institute efficient measures to abolish absolutely all dark rooms, to insure a fixed and sufficient amount of air space for each individual, to compel sanitary plumbing and draining of all tenements. Authority to condemn buildings that are hopelessly infected, and to compel their removal, should be vested by the state in the health officers of every community.

Not very long ago I read in a newspaper a letter from a priest, the pastor of a church located in the most infected part of one of our large cities. The proposition had been made to the health board to remove a whole block of houses that seemed to be irremediably infected with tuberculosis, and to leave the space open as a breathing place for the crowded tenement dwellers of that district. The priest wrote in protest, claiming that every room in his parish was overcrowded, and that the removal of an entire block meant that the occupants must be crowded into buildings already too full. This good man in his plea, as he supposed in the interests of his parishioners, was uplifting the hands of their oppressors. The average owner of tenements will give the least he can, and will crowd to any limit that the public will endure. The tenants are too poor to protest, but suitable laws on their behalf would soon better their condition. The business is too profitable. No legislation will drive it away from where it pays. If the law prohibited overcrowding suitable accommodations would appear just whenever and wherever there was a demand. It is not to be supposed that this abuse in tenement construction is confined to the very large cities. In places where land is much less expensive and there is no possible excuse for unsanitary construction the same evils are rapidly developing. The unprincipled landlord is determined, and commands the resources and the political influence to create a power that is not to be easily withstood. Intelligent and immediate legislation to control these evils is the duty of the state. No measure has a more powerful bearing upon the tuberculosis question, and probably no measure is more distasteful to the average politician. United and persistent effort is called for to correct the tenement house abuses.

Registration of Cases.—Registration of all cases of tuberculosis is another important factor in the management of the tuberculosis problem. This should be required by law in every community. It is singular that there should have been so much opposition to this requirement not only from the laity but from a large body of physicians. It has taken years to get at anything like a full report of cases in New York City.

Much tact and good judgment have been called for to secure the co-operation of physicians in reporting their cases. The impression that such a report is in some way a violation of professional confidence is mistaken. The object of registration is to secure some understanding of the destructiveness of the disease and of the measures required to cope with it wherever public care is called for. In private homes where the patients are under competent medical care no interference upon the part of the state or municipal authorities is called for or contemplated. In the crowded tenements the necessity for protecting those who are in good health is apparent, and this can only be accomplished when all cases of tuberculosis are known. There is another point of vast importance, and that is in the care that can be extended to the sick when their condition is known. The condition of the poor sufferers from consumption to-day as compared with their condition before any effort at systematic control was made is vastly improved. No greater charity exists than that extended by the free dispensary for tuberculosis, the district nursing, and the other measures for the care of the tuberculous that are familiar to us all. The state should require registration, and the requirement should not be allowed to go unheeded. No one questions reporting yellow fever, small pox, or other contagious diseases; why should any argument be called for in the case of a disease that destroys more than all other contagious diseases combined?

The Spitting Nuisance.—As to legal restraint upon the spitting habit, it is not necessary to dwell. We know that through indiscriminate expectoration more than in any other way tuberculosis is scattered broadcast. We know that the habit is filthy and inexcusable. We all know how much has already been accomplished in eliminating the evil practice that at one time was considered our chief national characteristic. Expectorating in public places should be legally prohibited, and the public should be made to respect the law.

Education of the Public.—The education of the public as to the nature of tuberculosis, its distribution, and the proper precautions to avoid infection has been so widely undertaken by the health authorities throughout the country that I need only mention it as one of the important duties of the state. Its importance is recognized, and as the distribution of health tracts does not come in conflict with any selfish interests in the community, little or no objection is raised in opposition to the work.

All of these measures for the protection of the public against tuberculosis of which I have spoken come rightly under the control of the state. Individual effort cannot successfully control influences that are so widely distributed and whose combined opposition is inevitably opposed to reform. All movements toward better sanitation have been met in our legislatures by violent opposition, and the unsatisfactory laws that we have to-day have been secured only after bitter and wearisome struggles on the part of a few broad-minded, disinterested citizens. It has always been so difficult to secure legislation to protect the public against their own filth, that

one is inclined to say, What is the use? The failures to secure laws of the utmost importance to the community simply because the politicians fear that in some way their personal interests may suffer are a trial to one's faith.

It is undoubtedly true that the reforms spoken of will surely come, not now, perhaps, but ultimately. Let us hope within a reasonable time. If the workers for such reforms feel disheartened, they can gain courage by looking back over the past twenty years. They will find that surely, if it has been slowly, the great work has been going on in the right direction. Ultimately pure water and milk, clean food, and sanitary tenements will be demanded by the public, and their demands will be respected. Legislatures will find that in serving the public interest they must recognize the duty of the state to guard the public health. State boards of health will ultimately be empowered to enforce sanitary regulations that are of manifest advantage to all and are opposed to-day through a false idea that in some way they conflict with the business interests of individuals. In enforcing the reforms alluded to the state will do much toward the elimination of tuberculosis, and at the same time elevate the moral and physical tone of every community.

State Care of Indigent Consumptives.—There is another phase of the subject in which the state has an important interest. I refer to the care of indigent sufferers from tuberculosis. Their name is legion. Thousands are to be found in every state who have already fallen by the way and have become a public charge or are dependent upon those who are utterly incapable of properly caring for them. Thousands more are gradually yielding to the insidious evil that slowly curtails their efforts and in the end leaves them helpless—a burden on friends, a menace to all about them. For this vast army some provision must be made.

It is idle to suppose that the state can provide sanatorium accommodations for such a host. The financial outlay that would be called for, if indeed it was practicable to house such a large number, would never be granted by any state government. It would not be right, and it is not necessary. If we have the general registration of all tuberculosis patients that I have already alluded to, it becomes a comparatively easy proposition to make a census of those who are properly classed as subjects for public care. These sufferers must be cared for by their own communities. All municipalities should be required by the state to provide suitable accommodations for their indigent tuberculosis patients, not crowded into ill-ventilated poorhouses in intimate association with the intemperate and otherwise vicious, but properly cared for in suitable wards and camps under the general supervision of non-political state tuberculosis boards. The extraordinary work that is already being accomplished all over the world through local tuberculosis dispensaries, district inspectors, and best of all district nurses, the distribution of food to the sufferers through these agencies, and the great betterment that is made in their condition through the instruction that is given as to the value of light and air and proper sanitary precautions, should be the work of municipal boards of health rather than of the state. The state should require of all communities this scientific and humane management of the tuberculous. It should not be left to local health boards to undertake or disregard the work as they may deem it to their interest to do.

The curability of tuberculosis without change of climate has been well established. There is not a city in our country that has not within easy access some suitable open space where the indigent consumptive can receive proper care and where he may possibly be restored to health. The public are slow to accept a statement that seems to them so radical. The long years of training in the belief that climate was the cause of tuberculosis and change of climate the only possible escape from death has left a firm impression upon the public mind. In fact, a large proportion of the practicing physicians, over forty years of age, are even to-day inclined to ridicule the modern conception of tuberculosis, and cling with blind confidence to their bottles of cod liver oil, creosote, and that long list of drugs that are worse than useless.

The report of the Phipps Institute should be accessible to the whole community. In it we read of the work of a hospital located in the poorest part of Philadelphia producing excellent results and contributing valuable scientific information to the world. If such work can be accomplished in an old Philadelphia house made over for hospital use, certainly places can be found in every community, as I have already said, where the tuberculous can be cared for properly.

It has been the custom in the past to confine indigent patients in the town poorhouses. This is cruel and unjustifiable upon sanitary grounds. The tuberculous should not be mixed indiscriminately with other inmates in such institutions. The cost of building in close proximity to such town houses suitable wards where the tuberculous can be cared for would be very trivial. Open tent wards with suitable rooms for dining and recreation can be put up at small cost.

I cannot refrain from a few words upon the question as to the expense of suitable accommodations for the tuberculous, even if it may seem somewhat aside from the subject of this paper. The public, and especially the private sanatoria now in operation in our country are, in the main, costly and in some instances luxurious establishments. This large financial outlay has come to be regarded as unavoidable, and has discouraged many who would gladly enter upon the work if such great expenditures could be avoided. People of wealth have shown much interest in the work and have given very freely for the construction of buildings, in most instances memorials of those who have been victims of tuberculosis. Such buildings are valuable, and there is no reason why they should not be as luxurious as the builders desire, but they are not necessary. In all parts of the country suitable provision for the care of the tuberculous can be made at very small cost and the results of the work under such conditions be equally satisfactory. It is the duty of those who are engaged in the work of construction to make every effort to reduce the expense of buildings and equipment to the minimum. To those who are

familiar with the beautiful buildings that have been erected about the country the simple shack erected at the cost of perhaps a hundred or two hundred dollars seems poor, but it can be made a suitable and scientific provision for patients. These shacks are equally comfortable and are better adapted to the treatment than many of the elaborate structures. The sanatorium treatment cannot be developed all over the country as it should be if there is not more attention paid to the question of economy. A simple farm house with shacks built about it at small cost is quite sufficient for the work. If there is money to spend, let it be expended for competent medical attendants and nurses that make for the good of the patients rather than for useless and too often offensive architectural ornamentation.

I have been told that the public would not submit to the treatment of indigent consumptives in municipal sanatoria; that the patients themselves would undoubtedly resist such treatment. As to the qualms of the sentimentally inclined philanthropist who would consider it a hardship to put the poor consumptives into the poorhouses, I would say that that is just where they have been put for time out of mind, and where they are now. I trust the day is near at hand when they will be properly housed away from the discomforts of such confinement. As to complaints of patients, I have no doubt that paupers would complain of the fresh air treatment wherever administered. It is a violent wrench from their crowded and ill-smelling rooms into cleanliness and pure air. In sanatorium work we find that it is the poorest patients who enter upon the open air treatment with misgiving and often hostility, but they are easily converted.

This possibility that many patients, especially the most ignorant, would decline to go to such institutions as I have spoken of raises the question as to enforced treatment. Should the authorities compel residence in a tuberculosis ward and detain the patient as long as it may be deemed advisable to do so? There is no possible doubt, if tuberculosis is to be controlled, that the health authorities should have the right to detain dangerous cases. In the acute contagious disease epidemies enforced detention has long been respected by the community as a suitable measure. With tuberculosis, owing to the very prolonged character of the disease, the necessity for detention is not so apparent. So long as suitable care, from whatever source, will keep the sufferer from becoming a source of danger to the public, no one would advise removal to special institutions. Detention is only called for in the case of the indigent and ignorant who are unable to care for themselves properly and are indifferent to the necessary restrictions. To protect the public these patients must be properly cared for. As the community must meet the whole expense, it has a right to say when and where patients should go for treatment.

What I would like to emphasize is the idea that in its effort to control tuberculosis the state should impose upon all communities the responsibility for their tuberculous citizens, and the institutions for their care and residence should be scientifically constructed and under the inspection of some non-political state board. If such provision for the care of the tuberculous should be made, the solution of the tuberculosis problem would be immediately simplified. When once established, it will be found that the vast majority of inmates of these town tuberculosis wards are hopelessly sick, offering no possibility of cure, and little for improvement. There will be some, however, who will improve rapidly and give promise of recovery. For such curable cases (I avoid the word incipient) the state should make special provision, and should assume some part of the cost.

Before entering upon a discussion as to the character of state institutions for the treatment of tuberculosis, it is proper to answer the question, why the state is under any obligation to build such institutions. In reading an address read before one of your State Medical Societies during the past year, I came upon this passage: "All sanitarians are agreed that among the most powerful means for the restriction and prevention of the communicable diseases are isolation hospitals." " I dwell upon the utility of a state hospital for consumptives, not for its benefit to a class of unfortunate citizens worthy of sympathy and of all possible aid to recovery, but especially as a means toward the restriction of tuberculosis." This quotation certainly conveys a very mistaken impression as to the purpose of a state sanatorium. No one can seriously propose to a state government the construction of buildings for the isolation of consumptives. Under present conditions the number of tuberculosis victims is so vast that the only possible method of caring for those who are indigent and helpless is by the method I have already suggested. All charitable sanatoria, public or private, justify their existence if they return to health and active work one-half of their beneficiaries. It is undoubtedly this phase of the sanatorium work that appeals with especial emphasis to the philanthropist. The highest claim, however, that such institutions have upon state support is not in their charitable but in their educational value. Patients are not only cured, but they are educated in the proper care of their person, and are led to appreciate the value of all essential sanitary precautions. They go home and abroad, missionaries to preach the gospel of fresh air, pure food, clean rooms. Their influence extends far and wide, and is respected by their associates where the instructions of the professional visitor may possibly be disregarded. The educational value of such institutions is now a demonstrated fact and constitutes a just claim and as I regard it, the chief claim upon the state for assistance. In what form is it desirable for the state to share in this work?

If it is to be in the form of a state sanatorium, built by a committee of the legislature, without the co-operation of medical men who have an intelligent and disinterested interest in the institution; if it is to be designed by partisan architects and constructed by political contractors; if such buildings are to be located with reference to the interests of some political party or boss; worse than all, if the attending physician must be politically acceptable and look to politicians for all he

needs; if, in short, a state sanatorium is to be a political institution, then I say don't build it. Such an institution would be a curse upon the cause it professes to serve. I am inclined to the opinion that it is not advisable to advocate the construction of sanatoria that are to remain under state control. I am aware that my views are not in accord with those of many earnest men interested in the cause. Massachusetts has maintained at Rutland a model state institution designed by masters in our profession and at all times under their supervision. With such a model before us, I hesitate to question the advisability of erecting state institutions. I have already said that the state has a very important relation to the development of the institutional treatment of tuberculosis, but I am sure that there is a method of meeting the demand that is much more efficient and can be relied upon to develop a higher scientific standard than is to be looked for in most state institutions.

When one reads the reports upon tuberculosis and learns that thousands of cases are developing every year, and then turns to read a petition to the legislature for an appropriation of $200,000 to build an institution with possibly 100 beds, the outlook for the sanatorium treatment of the tuberculous does not seem to be propitious. The vital question is, how can the sanatorium influence be extended without making unreasonable financial demands upon the state treasury?

I would reply that it can be extended by the building of small private sanatoria wherever they are called for. At the present time when the public is well aroused upon the question, I would advocate the formation of state anti-tuberculosis associations, embracing all, professional and lay, who are interested in the tuberculosis question, and I would have these associations directly responsible for the construction and maintenance of the local sanatoria. The rich and well-to-do are ready to give and to give liberally towards the construction of these institutions. I do not believe there is any section of our country where an appeal made for private assistance in such work will go unheeded. When a state association has determined upon a proper location for its buildings and has secured from citizens interested in the work the requisite funds for their construction, then let them ask of the state a bounty to launch the work and a subsequent annuity to meet the annual deficit that is inevitable in all such undertakings. By this plan you enlist the sympathy of the public, and the local sanatorium soon becomes a matter of interest and pride. This arousing of local interest is an important factor in all anti-tuberculosis work that may be developed in connection with the sanatorium. When men have given of their means for the construction of such an institution they do not look upon it as a state affair, located at some remote point and controlled by a committee of unknown legislators. It is their property, a home institution. They see its operation. They soon learn that it is a fact that many cases recover and practically all are greatly benefited. The sanatorium is near home, where one can send a needy friend and keep him under observation. It stands in the community as a sanitary schoolhouse, and is, in respect to the well-being of the public, of as much importance as the district school.

It would be impossible at the present time to go into any details as to the character of such sanatoria. Suffice it to say that where state aid is asked for these institutions should be exclusively for the treatment of hopeful cases of tuberculosis among those of moderate means or the absolutely poor. In short, they should always be strictly charitable institutions. It is not necessary, however, nor is it desirable, that they should be free institutions. Sanatoria are not "consumptive homes," but institutions especially required for the development of a wider and more intelligent conception upon the part of the public of the measures necessary to suppress tuberculosis. While the patients should be selected from those who are not able to command the comforts that are accessible to the wealthier sufferers, they should be carefully selected as to their intelligence and physical condition. An effort should be made to select from the mass of material at hand such patients as will have intelligence enough to appreciate the importance of the fresh air treatment and influence sufficient to develop a higher standard of living among their limited circle of associates after their return to work. I have already tried to outline the proper disposition of the vast army of indigent and ignorant consumptives, who should be removed to municipal institutions and should receive all proper consideration as to their personal comfort. These sufferers are in the main ignorant, prejudiced, many of them foreign born, and unfamiliar with and wholly indifferent to our social requirements. The duty of the state in the treatment of such is in the direction of humane isolation as a means of protection to those with whom they would otherwise come in contact. Such patients are, as a rule, unappreciative and ready to conceal their disease and resist interference. They are not suitable material for the state to receive into its institutions where the educational value of the work is the predominating idea. Wherever the attending municipal physicians recognize a case of unusual intelligence and giving promise of cure, such case should be transferred to the sanatorium and the cost be shared by the municipality and the state.

It may appear to some that under a possible excess of enthusiasm there may be an unreasonable development of sanatoria; that associations from all parts of the state may be calling upon the state for bounty. This is a simple business proposition. The organization of state associations embracing all local associations for the suppression of tuberculosis, would soon systematize the sanatorium work. All sanatoria should be incorporated and should cover in their work a territory containing a population of at least two hundred and fifty thousand inhabitants. Less populous sections should unite and their association should not receive state aid until they represent a population sufficient to justify the expense to the state.

The Ontario government offers a grant of twenty per cent of the cost of all municipal sanatoria, but no grant to exceed $4000. I was pleased to learn that the counties of Perth, Oxford, Wellington, and Waterloo had applied to the government for a grant to each county so that they could control $16,000 toward the erection of a sanatorium for their joint use. This union of counties comes so much within the line of my earnest effort as to be very gratifying.

Is this plan for the development of private sanatoria assisted by state bounty practicable?

I am happy to be able to say that it is not only practicable, but that such an institution has been in operation in our state for over a year. The Anti-Tuberculosis Association of New Haven County was the creation of a few lay and medical men who were deeply interested in the work contemplated. They associated with themselves as directors a number of men of the highest position in the county. The association was incorporated for the purpose of furthering every possible effort for the elimination of the scourge of tuberculosis.

The most formidable undertaking of our association was the construction of a sanatorium that should be up-to-date in every respect. The responses to the call for financial assistance were most generous. After a sufficient sum was secured a suitable farm was purchased and the construction of the sanatorium buildings commenced. The state was then asked for an appropriation of $25,000 in part to provide for the erection of barns and other buildings which would not readily appeal to the private donors; the balance to be used as capital to maintain the work until the sanatorium could make its own appeal to the sympathy of the public. As a result, there is in operation at the present time a very beautiful sanatorium containing fifty beds. I have no hesitation in saying that there is not a demand that can be made by this institution that the citizens of the county are not ready to meet. The important point as bearing upon the subject of my paper is that Connecticut has given to a private association a liberal bounty to start their work, and has recently granted $5000 a year for the next two years to meet the inevitable deficit.

Another institution has been built in Hartford County, to which the state has made similar grants. Thus it is seen that with an outlay of but $50,000 there are already one hundred beds in Connecticut. I hope ere long to see two more institutions of this character in our state. Two hundred beds in a state the size of Connecticut is ample for the purpose for which the state can justly be asked to contribute, and any further extension of the work should be left to private philanthropy. These Connecticut sanatoria are absolutely non-political, and their management is entirely under private control. Another sanatorium under private control with state aid is that most admirable institution at White Haven, Pennsylvania. Other instances might be mentioned, but it is unnecessary. If it can be done in Connecticut and Pennsylvania, it can be done everywhere.

Who will do the work called for in the development of a sanatorium? Will men accept such a responsibility that means many days of hard work, frequent periods of discouragement, and unfortunately much bitter criticism and misinterpretation of their motives? Yes, men will do it, do it gladly, and find their reward in the growth of the work and the good that it accomplishes. I trust that it may ever be one of the most important functions of our National Association for the Study and Prevention of Tuberculosis to arouse the public all over our land to an appreciation of the importance of organized effort if the disease is to be controlled. When the public is once aroused the private state sanatorium can be easily maintained.

I wish to read a letter that I received recently, written in response to one in which I had briefly outlined my views as to the proper form in which the public sanatorium work should be developed. It is from Dr. Trudeau, and I have his permission to read it. The doctor writes: " The more I think of the matter of state sanatoria the more I think that the plan of having every community build its own institution and receive support pro rata from the state is the best and most efficient plan of combating the disease and eliminating the evils of large political institutions. Each community will be more willing to pay, too, for its own consumptives than to pay tribute to support all the consumptives in the state institution to which, perhaps, none of the particular community's invalids may be able to gain access. Besides, each community likes to manage, as far as it may, its own affairs."

I have been asked, What should be done in a state where no interest was shown in the building of a sanatorium? There is a very simple answer. Let it go without. The day is at hand when to be without such provision for the public welfare will be a reproach.

It has been my endeavor to show that the relation of the state to tuberculosis is two-fold. Measures to prevent, by wise sanitary legislation. Measures to educate, and if possible to cure. I have outlined a plan for public sanatoria that I believe will develop the work for the best interest of the individual and the state.

To arouse the state government to a proper appreciation of the measures advocated calls for organization. Let there be anti-tuberculosis associations in every state. In these associations enroll the members of all societies working upon sociological problems. What helps one helps all in this crusade against unsanitary living. The time for action is at hand. The work is to be done. I have full faith that in time it will be done, and done well.

THE X-RAY DIAGNOSIS OF THORACIC ANEURYSMS.[1]

By F. H. BAETJER, M. D., *Assistant in Actinography.*

In the ten years that have elapsed since the discovery of the X-ray all branches of medicine have been benefited by this new diagnostic agent. Upon no one branch of medicine, however, has as much light been thrown as upon the chest and its diseases; especially true is this of the heart and its appendages.

Heretofore with the means at our disposal the diagnosis of aneurysm was often difficult and sometimes impossible. In the very early cases just when the most good could be done aneurysms would be overlooked and probably not recognized until their size would preclude almost any hope of doing good. Especially true is this in strong, muscular men at about the fourth decade of life who have degenerative processes in the walls of the arteries due to syphilis or alcohol. On the other hand, a diagnosis of aneurysm may be made which would of necessity cause an absolute change in a patient's habits and mode of living, and yet the subsequent history or possibly the autopsy would show that all the patient's care and anxiety were needless, as no such pathological condition had existed. Since the discovery of the X-ray this doubt and uncertainty has been removed and now we can practically make an absolute diagnosis both positive and negative.

The two methods at our disposal, radiographic and radioscopic, give us an accurate knowledge of the chest and its organs. Whereas the radiograph gives us a permanent record and reveals more detail, yet the examination by the fluorescent screen gives us a more comprehensive knowledge of the chest.

By means of it we can examine the chest from various angles and see the actual pulsations of the heart and its vessels. In this hospital the value of this method of examination has become so apparent that it has become practically a routine practice to examine thus every obscure chest disease.

Briefly, the method of procedure here is as follows: Before proceeding with the X-ray examination the patient is examined to see that there are no abnormalities as to the formation of the chest or spine due to some disease. For example, a diseased vertebra may push the aorta aside and the condition simulate that of an aneurysm. In rachitic children it is common to see a pulsating tumor to the left of the sternum simply due to the displaced aorta.

Having assured ourselves that no abnormalities exist, the patient is placed in a sitting position with his back to the tube. The tube is placed at the level of the third rib and from twenty to twenty-four inches away. At this distance there is very little divergence of the rays and consequently the image projected upon the screen is not materially enlarged or distorted.

After this examination has been made, the tube is placed in front at the same level and the patient is examined from the back. By means of these two positions we can locate the position of an organ by comparing the size of the shadows in each case, since the shadow is always larger the further it is removed from the screen. Now, by means of transverse, or slightly transverse illumination, we can· frequently tell whether the object has its attachment in front or behind. This is especially important in determining whether an aneurysm springs from the ascending or descending portion of the aorta.

[1] Read before the Johns Hopkins Hospital Medical Society, October 9, 1905.

Before leaving the chest it is well to make an examination both from the front and behind with the tube placed on a level with the end of the sternum. By having these fixed positions of examinations we get a composite normal and one soon learns to tell any variation from this normal.

The objection may be advanced that this method does not give an absolutely true picture of the chest because the tube and screen are not always in the same plane. By making the examinations at two different levels the objection is obviated and our composite picture is a true one as the records of the physical examinations and autopsy reports in this hospital have shown.

In a normal individual the fluorescent screen reveals the following picture. The lung substance being permeable to the ray gives us a clear view of the clavicles, scapulæ, and ribs. In the median line we have a dark band about two inches broad extending downward from the clavicular articulations to be lost in the shadow of the heart. This is caused by the spine and sternum. On the left side, low down, the pulsating heart can be readily made out, its shadow fusing into that of the diaphragm. On the right side is a slight pulsating shadow due to the right heart and beneath, the shadow of the right diaphragm. Since the aorta lies just above the spine its shadow is obscured by that of the spine and sternum and consequently no pulsation can be seen either to the right or to the left of the sternum. This practically always holds true. In very thin individuals, however, a slight pulsation of the arch may be observed occasionally, but this is rare. In only one per cent of the cases has this been observed. Abnormalities causing displacement of the aorta have already been mentioned.

From what has been said we can assume that any shadow existing either to the right or to the left of the sternum is abnormal. This may be due to a variety of conditions, such as:

1. New growth.
2. Enlarged glands.
3. Displaced aorta.
4. Dilatation of the aorta.
5. Aneurysm of the aorta.

In new growths and glandular enlargement the history of the case is important and then, too, the shadow cast is more dense than one cast by an aneurysm. Absence of pulsation is of value, but cannot always be relied upon, as frequently we get a transmitted pulsation which can scarcely be distinguished from that of an aneurysm. The two distinguishing features, however, are that the shadow is darker and the edges are more hazy and irregular.

A displaced aorta can be ruled out by examining the spine and chest to see that there are no abnormalities.

In dilatation of the aorta a distinct pulsation of the shadow can be seen, but the diagnostic point is that the shadow disappears between pulsations because the aorta contracts markedly in this condition and its shadow lies within that cast by the sternum and spine. In this connection I may say that especially in such cases is the examination by the fluorescent screen of more value than by the radiograph. The radiograph may show no shadow if taken between the pulsations or if taken during the pulsation show one. In either case a false interpretation of the condition would be made. Aneurysms where the sac is large and pulsating offer no difficulties as to diagnosis.

The detection of small aneurysms just when an early diagnosis is of such value to the patient is often difficult. The one point to bear in mind is that a pulsating shadow which does not disappear between pulsations should always be viewed with grave suspicion. Very small aneurysms can be diagnosed as evidenced by Case 74, which we will consider later.

Broadly speaking, aneurysms may be divided into two classes, namely, sacculated and diffuse. The sacculated ones offer but little difficulty of diagnosis. The shadow pulsates and stands out as a rounded mass from the sternum.

Diffuse aneurysms where the aorta is uniformly enlarged, are marked by a broad shadow extending down along the sternum, generally on both sides. The distinguishing feature, as spoken of before, is that the shadow persists between pulsations.

Naturally, the appearances vary greatly and depend upon the size and position of the aneurysm. Roughly speaking, the positions may be classified as follows:

1. Aneurysm of the ascending portion of the aorta usually casts a shadow more to the right than to the left of the sternum, above the heart, and by localization would be found to be nearer the anterior than the posterior wall of the chest.

2. Aneurysm of the arch casts a shadow slightly to the left of the sternum and this shadow extends well up into the neck and by localization would be found nearer the anterior chest wall.

3. Aneurism of the descending arch of the aorta casts a shadow to the left of the sternum and by localization is generally nearer the posterior than the anterior chest wall.

The above classification covers the common situation of aneurysms, though they may occur anywhere in the course of the thoracic aorta. The records of this hospital show one case where the aneurysm arose from the aorta just before it passed through the diaphragm. The heart was displaced upward and outward and just below to the left of the median line a large pulsating mass the size of an orange could be seen readily. The movement of the left side of the diaphragm was markedly inhibited. The interesting feature in this case was the fact that the patient had been sent to the hospital as a case of rheumatoid arthritis of the spine.

Since practically all obscure chest conditions are examined in this hospital as a routine procedure, we will not take into consideration those cases in which no aneurysms were found, but will confine ourselves entirely to those of aneurysms.

In the past four years there have been 104 cases in which a positive diagnosis of aneurysm has been made. These cases extended over a wide field; some were found by accident, in others the signs were suggestive, and in still others both signs and symptoms pointed distinctly to aneurysm.

A brief mention of some of the unusual cases may be of interest to this Society.

Case 68 is of interest on account of the absence of physical signs and a previous diagnosis of intercostal neuralgia. The patient was a man aged 45, who complained of pain in left side and loss of weight. The onset of his illness was one year ago with pain in right lower thorax radiating to the spine, worse on exertion and paroxysmal in character. This pain gradually increased in intensity and frequency of attack. He entered a hospital in one of the Southern States and there his disease was diagnosed intercostal neuralgia.

After he left the hospital his symptoms increased with the addition of weakness and some dyspnœa. He came to this city to consult Dr. Osler. The physical examination was absolutely negative for aneurysm. Dr. Osler referred the patient to me for an X-ray examination and a large, well-defined aneurysm of the ascending aorta, size of an orange, was discovered.

Case 71—Woman, aged 23.—Complained of shortness of breath. Onset of trouble five weeks ago with cough and shortness of breath. Symptoms increased, accompanied by severe attacks of dyspnœa. The patient was admitted to the hospital in the service of Dr. Osler. At that time marked respiratory distress and cyanosis. Physical examination of chest negative, except for harsh breath sounds due to labored breathing. Diagnosis: Some obstruction to trachea, either external or internal, due probably to a new growth.

An X-ray examination was made and a small aneurysm of the transverse arch of the aorta springing backward and causing tracheal pressure was found. The patient improved for a time, when she suddenly became worse and was unconscious, due to asphyxia. She was immediately seen by Dr. Halsted and, as the obstruction seemed below the larynx, he did a tracheotomy and introduced a rubber tube to a point 15 cm. below the tracheal wound, which gave immediate relief. Exploration of the mediastinum was deemed advisable. A portion of the sternum and ribs was removed and the mediastinum was well exposed, but a hasty exploration revealed no tumor. The patient died that afternoon and an autopsy showed a very small aneurysm coming from the transverse arch, going backward and pressing on the trachea.

Case 85 illustrates the bad results of a late diagnosis. The patient, a man of 65, complained of shortness of breath and respiratory distress. His illness extends over a period of ten years. He was seen seven years ago by a prominent consultant who diagnosed the case as one of asthma. He never improved to any extent. Two months ago his voice became husky and indistinct, due to a recurrent laryngeal paralysis. With the exception of the asthmatic condition, his chest was negative. An X-ray examination revealed one of the largest aneurysms I have ever seen. It practically filled the entire upper left chest.

Case 100 is interesting on account of the peculiar symptoms. A male, aged 57, complained of pain in back, side, stomach, and chest. Three years ago he had a gallstone operation to relieve these symptoms. No gallstones were found and his symptoms did not disappear. One year after the operation shortness of breath came on. He came to this hospital and the marked pain and rigidity of spine suggested spondylitis deformans.

The physical examination of the chest was practically negative. There was a slight pulsation in the second intercostal space which was attributed to an enlarged mammary vessel. To definitely rule out aneurysm, however, the patient was referred to the X-ray department, where a large aneurysm of the descending portion of the aorta was found.

The question naturally arises, In how many of these cases has the subsequent history proved the diagnosis of aneurysm to be correct? Of these cases 70 to 75 per cent were referred to the X-ray department by the medical side with a definite diagnosis of aneurysm. In these the position and size of the tumor as shown by the X-ray findings practically always agreed with the medical findings; in 20 to 25 per cent the diagnosis was doubtful, but in many of the cases the subsequent history proved the X-ray diagnosis to be correct. In 5 per cent of the cases the aneurysm was found by accident, there being no physical signs.

Of all these cases 18 per cent came to autopsy and the anatomical findings corresponded exactly with the X-ray findings.

Naturally, in the class of cases that come to a hospital many of them are finally lost sight of and final proof of the diagnosis cannot be obtained.

The value of the X-ray examination is so apparent in such conditions that it needs no one to urge its claims. Dr. Osler believes that an X-ray examination of the chest should be made in all cases.

In conclusion let me quote Williams, who sums up the situation so admirably: "X-ray examinations should always be made. Normal outlines in the upper part of the chest give us the best assurance that an aneurysm of the aorta is not present, though symptoms may obtain which lead the physician to suspect it. On the other hand, if an aneurysm be present, its outline will be demonstrated by the X-ray examination. An outline suggestive of aneurysm may be due to other causes, as new growth for example. But confusion of this kind is not common and we can in most cases convince ourselves by a careful examination whether or not it is an aneurysm which casts the shadow. X-ray examinations enable us to determine the extent of an aneurysm more accurately than the usual physical examination, and to detect its existence at a much earlier stage. Successive examinations enable us to determine whether or not it is increasing in size.

To make a definite diagnosis of aneurysm by the usual physical examination we may be obliged to wait for the development of marked signs and this delays treatment. On the other hand, if the physician begins treatment because the signs are suspicious, he runs the risk of subjecting his patient to unnecessary regimen. The advantages of X-ray examination when compared with the usual physical examination are evident. A definite diagnosis can be made in most cases before there are physical signs. Treatment can, therefore, be begun at an earlier and more hopeful stage, can be planned more intelligently as the knowledge of the position and ex-

tent of the aneurysm is more accurate, and its results can be better estimated because we can more accurately measure any change in size."

A METHOD OF ESTIMATING THE OPSONIC CONTENT OF BLOOD AND OTHER FLUIDS.[1]

By Charles E. Simon, M. D., and R. V. Lamar, M. D.

(From the Clinical Laboratory of Dr. Charles E. Simon, Baltimore, Md.)

(Under a grant from the Rockefeller Institute for Medical Research.)

Through the researches of Wright and Douglas it has been ascertained that phagocytosis by human leucocytes of various bacteria is essentially dependent upon the presence in the serum of substances which they term opsonins, and that the polynuclear neutrophiles when washed free from serum are incapable of taking up bacteria. If, however, bacteria are suspended in normal blood serum and subsequently exposed to the action of the washed leucocytes, phagocytosis promptly takes place. Hektoen and Rüdiger subsequently showed that similar conditions obtain in the case of phagocytosis by the leucocytes of various animals, such as the guinea pig, rabbit, dog, goat, white rat, and mouse. They showed, moreover, that sera of different animals may sensitize bacteria for phagocytosis by human leucocytes. In order to study certain phenomena of phagocytosis as influenced by the opsonins of the serum, investigators have hitherto largely used defibrinated blood to which, in the case of the rabbit and guinea pig, leucocytes derived from an aseptic pleural exudate are further added, as otherwise the number of polynuclear leucocytes is too small.

In connection with certain experiments which we have undertaken this method of procedure proved unsatisfactory, especially as it was necessary to have non-phagocytic leucocytes available at any time. At the same time it was found that Leishman's method of estimating the phagocytic power of leucocytes, while convenient in a general way and for certain purposes, was not well adapted to our ends. With this method equal parts of blood and bacterial suspensions are mixed and incubated for 15 minutes at 37° C. Smears are then prepared and the average number of bacteria pro leucocyte determined by actual count.

In the course of our experiments it was ascertained that human leucocytes, when washed with normal salt solution containing 0.1 per cent of ammonium oxalate, promptly lost their phagocytic power, but that this could be restored by the subsequent addition of normal serum. A method was thus given by which it is possible to obtain non-phagocyting leuco-

cytes in sufficient quantity for all ordinary purposes in a very convenient manner and with the least expenditure of time. To this end the blood is obtained from the finger or the lobe of the ear, as in ordinary clinical work. Approximately 0.5 cc. is drawn up into a calibrated tube, transferred to a washing tube of .5 cm. diameter, mixed with an excess of normal salt solution containing 0.1 per cent oxalate and centrifugalized. When the corpuscles have been well packed the supernatant fluid is twice replaced by normal salt solution, the tube inverted a few times, and again centrifugalized. The leucocytes after this are devoid of phagocytic action, and ready for use, when it is desired to determine the opsonic content of the second specimen of blood or other fluids. In the case of the blood a corresponding amount, as in the first instance, is obtained by puncture, placed in a drawn-out tube, and at once centrifugalized, until the corpuscles are firmly packed and the supernatant fluid is clear. With this serum dilutions are made with normal salt solution in varying proportions. Small tubes are charged with a few drops of diluted serum, inoculated with the microorganisms under consideration, so that a moderate milky turbidity results, further treated with a small quantity of washed corpuscles, and incubated for 30 minutes at 37° C. Smears are finally prepared on slides, and, when air-dry, stained with a strong solution of methylene blue, containing a trace of sodium hydrate. As index of the opsonic content of the blood under examination we then take that degree of dilution at which phagocytosis has practically become extinguished, or when the number of non-phagocyting cells exceeds 90 per cent. This we designate as the opsonic coefficient of extinction.

We have thoroughly tested the practical value of the method as just outlined and have every reason to regard it as established. It renders possible the investigation of various problems connected with the opsonins and phagocytosis which heretofore was beset with considerable difficulties. The results which we have obtained by its use we shall report on a future occasion.

TROPICAL SPLENOMEGALY.

By

W. E. MUSGRAVE, M. D.,

Pathologist, Biological Laboratory,
Physician-in-Chief, St. Paul's Hospital, Manila.

W. B. WHERRY, M. D.,

Bacteriologist, Biological Laboratory,

AND

PAUL G. WOOLLEY, M. D.,

Director, Serum Laboratory,
Pathologist, St. Paul's Hospital, Manila.

(From the Biological and Serum Laboratories, Bureau of Government Laboratories, Manila, P. I.)

Enlarged spleen is a constant manifestation in such diverse clinical and pathological pictures that, except in those in which the etiologic agent has been found and a distinct disease thereby separated and established, classification has been unsatisfactory, and clinical and pathologic descriptions confusing.

To students of tropical medicine this subject is still more complex, for in addition to the greater or less prevalence of the usually described types of this complex in temperate climates, we have to deal with a variety or varieties which have additional symptoms of enough significance to warrant considering them a class by themselves. This group is variously designated as tropical splenomegaly, kala azar, dum dum fever, kala dunkh, etc.

Splenomegaly is not uncommon among the Filipinos, and it is not difficult to find types corresponding with those described by Osler, Banti, and others in temperate climates. However, these do not concern us here, and we shall consider only that group that is, because of geographic distribution and certain well-defined features not seen in temperate climates, generally included under the term tropical splenomegaly. Since Leishman's discovery it seems possible that at least one etiologic entity may be separated from this clinical class, but since the parasite has not been found in all cases, it will be necessary at some future time when the exact zoological status of the Leishman body has been determined, to rechristen certain members of the group, and to allow the more ancient terms to apply to the purely clinical forms.

The principal features of tropical splenomegaly, which distinguish it from other types of similar disease in other parts of the world, and which are also seen in the tropics, at least in Manila, are the prevalence and character of the fever, the toxic disturbances, certain gastro-intestinal phenomena, and changes in the skin.

CASE I.—The first case observed by us in the Philippine Islands, which from its clinical manifestations belongs to the class of tropical splenomegaly, gave a history briefly as follows:

J. J. L., an American volunteer soldier, 24 years old. His family and previous history are unimportant. After about five months' residence in the Philippine Islands, a moderate diarrhea developed, which lasted for about two weeks, and which was accompanied by moderate remittent fever, and a peculiar macular eruption of the skin, distributed over most of the body but not on the face, hands, or feet. There were slight rheumatic pains, particularly in the knees and shoulders. The diarrhea continued intermittently during the eighteen months which were spent in the Islands, and until the time of death about three years after the first attack. The diagnosis of intestinal amebiasis was made about one and a half years after the original attack. A few weeks after the first diarrhea, fever of a remittent type developed and lasted for about two weeks and was accompanied by headaches, muscular and joint pains, and nausea in addition to the dysentery. During this attack the patient noticed that his spleen was enlarging, and it continued to increase in size during the next year. He suffered repeatedly from recurrent attacks of fever without definite chills. Eighteen months after his first attack of fever the spleen had attained an enormous size, and there was constant dragging pain in the left side. He became reduced from 160 to 105 pounds, was pale, anemic, and mentally depressed. Repeated blood examinations failed to indicate the nature of the disease. There were no malarial parasites or pigment, no agglutination of B. typhosus or M. melitensis, and in fact nothing in the slightest way diagnostic. The red blood corpuscles were 2,120,000, and the leucocytes 3,900, and there was nothing suggestive in stained specimens. The urine contained no albumen, sugar, or casts. Quinine had no effect upon the course of the fever, and physical examination simply supported the diagnosis of tropical spleen.

The patient was invalided home to the United States, where he lived in a country town, and there he died of rupture of the spleen and dysentery, three years after the beginning of his trouble.

CASE II.—A. A., a native of the Island of Mindoro, and about 25 years of age. About five years before coming under observation he contracted a severe fever which lasted about a month, and which was followed by enlargement of the spleen, which, he stated, is a common disease in his part of the country, where it is known as "cayana." During the four and a half years following the first attack he had several similar ones and the spleen continued to increase in size. Rheumatic pains were always present with the fever and to a less extent during the remissions. On several occasions he noticed edema of the feet and ankles, and he thought that the edematous looking skin-disease scattered over the feet, legs, arms, and chest developed coincidently with his second attack of the fever. Diarrhea was usually present with the fever and subsided during the intermissions. One month after entering Bilibid Prison to serve a life sentence, he was admitted to the prison hospital and was there treated, for eighteen days, for a remittent fever, which was not influenced by quinine. During this attack there were mild jaundice and slight rheumatic pains. The patient was returned to duty and remained fairly well for about three months, when he was again admitted to the hospital with a temperature of 39° C., cough, and labored respiration. Owing to the fact that there was an epidemic of pneumonia prevailing in the prison at the time, a diagnosis of this disease was made without further examination. We saw him for the first time a couple of days later and after examination the diagnosis was changed to kala azar. At the time of examination he was emaciated, anemic, and slightly jaundiced. There was an old eczematous condition on the legs, arms, and abdomen, and the feet and arms were edematous. The spleen was very much enlarged, extending below the costal arch, and well to the right of the median line. It was slightly tender on pressure, quite firm, and slightly rough. The liver was but slightly enlarged, and there was some tenderness over the region of the gall-bladder. The abdomen was tender along the colon, and there was quite active diarrhea. The superficial lymph glands, particularly those in the groins, were somewhat enlarged, and moderately firm (a condition very common among Filipinos). The temperature was intermittent in character, ranging from 37° to 40° C., and accompanied by dragging pain the left side and rheumatic pains in the shoulders and knees, and difficult respiration.

On May 19, 1904, a little more than three months after his first admission into the hospital, and two days before death, a splenic puncture was done and a syringe-full of fluid was withdrawn. Part of this was injected into the abdominal subcutaneous tissue of a monkey (*Macacus cynomalgus*), part was rubbed into the mucous membrane of the monkey's lips, and part was used to make smears for microscopical examination. The smears were stained with Wright's modification of Romanowski's stain, and with dilute (1-10) carbol-fuchsin. No Leishman bodies, no bacteria, and no malarial organisms were seen. The monkey never showed any signs of disease

following the inoculation, had no rise of temperature, and no palpable enlargement of the spleen or liver.

The patient died on May 21, 1904, and the autopsy was done by Dr. Brinckerhoff immediately after death.

The body, which was that of a well-developed but poorly nourished native, was still warm. Rigor mortis was present in the muscles of the jaws and fingers. The subcutaneous fat was 2 to 3 mm. thick. The muscles were of a beefy-red color. The surface of the peritoneum was smooth and shining. There were about 100 cc. of blood-stained fluid in the pelvis. On the lateral aspect of the spleen there was a fresh blood clot of about 100 cc., and this organ was adherent to the diaphragm. The appendix was normal. The mesenteric lymph nodes were normal. Both lungs were bound to the chest walls by old fibrous adhesions which partly obliterated the pleural cavities. The pericardial cavity was normal. The aortic valves presented thickenings of the cusps with irregular losses of substance and soft grey-red vegetations. The myocardium was normal. The other valves showed no abnormalities. The surface of the spleen was smooth and wrinkled. There was a punctured wound on the superior surface. Weight 600 grams. Upon section one old and one recent infarct were discovered. The consistence of the liver was increased but the organ was otherwise apparently normal. The intestines showed no marked change. There were some anchylostomes in the duodenum. The pancreas, kidneys, bladder, testes, and bone marrow were apparently normal. The brain showed some sub-pial edema. The cord was apparently normal.

Bits of the spleen, liver, kidneys, and cardiac vegetations were fixed in Zenker's solution. The brain and cord were, with the exception of specimens of the cord from three levels, which were fixed in 93 per cent alcohol, fixed in 10 per cent formalin.

Cultures from the spleen were made on —I glycerine agar and on —I plain agar and also in deep glucose-ascitic-agar stabs; and from the liver on —I glycerine agar and —I plain agar slants. The cultures on +I glycerine agar and —I plain agar remained sterile during forty days' observation. Those in glucose-ascitic-agar stabs showed a slight cloudiness near the upper portion of the stabs on the fourth day. A stained preparation (1-10 carbol-fuchsin) showed many minute coccus-like bodies, and also some few larger cocci. No growth appeared in transplants from this into +I sugar-free bouillon (aerobic), or in glucose-ascitic-agar stabs (anaerobic, pyrogallic). In the cultures from the liver a number of colonies of an organism diagnosed as Staphylococcus citreus appeared.

A small piece of the spleen was broken up, in an aseptic manner, in 10 cc. of an 0.8 per cent sodium chloride solution, and of this 3 cc. were injected into the peritoneal cavity of each of two guinea pigs (Nos. 603, 604), and 3 cc. into the right axillary subcutaneous tissue of the monkey (No. 712), which had been inoculated with the fluid from the splenic puncture. These guinea pigs died three and a half and four and a half months, respectively, after inoculation. Their spleens and livers were not enlarged but the splenic follicles were somewhat hypertrophied. Fresh smears from the organs showed an enormous number of sulphur-colored granules and rounded bodies varying from 1 to 5 microns in diameter, and often arranged in masses of considerable size. These were tinted a light green by Wright's stain and colored red with dilute carbol-fuchsin. They were present in a certain number of control pigs, but were also absent in some. They were in all probability simply an expression of abnormal pigment formation. Sections showed nothing abnormal. In all twenty-three guinea pigs were used, and two normal animals as controls were killed and their tissues examined microscopically. This number comprised one series of 10, all of which were injected with 1 cc. of a spleen emulsion and then killed after successive weeks. Nothing abnormal was found in smears or sections.

The tissues from the autopsy of the patient were imbedded in paraffin and sectioned. These sections were stained with methylene blue and eosin, Borrel's stain, Heidenhain's iron hematoxylin, and with Willyoung's picro-fuchsin-thyonin mixture. In spite of painstaking searches, no bodies presenting the features of those described by Leishman, Donovan, Wright, Christophers, or Marchand and Ledingham could be found. There did not seem to be any abnormal part played by the endothelium in any organ. The liver and spleen showed a moderate congestion. The liver presented some increase in fibrous tissue which was perilobular and minimal in amount. The centers of the lobules were not affected as in Christophers' cases. The spleen showed a chronic hyperplasia with congestion. The kidneys were the seat of a cloudy swelling. The adrenals were not abnormal. There was no sign of foreign bodies or of parasites in the cardiac vegetations.

CASE III.—This case, like the previous one, was a native of the Island of Mindoro, and from the same town. He was 30 years old. He said that when he was 17 years old he had a severe fever which lasted for more than a month and which was followed by rapid enlargement of the spleen. At the same time he was jaundiced. He also called the disease cayana and said that the complex of large spleen and fever was well known in his country. There have been repeated attacks of fever since the first one and jaundice has always been a decided feature. He has also noticed swelling of the feet and ankles, and occasionally of the abdomen (ascites).

The man was admitted to the hospital in Bilibid early in 1904 and has been under observation since that time. He never has suffered from pain. Since coming under observation there have been many attacks alternating between periods of apyrexia and others in which there was intermittent fever running from 38° to 39° C., and lasting from one to two or more weeks. He is fairly well nourished, but listless, and his muscles are very soft. There has been constant slight jaundice which becomes more marked with exacerbations of temperature. The skin is usually dry and scrawny and slight edemas of the legs and under the eyes have been noticed. The inguinal glands are decidedly enlarged and quite firm, but the other peripheral lymphatic glands do not show this change to any extent. When he first came under observation there was a small amount of fluid in the peritoneal cavity and this has increased somewhat. At the same time the spleen was very much enlarged but has not varied in size for many months. The liver is also considerably enlarged, extending below the ribs in the mammary line. The surface feels hard and slightly nodular. The patient states that the enlargement on the right side came on within the last five years. There are no evidences of heart lesions and the lungs are clear. Urine examinations on two occasions were negative for albumen, sugar, and casts. There was, however, considerable pus, probably from the urethra. There have been repeated attacks of diarrhea, but microscopic examinations of the stools, on several occasions, have been negative. The fever has not been influenced by repeated cinchonization.

Blood counts: August 16, 1904, red cells, 4,840,000; white, 8000.

	May 5.	June 8.	August 15.
Neutrophiles	33%	40%	63 %
Eosinophiles	48%	48%	25.5%
L. M.	7%	8%	6 %
S. M.	12%	2%	3.5%
Basophiles	—	2%	1 %

In feces a few ova of Trichocephalus dispar. No parasites in blood.

CASE IV.—A native man from the same island and town as the two above cases. Age 27. He states that the duration of his disease has been about six years. The mode of onset, the subsequent course, and present condition, very closely resemble those of Case III.

Blood examinations:

	May 26. 1904.	June 8.	August 16.
Neutrophiles	77%	81%	73.5%
Eosinophiles	8%	9%	11.5%
L. M.	7%	6%	7 %
S. M.	6%	2%	5.5%
Basophiles	—	2%	2.5%

August 16, 1904: Red cells, 3,640,000; white, 4000.

A few ova of uncinaria in stool. No parasites in blood.

From Cases III and IV some material was withdrawn by splenic puncture. This was mixed with potassium citrate and used in making smears and cultures (citrate solution of 0.01 per cent in physiological salt solution). In none of the smears were any parasites observed, and there was no malarial pigment seen. In smears from Case III there were some colorless granular materials of uncertain origin. With the citrated solution of the fluid obtained by splenic puncture flasks containing about 350 cc. of —I sugar-free bouillon were inoculated from each case and placed at 35° to 37° C. Cultures were also made in ascitic agar stabs (ærobic and anærobic), and on +I glucose agar (anærobic), and on +I glycerine agar slants. All were kept at 35° to 37° C. No growth occurred in any of the cultures.

CASE V.—A native of the province of Nueva Ecija, in Luzon, age 27 years. His first attack was while a boy. This lasted a long time and was followed by the appearance of a tumor in the left side. The patient stated that the disease is a common one in his part of the country and that it is known as "quisig," and that the common treatment consists in bandaging over the site of the tumor a flat piece of iron that has been chilled by remaining out of doors over night, and is still covered with dew. He also said that he had no further trouble after the first attack until about a year ago, when he had a very severe one, and with this he had swelling of the feet and rheumatic pains. He was admitted to the prison hospital suffering with remittent fever. The attack lasted about twenty days. Physical examination showed that the spleen extended about 8 cm. below the costal margin, and beyond the median line. The liver was not enlarged. The chest was apparently normal. Urine normal. Diarrhea present, but no parasites could be found.

Blood count: Red cells, 4,280,000; white, 8000.

Neutrophiles	71.3%
L. M.	5.6%
S. M.	19.3%
Transitionals	2.0%
Eosinophiles	1.6%

Splenic puncture on two occasions. Smears stained with Wright's stain and with carbol fuchsin (1-10) showed no abnormality.

CASE VI.—Patient is a male Tagalog, 24 years old.

Three years before coming under observation he had a severe fever which was followed by enlargement of the spleen. Since that time he has had repeated attacks of fever and the spleen has gradually increased in size until now it extends 7 cm. below the ribs. He gives no history or evidence of other disease. The course of the disease closely resembles that of Cases III and IV, but he has no pain. The urine is healthy. He had intermittent diarrhea, but no parasites could be found. He also had double chronic conjunctivitis, swelling of the legs, and remittent fever.

Blood count: Red cells, 3,820,000; white, 8000.

Neutrophiles	64.5%
L. M.	14.0%
S. M.	18.0%
Transitionals	3.5%
Eosinophiles	0.3%

Splenic puncture on two occasions. Smears stained with Wright's stain and with carbol-fuchsin (1-10) showed no abnormality.

CASE VII.—This case came from the same district as did Case IV. His history is practically that of the latter. He also gave a history of rheumatic pains which involved even some of the smaller joints. Since the second attack of fever the joint pains have been recurrent.

CLINICAL SUMMARY.

A clinical summary of this symptom complex as it occurs in the Philippine Islands shows that it is very closely related, if not identical with those forms occurring in other tropical countries, where it is variously known as kala azar, dum dum fever, etc.

In the Philippines as elsewhere young people from 15 to 25 years of age seem to be most susceptible.

The disease is almost invariably ushered in by an attack of remittent or intermittent fever which clinically resembles malaria or dengue, and is accompanied by enlargement of the spleen. Recurrent exacerbations of fever at irregular intervals occur throughout the course of the disease. This fever is not influenced by quinine and, in the Philippines, is recognized by the natives as a "cayana" or "quisig" and is held by them to be a distinct disease from malaria.

We have not visited any of the districts from which our cases came and can discover little more about them than we have stated, because in these districts there is an almost complete lack of medical attendance. However, the laity consider the disease as a very fatal one, and often of very short duration, but more often chronic, the patient living for several or many years.

The spleen usually enlarges quite rapidly, reaching its maximum size by the second or third attack of fever, and then very often no further change occurs, unless the idea of the natives is correct, that the organ grows harder. The liver may or may not be enlarged, but when it is that change is secondary to the splenic enlargement.

Jaundice, usually slight, but also well developed, is often present, sometimes even in those cases without enlargement of the liver. This fact accounts partly for the muddy pigmented appearance of the skin and mucous membranes, which is so commonly seen.

There seems to be a special tendency to involvement of the mucous membranes in this disease. This is shown by the frequent gastro-intestinal disturbances, conjunctivitis, etc. The natives say that it also causes discharges from the vagina and sometimes also abortion.

There is also a tendency to hemorrhages in both the mucous membranes and the skin. Three of our cases had epistaxis and bleeding from the gums. One showed hemorrhages into the conjunctiva, and two, old cutaneous remnants of hemorrhages. This tendency may be explained in some cases by the jaundice.

Edemas, at first transient, and later more marked and persistent, are common occurrences, and are more common on the legs and face. Ascites and pulmonary congestion may also be remarked.

Anemia, emaciation, and cachexia develop gradually in nearly all cases.

Pain is a frequent but by no means a constant symptom. It is manifested by headache, arthralgia, and myalgias, and is apparently more common in the early stages of the disease.

Clinically the condition seen in the Philippines is a fairly definite one, and is identical or closely resembles the kala azar of other tropical countries, and might from clinical findings alone be considered as a specific entity.

Our studies in the etiology of the disease have been negative,

and in view of the discoveries of Leishman and others in clinically similar conditions it seems best for the present, at least, to consider these cases as examples of tropical splenomegaly and to search for further etiologic data.

NOTES AND NEWS.

Dr. William S. Baer is Visiting Orthopedic Surgeon to the Cambridge Hospital, Cambridge, Md., and to the Union Protestant Infirmary, Baltimore. Address: 714 Park Avenue, Baltimore.

Dr. Lewellys F. Barker, Physician-in-Chief to the Hospital, resides at 6 East Franklin Street, Baltimore.

Dr. L. Clyde Bixler is associated with Dr. Lawrence Litchfield, of Pittsburgh, Pa. Address: 216 North Highland Avenue, Pittsburgh, Pa.

Dr. E. Bates Block is Professor of Mental and Nervous Diseases, Atlanta College of Physicians and Surgeons, and Visiting Physician to the Presbyterian Hospital, Tabernacle Infirmary and St. Josephs Infirmary. Address: 723 Empire Building, Atlanta, Ga.

Dr. George Blumer is Assistant in Medicine in the Medical Department of the University of California. Address: 369 Sutter Street, San Francisco, California.

Dr. Maurice B. Bonta is Resident Gynecologist, The Lakeside Hospital, Cleveland, Ohio.

Dr. John B. Briggs is Assistant in Physiology, Georgetown University Medical School. Address: 1718 Rhode Island Avenue, Washington, D. C.

Dr. Joel I. Butler is Assistant Surgeon to the Mercy Hospital, Springfield, Mass., and Medical Referee for Western Massachusetts for the Mutual Life Insurance Company of New York. Address: 164 St. James Avenue, Springfield, Mass.

Dr. W. J. Calvert is Assistant Professor of Internal Medicine in the University of Missouri. Address: University of Missouri, Columbia, Mo.

Dr. C. N. B. Camac is Visiting Physician to the City Hospital, Blackwell's Island, New York, Instructor in Medicine, Cornell Medical College, and Chief of Clinic, Cornell Dispensary. Address: 108 East 65th Street, New York.

Dr. Sydney M. Cone is Professor of Pathology and Professor of Orthopedic Surgery at the Baltimore Medical College. Address: 2326 Eutaw Place, Baltimore.

Dr. George W. Dobbin is Professor of Obstetrics and Gynecology at the College of Physicians and Surgeons. Address: 56 West Biddle Street, Baltimore.

Dr. Joseph Erlanger is Associate Professor of Physiology in the Johns Hopkins University. Address: 103 Jackson Place, Baltimore.

Dr. W. W. Farr is Physician to the Leamy Home. Address: 7432 Boyer Street, Mt. Airy, Philadelphia, Pa.

Dr. Simon Flexner is Director of the Laboratories of the Rockefeller Institute for Medical Research, New York. Address: 105 East 62d Street, New York.

Dr. W. W. Ford is Associate in Bacteriology, Johns Hopkins University. Address: 1134 Cathedral Street, Baltimore.

Dr. R. E. Garrett is First Assistant Physician to the Maryland Hospital for the Insane, Catonsville, Md. Address: Catonsville, Md.

Dr. H. Z. Giffin is an assistant in the Children's Hospital, Philadelphia. Address: 207 South 22d Street, Philadelphia, Pa.

Dr. Norman B. Gwyn is Instructor of Medicine in the University of Pennsylvania, and Registrar at the Philadelphia and Children's Hospitals. Address: 23 South 21st Street, Philadelphia, Pa.

Dr. M. L. Haviland is on the Assistant Staff of the Parks Hospital at Glens Falls, N. Y. Address: 5 Centre Street, Glens Falls, N. Y.

Dr. Josephine Hemenway, after January 1, 1906, will assume the position of Resident Physician at the Babies' Hospital, New York City.

Dr. August Hoch is First Assistant Physician at Bloomingdale Asylum and Instructor in Psychiatry, Cornell Medical School. Address: Bloomingdale, White Plains, N. Y.

Dr. Gerry R. Holden is located at Jacksonville, Florida.

Dr. G. L. Hunner is Associate in Gynecology, Johns Hopkins University, Professor of Genito-Urinary Diseases, Woman's Medical College, and Consulting Gynecologist to the Hebrew Hospital, Baltimore, the Frederick City Hospital, Frederick, Md., the Peninsula General Hospital, Salisbury, Md., and to the Brattleboro Memorial Hospital, Brattleboro, Vermont. Address: 1420 Eutaw Place, Baltimore.

Dr. Herbert M. Little is Medical Superintendent of the Montreal Maternity, and Senior Demonstrator of Obstetrics in McGill University. Address: Montreal Maternity, Prince Arthur and St. Urban Streets, Montreal, Canada.

Dr. Harry T. Marshall is Visiting Physician to the Hospital of the Home of the Friendless. Address: 5 West Chase Street, Baltimore.

Dr. Herman W. Marshall is Surgical House Officer at the Massachusetts General Hospital, Boston, Mass.

Dr. E. W. Meisenhelder, Jr., is in private practice in York, Pa. Address: 342 West Market Street, York, Pa.

Dr. Eugene L. Opie is Associate of the Rockefeller Institute for Medical Research, and Editor of the Journal of Experimental Medicine. Address: Rockefeller Institute for Medical Research, New York.

Dr. Mary S. Packard is attending Physician, North End Dispensary for Women and Children, Providence. Address: 425 Angell Street, Providence, R. I.

Dr. Charles D. Parfitt is Physician-in-Charge of the Muskoka Free Hospital for Consumptives, Gravenhurst, Ontario.

Dr. Jewett V. Reed is at present Demonstrator in Neuro-Anatomy and Pathology in the School of Medicine of Purdue University, and Visiting Physician to the Ednor Hospital for Children. Address: 35 Willoughby Building, Indianapolis, Indiana.

Dr. Robert Reuling is Physician-in-Chief of the Out-Door Clinic, Garrett Hospital for Children, and Demonstrator of Neuro-pathology in the University of Maryland. Address: 103 West Monument Street, Baltimore.

Dr. Theodore F. Riggs is First Assistant Resident Physician at the Union Protestant Infirmary, Baltimore.

Dr. Carey P. Rogers is Director and Consulting Surgeon, De Soto Sanatorium, Jacksonville, Florida, Consulting Surgeon, Seaboard Air Line Railway, and State Referee Mutual Life Insurance Company of New York. Address: Bisbee Building, Jacksonville, Florida.

Dr. John A. Sampson is Gynecologist to the Albany Hospital and Lecturer on Gynecology, Albany Medical College. Address: 180 Washington Avenue, Albany, N. Y.

Dr. Charles E. Simon is Professor of Clinical Diagnosis, Baltimore Medical College, and Clinical Microscopist to the Union Protestant Infirmary. Address: 1302 Madison Avenue, Baltimore.

Dr. J. Morris Slemons is Associate in Obstetrics, Johns Hopkins University. Address: 23 West Chase Street, Baltimore.

Dr. Charles N. Spratt is Visiting Ophthalmologist and Otologist, Minneapolis City Hospital, and to the Out-Patient Department, Asbury Hospital. Address: 305 Syndicate Arcade, Minneapolis, Minn.

Dr. Walter R. Steiner is Pathologist and Bacteriologist at the Hartford Hospital. Adddress: 4 Trinity Street, Hartford, Conn.

Dr. A. R. Stevens is assistant to Dr. H. H. Young. Address: 1005 North Charles Street, Baltimore.

Dr. Martin B. Tinker is Lecturer on Surgery, Cornell University Medical College. Address: The Clifton Springs Sanitarium, Clifton Springs, N. Y.

Dr. J. H. J. Upham is Adjunct Professor to the Chair of Medicine, Starling Medical College, Columbus, Ohio.

Dr. Otis B. Wight is Clinical Assistant and Lecturer in Medicine, Medical Department, University of Oregon, Secretary of the City and County Medical Society, Portland, Medical Referee for Oregon for the Mutual Life Insurance Company, and Medical Examiner for the Washington Life Insurance Company. Address: 509 The Dekum, Portland, Oregon.

Dr. Sarah D. Wyckoff is Lecturer in Domestic Science and Hygiene in the High School at Wilkesbarre, Pa., also examiner of pupils for gymnastic work at the Wyoming Seminary. Address: 68 West South Street, Wilkesbarre, Pa.

Dr. Charles W. Young is connected with the Mission of the American Board at Pekin, China.

PROCEEDINGS OF SOCIETIES.

THE JOHNS HOPKINS MEDICAL SOCIETY.

November 6, 1905.

Dr. W. G. MacCallum, president; Dr. C. H. Bunting, secretary.

Exhibition of Medical Cases. DR. THAYER.

Anomalous Cardiac Murmur.—The patient was a male, colored, 57 years old; admitted sixteen times, the first admission being in 1896. He gave a history of only ordinary children's diseases; lues was denied. On first admission he showed œdema of legs, shortness of breath, albumen in the urine, and a dilated heart, which symptoms cleared up under treatment. He had an attack of rheumatism of doubtful nature during the next year. On admissions to 1903 his heart was more and

more dilated with a systolic murmur at apex. At that admission the apex was in the seventh interspace with a systolic murmur. In the fifth interspace in the parasternal line there was a peculiar murmur of decreasing intensity beginning after a slight pause after the second sound, and ending just before the first sound. It was in every way similar to a diastolic murmur of mitral stenosis except for its position. The patient on exhibition had a greatly dilated heart with tricuspid insufficiency, systolic pulsation in veins of neck and in liver. The first sound was replaced by a soft systolic murmur, and the second pulmonic was louder than the second aortic. There was no suggestion of aortic valvular disease and no evidences of a true organic mitral lesion. The murmur was heard in area where murmur from tricuspid ought to be heard best when the blood is flowing from the right auricle to the right ventricle, but there was nothing that would point to tricuspid disease, and besides murmurs in tricuspid stenosis are very rare. Had there been an aortic lesion a faint murmur heard in this region instead of its usual area near the apex might be considered. The patient has a marked grade of sclerosis. Might not sclerotic atheromatous changes extending from the aorta to the anterior mitral curtains cause a slight interference to the passage of blood from the left atrium to the left ventricle by a thickening of the curtain? The sound began with a slight shock. The opening snap of mitral valve from relaxation of ventricle and pressure of blood from above might be caused by such a condition. The snap begins at the beginning of diastole. There was thought not to be mitral endocarditis, but a dilated and hypertrophied heart secondary to arteriosclerosis. There was a mitral and tricuspid insufficieney due to dilatation of the ring. The murmur was thought to be produced at either one or the other of these valves, most probably the mitral.

Marked Grade of Enteroptosis. DR. THAYER.

Patient was a colored woman, aged 45 years. She had a pulmonary tuberculosis involvement. The abdominal wall was remarkably relaxed. The liver edge was practically normal. Below it, just below the umbilicus, was a shadow descending on inspiration with peristaltic waves passing from left to right, which on dilatation proved to be stomach. The stomach was entirely below the ribs, the tympany of the fundus beginning at the costal margin. The right kidney was very movable.

The Significance of Casts in the Urine. DR. EMERSON.

Cylindruria is the presence of casts in the urine. It is "pure" if no albumen is present as tested by the ordinary clinical tests. *Varieties:* Epithelial casts are made up of cells with round nuclei. They are parts of the tubules below the loops of Henle and some have lumina which can be seen. In addition to these, and classed under the same name, are hyaline casts with one, two, or a few cells with round nuclei attached. Many of these cells have a perfectly clear protoplasm, though the kidney cells are granular. Those of the first type are rare. They occur in acute nephritis. Those of the second type are common. They can be found in bicycle riders and athletes, as can blood casts, not uncommonly after hard exercise, i. e., hyaline casts with a few blood cells attached. Blood casts which are clots of blood occur in hemorrhagic nephritis. A true pus cast occurs in purulent nephritis, but hyaline casts with pus cells attached are found in athletes. Coarsely granular casts are opaque with very coarse granules. They are not translucent and evidently are pus or epithelial casts gone to pieces. The next stage in the degeneration of this form is the waxy cast which occurs of two varieties, white and yellow, both of which tend to split transversely. The true hyaline cast is faint and watery and is seen only by shutting off the light. It may be found wherever albumen is expected and does not stain by iodine. There is a cast usually called hyaline, though it is not, which is not so refractile as the waxy casts, which occurs in nephritis or long-standing renal trouble, and stands between the waxy and hyaline groups. Associated with this intermediate group are very translucent fine granular casts. The waxy casts are the modified granular casts. These may be found in the last few cc. of urine secreted before death even though they were not formerly present. Also one can find waxy casts of all stages in the tubules. Fatty casts are covered with globules of fat. In the last five years every case with fine fatty casts in the Johns Hopkins Hospital was of malarial nephritis. However, often in nephritis the renal cells will be swollen with fat globules and all transitions between rows of single cells and fatty casts can be seen. There may be globules of myelin degeneration in the cells. These do not take osmic acid and may form a true myelin cast.

The autopsy records of all our cases with a clinical diagnosis of nephritis, also the clinical records of all with an anatomical diagnosis of nephritis were studied. In some cases of chronic passive congestion with a clinical diagnosis of nephritis, but no anatomical evidences, there were all varieties of casts. In some cases of cloudy swelling where there had been all varieties of casts there were no evidences of nephritis. Cases with fatty kidneys had been diagnosed nephritis. 109 cases of acute nephritis were studied. The diagnosis cannot be made from the urine alone, for acute nephritis and exacerbations of chronic nephritis cannot be thus distinguished. To make a diagnosis of acute parenchymatous nephritis, one must also have a history of the patient. Of chronic interstitial nephritis there were two types, the white kidneys and the red kidneys, the latter due chiefly to arteriosclerosis. In the cases of small red kidney the trace of albumen often persists longer than the casts which often disappeared first. In the small white type the albumen often clears up first. Of eighteen cases of amyloid kidney only one-fourth had large amounts of urine and albumen but very few casts. The more acute the attack the more epithelial, blood, and pus casts are present. In the chronic attacks these diminish and are replaced by waxy, hyaline, and granular casts. These cases can be followed by the casts alone.

Pure cylindruria occurs oftener than is generally supposed if the urine is examined fresh, centrifugalized, and carefully studied. A slight circulatory disturbance of the kidneys, or manipulation as bimanual palpation, may cause casts and no albumen, or the reverse, or both. The cases of chronic nephritis with history of small white kidney may have casts with no albumen.

Pure cylindruria may follow the use of drugs, e. g. sodium, salicylate, though the casts disappear as soon as the medicine stops. Alcohol in moderate doses will cause cylindruria in over one-half the cases; in others albuminuria. Ung. hydrarg. also may cause the presence of casts. Many of the acute diseases, as erysipelas, scarlet fever, tonsillitis, and diphtheria, show the symptoms of nephritis, but in some cases only casts can be found. The point to be emphasized is that the number of such cases is large.

"Showers" of casts may herald oncoming diabetic coma, sometimes without albumen; they appear suddenly. There are few epithelial or waxy casts, but those present are hyaline or finely granular. These showers occur in exacerbations of nephritis, after diuretics, or, as a terminal event, the last two or three days before death. In chronic constipation there may be found a pure cylindruria. It is an inflammatory or irritative process, not a degeneration, that causes casts. The greatest number of casts is produced by kidneys which are but slightly diseased or by the disturbance of a normal cortex. Fewer by a small granular kidney, and the least number when the cortex is most extensively diseased. The more normal the cell the better its cast-producing ability. The number and kind of casts are indications of the present condition of kidney epithelium. The specimen should be centrifugalized and examined carefully immediately after voiding. Epithelial, blood, and pus casts do not have as much significance as generally supposed. Cells of casts should be studied to determine whether they are epithelial or pus cells, for these casts are certainly present more often than recorded.

Dr. MacCallum in discussion said the reason there is a less abundant supply of casts in the contracted kidney is because the epithelial cells are gone. The active process is in the large kidney, where there is a greater mass of degenerating epithelial cells. The large white and the small kidneys should not be so carefully subdivided, for they represent conditions more or less severe in different stages. There should be some uniformity of the casts in acute kidneys and the kidneys in exacerbation.

Demonstration of the Spirochæta pallida. DR. KEIDEL.

Dr. Keidel demonstrated three specimens of Spirochæta pallida. He said the organism was found in nearly all lesions of primary syphilis. One of the specimens was gotten from serum from a primary sore; the others from condylomata. They were stained with eosin azure after Schaudinn's methods. The organism is not at all refractile. It is spiral, 4 to 10 microns in length, ¼ of a micron thick, with spirals about 1 micron apart. Spirochæta refringans can be easily differentiated from Pallida by being coarser, the spirals being flat, more irregular, and undulatory. Refringans also stains easier and is more refractile. Spirochæta pallida, which may be a protozoan, has not been cultivated on artificial media.

The Mosquitoes of Baltimore.

Mr. T. H. Coffin, who worked upon the distribution and classification of the mosquitoes of Baltimore last summer, preparatory to plans being made for their extermination, said that three factors influencing the prevalence of the summer pest should be taken into account. They were: first, climatic; second, topographical; third, local conditions.

Regarding climatic factors, Baltimore with its temperate climate, abundant rainfall, and hot summers, would be expected to have a number of species of mosquitoes. Of these some would be southern in their range with this locality a

northern limit, others are common to the more northern climates and can stand the cold, and others are of a wide geographical distribution. All three types have been found here. The Stegomyia fasciata, the yellow fever mosquito, is common to the South, being only occasionally found here. Culex pipiens, of wide geographical distribution, is the most common species in Baltimore, while Culex canadensis, a common species farther north, and which can withstand severe winter weather, was found here only in the spring. The malarial mosquitoes, the Anopheles, which are of wide geographical distribution, are by no means uncommon here.

From a topographical standpoint, such a region as Baltimore, being near the sea level where there are sluggish streams and marshlands with standing water, offers many advantages for the development of mosquitoes, particularly the salt marsh types, a number of species of which are found here.

The local conditions, i. e., the presence within the city of undrained pools, puddles, gutters, choked rain spouts, old tin cans, barrels, buckets, in short anything which will hold rain water for ten or twelve days, are responsible for the mosquitoes in the residence and business blocks of the city. Mosquitoes do not fly far from their breeding places; not more than a few hundred yards for the species found here. Jones Falls, a stream running through the center of the city, was thought by many to be a prolific breeding place, but investigations proved it the contrary. Mosquitoes were only found breeding there where the high water receding had left pools in the rocks at the side of the stream.

The habits of mosquitoes must be considered, as three of their four stages demand water for their development. Only the female bites. After a meal of blood is digested she lays her eggs, three or four hundred in number, in boat-shaped masses, in some species as Culex pipiens, and singly as in Anopheles. In about twenty-four hours the larvæ or wigglers emerge from the eggs and begin active life. During this stage they breathe through a caudal breathing tube. In a few days they shed the larval skin and become pupæ, during which stage they breathe through cephalic breathing tubes, feed but little, and rest quietly at the surface unless disturbed. The different species can be distinguished in these stages by their positions in the water and anatomical differences. Oil is so valnable in the extermination of mosquitoes because it forms a thin film over the surface of the water and prevents the breathing tubes being thrust through. In two or three days, if the pupæ are not suffocated or eaten by fish or aquatic insects, they emerge from their skin into full-fledged adults.

The most common mosquito found in Baltimore was Culex pipiens, a medium-sized brown species, and a persistent pest. The malarial mosquitoes were not uncommon in the city, though they were more numerous in the outskirts. Three species were found, Anopheles crucians, the daylight flyer, and A. maculipennis and A. punctipennis, which are night flyers. The many other varieties found are mentioned in the appended list. The differences in the morphology of various species and the distribution of breeding places in Baltimore were shown by lantern slides prepared from drawings and photographs. Among the most striking of these were the characteristic differences in the resting positions of *Anopheles* and *Culex*, the body of the former resting at an angle of from forty-five degrees to a right angle, and the body of the *Culex* resting in a plane parallel to the resting surface. As a result of this work the suggestions for extermination offered were:

1. The individual care and investigation of private premises.

2. The education of the public regarding habits and breeding places of mosquitoes.

3. Drainage of pools and marshes, grading vacant lots, use of oil where necessary.

4. Fumigation of cellars, outhouses, and stables during hibernating periods to kill adult mosquitoes.

Mosquitoes Found in Baltimore.

1. *Culex pipiens* .... House mosquito.
2. *Culex restuans* .... White dotted mosquito.
3. *Culex territans* .... Little black mosquito.
4. *Anopheles maculipennis*.. 4-spotted mosquito.
5. *Anopheles punctipennis*.. Mottled wing mosquito.
6. *Anopheles crucians* ...... Daylight mosquito.
7. *Culex sollicitans* .... White banded salt marsh mosquito.
8. *Culex salinarius* .... Unbanded salt marsh mosquito.
9. *Culex jamaicensis* ...... Spotted leg mosquito.
10. *Culex cantans* .... Brown salt marsh mosquito.
11. *Culex taeniorynchus* .... Small salt marsh mosquito.
12. *Culex sylvestris* .... Swamp mosquito.
13. *Culex atropalpus* .... Rocky pool mosquito.
14. *Culex triseriatus* .... Tree hole mosquito.
15. *Culex perturbans*........ Irritating mosquito.
16. *Culex serratus* .... Silver striped mosquito.
17. *Culex cantator* .... Brown woods mosquito.
18. *Culex canadensis* .... Woodland pool mosquito.
19. *Psorophora ciliata* ...... Giant mosquito.
20. *Janthinisoma musica* .... White footed wood mosquito.
21. *Megarrhinus rutilus* .... Curved beak mosquito.
22. *Taeniorynchus squamiger*. Scaly wing mosquito.

Note.—4, 5 and 6 malarial carriers: 7, 8, 9, 10 and 11 salt marsh species.

Discussion.

Dr. Kelly said that there is interest in the mosquito question in the city has been manifested by the newspapers and council. Maryland or Baltimore should have such a law as there is in New Jersey, which classifies mosquito breeding places among *ipso facto* nuisances, and if the owner does not take care of them the Board of Health acts and charges him with costs. In outlying districts the owner is notified that he is maintaining a nuisance, and if he does not attend to it the Board of Health goes ahead, the owner's negligence after notification giving them power to act without delay. Ridding a community of the pests increases the property values. The next step here is to get the necessary legislation.

November 20, 1905.

Adenocarcinoma of the Stomach. Dr. Sowers.

In the absence of Dr. Bloodgood, Dr. Sowers showed a case of adenocarcinoma of the stomach. The patient was a male, 43 years old; admitted to the Hospital in June, complaining of pain in the umbilical area, which had grown worse since Christmas. He had had discomfort for two years, and during the last year had lost forty pounds in weight. He had had six attacks of vomiting after attacks of pain and not associated with eating. He had quit work in December, and had taken no solid food for three months. On examination the patient's color was good, abdomen was scaphoid with pigmented areas over the epigastrium from plasters. Though weak, patient felt good except when he had attacks of pain, which were brought on by taking any solid food, and were worse in area of the umbilicus. The bowel felt firmer in the region of the splenic colon, otherwise the abdominal examination was negative. Patient was operated on by Dr. Bloodgood on June 29, the peritoneal cavity being opened by a median line incision from the ensiform cartilage to below the umbilicus. A carcinomatous growth was found on the lesser curvature of a moderately dilated stomach 3 cm. below the pylorus. Practically all the lesser curvature was removed together with an adjacent gland showing metastasis. All the fat was removed with lesser curvature, and adhesions binding the stomach to the pancreas were broken up, showing an area of induration in the central portion of the pancreas. The duodenal and stomach ends were united, a loop of the duodenum being anastomosed to the posterior wall of the stomach. The pancreas was left intact, an inflammatory induration of the pancreas, in cancer of the stomach, not indicating its removal as a cancerous involvement would. Patient left the Hospital on July 30 and has since gained 32 pounds in weight; he has had no vomiting or pain, and bowels are regular. After a test meal of 100 cc., 12 cc. were gotten an hour later. Pathologically, the tumor, which was a large fungus mass on the lesser curvature of the stomach reaching to within 3 cc. of pylorus, was an adenocarcinoma.

Stenosis of the pylorus in Infancy. Dr. Charles L. Scudder, of Boston.

A paper was presented based upon the review already published [1] of all reported cases of stenosis of the infantile pylorus. The facts discovered at autopsy and at operation were stated. The clinical picture of the disease was described. An analysis of the medical and surgical treatment hitherto employed was presented. A brief report was made of two operative experiences in cases of stenosis of the pylorus in babies during the past summer. In one instance the child was fourteen days old at the time of operation (a case seen first by Dr. Chas. W.

Townsend). In the second instance the child was twenty-four days old when operated upon. Both of these children are in good health now, three months after the operative treatment. These cases will be reported at a later date in detail. Lantern slides were shown illustrating the pathological findings in these cases of infantile hyperplasia of the pylorus.

The Relation of Dilatation of the Duodenum to Gastric Disturbances. Dr. Finney.

Five or six years ago upon opening the abdomen for a variety of conditions, particularly of the stomach, duodenum, and gall bladder, a condition was found which was not mentioned in the literature, *i. e.*, a dilatation of the duodenum with a patent condition of the pylorus. At that time pyloroplasty was done for want of something better. The patients gave a history of indigestion for months or years, of nausea and vomiting, and symptoms that were indefinite but distressing. Most of the patients had had medical treatment without results. In all the cases there was Glenard's disease. The symptoms presented by the patients were unsatisfactory for operation. When these cases were first noticed gastroenterostomy was in its infancy. Nothing that was done seemed to relieve the symptoms. The nearest to a description of the condition was a paper read by A. J. Ochsner in San Francisco this year, in which he reports 14 cases. Mayo, in a recent article on stomach diseases, refers to this condition. He says it is associated with enteroptosis, but does not say what to do for it. Four years ago, after an operation for gall stones, a patient began to vomit and vomited until she died. At autopsy there was found a dilated stomach and dilated duodenum, but no lesion could be found. Autopsies on forty-six post-operative cases, only one of which was recognized clinically, have been reported from Vienna. The duodenum passes behind the superior mesenteric vessels, the superior mesentery itself running down to the right iliac fossa. When the stomach is much dilated, filled with fluid, and has descended to the pelvis, there is a dragging on the mesentery and vessels. This is apparently the obstruction. To the proximal side the intestine is dilated, and at the distal side it is collapsed. Rokitansky in the Fifties suggested that this condition might exist. Glenard also suggests that dragging on the mesentery might obstruct the duodenum. In four of the forty-six cases from Vienna the stomach was not markedly dilated, though in most of the cases it had descended. The explanation is not satisfactory for the condition. The dilatation is the effect, not the cause, though it may be both. Two cases have been reported after operations other than abdominal, one being a breast removal and the other an operation on the elbow. Schnitzler suggests that it takes place after anæsthesia, particularly after chloroform.

Prevention, Prognosis, and Treatment.—Only one case was diagnosed before autopsy. A postural treatment has been suggested. Put the patient in the knee-chest position for fifteen minutes every two hours, or have her lie on the left

¹ Journal of the American Medical Association, May 27, 1905. Scudder and Quinby.

side with hips elevated. Lavage has been tried with some success. The condition generally occurs in nervous patients who are not well nourished and who have an enteroptosis. A jejunostomy may be done to get below the obstruction. In some of the cases the obstruction has been near the pylorus, in others below the papilla of Vater, for the patient vomits great amounts of dark, bile-stained fluid. This condition, with both the ante-operative and post-operative types, is a definite entity. No other observer has noted the circular, muscular bands around the duodenum, which Ochsner, who draws an analogy between a pylorospasm and a spasm at the iliocæcal valve, has described. Gastroenterostomy has been done several times and found wanting. In post-operative cases the postural method, or jejunostomy, might be tried.

Discussion.

Dr. Barker.—I should like to ask Dr. Finney whether or not, in the condition he has described, any additional information is gained by testing for the presence of pancreatic secretion when bile is present in the vomitus? Inasmuch as both secretions are emptied into the intestine through the one duct, it might seem that the presence of either of the secretions would indicate that fluid was being regurgitated from the level at least of the opening at the end of the plicæ longitudinalis duodeni. I can understand, however, the importance of the accessory pancreatic duct of Santorini, which opens at the papilla duodeni (Santorini) somewhat above and in front of the opening of the ductus choledochus and the main ductus pancreaticus; stenosis of the duodenum below this papilla duodeni of Santorini, but above the opening of the common bile duct, could prevent bile passing backward into the stomach, though it would not interfere with regurgitation of that portion of the pancreatic juice which is emptied into the intestine through the accessory pancreatic duct.

It is easy, of course, to test for the presence of pancreatic juice in the vomitus. One has only to neutralize any acid present, and make the fluid slightly alkaline, then place a flake of fibrin stained with Magdala red in it, and keep the tube in the incubator at the body temperature. Should the fibrin be digested the fluid will be colored red. The digestion of fibrin in an alkaline fluid cannot be due to pepsin, but must be due to some other proteolytic ferment, in the case under consideration almost certainly trypsin.

I should further like to ask Dr. Finney whether the wall of the duodenum in the cases he describes is hypertrophied, or is simply in a state of atonic dilatation? Does it take part in the peristaltic movements observed, or is peristalsis paralyzed? If no persistence is visible, can it be set up by mechanical stimulation when the duodenum is exposed?

I am wondering, too, since gastro-enterostomy seems to be of no avail in these cases, whether or not a duodeno-jejunostomy, connecting the lowermost part of the dilated duodenum with the closest available part of the jejunum, would be of any service. It is conceivable that, by permitting the onward flow of the bile, pancreatic juice, and duodenal secretion, as well as the chyme, some benefit might result.

THE JOHNS HOPKINS HISTORICAL CLUB.

October 16, 1905. (*Continued.*)

Association between Famous Artists and Anatomists. DR. FUTCHER.

As there has been considerable controversy concerning the origin of the excellent drawings in the famous anatomy of Vesalius, the paper was introduced by a brief sketch of this great anatomist and his monumental work, the Fabrica.

Andreas Vesalius was born at Brussels in 1514. He received his early education at Louvain and his medical instruction at the Universities of Montpellier and Paris. Owing to the popular antipathy in France against the dissection of the human body, he was forced to go to Italy, where more liberal views prevailed. In 1536 he studied anatomy in Venice. Before he completed this, his twenty-second year, he demonstrated publicly at the University of Padua. He was a professor in three universities and is said to have taught anatomy at Padua, Bologna, and Pisa in the course of the same winter. He was a person of marvellous industry. At the age of twenty-five he began to collect the drawings of his dissections for the publication of his Fabrica. He completed the task in 1543 when he was twenty-nine, and in that year—the year of its publication—he went to Basel to see his anatomy through the press. Soon after this he accepted an invitation as imperial physician at the court of Charles V and later, on his abdication, at that of his son, Philip II, at Madrid. The events that lead up to his death are not generally agreed upon, but they are believed to be as follows: While examining the body of a Spanish grandee it was observed that the heart, when incised, appeared to give some feeble pulsations. This so enraged the grandee's relatives that he was condemned to be tried by the Inquisition. Through the King's intercession he escaped this tribunal on promising to make a pilgrimage to the Holy Land. When he reached Jerusalem he received an invitation from the Venetian senate to accept the professorship at the University of Padua, rendered vacant by the death of Fallopius. He accepted and started to return to Italy. He encountered violent storms in the Ionian sea and was wrecked on the island of Zante, where he is said to have later starved to death in 1564.

There has been much discussion as to the source of the drawings with which the Fabrica is illustrated. It has been claimed by some that the originals were drawn by Leonardo da Vinci and that Vesalius used them for illustrating his work. Leonardo was born at Vinci, in Italy, in 1452 and died at Amboise, in France, in 1519. His biographers claim that so far as breadth of accomplishments and versatility are concerned he was the most remarkable individual that has ever lived. In addition to being the most accomplished painter of his generation, he was a distinguished sculptor, architect, anatomist, physiologist, mechanical engineer, botanist. chemist, astronomer, and geologist. As a painter we know him best for his "Christ's Last Supper," which adorns the refectory wall of the convent of Santa Maria della Grazie, in Milan. With the Raphael's "Sistine Madonna" and Michael Angelo's

"Last Judgment" it ranks as one of the three most celebrated paintings in the world.

At the height of his reputation Leonardo studied anatomy and dissected for ten years under Della Torre, Professor of Anatomy, at Pavia. During this time he was engaged also in making the illustrations for an anatomical work which was to have been brought out by Della Torre, but which for some unknown reason never appeared. His "Sketch Book," which was presented to Charles I of England by the Earl of Arundel, is now a part of the royal library at Windsor Castle. It contains several sketches of anatomical dissections, showing the muscles, vessels, etc., which he had made during his anatomical studies. These sketches are reproduced in Choulant's "Geschichte der Anatomische Abbildungen." The legends describing the drawings are in Italian and written from right to left. In other words Leonardo was a "mirror" writer and undoubtedly left-handed. His being left-handed is one of the arguments advanced in support of his being the person who executed the originals of the drawings in the Fabrica of Vesalius. A study of these will show that the light falls on the right and the shadings and shadows are on the left of the figures, the reverse of what is customary with right-handed artists.

It has been claimed by some that Titian made the drawings. This seems improbable, however, because in 1539, when Vesalius began to collect the material for the Fabrica, Titian was 62 years old and his reputation was already established and it is not likely that he would undertake this line of work. To Christoforo Coriolano has also been given the credit. He too can almost certainly be eliminated, as his earliest work did not appear until 1568.

Many biographers and critics hold that the drawings as well as the wood-cuts were made by Johann Stephan von Calcar. In support of this view is the fact that in one or two instances in the text Vesalius states specifically that von Calcar made a particular illustration. Von Calcar lived from 1499 to 1546. He was a pupil of Titian and perfected himself by studying Raphael. He imitated these masters with such skill as to deceive the most skilful critics.

Roth, who has written the best biography of Vesalius, is of the opinion from a careful analysis of the evidence that Vesalius himself made most of the illustrations for his work.

Michael Angelo (1474-1563) applied himself to the study of anatomy for twelve years during his developmental period. He is known to have studied anatomy with Realdo Colombo, a surgeon and well-known anatomist of his day. Some of his anatomical sketches are preserved and are reproduced by Choulant.

Sir Christopher Wren (1631-1723) is known best to the world as an architect, but is entitled to be mentioned with Leonardo and Michael Angelo, both of whom were also eminent as architects. He is known to have been a close friend of Thomas Willis (1621-1675), the famous physician and anatomist of his day. Willis gives Wren the credit for executing a number of the drawings illustrating his anatomical dissections, including those represented in his Cerebri Anatome. Richard Lower is also known to have made many of the dissections and illustrations.

Although Rembrandt (1606-1669) is not believed to have had any intimate knowledge of anatomy, his name will ever be associated with the subject for having painted " The Lesson in Anatomy," which represents Prof. Tulp, the anatomist, demonstrating the dissected muscles and tendons of the forearm to a group of seven students. It was painted in 1632 at Tulp's request for the Surgeon's Guild.

NOTES ON NEW BOOKS.

Malformations of the Genital Organs of Woman. By CH. DEBIERRE, Professor of Anatomy in the Medical Faculty at Lille. With 85 Illustrations. Translated by J. HENRY C. SIMES, M. D., Emeritus Professor of Genito-urinary Surgery and Venereal Diseases in the Philadelphia Polyclinic. (*Philadelphia: P. Blackiston's Son & Co., 1905.*)

In this little book, the author gives "a new history on this subject," having 'a two-fold purpose, " to interest, to instruct." He applies to this division of teratology the well recognized principle that anomalies of growth are due to arrested or perverted development. He takes up first the anatomy, to which about a third of the book is devoted. Then comes a short chapter on development. In the third and last chapter he considers malformations in the light of the preceding articles. The text is on the whole a concise and fairly clear statement. But there are passages which cannot be so described. The illustrations are numerous and rather clear, but not always well selected. There is no index. The date of the American copyright is 1905, but no date is given of the French edition from which the translation is made. The latest literature cited, however, is 1891, so one is not surprised at the absence of reference to the more recent contributions.

The "interesting" side of the subject has been taken up at needless length, with selections from lay writers, such as are not usually found in books of science. It is hardly necessary to say that the book does not fill the void in English medical literature for which the translator has destined it.

In closing, the author says, characteristically—" Conclusion— Our general conclusion from the study of the anomalies of the genital organs of women is that in nature nothing is unusual, and our ignorance alone gives power to the fetish gods and manitous of all times and of all countries! "

Gynecology, Medical and Surgical. Outlines for Students and Practitioners. By HENRY J. GARRIGUES, A. M., M. D. With Three Hundred and Forty-three illustrations. (*Philadelphia and London: J. B. Lippincott Company, 1905.*)

In this new book, the well-known author aims to give the "essentials of Medical and Surgical Gynecology," " in outline," "especially intended as a guide for beginners (medical students) and general practitioners." He begins with general considerations, discussing puberty and the climacteric in a separate chapter instead of under etiology which he next takes up. Then he thoroughly covers examination and treatment in two more chapters. Under " Metrorrhagia and Menorrhagia," little is said of the significance of these symptoms as suggesting possible malignant disease. Their importance cannot be too much emphasized, especially in a book of this kind, for it is the general practitioner who first sees such cases. This section otherwise covers the ground well. The general division is concluded with a chapter on leucorrhœa, merely a symptom, to be sure, but well considered by itself, as an important "chief complaint."

In the special division, diseases of the external genitalia are taken up first; the chapters on the vulva and vagina are especially complete. However, in the differential diagnosis of hernia exploratory aspiration is not generally recommended. In the diagnosis of gonorrhœa he rightly holds the presence of the diplococcus of Neisser to be the test, though dwelling on the importance of the symptoms as well. Under treatment he emphasizes prophylaxis and is not in favor of severe local treatment in the acute stage. Operation is advised for extension of the disease to the adnexæ, seemingly only when there are sacs of pus, or after several attacks of pelvic peritonitis, a conservatism which could be more widely practiced to advantage. The chapter on diseases of the uterus is not as satisfactory as the others. The histological pictures of the changes in the endometrium in membranous dysmenorrhœa and pregnancy are by no means clear. Of sarcoma he says—" the epithelial cells of utricular gland scrapings are unchanged in endometritis, while in sarcoma they break down into sarcomatous cells." We find under " perimetritic inflammation," subdivisions into " peritonitis," " cellulitis," " phlebitis," " lymphangitis and lymphadenitis." The difficulties of such a classification are evident in the description of the separate lesions, in which the anatomical changes refuse to correspond to the classification.

The consideration of ectopic pregnancy is not commensurate with its clinical importance. The closing chapters are devoted to the urethra, bladder, ureters, and rectum and anus. The book is to be commended for its concise and clear statement and for its rational and conservative therapeutics.

Serums, Vaccines and Toxines in Treatment and Diagnosis. By WM. CECIL BOSANQUET, M. D. (*Chicago: W. T. Keener and Co., London: Cassell and Co., Ltd., 1904.*)

There is no subject in medicine to-day in which such active work is being done as in that pertaining to the question of toxines, the use of serums and the whole problem of immunity. For the majority of the profession the subject is more or less obscure. New work appears with such rapidity, the work has become so complicated and there are so many new lines of thought to follow, that many of us feel hopelessly behind. In this work Dr. Bosanquet has given an account of the principal points which have been established in regard to these questions, and the general trend of speculation. This has been done to enable the practitioner to obtain a broad idea of the subject and to be able to follow more recent investigations.

The general problems of immunity are stated and the methods for the preparation and administration of the various serums are described. The infections for which serum treatment has been used are gone over in detail and the special points in regard to each are taken up in some detail. The style of the book is plain and clear—no easy achievement when the technical nature of the subject and the involved character of the majority of the articles on these questions are considered. We can recommend the work for those who wish some knowledge of the subject without being bewildered.

A Short Treatise on Anti-Typhoid Inoculation. By A. E. WRIGHT. M. D. (*Westminster: Archibald Constable and Co., Ltd. 1904.*)

One of the most important subjects in connection with the study of typhoid fever is the production of a curative serum. Equally interesting is the possibility of anti-typhoid inoculation. It is with the latter of these that this work deals and the name, of the author has been especially associated with this subject. In this book the general principles of protective inoculation are described and its special application to the production of immunity against typhoid fever. Then a brief account of the method of preparation of anti-typhoid vaccine is given, with a description of the method of injection and the clinical symptoms following this. The writer also discusses the statistics which are available in regard to the efficacy of the procedure. The descriptions throughout the book are clear, and it can be recommended as giving a very good summary of the present condition of the problem. The last word on this subject has not been said, and we may hope to have further publications from Dr. Wright on this work, which he has done so much to advance.

The Principles and Practice of Medicine. By WILLIAM OSLER, M. D. Sixth Edition. (*New York and London: D. Appleton and Company, 1905.*)

Kipling's "McAndrew's Hymn," represents an old engineer reflecting on the advances that had come in the construction of steam engines, and saying "We're creepin' on wi' each new rig." The writer felt in the same state of mind as he took down the first edition of this work and compared it with the present one, the sixth. Although the interval has been only thirteen years, it is interesting to note the changes, not only of addition but also of omission. The number of copies printed before this edition, reached one hundred thousand—a remarkable record and one which has probably not been surpassed. The work is used extensively in England and Australia, and without reflecting on the merits of other text-books of medicine may be regarded .as foremost in any language.

This edition means in many ways a new book and the changes made are most extensive. There has been alteration in the order of the subjects, the first section now being that dealing with diseases due to intestinal parasites, and that on the specific infectious diseases follows. Throughout there have been many alterations, certain of the articles being almost entirely re-written. To note these in detail would be to mention the greater part of the work.

Perhaps there is no text-book of medicine which contains so many references to unusual conditions. There may not be room for much discussion but a little is given. Throughout the work there is evidence of the literary tastes of the author. It may be remembered that a few years ago an ingenious London medical student got up an examination paper on the literary references in this book. No one was found who could answer all the questions, in fact, there was one which Dr. Osler himself is said to have been unable to answer.

To praise this book is not necessary. It stands as an example of the author's work and methods. Clear-cut descriptions, completeness, scientific accuracy, with the avoidance of speculation and diffuseness, are characteristic. To those of us who knew the early editions of the book before we knew the man, for a time often came the thought in his clinics "There's his book! " Now, knowing him, the feeling comes when reading the book "There's the man! "

Pathology and Morbid Anatomy. By T. HENRY GREEN, M. D. 10th American Edition, Revised and Enlarged by W. CECIL BOSANQUET, M. D. (*Philadelphia: Lea Brothers & Co., 1905.*)

Green's Pathology has long been a favorite with English and American students who desire a text-book that covers the essentials of the subject in a more thorough manner than is done by quiz compends, but without the discussions into the realms of theory which characterize the more extensive treatises on pathology. The tenth edition of such a work surely needs no extended introduction. The greater part of the work is of neces-

sity devoted to general pathology, with a short section on special pathology in which the defects of the work are most apparent. While the book may be recommended to students as an outline, it is not to be recommended to any one desiring an exact or thorough knowledge of any part of the subject of pathology.

The Accessory Sinuses of the Nose and Their Relations to Neighboring Parts. By GUSTAV KILLIAN. Translated by D. R. PATTERSON. (*Jena: Gustav Fischer, 1904; Chicago: W. T. Keener, 1905.*)

We cannot praise this fine work too highly. It supplies, in a most artistic way, what we have long lacked, an atlas illustrating the accessory sinuses of the nose as seen from all aspects. With its aid we get an accurate idea of the relative size of these cavities and their relationship to neighboring muscles, blood vessels, nerves and other structures.

The plates illustrating the close proximity of these cavities to the cerebral structures, as obtained from dissections from both without and within the cranium, are most instructive. The explanatory notes devoted to these plates, point out clearly the possible sequelæ in the central nervous system that might follow suppurative disease of these sinuses and indicate the routes that must be followed in their surgical treatment.

The explanatory notes are well written, the only possible objection being the nomenclature used. The author names the various cells of the ethmoid labyrinth from the embryological standpoint and we question whether this is advisable in a practical atlas such as this. It is much easier to consider these cells in groups which empty either into the middle meatus of the nose or into the superior meatus. With this as a basis the variations of the anterior ethmoidal cells (emptying into the middle meatus) and posterior ethmoidal cells (emptying into superior meatus) can be readily described.

SYLVAN ROSENHEIM.

A Manual of Diseases of the Nose and Throat. By C. G. COAKELY, A. M., M. D. (*New York: Lea Bros. & Co., 1905.*)

It gives us great pleasure to recommend this small manual both to students and practitioners of medicine. In it we have a clear and concise resumé of the subject, especially valuable to the student whose time for this work is very limited. The chapters on diseases of the accessory sinuses are especially full for a book of this size, and they contain the most approved methods of treatment.

We cannot agree with the author in his advice of the use of ether or chloroform anæsthesia for the removal of adenoid tissue in the nasopharynx. Anæsthesia with ethyl bromide or chloride is much safer and gives sufficient time for this short operation.

The book is excellently printed and illustrated and the chapters on treatment are very full.

A Guide to Anæsthetics for the Student and General Practitioner. By THOMAS D. LUKE, M. B., F. R. C. S. (Ed.). With 45 Illustrations. Second Edition. (*Edinburgh: Wm. Green and Sons; Philadelphia: J. B. Lippincott Co., 1905.*)

The second edition of this book is produced on account of the revision made necessary by the importance of ethyl chloride as a general anæsthetic, as it " bids fair in a few years to be the most frequently employed anæsthetic which we possess." The book has much to commend it. It is compact, well balanced and gives the essentials clearly. The author discusses chiefly nitrous oxide, ethyl chloride, ether, and chloroform. He favors chloroform, either alone or mixed with more than most anæsthetists in America. This is but natural for one of the Edinburgh school. At the same time he acknowledges the dangers of chloroform, and cautions against its use in unselected cases. The descriptions of the apparatus are clear, and the illustrations in general good, though in giving artificial respiration (Figs. 36-37) it is hard to see how the second position is derived from the first (position of hands of operator).

In the introductory chapter he emphasizes the importance of entrusting the administration of the anæsthetic to trained assistants only, and makes a plea for improvement in this side of medical education. Many think the anæsthetist has a responsibility less only than that of the operator. The value of the table of the number of deaths each year from an anæsthetic, would be increased if another table were added, showing the number of cases each year to which an anæsthetic had been given. This chapter contains also several paragraphs which every one giving an anæsthetic should constantly have in mind. As so

frequently the anæsthetic must be given by one who has had little experience, the brief chapter on Anæsthetic Apparatus in General Practice is not out of place.

Of the complicated pieces of machinery, the Dubois and Vernon Harcourt chloroform inhalers, which have been evolved in the effort to lessen the mortality in chloroform anæsthesia, he says " It is extremely unlikely, that they will ever take a very important place in practical anæsthetics." " While any attempt to develop accuracy of dosage of chloroform is in the right direction, by no means known to us at present, can this valuable but lethal drug be rendered as safe as ether "—a conclusion which will find wide acceptance.

The value of the book is enhanced by a brief summary of the History of Anæsthesia, an account of Anæsthetic Commissions and Investigations, and an excellent index.

BOOKS RECEIVED.

The Pharmacopœia of the United States of America. Eighth Decennial Revision. By authority of the United States Pharmacopœial convention held in Washington, A. D., 1900. Revised by the Committee of Revision and published by the Board of Trustees. Official from September 1, 1905. 8vo. LXXV + 692 pages. P. Blakiston's Son & Company, Philadelphia, Agents.

A Text-Book of Physiology, Normal and Pathological. By Winfield S. Hall, Ph. D. (Leipzig), M. D. (Leipzig). Second edition, revised and enlarged. Illustrated with 340 engravings and three colored plates. 1905. 8vo. 795 pages. Lea Brothers & Company, Philadelphia and New York.

International Clinics. Edited by A. O. J. Kelly, A. M., M. D. Fifteenth Series. Volume 2, 1905. 8vo. 310 pages. J. B. Lippincott Company, Philadelphia and London.

The Ready Reference Handbook of Diseases of the Skin. By George Thomas Jackson, M. D. With 91 illustrations and 3 plates. Fifth edition, thoroughly revised. 1905. 12mo. 676 pages. Lea Brothers & Co., New York and Philadelphia.

The Treatment of Diseases of the Eye. By Victor Hanke, M. D. Translated by J. Herbert Parsons, B. S., D. Sc., F. R. C. S., and George Coats, M. D., F. R. C. S. 1905. 12mo. 222 pages. W. T. Keener & Co., Chicago. Hodder & Stoughton, London.

International Clinics. A Quarterly of Illustrated Clinical Lectures and Especially Prepared Original Articles. By Leading Members of the Medical Profession throughout the World. Edited by A. O. J. Kelly, A. M., M. D. Volume III. Fifteenth Series, 1905. 8vo. 302 pages. J. B. Lippincott Company, Philadelphia and London.

Clinical Treatises on the Pathology and Therapy of Disorders of Metabolism and Nutrition. By Professor Dr. Carl von Noorden. Translated by Florence Buchanon, D. SC., and I. Walker Hall, M. D. Part VII, Diabetes Mellitus, its Pathological Chemistry and Treatment. 1905. 8vo. 211 pages. E. B. Treat & Company, New York.

The Diagnostics of Internal Medicine. A Clinical Treatise upon the Recognised Principles of Medical Diagnosis, Prepared for the use of Students and Practitioners of Medicine. By Glentworth Reeve Butler, Sc. D., M. D. With five coloured plates and two hundred and eighty-eight illustrations and charts in the text. Second revised edition. 1905. 8vo. 1168 pages. D. Appleton & Company, New York and London.

The Medical Epitome Series. Practice of Medicine. A Manual for Students and Practitioners. By Hughes Dayton, M. D. Series edited by Victor Cox Pedersen, A. M., M. D. 1905. 16mo. 324 pages. Lea Brothers & Co., New York and Philadelphia.

Practical Massage in Twenty Lessons. By Hartvig Nissen. With 46 original illustrations. 1905. 12mo. 168 pages. F. A. Davis Company, Philadelphia.

A Guide to Anæsthetics. For the Student and General Practitioner. By Thomas D. Luke, M. B., F. R. C. S. (Ed.). With 45 illustrations. Second edition. 1905. 8vo. William Green & Sons, Edinburgh. J. B. Lippincott Company, Philadelphia.

Anatomy, Descriptive and Surgical. By Henry Gray, F. R. S. Edited by T. Pickering Pick, F. R. C. S., and Robert Howden, M. A., M. B., C. M. New American edition, thoroughly revised and re-edited with additions, by John Chalmers Da Costa, M. D. Illustrated with 1132 elaborate engravings. 1905. 1600 pages. Lea Brothers & Co., Philadelphia and New York.

Neurotic Disorders of Childhood. Including a Study of Auto and Intestinal Intoxications, Chronic Anæmia, Fever Eclampsia, Epilepsy, Migraine, Chorea, Hysteria, Asthma, etc. By B. K. Rachford, M. D. 1905. 8vo. 440 pages E. B. Treat & Company, New York.

Medical and Surgical Report of Bellevue and Allied Hospitals in the City of New York. Volume I, 1904. Edited by Alexander Lambert, M. D., W. K. Draper, M. D., B. Farquar Curtis, M. D. George Woolsey, M. D. 1904. 8vo. 387 pages. Martin B. Brown Press, New York.

Surgical Aspects of Digestive Disorders. By James G. Mumford, M. D. in association with Arthur K. Stone, M. D. 1905. 8vo. 395 pages. The Macmillan Company, New York. Macmillan and Co., Ltd., London.

Indigestion. The Diagnosis and Treatment of the Functional Derangements of the Stomach. With an Appendix on the Preparation of Food by Cooking with Especial Reference to its Use in the Treatment of Affections of the Stomach. By George Herschell, M. D., Lond. Third edition, entirely re-written. 1905. 8vo. 293 pages. W. T. Keener & Co. Chicago. Henry J. Glaisher, London.

The Accessory Sinuses of the Nose, and Their Relations to Neighboring Parts. Illustrated by fifteen colored plates. By Dr. Gustav Killian. Translated by D. R. Patterson, M. D., M. R. C. P. 1904. Fol. Gustav Fischer, Jena, W. T. Keener, Chicago.

Clinical Methods. A Guide to the Practical Study of Medicine. By Robert Hutchison, M. D., F. R. C. P. and Harry Rainy, M. A., F. R. C. P., Ed., F. R. S. E. With upwards of 150 illustrations and 9 colored plates. Ninth edition. 1905. 16mo. 634 pages. W. T. Keener & Co., Chicago.

A Manual of Chemistry. Inorganic and Organic. Covering the Synopses of the Conjoint Board and the Society of Apothecaries. By Arthur P. Luff, M. D., B. Sc. (Lond.), F. R. C. P.; F. I. C. and Frederic James M. Page, B. Sc. (Lond.), F. I. C. Illustrated with 43 engravings. Third edition, revised throughout. 1905. 16mo. 555 pages. W. T. Keener & Co., Chicago.

Hygiene and Public Health. By B. Arthur Whitelegge, C. B., M. D., B. Sc., Lond., F. R. C. P., D. P. H., and George Newman, M. D., D. P. H., F. R. S. E. New edition, revised, enlarged, and in great part re-written. Illustrated. 1905. 636 pages. W. T. Keener & Co., Chicago.

A Manual of Diseases of the Nose and Throat. By Cornelius Godfrey Coakley, A. M., M. D. Third edition, revised and enlarged. Illustrated with 118 engravings and 5 colored plates. 12mo. 594 pages. Lea Brothers & Co., New York and Philadelphia.

The Principles of Bacteriology. A Practical Manual for Students and Physicians. By A. C. Abbott, M. D. Seventh edition, enlarged and thoroughly revised. With 100 illustrations, of which 24 are colored. 12mo. 689 pages. Lea Brothers & Co., Philadelphia and New York.

Biographic Clinics. Volume III. Essays Concerning the Influence of Visual Function Pathologic and Physiologic Upon the Health of Patients. By George M. Gould, M. D. 1905. 12mo. 516 pages. P. Blakiston's Son & Co., Philadelphia.

Therapeutics: its Principles and Practice. By Horatio C. Wood, M. D., LL. D. Twelfth edition. Thoroughly revised and adapted to the eighth edition (1905) of the United States Pharmacopœia. By Horatio C. Wood and Horatio C. Wood, Jr., M. D. 1905. 8vo. 907 pages. J. B. Lippincott Company, Philadelphia and London.

A Practical Treatise on Sexual Disorders of the Male and Female. By Robert W. Taylor, A. M., M. D. Third edition, thoroughly revised. With 130 illustrations and 16 plates in colors and monochrome. 1905. 8vo. 525 pages. Lea Brothers & Co., New York and Philadelphia.

Color-Vision and Color-Blindness. A Practical Manual for Railroad Surgeons. By J. Ellis Jennings, M. D. Second edition, thoroughly revised. With illustrations. 1905. 8vo. 132 pages. F. A. Davis Company, Philadelphia.

Methods of Organic Analysis. By Henry C. Sherman, Ph. D. 1905. 8vo. 245 pages. The Macmillan Company, New York.

Ophthalmic Neuro-Myology. A Study of the Normal and Abnormal Actions of the Ocular Muscles from the Brain Side of the Question. By G. C. Savage, M. D. Thirty-nine full page plates and twelve illustrative figures. 1905. 16mo. 221 pages. Published by the Author, Nashville, Tenn.

Dispensing Made Easy. With numerous Formulæ, and Practical Hints to Secure Simplicity, Rapidity and Economy. By William G. Sutherland, M. B. Aberd. Second edition, revised. 1905. 16mo. 105 pages. John Wright & Co., Bristol. Simpkin, Marshall, Hamilton, Kent & Co., Ld., London.

Pathology and Morbid Anatomy. By T. Henry Green, M. D., F. R. C. P. Tenth American, revised from the tenth English edition. Revised and enlarged by W. Cecil Bosanquet, M. A., M. D. Oxon., F. R. C. P. Lond. With a colored plate and 348 illustrations in the text. 1905. 8vo. 610 pages. Lea Brothers & Co., Philadelphia and New York.

The Practical Study of Malaria, and Other Blood Parasites. By J. W. W. Stephens, M. D. Cantab, D. P. H. and S. R. Christophers, M. B. Vict., I. M. S. [Second Edition.] 1904. 8vo. 396 + XLIV pages. The University Press of Liverpool, by Williams and Norgate, London.

The National Standard Dispensatory. Containing the Natural History, Chemistry, Pharmacy, Actions, and Uses of Medicines. Including those Recognized in the Pharmacopœias of the United States, Great Britain, and Germany, with Numerous References to Other Pharmacopœias. In Accordance with the Eighth Decennial Revision of the United States Pharmacopœia, 1905. By Hobart Amory Hare, B. Sc., M. D., Charles Caspari, Jr., Ph. G., Phar. D., Henry H. Rusby, M. D., Joseph F. Geisler, Ph. C., Edward Kremers, Ph. D., and Daniel Base, Ph. D. 1905. 4to. 1860 pages. Lea Brothers & Co., Philadelphia and New York.

Manual of the Diseases of the Eye. For Students and General Practitioners. By Charles H. May, M. D. Fourth edition, revised. With 360 original illustrations including 21 plates, with 60 colored figures. 1905. 12mo. 391 pages. William Wood and Company, New York.

Natural Science in Hygiene: or the Life-History of the Non-Bacterial Parasites Affecting Man. By James Rodger Watson, M. A., B. Sc., M. D. (Edin.). 1905. 16mo. 62 pages. John Wright and Co., Bristol. Simpkin, Marshall, Hamilton, Kent & Co., Ld., London.

The Principles and Practice of Medicine. Designed for the Use of Practitioners and Students of Medicine. By William Osler, M. D. Sixth edition, thoroughly revised from new plates. 1905. 8vo. 1143 pages. D. Appleton and Company, New York and London.

Board of Health of the State of New Jersey. Twenty-eighth annual report and report of the Bureau of Vital Statistics. 1904. 8vo. 494 pages. 1905. Paterson, New Jersey.

INDEX TO VOLUMES 1-16 OF BULLETIN.

A subject and author index of the first sixteen volumes of the Johns Hopkins Hospital Bulletin is now ready. As the edition will be limited, it is desirable that orders be sent in as promptly as possible.

Price bound in cloth is fifty cents.

Orders should be addressed to the Johns Hopkins Press, Baltimore, Md.

The Johns Hopkins Hospital Bulletins are issued monthly. They are printed by the FRIEDENWALD CO., Baltimore. Single copies may be procured from NUNN & CO. and the BALTIMORE NEWS CO., Baltimore. Subscriptions, $2.00 a year, may be addressed to the publishers, THE JOHNS HOPKINS PRESS, BALTIMORE; single copies will be sent by mail for twenty-five cents each.

BULLETIN

OF

THE JOHNS HOPKINS HOSPITAL

Entered as Second-Class Matter at the Baltimore, Maryland, Postoffice.

Vol. XVII.—No. 179.]　　　　　BALTIMORE, FEBRUARY, 1906.　　　　　[Price, 25 Cents.

CONTENTS.

A CLASS MODEL OF THE SPINAL CORD.

BY IRVING HARDESTY.

(From the Hearst Anatomical Laboratory of the University of California.)

The value of allowing the student in anatomy to model various parts of the body has been thoroughly proven and in the more modern methods of teaching is a plan quite frequently employed. In the teaching of osteology modeling has been resorted to for some years in the Johns Hopkins University and in the University of Chicago, and during the past four years it has been especially successful in this laboratory.[1] In class work in other branches of anatomy it has also been found of great help. The reconstruction of arrangements which are of unusual interest or of those whose relations in the third dimension are difficult to acquire, has proven a very valuable means of instruction.[2] Modeling in class of various parts of the central nervous system by the use of potters' clay and differently colored floss has also been tried and strongly advocated.[3]

Modeling an organ or part of an organ not only fixedly directs the attention of the student upon its relative size and proportional dimensions, but, in actually constructing them

himself, the more delicate inter-relations of the component parts and the finer details of contour are impressed upon him as in no other procedure. The only argument against the general application of the plan to all the parts of the body is the time it involves. Even those students who quickly develop considerable skill and rapidity in modeling and who possess a good sense of form would be unable to model anything like all of their dissections in the time usually alloted to the subject. The next best plan is to allow the modeling only of certain structures and arrangements whose mechanism and architecture are the more difficult to grasp. Even then the time will scarcely allow for each student of a class, or even each group of students working together, to model the same structures throughout the laboratory, for, since the regular dissection must precede, it means extra work for the student. In lieu of this, it should be found possible at least to have two or three students of a class spend a portion of their time in making a model of an important part, while the remainder of the class, keeping on with their regular dissection, watch the model grow from day to day. This they will do and with considerable interest, making intelligent comments and sug-

---

[1] Moody, R. O. Johns Hopkins Hospital Bulletin, Vol. XIV, March, 1903.
[2] Flint, J. M. Jour. Med. Research, Vol. VIII, Dec., 1902.
[3] Herring, A. P. Jour. Am. Med. Assoc., Vol. XLIII, Aug., 1904.

gestions and continually comparing the model with their own dissection, much to the profit of all.

In teaching microscopic anatomy with the usual and necessary sections on the slide, it is well known that one of the great difficulties lies in getting the student to realize third dimensions and to obtain an accurate mental picture of a structure in its entirety. In my experience in teaching this subject the modeling of a cell or group of cells, even off-hand, has often been of great aid in cases where the student has difficulty in obtaining morphology and relationships in perspective.

In teaching the microscopic anatomy of the central nervous system, I have tried to make it possible during the past years for some of the students of each year's class to make a model of the spinal cord showing the contour of the different levels comparatively, the position and changes in shape of the different columns of gray and white substance, and the origin, position, and functional direction of the principal axone pathways. The model has necessarily included one level of the inferior portion of the medulla oblongata, i. e., a level through the decussation of the pyramids. The spinal cord has been taken because its structure is simpler than that of the encephalon and because in the order of study of the system it is taken up first. An idea of the structure of the spinal cord in perspective once obtained, the student looks upon the various preparations of the encephalon from a different and more comprehensive viewpoint and obtains a picture of its architecture with greater accuracy and considerably greater ease.

In these attempts at models of the spinal cord the procedure has been quite simple. The students undertaking it were supplied merely with the following: (1) an inch thick wooden board for a base; (2) pieces of stout wire to be inserted into the base for upright supports of the model; (3) a piece of small brass tubing (usually curtain rod) to represent the central canal; (4) thick cardboard upon which the various sections of the cord were outlined under similar magnification, then cut out, and the gray figure of each and the localities of the various fiber tracts colored in with crayons according to a definite color scheme; (5) some beads of suitable sizes and colors to represent the cell bodies of the different neurones; (6) balls of differently colored twine to string through the sections to represent the course of the fiber tracts, the colors corresponding to those of the color scheme on the cardboard; and (7) some wax and mucilage for holding the parts in place. One of the pieces of cardboard, usually that representing the cervical enlargement, was taken of sufficient size to include an outline of the dorsal and ventral roots with the spinal ganglion and the beginning nerve trunk with its dorsal division and rami communicantes schematically represented. Upon one side of all sections projections of the cardboard were left to suitably represent small proximal portions of the dorsal and ventral roots. Most of the beads representing the various nerve cells were more conveniently attached to their positions on the cardboard before arranging the latter in position. The beads were either stuck in position with wax or sewed onto the cardboard with fine thread. The twine representing their axones was attached to them later. Then the pieces of cardboard were punched in the localities of the different nerve pathways with holes just large enough to carry the twine and the central canal was punched out, and through the opening representing the canal the sections were strung on the brass tube and made fast at regular intervals along it. The whole was then attached to the stout wire upright supports inserted into the wooden base board and in this position the running in of the colored twine representing the fiber tracts was begun. The segment retaining the nerve roots and spinal ganglion required an extra support. This was attached to the ganglion so as to hold the roots curved caudad in their natural position. The twine representing ventral root axones was attached to the appropriate bead in the ventral horn and then stuck to the cardboard along its efferent course. The axones attached to spinal ganglion cells were stuck to the coardboard as naturally as possible in the more or less coiled condition close to the cell and the T- and Y-divisions were made by simply tying on another piece of twine to represent the bifurcation. Collateral branches were made in the same way. All end brushes or telodendria of both ascending and descending fibers of long or short course or of association and commissural axones were accomplished by simply tying a knot in the twine a short distance from the end and the end frayed into its component threads and these stuck about the beads representing the appropriate cell bodies. The cells of the nucleus fasciculi gracilis and nucleus fasciculi cuneati were represented by beads similar to those for spinal ganglion cells but colored differently, while the beads for the nucleus dorsalis (Clarke's column) and especially those for Golgi cells of Type II were of smaller size. No attempts were made to show differences in size of axones and only the general and more accepted and fundamental arrangements were undertaken. The finer detail and disputed relations would have made the model too complicated for practical use, the chief purpose of the model being for the student to get accurate foundation ideas upon which to build correctly and easily the additional ideas obtained in his reading.

Sections from six different levels were usually represented in the model, namely, from the conus medullaris, the third lumbar segment, the mid-thoracic region, the sixth cervical segment, the first cervical segment, and the decussation of the pyramids.

In my class in microscopic anatomy of the school year just passed, there fortunately developed a disposition to consider the making of a model of the spinal cord more seriously than in the procedure above described. One of its members, Mr. F. M. Allen, kindly gave considerable of his spare time to it, and the result is a model of more permanent construction and of more permanent value. The plan of its construction required considerable thought and may be of interest to those having to face similar problems.

A photograph of this model in partial profile is here given in Fig. 1. The different segments represented are indicated in the lettering above each section. It is seen that there are eight different levels of the nerve axis involved instead of six as previously. A level through the beginning of the decussation of the lemnisci and the nuclei of the fasciculus gracilis and cuneatus is added in order to illustrate the central termination of the sensory neurones of the first order and the origin and beginning course of certain of the axones of the lemnisci or sensory neurones of the second order. The level is near the beginning of the decussation and therefore involves only the inferior tip of the nucleus of the twelfth nerve and of the inferior olivary nucleus and but a few of the fibræ arcuatæ externæ. Two levels of the thoracic region are represented instead of one, so that the contour of the thoracic decrease in diameter may be curved rather than angular and in order to obtain a greater extent of the nucleus dorsalis (Clarke's column) as well as to show structural variations found within this region.

The process of construction may be arranged in the following steps:

(1) Of the sections from the different regions used by the class, a set was chosen as perfect as possible as to preparation and normal appearances. Instead of using the dissecting microscope and millimeter ruler as used by the rest of the class for their laboratory drawings, each section of the set was enlarged to the same extent by means of the Edinger projection apparatus and both the periphery of the section, with its septa and ventral fissure, and the contour of the gray substance were carefully outlined on a sheet of smooth white paper and the paper labeled corresponding to the label of the slide. In the outline of the gray figure only the larger projections forming the reticular substance were undertaken, while the ingrowths of pia indicating the position of nerve fasciculi and the passage of root fibers were carefully reproduced.

(2) A mixture of 90 parts by weight of beeswax, 5 parts white rosin, and 1 part hard paraffin was used for the reconstructions, the rosin being added to increase the resistance of the wax to both handling and temperature. To make the plates this was melted and poured into shallow pans, and while melted each pan containing it was floated upon water. On the water the wax becomes level and cools with even thickness. In cooling it shrinks away from the sides of the pan and may be easily removed. The pan should be cold when the wax is put into it. A thin film of glycerine was sometimes used, but was not absolutely necessary.

(3) A sheet of the paper with the drawing of one of the sections upon it was then placed in position upon one of the plates and pressed down upon its smooth surface to insure against slipping and all the lines of the drawing carefully gone over with a hard pencil or smooth-pointed probe, thus transferring the drawing to the wax. Then for each section the paper was removed and the outline of the gray figure alone was transferred upon a second plate. Before cutting out the sections from the plates, the plates were placed in a thermostat raised to a temperature of about 45° C. for a few moments to soften. Then they were laid upon a smooth glass plate and cut out.

In cutting, a very narrow instrument is necessary in order to follow the finer details of contour. An ordinary steel dissecting probe ground flat and to an edge on one side was found the best adapted to the purpose. When cut out the first plate consisted of the peripheral contour of the whole section of the cord with the gray figure, septa, etc., outlined upon it, while the second consisted of the gray figure cut out separately. The gray figure thus cut out was fitted over its identical outlines on the first plate with all its features superimposed and pressed down firmly. Pressure will cause the two to adhere firmly, but to insure permanency of its contour, the edges of the gray figure were gone carefully around with a chisel heated sufficiently to melt the wax, thus smoothing the irregularities of cutting and cementing the two parts together more securely. Each section of the cord thus prepared was then compared in detail with the outlines of the original drawing and all irregularities and variations from the original contour were remedied by paring with a sharp, thin-bladed knife. Deficiencies in contour were easily remedied by fusing on bits of wax to complete them. The spinal ganglion (G, Fig. 1) with dorsal and ventral roots and beginning nerve trunk were schematically outlined upon and cut from a separate wax plate and were later fused to the section for which they were intended.

In climates subject to high temperatures in summer it would, perhaps, be advisable to use wood instead of wax for the sections. Either prepared basswood or the ordinary three-ply board used in furniture making would insure against warping and the outlines could be accurately followed with a scroll saw. Wood also would be less expensive. Wax was here used tentatively because of the ease with which the sections could be finished off and the ease with which the beads, etc., representing the various cells, could be attached. The beads had merely to be warmed, placed in position, and pressed slightly into the wax, where they stick. The wax also takes the paint, later applied, more accurately than wood.

(4) The choosing and placing in position of the representatives of the various types of nerve cells was next accomplished. While the cells can be quite readily put into the wax plates after they are arranged vertically in series, they can be more easily and uniformly arranged with the plates lying flat, face upward. Various sized beads were used to represent the cell bodies of all the types of neurones considered in the model except the large motor type of the ventral horn. In these alone an attempt was made to represent the external form of the type. The ventral horn cells were cast in Wood's metal. Two or three slightly varying models of cells were made in oil-softened modeling clay and molds made of them in plaster of Paris. Then from these molds a sufficient number of cells were made by first taking a piece of copper wire of the size used for axones in the rest of the model, placing it in the groove representing the axone in the mold with its end extended to the center of the mold, and then filling the mold with melted Wood's metal. The metal fuses upon the wire firmly, and upon cooling the cast may be removed by means

of it. These casts may be seen in position by examining Fig. 1 with a hand lens, and No. 7 in Fig. 2 is an illustration of one of them. The form of the spinal ganglion cell is closely approximated by the spherical beads. In lieu of a greater variety in the sizes of the beads, the same sized beads were used to represent the spinal ganglion cells of the Ranvier type, the cells of the nuclei of the fasciculus gracilis and fasciculus cuneatus and the recipient nucleus of the spinal tract of the trigeminus. Beads of smaller size were used for the nucleus dorsalis (Clarke's column), for the Dogiel spinal ganglion cell of Type II, and for the association and commissural neurones of longer course. A third and yet smaller size were used for the association and commissural neurones of short course, including Golgi cells of Type II, and for the portion of the nucleus olivaris inferior included in the model.

(5) The cells in position, the various sections were next painted according to a definitely prearranged color scheme. The back sides and edges of all the plates were painted black—the various structural details were contained on the cephalic or anterior surface of each section. The position, shape, and size of all the nerve fasciculi in their variations at the different levels were outlined with thin black lines which remained permanent, being used as limiting boundaries in the subsequent coloration of the parts. In outlining the fasciculi, Fig. 749 of Spalteholtz's *Atlas of Human Anatomy* was used largely as a basis upon which to build.

Several small holes were next drilled through each of the areas outlined for the fasciculi. These holes were of a size merely sufficient to carry the wire to be used in representing the fasciculi and attention was given to their uniform distribution in the areas of the different sections and to their increase or decrease in number at the different levels. Then the areas were painted their respective colors.

The color scheme employed throughout for the entire eight localities was as follows:

All cell-bodies were given a slightly different shade of the same color as that of the fasciculi with which they have to do.

Mass of gray figure of cord and gray masses of medulla.................grayish white.
General color of ascending cerebro-spinal fasciculi ....red.
General color of descending cerebro-spinal fasciculi ....blue.
General color of ascending cerebello-spinal fasciculi and bundles to brain stem at levels of cerebellum........green.
General color of descending cerebello-spinal fasciculi and bundles from brain stem at levels of cerebellum..yellow.
General color of all fasciculi proprii....dark brown.

Colors in Detail:

Fasciculus gracilis (Goll's column).....vermilion.
Fasciculus cuneatus (Burdach's column) or middle root zone..............maroon.
Lissauer's or postero-lateral root zone..crimson.
Dorsal root and spinal ganglion (cervical region) ....dark crimson.
Comma shaped tract (Schultze's)......scarlet.
Fasciculus cerebro-spinalis anterior (direct pyramidal) ....deep blue.
Fasciculus cerebro-spinalis lateralis (crossed pyramidal) ....deep blue.

Ventral root fibers and cells giving origin to them ....light blue.
Fasciculus cerebello-spinalis (direct cerebellar tract) and cells of nucleus dorsalis (Clarke's column) ....green.
Fasciculus anterolateralis superficialis (Gowers') ....green dotted with yellow.
Fasciculus from nucleus vestibularis lateralis or Deiter's nucleus and from nucleus ruber (mixed lateral zone).yellow dotted with green.
Fasciculus sulco-marginalis ....yellow.
Fasciculus marginalis anterior ....yellow.
Helweg's fasciculus ....light brown.
Fasciculus proprius lateralis and ventralis ....dark brown.
Fasciculus proprius dorsalis (anterior root zone of posterior funiculus) and fasciculus septo-marginalis (oval bundle) ....dark brown.
Neurones of Golgi Type II............blue black.
Tractus spinalis of the trigeminus......chrome orange.
Lemniscus and arcuate fibers joining it.light maroon.
Arcuate fibers arising in olivary nucleus ....chrome green.
Afferent sympathetic axone to spinal ganglion ....red orange
Dogiel spinal ganglion neurone of Type II ....purple.

Commissural fibers were colored according to the neurone to which they belong, whether axones or collaterals of associational, commissural proper, pyramidal, or dorsal root neurones.

(6) A baseboard (*B*, Fig. 1) was chosen of sufficient width and length and with a thickness of two inches to insure plenty of stability. Three upright supports, *A*, 8 inches in length, were made of ½-inch steel rod, one end of each threaded into flange bases with 3 screw holes in each flange, and the other end fitted with set-screw eyes of a caliber sufficient to carry the brass tube (*cc*) which represents the central canal. These uprights were screwed upon the base-board as shown in the figure. To prepare the supports indicated by *S*, Fig. 1, the sections were first strung upon the brass tube by passing it through the central canal, bored out in each section to fit the tube. While stringing on the sections the tube was at the same time passed through the set-screw eyes of the supports, *A*. The sections were then arranged equidistant along the tube and, held ventral side down, measurements were carefully taken of the distance between the baseboard and the ventro-lateral edge of both sides of each section and the measurements recorded for the right and left sides of each. Then the sections were taken down till the supports could be prepared. For these, ⅛-inch steel rod was cut into lengths, each 1½ inches longer than the measured distance for which it was individually intended. All the lengths of rod being cut, holes one inch deep were bored into the baseboard at the required places of such a fit that the rods would have to be driven into them. Then a malleable copper washer of a width about equal to the thickness of the wax plates was fitted upon each of the rods ½ inch from the end and soldered firmly in place. One of these rods is shown in Fig. 2, No. 1. The rods were next driven into their respective holes in the baseboard, the upper end of each bearing the washer. Holes of the same size as those in the baseboard were bored ½ inch deep into the ventral edges of each section at the points where its

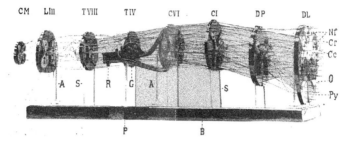

CM LIII TVIII TIV CVI CI DP DL

Nf
Cr
Cc

A S R G A S

O
Py

P B

FIG. 1.

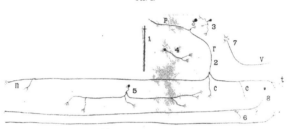

FIG. 2.

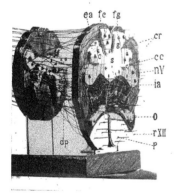

ea fc fg

cr
cc
nV
ia

o

rXII
P

dp

FIG. 3.

FIG. 1.—Photograph of model of spinal cord in partial profile. The Roman letters and numerals above the different sections indicate the regions and segments from which the sections represented were taken. C = cervical; T = thoracic; L = lumbar; CM = conus medullaris; DP = decussation of pyramids; DL = decussation of lemnisci; B = wooden base; A = upright supports to model with flange bases screwed upon wooden base with set-screw adjustments at top through which runs the brass tube CC (representing the central canal); S = upright supports of steel rod, two for each section (same as No. 1 in Fig. 2); G = spinal ganglion with dorsal and ventral roots and beginning nerve trunk with dorsal division; R = ramus communicans; P = projection of wooden base upon which support for ganglion rests; Py = pyramidal fasciculi; O = tip of inferior olive; Cr = restiform body; Nf = nuclei of fasciculi gracilis and cuneatus.

FIG. 2.—Photograph illustrating the construction of some of the constituent neurones used in representing the fasciculi of the model shown in Fig. 1. No. 2 = Afferent or spinal ganglion neurone with T-shaped division near its cell-body and the Y-shaped division of its axone within the spinal cord; p = a portion of its peripheral process; r = the axone as contributing to the dorsal root; c = collaterals with their telodendria; t = final termination of caudad division; n = termination in nucleus fasciculi cuneati, for example. No. 3 = Dogiel spinal ganglion neurone of Type II. No. 4 = commissural neurone of short transverse course in gray substance of cord. Forms similar to Nos. 3 and 4 were used to illustrate Golgi neurones of Type II. No. 5 = association neurone of medium long course. No. 6 = axone of pyramidal neurone, the majority of which in threading them into the model were bent across the mid-line at the level of the decussation of the pyramids; others were made to decussate at lower levels. No. 7 = motor neurone of ventral horn with ventral root portion of its axone (v). No. 8 = neurone of nucleus dorsalis (Clarke's column), the axone of which extends through fasciculus cerebello-spinalis lateralis to corpus restiforme. No. 1 = form of smaller support indicated by S in Fig. 1.

FIG. 3.—Photograph of section of model at level of beginning decussation of the lemnisci. cc = central canal; cr = restiform body; c = nucleus of funiculus cuneatus; fc = funiculus cuneatus; g = nucleus funiculus gracilis; fg = funiculus gracilis; dp = decussation of pyramids; ia = internal arcuate fibers and decussation of pyramids; ea = external arcuate fibers (in two colors); o = inferior tip of inferior olive; p = pyramid; $rXII$ = root fiber of XIIth nerve; s = central gray substance; nV = nucleus of spinal tract of trigeminus.

respective rods touched when it was held in place. The section was then fitted firmly upon the rods till the washers came in contact with the edge. The copper washers being malleable, they were bent with forceps beforehand so as to conform to the contour resting upon them. When all the sections were in their places on the supports, s, the tube cc was passed through them and through the eyes in the supports, A, at the same time and the set-screws were run down to grip the tube firmly and permanently. The section representing the conus medularis, Cm, does not necessarily require supports.

An extra support similar to the supports, A, was necessary for holding the spinal ganglion in position. Though the nerve roots were naturally flexed caudad, yet the spinal ganglion and beginning nerve trunk necessarily extended some distance from the line of the sections. To avoid a too wide and clumsy baseboard, a projection, P, was attached to the base for the support of the ganglion. The position of this and the position of the upright screwed upon it was best determined after the sections were in place. Then the nerve roots were fused in position upon the section and the whole was securely attached to the upright by means of staples of small copper wire driven through the ganglion and the ends twisted upon the upright.

(7) When the various parts were in position on the supports and arranged permanently, the model was ready for stringing in the nerve fasciculi. In constructing these, No. 18 copper wire was used for the axones, supplemented by No. 1 wire picture cord for the collateral branches and final terminations with their telodendria. The lengths of wire required varied, of course, according to the locality at which an axone in question originated or terminated. Practically no duplications were allowed lest the model should appear too bewilderingly complicated. Therefore, each axone was measured off, constructed, and fitted in individually. In representing collaterals, a piece of picture wire was cut the required length, twisted tightly, the threads at one end slightly frayed and clasped upon the axone wire and then soldered in place. Soldering them not only insured their remaining firmly in whatever position they were placed, but it improved the appearance of the result, and, if the solder resulted in a slight varicosity at the point of junction, such was considered nothing more than the frequent natural appearance of axones as seen after the Golgi method. The soldering process was very rapid and simple. Drops of molten solder were allowed to fall upon the table from a height of 12 or 15 inches, and upon striking they flattened out and cooled as thin plates. These were cut into narrow strips about half an inch long. The junction of the copper wire and the picture wire (clasped upon it) was treated with a touch of acid zinc chloride, then one of the strips of solder was wound upon the junction, and a second over a Bunsen flame was sufficient. When it was necessary for collaterals to occur on an axone on both sides of a section through which the axone had been strung, such collaterals had to be put on after the axone was in place. This was done by simply attaching the collateral in the same way, after the stringing in, and then holding a spirit lamp or Bunsen burner under the

point of junction. The final terminations of the axones were represented by soldering the piece of picture wire upon the copper wire end to end. These points of junction were dressed with a file and then could be easily passed through the holes in the sections, and so all were attached before stringing in, because it could be done much more easily when holding the two pieces upon the flat surface of the table. As is evident, the picture wire was used in order to represent the end-brushes or telodendria. No. 1 picture wire is composed of 8 strands. These could be frayed out, clipped, and bent so as to resemble any form of end-brush usually seen.

To represent bifurcations of the axone proper, as is the case in the spinal ganglion neurone, for example, an extra piece of copper wire was soldered on to the main portion of the axone and the junction bent in any angle desired. Bifurcations in the region of the final termination were accomplished by either soldering on an extra piece of picture wire or by dividing the threads of the terminal picture wire into two equal numbers, twisting each number into separate wires, and making end-brushes on each as before. The results of both procedures are shown in Nos. 2 and 5 of Fig. 2.

Axones of short course were made wholly of picture wire. For Dogiel spinal ganglion neurones of Type II, for example (No. 3, Fig. 2), the wire was doubled and then divided into as many branches as desired, each twisted into a separate wire and frayed at the end. Golgi cells of Type II were made in the same way. Connections of the sympathetic system were represented by a piece of picture wire passing through the ramus communicans into the nerve trunk and thence into the confines of the spinal ganglion, there to break up into divisions, one of which terminated about a Dogiel cell of Type II, others about spinal ganglion cell bodies of the ordinary Ranvier type. In response, a ventral root axone passes into the domain of the sympathetic via the ramus.

The small copper wire being very flexible, it could be drawn through the holes prepared for a given fasciculus with almost as much ease as string, and it is much better than string in that it and the collaterals remain as arranged. It does not sag and, combined, it adds considerably to the rigidity of the model. As shown in the illustrations of several of the types of neurones given in Fig. 2, Nos. 2 and 5 could not be used in the model, since they have certain collaterals that could only be attached after the wire has been threaded through the holes in the wax sections. Also, such axones as have their cell bodies within the spinal cord are shown in Fig. 2 as equipped with them, when, it will be remembered, the cell-bodies were attached to the sections before they were put up in series and the axones threaded in. The beads (cell bodies) are only added in Fig. 2 to complete the appearance of the neurones presented. In making the model each axone was threaded in bare of a cell body, was arranged as to its end of origin with special reference to its appropriate cell body, was then clipped the required length and the end inserted into the eye of the bead. To further insure both the end of origin and the bead remaining in position, a fine wire staple was placed astride the wire close up to the bead and driven into the wax section. When the wires were painted this staple became invisible. The ventral horn neurones alone were put in position with the cell bodies already attached to the axones. The end-brushes or telodendria were made to clasp appropriate cell bodies in a neurone chain by simply bending the twigs about a bead and pressing the ends of some of them into the wax and the arrangement held in place by the use of the fine wire staple when necessary.

Great architectural detail was necessarily avoided to maintain the simplicity and usefulness of the model. Only the simpler and most generally accepted arrangements of neurones were undertaken. In case of Helweg's fasciculus, which is claimed to be a spinal cord-olive connection but the locality of the cells of origin of which is uncertain, only plain, straight wires were used piercing the first section in the region of the olivary nucleus and extending into the cervical region of the cord where they were simply cut off without indications of either origin or termination. Fig. 3 gives an idea of the number of architectural arrangements undertaken at the more complicated level of the beginning of the olivary nucleus and the decussations of the lemnisci. The mere explanation of the figure will suffice for the description of the construction. The color detail is, of course, not brought out in the photographs, the different shades of red, yellow, green, orange, and brown all taking dark and not distinguished from the black outlines of the fasciculi, while the grayish white and the blue alone show light. Association neurones with both their cells and fibers brown on a brown background show scarcely at all. Neither does the lemniscus, for example.

After the construction of the model was completed, it was carefully gone over with paint. Each fasciculus of wires was painted the color of the corresponding fasciculus outlined on the wax sections through which the wires run. Associational and commissural neurones and ventral horn neurones were given their respective colors. Injuries incurred in threading in the wires were repaired and the areas indicating fasciculi on the sections were repainted or touched up, according to necessity. The baseboard was given a thick coat of light yellow to light up and give contrast to the structure above, and the upright supports were given a light metallic luster with a coat of silver paint. Then after all was dry, the whole model was given two coats of transparent varnish to protect the colors and facilitate in dusting the model.

In painting the wires fine globules of paint would form on the twigs of the end-brushes. These globules resemble closely the varicosities seen upon these when stained by the Golgi method or by methylene blue, and so no attempt was made to avoid them.

THE REVEREND GERSHOM BULKELEY, OF CONNECTICUT, AN EMINENT CLERICAL PHYSICIAN.*

By WALTER R. STEINER, M. D.

The interest aroused of late in the medical history of our own country has caused its study to throw much light on the early colonial period, and many former worthies have now become quite familiar to those of us, who cherish the past doings of our profession in the United States. There was, however, a class of eminent practitioners, flourishing chiefly in the seventeenth century, who have been somewhat slighted by Packard, Mumford and others. I refer to the clerical physicians, who were mostly to be found in New England. Some of these "there be which have no memorial," yet there are others of them, who "have left a name behind them that their praises might be reported," though, in many instances, their records are indeed quite fragmentary. In this latter group the name of Gershom Bulkeley stands out large and bold.

He was born in Concord, Mass., about the year 1635,[1] of distinguished parentage. For his father, the Rev. Peter Bulkeley, driven from England on account of his rigid nonconformity and "shut up"[2] in Concord, then a remote and inaccessible spot, was a man of great learning and piety, while his mother was the daughter of Sir Richard Chetwode. Reared, consequently, in the best of family surroundings, he was carefully educated and was graduated at Harvard College, with one other, in the class of 1655.[3] The Steward's book contains a full record of his expenses there from the time of his admission to the date of the rendering of his last quarter bill. Many interesting items are to be found in it, including one for "shoo-mending," and credits of rye, Indian "wheatt," "wheatte meall," butter, cheese, "appelles," "backen," "beaff," "turkey henes," "lambes," "sheepe," "on cow," "on oxe," "430 ft. bords," etc.[4]

Shortly after graduating he began to study for the ministry. He possibly, also, took up the study of medicine, but we

* Read before the Johns Hopkins Hospital Historical Club, April 11, 1904, and also published in the Med. Lib. and Hist. J., 1904, II, pp. 91-103.
[1] Chapin and Caulkins give 1636 as the year, while Shattuck and Chapman put it a year earlier, as above. Sibley cannot determine the exact date and says it was in 1635, 1636, or 1637.

[2] These were the words by which he expressed his seclusion. (See Shattuck. History of the Town of Concord, Mass. Boston, 1835, p. 158.)
[3] Sibley. Harvard Graduates. Cambridge, 1873, I, pp. 389-402.
[4] Sibley. Op. cit., pp. 389-390.

have no information as to who his instructor was in either of these branches, or where he resided at that time. We imagine his father had much to do with his training at this period. In 1661, after several months' trial, the people at New London, Conn., made a contract with him by which he was " to become the minister of the town on a salary of eighty pounds yearly for three years " with the stipulation that it would then be increased if circumstances would permit.[3] During his first term of years he was to have " all such silver as is weekly contributed by strangers, to help towards the buying of books "[4] and the many volumes that still remain of his library show that he probably expended all of the money that thus came to him. His pastorate appears to have been for some years an eminently happy one. The salary was increased in 1664 to six score pound a year,[7] and about this time he brought his mother to New London to live. Everything pointed to his long service in the ministry of this town, but shortly thereafter some friction seems to have arisen, due, it appears, to his opposition to the half-way covenant.[8] On February 25, 1665, the town voted that " they were willing to leave Mr. Bulkley to the libertye of his conscience without compelling or enforcing him to anything in the execution of his place and office contraye to his light according to the laws of the commonwealth,"[9] and, some months later, the town " understanding Mr. Buckley's intention to goe into the Bay " sent messengers to him " in order to know Mr. Bulckley's mynde fullye."[10] Unfortunately he was determined to go in spite of all entreaties to remain, although he consented to occupy the pulpit until a successor was obtained.

He was invited, on June 1, 1666, by the church in Wethersfield " to come and to be helpful to us, and to settle among us in the work of the ministry."[11] This call was accepted and he served them well until he was obliged to resign early in 1677, probably " by reason of weakness of his voice." His resignation was accepted with the utmost reluctance by the town, who had previously declared themselves " freely willing to provide another minister to assist him, and to be a comfort and help to him in that work, and did declare it to be their desire that their Reverend pastor would afford them his help and advise and direction respecting a meet person for that work, for which they shall be thankful to him and take it into serious consideration."[12]

After his dismission from this church he retired from the ministry and devoted the remaining years of his life largely to the practice of medicine. Chapin says that he removed at this time to the other side of the Connecticut River and

settled in the town of Glastonbury.[12] There seems to be some doubt as to this, as in his will he describes himself as from Wethersfield.[14] We know his favorite daughter Dorothy, the wife of Thomas Treat, lived in Glastonbury, and his long visits to her may have created the impression that he dwelt in the same town.

There is no record pertaining to his medical career before the time of King Phillip's War, but he must have had considerable attainments in medicine and surgery before this, as on October 20, 1675,[15] the Court ordered him " to be improued in this present expedition, to be chyrurgion to our army." He was also " ordered and impowered to be of the Council of War." Two months later the Colony's Council of War, showing its esteem for him, commissioned Major Treat, in command of the army, " to take speciall care of the Reverend Mr. Bulkly,"[16] and a little while later appointed two men to go to New London " to take care of and assist in the dressing of the wounded men there, whilst Mr. Buckly goeth forth with the army."[17] From January 26 to February 5, 1676, he was absent with Major Treat and his forces on an expedition against the Indians. About two weeks after their return another expedition was planned and Bulkeley was ordered " to hasten up to goe forth with the army."[18] While ranging through the woods, on ·this expedition, he was wounded in the thigh by the Indians, early in March, in the vicinity of Wachusett, now Princeton, Mass.[19] The wound, however, could not have been a serious one as Israel Channey, also a surgeon in the army, wishing to be relieved on account of sickness and death in his family, writes on March 27, " I hope my brother Bulkly provided he have an easy and able horse will attend the army on the present motion; only if it be expected he doth desire care may be taken for an easy horse, and that it may be sent him this night."[20]

Bulkeley seems to have gone on this third expedition, but must have returned to Wethersfield by May 13 for the Court, " then being informed that sundry wounded men are come to Mr. Buckly, desired Mr. Buckly to take the care and trouble of dressing the s[d] wounded souldiers till God bless his endeavoures with a cure; and Mr. Stone is desired and ordered to assist Mr. Bulkley in the works of the ministry so long as Mr. Bulkly shall be improved as before."[21] Two days later Connecticut raised a small number of men in the war against the Narragansetts and styled them an army with Major Talcott as their leader and Gershom Bulkeley as their

[3] Caulkins. History of New London. New London, 1852, p. 131.
[4] Caulkins. Loc. cit.
[7] Caulkins. Op. cit., p. 136.
[8] Sibley. Op. cit., p. 391.
[9] Caulkins. Op. cit., p. 137.
[10] Caulkins. Loc. cit.
[11] Sibley. Op. cit., p. 393.
[12] Adams. Historic Sketch of the First Church of Christ in Wethersfield. Hartford, 1877, p. 10.

[13] Chapin. Glastonbury for Two Hundred Years. Hartford, 1852, p. 40.
[14] Chapman. The Bulkeley Family. Hartford, 1875, p. 81.
[15] Conn. Coll. Records, II, p. 271.
[16] Conn. Coll. Records, II, p. 388.
[17] Conn. Coll. Records, II, pp. 399-400.
[18] Conn. Coll. Records, II, p. 409.
[19] Hubbard. The History of the Indian Wars in New England. Edited by S. G. Drake. Roxbury, 1865, I, p. 204.
[20] Fowler. Memorials of the Chaunceys. Boston, 1858, p. 280; and Conn. Coll. Records, II, p. 424.
[21] Conn. Coll. Records, II, p. 277.

"chirurgion." This time also Bulkeley was one of the army's Council of War.[22]

For these many services the Colony's Council of War showed its appreciation by allowing Bulkeley liberty, in 1676, to transport 60 bushels of corn to Boston "to purchass some necessaries and phissicall druggs"[23] and in the fall of the next year he was permitted to transport "two hundred of deere skins out of this Colony this next yeare, any law to the contrary notwithstanding."[24] He wished the liberty to do this so that he could exchange the skins for medicines. Besides the above esteem, which the Council showed for his services, they returned to him their "hearty thankes," January 2, 1677, "for his good service to the country, this present war," and did "order the Treasurer to pay unto him the sume of thirty pounds as an acknowledgment of his good service to the country, besides the sattisfying of those that have supplyed his place in the ministry."[25]

After the war he had trouble in collecting his pay from Massachusetts for his care of Jonathan Welles, a wounded soldier, as he would not accept this state's proffered amount[26] and sued Major John Pynchon of Springfield, at the Hartford County Court, on his engagement that due care should be taken for payment of charges, medicine, etc., for Welles and obtained judgment for forty-nine pounds.[27] Massachusetts subsequently complained of the allowance and countenance of this suit by Connecticut,[28] and we do not know if Bulkeley ever received his pay.

Four of his medical account books remain and they all bear witness to the fact that his practice was a large one. I have seen three of them. The first one which I have consulted was his ledger which covered the years from 1680 to 1684. The second book was examined by Dr. G. W. Russell, of Hartford, some twelve years ago and was merely a portion of his day book for 1688, consisting only of twenty-eight pages and dating from August to December 31 of that year. The third covers the period from 1708 to 1713, while the last book, in the library of Trinity College, is well filled with visits paid and medicines and services administered to his various patients from 1702 until August 7, 1713. All of them show he had the same trouble in collecting his bills as doctors now experience. One of his bills was settled twenty-four years later and caused him to make the following remarks:

"But at last we have Reckoned on Aug. 27, 4. An. Dom: 1707 & he hath given me a bond for five pounds money payable at or before ye first day of March next ensuing wch is in full of all accounts between me & ———— from ye beginning of ye world to this day: & he hath kept such poor Accounts yt I remitted between 3 & 4 pounds in money, partly out of good will to him & partly to make sure yt he might have no wrong by me. He had

[22] Conn. Coll. Records, II, p. 444.
[23] Conn. Coll. Records, II, p. 433.
[24] Conn. Coll. Records, II, p. 325.
[25] Conn. Coll. Records, II, p. 483.
[26] Conn. Coll. Records, V, p. 282.
[27] Conn. Coll. Records, III, p. 510.
[28] Mass. Records, V, p. 318.

no account of ye six pounds & nine shill. above mentioned, wch he had payed me by his brother Stephen, besides divers & many other other lesser particulars on both sides: but now this Account is all straightened & done well

G. Bulkley"

His patients came from a wide territory, as we find them consulting him from Wallingford, Farmington, Colchester, Killingworth, Middletown, Guilford, Hartford, New Haven, Haddam, Lebanon, Windsor, Wethersfield, Glastonbury, Rock Hill, New London and Derby in Connecticut, and from Springfield and Northampton in Massachusetts. The names therein entered show he treated some of the best families in the State, for we find mention of the Walcotts of Windsor the Griswolds of Lyme, the Pitkins, Hayneses and Wyllises of Hartford, the Hills of Guilford and many others.

The handwriting in these books is somewhat illegible and the various symbols, then employed, render it exceedingly difficult to decipher some portions. We learn he dispensed the "sovereigne remedy" Rubila of John Winthrop, Jr., but we doubt whether he knew its composition as its worthy maker was very careful in keeping its ingredients secret. In one place Bulkeley charges Mr. Peter Bulkeley 6 shillings for half an ounce of this medicine. As I have previously shown,[29] two grains was the average dose, and Peter Bulkeley must have obtained this quantity for several subsequent dispensings. The usual price for this remedy appears to have been two shillings per grain. On one occasion one patient was charged 2 shillings and 8 pence for 6 grains of the Rubila, and may have taken it as one dose, for Mrs. Davenport of New Haven once took that amount, although it was an unusual quantity. Another patient of Bulkeley's, however, holds the record for taking heroic doses of this drug. We read the following in a letter Fitz-John Winthrop wrote to his brother Wait about their sister Lucy:[30] "I found my poor sister ill with ye beginnings of a feavour wch every day encreased upon hir: thre dayes after I persuaded hir to take 10 graynes of rubila, wch wrought twice, but ye malignety of ye feavour was little abated; ye second day after she complayned of oppression at hir stomack, & desired a litle vomiting drink. I gave hir 16 graynes but did not work; an houre after she toock 5 more, wch wrought twice; at night she toock a potion of ye black powder & rested a litle; but ye feavour allwayes upon hir without any intermission, & she grew weaker every day. Thre dayes since I advised to send for Mr. Buckly who came ye next day & gave hir such things as he thought suitable but noething abated ye feavour & she is now quite gon to all hope, & can onely be recovered by a miracle from Heaven." Unfortunately this miracle was not forthcoming and she died five days later.

With all these patients, many of whom he treated before 1686, it seems strange that he was not licensed to practise medicine until October 14 of that year. The license then issued reads: "This Court being well acquainted with the

[29] Steiner. Governor John Winthrop, Jr., of Connecticut, as a Physician. Johns Hopkins Hosp. Bull., 1903, XIV, p. 302.
[30] V. Mass. Hist. Coll., VIII, p. 281.

ability, skill and knowledge of Mr. Gershom Bulckley in the arts of phissick and chirurgery, doe grant him full and free liberty and license to practise in the administration of phissick and chirurgerie as there shall be occassion and he shall be capable to attend." [21] It is hard to find a reason for this long delay, but it has been suggested that he might have been denied before this "the legal power to collect his professional fees, as he was not sanctioned by authority." [22]

His library is now much scattered and destroyed, but a number of books and manuscripts yet remain. Some are in the possession of Trinity College, while others are owned by Dr. G. W. Russell of Hartford. His manuscripts show that he was in the habit of making abstracts of important articles and books he did not own, and was constantly recording prescriptions and remedies said to be effectual by members of his profession or the laity. It will suffice to quote five of them.

Against the Wind Collicke
"A Receipt agt ye wind Collicke, sent by (my now ffather in Law) Mr. Charles Chauncey then of Situate, May 3, 1648, to my own ffather Mr. Peter Bulkeley of Concord, for my mother, who was wont to be much troubled with ye wind Collicke. The Recp. is this When she hath the fits in any extremity, Take a thicke toste of white bread, toste it thorwly & leisurely on both sides browne; in the meane time heate half a pint of muscadine or somewhat more (or for want thereof, of sacke) on a pewter dish upon a chafing dish of water, very hot, and put ye dry toste into it, & let it drinke up as mch of ye muscadine (or sacke) over ye coales as it will receive, & let this toste be applied as hot to her navill as she can possible endure it, & let it ly on till it be cold. Muscadine (if it can be gotten) is more effectual than sacke, & never failing in ye disease, yt I could find; but ye other (viz. sacke) gives speedy ease through God's blessing."

His other remedy for this affection does not sound so attractive.

℞ Wolfes gutts cleansed from ye filth, then washed over and over in odoriferous wine wherein wormwood hath been boiled, dry them in ye north wind, one dram of ye powder of ye guts, so prepared in 3iii of wine or more (after a clyster given) is an excellent remedy for ye extreme paines of ye wind Collicke.

Hysterical fits were thus treated:

℞ Wolfes flesh, salt it, 3i thereof dissolved in aqua hysterical & epileptical. q. s. is no less effectual against hysterical fitts, the pty then wearing a little piece of ye same about her.

For violent paine in the stomach and bowels, together with invincible costiveness, he employed this prescription, given him by a Hartford blacksmith.

Violent paine in the stomach & bowells together with invincible costiveness
℞ Elicampane, Licoras, brimstone & burnt alum, of each an equal quantity powder them & mix them with a little sallet oile & Rume to the thickness of an electuary, & take ye quantity of a small nutmeg, it is a singular remedy for ye violent paine of ye stomach and bowells accompanyed with invincible costiveness, loosen ye body & ease the paine when nothing

else yt could be gotten would do it, uti saepius pbatum a Josepho Nash Hartfordiensi fabro, a quo accepi.

The following remedy of Thomas Thacher's for indigestion is of interest, for he was the author of a "Brief Rule to Guide the Common People of New England. How to Order Themselves and Theirs in the Small Pocks or Measels"—the first medical publication in this country.

℞ a wine cup of Baume water in ye cold still drawn from ye herb a comon wine cup full, & of Brandy one spoonful in ye morning fasting: Then for breakfast two hours after take spring water a pint and dip in it a good slice of manchet: what bread & water you please thus soaked eat for breakfast, at dinner do ye same & at supper also, pr palpitatione Cordis prbatur, ex propria eperentia Mri Thomae Thatcher ecclesiae 3tiae Bostoniensis (in N. A.) Pastoris qui superaddit. Thus have I done twice since I came to Boston, & if I have any fit at night I take ye water and brandy in ye morning. I used no drugs. This receipt of Mr. Thatcher's I received from Mr. Bradstreete of N. London under Mr. Thatchers owne hand, this 3, 5, 1672. [23]

Bulkeley's breadth of view and diagnostic acumen are well shown in two instances which have come down to us. The first one relates to his opinion in regard to Mary Brown of Wallingford, who was being tried for the murder of her son. "She had been subject to paroxysms of insanity and the court and the jury were in some perplexity relative to their own course of proceeding." They consequently applied to Mr. Bulkeley, who showed his sound sense in the following: "If she were not compos mentis at the time of the fact it is no felony and consequently no willful or malicious murder; and if she be known to be a lunatic, though she have her lucid intervals, there need be very good and satisfactory proof that she was compos mentis for the law favors life." [24]

The second instance relates to Abigail Thompson of Farmington, who was accused of killing her husband by throwing a pair of shears at him, in a fit of anger, thus causing a wound from which he died. Bulkeley writes: "I find yt ye womans act was in ye nature of a chance medley, done in a quarrell, upon a sudden provocation; and also yt ye man lived 18 days after ye wound, was up and down, here and there, cut wood, dressed flax, &c., all weathers; and yt in all this time no care was taken of him by any of his neighbors or relations, his wound was never searched, no proper means at all used for his cure, nothing but a plaster applyed, wch skinned it over 3 or 4 days before he dyed; and in fine, nobody abiding in ye house with them night or day, but he was wholly left to the mercy, care and nursing of that bloody woman, who they knew had wounded him. Hereupon my little sense concludes that ye wound, penetrating into ye brain, was indeed such yt he might possibly dyed of it, but the neglect of it and ye (illegible) method of cure was such

[21] Conn. Coll. Records, III, p. 218.
[22] Russell. Early Medicine and Early Medical Men in Connecticut. Proc. Conn. Med. Soc., Bridgeport, 1892, p. 28. Dr. Russell gives an excellent account of Gershom Bulkeley.

[23] The above selections are taken from those given by Russell in his article previously cited. They are to be found in the original in a manuscript volume of Bulkeley's, now owned by Dr. G. W. Russell. I am greatly indebted to Dr. Russell, as he allowed me to consult this volume.
[24] Sumner. Address on the Early Physicians of Connecticut. Hartford, 1851, p. 28.

that he must of necessity dy of them, and tis impossible to make it evident yt he died of ye wound. I cannot say ye wound would have been cured if good means had been seasonably used; but I can say it is probable it might have been cured, because more dangerous wounds of ye brain than that have been cured. It neither is or can be evident that he died of ye wound; but I think tis evident yt he died of corruption, gangrene and suppuration of ye wound and brain, through ye neglect of means to prevent it, wch in an ordinary way of Providence, might have been done. Tis now endeavored to lay ye fault of ye neglect upon ye woman. I cannot excuse her, any more than ye man or his friends. I think y^y all are to blame; but besides else may be said to avoid it, tis certain she was not indicted, or brought to answer, on that account, and we must not indict upon one crime and evidence for another." [33]

His knowledge of chemistry was most profound and his laboratory was well stocked with apparatus and chemicals. "Even to alchemy with its visionary speculations, then so closely allied to chemistry, he seems to have paid considerable attention. He was master of several languages among which may be reckoned the Greek, Latin and Dutch." [34] Besides theology and medicine he was skilled in the knowledge of law and was a politician in the noblest sense of that word. He was on the losing side, however, for his loyalty was of the "high tory and passive obedience type " [35] so he was an ardent advocate of Sir Edmund Andross, by whom he was made a Justice of the Peace in 1687. [36] His pamphlets entitled "The People's Right to Election " and " Will and Doom " attest his firm belief in the divine right of kings, and when the Connecticut charter was resumed in 1689, his position on Andross' side caused him to lose much in public favor. He had previously refused to take the freeman's oath, so he was denied a seat among the deputies, although he was elected as one from Wethersfield in 1679. [37]

Ill health caused him to visit Antigua, in the West Indies, with his son Charles, in 1681. [38] Eight years later, in one of his pamphlets he speaks of his " bodily infirmity," [39] while in his will he says: " I have much more than twenty years walked upon the very mouth of the grave, under so great infirmity that I cannot but wonder how I have all the while escape falling into it." [40] Yet in spite of his ill health he was able to continue in the practice of medicine until his death, at the age of seventy-seven, on December 2, 1713. He was buried in the cemetery back of the Congregational Church in Wethersfield, and upon his tomb the following inscription can yet be deciphered:

[33] VI Mass. Hist. Coll., III, p. 399.
[34] Chapin. Loc. cit.
[35] Conn. Coll. Records, III, p. 389.
[36] Conn. Coll. Records, III, pp. 455 and 457; and Hoadley, Coll. Conn. Hist. Soc., Hartford, 1895, III, p. 73.
[37] Conn. Coll. Records, III, p. 26.
[38] Hoadley. Coll. Conn. Hist. Soc. Hartford, 1895, III, p. 71.
[39] Coll. Conn. Hist. Soc. Hartford, 1860, I, p. 59.
[40] Chapman. Loc. cit.

"HE WAS HONORABLE IN HIS DESCENT,
OF RARE ABILITIES, EXCELLENT IN LEARNING,
MASTER OF MANY LANGUAGES,
EXQUISITE IN HIS SKILL
IN DIVINITY, PHYSIC AND LAW
AND OF A MOST EXEMPLARY
AND
CHRISTIAN LIFE
IN CERTAM SPEM BEATAE RESURRECTIONIS REPOSITUS " [41]

His will was dated May 26, 1712, and in its first clause he states his occupation was that of a " practitioner of physick." In it we also find the following: " Item, to my grandson Richard Treat, (the son of Thomas and Dorothy) I give and bequeath all my books and manuscripts, which anyway concern medicine and chymistry, among which I include all Glauber's and Boyle's Books, which I have, whether in Latin or English, as also Georgius Agricola De Re Metallica and Lazarus, each re-translated by St. John Pettus called Fleeta Mina, or the art &c of Metalls; and the same St. John Pettus his Fodine Regales, and such like books, and also Littleton's Dictionary for the Latin tongue, and my Dutch Grammar for the Dutch language, together with my manuscript Dutch Dictionary which may help him to read and understand Hehwart's Degerend, &c., i. e. the Day Spring, a new resurrection of the art of medicine which book is in the Dutch language, and together with all my vessels and instruments useful thereabout, of glass, brass, copper, iron, stone or earth. All these I give to him, provided he hold and pursue his inclination to that study, but if by death or otherwise he be diverted or depart from it, then I give all to the next of his bretheren that will apply himself to the study, but if none of them, then I give them all to his mother (my daughter Dorothy) to dispose of at her discretion or to his father, in like manner, if he survive her." [42]

Various estimates are given of his character. Channey writes in 1721: " I have heard (him) mentioned as a truly great man, and eminent for his skill in chemistry" [43] and Benjamin Trumbull says "Mr. Bulkley was viewed as one of the greatest physicians and surgeons then in Connecticut." [44] Later writers as John Hammond Trumbull and Palfrey somewhat detract from previous estimates of him. The former states " he had few superiors in the colony in natural ability, professional learning or general scholarship" but adds " overweening self importance, obstinate adherence to his own opinions or prejudices, a litigious spirit and the peculiarities of his political creed, detracted from his usefulness, and kept him almost continually at strife with his parish, his neighbors or the government of the colony." [45] While Palfrey

[41] Tillotson. Wethersfield Inscriptions. Hartford, 1899, p. 30.
[42] Chapman. Op. cit., p. 84.
[43] Mass. Hist. Coll., X, p. 155.
[44] Trumbull. History of Connecticut. New London, 1898, I, p. 291.
[45] Conn. Coll. Records, III, pp. 388-389.

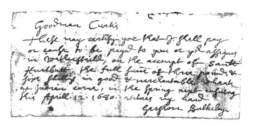

Holograph Note and Signature of Gershom Bulkeley.

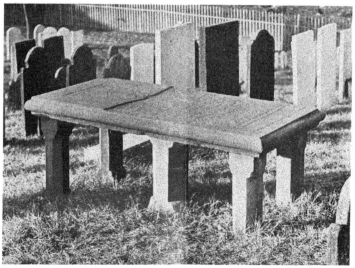

Table Monument, Gershom Bulkeley, showing the Coat-of-Arms of the Bulkeley Family.

notes " He was always a discontented and troublesome person." [a] A contemporary opinion of him is to be found in the Boston News Letter for December 28, 1713. Here we read " he was Eminent for his great Parts, both Natural and Acquired, being Universally acknowledged besides his good Religion and Vertue to be a Person of Great Penetration, and a sound Judgment, as well in Divinity as Politicks and Physick; having served his Country many years successively as

a Minister, a Judge and a Physician with great Honour to himself and advantage to others." [b]

I shall feel that my labors have been rewarded in thus bringing before you Gershom Bulkeley, numbered among those " Persons whose more declared Business was the Study of Divinity," [b] if he shall henceforth find, at least, slight mention in subsequent accounts of colonial medicine in this country.

---

[a] Palfrey. History of New England. Boston, 1864, III, p. 544.

[a] Sibley. Op. cit., p. 397.

[b] Mather. Magnalia. Hartford, 1853, I, p. 493.

A SKETCH OF THE LIVES OF A GERMAN AND AN AMERICAN MASTER OF SURGERY.[1]

By Martin B. Tinker, S. B., M. D.,

Formerly First Assistant Resident Surgeon, Johns Hopkins Hospital; Lecturer on Surgery, Cornell University Medical College, Ithaca, N. Y.; Surgeon to the Clifton Springs Sanitarium.

It has often seemed to me that the rewards in honor and lasting fame which we bestow upon our eminent men are not quite fairly distributed. The men who laboriously glean from accumulated knowledge the facts most important and useful in present day practice, who seek underlying principles, who simplify and systematize, are often far less widely known and honored than the men who make some discovery of relatively slight importance, describe some anatomical point, invent a new instrument, or devote their lives to the development of some one method of treatment. Some of our most truly great men who have deeply influenced their students, associates, and the ideals and practice of their day have not startled the world with anything new. What such men accomplish does not make their names immortal but they inspire others; they transmit less of their knowledge than of their enthusiasm and methods of work. A few facts about the lives of two men of this stamp I shall attempt to give this evening.

Bernhard Rudolph Conrad Langenbeck was born November 8, 1810, at Padingbüttel, a town located on the coast of the North Sea near the mouth of the Weser. His father was a clergyman of much ability, who also kept a private school in which Langenbeck was educated for the first seventeen years of his life entirely under his father's private teaching. His early studies were intended to prepare him for entering the ministry. After leaving his father's school he entered an advanced class in the gymnasium at Hildesheim where he further pursued studies in preparation for theology. On October 25, 1830, he matriculated in the medical department of the University of Göttingen, where his uncle was Professor of Surgery and Anatomy. He passed his examinations for the

doctorate *cum laude,* and April 17, 1834, presented for his graduating dissertation a paper on *The Structure of the Retina.* A further paper, *De Retina, Observationes Anatomico-pathologicae,* for which the Blummbach stipendium was awarded him in 1836, permitted him to take a scientific journey to Paris and England. After two years' study he returned and was made Privat-docent in physiology and pathological anatomy at the University of Göttingen, May 7, 1838. He gave instruction in both of these branches as well as in embryology for three years and with such success that in 1841 he was made Associate Professor of Pathological Anatomy. The change from physiology and pathology to surgery was influenced, Bergmann tells us, by three factors: In the first place he was offered a position as assistant to his uncle who at that time was Professor of Anatomy and Surgery in the University of Göttingen. The advantages for practical surgical work which he gained in that way were great and he developed a strong liking for surgery as well as an excellent foundation for it from a thorough study of anatomy. The second great influence which led him to take up surgery was his journey to England, where he saw the most eminent surgeons of that time and where he came into specially intimate contact with Astley Cooper. The collections in the museums of such hospitals as St. Thomas's in London were then unequaled in Germany and the brilliant sessions of the Royal Medico-Chirurgical Society greatly stimulated his interest in surgery. A third important factor was an acquaintance with Stromeyer, then Professor of Surgery in Erlangen, which Langenbeck made when attending the meeting of the National Natural History Society at Erlangen. Stromeyer was soon called to the chair of Surgery in Munich and he strongly recommended Langenbeck as his successor. Although he did not accept the chair at Erlangen this brought Langenbeck's name into prominence and, no

---

[1] Read before the Johns Hopkins Hospital Historical Club, February 8, 1904.

doubt, had an influence in securing him the professorship of surgery in Kiel one year later in 1842. During the six years spent in Kiel he established so high a reputation as an operator and teacher of surgery that at Dieffenbach's death he was called to Berlin as his successor. He spent thirty-four most productive years in Berlin, building up the Royal Surgical Clinic from a comparatively unimportant institution of twenty beds to one of the most important clinics in Europe, founding and editing the *Archiv für klinische Chirurgie*, founding and presiding over the German Surgical Association and teaching with such success that students flocked to his clinics and operative courses from many lands. When seventy-two years old, in 1882, Langenbeck resigned from active work and thought to spend the balance of his days in peace and comfort in his beautiful country place near the Rhine. But this was not to be: a severe eye disease (probably cataract) required repeated operations, and the death of members of his family filled his last days with trouble and sadness. He died at Wiesbaden in his seventy-seventh year, October 8, 1887.

As a surgeon he was noted for the perfection of his operative technic and his consideration for his patients. He is said never to have used an unnecessary or unkind word in his dealings with his patients or his assistants and nothing was looked upon lightly which concerned the comfort or welfare of his patients. His knowledge of anatomy and constant teaching of operative surgery on the cadaver no doubt contributed to his skill and accuracy as an operator. His constant endeavor was to simplify surgical methods and to learn general principles. As a military surgeon few men have had such wide experience or have used it so well. During the war between Germany and Denmark, in 1848, he served as surgeon in charge of the general army corps of the Dukedom of Schleswig-Holstein and then performed the first large series of joint resections in the history of surgery. He also served in the war between Austria and Prussia in 1866 and in the Franco-Prussian war of 1870. He was honored with numerous decorations and made many contributions of importance in military surgery, especially on matters concerning the sanitary arrangements of the German army, which may serve as a model on this subject for all time. In the Franco-Prussian War he organized a society of military hospital surgeons of all nationalities who met at frequent intervals and gave each other the benefit of their rich experiences. As an evidence of his success as a practicing surgeon it may be mentioned that when he entered the surgical clinic at Berlin there were scarcely twenty beds at his disposal; when he resigned his position to retire to Wiesbaden there was accommodation for over two hundred in his clinic and patients came to him from the entire civilized world.

Undoubtedly Langenbeck's influence was felt most strongly as a teacher. From the beginning, when in 1838 he was made privat-docent of physiology and pathological anatomy in Göttingen, his ability was recognized and this led to his promotion to ' *ausserordentlich professor* ' in pathological anatomy three years later, in 1841. In the spring term of 1842 he began his lectures in Kiel on Clinical, General and Operative Surgery, and while in Kiel he became widely known by the " worth and scientific spirit of his writing, his talent as an operator, and his gift as a lecturer on surgery." In the autumn of 1848 he began his clinical lectures in Berlin as successor to Dieffenbach and for thirty-four years he was the undisputed master of surgery in Berlin. He introduced the teaching of operative surgery on the cadaver, a training for students of even more importance than at the present, for in those days all operating had to be done without anesthesia. Bergmann says of his teaching that he was distinguished not so much by the brilliancy of his lectures as by their earnestness. In his clinical lectures he was most thorough and he presented the features of the case in clear and direct language which seldom failed to impress his hearers. His most gifted students were chosen as assistants and when once appointed they were never unkindly criticized but always praised for good work: lack of praise he said was as bad as the sharpest criticism. He frequently gave hints on problems for research but never extended advice, which he said ruined the individuality and originality of men.

The importance of his influence as a teacher is perhaps best appreciated when we mention the names of a few of his pupils and assistants who have attained eminence as surgeons and teachers of surgery: Bergmann, Gurlt, Sonnenburg; professors of surgery at Berlin, Trendelenburg at Leipzig, Küster at Marburg, Schede at Bonn, Lücke at Bern, and, master among masters, Billroth of Vienna. Of Langenbeck's surgical grandchildren, the pupils of his pupils, may be mentioned Lücke's student, Kocher of Bern, and Billroth's many students, including Mikulicz of Breslau, Czerny of Heidelberg, Eiselsberg and Gussenbauer of Vienna, Wölfler of Prag, Krönlein of Zürich and v. Hacker of Graz. In 1880, when he celebrated his seventieth birthday, his former assistants congregated from far and near and in the number were sixteen who were professors of surgery or directors of surgical clinics who had either previously acted as his assistants or had been his scholars. Through his activity in societies he was also a great teacher; he appreciated the great value of such meetings for interchange of ideas and was always prominent in their support. The founding of the German Surgical Society was entirely his work and he was its president for many years. For twelve years he was president of the Berlin Medical Society and when he left Berlin to take up his home for the last years of his life in Wiesbaden he was made honorary president of both of these societies.

Speaking of the character and influence of his work Bergmann, in his reminiscences of Langenbeck, says of him that he did not belong to the class of men who introduce startling new ideas or new methods of thought or who discover unsuspected treasures of knowledge. He deserves credit especially for emphasizing the bearing of the fundamental biological branches of medicine on surgery. In this way he stamped German surgery with a peculiar individuality and first placed it among the great schools of the surgery of the world. No other surgeon has had such an influence on investigation and the practical results following it as he. To understand the significance of his work it should be remembered that at the time of his appointment at Berlin the surgeons of Germany ranked far below those of France and England. Modern German surgery has outstripped its western neighbors largely as the result of the labors of Langenbeck. Until the beginning of the first decade of the nineteenth century the part which Germany had taken in the advance of surgery was very unimportant. It had no names to compare with Pare, Petit, Desault, Dupuytren in France, or of Potts, Cooper, and John Hunter in England. Even Dieffenbach's plastic method is called to-day the "French method" and with some right for it was first demonstrated in Paris and described in the French language. Küster also calls attention to the wonderful progress in the teaching and practice of surgery which began with Langenbeck's career, and states that up to that time all German surgeons were obliged to leave their own country to get the most advanced teaching to complete their surgical education. The present-day student at the University of Berlin has early pointed out to him the Langenbeck Haus, erected in his memory by his sovereign and the fellows of the German Surgical Association. This fine building, erected on the banks of the Spree, is the home of the German Surgical Association, of the Berlin Medical Society, and of a fine library which includes Langenbeck's collection. It is one of the finest memorials and perhaps the most fitting, ever erected to a member of our profession.

In an obituary notice Langenbeck's most eminent pupil, Billroth, said of him: "It is impossible to sketch briefly the significance of his work; this would be to sketch the history of surgery for the past forty years. There was a charm in his personality which captured all who came in contact with him. He was the inspired and inspiring leader, the embodiment of an ideal clinical teacher. He has left his name in golden letters not only in the book of the history of surgery but in the book of love of his scholars and friends."

I will now recall to your memories some facts regarding an American contemporary of Langenbeck. Samuel David Gross was born the eighth of July, 1805, on his father's farm within two miles of Easton, Pennsylvania. His grandparents had emigrated from the region of the lower Rhine, in Germany, and settled in Pennsylvania. His early years were spent on the farm, near which he attended school in a log-cabin school house. He tells us in his autobiography that as a boy he was careless and more devoted to amusement than to study. About the age of six years he conceived the idea of becoming a physician and from this purpose he never swerved. He was brought up in a German settlement where little English was spoken, and at the age of fifteen his knowledge of English was slight. At that time he had made considerable progress in the German language, so that he had read a number of books and was able to write German with some facility. At the age of seventeen he commenced the study of medicine

with a country practitioner, but finding that he had not sufficient education to enable him to understand the technicalities of medicine, he gave up his cherished plan and devoted two more years to preliminary study at the Wilkes-barre Academy and the Lawrenceville (New Jersey) High School.

When nineteen years old he began the study of medicine again with Dr. Joseph Swift of Easton, and soon afterwards he matriculated at the newly established Jefferson Medical College of Philadelphia. He was influenced to do this by the reports of the brilliant achievements of Dr. George McClellan, who was at that time professor of surgery, and soon after going to Philadelphia he became a private pupil of Dr. McClellan. As a student he states that he was very fond of practical anatomy and spent a large part of his time in the dissecting room. He graduated in 1828, when twenty-three years of age, devoting much care and labor to a thesis on *The Nature and Treatment of Cataract*. It is interesting to note that both Langenbeck and Gross were early interested in the eye, and both wrote their graduating thesis on subjects relating to ophthalmology.

Soon after graduation he opened an office in Philadelphia and for eighteen months eked out a livelihood, mainly by translating books from the German and French. He states that during the first year his income from practice did not exceed three hundred dollars and he labored night and day on his translations under the stimulus of both ambition and poverty. His different translations aggregated nearly fifteen hundred pages during this first eighteen months. At this time, in spite of his extreme poverty he married and returned to Easton, Pennsylvania, where he soon established a fair practice. During the two years and a half which he practiced in Easton he devoted his leisure time to the study of practical anatomy in a little dissecting room which he built at the foot of his garden. During the summer months he spent his time in composing a work on descriptive anatomy based on his dissection, which, however, was never published.

In 1833 through the help of Dr. Eberle, one of his college preceptors who had become professor in the Medical College of Ohio at Cincinnati, he obtained an appointment as demonstrator of anatomy and removed to Cincinnati, making the journey thence by stage, canal, and steamboat, in thirteen days. Soon after removing to Cincinnati he became a joint editor of the Western Medical Gazette, in which was published a review of Beaumont's treatise on *The Functions of Digestion*. In 1835 Gross was elected to the chair of Pathological Anatomy in the newly established Medical Department of Cincinnati College. Among his associates in the faculty of this school were Dr. Daniel Drake and Dr. Willard Parker, the latter afterwards professor of surgery in the college of Physicians and Surgeons of New York. A study of all the books on pathology which he could obtain and a large amount of practical post-mortem work enabled Dr. Gross to publish in 1839 his *Elements of Pathological Anatomy*. This was the first book on this subject in the English language and it passed through three editions and brought him fame and practice. Da Costa says of these two volumes that they did more to attract attention to the subject than anything ever done in this country, and Keen says, "It is strange to think that in a then small western town in America a young teacher in a new medical school should have published the first book in the English language on Pathological Anatomy." The work was fully recognized abroad and soon after the publication of the second edition Gross was made a member of the Imperial Royal Society of Vienna.

After declining an appointment to the chair of medicine in the University of Virginia and of anatomy in the University of Louisiana, Gross accepted in 1840 an appointment as professor of surgery in the University of Louisville, where he was again associated with Daniel Drake, also with Austin Flint and many other leaders in medicine at that time. He held this position for sixteen years, with the exception of the winter of 1850-51, which he spent in New York as the successor of Valentine Mott, in the chair of Surgery at the University of New York. During this time he carried out his extensive experimental studies on injuries of the intestines. He states that he devoted much of his time for over two years to this work, testing all the more important methods of treatment then in use by experimenting on over seventy dogs. The results of his work, which included his directing attention to the necessity for taking in the submucosa in intestinal suturing, were published in a volume of two hundred and twenty pages, which was illustrated by wood cuts and colored engravings. In 1853 he published a comprehensive monograph *On The Results of Surgical Operations in Malignant Diseases,* comprising one hundred and twenty-seven pages and embodying the experiences of the principal surgeons of all countries. Gross was the first to recommend the systematic removal of the nearest lymphatic glands and extensive excision in the treatment of breast carcinoma and other malignant disease. In 1856 he helped to found the Louisville Medical Review, of which he was senior editor, but owing to his appointment as professor of surgery in the Jefferson Medical College only six numbers of this journal appeared.

In the fall of 1856 he entered upon his career as a teacher in Philadelphia, which lasted for twenty-six years of active work, until he resigned his chair in 1882. It was during this time that he reached the zenith of his success. His reputation did much to draw students to Philadelphia and usually the names on the Jefferson Medical College catalogue represented all the states and territories in the Union, as well as a number of foreign countries. With him were associated John K. Mitchell, Robley Dunglison, Charles D. Meigs, Da Costa, Biddle, Bache, Pancoast, and many other men, whose names are famous in medicine. Soon after going to Philadelphia he established with his pupil, T. G. Richardson, the North American Medico-Chirurgical Review, in which he introduced a new feature in that various departments were entrusted each to a separate contributor, who furnished abstracts of the current literature, thus keeping its subscribers informed with regard to the latest discoveries and improvements in medicine. Dr. Richardson subsequently moved to New Orleans to become professor of anatomy and later of surgery in the University of Louisiana.

Three years after going to Philadelphia, Gross published his well-known System of Surgery, which, though much of its pathology and practical teaching are now obsolete, is still a mine of information. It was translated into several foreign languages and did much to establish his reputation everywhere that surgery was practiced. It passed through six editions, the last appearing only seventeen months before his death. That when almost eighty years old he was willing to throw aside prejudice and accept the newly introduced principles and practice of Lister, shows the progressive character of the man. Dr. Keen says of his work as an author "He blazed more than one new trail in the forests of surgical ignorance. In the early part, and even in the middle of this century (the nineteenth century) it was rare for Americans to write medical books; the most they did was either to translate a French or German work or annotate an English one. He was one of the earliest to create an American Medical Literature of importance." His text-book on surgery gave a position to American surgery abroad, which we can now hardly appreciate, while, as already related, his pathological anatomy was the very first work in the English language on that most important branch of medicine. He was always a champion of the American medical profession and did much to arouse the pride of Americans in the achievements of their fellow countrymen. At various times he wrote much on the history of American medicine and surgery, including a volume of nearly eight hundred pages on "The Lives of Eminent Physicians and Surgeons of the Nineteenth Century." Besides his own original writings, Gross's work in reviewing foreign surgical literature and bringing it before the profession in America deserves special mention as well as his translations of a number of important French and German books, and his labors as joint editor of the Western Medical Gazette and editor and founder of the Louisville Medical Review and the North American Medico-Chirurgical Review.

Gross also appreciated the importance of medical societies in spreading knowledge. He was founder and first president of the American Surgical Association, of the Philadelphia Academy of Surgery, and with Da Costa he founded the Pathological Society of Philadelphia. A medical writer and teacher of authority, both in this country and abroad, he never held himself aloof from his less progressive fellows, but his influence and example did much to elevate the standard of American surgery.

As a surgeon Keen speaks of him as painstaking, thorough, and careful in his investigations of a case. "Skillful as an operator and having so vast an experience and equally extensive acquaintance with the wide literature of his profession, he was scarcely ever perplexed by the most difficult case and rarely at a loss as to the proper course to pursue in the most unexpected emergencies." His study of wounds of the intestines led to much of the modern, rational, and successful abdominal surgery. He first advocated opening the abdomen in rupture of the bladder, amputation in senile gangrene, the immediate suture of tendons when divided in incised wounds, and extensive operation and excision of the nearest lymphatic glands in carcinoma. In his autobiography Gross says what few men of extensive practice can say, "I have never lost a patient upon the table from shock or loss of blood."

But he was perhaps at his very best as a teacher. I quote again from Professor Keen's address: " As a teacher, I can speak both with personal knowledge and enthusiasm. I can see his tall, stately form, his handsome face, his glowing features, his impressive gestures. He was earnestness itself. Filled to overflowing with his subject, his one desire was to impart to us as much of the knowledge he possessed as our young heads could hold. Repetition did not blunt the novelty nor time lessen the attraction of his theme. It always seemed as if he were telling us for the first time the new story of the beneficent work that surgery could do for the injured and the suffering. His whole heart was in his work. Especially did he inculcate the principles of surgery, for he was convinced, and rightly, that one who was thoroughly imbued with these could not go far wrong in his practice." The best evidence perhaps of the importance of his work as a teacher is the large number of his pupils and assistants who have attained eminence as surgeons and teachers of surgery in America. Among these should first be mentioned his own son, Samuel W. Gross, a surgeon of great ability and promise who died when he had hardly entered upon his career; Dr. T. G. Richardson, a pupil of Gross's at Louisville became Professor of Anatomy and later of Surgery in the University of Louisiana, New Orleans; David W. Yandell, also a pupil at Louisville, later occupied the chair of Surgery in the University of Louisville; Hunter McGuire, who left Jefferson College with several associates to join the Confederate Army at the outbreak of the Civil War, later became Professor of Surgery at Richmond, Va.; Clayton Parkhill was Professor of Surgery at Denver, Colorado; Phineas S. Connor occupies the chair of Surgery in the Medical College of Ohio at Cincinnati; Dr. W. L. Rodman, formerly a professor at Louisville, Ky., now holds the chair of Surgery in the Medico-Chirurgical College, Philadelphia; Drs. J. Chalmers Da Costa and W. Joseph Hearn are Clinical Professors in the Jefferson Medical College and Gross's eminent pupil Dr. William Williams Keen is his successor in the chair of Surgery at the Jefferson Medical College.

The urn in Woodland's cemetery, Philadelphia, in which Gross's ashes were placed after his cremation, bears this fitting inscription by Yandell:

IN MEMORIAM.

WITHIN THIS URN LIE THE ASHES OF

SAMUEL D. GROSS.

A MASTER IN SURGERY.

His life, which neared the extreme limits of the Psalmist, was one unbroken process of laborious years. He filled chairs in four medical colleges, in as many States of the Union, and added luster to them all. He recast Surgical Science, as taught in North America, formulated anew its principles, enlarged its domain, added to its art, and imparted fresh impetus to its study. He composed many books and among them

A SYSTEM OF SURGERY,

which is read in different tongues, wherever the Healing Art is practiced.

With a great intellect, carefully trained and balanced, he aimed with undivided zeal at the noble end of lessening human suffering and lengthening human life, and so rose to the highest position yet attained in science by any of his countrymen.

Resolute in truth, he had no fear; he was born tolerant and charitable.

Living in enlightened fellowship with all laborers in the world of Science, he was greatly honored by the learned in foreign lands, and deeply loved at home.

BEHIND THE VEIL OF THIS LIFE THERE IS A MYSTERY WHICH

HE PENETRATED ON THE

SIXTH DAY OF MAY, 1884.

HIS MEMORY

Shall exhort and his Example shall encourage and persuade those who come after him to emulate deeds, which great in themselves, were all crowned by the milk-white flower of

A STAINLESS LIFE.

It seems a pity to spoil such a climax but there are still a few points to which I venture to call your attention with regard to the lives of these men. You have already noticed a number of points of resemblance; a few moments further consideration will possibly serve to emphasize them: Both were for several years teachers of the fundamental branches of medicine; physiology and pathology in one case and anatomy and pathology in the other; both were teachers of surgery in two important medical schools of their respective countries; both were medical editors for many years, founders of national surgical societies, and the first real surgical leaders of their respective countries. Both had passed through the preliminary training which influences so greatly the character of every man's work and were well established in their profession before the introduction of anesthesia; hence they acquired the quick eye, ready judgment and rapid execution so essential to those days when every stroke of the knife meant agonizing suffering, "At that time a surgical procedure was a personal feat; the surgeon matched his courage, energy, and dexterity in an event. It was largely an attempt of the amphitheater in the mind of the surgeon, even if the spectators were few." Only the very rapid operator could hope to succeed. Now surgery has developed into a science, careful, painstaking, often wearisome to the spectators, rarely spectacular, as beneficial as it is laborious. Probably neither ever at all fully appreciated the significance of modern antisepsis in surgery nor practiced it, hence a great part of the most important modern surgery was entirely unknown to them. But Langenbeck by his resections, and Gross by advocacy of extensive excisions of malignant growths and removal of the lymphatic glands in carcinoma and his studies in intestinal surgery, laid the foundations on which are established much of our modern surgery of bones and joints, malignant disease and abdominal surgery. They were both students of surgery who not only mastered the principles and methods then approved but who took pains to keep informed of the advance of knowledge by closely following the surgical literature of all progressive nations: Langenbeck's biographers specially mention the important influence of English surgeons on his work and Gross frequently acknowledges his indebtedness to French and German surgeons. Not only did they profit by the work of others but as medical editors, writers, and founders of journals and societies they greatly aided the spread of knowledge and brought prominently before the world their own work and that of their countrymen.

Perhaps Langenbeck and Gross were at their best as teachers; they both possessed the rare gift of simplifying, systematizing, and imparting knowledge; more important than this they filled their students with enthusiasm for work, they inspired men so that their pupils and their pupils' pupils occupy the chairs of surgery in a large number of the leading medical schools of to-day.

Their assistants were chosen and retained not because of influence, wealth or whim, but because of recognized ability and industry. Few of them have failed to find honored positions in which they have spread the fame of their masters. Up to the time of Gross in America and Langenbeck in Germany the surgery of these countries was entirely patterned after and subordinate to the surgery of England and France. We often forget that Germany is much younger as a nation and little older as a scientific people than we in America. Until these men had established their reputations neither country had produced a surgeon whose name and achievements were known in all lands where scientific surgery was practiced nor whose teachings were widely followed, even by his own countrymen.

Both had such a grasp of every detail of their professional work; such an appreciation of the fundamental biological branches and their bearing on clinical practice; such discriminations as to the relative importance of acquiring, applying, and imparting knowledge; such sympathy and desire to help their students, assistants, fellow practitioners and their patients; such personal magnetism and force of character that they became acknowledged leaders in surgery, masters whose teachings still live, even though their names and the significance of their work are sometimes forgotten.

NOTE.—I am chiefly indebted for facts with regard to the lives of these masters in surgery and estimates of the importance of their work to the following sources: Obituaries of Langenbeck by Küster, Bergmann, Guttmann, Gurlt, Sonnenburg, and Billroth in the Berliner klinische Wochenschrift; Deutsche medicinische Wochenschrift; Münchener medicinische Wochenschrift; and Wiener klinische Wochenschrift, of 1887; to v. Bergmann's "Zur Erinnerung an B. v. Langenbeck," and to frequent references to Langenbeck and his work in the lectures of Bergmann and König while a student at Berlin; Gross's Autobiography; Keen's address at the unveiling of the Gross monument in Washington; Appreciations of Gross by Flint, Yandell, and others in the Journal of the American Medical Sciences; and to personal letters from Drs. Keen, Conners, Nancrede, and Rodman.

LINES READ AT A DINNER GIVEN IN HONOR OF DR. ROBERT FLETCHER, JANUARY 11, 1906, UPON HIS EIGHTY-THIRD BIRTHDAY.

If age means but the sum of leaves
   Time's calendars unfold,
Our honored guest must recognize
   That he is rather old.

If youth means elasticity,
   A ready wit and tongue,
A mind alert, a spirit gay,
   He's eminently young.

If age means stores of learning ranged
   On ordered shelves along,
Still crescent 'neath the nurture of
   A guardian sage and strong,

All centered in an index which
   Is hidden in the brain,
Our friend has surely reached an age
   We may not see again.

If youth betrays itself by vim,
   And broken bones, soon healed,
A constant tendency to pry
   In every secret field;

By always leading in the van
   Of life's long search for truth—
Why then, despite his years, he's but
   The prototype of youth!

So here's a glass to four-score years,
   To ripe and wise old age,
To all the gains which gen'rous time
   Scores on his record page;

And here's a glass to fervid youth,
   To supple limbs and mind
Wherein hope's rainbow arches o'er
   All doubts that low'r behind;

And here's a health to him in whom
   All these conditions meet,
Old in all virtues born of days,
   Young where'er youth is sweet.

Long may he live to taste alike
   Of age and youth the joys;
Old, yes, in years, but in his heart
   A boy among the boys!

          WILLIAM S. THAYER.

INDEX TO VOLUMES 1-16 OF BULLETIN.

A subject and author index of the first sixteen volumes of the Johns Hopkins Hospital Bulletin is now ready. As the edition will be limited, it is desirable that orders be sent in as promptly as possible.

Price bound in cloth is fifty cents.

Orders should be addressed to the Johns Hopkins Press, Baltimore, Md.

PROCEEDINGS OF SOCIETIES.

THE LAENNEC SOCIETY.

November 23, 1905.

Dr. H. B. Jacobs, President.   Dr. H. W. Buckler, Secretary.

Tuberculosis a Social Disease. Dr. S. A. Knopf, of New York.

The social causes of tuberculosis in infancy may be acquired, or direct and predisposing. Cases of acquired tuberculosis, and by this is meant post-natal cases, for there are only about forty hereditary cases on record, may be the result of mothers infecting children by carrying them in their arms and coughing over them, and by using the same spoon to taste the child's foods. As the child grows older and crawls it may become tuberculous, whether the mother is or not, because the father may have spit on the floor and the child may inhale bacilli or put its fingers into sputum and into its mouth, or its nails may not be kept clean. Foundling hospitals and nurseries often cause a spreading of infection by keeping all kinds of children together. Among the predisposing causes we find a physiological poverty transmitted from parents to children, which is not confined to tuberculous parents alone. Tuberculous persons should be prevented from marrying. Statistics covering a large number of cases of tuberculosis in which the history of the parents has been gotten, show very frequently that the patient was the seventh or eighth child of poor parents and that from age the parents were not able to transmit much vitality to their children, or owing to poverty were unable to care properly for so many children. We should believe in quality rather than numbers in offspring. Raising children on a bottle is a very frequent predisposing cause of tuberculosis. We should feel keenly on this subject, for when the mothers of one generation fail to nurse their children, the next generation has more difficulty. The majority of mothers can nurse their children, at least in part, and the female child will receive from such a mother the ability to nurse her child in turn. Although there may be some discussion as regards transmission to man of bovine tuberculosis, it is not safe to give milk to a child unless the cow has been found non-tuberculous.

A society in Paris has for its object the taking of children from tuberculous parents and placing them in homes and sanatoria for the sole purpose of preventing these children from contracting the disease while young. To prevent social and post-natal infections we need an education of the future mothers and an education for the school life of the children. A predisposing cause in school children is the overtaxing of their minds to the detriment of their physical beings. They are taught too much of the sciences and not enough of their own well being. Among the predisposing causes of tuberculosis in the college student, must be mentioned overdoing athletics. Statistics have shown that when the college athletes contract tuberculosis they go down twice as fast as others who had never heard of athletics. In the tenement districts little children go to school, often to stay all day, having for lunch only an apple or a couple of crackers. In Berlin a movement has been started to give each such little underfed child two sandwiches and a glass of milk for lunch, and all have increased in weight and done better school work. These results open a great field for philanthropy. Child labor is a great predisposing cause. Many poor girls and boys, while growing, and when they need all the fresh air and play they can get, are forced to remain indoors, and often in sweat-shops, from twelve to sixteen hours a day. It is a disgrace to the American people that some of the States permit this. Alcoholism among child-laborers is also a great factor in producing disease, for if children begin to take alcohol as a stimulant, not having the moral fiber to resist, they soon take it to excess.

Among the predisposing causes of tuberculosis in adult life are tenements, workshops, and alcoholism, under the last of which must be mentioned the use of patent medicines, for by their use a vast amount of alcohol is consumed. Over two hundred million dollars are spent annually for patent medicines, and the percentage of alcohol in a few of them may be seen in the following list: Green's Nervura 17 per cent; Hood's Sarsaparilla 18.5 per cent; Hoffman's Sulphur Bitters, 20.5 per cent; Lydia Pinkham's Vegetable Compound, 20.5 per cent; Paine's Celery Compound, 21.5 per cent; Ayer's Sarsaparilla, 25.6 per cent; Peruna, 28.5 per cent; Warner's Safe Tonic, 35 per cent.

Among the social causes of tuberculosis in adults is a lack of sanatoria for the treatment of tuberculous patients. We have no specific; but good food, fresh air, and plenty of water inside and out constitute the modern hygienic treatment. Sanatoria are necessities for consumptives among the poor and middle classes. We must aim to isolate the poor consumptives who are a menace to their fellow-men. We must have better medical attention. We must begin at the bottom of the problem, dealing first with the laboring classes, trying to provide better homes and places for Sunday recreation. We must make provision for the starving little ones. We make an appeal to the philanthropists who build churches, cathedrals, and libraries, to build model tenements where the laboring man can be happier, can frequent saloons less, and can sow less tuberculosis, for the man who serves his Creator in improving the conditions of his fellow-man serves his Creator best.

The Relation of the State to the Tuberculosis Question. Dr. J. P. C. Foster, of New Haven.

Dr. Foster advocated the inspection of milk and intelligent legislation to secure the production of milk under sanitary rules. Every farmer selling milk should have his premises inspected and should be licensed. The construction of tenement houses should also be regulated. The registration of tubercular cases should be enforced by the State for the protection of the well, and the better care of the sick who need help. Spitting in public places should be prohibited by law and the law should be enforced. The State cannot make provision for the care of all tubercular patients. They are too numerous. Each community through local, non-political boards should establish camps and shacks for the care of its own patients under the general supervision of State boards of inspection. The cost of constructing camps, shacks, and sanatoria should be reduced to a minimum and the money thus saved should be expended for nursing and competent medical care. The State, however, should share in this work by assisting local sanatoria intended for acute or incipient cases among the poor. Such local sanatoria should each represent a community of 250,000 persons and the State should aid them in a systematic manner. (The paper of Dr. Foster is published in full in the January BULLETIN.)

DISCUSSION.

DR. JOHN S. FULTON said: Not many years ago we were at the beginning of this work and the few hygienists who were interested made the mistake of applying procedures used in a different class of infectious diseases. In Maryland among measures to promote general prophylaxis are food inspection, inspection of milk supply, factory and child-labor inspection. There is also a State law against spitting but it mentions nothing about tuberculosis. As a special prophylaxis there is registration of tuberculous patients which has for its object a different purpose than the registration of acute infections. Many of the difficulties encountered elsewhere have not been met here. The registration began on the 27th of last April and during the first year cases have been satisfactorily registered. The registration in this State is guarded against public inspection. As a measure of domestic prophylaxis the consumptive must be reached at his home as soon as possible. This is done through the physicians who give advice and distribute sputum cups. The State pays a dollar and a half for each name turned in. Disinfection in Maryland is done by local boards of health, the law being mandatory. It is done with consent of the public or, if necessary, without it. The physician can do much by preparing the minds of the family to consent to disinfection after the patient's removal or death. About half the cases of tuberculosis in the State are not under medical observation.

DR. OWENSBY of the Bay View Asylum spoke upon the frequency of pulmonary tuberculosis in the insane. At Bay View it is five times more frequent than among the sane. Of 387 deaths at Bay View Asylum during the last eight years 75 were due to tuberculosis; 56 per cent of these were blacks and 44 per cent whites; 31 per cent of the patients gave tuberculosis as a cause of death in either parents, brothers, or sisters.

THE JOHNS HOPKINS HOSPITAL MEDICAL SOCIETY.

December 4, 1905.

DR. W. G. MacCallum, President.   DR. C. H. Bunting, Secretary.

Calcification of the Breast. DR. THAYER.

Dr. Thayer presented a colored girl, aged 16, who was admitted to the hospital on October 2, complaining of an illness which began eight days before with a chill, followed by pains in the bones, anorexia, diarrhœa, and occasional vomiting. Examination justified the diagnosis of typhoid fever. There was an absence of leucocytosis and a positive Widal reaction. The patient soon became very ill, the pulse rapid and slightly irregular, the blood pressure (maximum) between 80 and 90. On the 19th day of her disease there were several profuse hæmorrhages from the bowels. The condition of the patient was bad, the pulse at one time being as rapid as 164. ℞ Calcii lactatis 2. every four hours. At 11 a. m. an infusion with 500 cc. of a 1 per cent solution of calcium chloride was given under the left breast; the breast tissue was not punctured. The coagulation time of the blood on the following day was eleven minutes. There were several subsequent small hæmorrhages but the patient gradually improved. The administration of the lactate of calcium was continued for eleven days. On the 35th day of the disease the left breast was found to be the seat of a large fluctuating abscess which ruptured during examination. This was freely opened, a large quantity of thin brown pus with several large sloughs escaping. Cultures from the pus showed staphylococcus aureus and bacillus typhosus. Eleven days later it was noticed that the edges of the wound, especially about that side invading the breast tissue showed a bony hardness. This sclerotic rim extended back at least 4 om. from the opening of the wound. The pale granulation tissue contained numerous white spots and streaks which, when touched with the probe, felt like stone. These areas resembled closely the deposits of guanin in old ham. The probe introduced into the wound revealed the same sort of tissue wherever it could be passed.

Microscopical examination showed a granulation tissue with a fibrous basis containing many polymorphonuclear leucocytes, the lymphoid cells predominating. There were some epithelloid cells—a few giant cells—no tubercles. Areas of calcification were seen. No tubercle bacilli were found and there was no evidence of tuberculosis elsewhere. Examination of the calcified material showed that it consisted of phosphate of lime in some organic compound.

In addition to the calcification in the granulation tissue, there was a chain of hard nodules in the outer and upper part of the breast and a few small discrete nodules in the breast above the wound. There were a few enlarged glands in the left axilla which, however, were not strikingly hard. The calcium deposits had clearly diminished in size.

The condition appeared to be unique. The deposition of calcium in old tuberculous areas, in gummata, in atheromatous patches in arteries, in necrotic areas in general, and especially in areas of fat necrosis, is familiar. The so-called metastatic deposition of calcium in diseases of bone is well known. Kaufmann has described a case of osteo-porosis in which there was a calcified infarct as large as a child's hand. Animals in which the calcium content of the blood is normally high, such as rabbits, have a peculiar tendency to deposits of lime salts. Litten has shown that if the circulation in a renal artery of a rabbit be cut off for from one to four hours, extensive deposits of calcium may be found in that part of the kidney supplied by the occluded vessel. Certain poisons have been shown to favor the deposition of lime salts in the kidneys and in the liver. Especially notable are the salts of the heavier metals, lead, bismuth, and mercury, of the metalloids, iodine, of organic compounds, aloin and iodoform. These poisons probably produce degenerative changes in the cells of the kidneys and liver which are followed by the deposition of calcium; but not all poisons which produce necrotic changes predispose to these deposits. v. Kossa has shown that in animals in which the calcium content of the blood is artificially increased, calcification of the kidneys and liver may be induced by the administration of much smaller quantities of the predisposing poisons. Thus, in rabbits to which calcium chloride has been administered subcutaneously, relatively small doses of iodoform result in deposits of lime salts in the kidneys.

It is extremely interesting to note analogy between these experiments of v. Kossa and the condition which exists in this case. The patient had received 132 grammes of calcium lactate by the mouth during eleven days, in addition to 5 grammes of calcium chloride by subcutaneous infusion. A large abscess of bacterial origin developed during the time that the patient was receiving the calcium lactate. The cavity with its necrotic borders was packed with iodoform gauze, and iodoform is known to be a poison the absorption of which in animals favors the deposition of calcium. Wherever the gauze touched the wound there was a rim of calcium deposit. An attempt will be made to reproduce the condition experimentally in animals.

Yellow Fever. Remarks on the recent epidemic in New Orleans. DR. F. H. WATSON.

When yellow fever was discovered to be epidemic in New Orleans last summer it bid fair to outstrip the epidemic of 1878. For some time, with the histories of the past epidemies fresh in their minds and a realization of the paralysis of business and municipal demoralization that the known presence of yellow fever would cause, physicians have hesitated to diagnose and to report cases. Since 1897 there has been more or less yellow fever in New Orleans. The weather conditions of the past summer were most favorable. The first cases were reported on July 21. The city Board of Health immediately took hold and tried to cope with the epidemic until August 9, when, in response to a call, the United State Marine Hospital and Public Health Service sent assistance under the direction of Dr. J. H. White. The city was immediately divided into sections, the ward sec-

tions being under supervision and reporting to ward headquarters and these to central headquarters. The work consisted of: first, an educational campaign to convert the people to the mosquito theory; second, anti-mosquito measures for the destruction of breeding places. The *Stegomyia fasciata* breeds mostly in clear water, so all the cisterns and water barrels were oiled with a high-grade oil, as many of these were used to hold drinking water. All water-containing vessels were covered with netting or cotton sheeting. Stagnant pools were oiled, salted or filled in. Regular hours for fumigation were established, e. g., Sunday at 10 a. m., when with the sulphur furnished by the city, the buildings were fumigated. Next came a campaign against the spread of infection. All cases were isolated by covering the bed with netting and closing the room with netting. A preliminary fumigation was done, and, on or before the tenth day, the entire house and outhouses were fumigated. No methods other than those against the mosquito were used at any time. Every house was visited by the United States Marine Hospital authorities at least three times a week. When the fever was reported last July there were two hundred cases in the city, which is a greater start than the epidemic of 1878 had, in which later in the epidemic there were three hundred new cases a day. All former epidemics have died out with the approach of cold weather.

Practical points brought out by the epidemic:

The cistern should be absolutely mosquito-tight, and water barrels, troughs, etc., should be oiled or emptied daily. To prevent secondary cases seal the room to keep infected mosquitoes from escaping. Sulphur is the best insecticide, but it tarnishes brass and is injurious to pianos. Pyrethrum powder was used somewhat, but it does not kill, only stuns, and the mosquitoes have to be swept up and burned. If there are cases in a block the whole block should be fumigated. Yellow fever is a house infection, for Stegomyia is a house mosquito, going out only for water. It is not likely that it will fly as far as across the street, so one has practically only the infected house to deal with, unless there are other houses very close. Yellow fever does not necessarily mean black vomit, suppression of urine and death. There may be cases so mild as to last only twelve hours. The mild cases are very dangerous, for not being recognized or considered they are important in spreading the disease. Diagnosis is not positive until the fourth or fifth day, so all fevers should be reported immediately and the family physician held responsible. Thorough screening and fumigation prevent secondary infections. The concealed cases are the most difficult to deal with. These and the mild unrecognized cases go hand in hand, and the fight is successful only when both of these are cared for.

Studies from the Craig Colony for Epileptics with Biograph Illustrations. DR. W. G. CHASE, of Boston.

Dr. Chase gave a very interesting short talk on the development of photography from the wet-plate days of thirty-five years ago to the complex films and cameras used in the biograph of to-day. He spoke of the advantage of the biograph both in studying and in teaching medicine, and illustrated his remarks by throwing on a screen from fifteen hundred feet of films, pictures showing in characteristic movements and attitudes, in attacks, and characteristic gaits, cases of rhythmic idiocy, double nystagmus, grand mal, Jacksonian epilepsy, status epilepticus, athetosis, hemiplegias, etc. The pictures were very clear and showed patients in attitudes and movements that the average practitioner seldom sees.

Particularly interesting were the pictures showing complete attacks of epilepsy, those showing the sleeping positions of epileptics and the swaying movements of rhythmic idiots. The value of the biograph in clinical teaching was particularly emphasized, for these pictures could be thrown upon the screen to illustrate cases and for comparison at any time, whereas in most clinics such cases are not always available for exhibition and seldom for comparison.

SUMMARIES OR TITLES OF PAPERS BY MEMBERS OF THE HOSPITAL OR MEDICAL SCHOOL STAFF APPEARING ELSEWHERE THAN IN THE BULLETIN.

JOHN J. ABEL, and R. DE M. TAVEAU. On the Decomposition Products of Epinephrin Hydrate.—*Journal of Biological Chemistry*, October, 1905.

JOHN AUER, M. D., and S. J. MELTZER, M. D. On the rate of Absorption from Intramuscular Tissue.—*Journal of Experimental Medicine*, Vol. 7, No. 1, 1905.

WILLIAM S. BAER, M. D. District Nursing for Orthopedic Clinics.—*The Charities Record*, Vol. VI, No. 7.

CHARLES RUSSELL BARDEEN, M. D. The Development of the Thoracic Vertebræ in Man.—*American Journal of Anatomy*, Vol. 4, No. 2, 1905.

——— Recent Progress in Anatomy.—*Wisconsin Medical Journal*, April, 1905.

——— The State Society, the State University, and State Medicine.—*Wisconsin Medical Journal*, June, 1905.

LEWELLYS F. BARKER, M. D. Travel Notes.—*Journal of the American Medical Association*, September 3, 17, and 24, 1904; February 11, 18, and 25, 1905.

——— European and American Science.—*Science*, September 8, 1905.

———Methods in Medicine.—*Boston Medical and Surgical Journal*, September 21, 1905; also Medical Communications from the Massachusetts Medical Society, Vol. 20, No. 1, 1905.

E. BATES BLOCK, M. D. Albuminuria and Bright's Disease. Transactions of the Medical Associations of Georgia for 1905.

JOSEPH C. BLOODGOOD, M. D. Cysts of the Thyroid Gland.—*Surgery, Gynecology and Obstetrics*, August, 1905.

——— Review of Surgery.—*International Clinics*, Vol. I, 1905.

——— Anesthetics; Fractures; Dislocations; Amputations, Surgery of the Extremities and Orthopedics.—*Progressive Medicine*, December, 1905.

GEORGE BLUMER, M. D. A Case of Aleukaemic Lymphatic Leukaemia (Leukoblastoma) simulating acute Hodgkin's Disease.—*Albany Medical Annals*, April, 1905.

——— The Influence which the Acquisition of Tropical Territory by the United States has had, and is likely to have, on American Medicine. (Oration on State Medicine, Fifty-sixth Session of the American Medical Association.)—*Journal of the American Medical Association*, July 15, 1905; also *Texas Medical News*, September, 1905.

THOMAS R. BOGGS, M. D. The Influenza Bacillus in Bronchiectasis.—*American Journal of the Medical Sciences*, November, 1905.

JOHN B. BRIGGS, M. D. A recent Epidemic of Typhoid Fever.—*Medical Record*, January 7, 1905.

——— Certain Hypertensive Crises in Arteriosclerotic Subjects.—*American Journal of the Medical Sciences*, August, 1905.

THOMAS R. BROWN, M. D. Review in Medicine.—*Maryland Medical Journal*, January, March, April, August, September, December, 1905.

——— Dr. Osler as a Teacher.—*Maryland Medical Journal*, June, 1905.

——— Examination of the Leucocytes as an Aid to the Diagnosis and Prognosis of Disease.—*American Medicine*, November 4, 1905.

CLINTON E. BRUSH, M. D. Blood-Pressure Observations for the Practising Physician.—*American Medicine*, July 15, 1905.

WILLIAM J. CALVERT, M. D. Abdominal Systolic Murmur. —*Interstate Medical Journal*, Vol. XII, No. 6, June, 1905.

——— Diminutive Spleen.—*American Journal of the Medical Sciences*, Vol. CXXX, No. 2, August, 1905.

——— Cause of Pulsation in Empyema.—*American Journal of the Medical Sciences*, Vol. CXXX, November, 1905.

——— Blood Vessels of the Lymphatic Gland.—*Interstate Medical Journal*, Vol. 12, November, 1905.

C. N. B. CAMAC, M. D. Some Observations on Aneurysm and Arteriosclerosis.—The Mutter Lecture delivered before the College of Physicians, Philadelphia.

——— Laennec and his Stethoscope.—*Medical News*, May 20, 1905.

——— Medicine at Oxford.—*Medical Notes and Queries*, November, 1905.

THOMAS W. CLARKE, M. D., and EDWARD F. CUSHING, M. D., Copious Water-drinking and Polyuria in Typhoid Fever. —*American Journal of the Medical Sciences*, February, 1905.

—— and DAVID H. DOLLEY, M. D. A Case of Congenital Hepatoptosis, showing a Mesohepar.—*American Journal of the Medical Sciences*, December, 1905.

J. W. CHURCHMAN, M. D. Paraurethritis. An Anatomic Review, with report of two Cases.—*Journal of the American Medical Association*, January 14, 1905.

HENRY W. COOK, M. D. The Early Recognition of Hypertension.—*American Medicine*, January 14, 1905.

—— Chronic Arterial Hypertension.—*Journal of the American Medical Association*, January 28, 1905; also *Virginia Medical Semi-Monthly*, January 27, 1905.

THOMAS S. CULLEN, M. B. Cysts of Bartholin's Glands, with Brief Remarks on the Anatomy of the Normal Gland Structure.—*Journal of the American Medical Association*, January 21, 1905.

—— Large Carcinomatous Tumor of the Liver. Removal Seventeen Months after Nephrectomy for Carcinoma of the Left Kidney. Temporary Recovery.—*Journal of the American Medical Association*, April 22, 1905.

—— Uterine Elevator Forceps.—*Journal of the American Medical Association*. April 29, 1905.

HARVEY CUSHING, M. D. The Special Field of Neurological Surgery. *Surgery, Gynecology and Obstetrics*, October, 1905.

—— The Surgical Aspects of Major Neuralgia of the Trigeminal Nerve.—*Journal of the American Medical Association*, March 11, 18, and 25; April 1 and 8, 1905.

—— The Establishment of Cerebral Hernia as a Decompressive Measure for Inaccessible Brain Tumors; with the Description of Intermuscular Methods of Making the Bone Defect in Temporal and Occipital Regions.— *Surgery, Gynecology and Obstetrics*, October, 1905.

—— Concerning Surgical Intervention for the Intracranial Hemorrhages of the New-born.—*American Journal of the Medical Sciences*, October, 1905.

—— On Preservation of the Nerve Supply to the Brow in the Operative Approach to the Gasserian Ganglion.— *Annals of Surgery*, November, 1905.

—— Arterio-Venous Aneurism of the Occipital Vessels.— *New York Medical Journal*, November, 1905.

PERCY M. DAWSON, M. D. The Change in the Heart Rate and Blood " Pressures " Resulting from Severe Hæmorrhage and Subsequent Infusion of Sodium Bicarbonate. —*Journal of Experimental Medicine*, Vol. VII, No. 1, 1905.

WILLIAM RUSH DUNTON, JR., M. D. The Pathology of Epilepsy.—*Maryland Medical Journal*, February, 1905.

—— Note on the Mechanical Irritability of the Facial Nerve in Dementia Præcox.—*American Medicine*, July, 15, 1905.

ARTHUR W. ELTING, M. D. The Surgical Treatment of Tumors of the Brain.—*Albany Medical Annals*, February, 1905.

—— and HENRY L. K. SHAW, M. D. Pyloric Stenosis in Infancy.—*Albany Medical Annals*, January, 1905.

JOSEPH ERLANGER, M. D. A New Instrument for Determining the Minimum and Maximum Blood-Pressures in Man.—*The Johns Hopkins Hospital Reports*, Vol. XII, p. 53.

—— On the Union of a Spinal Nerve with the Vagus Nerve.—*American Journal of Physiology*, Vol. XIII, p. 372.

—— Vorläufige Mitteilung über die Physiologie des Herzblocks in Säugetieren.—*Centralblatt f. Physiologie*, Vol. XIX, p. 4, 1905.

—— On the Physiology of Heart-block in Mammals with Especial Reference to the Causation of Stokes-Adams Disease. Part I.—*Journal of Experimental Medicine*, November, 1905.

—— and A. D. HIRSCHFELDER, M. D. Vorläufige Mitteilung in Bezug auf weiteren Studien über die Physiologie des Herzblocks in Säugetieren.—*Centralblatt f. Physiologie*, Vol. XIX, 1905.

—— and D. R. HOOKER. An Experimental Study of Blood-Pressure and Pulse-Pressure in Man.—*The Johns Hopkins Hospital Reports*, Vol. XII, p. 145.

ROADES FAYERWEATHER, M. D. Infectious Arthritis.— *American Journal of the Medical Sciences*, December, 1905.

SIMON FLEXNER, M. D. The Etiology of Syphilis. Wesley Carpenter Lecture of the New York Academy of Medicine.—*Medical News*, December 9, 1905.

—— The Constituent of the Bile causing Pancreatitis. —*Transactions of the Association of American Physicians*, 1905.

—— The Action of the Colon-Typhoid-Dysentery Group of Bacilli upon Arabinose, Dulcit and Iso-dulcit.—*Journal of Experimental Medicine*.

—— and HIDEYO NOGUCHI. On the Occurrence of Spirochæta Pallida.—*Medical News*, June 17, 1905.

JOSEPH M. FLINT, M. D. The Framework of the Glandula Parathyroidea.—*American Journal of Anatomy*, Vol. 4, No. 1, 1904.

W. W. FORD, M. D. The Carbohydrate Reactions of the Paratyphoid or Paracolon Group (Preliminary Communication).—*Medical News*, June 17, 1905.

—— Antitoxin for Poisonous Mushroom Intoxication (Preliminary Communication).—*Medical News*, October 21, 1905.

HARRY A. FOWLER, M. D. Nephritis and Hæmaturia.—*New York Medical Journal*, December 2, 1905.

THOMAS B. FUTCHER, M. B. An account of the Dancing Mania of Europe and of Epidemic Convulsions in Kentucky.—*Old Maryland*, March, 1905.

THOMAS B. FUTCHER, M. B. A Clinical Report of Nine Cases of Diabetes Insipidus.—*Cleveland Medical Journal*, March and April, 1905.

—— On the Relations of some of the Metabolic Diseases to Intestinal Disorders.—*Medical News*, July 22, 1905.

—— Xanthelasma and Chronic Jaundice.—*American Journal of the Medical Sciences*, December, 1905.

NORMAN B. GWYN, M. D. Typhoid Fever. Accidental Infection with Bacillus Aerogenes Capsulatus or Bacillus of Malignant Oedema.—Proceedings of the Philadelphia County Medical Society, June-September, 1905.

—— and NORMAN MacL. HARRIS, M. D. A Comparison Between Results of Blood Cultures taken During Life and After Death.—*Journal of Infectious Diseases*, June 24, 1905.

WILLIAM S. HALSTED, M. D. Results of the Open-Air Treatment of Surgical Tuberculosis.—*American Medicine*, December 2, 1905.

NORMAN MacL. HARRIS, M. B. Bacillus Mortiferus (Nov. Spec.).—*Journal of Experimental Medicine*, Vol. 6, Nos. 4, 5, 6, 1905.

—— The Construction of the Thermostat-Room.—*Journal of Experimental Medicine*, Vol. 7, No. 3, 1905.

T. W. HASTINGS, M. D. A Method for Preparing a Permanent Nocht's Stain (Nocht-Jenner Stain).—*Journal of Experimental Medicine*, Vol. 7, No. 3, 1905.

AUGUST HOCH, M. D. A Review of Some Recent Papers Upon the Loss of the Feeling of Reality and Kindred Symptoms.—*Psychological Bulletin*, July 15, 1905.

GERRY R. HOLDEN, M. D. The Results of Ventral Suspension of the Uterus at the Johns Hopkins Hospital.—*American Journal of Obstetrics*, April, 1905.

—— Perineorrhaphy by Uniting the Borders of the Levator Ani Muscles.—*American Journal of Obstetrics*, October, 1905.

—— Dilation and Curettement for Dysmenorrhea. Report of 95 Cases.—*American Medicine*, November 4, 1905.

CAMPBELL P. HOWARD, M. D. Symptomatology and Diagnosis of Gastric Ulcer.—Proceedings of the Philadelphia County Medical Society, March 31, 1905.

GUY L. HUNNER, M. D. The Significance of the Urinary Examination in Women.—*American Medicine*, Vol. IX, 1905.

REID HUNT. The Influence of Thyroid Feeding upon Poisoning by Acetonitrile.—*Journal of Biological Chemistry*, October, 1905.

HOWARD A. KELLY, M. D. What is the Right Attitude of the Medical Profession Toward the Social Evil?—*Journal of the American Medical Association*, March 4, 1905.

—— The Treatment of Pyelitis.—*Medical Record*, April 8, 1905.

—— The Uterine Curette.—*American Journal of Obstetrics*, May, 1905.

HOWARD A. KELLY, M. D. Some Surgical Notes on Tuberculosis of the Kidney.—*British Medical Journal*, June 17, 1905; also *The Lancet*, June 17, 1905.

—— The Best Way to Treat the Social Evil.—*Medical News*, June 24, 1905.

—— The Treatment of Nonmalignant Strictures of the Rectum.—*American Medicine*, September 16, 1905.

—— Some Surgical Notes on Tuberculosis of the Kidney.—*Annals of Gynecology and Pediatry*, October, 1905.

HERBERT M. LITTLE, M. D. Der Bacillus Aerogenes Capsulatus im Puerperalfieber.—*Centralblatt f. Gynækologie*, No. VII, 1905.

—— The Bacteriology of the Puerperal Uterus.—*American Journal of Obstetrics*, December, 1905.

JOHN N. MACKENZIE, M. D. Remarks on Some Abuses in the Intranasal Surgery of To-day.—*New York Medical Journal*, January 28, 1905.

—— The Future of the Laryngoscope and the Study of Laryngology.—*Medical News*, July 22, 1905.

W. G. MacCALLUM, M. D. Die Beziehung der Parathyroiddrusen zu Tetanie.—*Centralblatt für Allgemeine Pathologie u. Pathologische Anatomie*, Band XVI, No. 1, May 31, 1905.

—— and C. F. DAVIDSON. Further Notes on the Function of the Parathyroid Glands.—*Medical News*, April 8, 1905.

J. W. MADISON, M. D. The Causes and Symptoms of Cardiac Insufficiency.—*Wisconsin Medical Journal*, October, 1905.

FRANKLIN P. MALL, M. D. On the Development of the Blood-Vessels of the Brain in the Human Embryo.—*American Journal of Anatomy*, Vol. 4, No. 1, 1904.

—— Wilhelm His. His Relation to Institutions of Learning.—*American Journal of Anatomy*, Vol. 4, No. 2, 1905.

HARRY T. MARSHALL, M. D. Studies in Hæmolysis with Special Reference to the Properties of the Blood and Body Fluids of Human Beings.—*Journal of Experimental Medicine*, Vol. 6, Nos. 4, 5, 6, 1905.

—— Therapeutic Value of Antitoxic Sera.—*New York State Journal of Medicine*, Vol. V, No. 8, August, 1905.

THOMAS McCRAE, M. D. Acute Lymphatic Leukæmia.—*British Medical Journal*, February 25, 1905.

G. BROWN MILLER, M. D. Post-Operative Complications Involving the Bronchi, Lungs, etc.—*American Journal of Obstetrics*, April, 1905.

GEORGE H. F. NUTTALL, M. D. An Address on Scientific Research in Medicine.—*British Medical Journal*, October 21, 1905; also *The Lancet*, October 21, 1905.

EUGENE L. OPIE, M. D. Enzymes and Anti-Enzymes of Inflammatory Exudates.—*Journal of Experimental Medicine*, Vol. 7, No. 3, 1905.

—— The Presence in the Bone-Marrow of Enzymes Resembling those of Leucocytes.—*Journal of Experimental Medicine*, Vol. 7, No. 6, 1905.

William Osler, M. D. Acute Tuberculous Pneumonia.—*Brooklyn Medical Journal*, February, 1905.

—— Valedictory Address at Johns Hopkins University.—*Journal of the American Medical Association*, March 4, 1905.

—— The Home in its Relation to the Tuberculosis Problem.—*Canada Lancet*, March, 1905.

—— Unity, Peace and Concord.—*Journal of the American Medical Association*, August 5, 1905.

—— The Student Life.—*Medical News*, September 30, 1905; also *St. Louis Medical Review*, September 30, 1905.

—— Aneurysm of the Abdominal Aorta.—*The Lancet*, October 14, 1905.

—— An Address on Sir Thomas Browne.—*British Medical Journal*, October 21, 1905.

Mary S. Packard, M. D. Two Cases of Chronic Anæmia with Splenic Enlargement.—*Providence Medical Journal*, January, 1905.

Charles D. Parfitt, M. D. The Selection of Cases for the Muskoka Free Hospital for Consumptives.—*Dominion Medical Monthly*, August, 1905.

Stewart Paton, M. D. The New Munich Clinic.—*Science*, September 8, 1905.

Clement A. Penrose, M. D. Sanitary Conditions in the Bahama Islands. Special Publication from The Bahama Islands, by Permission of the Geographical Society of Baltimore.—*The Macmillan Company.*

J. Hall Pleasants, M. D. Some Confusing Early Physical Signs of Pulmonary Tuberculosis.—*Journal of the Alumni Association of the College of Physicians and Surgeons*, January, 1905.

Jewett V. Reed, M. D. The Management of Prison Tuberculosis, with the Aid of Tuberculin, as a Diagnostic Agent.—*Journal of the American Medical Association*, February 4, 1905.

Robert Reuling, M. D. A Case of Sporadic Cerebro-spinal Meningitis with Pathological Studies of the Central Nervous System and Bacteriology.—*Maryland Medical Journal*, March, 1905.

Theodore F. Riggs, M. D. A Comparative Study of White and Negro Pelves, with a Consideration of the Size of the Child and its Relation to Presentation and Character of Labor in the two Races.—*The Johns Hopkins Hospital Reports*, Vol. XII, 1904.

—— Eine Vergleichende Studie ueber die Becken von Weissen und Negern.—*Centralblatt f. Gynaekologie*, Nr. 16, 1905.

Hunter Robb, M. D. The Early Diagnosis of Cancer of the Fundus, with Report of Cases.—*American Journal of Obstetrics*, Vol. LI, No. 1, 1905.

Hunter Robb, M. D. Inflammatory Conditions of the Appendix Accidentally Brought to Light in Pelvic Operations.—*American Journal of Obstetrics*, Vol. LII, No. 2, 1905.

Carey P. Rogers, M. D. The Need of Improved Surgical Facilities in Florida.—Transactions of the Florida Medical Association, 1905.

—— The Radical Treatment of Hemorrhoids.—*The Georgia Practician*, August, 1905.

John A. Sampson, M. D. Operations on the Lower Ends of the Ureters by the Inguinal Extraperitoneal Route under Local Anesthesia (Cocaine).—*Annals of Surgery*, February, 1905.

—— Cancer of the Uterine Cervix: Its Classification and Extension.—*Albany Medical Annals*, May, 1905.

—— The Importance of an Early Diagnosis in Cancer of the Uterus.—*Journal of the American Medical Association*, May 20, 1905.

Benjamin R. Schenck, M. D. Renal Hematuria of Unexplained Origin, Cessation after Nephrotomy.—*Journal of the Michigan State Medical Society*, January, 1905.

—— America's Part in the Progress of Surgery.—*Journal of the Michigan State Medical Society*, July, 1905.

Charles E. Simon, M. D. Ueber Futterungsversuche mit Monoæminosauren bei Cystinurie.—*Zeit. f. Physiol. Chem.*, Vol. 45, p. 357.

J. Morris Slemons, M. D. Metabolism during Pregnancy, Labor and the Puerperium.—*The Johns Hopkins Hospital Reports*, Vol. XII.

C. N. Spratt, M. D. The Use of Paraffin Spheres in Frost's Operation (Modified Mule's). With a Report of Twenty-three Cases.—*Archives of Ophthalmology*, Vol. XXXV, No. 2, 1905.

—— The Accurate Determination of Errors of Refraction, Without Cycloplegia, by means of Astigmatic Charts.—*St. Paul Medical Journal*, August, 1905.

Walter R. Steiner, M. D. Dermatomyositis, with Report of a Case which Presented a Rare Muscle Anomaly but once Described in Man.—*Journal of Experimental Medicine*, 1905, VI, pp. 407-442.

—— Two Medical Worthies Guilford Knew in Former Days.—Proceedings at Formal Opening of State Historical Museum, New Haven, 1905, pp. 37-42.

—— Some Remarks on Epidemic Cerebro-Spinal Meningitis.—The Second Annual Sanitary Conference of the Health Officials of Connecticut under the Auspices of the State Board of Health, New Haven, 1905, pp. 49-50.

Richard P. Strong, M. D. Some Questions Relating to the Virulence of Microorganisms with Particular Reference to their Immunizing Powers.—*Journal of Experimental Medicine*, Vol. 7, No. 3, 1905.

William S. Thayer, M. D. On Gonorrhœal Septicæmia and Endocarditis.—*American Journal of the Medical Sciences*, November, 1905.

WM. S. THAYER, M. D. On Some Public Duties of the Physician.—*Maryland Medical Journal*, November, 1905.

SAMUEL THEOBALD, M. D. The Genesis of Sympathetic Ophthalmitis.—*Journal of the American Medical Association*, January 28, 1905.

MARTIN B. TINKER, M. D. Bloodless Perineal Prostatectomy under Local Anesthesia.—*Journal of the American Medical Association*, February 11, 1905.

J. H. J. UPHAM, M. D. Recent Views on the Etiology of Diabetes.—*Columbus Medical Journal*, April, 1905.

—— Pernicious Anemia with Reports of Cases.—*Ohio State Medical Journal.*

ROY M. VAN WART, B. A., M. D. The Nervous Symptoms Accompanying Pernicious Anemia.—*Medical News*, January 14, 1905.

GEORGE WALKER, M. D. Transperitoneal Ligation of the Renal Vessels as a Preliminary to a Lumbar Nephrectomy in Tuberculosis or Malignant Growths of the Kidney.—*Journal of the American Medical Association*, November 25, 1905.

LOUIS M. WARFIELD, M. D. Erythema Multiforme Following Vaccination.—*Journal of the American Medical Association*, September 16, 1905.

LOUIS M. WARFIELD, M. D. Syphilis Hereditaria Tarda; Report of a Case.—*Archives of Pediatrics*, December, 1905.

STEPHEN WATTS, M. D. Loss of Entire Lower Lip.—*Annals of Surgery*, January, 1905.

F. H. WATSON, M. D., and others. A Preliminary Report on Cells Found in Yellow Fever Blood with Reference to their Etiologic and Diagnostic Significance.—*Journal of the American Medical Association*, September 23, 1905.

J. WHITRIDGE WILLIAMS, M. D. Contribution to the Origin of Adenomyoma of the Uterus.—*Annals of Gynecology and Pediatry*, January, 1905.

—— The Pernicious Vomiting of Pregnancy.—*Surgery, Gynecology and Obstetrics*, July, 1905; also *The Lancet*, October 21, 1905.

HUGH H. YOUNG, M. D. Conservative Perineal Prostatectomy.—*Annals of Surgery*, April, 1905; also *Journal of the American Medical Association*, February 4, 1905.

—— The Surgery of the Prostate.—*The Wisconsin Medical Journal*, November, 1905.

—— and J. W. CHURCHMAN, M. D. The Diagnosis of Urinary and Genital Tuberculosis.—*American Journal of the Medical Sciences*, July, 1905.

NOTES ON NEW BOOKS.

A Manual of Chemistry, Inorganic and Organic, for the Use of Students of Medicine. By A. P. LUFF, M. D., B. Sc. (Lond.), F. R. C. P., F. I. C., Physician to St. Mary's Hospital, and Lecturer on Medical Jurisprudence in the Medical School, and F. J. M. PAGE, B. Sc. (Lond.), F. I. C., Associate of the Royal School of Mines, Lecturer on Chemistry and Physics to the London Hospital Medical College, Examiner on Chemistry and Physics to the Society of Apothecaries, London, etc. Illustrated with 43 engravings. Third edition revised. 16 mo. 538 pages. (*Chicago: W. T. Keener & Co., 1905.*)

This book is intended as a guide to the study of chemical science for the use of students of medicine. The fundamental principles of chemistry are presented clearly and concisely, and the fact that a third edition was necessary, indicates that the book has found a field of usefulness. The first 332 pages are devoted to inorganic chemistry, while organic chemistry is presented in 154 pages. The difficult task of treating a subject of such magnitude in such a small compass has, as a whole, been accomplished successfully. We cannot here consider the individual chapters. It is evident that only little space can be devoted to physiological chemistry in a work of this kind. In the brief presentation of this part a few errors have crept in. Thus, in connection with the ferments we find preserved the old division into organized and non-organized ferments. Since it has been shown that the ferment activity of microorganisms is not dependent on their life processes this division has been abandoned. The general statement that putrefaction requires a certain amount of air to start the process is erroneous. These errors do not detract seriously from the value of the book since it does not pretend to treat fully of these subjects. The book can be recommended.   S. A.

Ophthalmic Neuro-Myology. A study of the normal and abnormal actions of the ocular muscles from the brain side of the question. By G. C. SAVAGE, M. D., Vanderbilt University. (*Nashville, Tenn.: Published by the Author.*)

This book serves to set forth the author's views regarding the influence of certain cerebral and basal centers which he has assumed exist, in the control of ocular movements. To quote from the preface, " The hypothesis on which Ophthalmic Neuro-Myology is founded may be stated as follows: There are eight conjugate brain centers in the cortex, by means of which the several versions are effected, and one conjugate center by which conveyance is caused. These conjugate centers act alike on orthophoric and heterophoric eyes, and when there is only one eye. Each of these is connected with two muscles, and the work done by the center and its muscles, under the guidance of volition is normal work. The conjugate centers have no causal relationship with the heterophoric conditions, nor have they any power for correcting them. There are twelve basal centers, each connected with only one muscle. If the eyes are emmetropic-orthophoric these centers are forever at rest, but when there is any form of heterophoria, one or more of these centers must be ever active during all working hours. These centers do not cause heterophoria but they stand ready to correct it. Under the guidance of the fusion faculty, each basal center stands ready to act on its muscle whenever there is a condition that would cause diplopia."

We cannot believe that there are basal centers which exist for the sole purpose of sending supplemental charges of what the author calls "neuricity" to weaker muscles when necessary. This would be at variance with established physiological facts, and we do not believe that nature has provided unique and special "safety-valves" to correct muscle errors in the eyes. Where the premises are hypothetical the conclusions must also be so, and the deductions made by the author are to say the least artificial and fanciful. The deductions are made at will by the author, but we do not believe that many of the ideas which he has arrived at will be established by facts, physiological, pathological, or otherwise. B. B. B., Jr.

An Introduction to Dermatology. By NORMAN WALKER, M. D. Third edition. (*Bristol: J. Wright & Co., 1905.*)

It is surprising how much has been comprehended within the 281 pages of this book.

There are about 100 illustrations. Of these the photographs are very much better than the colored plates, which are too highly colored and do not give a very good idea of the disease represented.

Classification of skin diseases is never easy, but the peculiarity of the author's arrangement can hardly be accounted for. There is no well-defined parasitic group and *pediculosis capitis* and *pediculosis pubis* are called infective inflammations, but *pediculosis corporis* is classed as an anomaly of circulation. The vegetable parasites are also grouped as infective inflammations, with the exception of *tinea versicolor* and *erythrasma*, for which a new class, saprophytes, is created.

There is more individuality shown in the contents than is usual in books of this class. The subject-matter is presented in an attractive way, and one does not tire easily in the reading.

The sections on treatment abound in excellent suggestions.

The book is well bound, the paper is good, and the type very clear.

Principles of Bacteriology. By A. C. ABBOTT, M. D. Seventh edition. (*Philadelphia and New York: Lea Brothers & Co., 1905.*)

Since the original appearance of Dr. Abbott's little book on the Principles of Bacteriology in 1891, so many advances have been made in our knowledge of this subject, that it requires considerable ingenuity in an author to include in one publication, the essential facts of the science. In the seventh edition Dr. Abbott has made a successful attempt to enlarge the scope of his previous editions, and he has, therefore, included a number of highly important advances in such subjects as the Morphological Classification of Bacteria, Bacteriological Technique, and Theories of Immunity. The present edition covers 700 pages and is a sensible, clear-sighted exposition of the subject. The chapter on Immunity is especially good from the historical standpoint and the author has not limited himself to any theory but gives in some detail the most important ideas which have been advanced to explain the complicated phenomena of serum-therapy. The names of the common species of microorganisms have been changed to conform to the accepted rules of botanical nomenclature, and some of the most recent investigations on species differentiation have been incorporated.

`As the book is now presented it is a valuable treatise not only for the beginner in bacteriology, for whom the first edition was intended, but also for the more advanced student of to-day who has ready access to well-equipped laboratories in almost any modern medical school.

It is unfortunate that Dr. Abbott has still adhered to the plan of the original edition in which somewhat simple directions were given the student for the performance of bacteriological experiments. Such directions now following such a philosophical exposition of immunity as Dr. Abbott has given are to say the least incongruous, and we venture the prediction that in the next edition Dr. Abbott will drop completely this heritage of the past. We would suggest also that the appendix containing a long list of useless laboratory supplies might well be left to the reader's

imagination. Could a few such drastic changes be made, the book would fulfill at once its present purpose, namely, to represent the entire subject of bacteriology in so clear, concise, and accurate a manner as to appeal to every student in our modern universities.

Practical Massage in Twenty Lessons. By HARTVIG NISSEN. (*Philadelphia: F. A. Davis & Co., 1905.*)

This book is a reprint of an earlier work of the author entitled, "Swedish Movement and Massage Treatment," published in 1889. Some small omissions are made, and about thirty or forty pages of new material, and twenty or more new diagrams and prints have been added throughout the text. The method of classification is also somewhat changed and improved.

But strictly speaking, the book should definitely be announced as an enlarged edition of an older publication. However unintentionally the impression is given, the book is practically offered as a new one, and the reader or student is not prepared to find that more than three-fourths of the two productions are word for word the same.

The title of the later book is hardly as accurate or comprehensive as the former one. In spite of a brief prefatory explanation as to the technical meaning of the term massage, the term will be misleading to the general mind, since the bulk of the book is given up to the consideration of physical exercises or medical gymnastics.

It is to be regretted too, that in revising the book, the author did not cite further and more recent illustrations of cases treated; those given being almost exclusively dated in the Eighties, that is, in the pioneer days of the Swedish Movement Treatment in America.

But although the book cannot be considered a new contribution, except in small degree as mentioned, it is a greatly improved edition of its former self, and taken as a whole, it is perhaps, a rather more concise and practical presentation of the general subject of mechano-therapy than has been made elsewhere.

The literary merit is not high. And the tone of the book in some minor respects lacks in dignity.

But it cannot be doubted that the author clearly knows whereof he writes from personal, practical experience, and this, which is the most important point of all, gives interest and weight to the questions treated in spite of the crudities of the book in general. H. C. BARTLETT.

Drink Restrictions (Thirst Cures) particularly in Obesity. By PROF. CARL VON NOORDEN and DR. HUGO SALOMON. Translated by BOARDMAN REED, M. D. (*New York: E. B. Treat & Co., 1905.*)

This monograph contains a very satisfactory historical review of all the conditions which have been treated by limiting the patient in his consumption of fluids and discusses the physiological changes which occur during periods of thirsting. The authors have studied especially the oxygen and nitrogen metabolism when the fluid intake is minimal and conclude that oxidation is not increased nor is the storage of nitrogen prevented. Whatever good results are obtained from "thirst cures" depend upon diminishing the work of the digestive and circulatory systems.

Manual of Chemistry. By W. SIMON, PH. D., M. D., Professor of Chemistry in the College of Physicians and Surgeons of Baltimore, etc. Eighth edition, with illustrations. (*Lea Bros. & Co., 1905.*)

This Manual of Chemistry is so well known to teachers of chemistry and students of medicine and pharmacy that an extended review of this, the eighth edition, is hardly necessary at this place. The work has been meritoriously popular from the first edition and still maintains its position as one of the leading text-books in American schools of medicine. We heartily congratulate Dr. Simon upon the continued success of his work.

C. E. S.

Hygiene and Public Health. By B. ARTHUR WHITELEGGE, C. B., M. D., and GEORGE NEWMAN, M. D., D. P. H. (*Chicago: W. T. Keener & Co., 1905.*)

This little book, dealing with the subject of hygiene and public health in a short six hundred pages, considers nearly every subject which could possibly have any relation to the science of medicine from the chemical and bacteriological standpoint. Mingled with a large amount of scientific information there is presented a complete system of the various enactments of the English government, regulating the duties and privileges of British officers of health. The information here presented gives a very practical insight into the practice of public health as it exists in England, and from a purely practical standpoint the book has value. The facts given are presented in a clear, concise, systematic manner, and it becomes a matter of considerable ease to inform oneself as to the usual conduct of matters pertaining to hygiene. Ten various enactments governing the sale of milk, meat, and other articles of diet, the laws regulating the proper construction of work-shops and tenement houses, the care of those sick with infectious disease and the disposal of the dead, together with such kindred subjects as disinfection and quarantine are considered at some length and in the main quite satisfactorily.

From the scientific standpoint, however, there are so many errors that the book could hardly be recommended to students or to practitioners unable to exercise a discriminating power of criticism. By way of example it is stated on page 364 that " milk has been abundantly proved to convey the diphtheria poison," on page 376 that " enteric or typhoid fever was differentiated from typhus in 1850 by Jenner," neither of which statements will pass unchallenged, especially .the latter.

Again, on page 433, in the discussion of yellow fever, half a page is devoted to a consideration of Sanarelli's claims for the *Bacillus icteroides* as the etiological agent of the disease, followed by the statement that the United States Army commission could not confirm Sanarelli's work but reported that the disease was conveyed "*probably* by mosquitoes." The names of Reed Carroll, Agramonte, and Lazear are not mentioned, nor are we informed that Guitéras has confirmed most of the commission's findings.

Finally, we read that a second U. S. Army commission reinvestigated the subject and found that a protozoan parasite *Myxococcidium stegomyiæ* was responsible for the spread of yellow fever and could be found in infected mosquitoes.

Further citation of errors is unnecessary as these examples but represent a mass of misstatements which rob the book of a large part of its usefulness.

Veterinary Pathology. By FRIEDBERGER and FRÖHNER. Vol. I, Infective Diseases of Animals. Translated by M. H. HAYES, F. R. C. V. S. (*Chicago: W. T. Keener & Co., 1905.*)

To the student of veterinary science Friedberger and Fröhner's Veterinary Pathology needs no introduction, the original German edition being universally employed in veterinary schools in Germany and Austria, and its French translation by Cadiot and Ries having been adopted as the highest authority in France. The present English translation by Hayes is of exceptional purity

and gives in a very remarkable way the clearest English expressions for somewhat complicated German ideas.

The various animal diseases are treated with that comprehensive grasp and conservative judgment so characteristic of the Teutonic mind and throughout the entire book the most recent studies in animal pathology and bacteriology are presented with accuracy and clearness.

The chapters on tuberculosis, anthrax, rabies, and distemper are especially good. The distinction between the disease of hog cholera as it exists in this country, and infectious diseases of swine in Germany has not been clearly grasped by the authors, who, therefore, fail to give proper value to the investigations dealing with the hog cholera bacillus. This error, however, if error it can be called, is one common to the German bacteriologist and in no way detracts from the great value of the book.

We feel that this first volume of the Pathology can be most highly recommended to all our students, especially in view of our present great and increasing interest in the diseases of animals.

A Manual of Practical Hygiene. By CHARLES HARRINGTON, M. D., Assistant Professor of Hygiene in the Medical School of Harvard University. (*Philadelphia & New York: Lea Brothers & Co., 1905.*)

We have already taken the opportunity in previous reviews of this text-book, of recommending its use by those who are especially interested in practical sanitation. The modern hygienist considers his subject usually from the standpoint of chemistry or bacteriology and Dr. Harrington has followed the former path to the understanding of sanitary problems. In the present edition however he has added a number of pages devoted to questions more purely of a bacteriological nature. Thus for instance he considers at some length the subject of Immunity and the Ehrlich theories, following this by a valuable account of an action of antitoxic sera in various diseases. The information presented throughout the book is given in a concise, systematic manner easily accessible to the reader. A few bacteriological errors have crept in, but they are mostly errors which are common to current literature. Such for instance is the consideration of *B. enteritidis sporogenes* of Klein as the etiological agent of summer diarrhœa, a claim by no means justified by the facts, since the organism obtained by Klein has been proved to be the *Bacillus aerogenes capsulatus* of Welch, which again has been shown to exist normally in the intestinal tract of nearly all individuals. The chapters upon the composition of food with a good discussion of their nutritive value appeal very strongly to clinicians who rely upon careful dieting in building up the strength of debilitated patients. Also the very excellent account of various epidemics of food poisoning with accurate data as to the number of cases, their symptoms and mortality, is another example of Dr. Harrington's habit of presenting his information in an easily-apprehended manner. Taken altogether the book is a very mine of information upon all sorts of subjects collateral to the science of medicine, and will prove of the greatest value in spreading our knowledge of practical hygiene. Finally we cannot forbear quoting from the section devoted to exercise, the statement that *golf* is " an ideal form of exercise for all ages above early childhood, and particularly for those whose lives are essentially sedentary or whose age precludes them from following the more violent games," a sentiment which will without doubt find ready acceptance in the Medical Faculty.

Neurotic Disorders of Childhood. By B. K. RACHFORD, M. D. (*New York: E. B. Treat & Co.*, 1905.)

This book is divided into two parts: In Part I, after discussing the physiological peculiarities of the child's nervous system, the author reviews some of the important factors concerned in producing the neuroses. One chapter deals with the temperature in childhood; a second with the gastro-intestinal toxæmias; a third with auto-intoxication, including acid intoxications and thyroid and biliary toxæmias. In the chapter on bacterial toxæmias, tuberculosis, rheumatism, malaria and syphilis are dealt with, and the subjects of chronic anæmia, reflex irritation and excessive nerve activity are each given one chapter.

Part II (Chapters X-XXVII), is devoted to the individual neuroses. The neuroses dealt with are fever, eclampsia, laryngismus stridulus, tetany, enuresis, migraine, recurrent vomiting, toxic epilepsy, recurrent coryza, chorea, hysteria, headaches, asthma, disorders of sleep, nystagmus, habit spasms and pica or dirt eating.

The first part is the more interesting. The author makes very clear the relation between the neuroses and the important etiological factors such as heredity, age and the various depressing influences which may be present. Tuberculosis, and chronic infectious anæmia, mal-nutrition and reflex irritation receive especial attention in this connection.

In Part II, the subjects most fully discussed are eclampsia, enuresis, migraine, recurrent vomiting and epilepsy. Rachford follows the modern tendency not to attempt to separate too widely the various neuroses and in a very interesting chapter he reports selected cases in which one neurosis was succeeded by a different one during the progress of the patient's career.

In a number of places, for example in the chapter on migraine, the author reaches well beyond the confines of pediatrics and works over into the field of general medicine.

From the nature of the case there is considerable repetition in the book. What is said in Part I in the general discussion of the etiology of the neuroses is repeated more or less fully in the subsequent chapters dealing with the individual neuroses.

The style is lucid and possibly a trifle too didactic, the matter is quite well systematised, and the book is a good up-to-date review of our knowledge on the subjects discussed.

There is an index at the end of the book.

The Physician's Visiting List (Lindsay & Blakiston's) for 1906. Fifty-fifth Year of Publication. (*Philadelphia: P. Blakiston's Son & Co.*, 1012 Walnut St.)

This handy memorandum book for physicians has been revised to bring it into harmony with the Eighth Decennial Revision of the U. S. Pharmacopœia. It is in compact form and easy to be carried, and contains such information as the physician needs to have ready at hand. It is to be recommended to all persons in the general practice of medicine.

HOSPITAL STAFF, JANUARY 1, 1906.

SUPERINTENDENT:
HENRY M. HURD, M. D.

PHYSICIAN-IN-CHIEF:
LEWELLYS F. BARKER, M. D.

ASSOCIATE PHYSICIAN:
WILLIAM S. THAYER, M. D.

SURGEON-IN-CHIEF:
WILLIAM S. HALSTED, M. D.

GYNECOLOGIST-IN-CHIEF:
HOWARD A. KELLY, M. D.

OBSTETRICIAN-IN-CHIEF:
J. WHITRIDGE WILLIAMS, M. D.

PATHOLOGIST:
WILLIAM H. WELCH, M. D.

ASSOCIATES IN SURGERY:
J. M. T. FINNEY, M. D.,   J. C. BLOODGOOD, M. D.,
HARVEY CUSHING, M. D.

ASSISTANT IN ORTHOPEDIC SURGERY:
WILLIAM S. BAER, M. D.

ASSISTANT IN ACTINOGRAPHY:
F. H. BAETJER, M. D.

ASSOCIATES IN MEDICINE:
T. B. FUTCHER, M. B.,   T. McCRAE, M. D.

ASSOCIATES IN GYNECOLOGY:
W. W. RUSSELL, M. D.,   T. S. CULLEN, M. B.

RESIDENT PHYSICIAN:
C. P. EMERSON, M. D.

ASSISTANT RESIDENT PHYSICIANS:
C. P. HOWARD, M. D.,   T. R. BOGGS, M. D.,
M. FABYAN, M. D.

RESIDENT SURGEON:
W. F. M. SOWERS, M. D.

ASSISTANT RESIDENT SURGEONS:
S. H. WATTS, M. D.,   R. T. MILLER, JR., M. D.,
J. R. CARR, M. D.

RESIDENT GYNECOLOGIST:
S. RUSHMORE, M. D.

ASSISTANT RESIDENT GYNECOLOGISTS:
H. T. HUTCHINS, M. D,.   DeW. B. CASLER, M. D.,
H. J. STORRS, M. D.

RESIDENT OBSTETRICIAN:
F. C. GOLDSBOROUGH, M. D.

ASSISTANT RESIDENT OBSTETRICIAN:
J. McF. BERGLAND, M. D.

RESIDENT PATHOLOGIST:
W. G. MacCALLUM, M. D.

ASSISTANT RESIDENT PATHOLOGIST:
C. H. BUNTING, M. D.

HOUSE MEDICAL OFFICERS:
K. H. BEALL, M. D.,   W. L. MOSS, M. D.,
J. A. CALDWELL, M. D.,   E. H. RICHARDSON, M. D.,
C. D. COWLES, M. D.,   F. P. ROUS, M. D.,
S. A. DODDS, M. D.,   R. B. SLOCUM, M. D.,
C. M. FARIS, M. D.,   D. VANDER HOOF, M. D.,
F. R. FORD, M. D.,   H. I. WIEL, M. D.

THE JOHNS HOPKINS HOSPITAL REPORTS.

VOLUME I. 423 pages, 99 plates.

VOLUME II. 570 pages, with 28 plates and figures.

VOLUME III. 766 pages, with 69 plates and figures.

VOLUME IV. 504 pages, 33 charts and illustrations.

VOLUME V. 480 pages, with 32 charts and illustrations.

CONTENTS:

The Malarial Fevers of Baltimore. By W. S. THAYER, M. D., and J. HEWETSON, M. D.

A Study of some Fatal Cases of Malaria. By LEWELLYS F. BARKER, M. B.

Studies in Typhoid Fever.

By WILLIAM OSLER, M. D., with additional papers by G. BLUMER, M. D., SIMON FLEXNER, M. D., WALTER REED, M. D., and H. C. PARSONS, M. D.

VOLUME VI. 414 pages, with 79 plates and figures.

Report in Neurology.

Studies on the Lesions Produced by the Action of Certain Poisons on the Cortical Nerve Cell (Studies Nos. I to V). By HENRY J. BERKLEY, M. D.

Introductory.—Recent Literature on the Pathology of Diseases of the Brain by the Chromate of Silver Methods; Part I.—Alcohol Poisoning.—Experimental Lesions produced by Chronic Alcoholic Poisoning (Ethyl Alcohol). 2. Experimental Lesions produced by Acute Alcoholic Poisoning (Ethyl Alcohol); Part II.—Serum Poisoning.—Experimental Lesions induced by the Action of the Dog's Serum on the Cortical Nerve Cell; Part III.—Ricin Poisoning.—Experimental Lesions induced by Acute Ricin Poisoning. 2. Experimental Lesions induced by Chronic Ricin Poisoning; Part IV.—Hydrophobic Toxæmia.—Lesions of the Cortical Nerve Cell produced by the Toxine of Experimental Rabies; Part V.—Pathological Alterations in the Nuclei and Nucleoli of Nerve Cells from the Effects of Alcohol and Ricin Intoxication; Nerve Fibre Terminal Apparatus; Asthenic Bulbar Paralysis. By HENRY J. BERKLEY, M. D.

Report in Pathology.

Fatal Puerperal Sepsis due to the Introduction of an Elm Tent. By THOMAS S. CULLEN, M. B.

Pregnancy in a Rudimentary Uterine Horn. Rupture, Death, Probable Migration of Ovum and Spermatozoa. By THOMAS S. CULLEN, M. B., and G. L. WILKINS, M. D.

Adeno-Myoma Uteri Diffusum Benignum. By THOMAS S. CULLEN, M. B.

A Bacteriological and Anatomical Study of the Summer Diarrhœas of Infants. By WILLIAM D. BOOKER, M. D.

The Pathology of Toxalbumin Intoxications. By SIMON FLEXNER, M. D.

VOLUME VII. 537 pages with illustrations.

    I. A Critical Review of Seventeen Hundred Cases of Abdominal Section from the standpoint of Intra-peritoneal Drainage. By J. G. CLARK, M. D.

   II. The Etiology and Structure of true Vaginal Cysts. By JAMES ERNEST STOKES, M. D.

  III. A Review of the Pathology of Superficial Burns, with a Contribution to our Knowledge of the Pathological Changes in the Organs in cases of rapidly fatal burns. By CHARLES RUSSELL BARDEEN, M. D.

  IV. The Origin, Growth and Fate of the Corpus Luteum. By J. G. CLARK, M. D.

   V. The Results of Operations for the Cure of Inguinal Hernia. By JOSEPH C. BLOODGOOD, M. D.

VOLUME VIII. 552 pages with illustrations.

On the rôle of Insects, Arachnids, and Myriapods as carriers in the spread of Bacterial and Parasitic Diseases of Man and Animals. By GEORGE H. F. NUTTALL, M. D., PH. D.

Studies in Typhoid Fever.

By WILLIAM OSLER, M. D., with additional papers by J. M. T. FINNEY, M. D., S. FLEXNER, M. D., I. P. LYON, M. D., L. P. HAMBURGER, M. D., H. W. CUSHING, M. D., J. F. MITCHELL, M. D., C. N. B. CAMAC, M. D., N. B. GWYN, M. D., CHARLES P. EMERSON, M. D., H. H. YOUNG, M. D., and W. S. THAYER, M. D.

VOLUME IX. 1060 pages, 66 plates and 210 other illustrations.

Contributions to the Science of Medicine.

Dedicated by his Pupils to WILLIAM HENRY WELCH, on the twenty-fifth anniversary of his Doctorate. This volume contains 38 separate papers.

VOLUME X. 516 pages, 12 plates and 25 charts.

Structure of the Malarial Parasites. Plate I. By JESSE W. LAZEAR, M. D.

The Bacteriology of Cystitis, Pyelitis and Pyelonephritis in Women, with a Consideration of the Accessory Etiological Factors in these Conditions, and of the Various Chemical and Microscopical Questions involved. By THOMAS R. BROWN, M. D.

Cases of Infection with Strongyloides Intestinalis. (First Reported Occurrence in North America.) Plates II and III. By RICHARD P. STRONG, M. D.

On the Pathological Changes in Hodgkin's Disease, with Especial Reference to its Relation to Tuberculosis. Plates IV-VII. By DOROTHY M. REED, M. D.

Diabetes Insipidus, with a Report of Five Cases. By THOMAS B. FUTCHER, M. B. (Tor.).

Observations on the Origin and Occurrence of Cells with Eosinophile Granulations in Normal and Pathological Tissues. Plate VIII. By W. T. HOWARD, M. D., and R. G. PERKINS, M. D.

Placental Transmissions, with Report of a Case during Typhoid Fever. By FRANK W. LYNCH, M. D.

Metabolism in Albuminuria. By CHAS. P. EMERSON, A. B., M. D.

Regenerative Changes in the Liver after Acute Yellow Atrophy. Plates IX-XII. By W. G. MACCALLUM, M. D.

Surgical Features of Typhoid Fever. By THOS. MCCRAE, M. B., M. R. C. P. (Lond.), and JAMES F. MITCHELL, M. D.

The Symptoms, Diagnosis and Surgical Treatment of Ureteral Calculus. By BENJAMIN R. SCHENCK, M. D.

VOLUME XI. 555 pages, with 38 charts and illustrations.

Pneumothorax: A historical, clinical and experimental study. By CHARLES P. EMERSON, M. D.

Clinical Observations on Blood Pressure. By HENRY W. COOK, M. D., and JOHN B. BRIGGS, M. D.

The Value of Tuberculin in Surgical Diagnosis. By MARTIN B. TINKER, M. D.

VOLUME XII. 548 pages, 12 plates and other illustrations. (Now ready.)

The Connective Tissue of the Salivary Glands and Pancreas with Its Development in the Glandula Submaxillaris. Plates I-III. By JOSEPH MARSHALL FLINT, M. D.

A New Instrument for Determining the Minimum and Maximum Blood-Pressures in Man. Plates IV-X. By JOSEPH ERLANGER, M. D.

Metabolism in Pregnancy, Labor, and the Puerperium. By J. MORRIS SLEMONS, M. D.

An Experimental Study of Blood-Pressure and of Pulse-Pressure in Man. Plates XI and XII. By JOSEPH ERLANGER, M. D., and DONALD R. HOOKER, A. B., M. S.

Typhoid Meningitis. By RUFUS I. COLE, M. D.

The Pathological Anatomy of Meningitis due to Bacillus Typhosus. By WILLIAM G. MACCALLUM, M. D.

A Comparative Study of White and Negro Pelves, with a Consideration of the Size of the Child and Its Relation to Presentation and Character of Labor in the Two Races. By THEODORE F. RIGGS, M. D.

Renal Tuberculosis. By GEORGE WALKER, M. D.

The Johns Hopkins Hospital Bulletins are issued monthly. They are printed by the FRIEDENWALD CO., Baltimore. Single copies may be procured from NUNN & CO. and the BALTIMORE NEWS CO., Baltimore. Subscriptions, $2.00 a year, may be addressed to the publishers, THE JOHNS HOPKINS PRESS, BALTIMORE; single copies will be sent by mail for twenty-five cents each.

BULLETIN

OF

THE JOHNS HOPKINS HOSPITAL

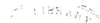

Entered as Second-Class Matter at the Baltimore, Maryland, Postoffice.

| Vol. XVII.—No. 180.] | BALTIMORE, MARCH, 1906. | [Price, 25 Cents. |

CONTENTS.

PERNICIOUS VOMITING OF PREGNANCY.[1]

By J. Whitridge Williams,

Professor of Obstetrics, Johns Hopkins University; Obstetrician-in-Chief, Johns Hopkins Hospital.

General History.

Slight degrees of nausea and vomiting in the early months of pregnancy have probably occurred from time immemorial, but according to Guéniot and Anquétin, the more severe forms of the affection were first described by Oribasius and Paul of Aegina, who, however, appeared to have no idea that it might end fatally. Similar views were held by Guillemeau, Mauriceau, and the obstetricians of the seventeenth and the greater part of the eighteenth centuries. Indeed, Dionis and many others considered vomiting a favorable sign, and thought that women subject to it were usually exempt from serious complications at the time of labor; or, as Rigby expressed it, nearly 150 years later, " a sick pregnancy is a safe one."

In 1789, Vaughan reported a case which he considered was saved from a fatal termination only by the employment of rectal feeding, so that it would seem that it was not until the latter part of the eighteenth century that it began to be recognized that vomiting of pregnancy might occasionally be so persistent as to lead to death from inanition.

As far as I can learn, Simmons in 1813 was the first to induce abortion for its relief, an example which was soon followed by Davis, Chailly-Honoré, Churchill, and others. The

justifiability of the procedure, however, was first brought prominently to the attention of the profession by a discussion before the Academy of Medicine of Paris in March, 1852, when Dubois and Danyau contended that the induction of abortion was not only justifiable, but urgently demanded in severe cases, while Cazeaux held that interference was unnecessary and even hastened death in some instances.

Dubois supported his contention by his own experience in fourteen severe cases, ten of which died without operation, while abortion was induced in the other four. Only one of the latter recovered; in two others the vomiting persisted until death; while the third died from infection. Notwithstanding these apparently poor results, which he held were due to the fact that interference had been delayed so long that death was practically inevitable no matter what line of treatment was adopted, Dubois contended that abortion was the rational treatment and should be induced before the patient's condition becomes absolutely hopeless, and was urgently indicated under the following conditions:

1. When the vomiting is incessant.
2. When emaciation is rapid and the patient so weak as to be obliged to keep her bed.
3. When she faints upon the slightest exertion.
4. When pronounced alterations occur in her features.
5. When there is marked and continuous fever and an

---

[1] Read in Abstract before the American Gynecological Society, Buffalo, May 26, 1905.

excessive acidity of the breath, which cannot be relieved by treatment.

The next important contribution to the subject was the monograph of Guéniot in 1863, in which the author collected from the literature 118 cases of pernicious vomiting with 46 deaths, and carefully analyzed them from the point of view of etiology and treatment. Concerning the former, his conclusions were not very satisfactory, but on the other hand he taught that the induction of abortion was urgently indicated in severe cases, and should be resorted to as soon as medicinal treatment proved unavailing and the patient was perceptibly losing ground.

The work of Dubois and Guéniot greatly stimulated the interest in the subject, concerning which an immense literature gradually developed. Unfortunately the contradictory statements of the various writers have simply served to accentuate the fact that their knowledge concerning the etiology of the condition was very fragmentary and imperfect; while the manifold recommendations as to treatment indicate that they either were practically worthless, or that several types of vomiting with varying clinical histories had been grouped together in a single category.

OBJECT OF ARTICLE.

In this paper it is my object to bring together the more important contributions to the literature of the subject, and, guided by my own experience, to set up certain well defined types of the disease, in the hope of establishing more satisfactorily its etiology and laying down more definite rules for guidance in its treatment.

Leaving out of consideration all cases in which the vomiting is dependent upon conditions which have nothing to do with pregnancy, and limiting our attention only to those cases in which it is apparently due solely to the pregnancy itself or to some lesion of the generative tract—in other words adopting the distinction of Matthews Duncan between vomiting in and vomiting of pregnancy—I hope to be able to show that the evidence at present available seems to justify the differentiation of three distinct types of vomiting of pregnancy, namely: reflex, neurotic, and toxæmic, each of which is dependent upon different etiological factors and demands especial methods of treatment.

FREQUENCY.

It is difficult to give definite figures as to the frequency of serious vomiting of pregnancy, since even the statements concerning the incidence of the ordinary morning sickness vary greatly. Thus Gardner states that the latter occurs in only 15 per cent of pregnant women, while Giles, Gerst, and Horwitz noted it in 47½, 66⅔, and 84 per cent of their cases respectively. My own experience leads me to believe that it is present in slightly more than one-half of all private patients. According to Pick and Lwow the pernicious type occurs about once in one thousand cases; but as their conclusions were drawn entirely from hospital experience, they do not neces-

sarily give a correct idea as to its incidence in private practice, in which it would seem to be much more frequent. This is clearly shown by my own experience at the Johns Hopkins Hospital, where only two out of 4500 clinical cases suffered from serious vomiting of pregnancy, while I have seen ten cases during the past two years in my private and consultation practice.

It would also seem, as Horwitz first pointed out, that there is a marked variation in its incidence in different countries, as it occurs much more frequently in France, England, and America, than in Germany or Russia; a fact which may possibly be explained by the greater frequency of neurotic conditions among the inhabitants of the former countries. Indeed many competent German authorities, such as Hohl, Lomer, Frank, and Strassmann, have stated that they have never seen a case of vomiting of pregnancy end fatally; while in this country there is hardly a general practitioner of extensive experience, who has not had one or more cases in his own practice. It is likewise interesting to recall the fact that Anquétin stated that the condition had apparently become more frequent in France after the abandonment of universal venesection.

ETIOLOGY.

1. *Reflex Vomiting.*—This variety of vomiting may be due to the presence of abnormalities of the generative tract or ovum, which existed prior to the onset of pregnancy, or are coincident with it. Among such conditions may be mentioned:

(a) Abnormalities of the uterus, particularly displacements.

(b) Certain cases of endometritis.

(c) Ovarian tumors.

(d) Abnormalities of the ovum, such as hydramnios, hydatidiform mole and certain cases of twin pregnancy.

The reflex character of the vomiting of pregnancy was recognized at an early period. Mauriceau attributed it to a sympathy between the uterus and stomach, as he believed that distinct nervous connections existed between the two organs, by which abnormal stimuli originating in the diseased uterus were readily transmitted to the stomach.

That uterine displacements may occasionally be the cause of the condition is apparently demonstrated by the fact that the vomiting sometimes ceases immediately upon the replacement of a retroflexed uterus. This conception was particularly elaborated by Graily Hewitt, who published extensive monographs upon the subject in 1871, 1885, and 1888, in which he clearly demonstrated that certain cases, at least, were due to displacements of the uterus and could be cured by restoring the organ to its normal position. At the same time, he probably erred when he concluded that anteflexion had a much more deleterious influence than retroflexion.

Owing to his extensive contributions, Hewitt is generally regarded as the father of this theory, although several earlier writers held similar, but not so pronounced, views; among whom may be mentioned Busch and Moser, Stolz, Brian-Moreau, Ulrich, and others. Following the publication of

Hewitt's last monograph, his view has never lacked supporters, as is evidenced by the teachings of Guéniot in 1889 and Lwow in 1900.

From my own experience, I can state without hesitation, that in exceptional cases, a retroflexed uterus may be the exciting cause of the condition, and in such cases vomiting ceases immediately after its replacement. At the same time it must be admitted that this is not a common etiological factor, since in the vast majority of patients with retroflexion of the pregnant uterus, even when symptoms of incarceration are present, vomiting is lacking or at least no more severe than in women with perfectly normal genitalia.

Dance, in 1827, in one of the earliest autopsies performed upon a woman dying from hyperemesis, noted an abnormal thinness of the uterine wall; and since then occasional advocates have been found for the belief that the vomiting is due to undue distension of the uterus, a view which was held in part by Schroeder. While it cannot be denied that such an explanation may occasionally hold good, as is apparently demonstrated in some cases of hydramnios and twin pregnancy, it must nevertheless be admitted that it is not of universal application, and even in those cases in which it appears most probable, conclusive evidence cannot be adduced in its favor.

Horwitz, in 1883, pointed out that in certain cases the vomiting appeared to be due to inflammatory conditions of the muscular wall of the uterus, which in several of his cases was associated with peritoneal involvement. Whether these lesions were really the cause of the condition, or should be regarded merely as accidental complications, cannot be decided, though the evidence at present available makes the latter probable. Tuszkai in 1895, rehabilitated the theory of peritoneal irritation with only partial success. At the same time there can be no doubt that abnormal conditions of the uterus certainly favor the occurrence of vomiting.

The uterine origin of vomiting was likewise advocated by Martin in 1904, who stated that the majority of cases should be attributed to hyperæmia of the uterus and its impaction in the pelvic cavity; while Evans of Montreal taught that the ordinary morning sickness was probably connected with the rythmical contractions of the organ.

In 1849, J. H. Bennett in his work on inflammation of the uterus directed attention to the part which he believed was played by inflammatory conditions of the cervix in the production of the vomiting of pregnancy, and ever since then this view has had numerous adherents; and he himself, in 1875, stated that more extended experience had only served to confirm his original views.

A little later Copeman invoked the influence of the cervix in another manner and assumed that the vomiting was due to an irritation resulting from its abnormal rigidity, particularly in the region of the internal os, and held that the vomiting could be cured by dilating the cervix. This view and the procedure dependent upon it was accepted by Rosenthal and many others and enjoyed considerable vogue for some years, but has gradually fallen into disrepute; although even as late as 1896, Kehrer reported a case which he considered demonstrated the correctness of such teachings. Cervical catarrh has likewise been considered to play an important etiological part, and Lwow stated that 75 per cent of the women suffering from vomiting of pregnancy presented this abnormality.

As far as I am able to ascertain, the causal relation between abnormalities of the cervix and the more severe forms of vomiting has not been conclusively demonstrated, nor do I think that it will be in the future; as it seems to me that a palpably accidental condition has been erroneously considered as causal. This contention is well exemplified by a case of Davis, in which several small cysts in the cervix were considered as the etiological factor; while autopsy showed marked lesions in the liver and kidneys; and still more forcibly by a case of Lang in which inflammation of the cervix was considered the essential factor, while autopsy demonstrated the presence of acute yellow atrophy of the liver.

Ever since 1827, when Dance at autopsy upon a patient dying from vomiting of pregnancy, found suppurative changes in the decidua, it has been considered that endometritis may play an important part in the production of the condition, a view which in modern times has been particularly insisted upon by Veit, Jaffé, Jaggard, Flaischlen, Goldspohn, and many others. Nevertheless it does not appear that its advocates have adduced conclusive evidence in its support, and it seems probable that endometritis when it occurs, should generally be regarded as an accidental complication, rather than an important etiological factor. At the same time it must be admitted that it may tend to exaggerate what might otherwise be only a minor complaint.

There can be no doubt that in exceptional instances the presence of tumors of the ovaries may accentuate or even cause serious vomiting. Such a connection was clearly demonstrated in a case of Krassowsky's, in which very severe vomiting ceased immediately after the removal of a small ovarian tumor, and in one of my own cases a similar result followed the removal of a small fibro-myoma of the ovary.

Clinical observation apparently shows that both hydramnios and twin pregnancies predispose to excessive vomiting, though whether this is the result of the mere overdistension of the uterus, or whether it is associated with some toxæmic condition has not yet been demonstrated.

Hydatidiform mole has a similar effect, and Bué has reported three cases in which the vomiting ceased immediately after the evacuation of the mole, and has collected a large number of similar cases from the literature. Likewise, in one of my cases the spontaneous expulsion of the mole prevented the induction of abortion for the relief of vomiting. But in this condition, as well as in twin pregnancy and hydramnios, the exact interpretation of the effect of the abnormality is not easy; as it is possible, on the one hand, that the vomiting may be merely the result of over-distension of the uterus, while on the other, it may quite as readily be attributed to a toxæmic condition, which may be due to abnormal metabolism on the part of the mother or fœtus, or to the formation of syncytiotoxins resulting from the presence of unusually large amounts of fœtal elements in the maternal blood. The latter conception has been particularly elaborated by Veit and Behm and will be considered in detail under Toxæmic Vomiting.

Chorio-epithelioma has likewise been invoked as a cause of the condition by Davis and Harris, although in their case it is questionable whether the vomiting was due to the presence of fœtal tissues in the growth itself, or merely to the mechanical action of the metastases which were found in the brain at autopsy.

2. *Neurotic Vomiting.*—Although the effect of pregnancy upon the mental, moral, and nervous equilibrium had long been recognized, and Anquétin, Tisserand, Duncan, Rosenthal, Ahlfeld, and others had pointed out that many cases of severe vomiting were neurotic or hysterical in origin, it was nevertheless not until Kaltenbach read his paper before the Berlin Obstetrical Society in 1890, that general attention was directed to this phase of the subject.

On that occasion he pointed out the necessity for narrowing the conception of the pernicious vomiting of pregnancy and confining it strictly to those cases in which there was no disease of other organs or of the generative tract to which it might be attributed. At the same time he emphasized the great paucity of positive autopsy findings, and commented upon the contradictory character of the lesions noted.

In this restricted sense, he held that the severe cases of hyperemesis were the result of an abnormal condition of the nervous system by which the reflex irritability was heightened and the reflex control lessened. This being the case, it could readily be understood how the irritation might be increased by diseased conditions on the part of the generative tract on the one hand or of the stomach on the other. Accordingly, he concluded that the vast majority of cases of vomiting of pregnancy were due to a neurosis, more or less allied to hysteria; although he was compelled to admit that many of the patients presented no evident manifestations of the latter condition. He therefore assumed that in many instances a hysteria, which had previously been larval, might become manifest under the influence of pregnancy. In view of its neurotic nature, he insisted upon the value of suggestion and the rest cure in its treatment, and held that if they were intelligently carried out, the field for the induction of abortion would be greatly limited, if not entirely obliterated.

This paper immediately gave rise to considerable discussion, and a number of authors, among whom may be mentioned Ahlfeld, Chazan, Rosenfeld, and others, claimed that they had antedated Kaltenbach's views by a number of years. As has already been indicated, this was undoubtedly true; but nevertheless it would seem that the credit rightly belongs to Kaltenbach, as he was the first to insist upon the importance of neurotic influences in their entirety. In this connection, it is interesting to note that two years later Mettler of Chicago

enunciated almost identical views, apparently without knowledge of Kaltenbach's work.

The neurotic origin of the condition was enthusiastically accepted by a number of writers, among whom may be mentioned Luez, Klein, and Graefe. Klein published histories of a number of cases and insisted upon the curative value of an absolute rest cure and attached less importance to the action of suggestion. He stated that the vast majority of cases could be promptly cured by putting the patient to bed, keeping her absolutely quiet, prohibiting all intercourse with her family and friends, and at the same time administering small quantities of iced milk at frequent intervals, and if this was not well borne to resort entirely to rectal feeding. If, however, such a course did not lead to the desired result within three or four days, he advocated the removal of the patient to a well regulated hospital, where she could be placed under ideal conditions for a very strictly conducted rest cure. Graefe expressed similar views in his original article in 1900 and reiterated them more strongly in 1904.

To anyone who has had considerable experience with this class of cases there can be no doubt that in many the vomiting must be attributed to some neurotic condition, as is manifested by the remarkable cures which sometimes follow all sorts of unphysiological procedures, as well as the mere threat to induce abortion, or a feigned attempt to bring it about. Only upon such a hypothesis can one explain the results obtained by Muret, Damany, and others. Thus the former observed a patient who had lost 49 pounds in weight as the result of incessant vomiting, which ceased immediately upon a single lavage of the stomach. In Damany's case equally satisfactory results were obtained by the use of an electrical battery, which was later found to be entirely out of order. Moreover, it is more than probable that the vast majority of cures following the application of leeches to the epigastrium or cervix, the dilatation of the latter by Copeman's maneuver, or the application of various drugs are susceptible of a similar explanation.

At the same time it should be borne in mind that it is possible that the underlying cause of the neurosis may be a mild toxæmia, but at present satisfactory evidence cannot be adduced in support of such a view.

When Graefe's first paper was read before the Leipzig Obstetrical Society in 1900, Winscheid stated in the discussion that the tendency to attribute all cases to neurasthenia or hysteria was too extreme, as he did not believe that such conditions could give rise to the extreme emaciation and cachexia which characterized the severe cases. To my mind, however, this objection does not necessarily hold good, as I have in several instances seen women, who had become markedly emaciated and were apparently dying from starvation, immediately cease vomiting after a vigorous lecture or upon the threat of inducing abortion, after I had unduly magnified its dangers.

3. *Toxæmic Vomiting.*—According to Mauriceau, one of the earliest theories concerning the production of the vomiting

of pregnancy was that it was due to the excretion by the stomach of humours resulting from the suppression of the menstrual function. As far as I have been able to ascertain, Fischl in 1884, was the first modern writer to suggest the toxæmic nature of the condition, being led to this conclusion after observing a woman, admitted to the hospital in a torpid condition with slight fever with a history of severe continuous vomiting, who was immediately cured by the evacuation of a densely impacted colon. As the result of his experience, he stated that the vomiting of pregnancy might be either essential or symptomatic, and held that the former would become more and more rare as the cases were more carefully investigated.

The following year (1885), Jolly reported two cases of paralysis which occurred in pregnant women suffering from the vomiting of pregnancy, and attributed the former condition to a neuritis which was probably caused by some toxic substance peculiar to pregnancy. Similar cases were soon described by Moebius, Whitfield, Desnos, Joffroy, and Pinard, and others, who expressed a similar belief concerning the inter-relation of the two conditions, but did not adduce absolute proof as to its correctness.

In 1892, Lindemann reported the autopsy findings upon a patient of Solowieff's, who died from multiple neuritis complicating hyperemesis, and stated that there were histological signs of parenchymatous neuritis as well as fatty degeneration and cloudy swelling of the liver and kidneys. As he found similar lesions in the organs of the fœtus, he was inclined to believe that he had adduced direct proof of the toxæmic nature of the condition, as the presence of lesions in both the mother and the fœtus could be due only to the circulation of some toxic substance.

Following Lindemann, a considerable number of cases of neuritis associated with vomiting were reported by Eulenberg, Stembo, Mader, Kühne, Kreutzmann, Bar, and others. Eulenberg gave a tabulated list of the cases occurring up to the time of his report, but thus far no one has advanced irrefutable proof in favor of the toxic nature of the two conditions, although each succeeding observation has rendered it more probable.

Additional support in favor of the toxæmic nature of the vomiting of pregnancy is afforded by its occasional association with jaundice. As early as 1879, Matthews Duncan suggested that the underlying factor in certain of the fatal cases, at least, was acute yellow atrophy of the liver, and supported his contention by autopsy in one case. This view was likewise advocated by Roughton in 1885, but obtained little if any recognition; although it is interesting to note that Lomer in his article upon icterus in pregnancy likewise suggested that possibly some connection existed between hepatic disturbance and the production of vomiting.

The toxæmic theory was likewise advocated in a modified form by Holladay who, in 1886, suggested that when the vomiting persisted after the fourth month of pregnancy it was probably due to the action of the secretion of an abnormally persistent corpus luteum.

Following these suggestions, there was a lull in the advocacy of the toxæmic nature of the condition, and it was not until the last years of the 19th century that other writers began to insist upon its possibility, when Allbutt and Bacon, in 1896 and 1897 respectively, expressed themselves in its favor upon purely theoretical considerations.

In 1898, Bouffe de Saint-Blaise in a long article upon the auto-intoxication of pregnancy, which was based in great part upon Pinard's hepato-toxæmia theory, made a tolerably clear case for eclampsia and the pre-eclamptic toxæmia; but when he attempted to apply the theory to the other complications of pregnancy the outcome was much less satisfactory.

With the exception of the positive autopsy findings of Lindemann, and several isolated cases of acute yellow atrophy of the liver, it was not until 1901 that Champetier de Ribes and Bouffe de Saint-Blaise reported definite hepatic lesions in vomiting of pregnancy. In a communication to the Society of Gynecology, Obstetrics and Pædiatrics of Paris, they briefly described the autopsy findings in a woman dying in convulsions at the end of pregnancy, who had suffered from vomiting throughout its entire course, and reported the presence of lesions in the liver, which they considered identical with those observed in eclampsia, and therefore concluded that the anatomical substratum was the same in both conditions. Unfortunately the promised report of the microscopical examination of their specimens has not yet appeared.

Since then an abundant literature has developed concerning the toxæmic nature of the condition, and four main theories have been advanced as to the source of the toxic materials giving rise to it:

A. Gastro-intestinal tract;

B. The ovum and its appendages;

C. Ovarian secretion;

D. Hepatic lesions.

A. Intestinal Origin.—The most consistent advocate of the intestinal origin of the condition is Dirmoser, who in 1901 summed up his observations in a monograph and two years later reiterated his experience in another article. He pointed out that in women suffering from the vomiting of pregnancy examination of the urine showed an increased amount of uric acid, indoxyl, skatoxyl, aromatic sulphates, phenols and nucleo-albumins; while the following abnormal substances were frequently noted—acetone, diacetic acid, peptone, urobilin, etc. From these observations he concluded that one had to deal with the absorption of toxic materials derived from the decomposition of carbo-hydrates in the stomach and proteids in the intestinal tract, which circulating in the blood brought about the neurosis, which, in turn, caused the vomiting. Moreover, he believed that the results of treatment still further substantiated this view, in that the administration of intestinal antiseptics and the copious employment of rectal irrigation frequently led to cure, or at least to a marked improvement in the condition of the patient. In his article of

1903, he added another link to his chain of evidence by demonstrating that the intestinal contents of such patients were more toxic than in normal individuals, as indicated by the fact that their administration to mice and rabbits was promptly followed by death, while control experiments gave negative results.

B. Fœtal Origin.—In 1902 and 1903 Veit, taking advantage of the fact that portions of the periphery of the ovum-chorionic epithelium and even portions of the villi are constantly gaining access to the maternal circulation during pregnancy, enunciated an hypothesis along the line of Ehrlich's side chain theory, which he believed capable of affording a satisfactory explanation for most of the abnormalities of pregnancy. He held that under normal conditions, the fœtal products gaining access to the maternal blood were readily rendered innocuous, but that when excessive amounts were introduced Nature was no longer able to fulfill her task and consequently cytotoxins were developed, which brought about lesions in the maternal organs and likewise led to hæmolytic changes in the blood.

Veit attempted to demonstrate the correctness of his theory by injecting into rabbits varying quantities of an emulsion of human placentæ; and, upon finding degenerative changes in the kidneys and the presence of albumin in the urine, contended that his point was proven. His conclusions naturally evoked the greatest interest, and similar experiments were promptly undertaken by Weichardt, Leipmann, Wormser, and others, with the result that considerable discredit was cast upon the syncytio-toxin theory. At present the general consensus of opinion seems to be that Veit's conclusions were based upon imperfect methods of experimentation, and that equally positive results would have followed the introduction of beefsteak or any other heterogeneous animal material. At the same time there is no doubt concerning the almost universal occurrence of "placental deportation," and accordingly it would seem rash to conclude that it may not give rise to abnormal conditions in some instances; but at the present time it would seem inadvisable to accept Veit's theory until further experimental contributions conducted along proper lines demonstrate its correctness.

Veit's theory has received a certain amount of support from the observation of hæmoglobinæmia and hæmoglobinuria associated with the jaundice and vomiting of pregnancy by Hirschberg, Schaeffer, Fellner, Brauer, von der Velden, and others. And it must be admitted in all such cases that the abnormal condition of the blood must be due to the action of some hæmolytic agent; but whether this is derived from fœtal cells or from other sources has not as yet been determined.

Shortly afterwards Behm reported to the Berlin Obstetrical Society that he had obtained excellent results in several cases of hyperemesis by the employment of abundant rectal injections of salt solution, and held that his results clearly indicated the toxic origin of the vomiting. He accepted Veit's syncytio-toxic theory in its entirety, and stated that the beneficial

results following the use of saline solutions could be readily explained by supposing that it served to wash out of the system the toxic agents which were produced after the entrance of abnormal amounts of fœtal tissue into the maternal blood.

While there can be no doubt as to the correctness of Behm's actual observations, the objections which have already been made to the acceptance of Veit's theory can be urged still more strongly against the theoretical deductions of the former. Moreover, it is interesting to note that the use of salt infusions in this connection was not original, as they had been employed by Condamin for many years prior to the appearance of Behm's communication. Following the teaching of Veit and Behm, not a few authors, among whom may be mentioned Clivio, Jardine and Kehrer have adopted more or less similar views.

C. Ovarian Origin.—Reference has already been made to the views of Holladay concerning the part played by the secretion of abnormal corpora lutea in the production of vomiting in the latter months of pregnancy. Pierrehughes in 1902, after carefully studying 6 cases, concluded that it was more than probable that in many cases, at least, the vomiting of pregnancy was due to some abnormality in the ovarian secretion. His argumentation was not at all conclusive and would apply equally well to abnormal products from the thyroid, liver, or other organs. It is interesting to note, however, that his conclusions were based in part upon metabolic observations by Meillère, who demonstrated in all his cases a decrease in the amount of chlorides in the urine and a diminished urea coefficient.

At the same time, Pierrehughes and Meillère made the interesting observation that while the amount of urea was found to be diminished when determined by accurate chemical methods, the urine nevertheless decomposed an amount of sodium hypobromite sufficiently large to indicate the presence of a normal urea content. The practical bearing of this observation will be dwelt upon when we consider the differential diagnosis of the several varieties of vomiting.

Somewhat similar views were advanced by Turenne in 1905, who held that the less severe types of vomiting were due to the suppression of the ovarian secretion during pregnancy, and that the condition might be alleviated or cured by supplying the deficiency by the administration of ovarian extract or tablets. He reported 24 cases in which excellent results were obtained by this means.

D. Hepatic Origin.—Reference has already been made to the views expressed by Matthews Duncan, Roughton, and Lomer concerning the possible part played by the liver in the production of vomiting, as well as to the autopsy findings of Lindemann, Champetier de Ribes and Bouffe de Saint-Blaise. The hepatic origin of the condition, however, was first brought prominently forward by Stone in 1903, who reported the autopsy findings in a fatal case of vomiting, in which the liver presented the lesions of acute yellow atrophy, in that the entire central portion of each lobule had undergone complete necrosis, while the peripheral portion showed signs of fatty degeneration, and only a few cells remained perfectly normal.

Stone's observations were confirmed by Ewing, who within the past few months reported finding similar changes in the livers of four women dying from the vomiting of pregnancy, one of whom had a convulsion immediately before death. As the result of his experience, Ewing concludes that both vomiting of pregnancy and eclampsia are closely allied conditions and are associated with similar hepatic lesions, and therefore should be grouped together under a common heading —toxæmia of pregnancy.

Edgar has advanced similar views, which are based upon Ewing's findings and not upon personal observation.

While there can be no doubt as to the correctness of the observations of Stone and Ewing concerning the association of lesions characteristic of acute yellow atrophy of the liver with certain cases of vomiting of pregnancy, I cannot accept their conclusions as to the identity of eclampsia and vomiting, as will be brought out more fully further on.

My own experience with the toxic type of vomiting of pregnancy dates from May, 1903, when I lost a patient after the induction of abortion at the 3d month. (Case I at end of article.) At the time the operation was undertaken her condition was fairly satisfactory and gave fair promise. of a successful outcome. The operation itself was not difficult, and immediately after its completion the vomiting ceased for eighteen hours, after which the patient began to eject at frequent intervals, large quantities of dark, coffee-ground like material without apparent effort. She gradualy passed into a torpid condition and later became comatose and died fifty-four hours after the abortion.

At the autopsy, which I was fortunate enough to obtain, we found changes in the liver, identical with those observed by Stone and Ewing, associated with intense degeneration of the secretory portion of the kidneys. (Fig. 1.)

This case made a deep impression upon me, as the patient clearly seemed to succumb to an intoxication rather than to starvation as is usually stated. But at that time I did not fully appreciate the significance of the hepatic lesions, for whose production I attempted to account by invoking one of the more common explanations, and, finding none, was inclined to regard it merely as an accidental complication.

Further experience, however, soon led me to change my opinion, for within the next year, I saw five other cases of severe vomiting of pregnancy, in all of which I felt compelled to resort to the induction of abortion. Two patients died, one just as the case mentioned above, and the other at the 7th month with the clinical symptoms characteristic of acute yellow atrophy. The remaining three patients were seriously ill, but recovered. Unfortunately, I was unable to obtain an autopsy in the fatal cases, but in two of the cases which recovered (Cases 2 and 3), I was able to make accurate metabolic observations, both before and after the induction of abortion. The results obtained were so surprising as to place the matter in an entirely new light and to force me to conclude

that the hepatic changes certainly played a most prominent part in the fatal issue. Since then I have had an opportunity to observe a fourth toxæmic case, as well as several neurotic ones, in which accurate metabolic observations were made, and which served to confirm me more fully in the view just mentioned.

In the three toxæmic cases (2, 3, and 4) in which careful metabolic observations were made, I found that the total nitrogen output was practically normal, while the urea nitrogen was considerably diminished, and the amount of nitrogen excreted as ammonia greatly increased, so that the so-called ammonia coefficient, instead of representing 3 to 5 per cent of the total nitrogen of the urine, reached 32, 38, and 46 per cent respectively. This condition clearly indicated a marked disturbance in metabolism and can readily be brought into relationship with the hepatic changes.[1]

Since observing my case of acute yellow atrophy of the liver accompanying hyperemesis, I have carefully searched the literature for similar observations and have found the following autopsy reports: one case each reported by Duncan, Roughton, Hirschberg, Lang, Beatty, Stone, Zaborski and four cases by Ewing, which together with my own make a total of twelve observations. Moreover, in five other cases reported respectively by Schmorl, Erismann, Lindemann, Davis, and Zaborski, marked fatty degeneration of the liver and kidneys was noted.

When one contrasts the extremely contradictory results obtained at autopsy upon women dying from the vomiting of pregnancy with the uniformity of the lesions observed in the seventeen cases just mentioned, one cannot fail to suspect that the association between the two conditions cannot be merely accidental, but that they must bear some direct connection to one another. Likewise, it seems very probable to me that many similar cases must have been overlooked in the past, for the reason that the majority of the autopsies were not performed in hospitals, but in private houses, and frequently by persons little skilled in pathological technique, and who, while searching diligently for lesions of the generative or intestinal tract, would very likely overlook so unexpected a change in the liver.

Moreover, when one studies the clinical history of acute yellow atrophy one cannot fail to be impressed with the marked relationship which it and the allied states of icterus gravis, typhoid icterus, etc., bear to pregnancy. According to Lebert, Kerkring in 1706 was the first to report the death of a pregnant woman from icterus gravis, and since that time everyone who has studied the condition has laid stress upon the association, as is. indicated by the writings of Horaczek, Ozanam, Budd, Rokitansky and all subsequent investigators. Thus, Thierfelder stated that 62 per cent of the 143 cases which he collected from the literature affected pregnant women; while Quincke estimates that more than 60 per

---

[1] Since writing the above I have observed three additional cases, with the same urinary findings. In each instance recovery promptly followed the induction of abortion.

cent of all cases occur in women, a majority of whom are pregnant.

Of course it is well known that ordinary acute yellow atrophy of the liver usually occurs in the second half of pregnancy and particularly after the 7th month; while the fatal cases of vomiting of pregnancy are much more common in the first half of gestation. At the same time, however, exceptions occur in both directions, Beatty and Le Masson having reported cases of acute yellow atrophy at the 6th and 8th weeks respectively; while occasional deaths result from vomiting in the second half of pregnancy. If it should eventually be demonstrated that toxæmic vomiting and acute yellow atrophy are really manifestations of similar toxic processes, it would seem difficult to explain their varying behaviour.

From our knowledge of the liver, it would seem that it is in a state of particular susceptibility during pregnancy, when it is much more prone to abnormal processes than at other times. Thus, Tarnier in his graduation thesis in 1857 stated that fatty degeneration of the liver was a usual concomitant of pregnancy and his contention was confirmed by Blot. Unfortunately these observations were made upon women dying from puerperal infection, and as similar observations upon normal pregnant women made in recent years are not at hand, it must remain doubtful for the present whether this condition of the liver is a characteristic accompaniment of pregnancy or merely a sequel of fatal puerperal infection.

At the same time there is no doubt that the liver in pregnancy offers a locus minoris resistentiæ, as is clearly shown by the occurrence of epidemics of catarrhal jaundice at that time. Thus, within the past one hundred years numerous such epidemics have been reported in which large numbers of the inhabitants in certain localities were affected. Under such circumstances the disease ran its ordinary course in men and in non-pregnant women; whereas in pregnant women it was remarkably fatal, as more than one-half the pregnancies ended in abortion or premature labor and many of the women died in coma and occasionally in convulsions. The most important of these epidemics were reported by Kercksig in Ludenscheid, 1794; Charpentier in Rubaix, 1854; Bardinet in Limoges, 1859; Saint Vel in Martinique, 1861; Meunier in Paris, 1871; Smith in St. Paul, Minnesota, 1873; Klingelhoefer in Heusenstamm, 1876 and Young in 1898.

In this connection it is interesting to recall the fact that pregnancy itself sometimes appears to be the etiological factor concerned in the production of the jaundice, as is well illustrated by the fact that certain individuals suffer with jaundice in each pregnancy. Such cases have been reported by Beking, Benedict, Schaeffer, Brauer, van der Velden, and others. In several instances it recurred in from four to six successive pregnancies, and was frequently associated with hæmoglobinæmia and hæmoglobinuria. In Benedict's case the same tendency was noted in two sisters.

Moreover, it should be borne in mind that other functions of the liver are more or less seriously interfered with during pregnancy. Thus, Payer has pointed out that alimentary

glycosuria is readily produced in 80 per cent of all pregnant women. And the investigations of Strauss have shown that the ease with which such a condition can be produced in non-pregnant individuals affords a valuable index as to the degree of hepatic insufficiency. Likewise, Charrin and Guillement have demonstrated that the liver cells of pregnant guinea pigs contain an unusually large amount of glycogen, thereby apparently indicating that less of it is consumed during pregnancy than at other times. They consider that such a condition renders more difficult the storing of additional quantities of glycogen, so that a considerable portion of the sugar ingested is promptly eliminated, instead of being converted into glycogen and stored for future use. If their supposition proves correct, it would afford a satisfactory explanation for the production of alimentary glycosuria.

When one attempts to explain the significance of the changes in metabolism noted in my toxæmic cases, one finds that it is difficult to do so satisfactorily. Ever since Schmiedeberg and Schroeder pointed out that ammonia was a forerunner of urea and was converted into it in the liver, it has been assumed that any condition which interferes with complete oxidation would tend to bring about an increase in the amount of ammonia excreted and a corresponding decrease in the urea output. Minkowski went a little further and showed that the actual precursor of urea was ammonium carbamate, which by oxidation was readily converted into urea. At first glance it would therefore seem permissible to suppose that the necrotic lesions observed in the liver might interfere with the complete oxidation of nitrogenous materials and thus lead to a marked increase in the ammonia coefficient at the expense of the urea. Moreover, such a conclusion would apparently harmonize with the urinary findings in acute yellow atrophy of the liver and acute phosphorus poisoning; since in both conditions there is marked destruction of liver tissue, associated with a considerable increase in the ammonia coefficient, though according to Neuberg and Richter, the latter does not reach so high a figure as in the cases of vomiting studied by me.

On the other hand it is probable that the relation between the liver changes and the high ammonia coefficient is not so direct, and that the increased ammonia output is not necessarily a manifestation of the destruction of liver tissue, but rather indicates that an excessive amount of acid material has been set free in the circulation and whose neutralization is absolutely essential if life is to continue. Thus, Münzer believes that such an explanation holds good for both acute yellow atrophy and phosphorus poisoning and, reasoning by analogy, there is no inherent reason why it should not apply to certain cases of toxæmic vomiting of pregnancy as well. Unfortunately it is extremely difficult at present to formulate a well defined expression of opinion in this regard, as the entire doctrine of acid intoxication seems to be still sub judice. Thus, while diabetes is considered the classical example of intoxication with oxy-butyric acid, and the increased ammonia coefficient accompanying it merely a manifestation of an attempt to neutralize it, it must nevertheless be admitted that our knowledge of the ultimate factors concerned in the excessive production of the acid is still very fragmentary.

Another example of excessive ammonia output is found in certain cases of gastro-enteritis in children, to which Czerny and Keller directed attention in 1897. They pointed out that in such cases the ammonia coefficient frequently rose as high as 30 to 52 per cent, and were in doubt whether it was a manifestation of an acid intoxication or was directly due to some disturbance in the function of the liver, probably resulting from absorption of toxic material from the intestines. Pfaundler on the other hand contended that neither view was correct, and held that the high ammonia output was attributable almost entirely to the presence of excessive amounts of fat in the food, which was decomposed in the intestines into its component acids, which were readily absorbed and required prompt neutralization. Plausibility is lent to his contention by the fact that the ammonia coefficient can be promptly lowered by simply decreasing the amount of fat taken with the food.

Moreover, Schittenhelm has shown that in adults a considerable increase in the ammonia coefficient may be brought about by arbitrary variations in the character of the diet and by other artificial conditions. Thus, he observed that an increase in the amount of fat ingested, or the administration of dilute hydrochloric acid, would readily bring about such a condition, which would promptly disappear upon the administration of an alkali, or a change in the character of the food. Moreover, he showed very clearly that various abnormal conditions of the liver were likely to lead to a similar change, and considered that variations in the ammonia coefficient of the urine might afford a fairly reliable index of the extent to which the hepatic function had become impaired.

That the absorption of toxic materials from the intestines may lead to changes in the ammonia output was shown by the experiments of Glaessner. This investigator, finding that none of the usual methods brought about prolonged constipation in dogs, exsected a portion of the intestine and replaced it in the reverse direction, so that its peristaltic movements were opposed to those of the rest of the bowel. This operation had the desired effect and the dog remained constipated for ten days to two weeks, at the end of which time an abundant stool would be passed, to be followed by another period of constipation. Careful study showed that the metabolism was of the ordinary type immediately following evacuation of the bowels, whereas the ammonia coefficient increased to double its usual value as the constipation became more marked.

To still further complicate the interpretation of the matter, Folin and Möner have shown that in individuals obtaining an insufficient amount of food, or who are actually starving, there is a marked increase in the ammonia coefficient, which in the cases studied by them reached 26.79 and 40 per cent respectively. Moreover, the former investigator showed that the substitution of a purely vegetable for a mixed diet was attended by a marked decrease in the urea and an increase in the ammonia coefficient, while some of the nitrogenous substances, such as kreatinin, underwent a still more marked distortion.

From the considerations just adduced, it would therefore seem evident that an increase in the ammonia coefficient may or may not afford conclusive evidence of the existence of an acid intoxication, and that in the present state of our knowledge, it would be inadvisable to dogmatise too strongly concerning its significance. This is particularly the case in my own observations, as acetone, diacetic, oxy-butyric acid, and allied substances were not found in the urine, and leucin and tyrosin were likewise absent in the two cases in which they were searched for. I did not attempt to determine the alkalinity of the blood, although it is hardly likely that notable changes would have been detected, even though an underlying acid intoxication were present, since an excess of acid would immediately have been neutralized by an increased production of ammonia and thus withdrawn itself from observation.

However, it seems to me that even had we been able to determine the presence of abnormal acids in the urine, the existence of an acid intoxication would not necessarily have been demonstrated, and while we might seriously consider its possibility we should nevertheless have been unable to advance a satisfactory explanation for its production. This being the case, I feel at present that I must remain content with demonstrating that in certain cases of toxæmic vomiting of pregnancy there is a marked disturbance in metabolism, which is manifested by a great increase in the ammonia coefficient, and that it must be left to future investigations to determine whether the change is directly due to the inability of the diseased liver to effect complete oxidation, or whether it is a manifestation of an acid intoxication or some other condition. Moreover, we are absolutely ignorant concerning the nature of the toxic material concerned, and whether it is derived from the fœtus or mother.

SYMPTOMS.

It is difficult to give a satisfactory definition of the pernicious vomiting of pregnancy, for the reason that the gradations between the ordinary morning sickness and the more severe forms of vomiting are often so gradual as to render it difficult to predict in a given case whether the condition may continue without injury to the health of the patient, or will pass into pernicious vomiting. Generally speaking it may be said that vomiting should be regarded as pernicious in character when it occurs so frequently as to interfere seriously with taking food, or leads to marked emaciation.

We are indebted to Dubois for the classical clinical picture of pernicious vomiting, which he divided into three stages. In the first the constant vomiting is associated with considerable emaciation and frequently with a troublesome dribbling of saliva. At the same time the urine becomes scanty and highly colored and the pulse somewhat accelerated. In the second stage the vomiting becomes still more severe, the emaciation more pronounced and the breath assumes a peculiar acid and fœtid odor. As the patient becomes worse, the pulse increases in frequency and eventually there may be a slight rise in temperature. Finally in the third stage there is an apparent amelioration in the symptoms for a short time, during which the vomiting sometimes ceases and the patient and her friends become encouraged as to the outcome. Unfortunately, this is merely a transient condition, and the patient soon passes into a delirious or torpid condition and dies in coma or convulsions. During the last period there is no hope for recovery, which was not out of the question in the preceding stages.

My own experience has led me to believe that the clinical picture drawn by Dubois cannot always be followed at the bedside, as pernicious vomiting may occur either in an acute or chronic form, the latter being more frequent.

In the acute type, which according to my experience is always toxæmic in character, death may occur within ten days or two weeks after the onset of vomiting. In such cases the patient, who was previously perfectly well, or simply suffering from what appeared to be ordinary " morning sickness," suddenly begins to vomit everything she ingests, and soon presents signs of considerable prostration. The condition is usually associated with but little elevation in the pulse rate and fever is absent. After it has persisted for a number of days the patient begins to eject at frequent intervals and apparently with but little effort considerable quantities of dark, brownish, coffee-ground like material, and soon passes into a torpid condition and later dies in coma, which is sometimes disturbed by convulsions. (Cases 1 and 4.) This variety of vomiting is not necessarily associated with great emaciation, as one of my patients (Case No. 4) died while apparently well nourished and with a pulse of 96.

In the early stages of this form of vomiting the ordinary tests show that the urine is apparently perfectly normal, though naturally it is diminished in quantity on account of the small intake of fluids. In the last stages of the disease, however, it contains albumin, blood, and various varieties of tube casts, though this may be noted only a few hours before death. As a rule the temperature is not materially elevated; but occasionally shortly before death, it may reach a considerable height, and in one of my cases, not reported in this article, it registered 108° immediately before the fatal outcome. Occasionally in the last stages of the disease the patient may present an icteric discoloration of the conjunctivæ or even a decided icterus, though the latter is exceptional.

In the chronic form on the other hand, which may be toxæmic or neurotic in origin, the vomiting may continue for weeks or months, during which the patient becomes more and more emaciated, apparently entirely as the result of the ingestion of insufficient amounts of food. Under such circumstances she gradually becomes too weak to pursue her ordinary avocations and eventually is forced to take to bed.

At the same time the pulse slowly increases in frequency, fever is usually absent and the black vomit of the acute variety is lacking until the very last stages of the disease. Consciousness is preserved until shortly before death, which is to be attributed in great part to inanition; while in the acute cases it is manifestly the result of an intoxication.

That inanition is the usual cause of death in the chronic variety has been generally recognized from the time of Dubois, and its importance was particularly insisted upon by Sutugin. Moreover, it is interesting to note that Frank in 1893, from the first study of the metabolism in this condition reached a similar conclusion, as he found that the quantity of nitrogen excreted by the urine was far greater than that taken in by the mouth.

In none of the cases which I have observed have the patients complained of disturbances in the olfactory sense, the so-called hyperosmia upon which Horwitz laid so much stress; though his observations in this regard are both interesting and significant.

The outline of the clinical history which I have just given applies particularly to cases of pernicious vomiting occurring in the first half of pregnancy. On the other hand, when it continues into the second half of pregnancy or originates in that period, the recognition of the significance of the condition becomes more difficult and the symptoms are frequently attributed to the typical pre-eclamptic toxæmia. Moreover, when the affection is associated with jaundice it usually presents the typical clinical picture of acute yellow atrophy; while if icterus is absent and the patient is only seen after she has passed into a comatose condition, it is quite natural to mistake the condition for eclampsia, especially as examination of the urine would show the presence of albumin, casts, and frequently blood.

DIAGNOSIS.

Hyperemesis, as indicated above, should be diagnosticated whenever the vomiting becomes so constant that the patient is unable to retain any considerable quantity of food, or presents considerable emaciation. Much more important, however, than the mere diagnosis of pernicious vomiting, is the determination as to whether one has to deal with its reflex, neurotic or toxæmic variety, since upon this point depends the treatment to be pursued.

Accordingly, whenever a woman suffers from serious vomiting, even though it may not be absolutely pernicious in type, a careful vaginal examination should be made for the purpose of detecting any abnormality of the generative tract or ovum. The existence of a displaced uterus, an ovarian cyst, or a pelvic inflammatory mass is readily detected by the usual methods; while an increase in the size of the uterus out of proportion to the supposed duration of the pregnancy should arouse suspicion as to the existence of a hydatidiform mole or hydramnios.

On the other hand, it is extremely difficult to diagnosticate decidual endometritis with certainty, although its existence should be suspected when it is known that the patient suffered from endometritis before conception, or when a dark brownish or brick-dust-colored discharge flows from the cervix. In the latter event, the occurrence of a spontaneous abortion may be expected.

If no abnormalities can be detected on the part of the generative tract or ovum, the diagnosis must lie between the neurotic or toxæmic types of vomiting. Unfortunately, as far as my experience goes, they cannot be differentiated positively by clinical symptoms, except at the terminal period of the affection, when it is too late to institute effective treatment, and therefore, our only resource lies in a thorough chemical examination of the urine, and the determination of the ammonia coefficient.

In order to make such a determination the entire amount of urine passed during the 24 hours should be collected, care being taken to place enough chloroform in the vessel to prevent decomposition. Then the total nitrogen should be determined by the Kjeldahl method and the amounts of urea and ammonia by the methods of Schoendorf and Schloessing respectively. In normal pregnancy, and even in neurotic vomiting, the ammonia coefficient varies from 3 to 5 per cent (Cases 5 to 7); while in the toxæmic type it may attain immense proportions, reaching 32, 38½, and 46 per cent respectively, as in cases 2, 3, and 4.

Thus far my experience with the toxæmic type of vomiting has not been sufficiently extensive to permit me to lay down definite rules as to the extent to which the ammonia coefficient may rise without particular danger to the patient; but at present it would seem that its increase to 10 or 15 per cent would justify the diagnosis of toxæmic vomiting, and would afford an urgent indication for the prompt termination of the pregnancy. In case 4 the ammonia coefficient was only 16 per cent when I first saw the patient, who did not appear to be seriously ill; and while it enabled me to make a diagnosis of the toxæmic origin of the vomiting, I felt justified in delaying interference and testing the efficacy of medicinal treatment. The outcome of the case, however, showed that I was in error, as the patient died in coma 48 hours after the induction of abortion with an ammonia coefficient of 46 per cent.

In addition to the determination of the total nitrogen and the urea and ammonia coefficients, it is if possible advisable to determine the other nitrogen subdivisions, as they may possibly throw still further light upon the nature of the condition. The urine should be likewise examined for the presence of leucin and tyrosin, which were absent in my cases, but were present in several of those examined by Ewing.

Unfortunately the determination of the ammonia coefficient cannot be undertaken by the ordinary physician in his office, but demands the services of a well trained chemist. In this connection it is extremely important to note that a rough estimate of the amount of ammonia cannot be made by determining the amount of urea by the Doremus apparatus, and assuming that a decrease in its amount indicates an increased ammonia coefficient, for the reason that with this test the ammonia as well as the urea is decomposed by the

sodium hypo-bromite. Accordingly it might readily happen that the test would indicate the presence of a normal amount of urea, when in reality it was markedly diminished and its place taken by ammonia. This fallacy was exemplified in case 1, in which a normal urea output, as determined by the Doremus method, and the absence of albumin and casts caused me to overlook the toxæmic nature of the condition until death was imminent. I have already mentioned that a similar observation was made by Pierrehughes.

Another complication is that the determination of ammonia by the Schloessing method requires the best part of 48 hours, so that the result cannot be known for two days after the urine has been placed in the hands of the chemist. It is therefore to be hoped that the method of distilling the ammonia in vacuo will prove thoroughly satisfactory, as under such circumstances the determination can be made within a few hours. At present, however, this is a matter for decision on the part of the professional chemist and need not detain us here.

In connection with the question of diagnosis it is important to direct attention to the condition of the pulse, as it is generally stated that some idea of the severity of the case can be obtained from its character and frequency. My experience, however, has led me to believe that this is not necessarily true, since in case 4 the patient died with a pulse of 96. Moreover, a rise in temperature is not nearly so common as was believed by the early observers, and many patients die without any manifestation of fever. The occurrence of the black vomit on the other hand, is a sign of the greatest value and indicates a most serious condition; and although it cannot be said that its occurrence is necessarily indicative of death, it must nevertheless be regarded as of most ominous prognostic import.

In view of what has been said concerning the connection between acute yellow atrophy of the liver and the toxæmic type of vomiting, the occurrence of jaundice in pregnant women suffering from hyperemesis should always be regarded as ominous, and as indicating some serious derangement of the liver, rather than as a manifestation of a simple catarrhal condition.

When discussing the symptoms of the vomiting of pregnancy, particularly in the latter months, it was pointed out how readily it might be mistaken for eclampsia, especially if the patient were comatose; and Ewing has gone a step further and stated that he considers both acute yellow atrophy of the liver and eclampsia as manifestations of one and the same toxæmia. This conclusion, however, is so absolutely opposed to my own experience, which has taught me that the two diseases differ radically, whether considered from a clinical, chemical, or histological point of view, that I cannot allow it to pass unchallenged.

Clinically, eclampsia is nearly always preceded by a characteristic pre-eclamptic toxæmia, which is usually associated with pronounced general symptoms and early evidence of serious disturbance in the renal and circulatory functions—scanty urine, containing albumin and casts, and œdema. In vomiting on the other hand, the urine is practically normal in amount until shortly before death, or at least is in direct proportion to the quantity of fluid ingested; whereas in the pre-eclampsia toxæmia it is always considerably diminished, notwithstanding the administration of diuretics and of large quantities of fluid by the mouth or rectum. Moreover, in vomiting, albumin and casts usually appear only in the terminal stage of the disease; while œdema is never present.

From a chemical point of view the difference is even more striking. In eclampsia there is usually a marked decrease in the total amount of nitrogen excreted, and while there may be a considerable diminution in the urea coefficient, pronounced variations do not occur in the ammonia coefficient, though occasionally it may rise to a slight extent. In vomiting, on the other hand, the total amount of nitrogen may be quite normal, while the amomnia coefficient becomes unusually high. (Compare charts 1 to 3 with 4 to 6.) My own experience would seem to indicate that an increase in the ammonia coefficient is of favorable prognostic import in eclampsia; whereas its significance is just the reverse in the vomiting of pregnancy.

From a pathological point of view, the lesions in the two conditions differ so markedly that I do not see how it is possible for anyone, who has once observed them, to consider that they are at all related. In eclampsia, as was first pointed out by Jürgens, Schmorl, and others, the lesion consists in hæmorrhagic necroses occurring in the portal spaces, dependent upon thrombotic processes in the smaller portal branches. At first they are sharply limited to the portal spaces, but as they enlarge, they invade the lobules from the periphery toward the centre; and are so characteristic that their mere presence justifies the diagnosis of eclampsia without any knowledge of the clinical history of the case. On the other hand, in the liver lesions accompanying the toxæmic vomiting of pregnancy the changes are purely degenerative in character, and begin about the central vein of the lobule and gradually extend towards its periphery. These differences are so sharply marked that it seems incredible to me that they could be confounded with one another.

After reading Ewing's article, I wrote to Schmorl, who has had the most extensive experience in the study of the liver lesions of eclampsia, and inquired whether he had ever seen the eclamptic lesions beginning in the center of the lobules. He replied in the negative and stated that they always began in the tissue about the periphery and only invaded the lobule itself secondarily. Moreover, Opie in his article upon zonal necroses of the liver, which was based upon material studied in the Pathological Laboratory of the Johns Hopkins University, stated that the lesions in eclampsia were highly characteristic, as it was only in that disease that they began at the periphery of the lobule, while in acute yellow atrophy the central or mid-zonal areas were the first to become involved. Therefore, from my own experience, as well as that of Schmorl, I cannot understand how it is possible for one to confound the lesions in the two conditions. Moreover, when one takes into consideration the difference in the clinical history and metabolism of the two diseases, the case becomes absolutely convincing.

From the evidence at present available, it would accordingly appear that we have to deal with at least two varieties of toxæmia of pregnancy, one giving rise to eclampsia or the pre-eclamptic toxæmia and the other to the vomiting of pregnancy and acute yellow atrophy, though it is quite within the range of possibility that further research will demonstrate the existence of still other varieties.

PROGNOSIS.

Generally speaking it may be said that the prognosis is excellent in the reflex and neurotic forms of vomiting, provided they are properly treated. At the same time it must be admitted that patients suffering from them may succumb to inanition if proper measures are not instituted in good time.

In toxæmic vomiting, on the other hand, in view of the serious organic lesions and changes in metabolism, the prognosis is most grave and it seems safe to say that death will be the universal outcome if the toxæmia is pronounced, unless the pregnancy is promptly interrupted. Thus far, six examples of the toxæmic type have come under my observation (Cases 1, 2, 3, and 4 and two others not mentioned in this article), in all of which I felt obliged to induce abortion, but notwithstanding it, death occurred in 4 instances, a mortality of 66⅔ per cent. Of course these figures are not sufficiently large to justify one in drawing very general conclusions, but at the same time they clearly demonstrate the great gravity of the condition.

TREATMENT.

The treatment to be pursued in a given case of vomiting of pregnancy depends entirely upon the variety with which one has to deal. It is assumed that medicinal treatment has been tried without avail before the medical adviser comes to regard the case as at all serious.

If any abnormality of the generative tract or ovum be found it should be remedied as far as possible; the retro-displaced uterus should be replaced and held in position by a properly fitting pessary; ovarian tumors should be removed and inflammatory masses treated by appropriate anti-phlogistic measures. On the other hand, if hydramnios or hydatidiform mole be diagnosticated the pregnancy should be promptly terminated.

If the toxæmic variety of vomiting be diagnosticated, abortion should be induced as soon as its nature is fully recognized, as it would seem to offer the only chance of saving the patient, since the lesions associated with it are apparently incompatible with life if far advanced, and especially as there is no reason to suppose that they can be materially influenced by medicinal or dietetic treatment. After the uterus has been emptied, the patient should be given abundant saline injections by the rectum or subcutaneously if the former are not well borne. The stomach should be washed out occasionally with a weak solution of sodium bicarbonate if the vomiting persists. No attempt should be made to feed the patient by mouth, and even ice should be withheld until the vomiting ceases, all reliance being placed upon the salt infusion and enemata and the employment of rectal feeding.

On the other hand, if the neurotic variety of vomiting is diagnosticated, the treatment will depend to a considerable extent upon the impressionability of the patient. In certain exceptional cases a vigorous moral lecture may prove all that is necessary. In other instances the patient should be assured that her condition will not terminate fatally nor require the induction of abortion, and that it will probably yield to intelligent treatment. She should then be given some harmless remedy and receive the most minute directions as to the character of her food and the manner in which it should be taken. If such mild methods do not suffice, the patient should be put to bed in charge of a sensible nurse and the family and friends excluded from the room; all feeding by the mouth should be stopped and its place taken by the administration of saline and nutritive enemata by the rectum. Occasionally it may be necessary to add small quantities of laudanum to the enemata, or to give an occasional hypodermic of morphia.

If, however, such treatment is not followed by improvement within three or four days the patient should be threatened with removal to a hospital, and if the threat does not prove effectual, it should be carried out actually and the patient placed in a private room in a well regulated hospital, where a rigorous rest cure can be instituted upon the most approved plan. In my experience such drastic measures are rarely necessary, as the modified rest cure, as outlined above, will usually be followed by the cessation of vomiting within a few days and the vast majority of patients will be on the highroad to recovery within a week. (See Cases 5, 6, and 7).

Of course it is possible that occasional cases may not be amenable to such treatment and under such circumstances it may become necessary to resort to the induction of abortion in order to prevent death from starvation; but I believe that with an accurate diagnosis and sufficient assurance on the part of the physician, such a resort will become less and less frequently necessary, and that the operation will be reserved almost entirely for the cases of toxæmic vomiting.

HISTORY OF CASES.

CASE I.—*Toxæmic vomiting. Mrs. P.* (Fig. 1.)

I first saw the patient on April 22, 1903, when she desired to ascertain whether she was pregnant. She was a tall, thin, delicate-looking woman, 28 years old, who had been married two years and had never been pregnant. Her last menstrual period occurred on February 10 and lasted five days, but in March and April there was a slight flow at the regular time, but much less abundant than usual. Prior to seeing me she had suffered a good deal from nausea.

On examination the uterus was found to be enlarged to the size of a two-months' pregnancy and softened, so that there was little doubt about the diagnosis.

A few days later I saw the patient again, when she was complaining intensely of nausea and vomiting, for which I regulated the bowels and ordered some capsules of pepsin and nitrate of silver. As these were without effect, various other remedies were employed with the same result. Gradually the nausea and vomiting became so intense that the patient was unable to retain anything at all, so that on May 6 I resorted to rectal feeding and ceased all attempts to administer food by the mouth. From this time she received two nutritive enemata daily consisting of 12 oz. of peptonized milk and 2 eggs, as well as a third enema of 750 cc. of salt solution. The enemata were borne extremely well and gave no discomfort, but nevertheless the patient grew weaker and more emaciated and still suffered severely from vomiting. Her pulse, which was 70 when I first saw her, slowly rose to 92.

On May 15 I asked her physician, Dr. W. F. Lockwood, to see her in consultation. At that time she was suffering intensely from profuse salivation and was constantly vomiting small quantities of a dark brownish-looking fluid and complaining of intense pain in the epigastric region. In spite of the comparatively low pulse, it was decided that the prompt induction of abortion was indicated, which was done on the afternoon of the 16th.

The cervix was dilated without great difficulty by means of Goodell's and Hegar's dilators sufficiently to permit the introduction of one finger into the uterus. The ovum was then detached from the uterine wall and broken up into small pieces, which were readily removed by means of ovum forceps. A douche of sterile salt solution was then given. During the attempt to introduce the finger into the uterus the outlet was considerably torn, so that it was necessary to repair it with three silk-worm gut sutures.

The patient stood the operation well and was put back to bed in good condition. For the following 18 hours her condition improved markedly, and the nausea and vomiting ceased entirely. At the end of that period they reappeared, however, and the patient constantly vomited small amounts of a coffee-ground-like material with almost no effort. This could only be checked by the administration of morphia hypodermically, which was continued throughout the 17th and 18th, but before its administration her condition became torpid and she gave the impression of suffering from a profound toxæmia.

Gradually the pulse became quicker and in spite of the administration of nutritive enemata, subcutaneous salt infusions, and the hypodermic use of digitalis and strychnia, it became more and more rapid. On the morning of the 19th it reached 119, and slowly increased in frequency until she died at 9 p. m. The temperature was normal until the morning of the day of death, when it reached 101.5°. During the last 12 hours of life the patient was absolutely unconscious and died without an effort.

The urine was examined several times during the illness and the day before the induction of abortion the 24-hour specimen amounted to 750 cc. and contained 30 grammes of urea as estimated by the Doremus ureometer. There was no trace of albumin, while microscopic examination was negative. No examination was made after the operation, so that it cannot be said whether albumin was present or not, though from the condition of the kidneys at autopsy, its absence would have been surprising. Unfortunately an accurate chemical examination of the urine was not made in this instance.

ABSTRACT OF AUTOPSY PROTOCOL. NO. 2110. DR. H. T. MARSHALL.

Anatomical Diagnosis.—" Recent laceration of the vagina with infiltration into adjacent tissues. Lacerated cervix. Portion of placenta adherent to and growing into uterine wall. Uterus of early pregnancy. Fatty degeneration, areas of necrosis and bile staining of liver. Fatty degeneration and bile staining of kidneys. Chronic adhesive pleurisy left side. Old latent tuberculosis of two-thirds of upper lobe of left lung. Scar at right apex."

Body of a well-built, sparely nourished woman. No œdema.

No jaundice. Pupils equal. Slight post-mortem discoloration of dependent parts. Subcutaneous fat slight in amount.

Peritoneal cavity negative.

Thorax.—Pleural cavities dry. Right pleural cavity is clear. On the left side dense adhesions between upper lobe and chest wall. Pericardial cavity clear.

Heart.—Apparently normal; valves clear. Myocardium is soft, opaque, yellowish, and apparently bile stained.

Lungs.—Upper lobe of left lung greatly reduced in size. Contains a few calcified and caseous foci. Small apical scar in right lung.

No structures, vessels, or glomeruli can be made out. The pyramids are pale and their periphery shows lines and areas of fatty appearance, which is particularly marked in their outer third. The renal pelves are normal.

·*Genitalia.*—Bladder normal. Tubes and ovaries normal. Uterus appears normal, and measures 11 cm. from fundus to cervix and 8 cm. between the insertions of the tubes. The external os is roughened and shows some superficial necrosis. On section the uterine cavity appears clear and normal, except a rough, shaggy, reddish area, which projects 6 to 7 mm. above the general surface on the posterior wall, near the fundus and extending to the right

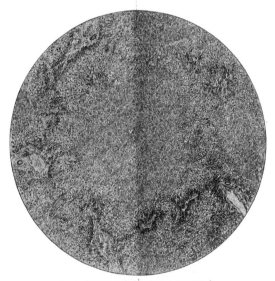

Fig. 1.—Showing Central Necrosis of Liver Lobule.

Liver.—Weight 1000 grammes. Is small and of a bright yellow color, with smooth surface and soft consistence. On section it presents a very fatty, bile-stained appearance, with areas of degeneration and necrosis evident to the naked eye. The capillaries stand out very prominently between the fatty and yellow strands. Except that the degeneration is not so extreme, the section suggests acute yellow atrophy. No nodules in liver. Gall-bladder normal.

Stomach.—Is small and contains about 500 cc. of dark fluid, containing blood cells, bile, and débris. Mucosa normal.

Intestines, spleen, pancreas, and *thyroid* normal.

Kidneys.—Both kidneys present an identical appearance and are considerably enlarged. The capsule strips off readily leaving a bile-stained, opaque, yellow surface, with no vessels showing. On section the cortex measures 7 to 8 mm., is very yellow, opaque, and granular and slightly raised above the level of the pyramids.

cornu. On section this presents a soft and somewhat friable appearance and extends some distance down into the muscular wall. It appears to be decidedly infiltrating, but no signs of it can be found outside of its original boundaries.

Microscopic Examination. Liver.—Under the low power, sections of the liver stained with hæmatoxylin and eosin present a remarkably mottled appearance, about one-half of the section being occupied by rounded and irregularly shaped areas which stain bright pink with eosin and are separated from one another by less brightly staining tissue. Upon closer examination it is seen that these areas correspond to the central portions of the liver lobules, all of which are involved in the process. The individual lobules are sharply marked off from one another and the interlobular spaces present a normal appearance with connective tissue, bloodvessels, and bile-ducts. Nowhere is there any hæmorrhage into the portal spaces, nor any trace of thrombosis of their vessels.

In each lobule three distinct zones may be distinguished: peripheral, midzonal, and central. The peripheral zone consists of one or two layers of practically normal liver cells with brightly staining nuclei and a faintly granular protoplasm. In places even this narrow zone of normal cells is imperfect, so that the cells of the midzonal layers of adjacent lobules abut directly upon one another. The midzonal portion of the lobules varies in thickness, but in general occupies one-half of the distance between the central vein and the periphery. It is made up of large, irregularly shaped cells, whose nuclei stain fairly well and whose protoplasm is almost entirely replaced by a number of vacuole-like structures nearly as large as the nuclei. These probably represent the location of fat droplets, which were dissolved out by the hardening fluids, but as osmic acid specimens were not available, positive statements cannot be made in this regard. In this layer, there is considerable engorgement of the intralobular capillaries. The connective-tissue elements are well preserved and in places appear somewhat increased in number. No leucocytes are present. The central portion of each lobule, which occupies at least half of its total area, is marked off from the midzonal layers by an irregular, wavy line, though in places it is perfectly apparent that the two portions merge into one another. The central portion stains brightly with eosin, and in many lobules is made up of absolutely necrotic cells with a coarsely granular structure, no nuclei of any kind being visible. In others an occasional connective-tissue nucleus can be distinguished, while in rare instances the degenerated nuclei of some of the liver cells take on an indistinct stain with hæmotoxylin. In some of the lobules there is a well-preserved central vein; in others its location is indicated by a mass of nuclei, while in still others all trace of it has disappeared. (Fig. 1.)

Kidneys.—Sections show that the glomeruli present a practically normal appearance. The secretory portion of the renal tubules on the other hand is almost entirely necrotic and the cells of the tubules are converted into irregular, coarsely granular, vacuolated masses, which contain only an occasional faintly staining nucleus. In many places the lumina of the tubules are obliterated, while in others they are more or less completely filled with granular material, which occasionally contains red-blood cells. The collecting tubules, on the contrary, appear to be perfectly normal and their cells stain in the typical manner. The connective tissue portion of the kidneys appears unchanged.

Uterus.—Sections through the projection at the fundus, which was noted at autopsy, show that it is composed almost entirely of fibrin, but immediately adjoining the uterine wall it encloses a few chorionic villi, which present a normal appearance. The decidua presents its characteristic structure, except that it appears richer in fœtal cells than is usually the case.

Placenta.—Sections through the placenta removed at the time of operation present the appearance characteristic of early pregnancy. The villi are covered by two layers of epithelium—syncytium and Langhans' layer—and present a myxomatous stroma, which contains but a few blood-vessels. Many giant cells are present in the intervillous spaces and occasional trophoblastic islands are seen.

CASE II.—*Toxæmic Vomiting. Mrs. A. Chart No. 1.*

The patient was seen October 26, 1903, in consultation with Dr. James Bosley, from whom I obtained the following history: 29 years old, has been married 7 years, but has never been pregnant; has always been perfectly healthy, although of a somewhat nervous disposition. The last menstrual period occurred on August 1, 1903. On September 9 she began to suffer from nausea and vomiting, which gradually became worse in spite of vigorous treatment. For the past two weeks the patient has been unable to retain food and has vomited almost constantly. She has lost approximately 20 pounds in weight. The day before I saw her

she had been seen in consultation by Dr. I. E. Atkinson, who recommended the induction of abortion.

Examination showed a very emaciated patient with eyes sunken far back in their orbits. She complained of intense pain in the epigastric region and stated that she vomited almost constantly. At the side of the bed was a basin containing a quantity of coffee-ground-like material which she had recently vomited. The patient looked extremely ill; her pulse was 132 and temperature normal. The heart and lungs were normal. There was apparently a slight

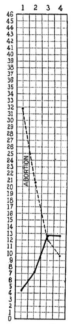

CHART 1.—Toxæmic Vomiting.

In this and the following charts, the solid line indicates total nitrogen and the broken line ammonia. Each square of the chart corresponds to 1 gramme of nitrogen and 1% of ammonia. The figures at top of charts indicate the day of observation.

diminution in the liver dullness, whose lower edge was two fingers' breadth above the costal margin. On palpation the fundus of the uterus could be felt just above the pubes.

In view of the serious condition of the patient it was determined that abortion should be brought on the following day. The delay was for the purpose of allowing the collection of a 24-hour specimen of urine. A trained nurse was procured and instructed to administer two rectal enemata of 500 cc. of salt solution during the next 24 hours. As soon as the first specimen of urine, which amounted to 500 cc. had been collected, the operation was proceeded with.

Examination at that time showed the vagina was short and the external os small, hard, and virginal. The cervix was dilated by means of Goodell's and Hegar's dilators until the index finger could be readily introduced into the uterus, which required about 25 minutes. The ovum was then separated from its attachment by the finger, its fragments being removed by means of an ovum

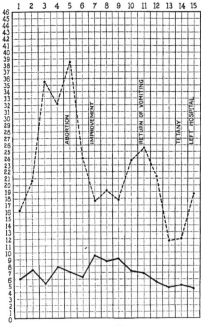

CHART 2.—Toxæmic Vomiting.

forceps. A uterine douche was then given and the uterus packed with gauze. The patient stood the operation well and was put back to bed in good condition with a pulse of 124.

She began to improve almost immediately after the operation, and within 24 hours the pulse had become slower, the nausea had practically ceased and a marked change in her general appearance was noted. After this convalescence was so rapid that it was unnecessary for me to see the patient after the 4th day. The pulse reached 72 on the 6th day after operation, and the highest temperature was 100.4° on the 2d day.

Chart No. 1 gives a graphic idea of the condition of the urine, which for the 24 hours immediately preceding the operation presented an ammonia coefficient of 32%. Albumin or casts were

at no time present. The specimen of urine examined one month later was perfectly normal, with an ammonia coefficient of 4%.

CASE III.—*Toxæmic Vomiting. Mrs. C. Obst. No. 1710, J. H. H. Chart No. 2.*

The patient was seen on February 25, 1904, in consultation with Dr. Geo. B. Reynolds, when I obtained the following history: 37 years old, married 14 months. One miscarriage at 2 months 8 months ago. Was in excellent health prior to the present illness. The last menstrual period began December 13, 1903. Four weeks later the patient began to suffer with indigestion, which was soon followed by nausea and vomiting, accompanied by violent pain in the epigastric region. For the past three weeks the nausea and vomiting has been intense, no solid food being retained for the past two weeks, and for the past two days even the blandest fluids cause immediate vomiting. During this period she has suffered almost constantly from severe headache, and has lost 15 to 20 pounds in weight.

On examination the patient was found to be a small, emaciated woman with a pale and haggard face. The lips and mucous membranes were without color and the tongue thickly coated. She was vomiting small quantities of clear fluid at frequent intervals. Auscultation revealed no abnormalities; pulse 120 and weak, temperature normal. The liver dullness was normal. The abdomen was not distended or painful on pressure. The fundus of the uterus could not be felt above the symphysis pubis. Vaginal examination negative, except for 8 to 10 weeks' pregnant uterus.

On account of her surroundings the patient was immediately transferred to the Johns Hopkins Hospital, where she was kept under observation for four days and nourished almost exclusively by the rectum and given copious enemata of saline solution. During this period the fluid intake and output were carefully measured and the amount of total nitrogen and the ammonia coefficient determined. At the end of this time her condition was worse rather than better, and as seen from the accompanying chart, the ammonia coefficient reached 35.5% on the 3d day.

In view of her condition it was thought best to attempt the induction of abortion by a bougie, which was readily introduced without anæsthesia at noon February 29, when her temperature was 99.2° and pulse 112. As the bougie did not bring on uterine contractions, it was removed the following morning and the uterus emptied by means of the finger and ovum forceps. The patient stood the operation well and was put back to bed in good condition.

Following the operation the patient improved slowly until March 5, when she became torpid and drowsy and gave the impression of being profoundly intoxicated. At the same time the nausea and vomiting, which had almost ceased, increased in severity. As seen by the chart this was accompanied by a rise in the ammonia coefficient from 18 to 25%. Following this there was improvement for several days until the 9th of March, when the nausea and vomiting reappeared and the patient developed a tetany, which continued for two days. During this period the nausea and vomiting were very severe and the patient impressed one as being desperately ill, the pulse varied between 88 and 100 and was of poor volume. By March 11 her condition had improved considerably, and the nausea had disappeared, so that she was able to take two meals of solid food during the day. As the patient had become dissatisfied with the hospital, she was allowed to go home at this time, although far from well.

She eventually made a good recovery and on returning to the hospital the following May had so improved in appearance that she was not recognized. The urinary examination at that time showed an ammonia coefficient of 4%.

At no time during the illness were albumin or casts present in the urine. The highest temperature was 100° F. on the day of abortion. Chart No. 2 gives a good idea of the relation between the total nitrogen and the ammonia coefficient.

CASE IV.—*Toxæmic Vomiting. Mrs. S. Obst. No. 2116. Chart No. 3.*

The patient was seen on March 20, 1905, in consultation with Dr. A. K. Bond, from whom I obtained the following history: 33 years of age, married October, 1904, no previous pregnancies. No serious illness, except typhoid fever five years ago. He was first consulted on the 13th of March, when the patient stated that she believed that she was two months pregnant, having menstruated last January 13, 1905. The next day she complained considerably of nausea and vomiting, which had begun February 20, 1905, and asked that something be done to relieve it. Simple remedies were administered without effect. By March 17, the vomiting had become so distressing that nothing could be retained by the stomach. The vomited matter consisted either of recently ingested food or of a clear, colorless, odorless and tasteless fluid. The only thing that seemed to give relief was morphia administered hypodermically. The bowels were constipated and resisted the strongest purgatives.

The patient is a large, well-nourished woman with a bright complexion and anxious expression, who is lying in bed and making almost constant efforts to vomit, but expelling only small quantities of clear fluid.

On examination the heart and lungs presented no abnormality; the pulse was 68 and of good volume. The liver dullness was apparently normal. No tenderness of abdomen on palpation. No jaundice. Vaginal examination showed a nulliparous outlet, the cervix virginal and quite hard; the uterus in normal position, soft in consistency, and enlarged to the size of an 8 to 10 weeks' pregnancy. Appendages normal.

I advised the stoppage of all attempts at feeding by the mouth and the daily administration of four high saline enemata of 400 cc. each. A trained nurse was obtained, who was directed to save a 24-hour specimen of urine. The first specimen measured a little over 500 cc. and contained 7.5% grammes of total nitrogen with an ammonia coefficient of 15.8%. Microscopic examination was negative except for the presence of amorphous urates.

A diagnosis of toxæmic vomiting was made on the strength of the high ammonia coefficient, but in view of the apparently satisfactory general condition of the patient, it was thought that immediate interference was not indicated.

Her condition continued the same on the 22d, but unfortunately the urine was not saved. On the 23d the vomiting became more intense and the matter vomited changed from a clear mucus to a dark greenish or brownish fluid material. The ammonia coefficient was 15.3%. When I saw the patient on the morning of the 24th, I recommended her removal to the hospital for the immediate termination of pregnancy, in view of the change in the appearance of the vomit and the continued high ammonia coefficient. Urine drawn by catheter just before the operation presented an ammonia coefficient of 21.3%.

The patient was anæsthetized by chloroform, and, after the usual preparations, the cervix was dilated with Wathen's instrument, followed by Hegar's bougies. It was so resistent, however, that only a No. 17 bougie could be introduced, after which the uterus was cleaned out by a dull curette and ovum forceps, followed by a hot intra-uterine saline douche and a pack of iodoform gauze. The patient stood the operation well and was put back to bed in good condition.

During the night following the operation the patient improved considerably, vomited but little and was very comfortable. When I saw her at 2 p. m. on the 25th she was looking better than before the operation, was in excellent spirits, and stated that she had not vomited since 10 o'clock the previous evening.

During the afternoon she became more uncomfortable and suffered so extremely from nausea that her stomach was washed out with a weak solution of sodium bicarbonate at 6.45 p. m. and a considerable amount of dark brown material removed, after which considerable relief was obtained. The patient passed a restless night, in spite of the administration of two hypodermics of ⅛ gr. of morphia. She became very restless about 3 a. m. March 26, when her stomach was again washed out and a large amount of apparently blood-stained material siphoned off.

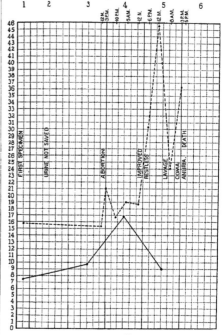

CHART 3.—Toxæmic Vomiting.

When I saw her at 11 a. m. her condition had changed markedly as compared with the previous day. She was very torpid and the pupils were quite tightly contracted, which it was thought was possibly due to the morphia. The pulse was more rapid than the day before and of poor volume, but did not exceed 100. The liver dullness was unchanged and there was no great tenderness over the lower abdomen. At this time a slight yellowish coloration of the conjunctivæ was noted. The stomach was again washed out and the material removed contained large quantities of brownish, reddish flakes, which under the microscope were found to be composed of blood cells. During the afternoon the patient became irrational and restless and tossed wildly in bed;

shortly afterwards she became comatose and remained so until she died at 6 p. m.

Prior to 3 p. m. as shown by the urinary chart, urine was excreted freely, but catheterization at that time yielded only 150 cc. of bloody urine, and at 5 p. m. only 4 cc. of apparently pure blood was obtained.

From the time I first saw the patient nothing was administered by the mouth, but large quantities of salt solution were given by

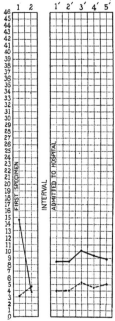

CHART 4.—Neurotic Vomiting.

the rectum, as well as occasional nutritive enemata after her admission to the hospital.

Before admission to the hospital the entire 24-hour specimens of urine were examined, but after the operation she was catheterized and the ammonia coefficient determined in each specimen, though the total nitrogen was estimated from the total 24 hours' output of urine.

From the accompanying chart (No. 3) it is seen that the ammonia coefficient remained between 15 and 16% for several days, but rose to 21.3% just prior to the induction of abortion, while the total nitrogen was practically normal. The high total nitrogen after the abortion was probably due, in part at least, to the involution of the uterus. As the patient became worse the ammonia coefficient rapidly rose and reached 45.5% 46 hours

after the abortion. The sudden drop immediately after this was probably due to the lavage with sodium bicarbonate, as it had risen to 36.5% in the specimen obtained three hours before death.

It is interesting to note that albumin or casts were not present until the day of death, the first trace of albumin being noted at 8 a. m., together with a few hyaline and granular casts. Seven hours later albumin was present in large quantity and casts were extremely numerous; while the last catheterized specimen consisted of only 4 cc. of blood. Leucin and tyrosin were not present.

At no time during the illness did the patient show any signs of emaciation, and just before death presented the appearance of a well-nourished woman with a ruddy complexion.

The temperature at no time was elevated, its highest point being 99.2° F. The pulse remained persistently low, and shortly before death, after it could no longer be felt at the wrist, was found to be 98 on auscultation.

CASE V.—*Neurotic Vomiting. Mrs. C. Chart No. 4.*

I first saw the patient November 14, 1904, when I obtained the following history: 28 years old, married 9 years, two children and one miscarriage. The labors were difficult but not instrumental. General health excellent, except in last and present pregnancy. The last menstrual period occurred September 5, 1904. Almost immediately after missing the October period vomiting began, which after a couple of weeks became so frequent and intense that she was hardly able to retain food of any description, and as a consequence has lost considerably in weight. Heart, lungs, liver, and genitalia normal. Pulse 96, temperature normal.

As shown by Chart 4, two 24-hour specimens of the urine examined at this time presented a normal ammonia coefficient. Shortly afterwards a slight, bloody discharge appeared and the patient believed that abortion was imminent. As long as this continued, she did not vomit; but as soon as the hæmorrhage ceased, the vomiting reappeared with its original intensity, so that I was urged to induce abortion, as the various remedies which I prescribed were without avail.

In the latter part of November the patient had a number of severe asthmatic attacks, similar to those from which she suffered throughout the second half of her last pregnancy. On December 1 her condition became so serious that she was transferred to the hospital. When I saw her shortly after admission she was sitting propped up in bed and gasping for breath, with labored respiration and a marked respiratory tug, and with loud rales over both lungs. The pulse was 116 and the temperature normal. She was considerably emaciated, with her eyes sunken far back in their orbits, and gave the impression of being desperately ill.

From the examination of the urine and the history of the case I felt convinced that a large part at least of the symptoms were neurotic in origin, and accordingly placed her under the care of a competent trained nurse and ordered a diet of measured quantities of water, milk, and egg albumin, and the saving of all urine. She was told that her vomiting was not of such a character as to necessitate abortion and would undoubtedly yield to treatment. As a result the vomiting ceased within 48 hours, while the asthmatic attacks became less frequent and severe. Improvement was so rapid that at the end of five days she was able to retain a more liberal diet, and left the hospital on the 10th day greatly improved. The second part of Chart 4 shows the condition of the urine during the first five days of her stay in the hospital.

The vomiting did not reappear after her return home, but within a short time the asthma grew worse and gradually became so severe as to appear to menace her life. Accordingly after consultation with her physician, Dr. Cary B. Gamble, she was once more removed to the hospital and abortion was induced on the 29th of December. With the exception of two days one week after the operation, the asthmatic attacks ceased with the administration of the chloroform. The convalescence was uneventful and the patient returned home in excellent condition.

CASE VI.—*Neurotic Vomiting. Mrs. McN. Chart No. 5.*

I first saw the patient February 12, 1905, when I obtained the following history: 25 years old, married 3 years, no children, one abortion at 2 months shortly after marriage. Last men-

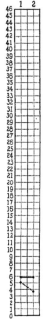

CHART 5.—Toxæmic Vomiting.

strual period December 21, 1904. She was perfectly well until February 1, 1905, when she began to suffer intensely from nausea and vomiting; for the past week she has vomited everything she has taken and has lost considerably in flesh and is extremely nervous.

Physical examination showed no abnormalities and the genitalia were normal, except for the pregnancy. Pulse 100, temperature normal. In spite of the administration of a number of remedies, the vomiting grew worse rather than better. Accordingly a 24-hour specimen of urine was saved on the 18th and 19th and found to be normal, as shown in Chart 5.

Having diagnosticated neurotic vomiting from the normal condition of the urine, I told the patient that there would be abso-

lutely no necessity for interfering with the pregnancy and that she would be promptly cured if she would implicitly follow my directions. I then put her to bed and gave very minute directions as to the character of her food and how it should be taken. When I saw her again on the 27th her condition had not improved. I accordingly told her that there was no doubt about her ultimate recovery, but that if she did not cease vomiting within three days, I should take her to the hospital, put her under a trained nurse, not allow her to see her family, and institute a rigid rest cure. Upon calling three days later to learn

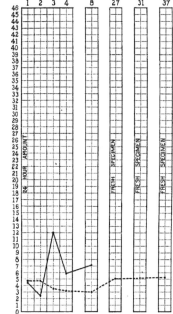

CHART 6.—Toxæmic Vomiting.

the effect of my threat, I found that the patient had not vomited since my last visit and had been able to eat three meals a day with great comfort ever since.

The vomiting did not recur and the patient improved markedly in appearance, so that one month later she was stouter than ever before in her life. She told me later that I could not have made a more fearful threat, as she had an abnormal horror of a hospital and would have done anything to escape going to one.

CASE VII.—*Neurotic Vomiting. Mrs. W. Chart No. 6.*

I first saw the patient April 12, 1905, in consultation with her husband, who is a physician. She was 21 years old, married 16 months, and had not been pregnant. The last menstrual period occurred February 5, 1905. She began to suffer from nausea and vomiting just after missing her March period. At first the vomiting occurred at regular intervals, but for the past three weeks it has occurred after every meal, sometimes at once and at other times not for several hours. Several days ago she fainted while vomiting. A week before I saw her she had gone to the seashore, but was not benefited by the trip. She has lost considerably in weight and complains of pain in the epigastric region.

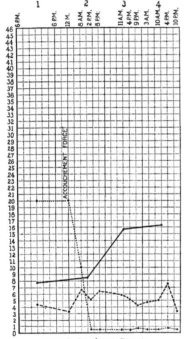

CHART 7.—Pre-eclamptic Toxæmia.

Dotted line represents albumen. Each square corresponds to one gramme per litre of urine.

She is very nervous and told me that her mother in all of her pregnancies had suffered with intense nausea, which on several occasions was so severe that the induction of abortion was considered.

Examination showed a small, thin woman, with no jaundice or œdema. The heart and lungs were normal; pulse 120, temperature normal. The abdomen was scaphoid and the liver dullness seemed slightly diminished, terminating 5 cm. above the costal margin in the mammary line. The genitalia were normal and the uterus enlarged to the size of a 7 to 8 weeks' pregnancy.

The patient was put to bed and a 24-hour specimen of urine collected, which, as shown by Chart 6, presented a normal ammo-

nia coefficient. Accordingly a diagnosis of neurotic vomiting was made. The patient was assured that she would recover promptly if she followed my directions, and a trained nurse was obtained and ordered to allow no one in the room but the husband and then only for a few minutes a day. She received saline enemata each day, but no food for the first 24 hours, and only albumin and water afterwards. Within two days the vomiting ceased and two days later small amounts of food were given by the mouth, and by the end of the week the patient was able to go about in comfort.

Her condition remained very satisfactory for nearly three weeks, when the vomiting returned and soon became more severe than before. The patient rapidly emaciated, and her husband felt that the only hope for her recovery lay in the induction of abortion. A more rigorous trained nurse was secured, the patient put back to bed and nourished only by the rectum and told that she could not see her friends nor receive anything by the mouth until the vomiting ceased; and that if that did not occur within a few days she would be taken to the hospital and completely isolated. On this occasion recovery was slower, but within 48 hours the nausea had become less violent, and the vomiting ceased two days later, although the patient still complained of great depression and felt that her recovery was merely temporary. Shortly afterwards she was allowed small quantities of solid food and began to move about the room. After this improvement was rapid, and a few days later when I telephoned to inquire how she was, I found she was dressing to go to the Horse Show. She rapidly regained her loss in weight and has since been in excellent condition.

CASE VIII.—*Pre-eclamptic Toxæmia. Mrs. C. Chart No. 7.*

Typical clinical history. Induction of premature labor. Compare this Chart with Charts 1 to 3 in cases of toxæmic vomiting.

I am under many obligations to my associate, Dr. J. M. Slemons, for the chemical examination of the urine in the cases here reported.

CONCLUSIONS.

1. The pernicious vomiting of pregnancy is not due to a single etiological factor, and occurs as one of three varieties, reflex, neurotic, and toxæmic.

2. The reflex type is dependent upon the existence of abnormalities of the generative tract or ovum and may be cured by their correction or removal.

3. The neurotic type is dependent upon the existence of a neurosis without demonstrable lesions and is more or less allied to hysteria. It is the most frequent variety of serious vomiting and can be cured by suggestion or a modified rest cure.

4. The toxæmic type is associated with characteristic changes in metabolism and in fatal cases, at least, with lesions in the liver analogous to those observed in acute yellow atrophy. It may occur in an acute or chronic form, the former causing death in 10 days or less, while the latter may persist for weeks or even months.

5. In reflex and neurotic vomiting there are no manifest changes in the urine, while the toxæmic variety is characterized by a marked decrease in the amount of nitrogen excreted as urea and a characteristic increase in the amount excreted as ammonia. The so-called ammonia coefficient rising from 3 to 5 per cent to as high as 46 per cent in one of my cases.

6. The toxæmic type is diagnosticated by the examination of the urine, the reflex by careful bimanual examination of

the genitalia, and the neurotic after the exclusion of the other two varieties.

7. The prognosis is excellent in reflex and neurotic vomiting, provided appropriate treatment is instituted, so that the termination of pregnancy is rarely indicated. In toxæmic vomiting, on the other hand, a fatal issue can be averted only by the prompt induction of abortion, and even then the prognosis is dubious.

LITERATURE.

Ahlfeld: Hyperemesis gravidarum, Ptyalismus, Hysterie. Centralbl. f. Gyn., 1891, 329-30.

Allbutt: Albuminuria in Pregnancy. Lancet, 1897, I, 579-82.

Anquetin: Les Vomissements incoercibles pendant la grossesse. Revue Médicale, 1865, II, 205-217, 275-89, 335-49, 398-407, and 467-78.

Bacon: The Vomiting of Pregnancy. Amer. Jour. Med. Sciences, 1898, CXV, 682-98.

Bar: Des Polynévrites et des mononévrites gravidiques. Bull. de la soc. d'obst. de Paris, 1904, VII, 180-85.

Bardinet: De l'ictère épidémique chez les femmes enceintes. L'union Médicale, 1863, XX, 260-63.

Beatty: A Case of Acute Atrophy of the Liver. New York Med. Record, 1895, XLVIII, 274-75.

Behm: Ueber Hyperemesis gravidarum mit Aufstellung einer neuen Intoxikationstheorie vom Wesen der Krankheit. Archiv f. Gyn., 1903, LXIX, 410-430.

Beking: Icterus gravidarum. Ref. Contralbl. f. Gyn., 1903, 787-89.

Benedict: Zur Kenntniss des Schwangerschafts-Ikterus. Deutsche med. Wochenschr., 1902, XXVIII, 296-97.

Bennett: On the Obstinate Sickness during Pregnancy. British Med. Jour., 1875, I, 769.

Blot: De l'ictère épidémique chez les femmes enceintes. Bull. de l'acad. imp. de méd. Paris, 1864-65, XXX, 55-66.

Bouffe de St. Blaise: Les autointoxications gravidiques. Annales de gyn. et d'obst., 1898, L, 342-72.

Braner: Ueber Graviditäts-Hæmoglobinurie. Münchener med. Wochenschr., 1902, XLIV, 825-26.

——— Ueber Graviditäts-Ikterus. Centralbl. f. Gyn., 1903, 787-89.

——— Eine Graviditäts-Toxonose des Zentralnervensystems. Münch. med. Wochenschr., 1904, LI, 1142-45.

Brian-Moreau: Note sur une cause peu connue des vomissements des femmes enceintes. Gazette hebdomadaire, 1856, III, 514-15.

Budd: On diseases of the liver. 3d Amer. Edition, 1857, 250-98.

Bué: Des Vomissements incoercibles et du curettage dans la mole hydatidiforme. La Presse Médicale, 1897, V, 29-30.

Busch and Moser: Handbuch der Geburtskunde. Berlin, 1843.

Cazeaux: Traité théoretique et pratique de l'art des accouchements. 3me. ed., Paris, 1850, 286-89.

Chailly-Honoré: Bulletin gén. de thérap., 1844, Oct., 288.

Champetier de Ribes et Bouffe de St. Blaise: Note sur un cas de vomissements incoercibles avec autopsie. Comptes rend. de la soc. d'obst., de gyn. et de paed. de Paris, 1901, III, 95-97.

Charpentier de Rubaix: Du danger de l'ictère chez les femmes enceintes. Revue med-chir. de Paris, 1854, XV, 268-70.

Charrin et Guillemet: Le glycogéne hépatique pendant la grossesse. Compte rend. de l'acad. de sciences, 1900, CXXX, 673-76.

Chazan. Ueber Hyperemesis gravidarum. Centralbl. f. Gyn., 1891, 541.

——— Zur Frage der Hyperemesis gravidarum. Centralbl. f. Gyn., 1896, 849-51.

Churchill: Theory and Practice of Midwifery. 2nd London Ed., 1850, 247-48.

——— Nausea and Vomiting. The diseases of Women. New Am. Ed. by Condie, 1852, 446-60.

Clivio: Das unstillbare Erbrechen der Schwangeren. Rassigna d'ost. e gin., 1901 (Ref. Contralbl. f. Gyn, 1902, 1037-8).

Condamin: Note sur un nouveau traitement des Vomissements incoercibles. Lyon médicale, 1902, XCVIII, 145-148.

Copeman: A novel treatment of obstinate vomiting in pregnancy. Brit. Med. Jour., 1875, I, 637-38.

Czerny u. Keller: Zur Kenntniss der Gastroenteritis im Säuglingsalter. Jahrbuch f. Kinderheilkunde, 1897, XLIV, 15-52, and XLV, 274-81.

Damany: Observation de vomissements incoercibles au début d'une grossesse. Gazette méd. de Paris, 1896, LXVII, 208.

Dance: Vomissements opiniâtres survenus au commencement de la grossesse, et paraissant dépendre d'un état morbide de l'utérus et du produit de la conception. Arch. gén. de méd., Paris, 1827, XIV, 245-52.

Danyau: Vomissements opiniâtres. L'Union Médicale, 1852, VI, 125-26.

Davis, D. D.: Elements of Obstetric Medicine. 2d Ed., London, 1841.

Davis, E. P.: Fatal nausea and vomiting of pregnancy. Trans. Amer. Gyn. Soc., 1894, XIX, 110-118.

Davis and Harris: Syncytioma malignum and ectopic gestation causing pernicious nausea. Trans. Am. Gyn. Soc., 1900, XXV, 364-81.

Desnos, Joffroy et Pinard: Sur un cas d'atrophie musculaire des quatres membres à évolution très rapide, survenue pendant la grossesse et consécutivement à des Vomissements incoercibles. Bull. de l'acad. de méd. de Paris, 1889, 3me S., XXI, 44-51.

Dionis: Traité général des accouchements, Paris, 1718, 143-47.

Dirmoser: Der Vomitus gravidarum perniciosus. Wien, 1901.

——— Ein weiterer Beitrag zur Autointoxikations-Theorie bei Hyperemesis gravidarum. Wiener klin. Wochenschr., 1903, XVI, 405-409.

Dubois: Quelques considérations sur l'avortement dans les cas de Vomissements. Bull. de l'acad. de méd., Paris, 1551-2, XVII, 557-83.

Duncan, Matthews: Clinical lecture on hepatic diseases in gynecology and obstetrics. London Med. Times and Gazette, 1879, I, 57-59; also Clinical Lectures on the Diseases of Women, 3d Ed., 1886, 293-305.

Edgar: Practice of Obstetrics. 2d Ed., 1904, 336-44.

——— Hepatic lesions in Obstetric practice. Jour. Amer. Med. Assn., 1905, XLIV, 1077-80.

Erismann: Beiträge zur Lehre von Hyperemesis gravidarum. D. I. Basel, 1890.

Eulenberg: Ueber puerperale Neuritis und Polyneuritis. Deutsche med. Wochenschr., 1895, 118-21 and 140-46.

Evans: On the etiology of the nausea and vomiting of pregnancy. Amer. Gyn. and Obst. Jour., 1900, XVI, 43-51.

Ewing: The pathology, anatomy and pathogenesis of the toxemia of pregnancy. Amer. Jour. of Obst., 1905, LI, 145-55.

Fellner: Die Beziehungen innerer Krankheiten zu Schwangerschaft, Geburt und Wochenbett. Leipzig u. Wien., 1907, 116-20.

Fischl: Zur Genese der Hyperemesis gravidarum. Prager med. Woch. enschr., 1884, IX, 222-24, 229-31.

Flaischek: Ueber Hyperemesis gravidarum. Zeltschr. f. Geb. u. Gyn., 1890, XX, 81-92.

Frank: Ueber Hyperemesis gravidarum. Prager med. Wochenschr., 1893, XVIII, 11-12 and 24-26.

——— Ueber Hyperemesis gravidarum. Centralbl. f. Gyn., 1898, 448-49.

Folin: Laws governing the chemical composition of the urine. Amer. Jour. of Physiology, 1905, XVI, 66-115.

Gardner: The diagnosis of early pregnancy. Amer. Jour. of Obst., 1897, XXXV, 54-63.

Gerst: Contribution à l'étude des vomissements de la grossesse. Thèse de Paris, 1903.

Giles: Observations on the etiology of the sickness of pregnancy. Trans. London Obst. Soc., 1893, XXXV, 308-33.

Glaessner: Experimentelles über die Obstipation. Wiener klin. Wochenschr., 1904, XVII, 1205-6.

Goldspohn: A unique case of circumscribed infection of the placenta and excessive vomiting. Amer. Jour. of Obst., 1904, L, 712-19.

Graefe: Ueber Hyperemesis gravidarum. Sammlung zwangloser Abhandlungen a. d. Gebiete der Frauenheilkunde und Geburtshilfe, 1900, III, Heft 7.

——— Zur Frage der Aetiologie der Hyperemesis gravidarum. Monatsschr. f. Geb. u. Gyn., 1904, XX, 23-39.

Guéniot: Des Vomissements incoercibles pendant la grossesse. Thèse de Paris, 1852, pp. 128.

——— Etiologie et traitement des vomissements incoercibles de la grossesse. Archives de Tocologie, 1889, XVI, 745-769.

Guillemeau: Du Vomissement qui vient aux femmes grosses. De la Grossesse et Accouchement des femmes, Paris, 1620.

Hewitt: The vomiting of Pregnancy: Its Causes and Treatment. Trans. London Obst. Soc., 1871, XIII, 103-17.

——— On the so-called uncontrollable Vomiting of Pregnancy. Trans. London Obst. Soc., 1885, XXVI, 273-324.

——— On the severe Vomiting of Pregnancy. Trans. Amer. Gyn. Soc., 1888, XIII, 218-58.

Hirschberg: Drei Fälle von acuter gelber Leberatrophie. D. I. Dorpat, 1856.

Hohl: Das Erbrechen der Schwangeren. Lehrbuch der Geburtshülfe., II Aufl., 1862, 222-25.

Holladay: Vomiting in Pregnancy. Lancet, 1897, I, 579-82.

Horaczek: Die gallige Dyscrasie mit acuter gelber Atrophie der Leber. Wien., 1843.

Horwitz: Ueber das unstillbare Erbrechen der Schwangeren. Zeltschr. f. Geb. u. Gyn., 1883, IX, 110-90.

Jaffé: Ueber Hyperemesis gravidarum. Volkmann's Sammlung klin. Vorträge, No. 305.

Jaggard: Notes on the pernicious Vomiting of pregnancy. Trans. Amer. Gyn. Soc., 1889, XIV, 441-61.

Jardine: Three cases of pernicious vomiting of pregnancy. Jour. of Gyn. and Obst. of the Brit. Empire, 1903, IV, 272-77.

Jolly: Ueber Paraplegie in der Schwangerschaft. Neurologisches Cen. tralbl., 1885, IV, 305.

Jürgens: Fettemboli und Metastase von Leberzellen bei Eclampsie. Berl. klin. Wochenschr., 1886, 519.

Kaltenbach: Ueber Hyperemesis gravidarum. Zeitschr. f. Geb. u. Gyn., 1891, XXI, 200-208.

Kehrer: Gazetamponade des Mutterhalses zur Stillung der Hyperemesis gravidarum. Centralbl. f. Gyn., 1896, 393-400.

Kehrer, E.: Die physiol. u. path. Beziehungen der weiblichen Sexualorgane zum Tractus intestinalis. Berlin, 1905, 92-160.

Kerckuig: Von einer epidemischen Gelbsucht. Hufeland's Journal der pract. Arzneikunde, 1799, VII, 3tes Stück, 94-109.

Klein: Hyperemesis gravidarum. Zeitschr. f. Geb. u. Gyn., 1893, XXXIX, 75-97.

Klingelhöfer: Beitrag zum Icterus epidemicus. Berl. klin. Wochenschr., 1876, XIII, 76-77.

Krassowsky: Les Vomissements incoercibles de la grossesse. Annales de gyn. et d'obst., 1894, XLI, 37.

Kreutzmann: Ein Fall von Hyperemesis gravidarum gefolgt von Polyneuritis in graviditate. New Yorker med. Monatsschr., 1900, XII, 101-108.

Kühne: Beitrag zur Lehre von der Hyperemesis gravidarum. Monatsschr. f. Geb. u. Gyn., 1899, X, 432-36.

Lang: Sur un cas de Vomissements incoercibles à 4 mois de la grossesse. Mort de la parturiente. Archives de tocolog. et de gyn., 1893, XX, 620-28.

Lebert: Ueber Icterus typhoides. Virchow's Archiv, 1854, VII, 343-96 and VIII, 147-91.

Le Masson: Les ictères et les coliques hépatiques chez les femmes en état de puerpéralité. Thèse de Paris, 1898, pp. 317.

Lindemann: Zur path. Anatomie des unstillbaren Erbrechens der Schwangeren. Centralbl. f. allg. Path. u. path. Anat., 1892, III, 625-630.

Liepmann. Ueber ein für menschliche Placenta specifisches Serum. Deutsche med. Wochenschr. 1902, 911-12; 1903, 80-81 and 283-85.

Lomer: Ueber die Bedeutung des Icterus gravidarum für Mutter und Kind. Zeitschr. f. Geb. u. Gyn., 1886, XIII, 169-85.

Luez: Hyperemesis des Vomissements de la grossesse, benins et graves reconnue d'origine nerveuse. Thèse de Paris, 1893.

Lwow: Hyperemesis gravidarum. Deutsche Medizinal Zeitung, 1900, XXI, 1013-15, 1025-27, 1037-39, 1049-51, 1061-63, 1073-75, 1085-87, and 1097-1100.

Mader: Zur Polyneuritis peripherica puerperarum et gravidarum. Wiener klin. Wochenschr. 1895, VIII, 537-39 and 555-59.

Martin: On the Vomiting of Pregnancy. Brit. Med. Jour., 1904, II, 1569-71.

Mauriceau: Traité des maladies des femmes grossesse. 6me Ed., 1721, I, 128-34.

McClintock: The Excessive Vomiting of Pregnancy. Dublin Jour. Med. Sciences, 1873, LV, 462-73.

Meillère: Sur quelques cas de rétention des chlorures. Comptes rendus de la Soc. de biologie, 1902, LIV, 1135-36.

Mettler: The Nervous Element in the Vomiting of Pregnancy. Jour. Amer. Med. Assn., 1892, XVIII, 160-64.

Meunier: Essai critique sur l'ictère des femmes enceintes à propos l'épidémie de Paris, 1871-2. Thèse de Paris, 1872.

Minkowski: Störungen des Stickstoffumsatzes in der Leber. Lubarsch-Ostertag. Ergebnisse der allg. Path. u. path. Anat. 1895, II Jahrgang, 726-31.

Möner: Quoted by Folin.

Münzer: Der Stoffwechsel des Menschen bei akuter Phosphorvergiftung. Deutsches Archiv f. klin. Med., 1892, LII. 199.
——— Die harnstoffbildende Funktion der Leber. Arch. f. exp. Path. u. Pharm., 1894, XXXIII, 164.

Muret: Hyperemesis gravidarum und Hysterie im Allgemeinen. Deutsche med. Wochenschr., 1893, XIX, 123-25.

Neuberg and Richter: Ueber das Verhalten von freier Aminosäure im Blute bei akuter Leberatrophie. Deut. med. Wochenschr., 1904, XXX, 499-501.

Opie: Zonal necrosis of the liver. Jour. of Med. Research, 1904, XII, 147-67.

Ozanam: De la forme grave de l'ictère essential. Thèse de Paris, 1849.

Payer: Ueber den Einfluss des Zuckers auf den Stoffwechsel der Schwangeren. Monatsschr. f. Geb. u. Gyn., 1899, X, 559-580 and 784-805.

Pick: Ueber Hyperemesis gravidarum. Volkmann's Sammlung klin. Vorträge. N. F., 1902, Nos. 325 and 326.

Pfaundler: Zur Frage der Säurevergiftung, etc. Jahrbuch f. Kinderheilkunde, 1904, LX, 719-30.

Pierrehughes: Étude critique sur les Vomissements incoercibles de la grossesse. Thèse de Paris, 1902.

Quincke: Acute Leberatrophie. Nothnagel's specielle Pathologie u. Therapie, 1899, XVIII, 294-315.

Rigby: A system of Midwifery: Philadelphia, 1841, 101-103.

Rokitansky: Die acute Schmelzung der Leber. Lehrbuch der path. Anatomie. 3te Aufl., 1861, III, 269-72.

Rosenthal: Ueber das Copeman'sche Verfahren zur Beseitigung des

hartnäckigen Erbrechens Schwangerer. Berl. klin. Wochenschr., 1879, XVI, 388-91.

Roughton: Pernicious Vomiting of Pregnancy. Lancet, 1885, II, 425-26.

Saint Vel: Note sur une forme d'ictère grave chez les femmes enceintes. Gazette des hôpitaux, 1862, XXXV, 538-39.

Schaeffer: Ein Beitrag zur Aetiologie des Wiederkehrenden Icterus. Monatsschr. f. Geb. u. Gyn., 1902, XV, 907-20.

Schittenhelm: Zur Frage der Ammoniakausscheidung im menschlichen Urin. Deutsches Arch. f. klin. Med., 1903, LXXVII, 517-39.

Schmiedeberg: Ueber das Verhalten des Ammoniaks zur Harnstoffbildung im Tierkörper. Arch. f. exp. Path. u. Pharm., 1877, VIII, I.

Schmorl: Path. anat. Untersuchungen über Puerperal-Eklampsie. Leipzig, 1893.
——— Zur Lehre von der Eklampsie. Archiv f. Gyn., 1902, LXV, 504-529.

Schroeder: Die Bildungsstätte des Harnstoffes. Arch. f. exp. Path. u. Pharm., 1882, XV, 364.
——— Lehrbuch der Geburtshilfe. 12te Aufl., 1893, 434.

Simmons: Quoted by Danyau.

Smith: A Synopsis of ten Cases of Jaundice occurring in Pregnant Women. Northwestern Med. and Surg. Jour., 1873-74, IV, 436-40.

Solowieff: Ueber einen Fall von Hyperemesis gravidarum, begleitet von Neuritis multiplex. Centralbl. f. Gyn., 1892, 429-97.

Stolz: Quoted by Hewitt, 1885.

Stone: Toxæmia of Pregnancy. Amer. Gyn., 1903, III, 518-50.

Strauss: Zur Funktionsprüfung der Leber. Deutsche med. Wochenschr., 1901, 757-9 and 786-87.

Sutugin: Hyperemesis gravidarum. Das übermässige Erbrechen der Schwangeren, Berlin, 1883.

Tarnier: Recherches sur l'état puerpéral, etc. Thèse de Paris, 1857.

Thierfelder: Acute atrophy of the liver. Ziemssen's Cyclopedia of the Practice of Medicine. Amer. Ed., 1880, IX, 242-305.

Tisserand: Du Vomissement nerveux. Thèse de Paris, 1865.

Turenne: Traitement rationnel de la toxémie gravidique précoce, et en particulier des Vomissements simples de la grossesse. Annales de gyn. et d'obst., 1904, 2me Sér., I, 657-85.

Tuszkai: Zur Frage der Hyperemesis gravidarum. Verh. der deutschen. Gesell. f. Gyn., 1895, VI, 766-87.
——— Ueber Indication zur Einleitung der Geburt bei Hyperemesis. Berl. klin. Wochenschr., 1903, XL, 803-805.

Ulrich: Lethaler Fall von Vomitus gravidarum. Monatsschr. f. Gebk., 1858, 92-97.

Vaughan: Case of Vomiting in Pregnancy successfully treated. Memoirs of the Medical Society of London, 1789, II, 125-32.

Veit: Ueber Endometritis decidua. Volkman's Sammlung klin. Vorträge, 1885, No. 254.
——— Ueber Albuminurie in der Schwangerschaft. Berl. klin. Wochenschr., 1902, 513 and 540.

Veit and Scholten: Syncytiolyse und Hämolyse. Zeitschr. f. Geb. u. Gyn., 1903, XLIX, 210-32.

Von den Velden: Icterus gravidarum. Hegar's Beiträge zur Geb. u. Gyn., 1904, VIII, 448-64.

Weichardt: Experimentelle Studien über die Eklampsie. Deutsche med. Wochenschr., 1902, 224-26.

Winscheid: Ueber Hyperemesis gravidarum. Centralbl. f. Gyn., 1900, 806-808.

Whitfield: Puerperal Neuritis due to the Vomiting of Pregnancy. Lancet, 1889, I, 627-28.

Wormser: Zur modernen Lehre von der Eklampsie. 1904, LI. 7-10.

Young: Simple and Malignant Jaundice of Pregnancy. Medical News, 1898, LXXVIII. 618-21.

Zaborski: Hyperemesis gravidarum. Monatsschr. f. Geb. u. Gyn., 1904, XX, 39-47.

INDEX TO VOLUMES 1-16 OF BULLETIN.

A subject and author index of the first sixteen volumes of the Johns Hopkins Hospital Bulletin is now ready. As the edition will be limited, it is desirable that orders be sent in as promptly as possible.

Price bound in cloth is fifty cents.

Orders should be addressed to the Johns Hopkins Press, Baltimore, Md.

PROCEEDINGS OF SOCIETIES.

THE JOHNS HOPKINS HOSPITAL MEDICAL SOCIETY.

December 18, 1905.

Dr. W. G. MacCallum in the chair.

Exhibition of Surgical Cases. MR. LANGNECKER, MR. HELMHOLZ, AND DR. CUSHING.

CASE I. RUPTURED BRACHIAL PLEXUS.—The patient presented by Mr. Langnecker came under Dr. Cushing's observation on October 10, with complete traumatic paralysis of his left arm. Examination showed great atrophy of the entire musculature of the arm and shoulder girdle. The muscles were flaccid and give the reaction of degeneration. The arm was anæsthetic to all forms of sensation over an area corresponding to the skin fields of the fifth cervical to the first thoracic segments inclusive. At no time following the injury had he suffered pain.

Operation.—On thoroughly exposing the plexus, which was found densely built up in connective tissue, the fifth and sixth roots were disclosed; the root of the seventh was missing; the root which had the appearance of the eighth was very much arched, and beneath this was a stump giving the appearance of the ruptured seventh. This stump was refreshed and sutured into the plexus at the region of the junction of the fifth and sixth roots which, after being freed from scar tissue, were found to have their continuity intact. The wound was closed and the patient made an uneventful recovery. Before operation there had been no sensation in the arm except on its post-axial surface just above the elbow (second thoracic field), and in the axillary region where there was some hyperæsthesia. The pupil on the left side was more contracted than on the right; the tension of the left globe was lower than the right; and there was a narrowing of the palpebral cleft. The under part of the arm was mottled and cyanosed; the member hung flail-like and the forearm was rotated inward and pronated. The humerus was very loose at the articulation and seemed merely to hang in the capsule. Since operation the patient has received daily massage and galvanism. The ocular symptoms have changed greatly but there still remains a trace of the sympathetic paralysis. There has been no return of motion in the arm, though there is slight voluntary action in the deltoid and pectoral muscles. Sensation has returned as far as the elbow, and there are points over the forearm and hand where the patient has some sensation. The muscles react well to the galvanic current, and the general appearance of the arm is much better. The rapidly returning sensation gives promise of further restoration of function.

There have been four other cases of ruptured brachial plexus in the hospital; the first was recorded in 1892. The patient had a complete rupture of the left brachial plexus. At operation the three main trunks were found encased in a firm, dense, fibrous tissue mass, which it was considered best not to dissect out. Three weeks later at the patient's request the arm was amputated. This was the usual treatment of total brachial plexus ruptures at that time, for the condition was regarded as hopeless, and the flail-like extremity was an encumbrance.

The second case was in 1893; the rupture of the plexus was not complete; the paralysis simulated Erb's type; the two upper cords were most affected. At operation much scar tissue was found around the trunks. After dissecting this away the stump of the posterior root was sutured to the main part of the plexus, but the patient was not benefited by the operation when last heard from.

The third case was in 1903. All cords of the right plexus were ruptured. At operation the scar tissue was found to be very extensive. A portion of the plexus was excised and an anastomosis made. The patient was benefited.

The fourth case in 1904, was similar to the third, only the fibrous tissue was more marked. The operation was extensive, a temporary resection of the clavicle being made. The nerve trunks were completely dissected out and several complex anastomoses were made. The spinal accessory was anastomosed into the upper cord of the plexus. The operation was successful in so far as the patient has already regained use of the upper arm and still continues to improve.

CASE II. VON RECKLINGHAUSEN'S DISEASE.—The patient shown by Mr. Helmholz was a white laborer, aged 19 years. Ever since the patient can remember he has had small patches of soft tissue on his body. The condition for which he was shown began twelve years ago, following a kick on the head by a horse. At this situation a tumor appeared and grew until it involved the whole left side of the head. It was painless. The great deformity brought him to the hospital. So far as he knows there has been one similar condition in the members of his family.

At examination his expression was rather dull and he seemed somewhat simple; he does not read or write. On the left side of his head was a soft, flabby tumor, reaching from the outer canthus back to the occiput and to within 2 cm. of the sagittal suture. The ear was dislocated downward far below its natural position and was folded on itself. The hair over the tumor was scant, coarse, and gray. Over the body were punctate as well as large irregular patches of pigmentation; small, bluish pin-point areas, looking like small bruises; congenital moles; and true fibromata mollusca. The patient was operated upon on November 9, by Dr. Cushing at a neighboring hospital, and a diamond-shaped piece of scalp, including the chief portion of the tumor, was removed from the side of the head above the ear. After removal of this tissue the closure of the wound has drawn the eye and ear back to their normal positions.

Pathologically the tumor removed was a piece of scalp 20 cm. long, 8 cm. wide, and from 1 to 1½ cm. thick. On the under surface was a nerve on which was a fusiform thickening 4 cm. long and 2 mm. in diameter, having a number of growths the size of millet seed, and with a number of thick fibers that could be traced into the œdematous tissue of the scalp itself. A neuroma which was in the scalp above the ear histologically was found to be full of intertwining bands of nerve fibrils. The sebaceous glands of the scalp were hypertrophied. The lower connective tissue layer of the scalp was composed of many whorls of connective tissue. In the midst of these concentric bands of fibrous tissue were a few nerve fibrils.

DR. CUSHING.—Brachial plexus ruptures are not uncommon in the adult. The lesions are the same as those which occur in the so-called obstetrical palsies in infants. In both instances the injury follows a violent separation of the head and shoulder. Mr. Langnecker's patient was a miner, and his plexus was ruptured by a mass of slate falling on his shoulder and causing extreme lateral flexion of the head.

Concerning the case of von Recklinghausen's disease he said: this plexiform manifestation of the disease is not uncommon, particularly over this cranial site. There have been many cases reported with various degrees of the same lesion. The first case of this type of the disease was reported by Valentine Mott in 1854, under the title of Pachydermatocele. Subsequently Paul Bruns called these tumors Ranken-neurome. In 1882, von Recklinghausen gathered together all the reported cases and made exhaustive studies, since when the disease in all of its various manifestations has been associated with his name. The pigmented patches often appear in the skin fields, representing segmental distribution.

DR. BARKER.—In regard to the case of plexus lesion and nerve anastomosis, has regeneration in the distal ends of the nerves been noticed? There is evidence that regeneration can occur in the peripheral nerves. In 1860, French observers claimed that there was at first degeneration, but after some months distal regeneration. Strobe later claimed that there was peripheral degeneration, but that no regeneration took place. The former theory was retracted, but in the last few years there has again been a leaning toward distal regeneration. If there is no connection between the distal and proximal ends, the distal end again degenerates. Bethe made these observations from work on young animals, but there should be the same tendency in older animals.

DR. CUSHING.—There are changes, doubtless reparative in nature, which occur in the distal ends of severed nerves and which are shown chiefly as a multiplication of the cells of the sheath of Schwann. This process has been regarded by almost all observers as a regenerative one but I do not think that those, who like Bethe have gone so far as to claim that the entire process of regeneration, including the reformation of axis cylinder processes, may take place in the distal segment alone, have proven their claim satisfactorily to all. Langley and Anderson have shown how technical errors not guarded against in Bethe's work, may have led to an erroneous interpretation of many of his experiments. It seems probable that

a double process must be at work in the regeneration of a severed nerve fiber—the well recognized peripheral changes and the outgrowing axone from the central cell; the former serving the purpose of a guide to the latter.

Experimental Arteriosclerosis and Myocarditis. DR. R. M. PEARCE, OF ALBANY, N. Y.

The term arteriosclerosis is here used in a tentative way to describe the changes occurring in the aorta of the rabbit as the result of the intravenous injection of adrenalin. The lesions thus produced are not identical with the arteriosclerosis of man but for purposes of experimental study they may perhaps for the present at least be regarded as arteriosclerosis for the rabbit. Previous to Josué's publication describing the production of vascular lesions in the rabbit by the use of adrenalin, all attempts to produce experimentally changes analagous to arteriosclerosis had been unsatisfactory. In the experiments about to be described Josné's methods were followed. A few minims of a one to one thousand solution of adrenalin chloride were injected into an ear vein of a rabbit on alternate days. In some instances considerably larger doses were given. The animals were killed after periods varying from a few days to eight weeks.

The vascular lesions produced were limited to the aorta and exhibited a more or less definite sequence. Rabbits receiving five to six injections showed no gross lesions but, histologically, important changes in the media were evident. These consisted of focal areas of degeneration in which the muscle fibers were destroyed without alteration of the elastica. Later the degeneration was more extensive and involved the greater portion of the middle zone of the media. At this time changes in the elastic tissue appeared; the fibers became swollen, stained irregularly and in some places appeared to be fused together. Special stains showed a small number of minute fat droplets in such areas. After 12 to 15 injections very definite lesions were evident macroscopically. The aorta was more or less distorted in shape, rigid and non-elastic. Irregular dilations alternated with elevated brittle areas of calcification. Distinct atheroma with ulceration was seldom seen. In the experiments, continued for six to eight weeks, the process became very diffuse and small dilations of the thinner portions of the aorta assumed the appearance of aneurysms. At this stage the destruction of the elastic fibers was extreme and all degenerated areas were infiltrated with lime salts. Cellular infiltration and repair about such areas were frequently seen in the late stages. In such there was also an extensive proliferation of the sub-intimal tissue. The aorta of the rabbit is a very delicate structure showing no sharp demarcation between the intima and the beginning of the media. There is no definite internal elastic plate and the endothelial cells are separated from the media only by a delicate layer, often not demonstrable, of fine elastic and connective tissue fibrils. In the proliferation in this part of the vessel it is difficult to differentiate between the part played by intimal and sub-intimal tissues. Certain it is that the endothelial cells proliferate not at all or to but a very slight extent. The proliferation of the intimal and sub-intimal tissue is always opposite areas of necrosis in the media and appear to be compensatory to such and is therefore of unusual interest in view of Thoma's well known theory concerning the development of arteriosclerosis in man. According to Thoma's view the most characteristic lesion of arteriosclerosis is a thickening of the intima compensatory to a weakening of the media. The condition in man is one acting slowly and over a long time. The experimental condition in the rabbit, although more acute and as far as the necrosis is concerned, more severe, is somewhat similar to the slighter changes which occur in man. A secondary degeneration taking place in the areas of compensatory hyperplasia is necessary, however, to make the condition more nearly analagous to arteriosclerosis in man.

The manner in which adrenalin produces these lesions has caused much discussion. Toxic action, the effect of increase of blood pressure and the part played by the vasa vasorum have all been considered. No unanimity of opinion exists. K. Ziegler has pointed out that owing to anatomical peculiarities certain portions of the inner and middle parts of the media of the aorta are not so well nourished as are the other portions and that therefore in such places the toxic substances more readily cause destruction. Although this theory may explain more or less the peculiar distribution of the lesion, it is not entirely satisfactory. It would appear much more probable that the disturbance of circulation is sufficient without a direct toxic action. At the time of arterial contraction caused by the action of adrenalin on the vasa vasorum a condition of local anæmia must exist; if to this we add the great strain on the vessel wall due to the greatly increased intravascular pressure, we have sufficient explanation it would appear for the disorganization of the media.

In the series of experiments just described, which were carried out with the aid of Dr. E. MacD. Stanton, little attention was paid to the condition of the heart. Certain degenerative and proliferative changes were, however, occasionally

observed and in order to determine the significance of these a second series of observations was undertaken.

In this second series of thirty-one experiments, degenerative changes in the myocardium were found frequently and connective tissue proliferation of greater or less degree in twelve. The primary effect of adrenalin is to produce severe circulatory disturbances. The animals generally recover from these though some die from extreme dilatation of the heart after one to five injections. In such, disorganization and degenerative changes are constant. Very frequently there is a marked œdema of the myocardium. In those having had four or five injections, areas of granular and hyaline degeneration of the fibers with complete loss of nuclei, a condition practically of anæmic infarction, were not infrequently present. Of twenty-two animals surviving seven to fifteen injections (initial dose of 0.1 cc. gradually increased every other day), twelve exhibited connective tissue proliferation of varying degree. In two the histological picture was that of a chronic fibrous myocarditis. The increase of connective tissue was partly diffuse and partly focal affecting all parts of the ventricle and to a considerable extent the papillary muscles. The focal areas were most frequent at the apex of the heart. As a rule extreme degeneration of muscle and proliferation of connective tissue occurred side by side.

The changes in the myocardium are not secondary to the changes in the aorta for in about half the animals very severe lesions in the heart were unaccompanied by vascular changes. In only one instance did vascular lesions involve the orifices of the coronary arteries. The theory put forth to explain the necrosis in the aorta would appear to be applicable also to the degenerative changes in the myocardium. The fibrous myocarditis represents an attempt to repair the degenerative lesion.

The conditions thus produced experimentally may not be the same as those occurring in man but work along these lines may eventually aid in elucidating some of the problems of vascular and cardiac pathology.

NOTES ON NEW BOOKS.

Operative Surgery. For Students and Practitioners. BY JOHN J. McGRATH, M. D., Professor of Surgical Anatomy and Operative Surgery at the New York Post-Graduate Medical School, Surgeon to the Harlem, Post-Graduate, and Columbus Hospitals, New York. Second edition, thoroughly revised, with 265 illustrations, including many full-page plates in colors and half-tone. (*Philadelphia: F. A. Davis Company, 1906.*)

The first edition of this book was published in 1902, under the title, Surgical Anatomy and Operative Surgery. The present volume is somewhat more voluminous than the first, and there are more and better illustrations.

Among the subjects not considered in the other edition, but now described, are operations for goitre and on the heart. There is still no mention of operations on the ureters, for aneurysm, for umbilical hernia, and others equally important. Some of the sections are practically unchanged, while others have been added

to and improved. This is especially noticeable in the section which deals with the stomach and intestines, where many of the latest methods are considered. The original Halsted operation for the radical cure of inguinal hernia is given, and not the modified method now used. Although the book is considerably improved in many respects, it is still incomplete and unsatisfactory.

A Text-Book of Clinical Anatomy for Students and Practitioners. BY DANIEL N. EISENDRATH, A. B., M. D., Professor of Clinical Anatomy, University of Illinois. (*Philadelphia, New York, and London: W. B. Saunders & Co.*)

This is a useful book and deserves to be in the hands of every student of medicine, surgeon, and general practitioner. It aims to supplement the study of gross and minute anatomy by giving a view of regional and topographic anatomy to the end that the various anatomical structures may be recognized in the living body. Directions are given for the various examinations required for purposes of accurate diagnosis. The diagnostic landmarks in different portions of the body are pointed out not only in the text but also by sections and schematic representations. The illustrations are numerous and of excellent quality and serve to elucidate the text and to render the meaning of the author more easily comprehended. The character of the book forbids an extended review of its contents. It is sufficient to say that the work bears evidence throughout of painstaking original work and can be commended as an excellent guide to all who have to do with surgery, neurology, or internal medicine.

Die Morphologie der Missbildungen des Menschen und der Thiere. Part I. *General Teratology.* By Dr. Ernst Schwalbe. (*Jena: Gustav Fischer, 1906.*)

This is the first volume of a text-book which the author has designed to be made up of three parts, the first dealing with general teratology, the second with twin and multiple formations, and the third with individual malformations. The last two volumes have not yet appeared; the first, which is here under consideration, is largely concerned with a discussion of the general conditions which bring about abnormal development.

The brief account which is given of the early literature and the history of monstrosities indicates the extreme ignorance which existed even as late as the seventeenth and eighteenth centuries concerning the cause of abnormal organisms. It was not until embryology became a well-established field of work, that rational studies were made of malformations; and the further development of experimental embryology gave finally an exact basis for what was called the science of teratology.

In Chapter IV the author gives a general review of experimental work which has been done in embryology and teratology, at the basis of which is the fact that the normal development of the egg is dependent upon certain definite external physical and chemical conditions and upon internal conditions of nutrition and assimilation. He cites Boveri's experiments in the production of abnormal larvæ from fragments of the ascaris egg in which there is an abnormally small number of chromosomes; and also the formation of monstrosities by double fertilization in which there is an increase of chromosomes. Among the external conditions which may cause abnormal development are changes in temperature and changes in the oxygen supply, especially lack of oxygen. Definite malformations occur in hens' eggs when the supply of oxygen is diminished. A change in osmotic pressure may cause abnormal development as shown in Loeb's production of artificial parthenogenesis in eggs which have been in concentrated sea water. Certain chemical changes in the surrounding media are of importance; abnormalities develop in calcium-free media, in solutions of lithium salts, etc. The lack of light retards development in frogs' eggs; and the regeneration of organs is also influenced by light. Gravity also has some influence on the development of a hen's egg.

The phenomena of regeneration in the various classes of animals are dealt with in considerable detail. Regeneration may be of all degrees of completeness, depending upon the species of animals and upon local conditions. On the other hand " super-regeneration " may take place when the regeneration is greater than the loss, e. g., lizards may grow two or more tails in the place of one which is lost. This is interesting in connection with the occurrence of polydactylous individuals. In relation to teratology, the heteromorphosis of Loeb is perhaps of special significance. The formation of a head in the place of a lost tail on tubularians and similar occurrences in other classes of animals suggest the possibility of this process playing a rôle in the production of monstrosities.

The special physiology of monstrosities depends largely upon the nature of the malformation. With many of these, intra-

uterine life is possible when extrauterine life is not. The great variety of malformations which may occur in the organs makes a corresponding diversity in physiological properties in the organism.

The period at which the malformation may originate in the life of the organism varies from the time of fertilization of the egg up to the time of birth. Malformations due to arrested development may occur also after birth. Various processes, such as abnormal fusion of organs, splitting of organs, hypertrophy and atrophy, degeneration of tissues, and inflammation may lead to malformations. The causes of malformations are discussed in further detail in Chapter X, where they are classified as mechanical, psychical, physical, and chemical, those due to fœtal disease or retardation of development, and amniotic malformations. A short account of the frequency, sex, and distribution of malformations completes this excellent volume, a notable feature of which is the application of the later results of biological experiment to the study of teratology. The great light which is thrown upon this subject by biological research is apparent in every part of the volume and we look forward with interest to the parts of this book which are yet to be published.　　　J. B. MacCallum.

Therapeutics: Its Principles and Practice. By Horatio C. Wood, M. D., LL. D., and Horatio C. Wood, Jr., M. D. Twelfth edition. (*Philadelphia and London: J. B. Lippincott Company, 1905.*)

A Text-Book of Practical Therapeutics. By Hobart Amory Hare, M. D., B. Sc. Eleventh edition. (*Philadelphia and New York: Lea Brothers & Co., 1905.*)

Organotherapy, or Treatment by Means of Preparations of Various Organs. By H. Batty Shaw, M. D., F. R. C. P. (*Chicago: W. T. Keener & Co., 1905.*)

Of works on therapeutics we have no lack, and the recent revision of the pharmacopeia has resulted in the necessity for new editions of the older books. The works written by Wood and Hare may probably be regarded as the most representative of American treatises on this subject. There are others which deal rather more with pharmacology and materia medica, but these two are essentially concerned with the subject of treatment. The attitude of the profession towards therapeutics has undergone some changes, but there are many of us who still believe that in too many cases treatment is regarded as meaning only the administration of drugs and not the supervision of many other things. We find in Dr. Wood's work that while 812 pages are devoted to the consideration of drugs only 59 are given to general measures, and 20 of these are concerned with electricity. This does not seem to us a proper division of space, too much attention being given to drugs and too little to other measures.

In Dr. Wood's book there is very slight consideration of massage, feeding, the employment of heat and cold, etc. The discussion of drugs is given under the headings of various classes, such as diuretics, alteratives, etc. Every one knows how difficult it is to classify all drugs under given headings, but this seems thus far perhaps the most satisfactory method. It is impossible to review such a work as this in detail and it may be said that as a rule the text is good. There are very full notes from the literature regarding many points and at the end of each section a good bibliography is given. Just by chance we selected the section on Jaborandi for examination. The discussion of this was rather disappointing as there is no mention whatever of the dangers of giving pilocarpine hypodermically. One cannot expect a writer to note every point but this seems one that should be discussed. The danger from pilocarpine is by no means slight but no reference is made to it.

The work of Hare is arranged in quite a different way, being divided into four parts, the first dealing with general considerations, the second with drugs, the third with measures other than drugs, and the fourth with the treatment of special diseases. Taking the space devoted to therapeutic measures we find 406 pages given to drugs and 94 to other procedures and feeding. As already remarked, the disproportion between these two should not be so great. In the discussion of the drugs they are considered alphabetically, which is perhaps in some ways the easiest method. In the section on pilocarpine the same criticism may be applied as was passed on the corresponding section in Dr. Wood's work. The discussion of remedial measures other than drugs is very good, but as already said there is hardly enough of it. In the section on diseases Dr. Hare again simply makes an alphabetical classification, which cannot be regarded as very satisfactory, although it is probably difficult to consider all the diseases of one system together. There is an elaborate index of diseases and remedies.

Dr. Shaw in his work takes up the subject of treatment by preparations of various organs. He has given us as satisfactory a work as the nature of his subject would permit, each organ being taken up separately and after a preliminary note of its anatomy and physiology the pathology and therapeutics are discussed. As might be expected the largest space is given to the discussion of the thyroid gland. It must be confessed that thus far we have not obtained the therapeutic results from the use of gland extracts which were expected. It is, however, probable that more may come out of it in the future, and if we have nothing more than the use of thyroid extract and adrenalin there is much to be thankful for. This work can be recommended as an excellent one for those who desire to obtain a good summary of this subject.

The Diagnosis of Diseases of Women. A Treatise for Students and Practitioners. By PALMER FINDLEY, B. S., M. D., Assistant Professor of Gynecology and Obstetrics, Rush Medical College. Second edition, illustrated. (*Philadelphia and New York: Lea Brothers & Co., 1905.*)

The appearance of a second edition of this work in two years from the publication of the first, indicates that it fills a place in the library of medical text-books. It covers the whole subject indicated in its title from the point of view of clinical manifestations and of gross and microscopic anatomy. Thoroughness is well carried out in all the chapters. Beginning with clinical history, it takes up different methods of examination, devoting separate chapters to the more common instruments used in diagnosis. Chloroform is preferred as an anæsthetic for curettage. This is contrary to the opinion of many surgeons and seems to add unnecessary risk to a slight operation. The chapter on mioroscopic examination of scrapings and excised pieces is useful and well written, giving a few good methods of preparing tissue for such examination. New chapters on blood examination and bacteriology are introduced on account of the importance of these subjects. The chapter on the blood is too brief for physicians not used to the methods described, and unnecessarily long for one familiar with blood examination. The plates of blood smears are good, but should give stains and magnification or be omitted. The chapter on bacteriology closes the general considerations. The diagnosis of uterine pregnancy is discussed fully. Extrauterine pregnancy receives the careful attention its frequency and importance demand. Chorio-epithelioma malignum, a subject as yet little understood, is treated in accord with the most recent views. An effort has been made to bring everything up to date. The diseases of the external and internal genitalia are taken up in order and discussed at length. While the cell-inclusion theory of the origin of ovarian dermoids receives careful description, no reference is made to the more recent contributions suggesting the ovulogenous origin of such tumors. The conditions, pelvic peritonitis, perimetritis, and parametritis

are described, and the points of difference noted; but the author says: "The distinction between perimetritis and parametritis is at all times difficult; . . . . it is to be remembered they can exist together." It seems hardly worth while to cling to the old nomenclature.

The book closes with chapters on diseases of the urethra, bladder, ureters, and kidneys.

The general make-up of the book is excellent; there are, however, a few typographical errors, as in the legends of Plates XLI and XLII. Clearness of description is sometimes wanting. The book has, however, much to commend it. It is profusely illustrated and well indexed.

The Treatment of Diseases of the Eye. BY VICTOR HANKE, First Assistant in the University Eye Clinic of Professor E. Fuchs in Vienna. Translated by J. HERBERT PARSONS, B. S., F. R. C. S., Assistant Ophthalmic Surgeon, University College Hospital, London, and GEORGE COATS, M. D., F. R. C. S., Chief Clinical Assistant, Royal London (Moorefields) Ophthalmic Hospital. (*Chicago: W. T. Keener & Co., 90 Wabash Avenue; London: Hodder & Stoughton, 1905.*)

This interesting volume of a little over two hundred pages will be found useful by the general practitioner. There are not a few works of exactly this character which are to be had nowadays, but Hanke's contribution holds its own with the best. At first sight one might be apt to regard it as more of a medical dictionary of the eye than a work which would be useful in the practice of ophthalmology, but a closer perusal shows that it is full of detailed and practical advice which emanates from no less a personage than Fuchs of Vienna. The book simply tells "what we do in the Royal Eye Clinic in Vienna," and it might justly bear this title. The chapter on the cornea will probably be found the most valuable. The cornea always brings out the best in writers of text-books on ophthalmology. We note that dionin is a favorite remedy in various forms of keratitis and we are convinced of its value in the more obscure forms in which the deeper parts are involved. Coming from such a source we look upon the work as trustworthy, a point of view which is strengthened by the fact that it is translated and presented to the English-speaking public by one of the leaders of British ophthalmology.

Surgical Aspects of Digestive Disorders. BY JAMES G. MUMFORD, M. D., Visiting Surgeon Massachusetts General Hospital and Instructor in Surgery in the Harvard Medical School, in association with ARTHUR K. STONE, M. D., Physician to Out-Patients, Massachusetts General Hospital and Assistant in the Theory and Practice of Physic in the Harvard Medical School. (*New York: The MacMillan Company, 1905.*)

This volume of 390 pages written by a surgeon and an internist, contains a great mass of interesting information. This association has enabled the authors to arrive at certain broad conclusions which we think are in the main justifiable.

Considerably over one-half of the work is devoted to diseases of the stomach and duodenum which are treated together. The conditions discussed are dilatation, ulcer, and carcinoma, with their diagnosis and medical and surgical treatment.

Short chapters follow on diseases of the gall passages, pancreas, and appendix vermiformis. Abdominal ptosis is also treated.

In addition to the above, the volume contains an appendix by Henry F. Hews, M. D., upon the diagnosis of gastric diseases including the ordinary methods of gastric juice analysis.

The authors do not think that diseases of the bile passages and gastric ulcer are purely surgical affections like appendicitis, but may become so in many instances, and they insist "that in all prolonged or severe disorders of such a nature a properly qualified surgeon should be sought."

We are glad to see this recommendation emphasized but are

disappointed to find no mention of it in certain diseases of the ileum and large bowel, for example, perforation of the bowel in typhoid fever, in which condition a similar association should be as close if not closer.

The work should constitute a connecting link between the views of internists and surgeons as to the subject discussed, and is a valuable contribution. The publishers have done their work well and the illustrations, although few in number, are excellent.

Progressive Medicine. A quarterly digest of advances, discoveries, and improvements in the medical and surgical sciences. Edited by Hobart A. Hare, M. D., Professor of Therapeutics and materia medica in the Jefferson Medical College, Philadelphia, etc., assisted by H. R. M. Landis, M. D., Demonstrator of Clinical Medicine in the Jefferson Medical College. Vol. III, September, 1905. (*Philadelphia and New York: Lea Brothers & Co.*)

This number contains a very good and complete review of the recent work on obstetrics, about one-third of the volume being devoted to that branch of medicine. There is, however, no marked advance in our knowledge of the subject.

A new classification of hyperemesis gravidarum is given by Williams and a method of differential diagnosis between the toxæmic and other forms. He divides the cases into the neurotic, reflex, and toxæmic, and shows that the ammonia output in the urine is normal in the first two and high in the third form, and advises induction of abortion when the ammonia coefficient is above ten per cent.

The section on artificial dilatation of the cervix gives the preference to instrumental methods for rapid dilatation, though a number of writers advocate vaginal cæsarean section. The combination of metal dilators and bags is advocated when the conditions are such that it is not necessary to complete the emptying of the uterus for several hours.

Van de Velde reports on several cases of hebotomy or extramedian symphysiotomy with very good results, and claims that this operation causes a permanent increase in the size of the pelvis.

There are several interesting and unusual cases reported.

The arrangement of the subjects under the headings pregnancy, labor, the puerperium, and obstetric surgery is very good.

At times it is difficult to tell from whom the author is quoting and one often needs to read several paragraphs before this point can be determined, and again there is sometimes confusion as to whether the author's or another's views are being given.

The Diagnostics of Internal Medicine. By G. R. Butler, Sc. D., M. D. Second revised edition. (*New York and London: D. Appleton & Co., 1905.*)

This is a very useful, compact work on medical diagnosis. Preceding the body of the text is a schedule for physical examination. The book proper is divided into two parts. The first, "The Evidences of Disease," comprises the larger portion of the reading matter, in it the various general symptoms are described and their possible causes enumerated; then follows the routine in the examination of the various systems, with a careful, though brief, description of all special physical signs, clinical methods, and instruments that are of aid in diagnosis. The second portion of the work is devoted to "Direct and Differential Diagnosis"; in it the main symptoms and physical signs of each disease are briefly presented, while the chief conditions from which the disease under discussion may be differentiated, are enumerated. There is a liberal use of italics and large type which may help to secure clearness of arrangement and promote ease of reference. Moreover, there is a good index and odd-page headings have been added. The plates are for the most part borrowed from other writers, but the diagrams appear to be original. The latter,

though useful, are perhaps a little too realistic in their execution, and may prove too diverting to the average student.

The book, in short, is quite up to date, and will prove of considerable value to the practitioner as well as to the student.
C. P. H.

Sexual Disorders of the Male and Female. By Robert W. Taylor, A. M., M. D., Consulting Genitourinary Surgeon to Bellevue and to the City (Charity) Hospitals, New York. (*New York and Philadelphia: Lea Brothers & Co., 1905.*)

The new edition of this work contains some added chapters on diseases and lesions of the female genital tract; many other sections have also been much amplified. The results too of the more recent studies of the secretions of the prostate and seminal vesicles have been incorporated.

It is only within very recent years that sexual disorders have been taken from the realm of theory and placed for the most part upon a firm pathological basis. The many, heretofore, so-called sexual diseases we now recognize as being most frequently but symptoms of definite pathological changes in the genital or urogenital tract. Hence, a treatise on sexual disorders resolves itself largely into a consideration of the inflammatory lesions of the urethral and genital tract, and so the author naturally gives considerable space to the subjects of chronic urethritis, prostatitis, etc.

The malformations and deformities, both acquired and congenital of the male genitalia, are gone into in some detail in addition to being well illustrated, while those troubles dependent upon a neuropathic condition receive but passing notice.

The work as a whole is treated in as complete and scientific a manner as the present state of our knowledge permits.

A Text-Book of Diseases of the Nose and Throat. By D. Braden Kyle, M. D. Third edition, revised and enlarged. (*Philadelphia, New York, London: W. B. Saunders & Co.*)

The third edition of this work can, on the whole, be recommended to students and practitioners interested in diseases of the nose and throat. We heartily agree with the author in his elimination of the word catarrh to designate inflammation of the mucous membrane, whether acute or chronic. This term is and has been used indiscriminately, not alone by the layman but also by the physician to designate inflammations of the nose and throat in general. As the author states, it is more proper to use a term that describes the existing pathological condition. He has classified these diseases on this basis, with a resulting clear and minute assorting of the various diseases.

The chapters treating of general considerations of mucous membranes and their pathology are highly interesting. The author thinks that by a study of the salivary secretion we can better judge the conditions of the chemical constituents of the system and determine the physiological and pathological processes going on within the body. He opposes all our knowledge of the chemistry of metabolism, when he states that a study of the saliva gives us more knowledge about these processes than an examination of the excretory secretions. He ascribes many diseases of the upper respiratory tract to an altered chemical condition of the saliva. In his discussion of hay fever, he does not even mention Dunbar's serum treatment.

The diseases of the accessory sinuses receives thorough treatment. The relationship of pathological processes of the nose and eye through the lachrymal duct are mentioned but the not infrequent class of eye troubles secondary to disease of the accessory sinuses of the nose is not spoken of. In the discussion of the treatment of deflections of the nasal septum, the author fails to describe the best methods of treatment, namely, the submucous operation as devised by Krieg abroad and Freer in this country.

The publishers deserve credit for the excellent appearance of the book.

The Johns Hopkins Hospital Bulletins are issued monthly. They are printed by the FRIEDENWALD CO., Baltimore. Single copies may be procured from NUNN & CO. and the BALTIMORE NEWS CO., Baltimore. Subscriptions, $2.00 a year, may be addressed to the publishers, THE JOHNS HOPKINS PRESS, BALTIMORE; single copies will be sent by mail for twenty-five cents each.

BULLETIN

OF

THE JOHNS HOPKINS HOSPITAL

Entered as Second-Class Matter at the Baltimore, Maryland, Postoffice.

Vol. XVII.—No. 181.]   BALTIMORE, APRIL, 1906.   [Price, 25 Cents.

CONTENTS.

ON SOME RECENT TEXT-BOOKS OF ANATOMY, WITH SPECIAL REFERENCE TO THE NEW AMERICAN EDITION OF GRAY.[1]

BY FRANKLIN P. MALL.

Judging by the numerous text-books of anatomy which have been published during the past century, it is quite clear that the authors have attempted to give the essentials of the subject, from one standpoint or another, for students of anatomy who are beginning the study of medicine. The book selected by the student usually makes a lasting impression upon him and in later years he frequently uses it for reference; for this reason it should be extensive enough to lead him into the literature upon the subject whenever it is demanded by special circumstances. Fortunately, during this period there has been a classic anatomy (Quain) in the English language, which has passed through numerous editions, having been revised successively by the greatest anatomists of England. This great work has guided many of our best students in their work, and has been made available to European students through numerous translations. However, the majority of students prefer a work which is more compact

and treats the subject from a more practical standpoint, that is, aids them to study anatomy in the laboratory, emphasizing especially those portions which bear directly upon practical surgery for the time being, leaving their own future development pretty well out of consideration.

Gray's anatomy fulfills this last requirement admirably. The first edition, which appeared in 1858, is a compact work well written and well illustrated from the standpoint of descriptive anatomy and its application to practical surgery. It immediately gained favor in England and in America, and with us has been viewed as a second Galen to which nothing could be added nor taken away, a view which hinders much the progress of any subject. New editions of the work rapidly followed one another, but in general they were revised but little for some 35 years, and on account of the very extensive use of the book by students, teachers, and examiners, it gained a position which made it heresy to question either its authority or its infallibility.

In looking over an old edition of Gray (1862) one is struck with the completeness and accuracy of the work to fit the knowledge of that time. For instance, the articles for the spleen and liver are excellent, being based upon the great works of Gray and Kiernan. Those upon the lung and in-

[1] Anatomy, Descriptive and Surgical. By Henry Gray, F. R. S. Edited by T. Pickering Pick, F. R. C. S., and Robert Howden, M. A., M. B., C. M. New American edition. Thoroughly revised and re-edited with additions by John Chalmers Da Costa, M. D., illustrated with 1132 elaborate engravings. (Philadelphia and New York: Lea Brothers & Co., 1905.)

testine, however, are meager in the light of our present knowledge of these organs. One reads there that "the villi are highly vascular structures covered with cylindrical epithelium and said to contain muscle which may aid in the propulsion of food." In the course of time Watney's work served as a basis for a revision of this statement. So until the 13th edition appeared we notice occasional changes here and there in the American edition; sometimes there is a chapter added on histology, or embryology, or on landmarks. In general the great bulk of the book remained unaltered until the 13th American edition appeared. However, this revision was not fortunate, and in the 15th edition we find the radical changes in it replaced in large part by the text from a previous English edition.

It is evident that the gradual and minor changes which we witness from edition to edition of Gray indicate that the science of anatomy is still developing, and any one familiar with its great literature would not hesitate to state that its development during the past 50 years has been very great. Anatomy can be viewed to advantage from other standpoints than the surgical, and its progress during the past century is due largely to those who have studied the subject from general, physiological, comparative, developmental, anthropological, and artistic standpoints. Furthermore, it is now questionable whether it is best for the student of medicine to study anatomy from the surgical standpoint alone, for it is probable that the greatest use to be derived from its study, outside of the discipline of a good laboratory course, is its value to the student in his subsequent study of physiology, pathology, and internal medicine, not to speak of the numerous specialties.

So if it is a fact that anatomy is growing and is of use to other branches of medicine than surgery, it follows that its scope should be morphological and general as well as descriptive. We should, therefore, not like to see Gray condensed and compact like Gerrish, but rather rewritten to include all of the modern work as has been done in an admirable way by Cunningham. Cunningham's anatomy is a clear-cut descriptive picture of the science of anatomy in 1902, as is Gray's of the science in 1850. The question now is whether the last revision, which is the only extensive one which has ever been undertaken, is thorough and complete and brings the subject fully up to date. Furthermore, the substance should be selected carefully, fundamental things should be emphasized, the growth of the science should be indicated, and enough references to the literature should be given to enable the student to find some of the important articles of the three or four thousand on anatomy which appear in some six hundred journals each year. This last point is extremely important, for if the work of the student of anatomy is to be of lasting value in later years he must come back to the subject from time to time and extend his knowledge in definite directions, and he naturally uses his old text-book which aids him if it has in it references to the literature which have been carefully and properly selected, as is the case in the

anatomies of Quain, Henle, Gegenbaur, Testut, and Poirier and Charpy. Then it is also to be remembered that the structures of the body are variable, some very much so, and an erroneous impression is left upon the student's mind if the book studied does not give the variations as far as they are known. In this respect Quain's and Henle's anatomies are satisfactory, for the variations are given in a very few words.

We read in the preface of the new Gray that in order to represent the world's best knowledge, American, English, French, and German text-books, monographs, and journal articles have been freely consulted, and that in every instance the aim has been to give proper credit to the author. It is further stated that the work is descriptive and surgical, histology and embryology having been omitted. From this standpoint then its work must be judged. We note especially in glancing through the pages that Gerrish, Cunningham, Toldt, Spalteholz, Poirier and Charpy, and Testut have been consulted freely, and to the extent in which this material has been blended with the original Gray the work has been markedly improved.

Numerous illustrations have been borrowed from the above-named sources and they have been carefully and beautifully re-engraved on wood in imitation of the illustrations retained throughout all of the former editions. However, the original pictures have a peculiar character which cannot be imitated easily by engravers unless they also have drawings made by Dr. Carter. In fact, these original illustrations are the best feature of the book, for the anatomy shown in them is simple, complete, and satisfactory, and their execution is concise and artistic (see, for instance, Figs. 648, 649, 650, 656, and 657 to illustrate the nerves of the lower extremity). The names of the parts are engraved in a delicate way on the original figures, a method used in Berenger's anatomy (1521), and from time to time since then. On the borrowed pictures in Gray the lettering is harsher and mars very much their beauty.

The original figures in Gray were pirated by Heitzmann, of Vienna, to form the major portion of his Atlas, which for many years was the favorite dissecting-room book in German laboratories. One of the inducements to produce the Atlas of Spalteholz was this pirated book, which was not adequate for the needs of German teachers, and it is a happy sequence that the book which indirectly stimulated the production of Spalteholz's Atlas should in turn be benefited by it. The great value of an atlas is that it enables the student to look ahead while making a dissection and to identify the parts as they are unraveled. Pictures of dissections true to nature aid the imagination of the student enormously and thus guide his work from the known to the unknown. It follows that the illustrations of an anatomical atlas must be typical, giving all the stages of a dissection from its beginning to its completion. The Atlas of Spalteholz meets this requirement, as does that of Toldt, and in a measure this may be said of the illustrations of Gray. In general older students and physicians leave the text and study the figures of Gray, and this fact speaks immensely in their favor. If a student's mental picture of the structure of the body is good, in later years good illustrations will enable him to recall his anatomy better than the text alone. I am sure that to look up a question of topographical anatomy Toldt's plates will prove to be of far greater value than Hyrtl's fascinating work, which contains no illustrations at all. A blending of the two makes a good combination, the method usually employed in Austria.

The only marked improvement which could be suggested regarding the illustrations in the new Gray would be to include more of Toldt's and of Spalteholz's pictures, but, of course, this is out of the question. A number of illustrations to represent the early growth of bone, as in the 2d edition of Cunningham, would improve the section on osteology. The wrist and ankle bones are not as well illustrated as in a number of other works. The muscles of the back need an additional illustration or two. A number of figures are not especially good, e. g., Figs. 396, 408, 426, 432, 433, 536, 602, 633, 670, 677, 684, 688, 693, 899, 978, and could be omitted to advantage. Also the following corrections may be made: Fig. 496 is after Poirier and Charpy; on Fig. 315 pectoralis major is called pectinius major, an error which appeared in the 13th edition; Fig. 503 is not properly copied; on Fig. 578 we read *knie* and *bein* : the legends of Figs. 112, 113, and 114, 115 are reversed; Fig. 842 is after Hertwig; Fig. 908 is after Ramon y Cajal; and Fig. 955 is not after Poirier and Charpy but after the late Dr. Hendrickson, of Philadelphia. Furthermore, the lack of uniform labeling of the figures is rather confusing to the beginner. An example is seen in Fig. 753, anterior auricular muscle, which in Fig. 755 is called attrahens aurem. In general the excellent progressive illustrations, with uniform lettering, in Cunningham makes these pictures more intelligible to the beginner, for the pictures fit into one another and the language is not confusing. In this book the old edition has passed into the new without a break in the illustrations, as is also the case with the new edition of Spalteholz; in both cases the character of the illustrations has been retained and improved.

The text of the new edition of Gray has been changed to a great extent, several chapters having been entirely rewritten. The task in blending the old Gray with a number of recent text-books is not an easy one and it is questionable whether a composite of this sort can ever bring a first-class result. As it is the editor has done remarkably well in dealing with the thousands of facts in anatomy, but we fear that this happy mean will be difficult for beginners to follow, and of little value to advanced students, for the literature of anatomy is not dealt with first-hand, but has only filtered in, mainly through Cunningham and Poirier and Charpy. Furthermore, no references are given to the many anatomical journals, with the one exception of the Journal of Anatomy and Physiology. At present there is an immense activity in anatomical research, even in this country, and we are rather inclined towards text-books which deal with the literature first-hand, for those who do this are most likely to give a clear, compact, and well-proportioned description of the subject. This is the

case with Cunningham, and to a more marked degree with Quain. In the latter book, for instance, osteology is treated in a most satisfactory way in half the space that is devoted to it in Gray, and we have here a well-written text which on account of its compactness and accuracy is to be recommended to beginners, and on account of its scientific attitude and its numerous references to the literature is the best book for the advanced student who wishes to extend his reading to monographs and journal articles. In general the text in Gray is involved and diffuse, and although it is built up from crystals it needs re-crystallization. We mean that it should be briefer, things scattered should be brought together, and irrelevant matter should be removed. It should be a well-proportioned, readable work like the second edition of Cunningham. Were we dealing with the first edition of Gray we would be more lenient, but a great work, which is in its 16th edition, must be criticized from a high standpoint.

Considering the number of pages in Gray, it is remarkable that there are so few references to the literature of anatomy. The anatomical journals are almost entirely ignored, but monographs are referred to occasionally. However, the article by Delamere, Poirier, and Cuneo is referred to 21 times (three times on one page) in the chapter on the lymphatics; once would suffice. When we consider that in Quain's Anatomy the same ground is covered in fewer pages than in Gray, that the descriptions are clear-cut, accurate and complete, and that the references are sufficiently numerous to lead the student into the whole history of anatomy, we feel disappointed over this omission.—Every part of the body varies, some parts so much that it is difficult to determine the normal, and the literature upon variation is so great that no book is complete unless it leads the student, who is so inclined, to the limits of our knowledge. That this may be done in a book smaller than Gray is shown in an admirable way in Quain. This work being an American edition, we naturally expect to see more of our own literature referred to. However, it is gratifying to see Miller's work upon the lung and Hendrickson's on the bile-duct creeping in through foreign books, probably Poirier and Charpy.

One of the greatest stumbling blocks in the study of anatomy is the nomenclature, and it has always been so. During the past century a number of attempts have been made to introduce a uniform terminology, however with little success until the work was undertaken by an international commission composed of many leading anatomists—Turner, Cunningham, and Thane representing England. After working six years a satisfactory report was rendered which is now generally accepted. That these terms are adopted as synonyms in Gray is to be commended, and adds immensely to the value of the book. However, the main point is missed by using the terms indiscriminately, for it is not *Latin terms* but *uniform terms* that the commission strove to introduce. In casting the new nomenclature 30,000 terms were reduced to 5000, and of these not over 250 differ from those used in older editions of Gray. For instance, in the new terminology (B. N. A.) in English a certain muscle of the ear is called the superior auricular, and to use in different parts of Gray the synonyms atollens auriculam, atollens aurem, auricularis superior only tends to confuse the student. Many more examples could be given; the worst we have noticed are the various synonyms (six) for colliculus superior. One name, best the new one, should be used consistently throughout the book, as is the case in Cunningham, with the synonyms in foot-notes, and if the anatomy is to be a book of synonyms, many more could be found than are given in this edition of Gray. Possibly, in its transition stage, it is well to treat this subject as it has been treated in Gray, but it seems to us a pity that the beginner should be tormented so much for a paltry 250 words when the many thousand synonyms could be pushed out of the main text into foot-notes, as in Henle, for those who wish to use them. They could then be brought together in an index, or in parallel columns, as in the "day-book" of the international commission, to form a second royal octave volume of a thousand pages and be of great service to advanced students.

What is said about nomenclature applies equaly well to measure. Most of the measures are given in feet and inches. but we often notice centimeters, millimeters, and microns. The metric system should be used throughout the work.

The section on osteology is one of the easiest to deal with in descriptive anatomy, and we find this subject treated in a satisfactory manner in the new Gray. The first fifteen pages are devoted to an excellent introduction to osteology and the rest of the chapter (over 200 pages) to a good description of the bones. We are of the opinion, however, that a large portion of the text might be omitted. for the description is already given in the many excellent illustrations. The question of ossification, which has always been well illustrated in Gray, is not quite up to date, as may be noticed by comparing it with the second edition of Cunningham and with the new Hertwig. X-ray pictures and Schultze preparations have given better data regarding the early ossification of bones, and we see other recent books taking advantage of these methods. We notice, for instance, that Gray states that the body of the vertebra has two centers of ossification, an error that is not to be found in the earlier editions. Why this mistake ever crept into the book is hard to explain for the double centers were exploded by Meckel in 1815 and have not been seen by any competent investigator since that time. The foot-note on this point shows that the English editor knows that the statement is out of harmony with the literature, and we may add with the facts which are correctly stated in the first edition of Gray.

Physical anthropology should also be considered more than it is, for there is no telling when a doctor is to be called upon to give an opinion regarding the age, sex, and race of a skull, and before he does it he naturally falls back upon his text-book. In this respect he will find Quain, Gerrish, and Cunningham adequate. We do notice that there is a brief account of the size and form of the cranium, copied from Cunningham, on page 146 in Gray. Unfortunately, the formula to determine

the cephalic index was not given correctly in the first edition of Cunningham, and it is taken over blindly with its blunder.

The chapter on the ligaments is greatly improved by the introduction of new figures and the revision of the text. However, it lacks the well-proportioned text found in Cunningham, and for this reason will not be as useful to students as that in some other books. The paragraph on the motions of the elbow joint, for instance, is diffuse, while that in Gerrish is shorter and gives more information. In Quain we also find a satisfactory description of the elbow joint and in addition a reference to the article from which the information was obtained.

The chapter upon muscles in Gray is considerably longer than that in Quain and twice as long as that in Cunningham, and does not contain any more information if we overlook the notes on surgery. Our experience is that the description in Quain is the most satisfactory and gives in addition numerous satisfactory notes on variations. Much space in Gray is devoted to the discussion of the relation of the muscles to one another, as well as to the surrounding parts, which might be greatly abridged, as well as aided by a number of transverse sections. The value of this method to illustrate relations and attachments is well shown in Fig. 295, giving a transverse section of the abdomen in the lumbar region. The descriptions of the individual muscles, while not especially full, are fairly good. In the introduction (p. 361) the descriptions of the muscle cells are far from lucid and accurate. In the next paragraph it is stated that the muscle fibers may be 10 cm. long, while on page 363 we read that those of the sartorius are nearly two feet in length. Several other minor errors are to be seen scattered through the chapter (pp. 368, 376, 394, and 481) ; however, such errors are not peculiar to Gray, for they exist in all books.

The sections on the vascular system are much in need of recasting, for the variations of the vessels are numerous and their position is of great interest to the surgeon. The general anatomy of the heart. arteries, and veins is meager and flavored somewhat with teleology.

In view of the recent important work upon the heart, this subject should be introduced with embryology, which gives a rational explanation of variations, and the heart musculature should be described according to MacCallum, who was the first to unravel this complicated structure successfully. The little bundle of His, Jr., which is of the greatest physiological and clinical importance, is also ignored. For the present the chapter on the musculature of the heart is better in Quain than in any other text-book, and it is not rash to predict that the newer work upon this subject will find a place in the next edition.

Within the last half century many studies have been made upon arterial variations, as may be witnessed by consulting the numerous articles in the anatomical journals. and some forthcoming book must incorporate this work. Not only must the extreme variations be recorded, but the types of distribution must be given also. For instance, Hitzrot has shown that the usual description of the axillary artery occurs in but 20 per cent of the cases. And very recently Bean has demonstrated that the branching of the subclavian artery, according to the description in Gray and Quain, is much more common on the left side than on the right, while according to the B. N. A. (Spalteholz and Toldt) the opposite is the case. Gray's description is found present in 27 per cent of all the cases studied, and the B. N. A. description in 30 per cent, leaving other types to account for the remaining 43 per cent. From these and other studies it is clear that the iron-bound description as followed by most anatomists is misleading to the student and injurious to the surgeon.

There is one other general item which requires reform; it is the description of the relation of the arteries to the surrounding structures. A round ring with names printed on four sides, as given in Gray, may possibly be of value, but when we see such excellent figures of sections as are given in Merkel's great topographical anatomy, or in Oskar Schultze's topographical atlas, we question very much their use. Furthermore, these latter figures are much better and are not misleading, for a circle has more than four sides to it and the surrounding structures are not of equal size. Gerrish, Merkel, and Schultze take advantage of the section to a certain extent, and the recent works of Jackson and Potter show what may be done with it with medical students in Missouri. Now that cross-section work has been well established in most of our leading medical schools, it·is to be hoped that books may be revised to meet our needs more than the ones that are at present at our disposal.

The chapter on lymphatics is very satisfactory, being based largely upon the excellent article by Poirier and Cuneo. The introduction, which should have more of Delemare in it, is unsatisfactory, for it has in it a vague notion regarding the extent of the lymphatic system. The description of the lymphnode is much too brief and inadequate. It is stated that the pleural, pericardial, peritoneal, and synovial cavities belong to the lymphatic system. Also that the valves are absent in lymphatic capillaries and seldom found in visceral lymphatics. These two statements show that the literature has not been consulted freely. However, it is a pleasure for us to note that the greatest progress in the study of the lymphatics in recent years has been made in America by Sabin and MacCallum, of Baltimore; by Lewis, of Boston and by Warthin, of Ann Arbor. The work of the first three investigators defines the extent of the lymphatic system morphologically and the last named author gives us the best description of the hemolymph-nodes in man. This work has received due recognition abroad, some of it is incorporated in the second edition of Cunningham, but none of it is mentioned in Gray.

One of the most difficult chapters to write is that on the nervous system, although we have a large number of excellent monographs to draw upon. Our standard is a book like Van Gehuchten or the recent excellent and "life-like" account given in the last edition of Edinger. A most satisfactory, complete, and modern account of the brain is given in the second edition of Cunningham. The facts in general appear to be correctly stated in the new Gray; some errors, however, have crept in.

The absence of a clear and systematic method in the presentation of the central nervous system renders the description of this complicated structure more confusing than is necessary. Isolated facts are given without sufficient correlation and without consistent sequence. One finds, for instance, the structure of the cerebrum, its commissural and association fibers described under the heading mid-brain (p. 913 ff.), together with those structures in the region of the aqueduct of Sylvius. Another striking feature is the absence of uniformity in the treatment of different regions. More than 16 pages are devoted to the surface markings of the cerebrum, which could have been largely shown with illustrations without any text; while the internal structure of the medulla receives but 6 pages. The pons, medulla, and cord all suffer for want of good illustrations showing cross-sections. There are but two of the cord, which, by the way, are wrong side up (pp. 838 and 844). No attempt is made to show the appearance of the various levels.

So many nerve-paths come together in the medulla and there is gradual transition of the medulla into the cord that for purposes of description and teaching it is much easier to pass from the cord to the brain than in the opposite direction. It follows also that the description of the medulla should be accompanied with numerous accurate pictures of sections at regular intervals, a method introduced by Stilling and followed in all of the great books on the brain. Such pictures are wanting in Gray. The gross illustrations (Figs. 604 and 606) of the floor of the fourth ventricle are crude and should be replaced by a new illustration from Retzius or by the excellent one from Streeter's article, which may be found in Edinger's Neurology. Furthermore, the description of this difficult region could be made clearer by Miss Sabin's reconstruction of the medulla, which shows the nerve paths in three dimensions.

It is stated on page 818 that neuroglia fibrils develop from the prolongations of neuroglia cells; the work of Weigert and of Hardesty is not considered. There is also a paragraph on complete fissures (865) which is based upon Cunningham's original article upon this subject. Later, in the first edition of Cunningham's Anatomy, less stress is placed upon the significance of these fissures, and since we have the results of Hochstetter and of Retzius it would be better to omit them altogether. On page 903 the posterior commissure is described as belonging wholly or principally to the inter-brain, and on page 905 the anterior pillar of the fornix is described as going through the optic thalamus. It would also be well, we think, to add the pulvinar to the diagram on page 1023.

The organs of special sense are treated in a satisfactory manner in Gray, taking up more space, however, than in Cunningham and in Quain. A brief description of the development of the eye and ear and of the gustatory organs would add to the clearness of this section. We make the same criticism of the section on the genito-urinary organs; they should be treated somewhat as is the alimentary canal on pages 1236-1245.

It would be well in describing the regions of the abdomen to give as well those recommended by Toldt and adopted by the international commission (B. N. A.), for they seem to be less variable and therefore of more value to the clinician. A more detailed description of the blood-vessels of the walls of the small intestine as well as the position of this organ is pertinent on account of frequent operations upon these structures. For this change space might be gained by omitting the paragraphs on the movements of the stomach and the intestines, which really belong to physiology. Five references to an article on the movements of the intestine are given on page 1323; one would suffice. The description of the structures of the liver and spleen have been excellent in all editions of Gray, one based upon the work of Kiernan and the other upon Gray's monograph. They illustrate well the advantage in compiling text-books from first-class studies, a method employed to great advantage in the various editions of Quain. At this point we go out of our way to mention Miller's work on the structure of the lung. He finally cleared up the relation of the air-cells to the terminal bronchus and to the blood-vessels, and his work has been incorporated in nearly all of the great European anatomies. It was he who introduced the term atrium, which we see mentioned on page 1378 of Gray. According to the index atria appear to be peculiar to the left bronchus.

We do not believe that a descriptive and surgical anatomy is complete without a chapter on superficial and relational anatomy. One may be found in Quain, in Cunningham, and in Gerrish, and for a number of editions Holden's Landmarks were published as an appendix to Gray. In recent years nearly three volumes of Merkel's great work have appeared, not to speak of the excellent atlas and text-book of Schultze and Stewart. Possibly the excuse for the omission of this important chapter from Gray is to be found in its large number of excellent new figures, as well as the wide distribution of Spalteholz, Toldt, and other atlases.

The above remarks, a little more numerous than are usual in an article of this kind, are made in the interest of anatomy. That a book like Gray, which has become so firmly established with us, is extensively revised and in part rewritten indicates that anatomy is developing in America. At present we are drawing heavily upon Germany, England, and France for light, and the new Gray comes forward to meet the demand.

We congratulate the editor and the publisher upon the many improvements of Gray in this edition, and hope that it will soon be given a new revision in which a uniform nomenclature is used, irrelevant matter cut out, the text made clear-cut and compact, and much of the new literature added, as is the case with each new edition of Quain. Possibly in a few years we may rise to the point of having real American anatomies, books good enough to export, like Minot's Embryology, and we should not be contented until this is the case.

A VARIATION IN THE SOLEUS AND PLANTARIS MUSCLES.

By D. H. DuPree.

(From the Anatomical Laboratory of the Johns Hopkins University.)

While dissecting in Dr. Mall's laboratory last winter I found the following variations, which he gave me permission to describe. The body in which they occurred was that of a negro male, No. 1217 in the collection. The variations consist in the absence of the plantaris in the right leg, and its peculiar insertion and size in the left leg, and of an extra slip in the soleus in the left leg.

The Soleus.—In the left leg of this cadaver the soleus consists of (a) a lateral head and (b) a median head, a deep groove running between them on the posterior aspect; and (c) of an *extra* slip anterior to the median head, which is inserted into the calcanean bone by a tendon of its own. The lateral head rises from the posterior surface of the head and upper third of the shaft of the fibula. Its origin is fleshy and tendinous, the tendon of origin running in the substance of the muscle and appearing on the anterior surface by its edge. The fibers are inserted into a broad aponeurosis on its posterior surface and thereby into the tendo Achillis, except some of its anterior fibers, which blend with the middle head

in the upper third of the leg. The median head arises from the inner border of the tibia in its upper third, and the oblique line of the same bone, and from the tendinous arch covering the posterior tibial vessels and nerves. Its fibers are inserted into an aponeurosis on its posterior surface and thence into the tendo Achillis. However, some of its fibers blend with those of the lateral head, as is seen on looking into the depth of the groove separating the two heads on the posterior surface. Moreover, in the upper third of the leg this part of the muscle is inseparable from the extra slip.

The extra slip rises in common with the median head. It lies on the anterior surface of the soleus and is blended with the median head in the upper part of the leg, as mentioned above, except for a shallow groove running between them along its lateral margin. In the lower two-thirds of the leg it is independent of the rest of the soleus. On its free posterior surface, i. e., below its separation from the median head, there is an aponeurosis from which fibers arise to be inserted into a tendon on its anterior surface. The tendon of insertion is broad above, but narrows as it approaches the ankle, and comes to lie on the mesial border of the muscle. It is inserted into the mesial surface of the os calcis near its posterior margin. This extra part of the soleus covers the posterior tibial artery and nerve throughout its extent. It is about the size of the middle head.

The blood supply of the median head comes from the posterior tibial artery. The extra slip receives four branches from the posterior tibial artery during its course under the muscle, and it also gets a branch from the peroneal just before this artery disappears under the flexors. The lateral head gets its blood from the peroneal artery.

The extra slip gets its nerve supply from a branch of the posterior tibial nerve in the upper third of the leg and it also receives a twig from a branch of the same nerve going to supply the median head. The lateral and median heads get their nerve supply from branches of this nerve.

The soleus is normal in the right leg of the cadaver.

In the embryo the mesenchyme of the hind limb differentiates into a central bony mass and a ventral and dorsal muscle mass, this differentiation progressing from the body distalward. The muscles become attached above first and later get their distal attachments to the bone. Hence it is easy to conceive that this extra slip of the soleus for some reason got separated from the rest of the muscle and extended on down the leg until it finally got attached to the os calcis by a tendon of its own.

Le Double says that in comparative anatomy this muscle is very variable in its development, and is absent in many species, among which are the kangaroo, the dog, etc. According to Quain, "the tibial head of the soleus is almost peculiar to man; among the lower animals it occurs, of small size, only in the gorilla and sometimes in the chimpanzee."

A number of anatomists have reported similar variations of the soleus. Henle mentions a "broad bundle going from the mesial surface of this muscle (soleus) to the mesial surface of the heel-bone."

Quain says that, "to the soleus an accessory portion is occasionally added at its lower and inner part; this usually ends on the inner side of the tendo Achillis, but it is sometimes attached separately to the os calcis, or to the internal annular ligament."

Turner, in writing on the frequency of the occurrence of accessories to the flexors in the region of the inner ankle, mentions "A long slip springing from the inner side of the soleus, and passing quite distinct from the tendo Achillis to be inserted into the inner concave surface of the os calcis."

L. Testut mentions the fact that the tibial head of the soleus is wanting in nearly all monkeys. He says that " one encounters sometimes, besides the normal soleus, a supernumerary soleus, which generally ends on the os calcis on its mesial surface," and arising from " the oblique line of the tibia, the soleus surface of the same, and the deep fascia of the leg, etc." He mentions a case in which he found " in the right leg a supernumerary soleus and a long accessory to the

flexors, both well developed and fused into a single muscle. This muscle covers entirely the peroneal and tibial arteries."

Le Double says, " one sometimes finds a supernumerary soleus muscle, small or large, situated in front of the soleus, having the same origin with it and inserted into the os calcis by a separate tendon." He quotes the references above to Quain and Testut. He says that Testut regards this accessory soleus attached separately into the os calcis as a variety

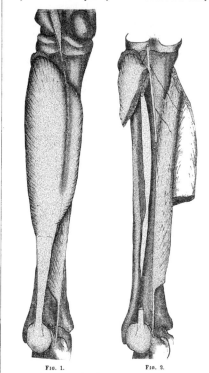

FIG. 1.   FIG. 2.

FIG. 1.—Dissection of left leg of No. 1217, showing attachment of extra slip of soleus to inner surface of os calcis, and the insertion of the tendon of the plantaris into the tendo Achillis at lower end of the middle head of soleus. The gastrocnemius has been cut away.

FIG. 2.—The soleus has been divided in upper third of leg and middle head and extra slip turned inward to show origin of extra slip and its relations to the rest of the muscle. The nerve exposed is the posterior tibial.

of plantaris, and disputes this view on the ground that it comes from the deep surface of the soleus and that it often co-exists with a well-formed plantaris.

The Plantaris.—In this subject the plantaris was entirely absent in the right leg. In the left leg it was very much reduced in size. Its origin was normal, but its slender tendon was inserted into the inner border of the tendo Achillis about half way between the knee and the ankle.

According to Quain, Gruber, and Le Double, this muscle is absent in man in about 7 per cent of subjects dissected. Le Double says that it is rarely absent in races of color. In anthropoids it is often absent also (Quain, Le Double).

The insertion of the plantaris is very variable and cases are mentioned in which it was found to end in the tissue separating the superficial from the deep muscles, the internal portion of the annular ligaments, the bursa or the os calcis under the tendo Achillis, or the plantar fascia (Le Double). Quain says that its tendon may be " sometimes enclosed in the lower part of the tendo Achillis."

In many of the lower animals the plantaris continued into the plantar fascia is a superficial flexor of the toes—the homologue of the palmaris longus. In man, using his feet only as a support to the body, the plantar fascia became attached to the os calcis and the plantaris is left only as a vestige (Le Double).

BIBLIOGRAPHY.

Henle: Vol. I, p. 309.

Quain: Part II, Vol. II, p. 264.

Wm. Turner: Transactions of the Royal Society of Edinburgh, Vol. XXIV, Part I, p. 175, Dec., 1864.

L. Testut: Anatomie Humaine, Vol. I, p. 740.

Le Double: Traité des Variations du Système Musculaire de l'homme.

Bardeen and Lewis: American Journal of Anatomy, Vol. I, 1901-2: " Development of the Limbs, Body-wall, and Back in Man."

THE PANCREATIC DUCTS IN THE CAT.

By George Julius Heuer.

(From the Anatomical Laboratory of the University of Wisconsin.)

The pancreas was known to the earliest investigators, and has been the subject of frequent study, especially with regard to its physiological and pathological significance. Whether it was known to Hippocrates is doubtful. Galen recognized the presence of the pancreas but was uncertain as to its significance. He thought that it served as a protection for the arteries, veins, and nerves which divided near it. As Galen was considered the authority by all following physicians and anatomists, his view was not questioned and it was not until the time of Vesalius, the founder of modern anatomy, that the authority of Galen was overthrown. Vesalius, although he overlooked the significance of the pancreas, made some important observations as to its attachment to the duodenum and its position in the omentum. After the time of Vesalius nothing of real importance was done on the pancreas until toward the middle of the seventeenth century, when Wirsung discovered a pancreatic duct in man, opening into the intestine in connection with the ductus choledochus. Other investigators, as Vesling, in 1664, and De Graaf, in 1671, showed that in man there were sometimes two ducts, the larger opening into the duodenum with the ductus choledochus, the smaller independently. These investigators, however, thought that the presence of two ducts was anomalous.

In 1775, Santorini established the presence of two ducts as the normal condition. He described the ducts in man and gave figures showing their relation. His work, however, seems to have been forgotten or ignored until the time of Bernard in 1846. Bernard called attention to the constant presence of two ducts in the adult and his observations, together with those of other prominent anatomists, established the presence of two ducts as the normal condition. Even after the time of Bernard, the presence of two pancreatic ducts in many mammals was overlooked. Chauveau states that in the ox, sheep, goat, pig, dog, and cat, the excretory duct of the pancreas is single and opens into the intestine at varying distances from the pylorus. Since the publication of this work, it has been found that instead of one duct there are normally two ducts in the ox, horse, dog, and cat, and it is probable that further investigation will lead to the same conclusion in many other mammals. Of the more recent papers on the ducts of the pancreas, Gage has described the ampulla of Vater and the pancreatic ducts in the cat, and Revell has described the pancreatic ducts in the dog.

The pancreas of the cat has been studied to a slight extent both from the embryological and anatomical standpoint. The fullest account of the development of the pancreatic ducts of the cat is that of Felix. He states that in embryos 9 mm. long there are two pancreatic anlages, one dorsal and one ventral. Later, in an embryo 11 mm. long, the dorsal bud is only slightly developed and thus it comes about that in the adult only one pancreatic duct is present.

Schirmer studied the ducts in the pancreas of the cat in 17 animals. He found that the form and size of the pancreas varied greatly. He described two ducts, a larger which opened into the duodenum with the ductus choledochus and a smaller which opened independently 3-7 cm. caudad to the first.

Gage, as already stated, worked on the ampulla of Vater and pancreatic ducts in the cat. He found two ducts, the larger opening into the duodenum with the ductus choledochus, the smaller independently.

From the study of the development of the pancreas in many mammals and vertebrates, the fact is well established at the present time that the pancreas arises from at least two anlages, one arising from the dorsal, the other from the ventral wall of the duodenum. More recently the presence of three pancreatic anlages has been found in man and in the chick, of which one is dorsal, the other two ventral. The two ventral anlages later fuse to form a single bud. The two anlages, the dorsal and ventral (whether single or formed by the fusion of two ventral buds) grow away from the duodenum and cross each other, fusing at the place where they cross. Correspondingly there are two ducts present which almost always anastomose with each other within that part of the gland which is formed by the fusion of the two anlages. The relation of these two ducts is subject to variation, but there is one type which occurs most frequently in each species and this type is called the normal. It was to find, if possible, this " normal " in the cat as well as to work out the distribution of the pancreatic ducts that the following work was undertaken.

The material used included, (1) 35 animals, of which 3 were fixed with formalin for the study of the topography. The pancreas of each of the 35 animals was examined with regard to its shape, the presence of an arm or bridge of pancreatic tissue (to be described later), the position of the opening of the ducts into the duodenum, and, with the exception of the 3 cases fixed with formalin, to the distribution of the pancreatic ducts as determined by the injection of a starch mass or by celloidin corrosions. (2) 3 animals were used for sections of the intestine through the ampulla of Vater; one for cross-sections of the duodenum and two for longitudinal sections, the two latter being at right angles to each other. (3) 2 animals were used for cross and longitudinal sections of the duodenum through the opening of the ductus accessorius.

Topography.—For the study of the topography of the pancreas, the animals were killed with chloroform, supported in their natural position and fixed by injecting a 10 per cent formalin solution into the carotid artery. After allowing the animal to remain for several hours or over night, the viscera were firmly fixed and hardened, and the position of the pancreas and its relation to the surrounding parts could be accurately determined (Figs. 1 and 2).

The pancreas in the cat is almost without exception cream-colored, of an elongated flattened form, being from 8-12 cm. long, 1-3 cm. wide, and .2-1 cm. thick. The size varies considerably even in animals of the same weight. It is made up of various sized lobes and lobules bound together by connective tissue. The free margins of the gland are irregular in outline.

At about its middle, the pancreas is bent acutely on itself, the straight lines including most of each half making an angle of about 45 degrees with each other. The apex of the angle lies dorsal to the pylorus. The right and left legs of the triangle were, in the 3 cases fixed with formalin, about equal in length. In examining other cases of fresh material, the left limb or cauda pancreatis sometimes appeared to be the longer.

The right limb or caput pancreatis (termed also the duodeno-dorsal portion) lies on the right side of the abdominal cavity. It follows the course of the duodenum, being attached to its median wall. In some cases it extends caudad as far as the U-shaped bend (pars horizontalis) of the duodenum; in other cases to within 1-2 cm. of the bend. The general direction of this limb is parallel to the antero-posterior axis of the animal.

The caput pancreatis is much flattened and has a dorsal and ventral surface. The dorsal surface lies ventral to the caudate lobe of the liver and the right kidney. The ventral surface is slightly hollowed. Into the hollow fits the dorsal wall of the ascending colon.

The left limb or cauda pancreatis (termed also the splenic portion) runs in the dorsal wall of the great omentum across the abdominal cavity, its long axis making an angle of about 45 degrees with the antero-posterior axis of the animal. It is narrower and thicker than the caput. The cephalic half of the cauda lies anterior to the transverse limb of the large intestine. Its anterior border lies dorsal to the greater curvature of the stomach. Its posterior surface is hollowed to receive the transverse colon. The posterior half of the cauda is flattened laterally and has a right and left surface. The left surface lies adjacent to the posterior portion of the spleen; the right surface is much hollowed to receive the descending colon. The cauda pancreatis as a whole. lies ventral to the left kidney and adrenal body and dorsal to the stomach and coils of the intestine.

Lying in the plica duodeno-jejunalis between the caput and cauda is a narrow strip of glandular tissue, the shape of which varies considerably (Fig. 2, *C*). It is characteristic in the cat, having been found in every adult animal examined. It occurs in two forms, either as a bridge connecting the caput and cauda, or as an arm or spur, that is, an outgrowth from the caput or cauda but not joining the two limbs. The former type is by far the more frequent. Of 35 cases examined, the bridge type was present in 25, the arm or spur type in 4, an incomplete formation in 5, while in 1 case, a young animal, the structure was absent altogether. When present as an arm, this strip of glandular tissue is clearly an outgrowth from either caput or cauda as the case might be. When present as a bridge it is apparently formed by an outgrowth from both caput and cauda, the two arms meeting and fusing to form the bridge. This is indicated in the 5 cases of incomplete formation of the bridge. In 2 of these there was an outgrowth into the plica duodeno-jejunalis from both caput and cauda, the two spurs approaching each other but still remaining widely separated (Fig. 3, I). In one.case the two arms had approached to within a millimeter of each other but were still distinctly separate (II). In 2 cases the two arms had slightly overlapped and between the two there had formed an extremely narrow strip of glandular tissue (III). This stage closely approximates the normal condition in which the fusion between the two arms is complete (IV). In all cases which were observed, the fusion of the two arms took place immediately dorsal to the arteria mesenterica superior and vena mesenterica superior which pass between the two limbs of the pancreas.

Pancreatic Ducts.—The pancreatic ducts in the cat were studied by dissections of hardened injected material and by celloidin corrosion preparations. The latter method was used in the majority of cases. The preparations were made by injecting celloidin into the ductus pancreaticus (Wirsungiania) with a hand syringe and then digesting the pancreas in pepsin (Fig. 4).

In describing the ducts the same general plan will be followed as was adopted by Revell in his description of the pancreatic ducts in the dog. The ducts then will be described in three parts:

(1) Intraglandular—lying within the gland.
(2) Free—between the gland and the wall of the duodenum.
(3) Duodenal—within the wall of the duodenum.

Ductus Pancreaticus (Wirsungiania).

(1) Intraglandular Part.—The ducts arise in the lobules as the intermediate ducts (called also intercalated ducts) formed by the union of the secretory capillaries of the end pieces of the gland. The intercalated ducts unite to form the interlobular ducts. The interlobular ducts unite usually like a letter Y. The stems of these Y's form the arms of larger similar Y's. The planes of successive Y's are at various angles to one another, being sometimes at right angles but oftener at angles less than 90 degrees. Very often instead of the Y form of union the ducts unite T-like. The union of the ducts is not confined to this Y-like or dichotomous form. It frequently happens that three branches unite at one point, all of which lie in different planes (Fig. 5, I).

The interlobular ducts unite to form the lobar ducts. Each lobar duct runs near the axis of the lobe toward the axis of the gland, being joined by lobular branches by which its diameter is constantly increased. The union of the interlobular ducts to form the lobar ducts continues to be dichotomous, especially in the case of the shorter ducts, and often is so up to the point of entrance of the lobar duct into the axial or main duct (Fig. 5, II).

In or near the axis of each limb of the pancreas runs the main or axial duct. It arises from the extremity of each limb by the union of the lobar ducts. Each axial duct runs toward the duodenum and in its course receives the lobar ducts from all sides and at varying angles of junction. The axial ducts receive also the branches from the bridge or arm of the pancreas. In the bridge type these branches are two in number. They arise together near the middle of the bridge by the union of small branches and pass in opposite directions, the

one joining the axial branch of the cauda, the other entering into the formation of the axial branch of the caput (Fig. 4, *A* and *B*). In most cases the two branches were distinctly separate at their point of origin. In three cases an anastomosis took place between the two branches, the union occurring in the portion of the bridge which lies dorsal to the blood vessels previously spoken of. This distribution of the ducts indicates also the way in which the bridge is formed. In the arm type there is a single branch which joins the axial duct of the caput or cauda as the case might be.

The axial branch from the caput meets that of the cauda adjacent, that is, to the left of the opening of the ductus choledochus, the union taking place toward the dorsal surface of the gland. From this point of union the duct continues toward the duodenum as a thick trunk from 4.5 to 9 mm. long which frequently receives a few short branches in its course. It emerges from the pancreas near its dorsal surface and continues toward the intestine as the free part of the ductus pancreaticus.

(2) Free Part of the Ductus Pancreaticus.—This is to be sought for on the dorsal side of the duodenum. It is near the anterior end of that part of the pancreas which is directly applied to the duodenum. The dorsal edge of the pancreas overlaps it and conceals its passage to the duodenum. The best guide to it is the ductus choledochus. This can easily be distinguished by its brownish or greenish color due to the bile within it and can readily be traced to its point of entrance into the wall of the duodenum. At this point the wall of the duodenum is slightly bulged out due to the ampulla of Vater. By lifting up the dorsal edge of the pancreas, the ductus pancreaticus will be seen as a whitish band (or other color if injected) passing from the pancreas to the wall of the duodenum and entering it immediately caudad to, and almost in contact with, the ductus choledochus. It is from 1 to 3 mm. long and 1.5 to 2.5 mm. in diameter. Its course toward the intestine is usually slightly caudad.

(3) Duodenal Part of the Ductus Pancreaticus.—This is from 2 to 3 mm. long and 1.5 to 2.5 mm. in diameter when distended. The duct enters the wall of the duodenum on its left dorsal side and curves around it toward its median dorsal side. Its course through the wall of the duodenum is oblique, the duct being directed caudad and making an angle with the longitudinal muscle coat of the duodenum which varies from 20 to 70 degrees. The duct opens together with the ductus choledochus into the ampulla of Vater, an enlarged space in the dorsal wall of the duodenum. The ampulla communicates with the lumen of the duodenum by a single opening which forms thus a common opening for both the bile and pancreatic ducts. This opening is situated at or a little caudad to the summit of a papilla which projects into the lumen of the duodenum from its dorsal wall. The papilla is the enlarged portion of a fold or ridge of the mucosa (plica longitudinalis duodeni) which extends caudalward from the pylorus along the dorsal wall of the duodenum. In a distended condition of the duodenum, the fold is nearly obliterated, but the

papilla remains quite prominent. It is often pinkish, due to the congestion of the neighboring blood vessels, and is frequently bile-stained. The opening, as before stated, is common to both the ductus pancreaticus and ductus choledochus. It is from 2 to 3 cm. from the pylorus.

The Ampulla of Vater.

As the ductus pancreaticus and ductus choledochus approach the duodenum their lumina lose their regular outlines due to the folding of the inner surfaces of their walls. Within the duodenal wall their lumina become still more irregular, and, in the undistended condition, are flattened antero-posteriorly. For a short distance the two ducts remain distinct, being separated by a wedge-shaped band of smooth muscle. Beyond the muscle band the two ducts lose their distinctness and continue as narrowed channels incompletely separated by folds of tissue. These channels open into the ampulla of Vater. The ampulla is likewise irregular in outline, being subdivided by folds of its inner surface. In the undistended condition these folds are arranged as shown in Figs. 6 and 7. In a distended condition the ampulla shows a different appearance. The folds now stretch across the cavity subdividing it into compartments as shown in Fig. 8. The folds thus present the appearance of a distinct valve. They may serve to prevent the contents of the duodenum from entering either duct and do aid in preventing the flow of the bile into the ductus pancreaticus or vice versa. This is shown by the results of injections. A number of unsuccessful attempts were made to inject the pancreatic ducts by introducing the needle of the syringe into the opening of the ampulla. A small quantity of celloidin passed into the ampulla, but none entered the pancreatic duct. It was necessary to break through the folds of the ampulla and have the needle enter the pancreatic duct before successful injection could be obtained. Again several attempts were made to inject the pancreatic ducts by closing the opening of the ampulla into the duodenum and then injecting into the ductus choledochus as Revell did in the case of the dog. Under ordinary pressure no celloidin entered the ductus pancreaticus at all, and under high pressure but very little passed into the pancreatic duct, so that successful celloidin injections could not be made in this way. With fluids, such as water or an aqueous solution of Berlin blue, the same results were obtained. Little, if any, of the fluids entered the pancreatic duct even under high pressure. That the folds are not always present or do not invariably prevent fluids from passing from one duct into the other was shown in one case in which regurgitation of the bile into the ductus pancreaticus had taken place. It is to be regretted that an examination of the ampulla was not made in this case.

The relation of the bile and pancreatic ducts to the ampulla was found to be quite different from that which Gage describes and figures. Beyond the wedge of smooth muscle, the two ducts, as before stated, lose their distinct walls and can be traced into the ampulla as narrow channels between the folds of mucosa. Two distinct ducts in the ampulla, of which

the bile duct extends up to within a short distance of the orifice, while the pancreatic opens about the middle of the ampulla, as is shown in Pl. XIV, Fig. 1, of Gage's paper, were not found in any instance.

Ductus Accessorius (Santorini).

(1) Intraglandular Part.—This portion of the duct lies within the pancreas ventral to the axial branch of the caput. Its direction is caudad and to the right, that is, as if it came from the cauda pancreatis. It is from 8 to 15 mm. long and from .4 to .7 mm. in diameter. It receives a varying number of branches which, as a rule, are small. The exact extent of the duct is not easily made out because of the difficulty in determining the point of anastomosis of the duct with the ductus pancreaticus. In some cases the extent of the duct could not be determined because of the fact that at one place the diameter of the ductus accessorius and the branch of the ductus pancreaticus with which it anastomosed was much reduced and increased from this place in both directions. This narrow portion that marked the boundary of the two ducts. The anastomosis between the ducts is subject to variation. The ductus accessorius may be connected by anastomosis with one of the small branches of a lobar duct belonging to the ductus pancreaticus, or it may be connected by anastomosis with the main stem of a lobar duct instead of with one of its smaller branches. In this case the duct has more nearly the form of a side channel from the main duct to the wall of the duodenum. Again, the branches of the ductus accessorius may anastomose freely with those of a lobar duct giving rise in some instances to quite a complicated network (Fig. 10, IV and V).

(2) Free Part of the Ductus Accessorius.—This is to be sought for on the ventral side of the duodenum, a little caudad to the ductus pancreaticus. The ventral edge of the pancreas overlaps it and conceals its passage to the duodenum. By pushing back the ventral edge of the pancreas and testing the attachment of the latter to the duodenum, a whitish band will be found which is firmly inserted into the wall of the duodenum and which can be traced to the point where it enters the substance of the gland. This whitish band is the free part of the ductus accessorius. It is from 1 to 2 mm. long and about .5 mm. in diameter. Its course toward the duodenum is usually at right angles to its wall.

(3) Duodenal Part of the Ductus Accessorius.—This measures from 1.5 to 2.5 mm. long. Its course through the wall of the duodenum is not in any constant direction, but is in some cases at right angles to the longitudinal muscle coat, in other cases directed either caudad or cephalad. On reaching the mucosa the duct usually enlarges somewhat in diameter. It opens into the duodenum at the papilla duodeni. This is situated 5 to 12 mm. caudad to the opening of the ductus pancreaticus and from one-fourth to one-third of the distance around the intestine to the left. In 3 cases the opening was at the same level as that of the ductus pancreaticus. The papilla duodeni is frequently very indistinct in fresh material,

but more prominent in material hardened in alcohol. This papilla is the slightly enlarged portion of a fold which extends from the pylorus caudad, running parallel to the plica longitudinalis duodeni. The opening can often be found by running a seeker along the fold toward the pylorus. The fold is, like the papilla, often indistinct and sometimes absent. From these facts it is seen that the determination of the position of this opening is often somewhat difficult. The best and surest way to find its location is to inject some thin mass into the ductus pancreaticus and force it around through the ductus accessorius so that it flows into the duodenum.

Note on the ductus accessorius.—Within the wall of the duodenum the duct loses its distinct wall although still lined by a layer of epithelium. The mucosa dips down between the muscle coats and the duct and is abundantly provided with glands which open into it. In the mucosa an enlargement of the duct usually occurs, this enlargement corresponding in some degree to the ampulla of Vater. Cross and longitudinal sections of the duodenum show that this part of the duct is subdivided by folds of the mucosa. In two cases, one of longitudinal sections, the other of cross-sections of the duodenum through the duct a reservoir was found in the mucosa which had a distinct epithelial lining and which was in connection with the ductus accessorius (Fig. 9). As these were the only two cases in which serial sections were made, its significance and the frequency of occurrence were not determined.

Communications between the Ducts.—Due to its small size and also probably to the thickness of the injection mass, the ductus accessorius was not injected in every instance. In a number of cases the duodenal part of the ductus accessorius was not injected. Whether this was due to the contraction of a sphincter muscle around the duct or to the atrophy of this part of the duct was not determined.

In the large majority of cases both the ductus pancreaticus and ductus accessorius were completely injected. A study of these showed that the communication between the two ducts is subject to great variation. All cases examined, however, could be reduced to one of four types (Fig. 10, I, II, III, and IV). In the first type the ductus accessorius communicates by anastomosis with a single branch of a lobar duct belonging to the axial branch of the caput. In the second type the anastomosis is single as in the first, but the lobar duct joins the axial branch of the cauda. In the third type several anastomoses are formed between the branches of the ductus accessorius and lobar duct, the lobar duct joining the axial branch of the caput as in type I. In the fourth type the number of anastomoses is greater than in the third, the lobar duct joining the axial branch of the cauda as in type II. Of the four types, type I was most frequently found and for this series may be called the normal. Fig. 10, V, shows how freely the branches of the ductus accessorius and those of a lobar duct may anastomose with one another. The variation in the communication between the two ducts indicates that, in a larger number of specimens, other types might be met with.

Remarks.—Variations in the shape of the pancreas were quite frequent and, as far as noted, were confined exclusively to the caput and to the strip of glandular tissue between the caput and cauda.

Of the five types of pancreatic anomalies described by Ruediger in man, none were found which exactly corresponded in the cat. Two cases of pancreatic anomalies, however, were met with. In the first case, a band of glandular tissue, apparently an outgrowth from the caput, passed cephalad, following the ductus choledochus and cystic duct and partly covering them on their ventral side. It extended to about the middle of the gall bladder, where it fused with the connective tissue around the latter. It had a duct which passed down its entire length and joined the axial branch of the caput. In the second case, Fig. 11, a similar though slightly narrower band of glandular tissue extended from the caput alongside the ductus choledochus and cystic duct. It then continued along the left side of the gall bladder to the posterior part of the liver, where it enlarged into an oval nodule about 1 cm. in its long diameter. This nodule occupied a hollow in the right central lobe of the liver to the left of the gall bladder. A duct was present which extended from the nodule down the middle of the band, joining the axial branch of the caput as in the previous case.

These two cases suggest an explanation of the formation of the pancreatic bladder, six cases of which have been reported by Miller. In the first case the strip of pancreatic tissue has not extended so far from the body of the pancreas and may be considered as an intermediary stage represented in completed form by case two. In both cases a duct was present. If in case two, one imagines the persistence of the duct with a bulbous dilatation of that portion of it contained in the nodule of pancreatic tissue and atrophy of the glandular substance, he will have a pancreatic bladder similar in every way to those which have been described.

With regard to the relation of the ducts to the gland, it will be seen that there is necessarily a close correspondence between the form and size of the ducts and the shape and lobulation of the gland. Thus the gland is long and so are the axial or main branches. The gland is narrow and consequently the lobar ducts are, as a rule, short. An exception to the latter statement occurred in four or five cases in which distinctly long lobar ducts were present. They appeared especially in the cauda and ran more nearly parallel to its axial branch than the other lobar ducts. The dichotomy of their branching was also less apparent and they resembled more nearly the axial ducts.

Of the five varieties of abnormalities of the excretory ducts described by Sappey in man, namely, (1) the accessory duct of Santorini entirely absent; (2) the duct of Santorini the main excretory duct; (3) the ductus pancreaticus not passing through the ampulla of Vater, but opening into the duodenum independently; (4) the presence of two excretory ducts of about equal size which run parallel to each other throughout the entire length of the gland, and (5) the presence of three excretory ducts, no distinct case was found in the cat. The

PLATE III.

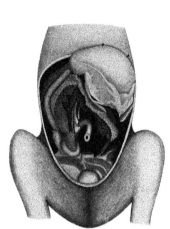

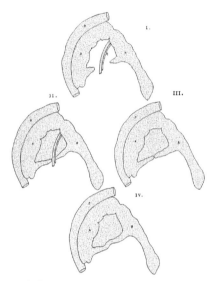

Fig. 1.—The coils of the intestine have been removed so that there remains only the duodenum and a small portion of jejunum and the rectum. The entire pancreas is seen in its normal position. The right limb is attached to the duodenum and extends down to the pars horizontalis. The left limb runs across the abdominal cavity posterior to the stomach. It lies ventral to the left kidney and its tip covers the left ovary on its ventral side. The spleen does not occupy its normal position but has been drawn forward by the displacement of the stomach. The right ovary lies in this case ventral to the pars decendens of the duodenum. In the posterior part of the drawing are seen the furrows in the fat mass occupied by the coils of the intestine.

Fig. 3.—Semidiagrammatic drawings to show the formation of the bridge. As is stated in the text, five cases of such incomplete formations were met with. In I a spur of tissue from both caput and cauda is approaching the blood vessels (superior mesenteric artery and vein). In II the two spurs have reached the blood vessels. In III the two spurs are almost in contact and between them there has formed a narrow bit of tissue. In IV the fusion between the spurs is complete and the bridge is formed. The fusion of the two spurs takes place dorsal to the blood vessels. A, caput pancreatis; B, cauda pancreatis; C, superior mesenteric artery and vein; D, portion of the duodenum.

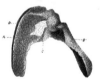

Fig. 2.—The pancreas from an animal fixed with formalin and drawn in its normal position, from its ventral aspect. A, caput pancreatis; B, cauda pancreatis; C, bridge of tissue connecting caput and cauda; D, groove along which the pancreas is applied to the duodenum.

PLATE IV.

THE JOHNS HOPKINS HOSPITAL BULLETIN, APRIL, 1906.

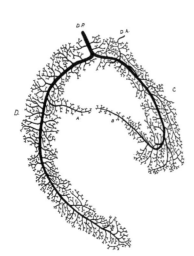

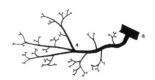

II.

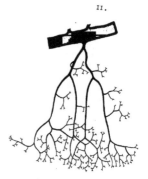

Fig. 4.—The pancreatic ducts in the cat. Drawn from a corrosion preparation. Dorsal view. *DP*, ductus pancreaticus (Wirsungiania); *DA*, ductus accessorius (Santorini); *C*, axial branch of the caput pancreatis; *D*, axial branch of the cauda pancreatis; *A* and *B*, branches of the bridge of the pancreas.

Fig. 5.—I. A lobar duct showing three branches, all lying in different plains, joining at the common point *A*. *B*, axial duct. II. A lobar duct showing dichotomous branching throughout. Usual type.

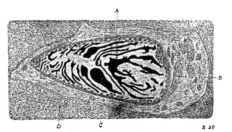

Fig. 6.—Transverse section of the ampulla of Vater. The ampulla was injected under low pressure with blue gelatin which filled the spaces between the folds of the ampulla represented by solid black in the figure. The section is the same as one which would be obtained if it were cut along the line *mn* in Fig. 7. *A*, folds in the ampulla; *B*, smooth muscle; *C*, space between the folds; *D*, glands of the mucosa.

PLATE V.

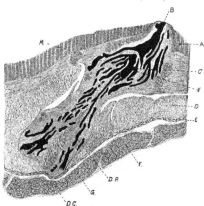

Fig. 7.—Longitudinal section of the ampulla of Vater. The ampulla was injected with blue gelatin as in Fig. 6. A, glands of the mucosa; B, opening of the ampulla of Vater into the duodenum; C, ampulla; D, circular muscle coat; E, longitudinal muscle coat; F, lobule of the pancreas; DP, ductus pancreaticus showing its opening into the ampulla; DC, ductus choledochus cut along one wall showing outfoldings filled with blue gelatin. By these the continuation of the ductus choledochus into the ampulla can be traced; G, wedge of smooth muscle between the ductus pancreaticus and ductus choledochus.

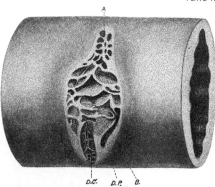

Fig. 8.—Drawing showing the ampulla of Vater in a distended condition. The opening of the ampulla into the duodenum was closed and then the ampulla was injected with celloidin under high pressure. After hardening in alcohol, the dorsal wall of the ampulla was removed and the celloidin carefully picked out of the spaces between the folds. A, position at which the ampulla opens into the lumen of the duodenum; B, folds subdividing the cavity of the ampulla into compartments; DC, ductus choledochus; DP, ductus pancreaticus.

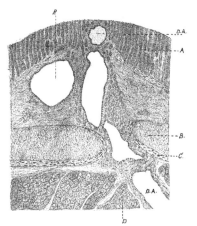

Fig. 9.—Section of the duodenal wall showing the duodenal portion of the ductus accessorius in longitudinal section. A, glands of mucosa; DA, ductus accessorius. The duct had a slightly tortuous course which makes it appear discontinuous in section.; B, circular muscle coat; C, longitudinal muscle coat; D, lobule of the pancreas; R, reservoir having a distinct epithelial lining. This reservoir opened into the ductus accessorius.

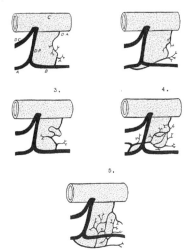

Fig. 10.—Diagrams showing the types of communications between the ductus pancreaticus and ductus accessorius. The same lettering applies to all of the diagrams. A, axial branch of the cauda pancreatis; B, axial branch of the caput pancreatis; DC, ductus choledochus; DP, ductus pancreaticus; DA, ductus accessorius; C, portion of the duodenum.

PLATE VI.

THE JOHNS HOPKINS HOSPITAL BULLETIN, APRIL, 1906.

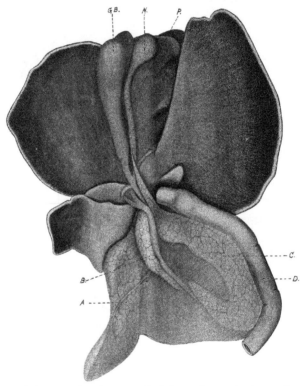

Fig. 11.—Drawing showing an anomaly in the pancreas. The duodenum and pancreas have been turned over to the left side so that their dorsal surfaces are seen. The strip of tissue *P* extends cephalad, terminating in the nodule, *N*. *GB*, gall bladder; *N*, nodule of pancreatic tissue; *P*, strip of pancreatic tissue; *A*, cauda pancreatis; *B*, arm of pancreatic tissue; *C*, caput pancreatis; *D*, portion of duodenum.

ductus pancreaticus was in every instance the larger, the ductus accessorius the smaller duct. The ductus pancreaticus in every case passed through the ampulla of Vater. The only resemblance to any of the varieties was one case in which two ducts of about equal size were present in the caput. They ran parallel to each other and joined the axial branch of the cauda at a common point. This case resembles variety four of Sappey.

The relation of the blood vessels to the ducts was found to be in general the same as Revell described in the dog. The artery (arteria pancreatico-duodenalis superior) runs caudad in the caput between the axial duct and duodenal wall. In its course it passes between the ductus pancreaticus and ductus accessorius, showing that the two or three pancreatic buds grow out and fuse over the blood vessel.

A comparison of the ducts as found in the cat with the normal ducts in other mammals, as man and the dog, shows a considerable variation. In the cat the ductus pancreaticus is the larger and opens into the duodenum with the ductus choledochus; the ductus accessorius is the smaller and opens into the duodenum independently a short distance caudad to the ductus pancreaticus. In man the ductus pancreaticus is the larger and opens into the duodenum with the ductus choledochus as in the cat; the ductus accessorius is the smaller but opens into the duodenum anterior to the ductus pancreaticus. In the dog the ductus pancreaticus is the smaller and opens into the duodenum with or immediately caudad to the ductus choledochus; the ductus accessorius is the main duct and opens into the duodenum caudad to the ductus pancreaticus.

In conclusion I wish to express my obligations to Dr. W. S Miller, under whose direction the work was done.

BIBLIOGRAPHY.

1. Chauveau: Comparative Anatomy of the Domesticated Animals, New York, 1873.

2. Ellenberger und Baum: Anatomie des Hundes, Berlin, 1891.

3. Ellenberger und Baum: Vergleichende Anatomie der Hausthiere, Berlin, 1900.

4. Felix: Zur Leber und Pankreasentwickelung, Archiv für Anatomie und Physiologie, Anat. Abth., 1892.

5. Flexner: Experimental Pancreatitis, Johns Hopkins Hospital Reports, Vol. IX, 1900.

6. Gage: The Ampulla of Vater and the Pancreatic Ducts in the Domestic Cat, American Quarterly Microscopical Journal, 1878.

7. Oppel, A.: Lehrbuch der vergleichenden mikroskopischen Anatomie, Bd. 3, Jena, 1900.

8. Owen: Anatomy of Vertebrates, London, 1868.

9. Revell: The Pancreatic Ducts in the Dog, American Journal of Anatomy, Vol. I.

10. Ruediger: Accessory Pancreas, Journal of the American Medical Association, Vol. XL.

11. Sappey: Traité d'Anatomie Descriptive, Paris, 1899.

12. Schirmer: Beitrag zur Geschichte und Anatomie des Pankreas, Basel, 1893.

13. Miller: Amer. Jour. of Anat., Vol. III, No. 3.

ON THE SCHULTZE CLEARING METHOD AS USED IN THE ANATOMICAL LABORATORY OF THE JOHNS HOPKINS UNIVERSITY.

By Eben C. Hill.

Before the invention of the microtome, the earlier embryologists studied embryos by gross dissection, and it naturally followed that they compared their dissections with those of the adult. Such a procedure often gave excellent results as may be seen in the great work of von Baer. Many questions, however, could not be answered by this relatively crude method, and it was not until sections of hardened embryos were made that more satisfactory results were obtained. Then followed methods by which very thin sections were easily made by the thousand and for a time it appeared as if what was studied with the microscope could not be brought into relation with our knowledge of human anatomy. However, this difficulty was soon overcome by His, who by graphic reconstruction combined numerous sections and thus demonstrated the relation of organs and tissues of the smallest embryos. This method was soon improved by Born, who substituted wax plates for the primary drawings of His, and thereby made concrete wax models on an enlarged scale. This method has been extensively used in this laboratory as well as elsewhere.

For sometime, however, there has been a tendency to abandon these slower reconstructive methods which present so many possibilities for error in the histological technique and in the subsequent construction of wax models, and to adopt instead such methods as will especially emphasize by staining and clearing reagents those tissues and systems which are under investigation. Besides the saving of time and energy, and the lessening of the chances for inaccuracy in interpretation and technique, Dr. Mall informs me that in the case of certain tissues these differential methods of staining and clearing give results which can be obtained by no other means. For instance, in the study of the cranial ossification centers of human embryos, Dr. Mall found that these centers were clearly demonstrated by staining and clearing at times when the ordinary histological methods gave no evidence of this ossification.

Schultze Method.—Schultze, in 1897, was the first to advocate the use of potassium hydroxide as a method for demonstrating the development of the skeletal cartilages, though, as he points out, Beale in 1853 and later Theodore Koelliker made use of this reagent to render transparent the softer tissues of embryos. Schultze advises that embryos ranging from five to ten centimeters in length be placed for from three to eight days in 95 per cent alcohol which should be frequently changed. Then follows a treatment with a 3 per cent aqueous solution of potassium hydroxide, which may be renewed on the following day. When the skeletal cartilages are apparent the specimen is placed in 25 per cent glycerine to which a small amount of .5 per cent formalin has been added in order to prevent the growth of moulds. A greater percentage of formalin tends, he says, to harden the embryo and cause opacity. Larger embryos receive the same treatment except that openings are made into the abdomen, thorax, and cranium so as to permit free access for the reagents. By following these methods of procedure, specimens demonstrating the development of the bones are easily obtained, but the best results may be had, he suggests, by the use of a 3 per cent alcoholic solution of potassium bichromate followed by treatment for several days with 95 per cent alcohol. The specimens are then placed in a mixture of one-third pure glycerine, one-third concentrated potassium hydroxide, and one-third distilled water; or equal parts of pure glycerine and concentrated potassium hydroxide may be used. Upon clearing, the bones appear brown. Schultze suggests the possibilities of injections of cinnabar but does not mention any results that he has obtained from such injections.

Van Wijhe Method.—In 1902 Van Wijhe published a method for demonstrating the development of the skeletal cartilages which differed materially from that of Schultze. His method depends upon the well-known quality of cartilage to retain aniline stains. Van Wijhe advocates 5 per cent sublimate solution, 10 per cent formalin or Zenker's fluid for fixing the specimens, after which they are placed in alcohol (percentage not given but presumably 95 per cent) in which is a trace of hydrochloric acid. The specimens are then placed in an alcoholic solution of methylene blue to which 1 per cent hydrochloric acid has been added; (one-quarter gram of methylene blue in 100 cc. of 70 per cent alcohol). After staining, the intensely blue objects are treated with 95 per cent and 70 per cent acid alcohols alternately, until there is no longer any trace of stain in the alcohols. So resistant is this aniline stain to the action of acid alcohols that specimens may remain a year or more in these media without the cartilage losing its stain. The objects are removed to absolute alcohol until completely dehydrated and are then placed in a mixture of two parts absolute alcohol and one part xylol. After this they are placed in a mixture of one part absolute alcohol and two parts xylol, which is then followed by pure xylol. They may then be permanently mounted in Canada balsam of a melting point of 60° C.

Lundvall Method.—Two years after the publication of this method Lundvall in his article treating of the staining and clearing of embryonic skeletal cartilages commends Van Wijhe's method for small objects, but pronounces it to be useless for larger specimens. He reiterates the advice of Schultze about removing the brains and viscera before proceeding with the clearing, and advises against the use of certain of the reagents which Van Wijhe especially recommends.

His method, in brief, is to fix the specimens in 10 per cent formalin for at least forty-eight hours. They are then placed in 95 per cent alcohol for a similar length of time, after which they may be stained in toluidin blue. This stain Lundvall considers is far superior to methylene blue in cases of medium-sized and large objects, maintaining that its action is more rapid and that the stain produced is more intense. This staining fluid is composed of .25 g. of toluidin blue in 100 cc. of 70 per cent alcohol which contains .5 per cent hydrochloric acid. Then add .5 cc. of hydrochloric acid and after standing twenty-four hours, filter. To obtain the best staining, specimens should be placed in this solution in a thermostat at 40° C. for one day. As suggested by Van Wijhe, the success of the decoloration is best assured if 95 per cent and 70 per cent acid alcohols are used alternately. Canada balsam and xylol Lundvall contends are useless because, according to his experiments, the specimens are rendered cloudy. So after removing the stain from all of the tissues except the cartilage he places the objects in 95 per cent alcohol for a day or so, and then removes them to absolute alcohol in which are placed a few crystals of copper sulphate to guard against the presence of water. After two days of dehydration the specimens are removed to a mixture of one part benzol and two parts absolute alcohol for from twelve to twenty-four hours, are then removed to a mixture of two parts benzol and one part absolute alcohol for twice that length of time, and are later placed in pure benzol. Finally they may be indefinitely preserved in carbon bisulphide. On account of the high refractive index of this preserving fluid the specimens should not be placed for study in round tubes or jars. Four-sided vessels are preferable, and to avoid the dangers of evaporation or explosion the tops should be held in place with sodium silicate.

Uses of Clearing Methods.—In the anatomical laboratory of the Johns Hopkins University the advantages of a method which would obviate the tedious cutting of sections and modeling and would in the end give the real object in its natural relations instead of an imitation, were readily appreciated, and since the first appearance of this article by Schultze, experiments in staining, injecting, and clearing have been carried on. The methods advocated by Van Wijhe and Lundvall have not received as much attention as the earlier method because of their more recent appearance and because the older method has been so perfected that it meets all of the requirements.

Schultze is the only one of the three who has hinted at the possibilities of the clearing method for other than the investigation of bone, and in his communication he does not mention any results that he has obtained from injections or partial clearings. Van Wijhe and Lundvall advocate their methods solely for cartilage and do not indicate any other uses to which they may be put. In reality this study of the skeletal system is but one of the many embryonic investigations which are greatly facilitated by clearing methods. The one objection to the use of the Schultze method for other than resistant bony tissue has been its unreliability. At times beautifully cleared specimens of the arterial and lymphatic systems were obtained by following one of the three procedures outlined by Schultze, but the uncertainty of obtaining good results and the possibility of destroying valuable material have kept it from gaining the popularity which with its present modifications it now deserves. These modifications have been introduced after many experiments in injecting, staining, and clearing human embryos and embryo pigs, and at the present time with reasonable care no specimen should be injured.

Before discussing the changes which it has been necessary to introduce into this method it may be better to first consider the uses to which it has been applied in this laboratory. On account of the large numbers of uteri of pregnant swine which are delivered each day immediately after removal, injections and clearings have been made which have greatly simplified the study of the development of the arterial, venous, lymphatic, and other tubular systems.

By staining and clearing human embryos Dr. Mall has demonstrated the earliest appearance of the ossification centers in the skeletal system. Injections which were subsequently cleared have shown the development of the vascular system of the brain,[10] the lymphatics of the intestines, the superficial lymphatics of the skin,[11] the semicircular canals, the arterial supply to the Wolffian body and kidney,[12] and the bile-ducts of the liver.[13]

Method of Injections.—In all of the problems except that of the development of the bone and cartilage the procedure has been essentially the same. There must be an injection fluid which will not distort the tissues by its chemical action or by the force necessary to cause its entrance into the ducts and capillaries. This fluid must also be unaffected by those reagents which are to render the tissues transparent. India ink furnishes such a medium and this has been the fluid which has been used in nearly all of the injections. Heuer, by injections into the thoracic duct and into the mesentery of embryo pigs followed by clearing the specimens according to the Van Wijhe or Schultze methods, succeeded in demonstrating the development of the lymphatios in the small intestine. In investigations of the respiratory system injections into the trachea with India ink were found upon being cleared to fill the alveoli of the lungs of a 30 mm. pig. By injections into the stomach the bile

capillaries of the liver have been demonstrated in the 100 mm. stage, and have been traced in this manner until the time of birth. In this case the stomach acted as a pressure bag and the injection mass after a short interval was seen to fill the gall-bladder, and its subsequent course through the bile-ducts and capillaries could be followed by noting the darkened areas. So constant was the pressure maintained by this method that upon microscopic examination few areas of extravasation were found, and yet in almost all of these experiments the pressure was sufficient to force the injection into the esophagus as well as through the loops of small intestine into the colon and later out of the rectum. Upon clearing the entire embryos, very instructive specimens were obtained. Injections into the urinary bladder demonstrate the uriniferous tubules of the kidney and Wolffian body. So far attempts to inject and clear the pancreatic ducts have not proved to be especially fruitful. Injections of the spinal canal gave beautiful pictures if the injection fluid was started from one of the ventricles of the brain.

The relations of the arterial and venous circulations in the placenta may be readily made out by injections into the umbilical arteries or vein. Upon ligation of the placental end of the cord and after a ligature has been passed around the body of the embryo just posterior to the heart, an injection into either of the umbilical arteries results in an arterial injection of the abdominal vessels as well as of those of the hind legs, which upon being cleared by the Schultze method demonstrate not only the larger vessels but even the small nutrient arteries of the bones. Because of the ductus arteriosns the ligature around the body of the embryo at the position indicated is essential to prevent an injection of both the arterial and venous systems. If small embryos are still alive when brought to the laboratory, as frequently happens, injections into the liver direct are soon forced to the heart which pumps the fluid through the entire arterial system.

In making the injections India ink diluted to one-third of its commercial strength has been used. The use of distilled water for injections at times causes a precipitation, but this may be easily remedied by the addition of a small amount of weak ammonia. Lamp-black solutions have proved to be most unsatisfactory because of the difficulty of obtaining solutions of similar consistency. Frequently also this injection-mass clogs the needle of the hypodermic syringe. The injections of the smaller embryos are carried on in warm water with the membranes still intact.

Clearing.—After the injections have been completed all unnecessary tissues surrounding the parts under investigation are removed and the specimens are placed in 95 per cent alcohol. The removal of this adventitial tissue is most important, though entire embryos may be successfully cleared if openings are made into the abdomen, thorax, and cranium. In large embryos ranging above 15 cm. it is still better to make sagittal sections of the hardened specimens and clear in halves The alcohol should be frequently changed and large quantities should be used. In order to obtain transparent specimens the tissues must be completely shriveled before removal from the alcohol, and the length of time necessary to accomplish this result depends, of course, upon the size of the objects. For very small specimens at least three days should be allowed while for large objects the time should not be less than one week. Experiments with absolute alcohol instead of 95 per cent alcohol gave no better results and its use is an unnecessary expense. The coagulation of the proteids occurs almost as rapidly in one percentage as in the other.

After the specimens have been sufficiently shriveled they should be placed in 1 per cent potassium hydroxide. When a higher percentage is resorted to, so rapid is the action that the safety of the specimen is endangered, and it was the use of the strong solutions advocated by Schultze which caused the loss of much valuable material. In this weaker solution the tissues become transparent in from four to forty-eight hours, depending upon the size of the objects. From this medium they should be transferred to 20 per cent glycerine in which clearing continues and a certain amount of hardening occurs, rendering the tissues firm enough to permit of dissection. Should the specimens be as transparent as is desired, they may then be transferred from time to time to higher percentages of glycerine till at last they are permanently stored in pure glycerine. A certain amount of shrinkage is noticed in some organs after an immersion in this fluid for a year or more, but when the specimens are studied immediately after being cleared the measurements are the same as in the fresh tissue. We have also found that embryos hardened in formalin can be cleared in 10 per cent potassium hydroxide in the course of several weeks or months. However, in order to show the ossification centers the specimens are not to remain in the formalin solution very long for it decalcifies the bone.

Blood pigment in all cases will not be removed entirely by this process alone and in organs such as the kidney transparency can sometimes be obtained only by a secondary treatment. After passing through the 1 per cent potassium hydroxide and being placed in the 20 per cent glycerine as outlined above, the specimens containing the objectionable pigment are treated with a mixture of equal parts of 50 per cent ammonium hydroxide and 1 per cent potassium hydroxide. In this solution there is comparatively little danger to the specimens as the hardening produced by the 20 per cent glycerine clearing reagents. Indeed, in cases where it is deemed advisable to stop the clearing action or for any reason it is found to be more convenient to continue the process at some future time, the specimens may be removed to this 20 per cent glycerine and retained in this medium until a more fitting time when much higher percentages of caustic solution may be resorted to without danger to the objects.

Method of Staining and Clearing the Skeletal System.—In demonstrating the development of the skeletal system Dr. Bardeen advocated the use of alum-cochineal in place of the stains advised by Schultze, Van Wijhe, and Lundvall. The specimens are placed, without previous fixing in formalin, in 95 per cent alcohol until shriveled. Then follows staining for twenty-four hours in alum-cochineal, after which they are cleared in the 1 per cent solution of potassium hydrate. Embryos treated in this way give beautiful specimens with the bone stained red.

Mounting Specimens.—Until recently the method of Van Wijhe had the advantage of permanently mounting the specimens in Canada balsam, which seems impossible in cases of tissues cleared with potassium hydroxide, but Bardeen has devised a method by which specimens may be mounted upon glass slides and placed in any desired position in jars of glycerine. This method, in brief, is to remove the specimens from pure glycerine, wipe, and quickly wash. They are then placed in a little thick gelatin solution and are laid upon a warm glass slide. As soon as the gelatin is hardened the specimens are returned to the pure glycerine without any danger of coming off. The purity of the glycerine should be assured, else the presence of foreign substances, such as water, may tend to soften the gelatin.

SUMMARY.

1. Specimens are placed in 95 per cent alcohol until completely shriveled. Three to seven days.

2. Are then removed to 1 per cent KOH until transparent. Four to forty-eight hours.

3. Placed in 20 per cent glycerine for forty-eight hours or more.

4a. If cleared, place at intervals of two or three days in ascending percentages of glycerine.

4b. If not clear, place in equal parts of 1 per cent KOH and 50 per cent ammonium hydroxide for five to seventy-two hours. Then place in 20 per cent glycerine for forty-eight hours or more, and continue treatment as outlined in 4a and 5.

By following this method the systems of bones, cartilages, arteries, veins, lymphatics, and various ducts can be demonstrated with a transparent embryo or with large sections of adult tissue without any distortion of the structures.

REFERENCES.

1. Mall, F. P. "Ueber die Entwickelung des Menschlichen Darmes und seiner Lage beim Erwachsenen." pp. 403-434. Arch. für Anat. u. Phy., Supplement, Band 1897.

2. Bardeen, C. R., and Lewis, W. H. "Development of the Limbs, Body Wall, and Back in Man." Am. Jour. Anat., Vol. I, pp. 1-35.

3. Lewis, W. H. "The Development of the Arm in Man." Am. Jour. Anat., Vol. I, pp. 145-183.

4. Flint, J. M. "The Blood Vessels, Angiogenesis, Organogenesis, Reticulum, and Histology of the Adrenal." Johns Hopkins Hospital Reports, Vol. IX.

5. Sabin, F. R. "Model of the Medulla, Pons, and Midbrain of a New-Born Babe." Johns Hopkins Hospital Reports, Vol. IX.

6. Streeter, G. L. "The Development of the Cranial and Spinal Nerves in the Occipital Region of the Human Embryo." Am. Jour. Anat., Vol. IV, pp. 83-116.

7. Schultze, O. "Ueber Herstellung Und Conservirung Durchsichtiger Embryonen Zum Studium Der Skeletbildung." Verhandlungen der anatomischen Gesellschaft, 1897, Band 13.

8. Van Wijhe, J. W. "A New Method for Demonstrating Cartilaginous Mikroskeletons." Kononklijke Akademie van Wetenschappen Te Amsterdam, 1902.

9. Lundvall, H. "Ueber Demonstration Embryonaler Knorpelskelette." Anat. Anz., pp. 219-223, Band XXV.

10. Mall, F. P. "On the Development of the Blood Vessels of the Brain of the Human Embryo." Am. Jour. of Anat., Vol. IV.

11. Sabin, F. R. "On the Development of the Superficial Lymphatics in the Skin of the Pig." Am. Jour. Anat., Vol. III, pp. 182-195.

12. Hill, E. C. "On the First Appearance of the Renal Artery, and the Relative Development of the Kidneys and Wolffian Bodies in Pig Embryos." Johns Hopkins Hospital Bulletin, Vol. XVI, No. 167.

13. Mall, F. P. American Journal of Anatomy, Vol. V.

ON THE EMBRYONIC DEVELOPMENT OF A CASE OF FUSED KIDNEYS.

By Eben C. Hill.

(From the Anatomical Laboratory of the Johns Hopkins University.)

At an autopsy recently held at Bay View Asylum in Baltimore, Dr. Bunting discovered an interesting case of fused kidneys which he kindly allowed me to study. Although this anomaly is by no means infrequent, the manner of fusion of the two organs and the relative positions of the ureters and blood vessels so clearly emphasized certain developmental conditions that a short description and an attempted explanation is permissible.

History of Case.—It was demonstrated at the autopsy that death was not due to fusion of the two kidneys, though certain pronounced lesions were found which indicated nephritis. Indeed, no cases are recorded in the autopsies of the Johns Hopkins Hospital where fusion of these organs had caused death. The kidneys seem quite as capable of properly functioning when fused and misplaced as when normally developed and located.

Extracts have been taken from those sections of the autopsy report which in any way apply to the location and arterial supply of this anomaly and its possible pathological effect on the surrounding tissues and organs.

Autopsy No. 2465. James C. Aet. 28 years. Autopsy by Dr. Bunting.

Anatomical Diagnosis.—Congenital malformation of kidney, chronic nephritis, cardiac hypertrophy and dilatation; general anæmia of organs; disseminated tubercles in liver.

Abdomen.—The peritoneal cavity is negative, no excess of fluid, and no adhesions.

Thorax.—The pericardial cavity is free from adhesions or from excess of fluid. The surfaces are smooth and glistening throughout. The heart is large, the hypertrophy being most marked in the left ventricle. The right side is dilated. Over the right ventricle there are one or two areas of thickening and opacity in the epicardium which are irregular in size and shape.

Heart.—The right auricle is practically free from clot, and is slightly dilated. The tricuspid orifice easily admits the tips of four fingers. The tricuspid valve is delicate and normal. The pulmonary valves also are delicate and normal. The right ventricle is somewhat dilated, its wall is not especially hypertrophied, averaging 5 to 6 mm. in thickness. The left auricle is somewhat dilated and has a hypertrophied wall. The mitral valve shows very slight thickening along the line of closure, has a fairly delicate free edge. The left ventricular wall is considerably hypertrophied, varying from about 22 mm. at the base to about 12 mm. at the apex of the heart. The papillary muscles are well formed, rounded, and show minute fibrous plaques of translucent greyish color. The muscle of the left ventricle is firm, rather pale, showing a few streaks, apparently of increase in connective tissue about the vessels. The aortic valves appear normal, and show no thickening, and are apparently competent. The coronary vessels are free throughout and show no sclerosis. The base of the aorta is practically free from sclerosis. The foramen ovale is open as an oblique slit. Apparently, functionally, it is closed.

Lungs.—Left lung shows a smooth and glistening pleura which is very pale in color, and which shows numerous emphysematous vessels, especially over the posterior portion of the upper lobe and some depressed areas in the posterior part of the lower lobe. On section the lung has the same pale, greyish-pink color, is quite dry except in the dependent portions, where it is somewhat congested and somewhat more moist. There is a slight yellowish cast to the cut section. The lung is apparently air-containing throughout, and feels somewhat more elastic than the normal lung. The right lung resembles the left. It also resembles the left on section, being particularly dry.

Spleen.—Measures 11.5 x 7 x 4 cm., and weighs 170 gm. The capsule is but slightly thickened and somewhat opaque, and shows beneath it a rather dark greyish-purple organ which feels softer than normal. On section there is slight thickening of the trabeculæ. The Malpighian corpuscles are large, but distinctly visible. The pulp is slightly increased in amount; however, it does not scrape off easily with the knife, and does not obscure the architecture of the organ. It has a slightly rusty tint.

Liver.—Measures 27 x 20 x 9 cm., and weighs 1970 gm. The surface is uniform and of a dark purple color except for three small nodules which are of a bright yellow and which lie over the middle part of the right lobe. The edge is sharp and straight, and the surface is smooth. The cut surface shows a dark brownish organ which is distinctly cloudy, and shows one or two areas of localized congestion. In general the central veins are but slightly congested, the parenchyma of the organ being brownish-yellow in color. The peripheries of the lobules are not distinctly marked out. The light yellow areas mentioned are found, on section, to be caseated masses resembling tubercles and with concentric arrangement of tissue about their periphery. The gall-bladder contains a thick greenish bile. Bile-ducts are patent.

Stomach.—Contains a large amount of greenish fluid and also some clot of milk. The mucous membrane is very pale, and has a slightly mammillated appearance toward the pyloric end. The rugæ are well marked.

Pancreas.—Is of a good size, somewhat pale, but appears normal.

Bladder.—Is very pale, but otherwise appears normal.

Prostate.—Appears normal.

Intestine.—Is free from lesions throughout, and rather pale.

Microscopical Notes—Heart.—The muscle fibers are all ex-

tremely hypertrophied, many of them contain large, swollen nuclei. There is an increase in the cells of the interstitial tissue. The stroma is also quite œdematous.

Kidneys.—Show marked degeneration of the epithelial tubules, many of which are compressed or have entirely disappeared. Those remaining are chiefly dilated, show a granular epithelium, and contain granular detritus and numerous hyaline casts. The glomeruli are clumped close together and are in the main in various stages of hyaline obliteration. There is very marked increase in the interstitial tissue which is firm and fibrous.

Macroscopic Description of Kidneys.—The left kidney is found in nearly its normal place but there is an L-shaped mass of kidney substance extending from just beneath the diaphragm in the left hypochondriac region about 16 cm. to just above the brim of the pelvis and then crossing the spinal column, the transverse portion measuring about 9 cm. The ureter from the upper portion of the kidney extends over the mass and crosses the iliac vessels about 5 cm. to the left of the median line, crosses the mid-line at the brim of the pelvis, and runs to the right side of the bladder. Both ureteral orifices are easily probed, and are apparently patent throughout and normal in position.

After fixation the fused kidneys show an L-shaped mass, the long arm of which is 16 cm. in length, the short arm 8½. The greatest width of the kidney is 5.5 cm., the greatest thickness about 3 cm. About 10.5 cm. of the long arm apparently corresponds to the left kidney, while the angle and short arm correspond to the right kidney. The pelvis of the right kidney is directed anteriorly and the calyces are somewhat distended. The pelvis of the left kidney is directed but

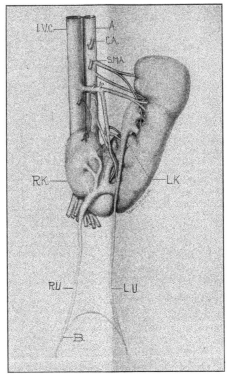

DESCRIPTION OF THE FIGURE.

Fused kidneys. *A.*, aorta; *I. V. C.*, inferior vena cava; *C. A.*, cœliac axis; *S. M. A.*, superior mesenteric artery; *R. K.*, right kidney; *L. K.*, left kidney; *L. U.*, left ureter; *R. U.*, right ureter; *B.*, bladder wall. Point of fusion of two kidneys indicated by dotted line.

slightly anteriorly. Its ureter crosses the kidney mass at about the angle of the L, also crossing one of the calyces of the right pelvis. The upper portion of the kidney received two arterial branches from the aorta, the first arising opposite the superior mesenteric, the second 1 cm. below the first. About 1 cm. below the second is given off a branch from the front of the aorta which is distributed to the extreme right of the short arm of the kidney. About 3 cm. below this branch are given off two branches of the aorta, one from the left side which is distributed to both the long and short arm of the kidney, one branch dividing about the lowermost calyces of the pelvis of the left kidney, the other about the uppermost calyces to correspond to the right pelvis. The second branch given off at this level is distributed to about the central portion of the short arm of the L. The capsule of the left portion of the kidney is thickened and adherent. On removal it leaves a finely granular surface, the projecting granules being light and opaque in color. On section of the organ the cortex is found to be from 4 to 5 mm. in width; its striation is somewhat irregular. The parenchyma is apparently diminished in amount, and here and there are opaque, yellow areas. The lower part of the kidney, the short arm, also has an adherent capsule and its surface is finely granular. The granules appear somewhat further apart and are separated from each other by a translucent firm tissue. The whole organ is much firmer than normal. The small arteries going to the kidney have thickened walls and stand wide open. The ureters are not distended and the bladder seems normal.

Probable Causes of Malformation.—From these extracts it will be seen that a general adjustment has taken place in order to accommodate this anomalous formation. The left anterior horn of the kidney is almost in normal position, but the lower border rests upon the brim of the pelvis and completely covers the body of the fourth lumbar vertebra. This position has crowded to one side the aorta and vena cava, and the spermatic and inferior mesenteric arteries are found coming off at higher levels. The peculiar manner in which the kidneys received their arterial supply is interesting, but it is impossible and impracticable to advance any theories as to the forces which caused them to so deviate from their normal courses. The renal artery to the left pelvis leaves the aorta at a slightly higher level than normally, but otherwise is not unusual. Probably the vessel entered after this portion of the organ had rotated and represents the left renal artery. The next lower artery to this might have been the right renal artery judging from the size and general location, but this is merely surmise. What seems quite plausible, however, in regard to this anomaly is the theory advanced by Pohlman which explains the frequent malformations of these organs, and this present case gives strong evidence to substantiate this theory.

Before presenting this hypothesis, however, it would be well to review briefly the embryonic development of the kidney. It will be sufficient to recall that the kidney arises as a tubular diverticulum from the Wolffian duct near its entrance into the cloaca. These renal buds penetrate the surrounding mesoderm and broaden at their distal ends, forming the renal pelvis while the tubular portion becomes the ureter. Growth continues cephalad until the human embryo has attained a length of 14 mm.[1] (Embryo 144) at which time the rotation begins; the kidneys changing from a dorsal to a lateral position in relation to the ureters. Complete rotation is found at 16 mm.[1] (Embryo Mall 43). The vascularization occurs after this rotation sometime between the stages of 22.0[1] and 24.0[1] mm. At the time that the renal buds appear and for a short time afterwards they lie only fifty microns apart and are separated by a thin layer of mesoderm. According to Pohlman,[2] whose theory has so satisfactorily explained the many renal anomalies recorded by Morris and others, it is this close proximity which accounts for the congenital malformation known as "horse-shoe" kidney. Through some cause unknown the two renal buds come into contact and in their upward growth absolute fusion occurs.

In the present case the upper pole of one and the lower pole of the other touched and the end-to-end fusion occurred at the point represented by the dotted line in the accompanying drawing. From the gross and microscopic structure of the specimen it would appear that the right renal buds had been displaced so far to the left as to touch by both the upper and lower poles the lower poles of the left pelvis. Growth continued till the time when rotation should normally occur, when the fused mass attempted to assume its proper position. The upper pole of the left-hand kidney being freer succeeded in rotating and consequently holds a normal position in relation to its ureter and pelvis.

The remainder of the mass, being more firmly bound and having no axis of rotation, remained in the position in which it had grown from the early embryonic state and still retains the ureter upon its ventral surface. Both ureters have worn deep grooves where they have lain on the cortex and the vertebral column has also made a deep depression.

There is no communication between the pelvis of what was probably the right and left kidneys. The lower part of the mass presents an interesting example of the not uncommon multiple pelves.

---

[1] These measurements refer to the collection of human embryos belonging to Dr. Mall.

[2] Pohlman, A. G., " A Note on the Developmental Relation of the Kidney and Ureter in Human Embryos." J. H. H. Bull., Vol. XVI, No. 167. Pohlman, A. G., " Concerning the Embryology of Kidney Anomalies." American Medicine, Vol. VII, No. 25.

THE JOHNS HOPKINS HOSPITAL BULLETIN.

The Hospital Bulletin contains details of hospital and dispensary practice, abstracts of papers read, and other proceedings of the Medical Society of the Hospital, reports of lectures, and other matters of general interest in connection with the work of the Hospital. It is issued monthly.

Volume XVII is in progress. The subscription price is $2.00 per year in the United States, Canada, and Mexico; foreign subscriptions $2.50. The set of sixteen volumes will be sold for $77.00.

A REVIEW OF SOME RECENT WORK ON THE MUSCULATURE OF THE HEART.

By WALTER A. BAETJER.

(Anatomical Laboratory, Johns Hopkins University.)

The difficulty in gaining a clear conception of the development and arrangement of the muscular layers of the heart is readily appreciated in reviewing the literature of the subject. That the descriptions in the text-books of anatomy are confusing is due to the fact that the one article amongst the recent publications on the musculature of the heart which is clear and concise in outlining the arrangement of the layers of cardiac muscle, has not yet been incorporated in any text-book. At the suggestion of Professor Sabin I reviewed the recent literature for the Anatomical Seminar and wrote this brief resumé of the researches of Ludwig, Krehl, Quain, Mac-Callum, His, Jr., and Retzer, who have made the most valuable contributions to this subject.

Before the publication of Ludwig's article in 1849 little was known regarding the arrangement of the muscular layers of the heart. In this paper, Ludwig states that the fibers on the outer surface run at right angles to those on the inner and between these two there are fibers in regular order showing all the transitions from one direction to the other. The fibers on the outer surface he divides into: (1) those arising in the right ventricle and ending in the left; (2) those arising in the left ventricle and ending in the right; (3) those which begin and end in the right ventricle. The deep muscles arise on the inner circumferences of the openings at the base of the heart and from the papillary muscles.

In 1891, Krehl published a similar work in which he emphasized the existence of a basket of muscle fibers in the left ventricle and at the same time called attention to a band of tendon along the posterior surface of the *conus arteriosus* between it and the aorta. By his discovery of this band of tendon, he was able to distinguish three tendinous points at the base of the heart in which it is possible for fibers to arise, the other two points being the circumferences of the two atrio-ventricular rings as shown in Fig. 1. The fibers of the left ventricle he divides according to their direction and insertion. Under the former classification he distinguishes three layers: the first arising on the upper surface to the right and passing to the lower surface on the left; a thicker one taking the opposite direction; and lastly, a layer of fibers taking an almost spiral course parallel to the long axis of the chamber. He distinguishes two layers according to insertion: the outer and inner ones ending in tendons; and the middle one which, as he expresses it, " ends in itself." The fibers one coming from the left ventricle, the septum, and the aortic of the right ventricle are divided into two layers: an outer ring; and an inner net-like layer. He describes also two other bands of fibers, one of which arising in the upper part of the

septum pursues a vertical course downwards in it, while the other belongs entirely to the conus.

Later Quain[1] describes the superficial fibers as composing a distinct layer arising from the tendinous points at the base of the heart and inserted in the left ventricle, chiefly into its anterior and posterior papillary muscles. Those crossing over the front and left side of the heart, he says, can be traced to the posterior papillary muscle, while passing over the back and right side help to form the anterior papillary muscle. Many of the superficial fibers, however, form an inner vertical layer which passes upward to be attached to the tendinous rings at the base of the heart.

The deeper fibers of the left ventricle, composing the thickness of its wall, he describes as arising from the tendinous rings at the base of the heart. From here they all pass obliquely downwards on the anterior and posterior wall toward the apex, where they turn abruptly toward the front of the septum. At this point he divides them into three layers: the first passing obliquely upwards to be attached to the central fibro-cartilage, thus forming V-shaped loops around the lumen of the left ventricle; those composing the second layer pass to the posterior wall of the right ventricle becoming partly continuous with the posterior papillary muscle; the third layer passes nearly horizontally into the posterior wall of the left ventricle and takes an annular course in it. But many of these are continuous with the deeper fibers of the right ventricle.

The right ventricle Quain regards as an appendage of the left, its superficial fibers being continuous with the posterior papillary muscle of the left ventricle and its deeper fibers also passing into continuity with those of the same ventricle. Attached to the right atrio-ventricular ring the anterior fibers of this layer pass backward in the septum to the posterior wall of the left ventricle, while the posterior fibers pass in the opposite direction to its anterior wall. The middle layer enters the lower part of the septum and passes upward to be attached to the central fibro-cartilage. Finally a number of fibers pass directly across the septum and encircle both ventricles.

In these articles we find layers of muscle described as belonging to one ventricle or the other, but in neither is there any mention of the deep layers as being continuous in both ventricles, thus forming the septum in their passage between the two as demonstrated by MacCallum's researches.

The investigations of MacCallum differed essentially from those of his predecessors in that he began his studies with embryonic rather than adult hearts. The tissues were macerated to facilitate the separation of the muscle layers, after which the auricles, in certain of the earlier stages of development, could be lifted away leaving the ventricles.

With the exception of two layers, all the muscles, both superficial and deep, are inserted into the papillary muscles of either the right or left ventricle. Those in the left ventricle are divided into three groups, viz.: a posterior and an anterior papillary muscle and a third group composed of many small muscles, forming the papillary muscles of the septum. A division, similar though less marked, is found in the right ventricle. Here the three groups are attached to the segments of the tricuspid valve.

Superficial Layers.—By their places of origin and insertion, MacCallum shows that the superficial layers can be divided into four groups, all of which arise superficially from one of the tendinous points at the base of the heart and end deeply in the papillary muscles of one of the ventricles. Three of these layers arise from the right side of the base of the heart and pass diagonally around the left ventricle to be inserted into one of its papillary muscles, thus offering an explanation for the greater thickness of its wall. Without exception these superficial layers all pass uninterruptedly across the inter-ventricular line.

(1) The fibers arising from the lower half of the tendon of the conus (Fig. 2, *B*) pass around the right ventricle to the ventral side of the heart, then, taking a diagonal course, they cross the inter-ventricular line passing downwards around the apex of the left ventricle where they turn up and in to be inserted into the anterior papillary muscle of the left ventricle.

Course.—From the posterior half of the tendon of the conus in the right ventricle to the anterior papillary muscle of the left ventricle, as shown in Fig. 2, *B*.

(2) The layer originating in the anterior half of the tendon (Fig. 3) passes upward around the conus to the ventral surface of the heart. From here it runs downward toward the apex just above the preceding muscle, where, after almost completely encircling both ventricles, it turns up and in from the ventral surface to be inserted into the papillary muscles of the septum in the left ventricle and to a slight extent into its posterior papillary muscle.

Course.—From the anterior half of the tendon of the conus in the right ventricle to the papillary muscles of the septum and posterior papillary muscle of the left ventricle, as MacCallum has shown in Fig. 3.

(3) The strands of muscle arising from the right auriculo-ventricular ring take a diagonal course around the posterior surface of the right ventricle to its ventral surface where they pass underneath the fibers from the lower half of the tendon, thus ceasing to be superficial. Continuing in their diagonal course underneath this layer, they cross the inter-ventricular line and wind about the apex to be inserted into the posterior papillary muscle of the left ventricle.

Course.—From the right auriculo-ventricular ring to the posterior papillary muscle of the left ventricle.

(4) The fibers arising in the left auriculo-ventricular ring

(Fig. 2, *A*) pass diagonally over the posterior surface of the heart across the posterior inter-ventricular line to the right ventricle where the deepest fibers of this layer begin to turn into the right ventricle to their insertion in its papillary muscles. This turning in of the deeper fibers is a continuous process all the way around the right ventricle to the anterior inter-ventricular line where the most superficial strands of this layer turn in and end in a similar manner.

Course.—From the left auriculo-ventricular ring to the papillary muscles of the right ventricle.

All these layers have a superficial tendinous origin in one ventricle and a similar deep insertion in the opposite one. There is also a small band of fibers crossing the posterior inter-ventricular line near the base of the heart and attached to the left atrio-ventricular ring.

Deeper Layers.—If the layers just described be removed, it will be seen that the deeper fibers all turn in at the inter-

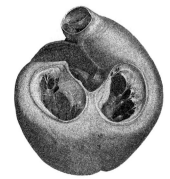

Fig. 1.—The tendinous points at the base of the heart. After Krehl.

ventricular line as though belonging distinctly to one ventricle or the other, which is in fact the generally accepted view. If, however, the left ventricle be gently unrolled from the right, the fibers from the latter are found to cross in the septum to the opposite surface of the left ventricle where they unite with those of the superficial layers to form the papillary muscles of the left ventricle. This process of unrolling is seen in Fig. 4.

These deeper fibers MacCallum divides into three layers according to their insertion in the left ventricle.

(1) The first layer arising most superficially in the right ventricle, *i. e.*, farthest from the lumen (Fig. 5, *A*), runs almost completely around this ventricle and crosses in the septum to the left ventricle where its course is closest to the lumen. It unites with the superficial layer from the right atrio-ventricular ring to form the posterior papillary muscle.

(2) The fibers composing this layer arise closer to the lumen of the right ventricle (Fig. 6, B) than the preceding layer where they follow a shorter, though similar, course across the septum to the left ventricle. Here their course is more superficial and longer than the preceding layer, passing about three-quarters of the way around the left ventricle to unite with the superficial fibers from the anterior half of the tendon of the conus to form the papillary muscles of the septum of the left ventricle.

(3) These fibers (Fig. 7, C) arise closer to the lumen and have a shorter course in the right ventricle than either of the preceding layers. They follow a parallel course, however, across the septum to the left ventricle where their course is the farthest from the lumen as well as the longest of the three layers. They pass almost entirely around the left ventricle where they unite with the superficial layer from the lower half of the tendon of the conus to form the anterior papillary muscle.

Intermediate Layers.—Besides the muscles just mentioned, MacCallum speaks of two other bands which do not fall in either of the above divisions. Contrary to those just described, these two muscles send no fibers to the papillary

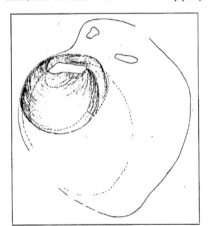

muscles. The first layer (Fig. 8) arising in the right auriculo-ventricular ring, crosses over in the septum to the left ventricle which it completely encircles, and, after again entering the septum, it coils about the deeper layers ending finally in the left auriculo-ventricular.

The other layer seems to belong entirely to the left ventricle.

Arising from the posterior border of the auriculo-ventricular ring (Fig. 9) it passes forward and to the left making one complete revolution and is then inserted above the fibers of origin.

In thus describing the musculature of the heart, MacCallum emphasizes the fact that while, in general, this is the arrangement of the fibers, it is impossible to make any abso-

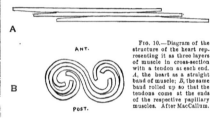

Fig. 10.—Diagram of the structure of the heart representing it as three layers of muscle in cross-section with a tendon at each end. A, the heart as a straight band of muscle; B, the same band rolled up so that the tendons come at the ends of the respective papillary muscles. After MacCallum.

lute mathematical division between the various layers. Those of the left ventricle, for instance, are separated chiefly by their points of origin and insertion, the division made being mostly for clearness in description.

The simplest conception of the heart can be gained, he suggests, by regarding it as simple band of muscle with three tendons at each end corresponding to the three groups of papillary muscles in each ventricle; and the whole thing wound into a scroll and surrounded by a superficial band of muscle divided into several layers according to their places of origin. In Fig. 10, A the heart is seen in cross-section as one band of muscle with three tendinous points at each end. In Fig. 10, B this same band is shown rolled up so that the tendinous points assume the relative positions of the papillary muscles of the two ventricles.

MacCallum also noticed that the muscular band comprising the deeper layers of the heart was comparatively thin in the middle and thicker at the two ends, thus indicating that the growth of the walls takes place at these two points. By a microscopic study of the heart in cross-section this was found to be the case. The younger cells, i. e., those with a simple protoplasmic network, are all found close to the lumen of the ventricle.

A further proof of this is the fact that the karyokinetic figures are all seen to be located on the inside of the ventricle close to the lumen.

Conclusions.—The chief things which MacCallum proves regarding the structure of the heart are:

1. The outer wall consists of several layers according to their places of origin and insertion, each of which begins superficially in the tendon of one ventricle and ends deeply in the papillary muscles of the opposite ventricle. The fibers composing these layers all pass uninterruptedly across the inter-ventricular line to the opposite ventricle.

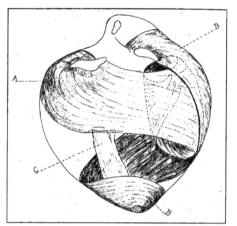

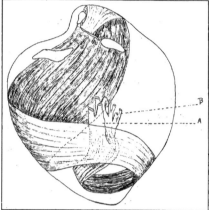

Fig. 2.—Diagram of the course of the superficial muscle layers originating in the left auriculo-ventricular ring and in the posterior half of the tendon of the conus. After MacCallum.

Fig. 3.—Diagram of course of superficial muscle layers originating in the anterior half of the tendon of the conus. *A*, posterior papillary muscle; *B*, papillary muscles of septum. After MacCallum.

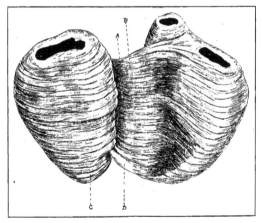

Fig. 4.—Posterior view of the heart showing left ventricle being unrolled from the right. *A* and *B* fibers passing directly from the right ventricle to the left. After MacCallum.

PLATE VIII.

THE JOHNS HOPKINS HOSPITAL BULLETIN, APRIL, 1906.

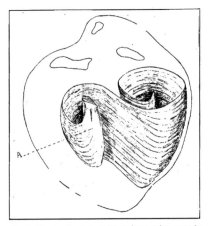

Fig. 5.—Diagram of course of deepest layer of left ventricle; A, posterior papillary muscle. After MacCallum.

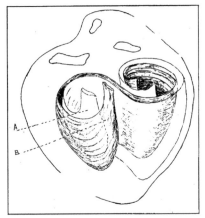

Fig. 6.—Diagram of course of layer superficial to that in Fig. 5. A, posterior papillary muscle; B, papillary muscle of septum. After MacCallum.

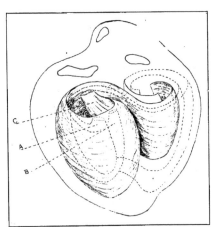

Fig. 7.—Diagram of layer still more superficial, ending in the anterior papillary muscle. A, posterior papillary muscle; B, papillary muscle of septum; C, anterior papillary muscle. After MacCallum.

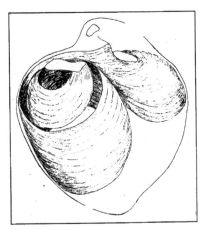

Fig. 8.—Diagram of muscle layer originating in tendon of conus and upper part of right ventricle. This surrounds the layers represented in the left ventricle in Figs. 5, 6, and 7. After MacCallum.

2. The deeper muscles consist of a simple band of fibers divided into three layers, each of which arises in the papillary muscles of one ventricle and takes an S-shaped course to be inserted into a similar structure in the opposite ventricle. Contrary to those forming the superficial layer, these fibers all turn in at the inter-ventricular line passing in the septum, across to the oposite surface of the other ventricle.

The most recent contribution to the anatomy of the heart has been the discovery of an atrio-ventricular band found by His and worked out by Retzer. This is a band of fibers about 18 mm. long which arises from both sides of the inter-ventricular septum. The fibers from the two sides then unite and run backwards over the muscular portion of the septum, to be inserted into the right half of the inter-atrial septum and. partly into the mesial leaf of the tricuspid valve.

The importance of the His bundle physiologically has been shown by Erlanger, who has produced heart-block by clamping the bundle.

LITERATURE.

1. Krehl: Abhandlungen d. math.-phys. Classe d. Königl. Sächsischen Gesellschaft d. Wissenschaften, Bd. XVII, 1891.

2. Quain's Anatomy, Vol. II, Part 2.

3. MacCallum, J. B.: Johns Hopkins Hospital Reports, Vol. IX.

4. Retzer: Arch. f. Anat. u. Phys. Anat. Abth., 1904.

NOTES ON NEW BOOKS.

A Manual of Materia Medica and Pharmacology. By DAVID M. R. CULBRETH, PH. G., M. D. Fourth edition. (*Philadelphia and New York: Lea Brothers & Co., 1906.*)

In this, the fourth edition of the work, there has been very thorough revision and in some parts a complete rewriting. Many of the changes have been made necessary by the eighth revision of the Pharmacopeia. To try to review such a book as this in any detail is much like attempting to do the same for a dictionary. As in the consideration of a dictionary, one is chiefly impressed by two things; first, the great number of points which he does not know—by no means an undesirable state of mind for a reviewer—and, second, the tremendous labor involved in colleeting and verifying all the information given. This work impresses us as being very carefully done. The drugs are arranged on the principle of associating those which have a common or allied origin. This applies to the vegetable drugs in their botanical relationships and to the organic drugs in their chemical affinities. The doses are given both in the metric and apothecary systems. In addition to the discussion of the pharmacopeial drugs there is a section on certain of the synthetic compounds which are used as remedies. There is an appendix dealing with poisons and their antidotes, and also with weights and measures and prescription-writing.

Reviewing a work on materia medica is very apt to lead to questions as to the usefulness of many of the drugs. The presumption is that somebody employs them, but we wonder, for example, how many men now use stillingia, or how frequently xanthoxylum is called for, or how much of a want would be felt if berberis or phytolacca had been accidentally left out? Doubtless there are men here and there in the profession who are attached to these old drugs but it seems as if many of them might well be dropped. However, to return to Dr. Culbreth's book, we can only repeat the opinion that it seems to be exceedingly carefully prepared and should be especially useful for students of pharmacy as well as for those in medicine.

The Ready Reference Hand-book of Diseases of the Skin. By GEORGE THOMAS JACKSON, M. D. Fifth edition. (*Philadelphia and New York: Lea Brothers & Co., 1905.*)

The feature of this book is the arrangement in alphabetical order of the various diseases of the skin. While this is not scientific it is eminently practical, and that it is popular is shown by the fact that the fifth edition is now in use.

The chapters on anatomy, physiology, diagnosis and treatment are concise yet complete. Under the heading, "Dermatological Don'ts" the author has offered about forty suggestions, which will prove invaluable to the practitioner.

Crocker's classification of skin diseases is the one followed. This is the most practical one in use and opposite each disease gives its prominent feature.

The material of the book is arranged to suit the needs of students, and while not exhaustive, is sufficient for that purpose. The illustrations, however, must be excepted. These are not sufficient for the requirements of a text-book either in variety or in number, and greater care could have been exercised in their selection, though much of the detail may have been lost in the printing.

An appendix contains many formulæ from various sources which should prove useful.

In the endeavor to keep the book abreast of the times new sections on eighteen diseases and eleven illustrations have been added.

Surgical Diseases of the Abdomen. By RICHARD DOUGLAS, M. D. (*Philadelphia: P. Blakiston's Son & Co., 1905.*)

The book comprises 866 pages. The type is sufficiently large and distinct to make the reading very pleasant and easy. There are 20 full-page illustrations, most of which are originals. Those representing kidney lesions are beautifully clear and accurate.

The author states in his preface that it has been his aim to elucidate the difficulties of diagnosis rather than to describe operative technique.

Considerable space is devoted to the consideration of the various surgical diseases of the kidney and of the female genital organs. Some of the latter are discussed at length. For instance, ectopic pregnancy is given 50 pages.

Appendicitis is discussed very fully. In attempting to distinguish various forms of the disease, the author, after making his divisions from a pathologic view-point, gives a separate heading to each and tries to elaborate a distinct train of symptoms. The general effect, however, is not happy, and as a consequence the reader is left with a somewhat confused idea of appendicitis as an entity.

In some chapters, a fuller treatment of the pathology would have been desirable. This is particularly true of the discussion of carcinoma of the stomach. The author's views in regard to the predisposing cause of cancer of the stomach are at variance with those so lately insisted upon by Mayo. The statement that ulcer is an unimportant etiological factor will certainly not meet with general acceptance.

The chapter on perforating typhoid ulcer is short but, on the whole, fairly complete.

Pancreatitis is dealt with at some length. The author favors the view of Opie as to its etiology.

Surgical diseases of the kidney occupy 112 pages. In regard to the formation of renal calculus he favors the view that it depends primarily on the presence of an underlying albumenoid cement substance. The section on renal tuberculosis might well have been fuller, but in general the text is well discussed.

The style is good and in the main clear, but occasionally the meaning is obscure. For instance, in the chapter on cancer of the pancreas, under prognosis, the following occurs: "The course of the disease is progressively downward, and the prognosis absolutely hopeless. Five months after supposed complete extirpation of the pancreas for a large carcinoma, Ruggi's patient was in perfect health." There is to be noticed also an occasional use of unusual words where simpler ones would appear to be preferable, as, for instance, *vespertine* instead of evening temperature.

To sum up, it may be said that the author discusses the various subjects from the standpoint of a study of the literature rather than from his personal experience. A personal imprint and personal views are lacking, and in many chapters, merely the opinions of others are given. Moreover, in some instances, without previous knowledge of the subject, it would be impossible for the reader to decide which view is the one most generally accepted.

On the whole, the book contains a valuable résumé of the subject, but as is the case with most text-books, very little original material.

Progressive Medicine. A Quarterly Digest of Advances, Discoveries, and Improvements in the Medical and Surgical Sciences. Edited by HOBART AMORY HARE, M. D., and H. R. M. LANDIS, M. D. Volume II. (*Philadelphia and New York: Lea Brothers & Co., June, 1905.*)

This volume of Progressive Medicine contains the usual good review of the progress of medicine and surgery during the past year.

Coley reviews the subject of hernia, while Foote takes up abdominal surgery, exclusive of hernia. Both of these articles are interesting and give many valuable references. Coley claims to get better results in operations for inguinal hernia by trans-

planting the spermatic cord rather than by leaving it *in situ.* He advises against operating for hernia with undescended testis in children before they are 8-10 years of age, unless there is some special indication for operating. It seems surprising that he gives so much space to McArthur's autoplastic method of suture in hernia operations.

The progress of gynæcology is reviewed by Clark, who discusses cancer of the uterus and myoma uteri at some length.

Stengel reviews diseases of the blood, diathetic and metabolic diseases, diseases of the spleen, thyroid gland, and lymphatic system.

Nervous and Mental Diseases. By ARCHIBALD CHURCH, M. D., and FREDERICK PETERSON, M. D. With 338 illustrations. Fourth edition, thoroughly revised. (*Philadelphia, New York, London: W. B. Saunders & Company, Publishers.*)

A previous edition of this work has been reviewed in the BULLETIN and it seems only necessary to refer to the new features of the present edition. The size of the book has been materially increased by the addition of several topics and the insertion of new illustrations. The portion on nervous diseases, written by Dr. Church, presents considerable new matter and many careful revisions. The more noticeable additions relate to nerve regenerations, intermittent limping, herpes zoster, and myoclonus epilepsy.

In the latter portion of the book, prepared by Dr. Peterson, a wholly new chapter appears from the pen of Dr. Adolf Meyer, entitled a "Review of Recent Problems of Psychiatry." It is in fact a complete monograph and contains a carefully prepared, critical, and analytical review of the work of Wernicke, Kraepelin, and Ziehen. The work is discriminatingly done but seems adapted to the requirements of the expert in psychiatry rather than to the "medical student and practitioner" for whom we are told in the preface that the work has been written. The writer points out the excellencies of each of these masters in psychiatry and above all the fact that they make a "conscientious effort to start in the first place from sets of patients and to adapt their descriptions and terms to what they see without any unnecessary regard for traditional classification of words." This is the key-note of their work and the faithfulness with which they have adhered to this ideal is the standard by which the writer estimates the relative value of their work. This chapter is unquestionably the leading feature of the present edition and should be read by every modern student of mental diseases. It is both illuminating and stimulating. The whole work deserves continued praise.

VOLUME XII OF THE JOHNS HOPKINS HOSPITAL REPORTS

This volume includes 548 pages, with 12 plates and 54 other illustrations. The price in paper is $5.00; in cloth, $5.50. It contains the following papers:

Orders should be addressed to **THE JOHNS HOPKINS PRESS, Baltimore, Md.**

The Johns Hopkins Hospital Bulletin are issued monthly. They are printed by the FRIEDENWALD CO., Baltimore. Single copies may be procured from NUNN & CO. and the BALTIMORE NEWS CO., Baltimore. Subscriptions, $2.00 a year, may be addressed to the publishers, THE JOHNS HOPKINS PRESS, BALTIMORE; single copies will be sent by mail for twenty-five cents each.

BULLETIN

OF

THE JOHNS HOPKINS HOSPITAL

Entered as Second-Class Matter at the Baltimore, Maryland, Postoffice.

Vol. XVII.—No. 182.]   BALTIMORE, MAY, 1906.   [Price, 25 Cents

CONTENTS.

INSTRUCTION IN OPERATIVE MEDICINE.[1]

WITH THE DESCRIPTION OF A COURSE GIVEN IN THE HUNTERIAN LABORATORY OF EXPERIMENTAL MEDICINE.

By HARVEY CUSHING, M. D.

As a preface to my entitled subject, some words, not altogether novel perhaps, but explanatory of my theme, may be permitted regarding the position in the medical fraternity that the surgeon proper has held in the past and holds today. It seems essential at the outset to make clear in what respect, if any, ' surgery ' is distinct from ' medicine ' in order that you may have a fuller understanding of the ideals that have led to the establishment of the operative course to be described. Finally, I trust, a brief explanation of the purposes of the building in which this work is now being conducted will render you more lenient toward the innovations in some time-honored methods of teaching therein practised.

The casual observer of present-day conditions might infer that something fundamental distinguishes the attributes of the physician from those of the surgeon—a distinction supposedly indicated by a sharp line of demarcation between their practices. Surgery, all will agree, is no more or less than a manual form of treatment; it is the craftsman's share of the therapeutic art, embracing measures to which the pure physician supposedly does not put his hand. Yet the prescribed course of training for the prospective physician as well as surgeon is the same; they have had the same scientific grounding; they have been taught alike what is known of the causation, the pathology and the symptoms of disease; they have learned from clinical evidence how to recognize its seat and nature. But from this point their paths are supposed to diverge, and in matters of therapy they are branded as unlike.

---

[1] An address before the Yale Medical Alumni Association at New Haven, February 23, 1906. Printed simultaneously in the Yale Medical Journal.

The almost superstitious devotion to Galenism—the Aladdin's lamp for medicine, which hanging unused through the dark ages, rusted for almost fifteen hundred years—has proved a fetish, the traces of which still linger in the minds of profession and laity alike; and practices essentially manual are still held to be a trifle less dignified than those of other kinds. As I shall endeavor to show, the surgeon to no small extent has himself to blame for the perpetuation of such a feeling.

In our great centres—for I cannot include the purer type of Aesculapian who in rural districts must perforce practise all kinds of therapy—a physician 'caught' operating for appendicitis, or a surgeon 'found' treating a case of typhoid fever would be more or less an object of ridicule, and yet either of these maladies may at times urgently demand operative intervention; in either of them recovery may ensue without the employment of surgical measures.

A physician will go so far as to puncture the lumbar meninges, to aspirate the pleural or pericardial sac for diagnostic or therapeutic purposes, or to perform venesection—all delicate manual procedures demanding rigid observations of 'surgical' cleanliness. He may even give an anæsthetic, yet he halts at a laminectomy, the excision of a rib or opening the abdomen, should more radical measures be demanded for the same maladies in which he has done the minor operations. It is merely a question of degree; and only in the dosage, as it were, in which they administer operative therapy are physician and surgeon apart.

The man, whose special bent inclines him to the practice of handicraft in matters therapeutic and who chooses to develop this special gift, should be no less capable of recognizing and alleviating conditions of disease than the 'internist,' unless he has neglected his educational opportunities, or has had none. By our collegiate degrees we are—in this country at least—all Doctors of Medicine, and should a surgeon's hands become maimed he surely could continue the practice of medicine. On the other hand, it is highly essential for the one who is disinclined to operate 'in large doses' to have just as thorough an understanding of the limitations and possibilities of major surgical procedures as the operator himself possesses; for a knowledge of surgery does not necessarily entail its practice. You will recall that in the medical past there have been many, like Albrecht von Haller, who have taught and written much of value upon surgical topics though they never operated upon their human kind. Nevertheless, unquestionably there are more physicians who are unaware of what may be accomplished for their patients by surgical measures than there are surgeons ignorant of the possibilities of medical treatment: more physicians who regard surgeons as incapable of caring for disease in any other way than by operating, than surgeons who, knowing how simple a thing their craft is when its technique has been acquired early, regard physicians as incapable of practising it.

It seems to me absurd, however, for surgeons to say that the physician has finally had to surrender the appendix, and reluctantly the gall-bladder, and must soon give up the treatment of many diseases of the stomach. On the contrary, the real change has been that the physicians are themselves carrying out manipulative measures which by actual investigation have proven to be more efficacious in relieving certain maladies than the medicinal ones heretofore employed. At the same time we must recognize the fact that he who thus operates safely and can learn by direct use of his senses, rather than by inference, the varying conditions of "living disease" has of course a vantage ground of understanding that is denied to the pure internist, whose pathology must often be that of the terminal stages of disease at the autopsy table. And assuredly the non-operating physician, be he an internist pure and simple, a gynæcologist, neurologist, or a special worker in any field, must 'surrender' certain conditions to the physician who does so use his hands. It is all operative Medicine—and following the example of Clifford Allbutt, I shall use the term Medicine in its Hippocratic sense with a capital M, to distinguish it from inner medicine.[1]

In order to reassure us of the oneness of Medicine, apparently now become so dismembered into specialties, it would be ideal could we some day see a Medical Faculty united in supporting a professorship of Medicine in its broad sense, the key-stone of the professorial arch; a position to be held by one with a wide comprehension of the under-lying general processes of disease, the Hippocrates or the Virchow of his time and place, who need not wear the badge of the stethoscope, the scalpel, forceps or microscope, to indicate his particular manipulative stock in trade, but under whom all clinical departments, which differ chiefly in their variety of therapy, should be subordinated.

Under the present system we are perhaps unconsciously inclined to favor too strongly the possibility of our particular form of therapy. Thus the stigma that attaches itself to surgeons is their operative furor, and in many respects this is a deserved blot on their good name. For in becoming operators pure and simple we are apt to lose sight of Medicine; we make little pretence of studying disease at the bedside or of any great familiarity with clinical methods. The expert diagnosis of our patients' maladies in most cases must be left to others, and we have come even to fight shy of an examination of the heart, lungs or nervous system; our presence is almost unknown to the investigators who work in the laboratories. There is perhaps reason for all this in the fact that the internist's therapy takes comparatively little time, rarely needing even personal supervision, so that he has greater leisure for the actual study of disease in its varying aspects; whereas the therapy of the scalpel on the other hand is hedged about with countless responsible details of preparation; is time-consuming and exhausting. He, who is drawn

[1] From Clifford Allbutt's address (The Historical Relations of Medicine and Surgery, Macmillan & Co., 1905) I have borrowed much and would gladly add more did I not believe that all, who perchance may look over this essay, will assuredly have read and probably re-read his volume to the end.

into devoting eight hours a day to the operative treatment alone of maladies, must needs grow rusty in his familiarity with disease at the bedside and in the laboratory. But is a surgeon of this type very far removed, except in his possibilities of accomplishment which he owes to Lister and to anæsthesia, from the cutter for hernia or stone of a few centuries ago?

Of the Aesculapian who does not operate it may be said that from the beginning he more often has a finer, a keener and a more receptive mind than has he whose activities by nature run to things manual, and this perhaps may make him the more impatient with the essential handicraftsman. But however this may be, the point I wish most to emphasize is that the physician himself today is doing his own operating, although he may be unwilling to recognize himself in this disguise; and so it is with operative Medicine that I treat.

It will be remembered that when Medicine was one, Hippocrates had his surgery—its description constitutes an important chapter in his writings—and though, through the dark ages and well into the morning of the new era, manual occupation was thought worse than undignified, even debasing, nevertheless throughout this period, even though groping in darkness, hands directing the scalpel were being used to relieve suffering and to further knowledge, until finally the despised, often indeed uncouth and ignorant manipulators, forced through public opinion the recognition of their practices upon the pure physician. But the very differentiation today of practitioners of the healing art into physician and surgeon is a relic of this long-enduring and unnatural prejudice against manual occupation.

But though this academic recognition, as it were, of surgery —and of surgery as though it were something apart from Medicine—has been of so short duration, the entire character of operative work since the surgeon came into his own, has changed. For reasons not far to seek, it was, until the present generation, a craft dependent for its success wholly upon anatomical knowledge. The chairs of surgery and anatomy were linked, and even today the dissecting-room in many communities remains the stepping-stone to a surgical career. An accurate knowledge of the old-time descriptive anatomy made the rapid operator, at a period when speed in his work was of paramount need: and one, who could 'drop a limb' in the fewest number of seconds; who could make the 'unerring thrust' through the perineum for stone; who in the fewest strokes could control hæmorrhage by the exposure and ligation of an artery 'high, low, or in its middle course,' was the better surgeon.

More than traces of all this remains in our work and especially in our teaching today, despite the changes wrought through the discovery of those mysterious substances that produce, what Oliver Wendell Holmes christened Anæsthesia, and despite the fact that, as Edmund Owen puts it, "Lister has entirely altered the map of the surgical world." For, thanks to Lister and to anæsthesia, surgery today has become more and more based on physiological principles and con-

centrates its attention upon disturbances chiefly of visceral function: whereas formerly anatomical knowledge was the main requirement, and the art did not go far beyond the cutting off or out of undesirable or unnatural tissue appendages.

Hence much more than before, the surgeon's requirements of ready information have become those of the physician— he has become an operating physician; or, to look again on the other side of the glass, those physicians who have a facility for craftsmanship are making use of operative therapy. And so in all special lines of work, in internal medicine—for the internist, so-called, is but a specialist—and in the lesser branches, in gynæcology, the specialties dealing with eye, ear or throat, in neurology, in obstetrics, in orthopædics and other lines, there are those who exclusively practice surgery and those who refrain from it altogether; but the latter are constantly becoming fewer, and the chief number of those who are not inclined or trained to use operative measures are largely grouped in internal medicine, where still remain the chief opportunities for the alleviation of suffering by measures other than manipulative.

If the contention be granted that there is no special difference between the species surgeon and the species physician, why is it that as types they continue to stand so apart? It is, I think, simply a matter of their up-bringing, and from an educational diet that leads to antipathetic rather than to sympathetic understandings, a diet too often seasoned by the belittlings—in good nature though they be—of one another's resources. Again, the very nature of the individual, who finds that he thinks and acts better through the medium of his hands, is such that he disregards, may even have a measure of disrespect—and this surely is turning the tables upon the physician—for the less tangible, the more obscure and the more difficult subjects and problems supposed to be relegated to the unhandy man with a more theoretical mind; while, on the other hand, in too many localities the latter may think, if not speak, disparagingly of the measures of his surgical colleague and hold back to the last his patient from "falling into surgical hands."

The physician is apt to regard the surgeon as a carpenter pure and simple in Medicine; and likely enough this is the surgeon's desert, for he too often 'carpenters' to the exclusion of all else. The apprenticeship to his craft has been long and expensive and arduous, and when once launched on the top wave of activity his operating life is, in the natural course of things—as eyes fail and fingers stiffen—brief. Thus it may happen that losing touch with general Medicine, except as a skilled manipulator for other and non-operating physicians, he hardly deserves the academic trust that has given him his post, and he becomes the modernized prototype of the peripatetic cutter-for-stone of a few centuries ago—differing from him chiefly in the fact that the patients now play the peripatetic role. It certainly cannot be denied that this relation holds true today in some particular fields of work in which the surgeon, making no pretense to familiarity with the symptoms or pathology of the malady, operates under the specialist's direction.

How may some of these unnatural relations be avoided? How can the "born physician" be brought to better appreciate and have the more patience with operative measures? How can the natural craftsman, on the other hand, be made to realize that he is likewise a physician and be led to moderate his activities within bounds, so that he may become more worthy of the position that his successes have forced from the medical faculties of earlier times? These results, I think, may in a measure be brought about by a different method of presenting the subject to the student; by making him realize that surgery is only a form of therapy—a form of therapy entailing great responsibilities and therefore not a thing to be made a show of before a crowded amphitheatre—and that the operator's duties and his relations to Medicine and to his patient are the same as those of the ' physician,' with whom he must share alike an understanding of the general pathology of disease and the recognition of its symptoms; that he owes it to his profession not to make his chosen branch of it a trade; and furthermore by urging upon those, who by nature are not particularly fitted for and have no leaning whatsoever toward manipulative practices in medicine, their even greater need of acquiring, during their student days, as much familiarity as possible with this branch of the healing art. I can conceive of no benefit so great to a practising internist as the experience that would have come, and has come in many instances, from a year or more of training as an apprentice to a surgeon or an assistant in an active hospital surgical service. It would be well were every prospective physician made to pass the most rigid examination in the surgical therapy of Medicine and perhaps none in his intended line of practice; and contrariwise, the surgeon should be subjected to as rigid a test in the recognition and treatment of diseases and conditions of diseases lying strictly on the medical side of the supposed border-line. Nor is this border-line easy to demarcate, for the overlapping, like that of the segmental skin-fields, is so wide that the loss either of the surgical or its adjoining medical segment leaves no total blank so far as the therapy of most maladies is concerned.

Generally speaking there have been in the medical past—and I will use the conditions in this country as a text—what we may recognize as three systems of instruction, under which young men have grown up into the practice of surgery. First of all, and by no means the least desirable, was that of the apprenticeship to an active practitioner; for under the immediate supervision of an interested master, a capable pupil could acquire facility, particularly in the manual practice of his art, better than in any other way. And it was largely the result of such a training that men were found in number and ability sufficient to fill, so ably as they did, the posts of responsibility when our schools of medicine began to be established a century ago. Among these men were many whose names remain illustrious in our annals of medicine; men of the type of Nathan Smith, who, already having founded one medical

school—Dartmouth, 1787—became a member of the original Faculty at the establishment of your school here in New Haven, where, please observe, he was Professor of the Theory and Practice of Physic, Surgery and Obstetrics, and occupied the chair—a sofa, Dr. Holmes would have called it—for sixteen years until his death in 1829. Here was a man who was far ahead of his day and generation, and to whom the medical profession has slowly been catching up.[3] His three years of apprenticeship under Dr. Goodhue probably did more for him than the subsequent courses of lectures at Harvard and Edinburgh, and he not only taught the practice of medicine and surgery at the same time, but made to both branches written contributions that remain classics.

With the establishment of the schools, however, there began a different system, not so desirable in some respects for the many—unless supplemented, as it often was, by apprenticeships during the long inter-semester vacation—for as classes grew the personal element of instruction must soon have been lost, and there was little place or material for practical work. Indeed it would seem as though the need for it was not recognized.

There are some destined to be leaders in their profession, who, by their own initiative, progress to the top under any system. Such a one graduated here ten years after the New Haven school was founded, and there was much of his father in him. For the father was not to be the last to teach both physic and surgery, though the son, by the titles of the posts he held, shows in what direction the tide was setting; for surgery, in imitation of what had happened in older countries, was forming its natural alliance with anatomy—a proper one at least for the surgery of the times.[4] And so Nathan R. Smith—a name it is pleasant for me to recall, as it makes a link between New Haven and Baltimore—held various chairs in succession—that of surgery and anatomy in the University of Vermont, of anatomy at the newly founded Jefferson school in Philadelphia, of surgery in the University of Maryland; later for three years in the justly celebrated Transylvania school he was Professor of the Theory of the Practice of Medicine, showing that the old association was not quite dead; and finally he returned to Baltimore to fill again the chair of surgery that he had vacated.

The teaching of surgery long continued to be carried on largely by didactic exercises, the only opportunities of acquiring manual facility being those afforded during anatomical instruction in the dissecting-room. Traces of the close association between these departments are to be seen in the surgical addenda in many of our text-books of anatomy, even in some whose first editions appeared subsequently to this period. With greater profit to us today—if the custom is at all a profitable one—we would well have similar addenda to our text-books of physiology; and though the times perhaps

---

[3] William H. Welch, The Relation of Yale to Medicine, Yale Medical Journal, 1901.

[4] See Billroth's " Lehren und Lernen." Wien 1876, p. 27.

are not yet ripe, the position of anatomy as the surgeon's sole hand-maiden is no longer unassailable.

It was Langenbeck, I believe, who first added to the curriculum of surgical exercises, which before had comprised didactic instruction with the opportunities of on-looking alone, the requirement of a practical operative course on the cadaver. His example was soon widely followed, and it has been under such a combination of exercises that the younger generation of today has for the most part been launched into practice.'

In my own under-graduate days—not so long ago, though long enough to make me wish them nearer—we were taught in large classes without much personal supervision, except perhaps for the favored few who were usually given the plums when teaching was done *en masse* and material was not superabundant. Our most important exercises were didactic; we saw cases diagnosed and handled by our instructors, and from an amphitheatre watched them operate; these hours of note-taking were supplemented by an excellent though brief operative course on the cadaver. I doubt if a better course was offered in any school or by better or more loyal instructors; but I cannot help thinking that even for the time—fifteen years ago—it was based on utterly wrong principles. For I doubt if many could have been trusted, when made doctors of medicine, to conduct with technical safety even the simplest operation on the extremities, not to mention the opening of an abdomen, a performance which some of us might have been called upon very soon to undertake in an emergency, inasmuch as a large number were going directly into rural practice. Was not the apprentice, with less of theory, but with a three year's practical training, even without a degree, better able to meet the medical needs of his community?

And as I earnestly believe that the one and only important distinction between surgery and medicine lies in the manual character of the operator's therapy—a part I have endeavored in this long preamble to make clear—this, being a manipulative practice, is not a thing to be taught by lectures. Lectures, recitations and clinics upon disease, whether given by the instructor in medicine or surgery, are chiefly means of presenting the theory of Medicine; and though there are some topics which for therapeutic reasons alone make them seem more ' medical,' as others seem more ' surgical,' yet the majority of the live topics today are border-line, and there should be no widely different point of view in their presentation. Looking back, for example, on a year's experience of my own, it would be hard to tell whether an attendance on Prof. Kocher's or Prof. Sahli's clinical exercises would be the more valuable for the graduate in medicine or the graduate in surgery, and it would be well if the same could be said for corresponding exercises in all other schools. Thus it is that the best text-book of general medicine (barring its therapeutic

aspect, which rarely is its strong point) today has become one's best work on general surgery; and I can see no reason why maladies whose management is largely operative should be excluded from such a work.

But when we come to treatment, it is a different matter. A student may read surgery, may hear and see surgery; and yet, without having himself practised operations and those on the living body, he remains totally incapable of carrying out those measures which alone distinguish this branch of medicine. One would not expect to play the violin after a course of lectures on music and merely by watching a performer for a few semesters. Just so with the looking-on at operations—an occupation that so far as the surgery (I do not include the pathology) of it is concerned, can be profitable to those alone who have already performed operations themselves, and who may learn something by observing the methods and technique of another man who may be a workman in some ways more dextrous and experienced than themselves.

It was in the endeavor to compensate for this defect in the presentation of a manual craft that the operative course on the cadaver was first introduced; but for present-day needs this method of teaching largely fails of its end, even if it be not altogether undesirable: since on the cadaver, in surroundings most unsurgical, we are taught operations before we know the first principles of operative technique, and as a result in the absence of the foundation stones of method a superstructure of knowledge is built on a very quicksand, ready to engulf a would-be surgeon with his first patient.

To send out from a school a man who has done, for example, the Chopart's and Lisfranc's, Forbes' and Hey's, Syme's and Pirogoff's with other amputations at and about the ankle-joint, without having had any experience with the only safe methods under which one of these relatively simple (though rarely performed) operations could in case of necessity be conducted, is to make of his little knowledge truly a dangerous thing. Contentment with such methods could be justifiable only in the pre-Listerian era of anatomical surgery— the surgery of Langenbeck's early days,' for it was really not until the remarkable contributions were made to abdominal Medicine by his pupils in the early eighties that surgery paid serious court to physiology. But though the surgery of today must be recognized as the child of this latter parentage, it is

---

* In his "Lehren und Lernen," Billroth mentions the need of "Localitäten fur Aufbewahrung und Pflege von Experimental- thieren" in addition to an abundance of cadavers for operative exercises though it is not apparent that he proposed to use the former for teaching purposes.

' I do not mean to intimate that von Langenbeck regarded work on the cadaver as an all sufficient training. Far from it. He began his actual career as a teacher before the days of modern surgery: and having been chosen a surgeon after an unusual experience as a physiologist and experimental pathologist, he appreciated full well the importance of experimental research. The influence of his teaching is everywhere shown in German surgery to-day—now two generations away from him. " So grunden sich auch alle die neuen Operationen, welche aus Langenbeck's Schule und namentlich deren Wiener Zweige hervorgingen, auf die Ergebnisse wohl überlegter und strengdurchgeführter Thierver- suche." (von Bergmann's Zur Erinnerung an Bernhard von Langenbeck, Berlin, 1888.)

still sent off to school to be brought up under the traditions of the old ways.

It was then, with a view of teaching our students of Medicine the first principles of operative technique, of which the all-important element is asepsis—for a surgeon's most active reflex must react to uncleanliness—at the same time that they were learning as much as possible of the diseases which in themselves or through their complications are supposedly amenable to operative measures, that this operative course was first inaugurated five years ago.

There has been no desire to turn out a multitude of operating surgeons—or physicians, as you will—any more than the aim of the manual training departments in some of our modern preparatory schools is to turn out finished cabinet makers or iron-workers, but rather to teach through simple living problems the proper and safe use of tools and fingers and respect for the material tissues on which they are to work.

DESCRIPTION OF A COURSE IN COMPARATIVE SURGERY.

An Extra-mural Course for Third Year Students.—It may, in the first place, be said that this is an elective subject, and one for which no examinations are held.[1] The course is offered to students who have just finished their first two years of detailed laboratory work, and in the clinical game—which we play in all seriousness—the instructor endeavors to keep fresh in their minds the anatomical, physiological and chemical principles that govern the rational study and treatment of such maladies as are brought up for consideration. An attempt is thus made to bridge over the gap that often yawns so widely between the laboratory and the clinical years of undergraduate life. At the same time, as the course is designed to prepare the students for the more advanced instruction to be offered them later on in the hospital, the exercises are modelled as closely as possible on the general methods of handling cases therein observed.

Students until late in their course (and then only in those few schools in which they are given the privilege of caring for and of following up cases themselves) rarely get a consecutive idea of any disease. On the contrary, glimpses of diseases are usually presented on the 'snap-shot' principle—a physical examination here, an operation there, or the ultimate result of the treatment in another instance. An effort is made in these exercises, even though the patients' maladies are conjectural ones, to stamp on the student's mind a moving picture of the disease and its treatment from start to finish—the biographic versus the snap-shot principle.

---

[1] It perhaps would not be a bad system if all of the associates who in our schools occupy positions analogous to the German Privat-docenten were not only privileged but expected to offer such extra-mural courses; for no opportunity serves to make an instructor put forth greater efforts, and there could be no more definite an index of the comparative value of a number of such courses than the student's selection therefrom.

Groups: Staff Units: Duties of Individual Members of These Units.—A group of ten students comprises as large a number as can well be overseen by one instructor, and until the present year, without the larger facilities now offered by our new laboratory, the number to whom the course could be offered was necessarily limited. Formerly, therefore, the instructor himself selected from the student body certain members of the class, who were given the opportunities for this work. At present in our new building, thanks to Dr. P. K. Gilman, a voluntary assistant, it has been possible to take at each exercise double the number, and thus by a quadruple repetition (the present third year class contains 80) to give all of the students in our comparatively small classes the privileges of the course. Much more could be done for a single group carried through the year, but, even as the work is now arranged, some of those students who show usual aptitude are encouraged to continue with special research problems.

These twenty men are divided into units of five, and each of these units comprises a non-operating physician, an operator, his first and second assistant and an anæsthetist. At each succeeding exercise the members rotate in these positions; the "family physician," for example, becoming the surgeon, the surgeon the first assistant, and so on.

The main exercise, held on Fridays, is a long one, consuming a large part of the day; this is supplemented by a shorter, preliminary (Wednesday) exercise at which preparations are made for the actual work to be done two days later.

Consultation upon Cases taken from Hospital Records.—At each Friday exercise the four family physicians present histories of their cases to the respective surgeons whom they are supposed to have called in consultation. These histories are discussed and the appropriate operative treatment, if any, is decided upon. In more detail: the four family physicians are told on a Wednesday what the subject for the following exercise will be, let us say, for illustration, lesions of the œsophagus, for which the establishment of gastric fistulæ for feeding purposes might be demanded. They have access to the records of Dr. Halsted's surgical service, and from them such histories of former hospital patients are chosen as may promise to furnish interesting subjects for discussion. Thus, by the perusal and study of real working histories, they learn to differentiate well-kept from untidy records, good from bad methods of portraying clinical pictures. Students are not restricted, however, to this source of supply alone, for they may make up hypothetical histories if they desire, or may select them from the current literature. The physician must have a clear idea of and be well posted in regard to his patient, for unexpected questions may be put to him, and there may prove to be sad omissions in the hospital histories if he has depended upon them alone for all of his information.

A concise and orderly anamnesis, together with complete notes in regard to the physical examination of the patient, is written out on hospital history sheets, in order that the student may acquire an early familiarity with the local way of keeping records. This history is brought to the Friday exercise without the surgical staff being aware even of the subject for discussion. Thus, to continue with my former example, in a recent exercise, aiming to take up the subject of gastrostomy, the following conditions were presented: one of cancer of the œsophagus in an adult; one of simple stricture following typhoid fever; a pharyngeal pouch; a patient with a foreign body lodged in the œsophagus.

One of the physicians then presents, without making the diagnosis self-evident, such data from his patient's history as he chooses to furnish. He is questioned by the consulting surgeon and the condition is discussed back and forth until the hearers are able to visualize the patient as clearly as though he were before them, and to have in mind his symptoms, past and present. When it has been determined where in all probability the lesion producing the symptoms lies, and what in all probability its nature is, a conclusion is reached as to the proper line of treatment—not always, it may be said, the same conclusion that was arrived at in the hospital. For when the consultation has been closed the physician tells what, according to the history, was the real outcome of the case.

And so in turn the other histories are taken up and discussed by the remaining three staff units. In this way, as can be seen, more than the usual advantages derived from the "case system" of teaching are brought into play. The mental training of this part of the exercise is valuable for instructor and students alike, but the latter are especially benefited by learning to present tersely and well an individual history of disease.

Didactic Part of Exercise.—During the above seance the instructor has played the part merely of middle-man, to direct if necessary the discussion during the presumed consultation. It then becomes his duty in a short talk to describe briefly the various affections to which the œsophagus is prone (the diagnostic symptoms of which are, for the most part, already well in the students' minds); to dwell more particularly upon those that are amenable to surgical therapy and upon the measures devised to relieve them. Thus, for this particular exercise, the various mechanical means of recognizing and of dealing locally with œsophageal lesions should be considered; and finally a review of the progressive steps in the development of the procedure to be undertaken (from Beaumont's experience with Alexis St. Martin's accidental gastrostomy, through the long series of purposeful attempts to establish a similar fistula, down to the more modern ways of performing the operation), should be illustrated by diagrams or free-hand drawings on the black-board. Furthermore, as many as possible of the original monographs which deal with the subject are brought to the exercise and put before the students, so that what their text-books have to say on the matter they may subsequently be able to read as they run. We may well cogitate upon the epigram of D'Israeli that "reading has ruined education."

The Practical Exercise.—After the instructor has thus presented the subject from the view-point of manipulative therapy, the students, practically undirected, select from among the various procedures that have been described the method of treatment that they wish to follow. The animals, picked out the day before by the physicians as substitutes for their patients, should have received a bath and have been kept in clean cages. Their breakfasts should have been omitted. A physiological dose of morphin, according to body weight, and given one-half hour before the operation, not only answers the purpose of the usual purge and enema administered in the hospital, but serves to make the animals so sleepy that they are indifferent to the subsequent proceedings. The patients are put on the tables, shaved and prepared for operation by the physicians, each of whom from this time on plays the part of general attendant, helping at the operation in a variety of ways, such as by keeping track of their particular animal's general condition, making blood examinations, washing out the stomach, furnishing needed supplies, reboiling instruments, etc., etc. The animal, as a rule, requires no general anæsthetic until the final stages of the preparation, when alcohol and antiseptic solutions are to be used upon the freshly shaved surface. If well morphinized, he objects not even to this, and indeed many of our operations are carried out under local anæsthesia.

In the meantime the assistants are cleaning up, preparing the instrument table, opening the sterilized packages of sponges, towels, gowns and other dry goods. The second assistant has selected the instruments and put them to boil; the anæsthetist has made an ether cone and commenced a chart which is to register the pulse and respiration, and sometimes the animal's temperature during the operation. Finally, in his turn the surgeon cleans up so as to be ready at the moment when the field of operation has been finally prepared; for there must be no delays with a patient under an anæsthetic.

The rivalry of the four groups becomes such that good 'team work,' which is an essential for group performance of any kind, is quickly acquired, and the preparations as a rule run smoothly after one or two exercises. Every effort is made to preserve the animal's warmth, to avoid discomfort and to prevent him from being frightened at his surroundings. There is as much chance, on the part of the anæsthetist, for the exercise here of moral control over his patient as in the hospital when an unreasoning child, for example, is being prepared for operation.

Operation.—As our aim is to teach proper methods of operating in general rather than the details of particular operations, the attention of the instructors is centered principally upon the strict observance of an aseptic technique. For when proper surgical reflexes have been acquired the individual procedure can safely be done perhaps in a variety of ways; and indeed by watching a handy student, unguided, devise means of overcoming such mechanical difficulties as may arise, the instructor himself may receive many valuable suggestions.

The students from the first usually wear gloves, and rapidly acquire the peculiar dexterity which comes to an operator who has learned to work with gloved fingers, an acquirement which makes the naked hands seem in a measure awkward. They are gowned and wear a combination of cap and mask, a very excellent model of which has been designed by one of this year's class. An operator, who has thus begun his surgical life, properly covered, is ever after uncomfortable when not so protected.

The instructors do little more than direct the students in the proper methods of using the scalpel; of applying clamps and other instruments; in proper ways of handling living tissues; of avoiding needless injury to nerves and blood vessels and of controlling hæmorrhage when it occurs; in the proper use of gauze for sponging and walling off; in ways of tying ligatures, of placing of sutures, etc., etc. And, whatever operation the student may be attempting, it is extraordinary how rapidly even the awkward man learns to do well and safely these simple things, and to keep surgically clean while doing so.

When the operation is finished all traces of it are removed. Even their instruments are scrubbed, wiped and put away, each group being responsible for a full set of them; and thus, as there is no place in surgery for a "Struwwelpeter," the students are made to observe every detail in preparation for and in completion of their work. They are supposed to be operating, for example, in a private house, and the room in which they have been working should be left as unsoiled and as tidy as when they arrived. A slovenly operator is known by his sloppy surroundings: and neatness in their work in every respect is expected of the students from the beginning.

Post-operative.—At the end of the operation the animals are taken in charge by their physician; they are put in their cages and kept warm. During the first few succeeding days the physician pays them regular visits; keeps track of their general condition and the state of the wound; directs the feeding; and administers such medicines as may be needed.

In case of a fatality a formal autopsy is held by the physician, the surgical staff being present; and should the cause of death not be clear, or should there be any evidence of pathological changes of interest, sections are cut and a complete histological report is added to the records. Unquestionably one learns more from his mistakes than from his successes, and some of the most important lessons for the students are those which the experiences of the autopsy-room have brought home to them. Thus not only many of the common causes of post-operative death, but many of the more unusual ones are encountered—to mention only a few, death from acute post-operative dilatation of the stomach, from intussusception, from hæmorrhage owing to a badly placed mass-ligature, from ulcer after certain forms of gastro-enterostomy. Nature hits back at the meddlesome surgeon, often in most unexpected ways, and the earlier in his career this fact is appreciated and taken into account, the better for his patients.

The Preparatory Exercise.—On Wednesday afternoon the students gather again in the laboratory for a short exercise. The patients of the previous Friday exercise are exhibited, their wounds are dressed and their condition is discussed. In case an autopsy has been held, the pathological tissues are demonstrated: and the completed history (containing the surgeon's descriptions of the operation, illustrated by as many diagrams as possible, together with the physician's post-operative notes) is indexed and added to the laboratory records.

At this same exercise the materials required for the next operative seance are prepared. The gauze is cut up and made into sponges and bundled for sterilization; the towels, gowns and caps which have been returned from the wash are also prepared; ether cones are folded; the sterilization of suture material which may take some time is gotten under way; and the prospective family physicians are made aware of the next subject to be taken up.

The value of such a preliminary exercise will be apparent to all operators, for few of us in our student days had anything to do with the details of preparation which lead up to and assure reasonable safety to our brief manipulations. These matters are usually left to a nurse or orderly, and supplies are ready at the hand of the hospital interne almost without his knowing whence they have come; so that when he goes out to actual work he must either take with him some one who has been trained to make up supplies, or must learn this fundamental part of his work "carefully and with tears" later instead of at the beginning of his surgical experience.

List of Exercises.—Some of our exercises—and there is no limit to the number and variety that may be offered—have been as follows: Gastrotomy for the removal of a foreign body inserted into the stomach; gastrostomy, as described above; pyloric operations for benign obstructions, as for instance a Finney pyloroplasty, an ideal operation for training in animal work; pylorectomy; the gastro-enterostomies in all their variety; intestinal resection with various forms of anastomosis: removal of the coiled cæcum of the dog for a chronically inflamed appendix; extirpation of the spleen, of the gallbladder, of the large mesenteric glands, an operation which has led to an interesting study concerning the method of their regeneration; major amputations at the hip or shoulder girdle; laminectomies; exploratory craniotomies with cortical stimulation; hysterectomies; operations on the heart and blood vessels; laparotomy for gunshot wounds.

Thus the possibilities of varying the exercises are so great that the instructor may keep his own interest from flagging in a course that must needs be repeated for different groups of students, for, to emphasize again what has been already said, it is not the operation in itself, but the observance of operative methods in general upon which chief stress is laid.

Research.—In a properly conducted hospital clinic, the work should not end with the taking of the history, the examination of the patient, the operation, and recovery or failure to give benefit as the case may be; but each condition that is in any respect out of the ordinary should suggest investigation to further broaden our knowledge. Many of the complications that have arisen in these patients of ours have led to researches, always of value to the investigator, and sometimes resulting in contributions in a small way to our knowledge. Moreover, in addition to our own special research problems, the surgical share of not a few investigations carried out in other laboratories has been conducted by the students while at the same time they are being trained in handicraft. Thus there may be an actual saving of animal life, for the conditions in most laboratories are not conducive to a high percentage of surgical recoveries; and Pawlow, perhaps more than anyone else, has shown the part which modern surgical technique may play, particularly in physiological research.

Veterinary Aspects of the Course.—For the conduct of exercises such as those already described, it is necessary to assume in normal animals the existence of lesions which correspond with those of the patients whose histories have been presented by the group physicians; and though we earnestly believe that our experimental work is done in a very good cause and with the infliction of a minimum of discomfort, it may be objectionable to those who disapprove of putting live animals to any such use.

There is consequently another feature of the course which we are anxious to encourage, and which is slowly developing from some small beginnings: one against which these objections surely can not be raised. This, for lack of a better term, we may designate as the 'veterinary' part of our work: and it is anticipated that some day the number of animals sent to us for the treatment of actual maladies may be sufficient to obviate any such necessity as exists under our present scheme of subjecting supposedly healthy vagrant animals to operations for conjectural lesions. The present laboratory may thus grow, as I hope to see it, into an actual Veterinary Department of the University, when opportunities for the study of unexperimental comparative pathology may be utilized, not only for purposes of organized research, but also for teaching surgery to medical students.

Veterinary surgeons—in this country, at least, for such a reproach can hardly refer to the graduates of the splendid schools that have arisen in London, Berlin and elsewhere—have rarely been brought up to realize that the surgery of animals, to be successful, requires the same care and detail that now belong to operative procedures on human beings. In consequence, surgical measures for very serious maladies are rarely attempted by them, and when they are undertaken, the mechanical means utilized are often crude in the extreme and such as would not for a moment be tolerated for the treatment of corresponding lesions in man. Hernias, tumors, goitres, prolapses and allied gynæcological conditions, obstetrical complications, ophthalmological lesions, as cataract—and the list might be enlarged almost indefinitely—are as common in our canine population as among their masters, all representing conditions not only amenable to, but for the most part urgently calling for surgical intervention.

As yet, however, the number of these patients is not large enough to furnish operative material for all; so that the students, who have themselves brought in the sick animals, or who in their other work may have demonstrated sufficient surgical ability to justify the choice, are selected to take charge of them. Histories are taken and physical examinations recorded as in the case of a patient entering the general hospital.[*]

In illustration a particular instance from among this year's experiences may be briefly cited:

A large animal of a mongrel Newfoundland type was brought to the clinic suffering from an extraordinary degree of general anasarca with ascites. A physical examination led to no definite conclusion as to the underlying cause of the trouble though suspicion was aroused by the detection of an indistinct cardiac murmur.

After the animal had been under observation and the object of study for some days, the student in charge having administered morphin, tapped the peritoneal cavity and withdrew several litres of bloody ascitic fluid. This led us to suppose that we should find a malignant abdominal tumor; and, sure enough, when the fluid was in large part withdrawn, an irregular, hard, movable mass became palpable in the left side of the abdomen, giving a definite ballottement, through the layer of fluid still intervening, when pushed with the fingers.

Two days later the animal was operated upon and our 'malignant tumor' was found to be a large, stony-hard, fæcal impaction almost filling the descending colon. This was broken up and removed bimanually; the remainder of the abdominal fluid was evacuated and the abdomen closed. Can anyone imagine a more valuable experience for students than this unnecessary operation? Would not many a surgeon who has made a similar mistake, or house-officer who for the first (and last) time has failed to recognize the presence of a fæcal impaction in a patient under his care, have been glad to have had such a lesson early in his career and not at the expense of human suffering?

But this is not all. The patient made an uninterrupted recovery from the operation; the wound healed by primary union; the animal for some time was benefited, but ultimately succumbed to the reaccumulation of fluid and its pressure effects. At the autopsy an extensive valvular lesion with dilated heart and cardiac insufficiency, leading to marked stasis phenomena, was found to have been responsible for the symptoms.

Bloody ascites from simple passive congestion being unknown to us, an effort has been made to reproduce this condition by the operative establishment of valvular lesions—a piece of experimental work on surgical lines the possibilities of which were suggested to us by Dr. William G. MacCallum's investigations on the immediate effects of injuries to the valves. Miss Henry, who had this animal in charge, and her colleagues have thus been able by intra-thoracic operations to reproduce most of the typical valvular lesions with subsequent recoveries from the operation, so that the consequences of these lesions, when of long duration, may be studied.

[*] Reference may be made to the series of papers by members of last year's class, reported in the Johns Hopkins Hospital Bulletin for May, 1905, under the title of "Comparative Surgery."

It has furthermore been possible for us through this investigation to overlap another university department, that concerned with the teaching of physical diagnosis, for these animals have been repeatedly used for the study of cardiac murmurs which are the outcome of a known rather than a presumed valvular lesion.[*]

Thus with proper laboratory facilities the subject of surgery, in so far as it differs from inner medicine, may be grasped by students early in their clinical course: whereas under other circumstances it would be long before they could be allowed, with justice to patients, to take an equally active part in its actual practice.

I am far from claiming that this method will make more surgeons out of a body of students, but it will, I believe, make the future physician more appreciative of the surgical point of view; more capable of understanding when handicraft may with propriety be called for, and the only safe methods of applying it; able, too, in case of need, to put his own hands to the work.

It will make of the students better and more trustworthy assistants when, later in the curriculum, they are privileged to take part in the more responsible operations on man—occasions when slips in technique must not occur. It will enable them, too, more easily and more intelligently to grasp the more serious surgery presented to them subsequently as hearers and more particularly as on-lookers, because, until they have once had their own hands in similar work the looking-on at another's operations, especially from the distant seats of an amphitheatre, is a comparatively unprofitable expenditure of time.

They learn, at the same time, to keep records; to present and discuss case histories intelligently; to visualize from such a history the actual condition of the patient. They learn to prepare all of the supplies necessary for an operation and by actual experience the way of conducting it. They learn to appreciate the risks of anæsthesia, and the need of untiring concentration upon his task by the administrator thereof. They learn to care kindly and properly for a living patient, in whose uneventful recovery as great personal pride will be taken as chagrin will be felt in case of complications for which some unavoidable error or neglect may have been responsible. They learn to describe their own operative procedures, to look up the literature of the subject, and are supplied with a stimulus for investigating experimentally the causes of such conditions as may still have an obscure etiology.

---

[*] Prof. Salomonson, "General Pathology as a University Subject," Festskrift ved Indvielsen af Statens Serum Institut, Copenhagen, 1902, in outlining a course in pathological physiology for students, says: "There is no better means for making them understand how difficult it is to account for the cause and development of a morbid state; or how momentous the part of experimental investigations has been in interpreting the observations made both clinically and in the post-mortem room." And I may add from the preface to Prof. Krehl's "Pathologische Physiologie" this, his concluding sentence: "Wirksamkeit, Bedeutung und Ansehen des "ärztlichen Stands in dem gleichen Maasse Sinken . . . . wie der Arzt aufhört Naturforscher zu sein."

THE HUNTERIAN LABORATORY OF EXPERIMENTAL MEDICINE.

The hospitality of the anatomical department for four years was sadly taxed in giving us even cramped quarters for the furtherance of this work; but now, thanks to the generosity of the University Trustees, we are happily quartered in a laboratory which may deserve some words of mention, for only in our present surroundings has it been possible to enlarge the scope of this operative course.

In drawing up the plans for our present quarters I was fortunate in being associated with my colleague, W. G. MacCallum, who assumes the responsibility of conducting work in half of the building, and who offers there an elective course for students in experimental pathology, which I trust he will fully describe elsewhere.

It was intended that the building should not only give facilities for our work as instructors, but should serve at the same time as the centre for work by those seriously inclined to undertake investigation along the lines of experimental surgery or pathology. Thus, as the floor plans indicate, Dr. MacCallum has partitioned off the upper floor of his end of the building into several private rooms for research. It was designed also that the laboratory should serve as the receiving station and centre for distribution of all animals that are used for investigation or for class work in the various university departments immediately connected with the medical school. Thus we hope in the course of time to provide not only accommodations suited to the comfort and humane care of all varieties of animals that may be needed for research, but also special cages and kennels for such privately owned animals as may be brought to us for treatment.

As the plans show, we have partitioned off the space on the ground floor into twelve units, quartered by separate hall-ways. The rooms on the western side of the building, designed for the accommodation of dogs alone, are connected with a large paddock where the well and convalescing animals may have sun-light and exercise. The paddock is divided so as to keep the sexes apart, and this provision has practically put a stop to their quarrelsomeness and noise. For newly operated animals, cages on the dormitory plan have been constructed in such a way that tops and sides can be readily taken apart and stacked up when not in use, and so be more easily kept clean. A receiving-room with bath, a work-shop and an autopsy-room, line the opposite side of the hall-way. The well animals are kennelled during inclement weather in the open rooms which are free from cages, and they are rotated in these quarters in such a way that one room may always be kept empty and aired after a thorough cleansing. Each of the rooms has a large central drain and can be easily flushed out. In fact, the drainage, light, heating and ventilation were the details to which we gave the most attention; otherwise the building was constructed as simply and cheaply as possible. It promised to be no small matter to house fifty dogs—the average number under our care—on the ground-floor of a building 80 by 40 feet, the upper story of which was to be

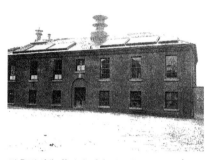

ast Front of the Hunterian Laboratory for Experimental
Medicine.

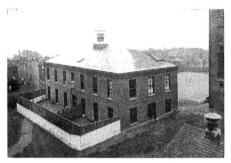

The Hunterian Laboratory. View from Anatomical Building
looking into Paddock.

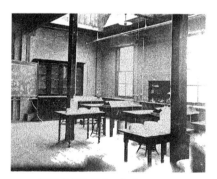

Corner of Students' Operating Room.

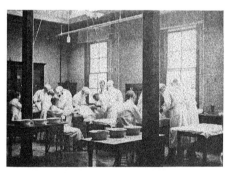

Three Surgical Staffs at Work in General Operating Room.

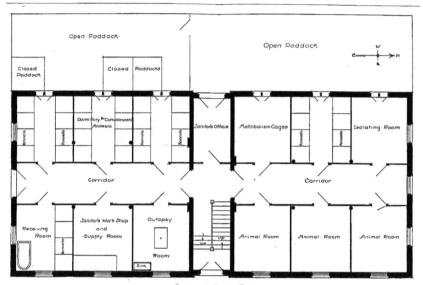

Ground · Floor · Plan ·

Scale

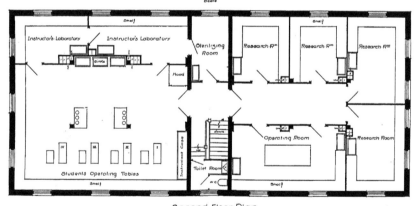

Second Floor Plan

Scale

used for teaching and needed, consequently, to be quiet, clean, free from odors, well warmed (from an adjoining building) and sufficiently well lighted for operative work. So far as we have gone our apprehensions lest we should fail in meeting these needs have been groundless.

Partly from lack of funds, partly because I do not feel that they are absolutely essential for safe surgery, we have made no such elaborate arrangements in the matter of operating and preparation rooms as Pawlow has had installed in the well-known Institute for Experimental Medicine in St. Petersburg. Though every one must agree with all that he says in regard to the importance for experimental physiology of the best surgical technique, I feel that, at the wound, operative asepsis—a matter in which there are no degrees—can be as certainly observed in the kitchen of a farm-house as in a glass and tile operating-room, and students should learn such precautions of cleanliness as would serve them in the humblest surroundings in which water can be made to boil.

In the establishment of this operative course, which, from its small beginnings in the fall of 1901, has grown like most things to which attention is paid, I can make no special claim for originality. Operative work on animals has been used before as a means of instruction in many localities, though I do not know that heretofore it has been made a part of the curriculum in this way, nor with just the same objects in view. The idea of its practicability possibly arose from my fortunate association, as an assistant to Dr. Halsted, in an experimental investigation he was conducting when I first came to Baltimore; its desirability was impressed upon me by the more recent experience of working for a few semesters in physiological laboratories abroad, during which time, it seems to me, I acquired more of real value for my surgical work than in my previous six years service as a hospital interne.

I have endeavored to make clear in this address that whatever its side issues may be, the primary aim of this work is to enable students to gain what Huxley called 'practical finger-end knowledge' of the underlying principles of modern surgical work, and early in their clinical course to become so familiar with the safe-guard of asepsis, the main essential to surgical success, that its observation becomes almost a second nature. Emphasis is laid at the same time upon the fact that the operation is not the beginning and end of surgery, but a therapeutic measure alone; and that those employing this manner of treatment must have the same knowledge of disease, the same ability to make examinations, the same instincts to follow pathological material to the laboratory and to investigate there the causes and symptoms of disease, as should characterize any other well-trained members of the body medical.

SUPRA-PUBIC HYSTEROTOMY AS A MEANS OF DIAGNOSIS AND TREATMENT OF THE UTERUS.

By WILLIAM WOOD RUSSELL, M. D.

Associate in Gynecology in the Johns Hopkins Hospital, Associate Professor of Gynecology in the Johns Hopkins University.

It is not necessary to enter into a discussion relative to the safety of an incision into the uterus deep enough to lay bare to examination and touch the entire uterine wall and cavity after the abdomen is opened and the uterus exposed. All that is needed is, I think, to demonstrate the utility of such a procedure in order to commend it to the surgeon for use on suitable occasions.

Vaginal exploration by splitting the anterior cervical and uterine wall, after separating the anterior cul-de-sac and the bladder, admits of palpation, but is unsatisfactory in a certain class of cases.

My experience with the first case reported in the list caused me to select the supra-pubic route. The result was most gratifying and since then, in carefully selected cases, my associates and myself have been similarly impressed with its value.

The procedure is as follows: A uterus which is suspiciously enlarged or which has given rise to intractable, unexplainable hemorrhages, is exposed, either in the course of an abdominal operation for other purposes or in the course of a purely exploratory operation where the abdomen has been opened for the particular purpose of doing a hysterotomy. After the pelvic organs have been examined, the uterus is drawn out of the abdominal opening as far as the cervical portion and surrounded by gauze on all sides. It is then grasped below on both sides by an assistant who lifts the body well up while the operator boldly splits it in the median line on the anterior wall, half way down towards the neck, as well as through the fundus to the posterior surface. The entire thickness of the uterine wall is divided for a distance of two or more centimeters down into the cavity, the mucosa can then be inspected at every point, the finger can be inserted and the whole cavity felt and if there are any nodules in the wall, they can be palpated.

If the mucosa is diseased, it can be scraped away with surprising ease and with the certainty of reaching all points efficiently, even in the cornua about the entrance of the tubes, a procedure which is almost impossible by the cervical route. This is of particular value as in some of our cases, delicate polypi were found which had not been reached by previous curettings. The bleeding is only moderate and it has not been necessary to put ligatures around a vessel.

The wound in the uterus is closed with interrupted catgut sutures passed from the peritoneal surface down to the mucous membrane. These are placed about one-half cm. apart, leaving the detail of closer approximation to fine catgut sutures. Catgut sutures may, if properly sterilized, be employed with safety in cases where there is not history of infection, otherwise fine silk is preferable.

Supra-pubic hysterotomy is of conspicuous service in cases of persistent uterine hemorrhage which is not controlled by any form of treatment and in which bi-manual palpation of the pelvic organs has given an absolutely negative diagnosis. In not a few instances the mucous membrane will show, by microscopical examination, a polypoid change, yet thorough and repeated curettings do not stop the irregular bleeding. This is explained, as already mentioned, by the fact that the growth is in the uterine cornua and also because none of the instruments devised will successfully reach these areas.

Small sub-mucous and pediculated myoma, which do not affect the size or contour of the uterus, but which may be the source of dangerous hemorrhage, are easily detected and removed by this method. Where the abdomen has been opened for some other purpose, and no explanation has been found for the uterine hemorrhage, I would then also advocate its application.

No deaths have occurred in the thirty-two cases here reported, notwithstanding the fact that many of these were complicated by other serious abdominal or pelvic disturbances, proving quite conclusively the slight danger attending the operation.

The following list comprises the cases which have been operated upon by Doctors Kelly, Cullen, Ramsay, Miller, Stokes, and myself, and which represent the various conditions found in the uterus where the operation is applicable. The histories are greatly abbreviated, only the salient points being given.

SUMMARY OF CASES.

CASE 1, No. 5372.—Miss L., aged 21, white, admitted to tue Johns Hopkins Hospital, July 18, 1897. Menstruation began at fifteen and has always been free and regular. Present illness began at seventeen years of age. She has lost blood for a month at a time and for this was curetted four times; the actual cautery being used twice. She suffers no pain but feels weak.

Physical examination reveals an outlet only moderately relaxed. Cervix slightly enlarged, but uterus of normal size, freely movable and in posterior position. No disease detected in tubes.

Operation.—Dilatation and curettement; cervix widely dilated and uterine cavity curetted. Several pieces of necrotic polypi brought away.

Second operation.—October 12, 1897. As the patient remained well only two months after the first operation, and bleeding persisted, a low median incision was made in the abdomen and after a careful examination of the tubes and ovaries, which were normal, the uterus was delivered and surrounded by gauze. It was then split anteriorly in the median line from the fundus

to about the internal os. Several polypi were found in the uterine cornua at the entrance to the Fallopian tubes and the membrane elsewhere was somewhat thickened.

After the mucous membrane had been removed and the polypi thoroughly curetted away, the edges of the wound in the musculature were sutured together with interrupted catgut sutures, the uterus was dropped back into the pelvis and the wound closed.

Result.—Recovery.

CASE 2, No. 523.—Mrs. W. L. K., aged 24, white, admitted to a private hospital, November 30, 1897. Menstruation began at thirteen years of age with dysmenorrhea until nineteen. Present illness began two months ago with irregular and painful menstruation. Pain comes on four or five days after the flow begins, and the patient takes morphine for relief. She has been treated with tampons and curettement.

Operation.—Hysterotomy and dilatation and curettement; Suspensio uteri. Large soft uterus dilated and curetted per vaginam. Abdominal incision, uterus opened in median line on anterior surface down into cavity, and finger inserted to explore it. The walls were found to be about 2 cm. thick. The bleeding was only moderate and the incision was closed by ten interrupted catgut sutures. After suspending the uterus in the usual manner, the abdominal incision was closed.

Result.—Patient recovered slowly, but had dysmenorrhea at first menstruation after operation.

CASE 3, No. 6637.—Miss L. H., white, aged 36, admitted to the Johns Hopkins Hospital, January 14, 1898. Menses began at fourteen and have always been regular, every four weeks until present illness began, two years ago. She has always had dysmenorrhea. Flow is now profuse, clotted, and rather offensive. She is always confined to her bed during the time, and has fever. Leukorrhea is profuse, just before and after menstruation.

Examination.—Hymen intact; vaginal mucosa bleached. Cervix in mild degree of descensus; uterus retroverted, lying low in pelvis, and normal in size.

Operation.—Hysterotomy, suspensio uteri, removal of cyst. Uterus lifted out through abdominal incision and split open down to mucosa, which was normal. Incision closed with interrupted catgut sutures, and uterus suspended with silk ligatures. A small cyst was removed from right tubal fimbria.

Result.—Recovery.

CASE 4, No. 6336.—Mrs. A. McK., aged 28, admitted to the Johns Hopkins Hospital, September 3, 1898. Menstruation was induced by medicine, and appeared at seventeen; for a few months the flow was regular, but profuse and clotted, lasting from three to four days with pain. After marriage at twenty, her menstrual periods were normal, but at present she is suffering from dysmenorrhea and a lumpy, offensive discharge. She has been losing flesh for eight months and has lost blood almost continually, which is in flesh-like clots at menstrual periods.

She has had two children, but no miscarriages.

Physical examination of pelvis, negative, except for a somewhat enlarged fundus.

Operation.—Dilatation and curettement were done for diagnosis, and only a small amount of curettings obtained. No relief being obtained from this operation, she consented to a second.

Second operation.—Hysterotomy. The uterus was drawn out of the incision and surrounded by gauze and split open. The mucous membrane was found to be rather thickened and dark red, but the cavity was not enlarged, and no polypi were found. Having thoroughly curetted the cavity, the wound was closed by first putting in four sutures to draw the mucosa together, the knots being tied so as to come within the uterine cavity. No. 3 catgut sutures were used.

Result.—Convalescence was very slow, patient being very weak and requiring feeding per rectum for four days after the operation.

CASE 5, No. 754.—Mrs. R., white, aged 23, admitted to a private hospital, April 26, 1899. Menstruation has always been regular but profuse. She has been married three years.

Present illness.—The complaint made was of sterility. Patient suffers with pain in lower abdomen and back beginning with flow. She has been treated with dilatation, and symptoms have been worse ever since. Her menstruation is severe and recurs three times in the month.

Operation.—Hysterotomy and curettement, ligation of right and left uterine artery. Uterus delivered and surrounded by gauze, then grasped firmly with the fingers and split about 5 cm. down the anterior face almost to the cervix into the cavity. Two large, flabby polypi extruded from the fundus on each side and were thoroughly curetted away. Wound was closed with interrupted catgut sutures. Hemorrhages were stopped and the arteries ligated.

Result.—A good recovery.

CASE 6, No. 6949.—Mrs. M. I., white, aged 28, admitted to the Johns Hopkins Hospital, May 26, 1899. Menses began at thirteen and have been regular every four weeks, and painless, until last December. Since then she has been suffering from pain and soreness in the right side of abdomen under the lower ribs, with at times pain in the back and lower abdomen.

Marital history.—Patient has been married eight years and has had three children.

Operation.—Hysterotomy. Abdomen was opened and a large uterus was found, brought out of incision and split open 4 cm. anteriorly and 3 cm. posteriorly. The cavity of uterus was then curetted and an abundant amount of endometrium was removed. The uterus was then sewed up with catgut sutures and all bleeding checked.

CASE 7, No. 6950.—Mrs. C. H., white, aged 41, admitted to the Johns Hopkins Hospital, May 27, 1899. Menstruation commenced at the age of thirteen, and the flow has always been very profuse, coming every three weeks. Leukorrhea is present but not troublesome.

Present illness.—Three years ago the patient had a uterine hemorrhage which came on at night and since then she has had hemorrhages at intervals of from one to four months.

Marital history.—The patient married at sixteen, and had one child at seventeen. Since then three miscarriages, the last one of seven months' pregnancy. A severe hemorrhage followed these miscarriages. She has been treated for years for erosion of cervix. She has pain in ankles and limbs.

Examination.—Vaginal outlet moderately relaxed, admitting two fingers. The cervix was found far back with patulous os and hypertrophied lips. The mucous membrane was everted but not friable or indurated. The fundus was sagging in the pelvis, movable, and its anterior surface irregular in outline.

Operation.—Hysterotomy. An abdominal incision was made, exposing a normal fundus lying in anteposition which was delivered through incision, surrounded by gauze, split open and curetted. A small myoma, the size of a marble in anterior wall was discovered and removed.

Result.—A good recovery.

CASE 8, No. 7022.—Mrs. K. W., white, aged 30, admitted to the Johns Hopkins Hospital, June 25, 1899. Menses began at fifteen years of age, coming regularly every month and lasting from six to eight days. Since July the hemorrhage has been profuse, last-

ing often for two, three, or four weeks, with intervals of two and three weeks. No pain accompanies the hemorrhage, which is clotted. There has been more or less leukorrhea since catamenia began.

Present illness began in July, 1899, when the flow became more than usually profuse and somewhat clotted.

Ether examination.—Outlet admitting two fingers; cervix found in axis, pointing outward; os uteri patulous; the fundus enlarged and in retroposition.

Operation.—Hysterotomy, suspensio uteri. A median line incision was made and the fundus was found hard pressed upon rectum; enlarged but not adherent. The right ovary had been converted into a cyst the size of an egg, thin-walled and transparent. All other structures were found normal.

Fundus was brought out of incision and split anteriorly; the uterine cavity was thoroughly curetted, bringing away considerable polypoid endometrium, mostly from left uterine cornu. The incision in the uterus was then closed with interrupted catgut sutures, and suspended with two silk sutures in the usual way. The peritoneal cavity was flushed with normal salt solution and the abdomen was closed.

Result.—Patient discharged well.

CASE 9, No. 7753.—Mrs. M. T., white, aged 37, admitted to the Johns Hopkins Hospital, June 27, 1899. This patient was operated upon in this hospital in 1895 for the repair of a relaxed vaginal outlet.

Marital history.—Two miscarriages when first married, in little over one year, but no full-term children.

Present illness.—Since the operation mentioned the patient has found little change in her condition. She complains of burning in pelvis and severe backache, with pain in left side of abdomen. These discomforts are worse when standing. She suffers also from severe headache which is worse during periods, and she is extremely nervous and unable to lead an active life. Menstruation is regular, lasts four days, and is less painful since the operation.

Examination.—Uterus found to be one and one-half times normal size, freely movable. A small myoma is found on the posterior surface.

Operation.—Hysterotomy, myomectomy. A median line incision was made in abdomen and the uterus was delivered and surrounded by gauze. It was then split open on anterior surface to cavity. The polypoid endometrium was curetted away and a small myoma shelled out of fundus; after which the wound was closed with catgut.

Result.—On recovery from this operation the patient was transferred to the medical side of the hospital for treatment of nephritis.

CASE 10, No. 7246.—Miss C. R., white, aged 24, admitted to the Johns Hopkins Hospital, September 20, 1899. Menses began at fourteen years of age, and have never been regular; the periods are delayed, coming every six weeks and again every seven and eight weeks, lasting five to eight days; they are normal in amount. When the patient is tired she has some leukorrhea.

Present illness.—The patient has worked steadily as a trained nurse since June, 1893. She has been suffering from dysmenorrhea but has felt fairly well until three years ago, when she began to have bearing-down pains and backache. These pains have been intense ever since, but are lighter at times than at others. In April, 1897, a dilatation and curettement was done, and for a considerable period she felt better, and menstruation was regular. She wore a pessary for five months which set up an irritation and was removed. She has gradually been getting worse.

Operation.—An abdominal incision was made and the uterus delivered and split open. All redundant mucosa was peeled away from the upper half of the fundus. No discharge or tumor was noted. After thoroughly curetting the uterine mucosa, the wound was closed with interrupted catgut sutures.

Result.—Recovery uneventful.

CASE 11, No. 7337.—Mrs. A. L., white, aged 28, admitted to the Johns Hopkins Hospital, November 1, 1899. Menstruation began at fifteen years of age, and has been regular, lasting five days. Discharge profuse, using six to eight napkins a day.

Marital history.—Married seven years. The flow always increased after child-birth, but the patient does not menstruate during pregnancy or lactation.

Present illness.—Profuse flow and free catarrhal discharge, with constant pain in hypogastric region.

Operation.—Hysterotomy and curettement. An abdominal incision was made. Uterus delivered and surrounded by gauze, split on anterior surface, and curetted. The wound was closed in usual way.

Result.—Patient discharged improved.

CASE 12, No. 7442.—Mrs. E. D. E., white, aged 37, admitted to the Johns Hopkins Hospital, December 12, 1899. Menstruation began at twelve years of age, with profuse flow soiling four napkins daily, but no pain. The flow is clotted. Leukorrhea has been slight for three years and of a yellow color.

Marital history.—Married fourteen years and has had three children. No miscarriages.

Present illness began four years ago. At that time the flow became hemorrhagic in character, and has continued for one year occurring every other day. For this she was curetted in 1896. She suffers from pain and burning sensation in back and loss of weight and strength, with occasional palpitation of the heart and shortness of breath.

Examination reveals the external genitalia normal; at hymen on the right side is a cyst the size of a pea. The cervix is low in the vagina, pushed forward, and is somewhat softer than normal. The external os is patulous, admitting the tip of the index finger. Rectal examination shows a large retroverted uterus one and one-half times normal size.

Operation.—Repair of vaginal outlet, hysterotomy, dilatation and curettement; suspensio uteri. Small amount of curettings obtained. Resection of vaginal outlet required extensive denudation. Abdomen opened in median line, uterus delivered and an incision made in anterior face through fundus in median line 7 cm. long, but nothing found in uterus to account for bleeding. The incision was closed with interrupted catgut sutures, and the uterus suspended in the usual manner.

Result.—Recovery.

CASE 13, No. 7594.—Mrs. I. C. H., white, aged 37, admitted to the Johns Hopkins Hospital, February 19, 1900. Menstruation began at eleven or twelve years of age, and has been regular until four years ago, since which time the periods have come every three weeks and last ten days. Sometimes she misses six or nine weeks. Leukorrhea has been slight. She was curetted in January, 1900, following which she has had constant flooding.

Present illness began nine months ago. Patient suffers from pain on left side, sometimes dull, sometimes sharp or labor-like in character.

Operation.—Hysterotomy, dilatation, and curettement; double salpingo-oophorectomy, suspensio uteri; dilatation of cervix per vaginam. Moderate amount of endometrium obtained with curette. The abdomen was opened and the uterus delivered, surrounded by gauze and split open. The previous curetting seemed to have been well done except in right cornu. The uterus was sewed up with catgut. The tubes and ovaries were removed for a large Graafian-follicle cyst and the uterus suspended to anterior abdominal wall.

Result.—Recovery.

CASE 14, No. 901.—Mrs. W. D. D., white, aged 34, admitted to a private hospital, February 26, 1900.

Present illness.—Patient had one child and dates present illness from its birth. For several years she has suffered from pain in back which is exaggerated by exercise and during menstruation. There is often a weight and bearing-down pain in lower abdomen. Leukorrhea is constant.

Examination.—Outlet moderately relaxed. Tear in the cervix. The fundus found in retroposition and medium size. Appendages adherent.

Operation.—Hysterotomy, salpingectomy, repair of vaginal outlet. Vaginal outlet repaired in the usual way. A median line incision made in the abdomen, and uterus delivered and split in anterior surface into cavity. The mucous membrane was curetted away. Both tubes having a nodular salpingitis, they were removed with a small portion of the ovary.

Result.—Patient made a good recovery.

CASE 15, No. 924.—Mrs. J. L., white, aged 30, admitted to a private hospital, April 1, 1900. Menstruation began at twelve years of age, flow has always been regular, and lasted from four to six days.

Marital history.—Married seven and a half years, and has had two children. Both labors instrumental.

Present illness began at birth of second child. Patient had a complete tear at first confinement. She suffers with acute pain in lower abdomen. Menstrual flow lasts three weeks. There is considerable leukorrhea.

Operation.—Dilatation and curettement, resection of vaginal outlet. Incision made in abdomen, in median line. A small ovarian cyst was removed. No adhesions were found. Uterus delivered and incision made in the median line down to uterine cavity which was explored with curette, not very much endometrium obtained. Uterus closed in the usual way, and suspended to anterior abdominal wall.

Result.—Patient recovered without interruption.

CASE 16, No. 1085.—Mrs. T. L., white, aged 43, admitted to a private hospital, January 23, 1901. Menstruation began at fourteen years of age, and has always been normal.

Marital history.—Has had four children and six miscarriages. Patient was previously operated upon by Dr. Kelly for adherent placenta.

Present illness.—Three weeks ago patient began to have constant floodings with passage of large clots. Has not been troubled with leukorrhea or dysmenorrhea.

Operation.—Dilatation and curettement in the usual manner, obtaining half ounce of non-malignant endometrium. Hysterotomy, and suspensio uteri. An abdominal incision was made in the median line and a soft, flabby uterus delivered, and incised 7 cm. through the fundus in the median line, exposing a cavity in which the mucous membrane was found smooth and normal. Uterus was closed and suspended in the usual manner and the abdominal wound closed.

Result.—Patient had a long and tedious convalescence.

CASE 17, No. 8489.—Miss R. H., white, aged 24, admitted to the Johns Hopkins Hospital, February 1, 1901. Menstruation began at twelve years of age, normal in amount and interval. Pain occurs on first day with backache. There is occasional but slight leukorrhea.

Present illness began three years ago, when dysmenorrhea became pronounced. Patient suffers with pain between shoulders and in left lower abdomen. General condition only fair.

Operation.—Hysterotomy, suspensio uteri. Abdomen opened and fundus found very large and retroflexed. Lateral structures normal. Median line incision made in abdomen, and uterus delivered. Incision through anterior face of fundus down to cavity. Walls of fundus found slightly thickened, but cavity of normal length. Mucous membrane thickened, and on curetting, membrane came off in thick strands. The wound was closed in the usual manner, and the uterus suspended to anterior abdominal wall.

Result.—Convalescence prolonged by badly nourished condition of patient.

CASE 18, No. 8586.—Mrs. M. L. F., white, aged 35, admitted to the Johns Hopkins Hospital, March 16, 1901. Menstruation began at thirteen years of age, and has been normal until six years ago, since when the flow has lasted for six and eight days at a time. Patient was curetted for this four years ago when a large amount of fungoid growth was removed. After this operation the flow lasted for three weeks. The last severe hemorrhage appeared at the regular time of the menses, and continued throughout the month. Patient suffers with leukorrhea, which has troubled her since catamenia began.

Marital history.—Patient has been married seventeen years and has five children, all labors normal, and no history of miscarriages.

Examination.—Cervix in moderate descensus, large and lacerated. Uterus in anterior position and normal in consistency and size. Lateral structures apparently normal.

Operation.—Vaginal hysterotomy. The anterior lip was bisected and a uterine polyp removed, and in addition to the ordinary curetting, the uterine cavity was explored with the finger.

Second operation.—Hysterotomy, suspensio uteri, removal of herniated corpus luteum. A median line incision was made in the abdominal wall, the uterus delivered, and surrounded by gauze and split through anterior face to cavity. An abundant overgrowth of endometrium was removed by the curette. A polyp on the posterior wall, which would not yield to curette was excised with scissors. A tag of tissue, probably the pedicle of the polypus removed by vaginal route, was scraped away. Wounds closed in usual way and uterus suspended to abdominal wall.

Result.—Convalescence prolonged from neurasthenia.

CASE 19, No. 1307.—Mrs. P. H., white, aged 28, admitted to a private hospital, February 3, 1902. Menstruation began at fourteen years of age and has always been profuse, lasting from three to five days. Lately the flow has lasted eight days and occurs every three weeks. Leukorrhea has always been present.

Marital history.—Patient has been married four years and has had two children, and two miscarriages. Labors have always been difficult, and the patient was lacerated at the birth of the first child.

Present illness began before the second child was born, when patient had puerperal mania. She is now very nervous, and becomes rigid. Head gets "muddled." She often loses consciousness, and suffers a great deal with backache and intense bearing-down pains.

Operation.—Repair of vaginal outlet and removal of tumor from left leg. Hysterotomy. An abdominal incision was made, and the uterus delivered and split in anterior surface. Polypoid endometrium scraped away. Uterus and abdomen closed in usual manner. The ovaries were found to be normal.

Result.—Recovery.

CASE 20, No. 8583.—Mrs. A. E. C., white, aged 36, admitted to the Johns Hopkins Hospital, March 18, 1901. Menstruation began at thirteen years of age, has always been regular, occurring every twenty-eight days, and lasting three days. Patient suffers continually from leukorrhea, which eleven years ago was very offensive and profuse for a time.

Marital history.—Patient has been married thirteen years. She has four children and has had two miscarriages. Labors were normal with the exception of first, when the child was premature.

Present illness began with birth of the first child and came on gradually. Patient exercised very actively up to birth of child and has ever since declined in health. She complains of dull pain in left loin and occasionally in lower abdomen on the right side, especially when fatigued.

Examination.—Tenderness in right kidney region. Considerable hypertrophy of anterior vaginal wall immediately under urethra. No infection. Outlet relaxed. Cervix high in vagina, pointing dorsally. Fundus somewhat enlarged and soft, resting against bladder, and tender on palpation. Lateral structures not well outlined, but there appears to be thickening on the side.

Operation.—Hysterotomy, suspension of right kidney, removal of cyst of right ligament. An abdominal incision was made in the median line, the uterus delivered and split anteriorly. Polyp growing from mucosa, and a general polypoid endometrium scraped away. Cervical canal dilated. Small cyst removed from right broad ligament.

Result.—Recovery.

CASE 21, No. 8698.—Mrs. L. M., white, aged 38, admitted to the Johns Hopkins Hospital, April 27, 1901. Menstruation began at twelve years of age, normal, five-day type.

Marital History.—Patient has been married thirteen years and has had no children and no miscarriages.

Present illness began eight months ago, the menstrual flow lasting from ten days to two weeks. Patient suffers with pain in the back and sharp pain and burning sensation in the left side. She also has slight leukorrhea.

Examination shows a large fundus in retroflexion. Immediately at the cervical and uterine junction on the right side, a hard nodule is felt.

Operation.—Hysterotomy, dilatation and curettement. An abdominal incision was made in usual manner and the uterus was delivered and split. A myoma was removed from the posterior wall of fundus. Small cervical sub-mucous myoma 2 x 15 cm. removed with curette. The incision in the uterus was closed with catgut sutures, about fourteen in all, which passed down to the mucosa to control hemorrhage.

Result.—Recovery.

CASE 22, No. 8726.—L. D., mulatto, aged 37, admitted to the Johns Hopkins Hospital, May 5, 1901. Menstruation began at fourteen years of age, and up to the past year has been regular.

Marital history.—Patient has been married eighteen years and has had two miscarriages, but no children.

Present illness.—For a year the menstrual flow has been profuse and clotted, accompanied with labor-like pains. Periods last from five to seven days. She complains of backache and pain in the lower and upper sacral region, which is exaggerated during menstruation. Patient has had leukorrhea for fifteen years, very profuse, and soiling four or five napkins a day. It is somewhat offensive, but not irritating, and most profuse following menstruation.

Examination.—External genitalia normal. Vaginal outlet not markedly relaxed, cervix deep in vagina, moderate size. Uterus in second degree of retroflexion, but movable.

Operation.—Myomectomy, hysterotomy, appendectomy, suspensio uteri. In the median line an abdominal incision was made, and the uterus delivered. Six small myomata were found at various points on the uterus, and enucleated. The uterus was split on its anterior face, down to the cavity. No diseased mucosa was found, but the cavity was curetted and the wound closed with interrupted catgut sutures. The fundus was then suspended after the usual method. The appendix, which was slightly adherent, was removed.
Result.—Recovery.

CASE 23, No. 9020.—Miss L. C., white, aged 38, admitted to the Johns Hopkins Hospital, August 30, 1901. Menstruation irregular for fifteen years.
Present illness.—Patient has been bleeding for nine weeks. She suffers with dysmenorrhea, and complains of pain in the back and thighs, and across the abdomen. Patient has no leukorrhea. In July at this hospital, she was treated with dilatation and curettement, after which her symptoms were good for three weeks, when the flow began again, sometimes clotted, sometimes free. There is pain just above the symphysis which she describes as unbearable at times.
Examination.—Outlet bathed in fresh blood. Cervix low in the vagina. Fundus lies against rectum in Douglass' cul-de-sac, small, and rather soft on its posterior wall.
Second operation.—Hysterotomy. Median line incision in abdomen. Uterus delivered and split to cervix. The mucous membrane was found apparently normal, but was curetted away through incision. The wound in the uterus was closed with interrupted catgut sutures. The abdominal incision was closed in the usual manner.
Result.—Convalescence uninterrupted.

CASE 24, No. 1240.—Mrs. V., white, aged 24, admitted to a private hospital, October 23, 1901. Menstruation has been irregular for nine months.
Marital history.—Patient has been married twenty-two years and has had two children and two miscarriages. Both labors were instrumental. Patient complains of frequent pain in various parts of the body, and general nervousness and anemia.
Present illness began nine months ago, with irregular and profuse menstruation. For this the patient was curetted in January. She suffers much pain during menstruation.
Operation.—Hysterotomy, myomectomy. An abdominal incision was made, the uterus delivered, surrounded by gauze and split through the anterior face down to cavity. A sub-mucous myoma, the size of an almond was found in the posterior wall and removed. The mucous membrane was thoroughly curetted and the wounds were closed in the usual manner.
Result.—Recovery.

CASE 25, No. 8531.—Mrs. R. R., white, aged 50, admitted to the Johns Hopkins Hospital, November 25, 1901. Menstruation began at sixteen years of age, lasting from two to three days. The flow has been very free and sometimes clotted.
Marital history.—Patient has been married twenty-eight years, and has had ten children and one miscarriage. Labors were all normal.
Present illness.—Patient complains of dragging sensation in lower abdomen. During the last three years there has been a mucoid discharge at the end of menstrual flow and headache before flow begins. The last menstrual flow lasted three weeks.
Examination.—Relaxed vaginal outlet, tenderness in left lower quadrant of abdomen, uterus far back and considerably enlarged but movable.
Operation.—Hysterotomy, dilatation and curettement, removal of polypi, radical cure of hemorrhoids by clamp and cautery.

An abdominal incision was made in the median line and the uterus delivered. Fundus split on anterior face into the cavity. A large polypus on the anterior wall about mid-way in the cavity twisted off, and excessive endometrium was scraped away with a sharp spoon curette. The incision was closed in the usual manner, and the fundus suspended to the anterior wall of abdomen. Repair of vaginal outlet after Emmett's method, and curettement per vaginam, bringing away a small polyp.
Result.—Convalescence slightly prolonged by hemorrhage of perineal stitches.

CASE 26, No. 1263.—Mrs. W. W., white, aged (?), admitted to a private hospital, December 2, 1901. Menstruation began at fourteen years of age; has been regular and lasts from three to five days, accompanied by severe pain.
Marital history.—Patient has been married three and a half years, and has three children. Two labors were spontaneous, but the last one was very difficult, complicated with laceration.
Present illness.—About eight years ago patient began to suffer with dysmenorrhea and abdominal pain upon exertion of any kind. She also suffers with backache and headache.
Examination.—Uterus retroflexed, kidney movable.
Operation.—Hysterotomy, suspensio uteri, suspension of kidney. An abdominal incision was made, exposing the uterus which was split 3 cm. in the median line anteriorly. No tumor was found, but a large amount of thick endometrium was removed by a curette. The vaginal outlet was repaired and the kidney suspended in the usual manner.
Result.—Recovery slow.

CASE 27, No. 9648.—Mrs. Z. G., white, aged (?), admitted to the Johns Hopkins Hospital, May 17, 1902. Menstruation did not begin until after marriage at the age of twenty. Flow was regular but excessive, and at times clotted.
Marital history.—Patient has been married five years, and has had one child, and two miscarriages.
Present illness.—For nine months patient has been flowing most of the time. She has a burning sensation in vagina, with constant desire to urinate.
Examination.—Fundus of normal size, lying in normal position. Outlet markedly relaxed, cervix slightly lacerated.
Operation.—Repair of vaginal outlet and curettement per vaginam; suspensio uteri, hysterotomy, appendectomy. Upon curetting, the uterine cavity was found so irregular that a hysterotomy was decided upon. A median line incision was made in the abdomen and the uterus delivered, surrounded by gauze and split about 6 cm. somewhat through anterior face. The mucous membrane was found adherent and lacerated by previous curetting. No disease found. The incision was closed by through and through catgut stitches. The appendix was released from adhesions and amputated. The uterus was then suspended in the usual manner.
Result.—Discharged improved.

CASE 28, No. 1425.—Mrs. M. D., white, aged 27, admitted to a private hospital, October 24, 1902. Menses began at thirteen years of age, and have been regular until two years ago.
Marital history.—Patient has been married seven years and has one child.
Present illness.—Six months ago the periods began to occur every four weeks, and lasted two weeks. In September the patient was packed for bleeding. Flow now lasts from ten days to two weeks. There has been a slight leukorrhea for two months.
Examination.—Uterus enlarged, fundus in retroflexion.
Operation.—Repair of vaginal outlet, hysterotomy and curettement of uterine mucosa, suspensio uteri, repair of vaginal outlet. Abdomen incised through median line and uterus delivered,

surrounded by gauze and split in median line on anterior face down to cavity. The mucosa was found to be 5 cm. thick and numerous small polypi were projecting from it. Polypi dug out with sharp spoon curette and the greater part of the thickened membrane removed. The uterus was suspended to the anterior abdominal wall in the usual manner.

Result.—Recovery.

CASE 29, No. 1458.—Mrs. E. W., white, aged 32, admitted to a private hospital, October 27, 1902. Menstruation began at twelve years of age, and has always been irregular, accompanied with more or less dysmenorrhea; the flow is clotted and lasts from six to seven days.

Marital history.—Patient has been married fourteen years and has had two children and two miscarriages. Labors were difficult and instrumental. Patient was lacerated both times.

Present illness.—Since March the patient has suffered with pain in the back and bearing-down sensation. She suffers from an annoying leukorrhea.

Examination.—Uterus retroverted, enlarged, and boggy. A dense, rounded tumor, giving somewhat the signs of a bi-cornate uterus is felt to the right. Cervix in descensus. Right ovary and tube not palpable.

Operation.—Hysterotomy, suspensio uteri, myomectomy. Plastic operation on Fallopian tubes. An abdominal incision was made in the median line, exposing uterus bound down with dense adhesions to the pelvic floor. These were cut with scissors. Right tube loosened, leaving a fimbriated end free and open. The right ovary was bound in a bed of adhesions to the posterior sheath of broad ligament, but was not disturbed. Left tube was loosened and an opening was made in its distal end, 3 cm. long. Uterus delivered and split on anterior face and curetted. A considerable amount of endometrium was removed. The cervical canal was dilated from above. Closure as usual. Uterus suspended with silk sutures and utero-sacral ligament shortened. Small myoma removed from broad ligament.

Result.—Patient discharged improved.

CASE 30, No. 1486.—Mrs. J. W. G., white, aged 26, admitted to a private hospital, December 3, 1902. Menstruation began at eighteen years of age, and has always been irregular and profuse, often coming every three weeks, and lasting from a week to ten days, at times amounting to floodings.

Marital history.—Patient has had children, but no miscarriages. Labors all difficult.

Present illness.—Patient complains of profuse and irritating leukorrhea, with menstrual disturbances noted above. Ten and four years ago she was curetted for the floodings.

Operation.—Myomectomy and hysterotomy, with ligation of

both uterine arteries. An incision was made in the anterior median line of abdomen, and the uterus delivered, surrounded by gauze and split. Two small myomata removed from uterine wall. Condition, otherwise, was found negative.

Result.—Convalescence interrupted by hysteria and nervousness. Period after operation was free, but painless.

CASE 31, No. 10,278.—Miss Z. G., white, aged 30, admitted to the Johns Hopkins Hospital, February 24, 1903. Menstruation has always been regular but profuse, accompanied with dysmenorrhea.

Examination.—Outlet marital. No signs of infection. Uterus small, movable, and in retroposition. Ovaries normal.

Present illness.—One year ago patient was curetted and menstruation afterwards was perfectly normal for three periods, but this was followed by a profuse flow which lasted seventeen days. Local and general treatment were tried without avail. Patient complains of general weakness and nervousness, and poor circulation.

Operation.—Hysterotomy and suspensio uteri. A median line incision was made through thick walls, and the uterus delivered, surrounded by gauze and split anteriorly. Considerable membrane was curetted away, and the wound in the uterus was closed by through and through catgut sutures. Suspension of uterus in usual manner.

Result.—Recovery.

CASE 32, No. 2379.—Mrs. M. W., white, aged 36, admitted to a neighboring hospital, February 8, 1904. Menstruation until October last was regular and normal in every respect.

Marital history.—Patient has been married two months.

Present illness.—About two months before marriage patient began flowing. This lasted six weeks, and at times was very free. She was kept in bed for two or three weeks, but the flow persisted. There was no pain of any description. One month later she was curetted, after which the flow ceased for two weeks, but began again, and has continued up to the present time. She has absolutely no other symptoms.

Examination.—Lower genitalia normal; the fundus in retroflexion and slightly enlarged, but no irregularities found. Tubes and ovaries normal.

Operation.—Hysterotomy and suspensio uteri. A median line incision was made in the abdomen, and the uterus delivered, surrounded by gauze and split on anterior face down to cavity. Numerous small polypi were found about the tubal openings. These were thoroughly curetted away and the wound in the uterus closed with interrupted catgut sutures, after which the fundus was suspended in the usual manner.

Result.—Convalescence was uninterrupted.

THE "HOME SANATORIUM" TREATMENT OF CONSUMPTION.[1]

By JOSEPH H. PRATT, A. M., M. D.,

Physician to Out-Patients, Massachusetts General Hospital,
Assistant in the Theory and Practice of Physic, Harvard University.

Some one has said, " There are two kinds of consumption— that of the rich and that of the poor. The former is sometimes cured, the latter never." This still indicates the feeling of most physicians. The attempt to cure tuberculosis in the

homes of the poor has seemed well nigh hopeless. Here and there, however, solitary workers like Dr. Flick, of Philadelphia, have obtained admirable results even in the slums of a great city.

As Dr. Osler said in his lecture before the Phipps Institute, " The problem of tuberculosis is in its most important aspect

[1] Read before the Johns Hopkins Hospital Medical Society, January 23, 1906.

a home problem. The vast majority of all tuberculous patients must be treated in their homes." [1]

The success of the sanatorium and climatic treatment of consumption is universally recognized. Yet the essential feature of the sanatorium treatment is careful regulation of the details of the daily life, and the essential feature of the climatic treatment is life in the open air.

In warm climates and in cold, at low altitudes and at high, consumption has been successfully treated wherever the out-of-door life has been adopted, and the modern method of treatment followed.

Since 1891 Dr. Bowditch has been demonstrating at the Sharon Sanatorium that consumption can be successfully treated in this supposedly unfavorable climate.

Dr. Millet, of East Bridgewater, was the first to advocate out-of-door sleeping in a harsh climate. In January, 1900, he published an important paper which bore the significant title, "The Night-Air of New England in the Treatment of Consumption." [2] It would be well if the truths contained in Dr. Millet's paper could be impressed upon every physician called upon to treat this disease.

Last winter I became acquainted with the methods used by Dr. C. L. Minor, of Asheville, N. C., in carrying out the hygienie-dietetic treatment among private patients outside of a sanatorium. The regulation of the daily life, the discipline enforced, and the results obtained by Dr. Minor compare favorably with those of the best sanatoria.

I became convinced that it was possible to carry out the same system in the homes of the poor even in a crowded city. For the opportunity to submit my plan to a practical test I am indebted to the Rev. Elwood Worcester, and to Emmanuel Church for financial support.

The reason that the results of home and dispensary treatment have been on the whole unsatisfactory is due to the lack of the careful supervision, and the lack of the strict discipline maintained in sanatoria. The tuberculosis dispensarles have been a potent factor in preventing the spread of the disease, and in educating the patients and the general public. But, I believe, relatively few cases treated by dispensary methods have been cured. This has certainly been the experience of my colleagues and myself in the out-patient department of the Massachusetts General Hospital, where the dispensary methods with the aid of the District Nursing Association have been employed for several years. The difference between our method and that of the tuberculosis dispensary is essentially this: that the tuberculosis dispensary

gives a relatively small amount of care to a large number of patients, while we give a large amount of care to a small number of patients.

Our organization is known as the Emmanuel Church Tuberculosis Class. We sometimes speak of it as a "home sanatorium," and it bears much the same relation to a sanatorium that a correspondence course does to a college course. Every detail of the daily life is supervised and strict discipline maintained. A nurse is employed who devotes her time to visiting the members of the class. I prefer the term " friendly visitor " to nurse, because it describes more exactly the nature of her duties. She should be the family's wise counselor, kindly and tactful, yet a good disciplinarian.

The class should number but a few members, I think the maximum limit should be twenty-five.

It should never be forgotten that it is the individual, not the disease, that needs treatment. We have been fortunate in having a small class, and so we have come to know our patients not simply as " this case of fibroid phthisis," and " that of pyopneumothorax," but as, " Elmer and Patrick."

The class was organized the first of July, 1905. Most of the applicants for membership were referred to us by the Out-Patient Department of the Massachusetts General Hospital. The rule was established that no one would be accepted until the clinical diagnosis was confirmed either by finding the tubercle bacilli or by a positive tuberculin test. There has been, however, no difficulty in demonstrating tubercle bacilli in the sputum of all our patients on admission to the class.

Our aid has been refused to none. Those who were too ill for home treatment have been visited by our nurse until admission could be secured to some hospital or until transferred to the District Nursing Association. We have placed consumptives in the Carney Hospital, the House of the Good Samaritan, and the Free Hospital for Consumptives.

Admission to the class has not been limited to favorable cases. In fact, only two of our patients were in the incipient stage of the disease.

All of our patients have been poor. None could afford even the $4.00 per week charged at the State Sanatorium. Not all the members are intelligent. Several are unusually stupid. In the family of Zelek P., a Russian Jew, no one can write English, and his wife cannot speak English.

Before admission to the class is granted the applicant must promise to give up all work, to live the out-of-door life, and to obey all the rules of the class. The truth of Brehmer's motto that " The most profitable work for a sick man is to get well," is impressed upon the patient. After the decision to join the class has been made a clinical history is taken and a complete physical examination made and entered on the clinical records. Once a month the lungs and sputum are re-examined. The patients are visited by the nurse as soon as they enter the class. Often before the decision has been made the nurse is sent to discuss the question with the invalid and his family, and to determine whether it will be possible to carry out the open-air treatment in their home. If there be

---

[1] Few if any states have greater facilities for sanatorium treatment than Massachusetts. It has been estimated that there are at the present time no less than 14,000 consumptives within its borders. For these 375 beds are available. In other words, about 3 per cent can be treated in the state sanatorium. As consumption is a disease of the poor, it is evident that most of the cases comprising the remaining 97 per cent must be treated in their homes, if they are to be treated at all.

[2] *Maryland Medical Journal*, January, 1900.

no roof, balcony, piazza, or yard available for the rest treatment in the open air, the family must move to a tenement that will enable the tuberculous invalid to spend the entire day and night out-of-doors. Our friendly visitors have spent much time in seeking satisfactory tenements for the members. At the first visit the nurse examines the house and locality, obtains the social history of the case, ascertains the exact financial condition, and gives what instruction may be necessary to prevent the spread of the disease. The first visit usually requires two hours or more. A detailed report of this is at once given to the physician in charge. Subsequent visits by the nurse are made as required. Usually the patient is visited daily or at short intervals, until the details of the treatment are understood and followed. It has been found that repeated visits are often necessary before some of the simplest rules are fixed in the minds of the invalid and his friends.

On January 5th, 1906, the class numbered fifteen members, and all but one were sleeping out-of-doors. The single exception is a patient who would have done so had his landlord not prevented him from putting up a tent on the roof. At present he sleeps with his head out of the window of his bed-room. One of our class sleeps on a balcony, the others in tents placed either on the roof or on the ground near the house. The tents have generally been loaned—as few of the members could afford to buy them. An ordinary 7' by 7' wall tent with a fly has been found satisfactory. This costs only $7.25. Except the time taken for meals, bath and exercise, the entire day is spent in the recumbent or semi-recumbent posture. A comfortable reclining chair is furnished each patient.

The prescribed diet consists chiefly of milk, bread, fruit, butter, and oil. Most of our patients drink two to three quarts of milk a day. In a few instances unsalted butter has been furnished free. Cotton-seed oil has been found to be a satisfactory and inexpensive substitute for olive oil.

For the first few weeks no exercise is allowed, and later only when the temperature is normal the entire day. Then the exact amount of exercise is prescribed. The patient begins by walking five minutes in the morning and five in the afternoon. It is required that a watch be carried and the exact duration of the walk noted in his record book. After exercising the temperature is taken and recorded. If rise of temperature occurs or if the patient becomes tired the amount of exercise is diminished. If the patient continues to improve, the exercise is gradually increased. Some of our patients now walk several hours daily. During the summer and fall our fever-free patients enjoyed the privileges of the Parker Hill Day Sanatorium.

An important aid in maintaining our strict hygienic regimen is furnished by the individual record book. The form of record adopted is that devised by Dr. Minor, of Asheville. Every detail of the day is recorded: The food eaten, including the total amount of milk and oil taken; the number of hours out-of-doors. The temperature and pulse-rate are entered and the quantity and character of the expectoration. The

patients now keep out-of-door life charts. This keeping of records serves to impress upon the members the importance of attention to detail in the treatment. It helps them to persevere in their monotonous life. We have found that it does not depress their spirits or cause introspection. It serves rather to keep up their courage. Most of the class take great pride in their records. Of course if a patient were doing badly, and losing weight rapidly, the individual record would be omitted.

A weekly meeting of the class has been held on Friday afternoons, formerly in my consulting room, now at the Massachusetts General Hospital. The record books are then inspected, and the patient's weight, temperature, pulse, and vital capacity are taken.

Expenses.—Emmanuel Church has paid for a special nurse, furnished tents, reclining chairs, and all other necessary supplies. To a few of the members a small amount of money has been loaned, and aid has been offered when it was necessary for a family to move to another tenement. A nominal fee of $2.00 a month is required from each patient. In some instances this has been remitted. The total expenses for the first six months ending January 1, 1906, were $513.00.

Miss Isabel Strong, acting as friendly visitor, gave her entire time to the work without pay during July and August. Dr. J. B. Hawes has assisted me in the medical work since the organization of the class. Recently Dr. C. S. Millet and Dr. N. K. Wood have associated themselves with us, and Dr. C. L. Tobey has taken charge of the laryngological work.

Old tuberculin has been used in a number of cases with apparent benefit. Pharmacotherapy has not been employed except for special conditions, such as constipation or diarrhœa. A few patients have been given creosote. Hydrotherapy has been found of value in every case. *Theilwaschungen,* full baths, chest compresses were the procedures selected.

Results.—Of the nine patients who have been members of the class for three months or more all show a gain in weight and all but two improvement in their general condition. One patient's weight has increased 40¼ pounds. In five of the nine cases the disease has been arrested. The term "arrested" is used in the sense in which it is employed by the Committee on Nomenclature of the National Association for Study and Prevention of Tuberculosis in their proposed classification.

WEIGHT-TABLE OF ALL WHO HAVE BEEN MEMBERS OF THE CLASS FOR THREE MONTHS OR MORE.

Name	Date of Admission	Weight	Last Examination	Weight	Gain	No. of Weeks
1. Minnie E.. .July 3		102¾	Jan. 12	114¼	11½	27
2. Elmer C....July 12		106	Jan. 5	130½	24½	25
3. Zelek P......July 12		131½	Jan. 12	171	39½	26
4. John H......July 18		131	Jan. 12	153¼	22¼	25
5. Samuel T....July 27		142	Jan. 5	165¼	23¼	24
6. Maria F... July 29		117	Jan. 12	138½	21½	25
7. Samuel H...Aug. 7		125½	Jan. 12	132½	7	22
8. William F...Sept. 2		145	Jan. 12	166¼	21¼	19
9. Patrick C....Sept. 15		120⅛	Jan. 12	124	3⅞	17

Average gain, 19.4 pounds.

Abstracts of the Clinical Records of all who have been members of the Class three months or over.

CASE No. 1.—Minnie E., aged 28, housekeeper. Ill since May, 1904. Cough; night sweats; loss of weight and strength; loss of appetite; frequent vomiting. Went to the Massachusetts General Hospital in January, 1905. Weight then 106½ lbs. Tubercle bacilli present in sputum. Joined the class July 3, 1905. Temperature at time of first examination 99.8°, pulse 100, respirations 26, weight 102¾. There was dullness at the right apex, bronchovesicular breathing, and many fine moist rales. At the right base crackles were heard. In the left interscapular region slight dullness, bronchial breathing, and rales at the end of expiration. January 12, 1906. Weight 114¼ lbs., temperature 98.6°, pulse 84. She now feels strong, and complains only of occasional nausea and vomiting. Practically no cough and no expectoration. No fever for four months. At the last examination of chest January 9, only a few rales were heard, and these were sticky in character. They were present at both apices." On December 22 sputum contained tubercle bacilli—Gaffky scale, No. 2.

CASE No. 2.—Elmer C., aged 56, painter. Came to Dr. Pratt's Clinic at the Massachusetts General Hospital in July, 1905, complaining of loss of appetite and pains in the chest. He has had a dry cough for five years, and expectorated some blood one year ago. For the week previous to visiting the hospital he had been troubled with night sweats. There had been some loss of weight and strength.

Status præsens: Thin man; bony framework prominent; weight 106 lbs. Temperature 99.6°, respirations 18, pulse 92. Mucous membranes somewhat pale. Chest rather long and narrow. Dullness over the left upper lobe in front, and flatness behind. Over both sides of chest above spine of scapula breathing is bronchovesicular with prolonged expiration. Kroenig's isthmus is 2 cm. wide at the left apex and 3 cm. at right apex. Vital capacity is 2225 cc. Many medium-sized moist rales over both upper lobes during both inspiration and expiration. More numerous on left side. No rales, over middle or lower right lobes. Over lower half of left scapula, especially near angle of scapula are a few crackles. Sclerosed radial arteries; tortuous brachials. Urine is free from albumin and sugar. Suggestion of diazo reaction. Sputum is mucopurulent. Tubercle bacilli present. Gaffky scale, No. 3. Fluoroscope shows a shadow over the entire left lung, darkest at the apex. Right lung is clear.

He regained strength rapidly, and the cough entirely disappeared. Tubercle bacilli have not been found in the sputum for three months. January 5, 1906. Patient looks healthy, skin ruddy, and mucous membranes are of good color. Weight 130½ lbs., temperature 98°, pulse 78, vital capacity 2500 cc. He feels better than he has for years, and weighs more than ever before. He walks four to five hours a day. Last physical examination December 14, 1905. Moderate dullness at left apex. No impairment of resonance over the right lung. At left apex expiration is prolonged but not distinctly bronchovesicular. After coughing a few subcrepitant rales were audible above the left clavicle, none were heard elsewhere.

CASE No. 3.—Zelek P., age 35, tailor, came to Dr. Pratt's Clinic at the Massachusetts General Hospital in July, 1905, complaining of cough and pain in the right chest. For several months he had been troubled with a cough and increasing weakness. He had lost a few pounds in weight since January. On examination he was found to have a temperature of 101.4°, respirations were 30 to the minute, and the pulse 80. There was dullness over the right side of the chest, front and back, shading into flatness at the apex. Breath sounds were bronchovesicular over the right

upper lobe, where a few fine rales were heard. The rales were increased by coughing. Sputum contained many tubercle bacilli—Gaffky scale, No. 7.

He gained steadily during the summer and fall. He slept and lived on his roof in the crowded West End of Boston. For ten weeks he was allowed no exercise. His temperature became normal in September, and has remained so. On January 12, 1906, he weighed 171 pounds, temperature was 98.2° and pulse 84. He has been free from all subjective symptoms for several months, but in the scanty expectoration tubercle bacilli are still demonstrable. Examination December 30 showed dullness, bronchial breathing, and intense bronchophony. A few rales were heard here; none elsewhere. Tubercle bacilli were absent from the sputum during the fall. After a severe tuberculin reaction in December they were again demonstrable. On January 12 very few were present. Gaffky scale, No. 1.

CASE No. 4.—John H., age 22, brass finisher, came to the Clinic in July, 1905. He had had a cough with considerable expectoration for three months; at times sputum had been streaked with blood. He had not lost weight; his appetite was good, and aside from the cough felt perfectly well. There were slight signs at the right apex, and the fluoroscope showed a shadow extending down as far as the third rib on the right side. There was a reaction to tuberculin, and then for the first time Dr. Hawes found tubercle bacilli in the sputum. Examination January 2, 1906, revealed slight dullness and bronchovesicular breathing at the right apex. No rales were heard. He looked strong and healthy, and had had no cough for two months or more, and tubercle bacilli had not been found in his sputum since September. On January 5 he weighed 153 pounds, a gain of 22 pounds, since joining the class. His temperature was 97.4°, and his pulse 104.

CASE No. 5.—Samuel T., aged 37, motorman. Cough of six months' duration. One attack of hæmoptysis. A few night sweats. Lost 70 pounds in weight during the past two years. Definite signs of phthisis were found at the right apex, and the sputum was loaded with tubercle bacilli. At the time of examination July 27, 1905, his weight was 142 lbs., temperature 98.2°, and pulse 116. Improvement followed treatment. He remained in the class six weeks and gained 14½ lbs. He then returned to his old home in New Hampshire, where he remained a month. While there he over-exerted himself, and the tuberculous process was lighted up. He rejoined the class on October 27. He was then having afternoon fever, and had lost ten pounds of weight in three weeks. He continued to have fever for six weeks. On January 5 his temperature was 98.8°, pulse 93, weight 165¾ lbs. He was then feeling much better. On December 26, the last physical examination was made. Kroenig's isthmus was found narrowed at each apex. The excursion of the diaphragm was greatly limited on the right side. Bronchovesicular breathing over right upper lobe. Numerous fine moist rales above the right clavicle and over entire right back. Rales also present in middle of left interscapular space.

CASE 6.—Maria F., aged 40, housework. She came to Dr. Lord's Clinic in July, 1905, complaining of a cough of one year's duration. For several months she had been short of breath on exertion. She had lost much weight. Over the left apex as far as the third rib in front and the spine of the scapula behind there was dullness, increased vocal and tactile fremitus, and fine moist rales. Weight 117, temperature 99.6°, pulse 104. Tubercle bacilli were found in the sputum. January 12, 1906. Temperature 104°, weight 138½ lbs. Cough and expectoration, although lessened, still persists. She raises about 10 cc. of sputum daily. Her general condition is much improved. Last chest examination December 26. Dullness at left apex and bronchial breathing. Scattered rales heard over entire left upper lobe.

CASE No. 7.—Samuel H., aged 27, rubber-worker. He visited Dr. Cabot's Clinic at the Massachusetts General Hospital in August, 1905. In July, 1904, he raised some blood at night; this was soon followed by a cough and increasing weakness. Many night sweats. Slight loss of weight. At the right apex there was slight dullness, bronchovesicular breathing, increased tactile and vocal fremitus, and fine moist rales. He has done badly. The constitutional symptoms have increased, and there have been repeated febrile periods.

The exertion of coming to the class always produced some rise of temperature. The physical signs remain practically the same except rales are now present at the right base as well as the right apex. On January 12, 1906, weight was 132½ lbs., temperature 100.4°, pulse 128. Many tubercle bacilli in sputum—Gaffky scale, No. 7. An effort will be made to place him in a hospital for consumptives.

CASE No. 8.—William F., aged 28, referred to the Emmanuel Church Tuberculosis Class by Dr. Cabot in September. Pleurisy January, 1905. Slight hæmoptysis also in January, but none since. In July, 1905, cough began. Occasional night sweats, some pain in the chest. He had lost about twenty pounds in weight, and felt weak and sick. Weight 145 lbs., temperature 101.5°, pulse 104. There were signs at the right apex, and tubercle bacilli

were found in the sputum. He has improved steadily under treatment. On January 2, 1906, slight dullness was found at the right apex; no definite rales heard. January 12, weight 166¼ lbs., temperature 98°, pulse 104. Slight cough, persists; general condition good. Sputum examined on December 22, contained numerous tubercle bacilli.

CASE 9.—Patrick C., aged 33, machinist, came to Dr. Cabot's Clinic at the Massachusetts General Hospital in August, complaining of shortness of breath. He had had a persistent cough since last winter. While in New York this spring he was suddenly seized with great shortness of breath, high fever, and prostration. He has been sick ever since. Patient was emaciated. On examination there was found to be a pyopneumothorax of the left side, and signs of phthisis at the right apex. Weight was 117, temperature 100.5°, pulse 84. An incision was made in the left side, and considerable pus, containing tubercle bacilli removed. In September he was referred to the Emmanuel Church Tuberculosis Class. On October 13, 450 cc. greenish pus were removed, which greatly relieved the dyspnœa. Temperature 100°, pulse 108. On October 27, 1080 cc. of fluid were aspirated, and again on December 19, 500 cc. were removed. He has continued to have slight fever. The physical signs have remained nearly stationary, but he has been weak, and had very little appetite. January 12. His lips looked bloodless. Left side of chest remains distended and flat. Weigh 124 lbs., temperature 98.6°, pulse 92, vital capacity 1100 cc.

TUBERCULOSIS IN PENAL INSTITUTIONS.[1]

By J. B. RANSOM, M. D., *Dannemora, New York.*

MR. PRESIDENT, LADIES, AND GENTLEMEN.—It is with more than ordinary pleasure, and, I may say, confidence, that I speak to you this evening upon a subject which concerns the general public, and both the State and Municipal Governments; speaking, as I am, in this marvellously virile city of Baltimore, surrounded by an atmosphere surcharged with encouragement to things altruistic and progressive, especially so, in that I am speaking to a Maryland audience, to whom history and tradition have alike assigned the first place in works affecting the public good.

Maryland was among the first to develop a thrifty colonial life; among the first to take up the sword in defence of the divine right of individual liberty; first to develop a practical scheme of internal improvements; and we have but to mention the name of Johns Hopkins to place her first in affording an opportunity for the higher education, and the broadest medical culture of our time. And coming a little closer to my subject of the evening, I know of no more striking illustration of her public spirit, her appreciation of what the needs of humanity are, than is shown in her recently-built penitentiary which represents in its construction the most modern and humane ideas of what a prison should be, and one of which any state should be proud.

[1] An address delivered before the Laennec Society for the Study of Tuberculosis, Baltimore, Md., January 25, 1906.

It is, therefore, with a ready optimism that I approach the subject of my remarks this evening, though they are upon a subject which by reiteration has perhaps become wearisome; yet, this subject of tuberculosis is so important, is so knit with the weal and woe of the human race, that we cannot allow it to slumber, we cannot afford to treat it with indifference.

Tuberculosis is undoubtedly the most widely diffused and common of all diseases. In fact, we may say that to be human is to be tuberculous. It is impossible to say just what per cent of the human family has been infected by tuberculosis in some degree. If we are to give credence to the arguments of more recent investigators, the percentage is very high. In fact, their conclusions would go to show that it would be easier to state the proposition in this way: What is the per cent of humanity that escape tuberculosis?

The question as to how this excessive diffusion has come about is one that reaches far back into the early life-history of the race, and in some degree, is impossible of solution. There are, however, certain well-established elements that have operated to bring about so general an infection; indeed, enough is known to lay the cause largely at the door of man himself.

Man was born out in the open—out under the stars,—and was predestined to the free use of his muscles and lungs in earning his daily bread. But what a contrast between the natural state of man and that which for centuries has been the life of man, especially in our great centers of population! We have shut out from our streets, our homes, our places of business, our manufactories, more especially from our institutions; in fact from our very lives, not only God's pure and life-giving sunlight, but much of his fresh air. This deprivation of a natural element, and an enervated nervous system consequent upon too strenuous a life, have brought about a general constitutional susceptibility. Figuratively speaking, the human family may be said to represent a vast culture medium ready to receive the initial stab of the bacillus.

Tuberculosis, therefore, is a disease of the life complicated—primarily not of the upper stratum, but essentially one of the sub-stratum of society. Its growth and development are not from above downwards, but from below upwards. It finds its richest sustenance in the lower walks of life; in crowded tenements; in the damp, dark, and narrow streets of large cities; in the unsanitary habitations of the poor; in the darkened rooms and damp corridors of our eleemosynary institutions, and within the gray walls and narrow cell-limits of our penal institutions.

While no age, class, or race, is exempt from this disease, we believe it would be short-lived indeed if these conditions of ill-living were eliminated. And to eliminate such features of unsanitary life is the burden of the hour. That it means work, well-directed and intelligent work, there can be no doubt; for many of the causes that lead to these life conditions are deeply rooted in the habits of the people, and have for their sustenance local and general conditions which involve the whole machinery of government—national, state and municipal. To dislodge so formidable and so long-established an enemy cannot be done by simply getting together and talking about it. It is a work that requires the most perfect type of organization. It must be extended to every department of human activity, industry, and life.

In reviewing the progress already made in this direction it may be said that a great deal has been accomplished. Much of the pioneer work has already been done. Many trails have been blazed through the undergrowth of superstition, ignorance, and misconception. One could not attend the Tuberculosis Exhibit so recently held in New York City without having his eyes opened to the vast amount of work that has been done. Progress was everywhere manifest, and nearly every department of human activity had been reached by the workers in this field. Especially was this true of the tenement house districts of our large cities. The work accomplished in attacking the disease in these strongholds was highly gratifying. There was one field, however, which apparently had been little worked, viz., the institutional, and more particularly, institutions of a penal nature; so far as I know, only one penal institution being represented in the exhibit, and that, Clinton Prison.

Turning to the directory of the Charity Organization of the City of New York, I find only eight penal institutions mentioned as taking any precautions against this disease, or giving any special attention to its management, and only two

of them could be said to have any comprehensive scheme for the proper care of this class of patients.

In my work of gathering statistics from all the penal institutions of the United States for the purpose of making a report to the Fifty-eighth Congress, for transmission to the Eighth International Prison Congress, on tuberculosis in penal institutions, I found very little evidence of systematic work in the way of special care of the tuberculous prisoner. There was evidence of a general awakening to the necessity, but only in three or four instances, had much been accomplished. Since that time, however, several states have taken up the task in earnest. In Illinois, special wards, and a roof-garden for open-air treatment, have been constructed in connection with one of its penal institutions. Fort Leavenworth has also erected a tuberculosis annex, and the state of Massachusetts has appropriated $25,000 for the purpose of building an institution for the care of tuberculous prisoners.

The populations of penal institutions of whatsoever nature, whether jails, workhouses, juvenile asylums, reformatories, penitentiaries or prisons, are especially vulnerable to infection by this disease. It is a well-established fact that prison environment and life are especially favorable to its development. The mortality from this disease has been variously estimated at from 40 to 60 per cent of all deaths in the prisons of the world. There are many isolated cases, however, where the mortality has reached a much higher per cent, even as high as 80 per cent. It is patent, therefore, that in these institutions there lies a wide field for effort, and one that not only demands attention, but must appeal to every one interested in this work.

I have been asked to speak this evening upon institutional tuberculosis as especially related to penal institutions, with which my work has largely been identified. I shall be pardoned, therefore, if I dwell almost exclusively upon the history of the work in the institution with which I am, and have been, connected for the past twenty years; namely, Clinton Prison, New York.

The work which is now in progress in that institution had its initiative in the then terrible mortality from tuberculosis in the prisons of the state of New York. When I began my medical service at Clinton Prison in 1889, I found on inspection of the hospital that it was filled to its utmost capacity with sick men, the majority of them ill from tuberculosis. These men were all in a common ward, mixed indiscriminately with those suffering from other diseases. The care given them would now be considered very inferior, and of a kind that was at that time given to those without hope. A rather superficial examination of the population showed 126 to be suffering from tuberculosis in a total population of 867. Coupled with the prevalence of this disease was an almost entire lack of any means of caring for these cases, either in isolation, bathing, working, or feeding. There was absolutely no distinction made between the tuberculous prisoner and any other. They worked, ate, and were locked together, and, when under hospital treatment, were mixed heterogeneously. A survey of the whole field revealed the fact that the only saving element in the past, which had acted as a preventive to an almost utter annihilation of the population, was the large amount of out-door labor which was then afforded. When a change came from out-door to shop work, a rapid increase in the number of tuberculous cases was apparent.

In my annual report of 1890, I reported 75 per cent of the deaths of that year to be due to tuberculosis. I earnestly called the attention of the Prison Department to the necessity for isolation, and the special treatment of this class of cases. This, however, had little or no effect, and no apparent effort was made to improve conditions.

At this time the disease was little understood. The idea of isolation was new, and met with determined opposition on the part of many. It was even difficult to obtain the ear of the medical profession, to say nothing of those most closely identified with prison management. The disease spread and showed increased virulence. These conditions were even worse in the other prisons of the state. In one prison alone, 44 deaths were reported as due to tuberculosis in one year; and during the period of five years from 1891 to 1895, inclusive, there were reported 253 deaths from tuberculosis in the three prisons, viz., Sing Sing 86, Auburn 133, Clinton 34.

At this time began the more or less irregular transfer of the more advanced cases to Clinton Prison. There was, however, no special provision made for them, and no systematic endeavor to place these transfers upon a rational basis. Continued agitation, and the excellent results which were obtained in the cases transferred, led to an awakening to the necessity for better sanitary conditions in the prisons. A change to the present system of manufacture, together with improved methods of administration in all the prisons of the state, especially in their medical departments, a more systematic transfer system, and a special line of treatment adopted, resulted in a great reduction of the death rate from tuberculosis. The five years from 1896 to 1901, inclusive, showed a total death rate of but 72 in the three prisons as against 253 in the previous period of five years—a gain of 71 per cent.

These results were encouraging. In 1901, at the earnest solicitation of the superintendent of prisons, Hon. C. V. Collins, the legislature appropriated the sum of $2500 for the purpose of constructing a ward for the treatment of tuberculous prisoners. This ward, though simple in construction, observed the chief sanitary requirements for the use to which it was to be put, and was well equipped for the care of this class of patients. This made it possible to provide suitable accommodations for the advanced cases and those positively requiring ward treatment. We already had a ward devoted to the treatment of the more advanced cases, which accommodated eleven patients. This gave us a total capacity of fifty-four. Prior to, and up to, this time, the only treatment that could be given to any but the most advanced cases, was in cells.

The ward went into operation on July 8, 1902, and proved to be of great advantage to the work, clearly demonstrating the practicability of the treatment of all classes of prisoners without reference to the nature of their crime or the lengths of their sentence, without violence to prison discipline. It was at first feared that the turning loose of so many men of this character in one open ward might lead to insurrection and breaks for liberty; but such has not been the case, and I believe that the number of serious infractions of the prison rules has averaged less than with the same number of men of the same class locked in regular cells.

Since 1902, additional construction has increased our capacity until at the present time the Tuberculosis Annex consists of three extensions to the main hospital, radiating from a central court, and occupying a floor space of 20,000 feet. The south extension, 75 x 55 feet, is devoted to the treatment of the far-advanced cases, and accommodates over forty patients. The eastern extension, 20 x 55 feet, forms the special diet kitchen and laboratory, while the northeastern extension, 70 x 150 feet, is devoted to the treatment of cases in the early and somewhat advanced stage and accommodates over 100 patients. The main ward is constructed with a high vaulted roof ceiling extended upward by a clear-story to a distance of thirty-five feet, thus affording a large air and light space. The building is windowed on all sides as closely as safe architecture permits, the clear-story being entirely set with windows opening and closing by a mechanical device. In connection with this ward are modern lavatories, toilet facilities for spray and tub baths, rooms devoted to the treatment of patients by the incandescent and arc lights, and a disinfecting room. It has a hard-wood floor, waxed and polished, and is heated by steam and lighted by electricity. Adjoining this ward is a dining-room that will seat 120 persons, the food for whom is supplied from the special diet kitchen. The ward is cheerful, light, and airy, and admirably meets the purpose for which it was designed. Each patient in this ward has a white enamel iron bed, furnished with woven wire springs, fiber mattress, feather pillow, sheets, woolen blankets and a counterpane. At the head of each bed is a white enameled steel bedside table with glass top and steel shelf, while at the foot is a comfortable arm-chair. The patients are also supplied with a porcelain-lined drinking-cup, and a different form of sputum-cup. The ward devoted to the treatment of the far-advanced cases is similar in most particulars.

The diet kitchen, an important factor in this work, is equipped with a 9-foot French steel range, a large porcelain-lined refrigerator, and all the necessary appurtenances for preparing food according to modern methods. During the twelve months ending September 30, 1905, there were served from this kitchen 108,301 meals.

The greater number by far of the men treated in this institution are received by transfer from the other prisons and reformatories. The method of procedure in transferring is as follows:

When the physician of any of these institutions finds by examination that an inmate is suffering from tuberculosis, he places him under special observation and isolates him from the rest of the population until such time as the number of cases warrants an application for their transfer. He then applies to the superintendent of prisons for a transfer order, and the physician to the tuberculosis hospital visits the institution and determines by examination the cases likely to be benefited by the special treatment afforded at Clinton.

Upon transfer to Clinton, the convict thus admitted is bathed and given a careful physical examination, and if it is determined that he is suffering from tuberculosis, he is given a special examination, and his sputum is subjected to a searching study. His case is then recorded on a filing-card which details his previous environment, family history, source of infection, duration of disease, and all questions pertaining to his disease that could be of value, together with a chart of the chest with the diseased areas indicated in colors. If he is found to be in an active stage of the disease, or in a weak or exhausted condition, he is at once admitted to the hospital. He is then assigned a bed and hospital clothing, and a careful daily record of his condition is kept thereafter. He is also instructed as to the hospital regulations governing his personal habits; the care of his sputa, his teeth, his hair, and his clothing. He is required to deport himself in an orderly manner, and is permitted as much liberty as is consistent with hospital discipline.

The treatment of the patient is physical, medicinal, and dietetic. The physical treatment usually consists of simple calisthenics and out-door exercise. The exercise ground is provided with seats, elevated cuspidors containing antiseptic solutions, a toilet room, a crematory for sputa, and running spring-water. The patient is required either to sit or exercise out-doors each day whenever the weather permits.

The medicinal treatment, while subordinated to the physical and dietetic, is nevertheless considered a feature, and most patients do better with some medicinal treatment than without it. In addition to the usual medical treatment, we use the ultra-violet X-ray, the incandescent light treatment, and the sub-cutaneous injection of olive-oil.

The diet of these patients is prescribed daily by the physician, and is furnished from the diet kitchen on his order. It is aimed to make this diet as nutritious as is consistent. It includes principally cereals, fruits, milk, eggs, meats, and fish.

It is not, however, to the mere treatment alone that improvement is due, but to the general training of the patient, and his opportunity to be out in the open air in a favorable climate. It is, however, impossible under prison conditions to give the tuberculous patient the amount of open air that his case requires, and herein lies a great drawback to the work. Notwithstanding this, it is gratifying and sometimes astonishing to see how these men improve under this treatment. They come to us emaciated, anæmic, exhausted, and apparently to live but a short time. A few weeks' treatment makes a manifest improvement in them. If they have an elevation of temperature, it gradually subsides; they soon begin to take on color and weight, many of them gaining a large number of pounds.

The total number of recorded cases transferred to Clinton for treatment up to January 12, 1906, is 1137. During the period between October 1, 1902, and January 12, 1906, the total number of cases treated in the hospital was 596. Of this number, 313 were discharged from the prison, leaving 279 now in the hospital. Of the number remaining, 188 are under treatment and 91 are assigned to labor of different kinds best suited to their individual cases. In a majority of these 91 cases the disease is apparently cured.

No results are given of men discharged from hospital to cells, but only of those discharged from the prison, thus affording a most excellent opportunity of judging of ultimate results: a man often serving several years after his case has been arrested or cured at such labor as his physical condition will permit. Of the 313 cases discharged from the prison during this period, the results were as follows:

    Apparently cured 16.93%
    Disease arrested 40.26%
    Improved 38.98%
    Negative 3.83%

The mortality in the tuberculous population during the same period was 2.16 per cent. Simply to show what it is possible to accomplish in connection with a prison in this work, a comparison with Clinton of seven other representative institutions admitting the patients of the same class, i. e., in all stages of the disease, shows an average death rate of 18.46 per cent; the lowest mortality being 5.20 per cent, and the highest 29.68 per cent; while Clinton's, as before stated, was 2.16 per cent.

These results have not been accomplished by the usual routine work of the prison. It has been a long and hard struggle on the part of the prison department against great odds. With no precedent to guide them; with prejudices to overcome, and with small means at their disposal, this problem has been gradually solved.

The total appropriations made by the Legislature for the building and equipment of the plant now in use are about $50,000. Thus far, no special appropriation has been made for the maintenance of this work, the expense being paid from the maintenance fund of the prison proper. It is, however, expected that a special appropriation will be soon made for the separate maintenance of this department. We estimate that the cost per capita per annum will reach beween $175 and $200, which is much below the cost of outside institutions of this nature.

The work in the State of New York has progressed to a point where highly satisfactory results are being obtained. These results are being shown in the decreased death rate from tuberculosis in the several prisons of the State to a minimum as compared with former times; in improving the personnel of the men in habits and physique, and permitting of their discharge in a condition making it possible for those to earn a livelihood who otherwise would have either died in prison, or have gone out in ill-health, fit only to become paupers or dependents, and carriers of infection.

Though the work has been thus placed upon a substantial footing, it is still in its infancy. It is hoped to extend it and increase its capacity to a point which will admit the transfer of all cases of tuberculosis from all the penal institutions of the State, including the jails; for it is during the jail life of the prisoner that much of infection takes place. I know of but one State that has made provision for the tuberculous prisoner in this respect, and that is the State of Texas. In 1895 the Wynne Farm at Huntsville, Texas, was established, to which are sent all tuberculous subjects from all the penal institutions, including the jails, of the State. The results in the third year of its establishment showed a decrease in the number of consumptive prisoners of one-half, and the results to the general prison population were highly beneficial.

I believe that in every State there should be a special institution or farm for the care of tuberculous prisoners. This work should include all the juvenile institutions; for it is often among the juveniles that infection takes place. In connection with this, I believe that there should be a mandatory examination by a competent physician, and the recording of all cases of tuberculosis in all penal and reformatory institutions. As before intimated, it is in the sub-stratum of society that this disease finds its richest pabulum; and if we are to eradicate it we must include in our field of work all institutions, especially penal institutions. For not only are the populations of these institutions especially subject to this disease, but they are so largely made up of the indirect results of it themselves. Much of pauperism, dependency, insanity, and crime, can be traced to tuberculosis as a first cause; not only by its interference with the physiologic functions and the lowering of the vital resistance, but also to its incapacitating effect upon the individual; unfitting him for the arduous toil and the sweat and heat of the life struggle. These mental and physical weaklings are easy preys to criminal influences and thus our penal institutions are especially the homes of the tuberculous refugee.

At first thought it may appear of small importance to the general public as to what is being done in penal institutions so long as the prisoner is kept safely until the expiration of his sentence, not absolutely injured, or subjected to cruel or unusual punishment. A little reflection and investigation of the subject, however, will quickly convince one that a prison population is essentially as much a part of the community as any other class. In the first place, putting a man behind prison bars, and dressing him in stripes does not relegate him to another species. He is still a man, and, like other men, subject to the laws of life, health, and emotion. As Joaquin Miller puts it:

> " In men whom men pronounce as ill,
>   We find so much of goodness still;
> In men whom men pronounce divine,
>   We find so much of sin and blot;
> We hesitate to draw the line
>   Between the two, when God has not."

Neither does this temporary incarceration entirely divorce him from the ties of family, home, and friendships; nor does it always deprive him of social and political influence. He must, therefore, be reckoned with as a social factor, and society is morally, as well as legally, bound to protect him in all that appertains to his bodily and mental vigor. But this is not the only or chief reason why society and the immediate community are, or should be, interested in the conduct of penal institutions and the welfare of their populations.

Penal populations are always tidal populations, with an outgoing as well as an incoming tide. In the State of New York alone, 12,000 prisoners are annually discharged upon the public from all classes of penal and reformatory institutions; and between these tidal populations and the populations inhabiting the crowded areas of our large cities, there is a constant intercourse, and thus is afforded an opportunity for infection and reinfection. It, therefore, means much more to the community as to what a man is when he comes out of prison than when he goes in; for he then becomes a local factor in the social problem and what he is as a man, his individuality, his personality, and both his moral and physical condition are important; he then becomes a menace, a real danger to the community to which he is discharged, or has within him the possibilities of becoming a useful citizen.

So complex is the problem of the moral reform of the incarcerated criminal, that there may be more or less doubt as to just how far our present prison methods go toward making good citizens of those convicted; but when we come to the bodily health, we have a feature which is as clearly and positively within correctional lines as is the health of any other body of citizens. Disease is no respecter of persons. A prisoner can, with few exceptions, be discharged with a degree of health which will at least prevent his becoming a menace and a burden to the community in which he is to reside, and place him in a much more favorable attitude, both as to his moral probabilities and his working capacities. This is especially true of the consumptive.

Should there be doubt on the part of any as to the propriety of the States thus protecting the incarcerated criminal in such measure as is here proposed, let it be remembered that the exercise of this function by the State is not sentimental or paternal, but is its legitimate prerogative, which is inherent in all constitutional governments, and appeals both to the reason and common sense. The exercise of the State's authority in convicting a man of crime does not imply the cutting off of his opportunity for future usefulness; for if this were the object and the function of the law, there could be no sentence short of life or of the death penalty.

When a man is given a sentence of ten years, the inference is that not only will society be rid of his presence for that length of time, but that he will be returned to society more or less cured of his moral infirmity, and better fitted to assume the life of a useful citizen. In view of this, if for no other reason, the State is bound by every principle of self-interest, to say nothing of fairness, justice, and right, to clearly define the relations which exist between itself and its institutional population as that of guardian and ward, and the claims of such a population upon the State's interest and protection from incapacity engendered by disease take precedence over its interest in this regard in outside communities, which are so largely protected by town and municipal regulations. That the State should not withhold its powerful aid to the general community in a manner calculated to make for a healthier people is patent; but neither should it deny such assistance to those who are its legal wards. This is, indeed, not only its rightful legal function, but it is its privilege to thus lend itself to the betterment of its institutional populations, no only for their own safety, but for that of the community at large.

The means which I believe most likely to secure the best possible results may be briefly summarized as follows:

(1) Improved construction, housing, and working environment.
(2) The recognition of the prisoner's receptivity to infection.
(3) The absolute separation from the prison population proper of all tuberculous subjects.
(4) Special wards for the treatment of all active cases.
(5) A compulsory law enforcing the examination of every criminal admitted to every penal institution for the purpose of an early detection of the disease.
(6) The construction in every State of a special hospital or sanitarium, and the transfer thereto of all tuberculous cases from all the penal institutions.
(7) Provisions for out-door employment, such as farming, light gardening, etc.

It is coming to be recognized by nearly all those engaged in prison work that not only are these things necessary to the prevention and cure of a special disease, but they are essential to a sound and satisfactory penal administration; for it cannot be said that the presence in an institution of a population afflicted in any degree with a communicable disease, which impairs the usefulness of so many inmates, is compatible with a prosperous and economic administration.

Applying the same principle to the work in general, it may be said that the exercise of the legislative function by the State in providing for the recognition and treatment of tuberculosis in any department of society, be it town, municipality, or eleemosynary institution, is of a high order of statesmanship, and appeals to the intelligence as well as to the conscience; it is practical, self-preservative, and self-compensating.

It is manifestly time that every function of government, every organized body of citizens, of whatsoever nature, as well as individuals, do their part in this work for the eradication of tuberculosis; and we appeal to every executive officer, to every legislator, and to every individual to do his part, and in some way help on this great work. We want your help; we must have your help if we are to succeed. We have been unconsciously too tolerant of this disease. We have housed it, condoned it, and belittled it. It is very difficult for human nature to believe what it cannot see, and much of this toleration and submission to the disease has arisen from a lack of appreciation of its nature and effects. To no other reason can we ascribe the fact that this great harvest of death that has gone on, and is still going on with but lessened destructiveness has not aroused the people to a keener appreciation of the true situation.

With what horror the people look upon the carnage and fatalities of war! And yet, tuberculosis destroys more lives by far in a single year in this country alone than were slain altogether in our late civil war! The people are in consternation at the presence in their midst of an epidemic disease; they are aghast at the long roll of deaths from railroad, steamship, and other disasters; when the fatalities from all these compared with those of consumption are insignificant.

Strangely enough, the same people, so fully alive to the every-day accidents of life, will resignedly see neighbors, friends, and loved ones succumb to tuberculosis and hardly ask the question: Why? And death is only a single feature; for there remain the deformities, insanity, incapacity, pauperism, and crime, for which this disease is directly and indirectly responsible. At what a cost to humanity in health, in life, and in achievement, has this inertia of resignation been purchased! At what a cost in heart history! What a burden of grief, disappointment and discouragement has come to the human family through and of it! This disease that is always with us. What a grave-yard to human hopes! If they could be brought within the scope of our vision, what a multitude of whitened shafts would rear heavenward in solemn protest; marking the sepulchres of not merely the humble, useful citizen, but also of the great man, the poet, the musician, the artist, and an unnumbered host of the character beautiful, of whom may it well be said in the words of Gray:

"Perhaps in this neglected spot is laid,
   Some heart once pregnant with celestial fire:
Hands that the rod of empire might have swayed,
   Or waked to ecstasy the living lyre."

But this host of unnumbered dead has not altogether perished in vain. There is an awakening and an army of workers is following the lead of the men who have breasted the storm of early opposition, and who, through long weary years of unremunerative toil, have sustained the conflict; solved many of its problems, and established the work upon a firm and progressive basis. On every hand and in every department of life, the importance, yea, the absolute necessity, of this work is fast coming to be recognized. This work is not the mere frothing or effervescence of a handful of enthusiastic theorists; it is the grand work of rejuvenating humanity; of returning man to his pristine condition of physiologic integrity. To take an indifferent view or an inactive course in this God-like work is to be in the rear of progress; and let him who casts a straw or even a molecule of obstruction against it, in whatsoever way, know that he might as well attempt to side-track the destiny of the race. To do this would be as futile as was the effort to strangle the principle of individual liberty in 1775, or as would now be the attempt to check the wave of patriotic feeling enkindled in every American heart by the inspiring strains of the " Star Spangled Banner," which so fitly found its inspiration and voice off the sunlit shores of Maryland.

PROCEEDINGS OF SOCIETIES.

JOHNS HOPKINS MEDICAL SOCIETY.

January 8, 1906.

Report of Cases. DR. THOMAS S. CULLEN.

CASE I.—*Early Tuberculosis of the Kidney.—Diagnosis of the tuberculous process made from thickening of the ureter detected on vaginal examination.*

Miss E. Q., aged 24, seen in consultation with Dr. Fenby and admitted to the Johns Hopkins Hospital, October 26, 1905. The patient complained of pain on urination. The family and personal histories were not important, except that she had been suffering with diarrhœa and complained of slimy stools with pain in the rectum on defecation. She had had dysmenorrhea.

Present trouble.—For eight months she has had pain at the end of urination. This is her chief complaint at present. At first the pain was cutting and almost intolerable. At present she has to void small quantities every ten or fifteen minutes. There is no history of hæmaturia. Five or six days before admission her trouble became very acute and she noticed shreds in the urine. Recently she has had chills and fever. She has always had pain and tenderness on the left side just above the hip and in the flank.

General examination.—The heart action is weak and irregular. The lungs are clear.

A cystoscopic examination shows well-defined ulcers scattered throughout the base of the bladder; in numerous places near the ulcers are small tubercles. The inflammation is especially noticeable around the left ureter. The urine contains pus, but no tubercle bacilli can be detected. On further examination the left ureter can be palpated through the vagina, and is recognized as a hard pencil-like cord passing upward along the left side of the pelvic wall.

Operation, October 28, 1905.—Left nephrectomy; partial ureterectomy. On cutting down on the kidney the capsule was found adherent and definite tubercles were easily made out.

After tying the renal vessels separately the ureter was freed as far as possible, but as the patient's pulse was 140 when we started and became weaker it was impossible to take time enough to remove the entire ureter. The ureter was freed as far as the pelvic brim, tied with Pagenstecher thread, and then cut across with the Pacquelin cautery. A small drain was inserted. The patient did well after oper-

ation and rapidly grew stronger, although she had intense bladder pain.

Second Operation, November 11.—Ureterectomy. Cystoscopic examination still showed considerable cystitis, but there had been a moderate improvement. It was consequently decided not to make a vesico-vaginal fistula, but rather to see if the bladder symptoms would not clear up after removal of the ureter. An incision was made parallel to Poupart's ligament, from the anterior superior spine almost to the symphysis. A gridiron incision was made in the muscles and the peritoneum pushed toward the median line. The thickened ureter immediately came into view. The upper part was loosened without much difficulty; the ureter was freed down to the uterine vessels. The uterine artery and veins were then tied on both sides and cut as in a Wertheim operation. An artery clamp was then introduced into the vagina and pressed upward. It was seen that nothing but the vaginal mucosa lay between the field of operation and the vagina. The forceps was then cut down upon, the vagina opened, and the ureter drawn through into the vagina. The lateral incision was now partially closed. After a small drain had been carried down to the bottom of the incision the ureter was excised. Where cut across it showed no thickening. There was a slight leakage from the vagina for several days.

November 25.—The patient still has dysuria, but her general condition is greatly improved.

January 6, 1906.—During her stay in the hospital she gained fifteen pounds and at present looks very well. Micturition is still frequent and last night she had to get up at least eight times. There is now much less tenesmus, whereas formerly just a few drops of urine in the bladder were sufficient to bring on a desire to void. The site of the left ureteral orifice looks puckered. From the right ureteral orifice spurts of urine can be seen and a tendency to eversion of the ureter. The bladder mucosa looks somewhat injected but the ulceration has apparently disappeared.

Pathological report.—The kidney is normal in size. At its upper pole there is an area of softening, 2 by 3 cm. At this point beneath the capsule numerous fine yellowish-white tubercles are detected. On section the capsule of the kidney can be easily stripped off. Near the point at which the tubercles were noted is a cavity 2.5 by 2 cm. Lining this are numerous minute tubercles. The cavity is filled with a rather grumous material. The cortex between the cavity and the surface is everywhere studded with tubercles. The greater part of the kidney is comparatively free from the growth, but near the middle a few isolated tubercles are visible, and at the lower pole several can be detected. A small portion of the ureter is present. It is 6 mm. in diameter and very firm.

On *histological examination* of the area where the tuberculosis was macroscopically unmistakable there is a great deal of alteration. The tissue is markedly infiltrated with small round cells. There is an obliteration of the usual landmarks and many tubercles are seen, sometimes lying in groups of epithelioid cells; in other places are large masses of epithelioid elements. There is little tendency toward the formation of giant cells. In some places the process has gone to caseation. The wall of the cavity in the upper part of the kidney is composed essentially of tuberculous tissue, and the cavity itself contains quantities of polymorphonuclear leucocytes.

The outer coats of the ureter are for the most part normal. Here and there, however, a small tubercle is seen. The tissue directly beneath the mucosa shows slight invasion with tubercles, but the epithelium lining the ureter is intact. Sections from the lower part of the ureter show that the epithelium has entirely disappeared, the cavity being lined almost entirely by typical tuberculous tissue.

This case demonstrates very well the pronounced vesical symptoms which can exist with a very small amount of renal tuberculosis and the great disintegration of the ureter that may take place when so little renal substance is implicated.

The cord-like ureter detected on vaginal examination is practically pathognomonic of tuberculosis of the kidney even without an examination of the bladder or of the urine.

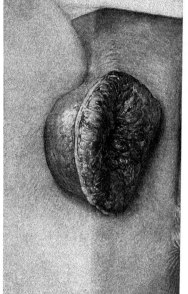

CASE II.—A very rapidly growing squamous-celled carcinoma of the inner side of the thigh.

CASE II.—*A very rapidly growing squamous-celled carcinoma of the inner side of the thigh.*

Gyn. No. 12.330. Mrs. B. F. Admitted to the Johns Hopkins Hospital August 29, 1905, complaining of a lump in the right side of the thigh. The patient is 53 years of age, white. The menopause occurred at 52, a year before the onset of this trouble. The patient has been married 29 years; had one child 28 years ago, no miscarriages. Ten years ago she noticed a pimple in the groin. This has been growing larger ever since and recently there has been a watery discharge from it. Pain has sometimes been present when she was sitting up. The tumor had increased only gradually, but since the last fourteen days the growth has been very rapid. The ulcerated surface is painful to the touch; the non-ulcerated or outer portion is not.

Operation September 24.—Excision of the fungoid tumor. The tumor was carefully covered over with gauze, then drawn up and excised without exposing the area of ulceration. There was little or no bleeding. The tissues were brought together with ease.

Oct. 17.—Patient discharged. Incision well healed. The outlook is of course most gloomy.

Path. No. 8194.—Just to the right of the vagina with its long axis parallel to that of the vulva is a somewhat pedunculated tumor which rises about 6 cm. above the skin. It is 8 cm. in length, 4 cm. in breadth. Its outer surface, that is, the portion nearest the thigh is covered with brawny, glistening skin, bluish-purple in appearance. The inner or median half is ulcerated and presents a most sickening appearance; the color is reddish-blue, greenish, or yellow; the picture varying greatly in different parts according to the amount of discharge and the distribution of the areas of necrosis. On its surface as one passes up toward the inguinal region the tissue is somewhat raised, has a reddish hue and there has evidently been an infiltration of the lymphatics upward toward the inguinal glands on the affected side.

On *histological examination* the skin a short distance from the growth is unaltered. In the vicinity of the growth it shows a definite tendency to project downward, although the individual cells still retain their usual appearance. The underlying connective tissue, however, shows a great deal of infiltration with small round cells, particularly abundant along the course of the blood-vessels. The growth itself is made up entirely of epithelial cells. These have vesicular nuclei. They are not, however, uniform in size. There are masses of protoplasm containing two, three, or more nuclei. Nuclear figures are abundant and here and there are masses of deeply staining chromatin. The nuclei are sometimes so arranged as to form large mulberry-shaped masses. The growth is a very cellular one. There is very little intervening stroma. Scattered abundantly throughout the superficial portions of the growth and also at various places deeper down are large numbers of polymorphonuclear leucocytes. The superficial portions of the growth have undergone complete necrosis. There are fragmentations of nuclei and deposits of fibrin.

Diagnosis.—A very rapidly growing squamous-celled carcinoma on the inner side of the thigh.

CASE III.—*Early tuberculosis of the appendix.*

Mrs. D. Seen in consultation with Dr. Mayer, September 8, 1905. The patient is 30 years of age and has had several definite attacks of appendicitis within the last year. I saw her in a subacute attack with the temperature just a little above normal, pulse normal, but a definite tenderness over the appendix. On opening the abdomen we found the appendix partly bound down by adhesions. At its center was a swollen patch that formed a ring around the appendix. The right tube and ovary were partially bound down by adhesions. The pelvis was filled with clear fluid. We did not obtain any history of tuberculosis.

Path. No. 9040.—The appendix is bulging at the tip. There is some injection of the vessels. Apart from the annular thickening and the slight bulging at the tip little was to be made out macroscopically.

Histological examination.—The surface is covered with quite a number of adhesions which are recent and very vascular. In one of the adhesions is a typical tubercle. The muscular walls are for the most part normal, but at one point a tubercle is to be seen. Scattered throughout the lymphoid tissue are many tubercles, some of them typical, others consisting of epithelioid cells; at numerous points caseation has already taken place. The mucosa of the appendix is for the most part intact and normal. The lumen of the appendix contains a great number of polymorphonuclear leucocytes, and in the wall of the appendix, at one point, is a fairly large abscess.

In this case we did not for a moment suspect tuberculosis. Such instances emphasize the necessity for a routine histological examination in all cases. On questioning the patient carefully after operation we learned that she had been under treatment within the last year for incipient tuberculosis of the left lung.

CASE IV.—*Tuberculosis of the appendix, cæcum, colon, and small bowel.*

Mr. M. Seen in consultation with Dr. Mayer and admitted to the Church Home, November 13, 1905. The patient is 34 years of age and for several months has been under the care of Dr. McConachie for ulceration of the larynx. His symptoms were relieved, but the exact cause was not determined.

The patient has also been suffering from tuberculosis of the left lung. During the last six weeks he has lost twelve pounds and has complained of a great deal of pain in the pit of the stomach. On palpation a definite thickening can be made out over the pyloric orifice. He has had some fever. Yesterday it was 102° F.

It was deemed wise to do an exploratory laparotomy. An incision was made over the appendix as there was also some thickening at that point. The appendix was found to be more than twice its natural size. The cæcum in the vicinity showed much induration, especially around the base of the appendix. The area of thickening detected on clinical examination proved to be in the transverse colon. Here over an area fully 5 cm. long the bowel was greatly thickened. Over its surface was a leash of blood-vessels, and beneath its peritoneum a few definite tubercles could be detected. On further examination I found that the small bowel at intervals of from six to eight inches was encircled by bluish-red areas fully 1.5 cm. in breadth—annular ulcerations. These were abundantly dotted with small tubercles and along their blood-vessels were little beads of tubercles. In many places along the convexity of the intestines were little streaks, evidently dilated lymphatics. It looked very much as if one had gone over the surface here and there with a fine brush and white fluid making delicate streaks. All gradations of the early tubercles could be detected, but at no point was there evidence of caseation. We removed the appendix and closed the abdomen. There was no apparent involvement of the omentum or of the abdominal peritoneum. The patient improved very much. His temperature remained normal for at least a weak. Later on he was put on tuberculin. Just prior to leaving the hospital his temperature again arose and he rapidly lost ground.

Path. No. 9209.—The appendix is 6 cm. long and varies from 7 to 12 mm. in diameter, the end being considerably distended and blunt. It is covered with delicate shaggy adhesions and its vessels are very much injected. At no point is there any evidence of stricture. On section the lumen is found to be filled with greenish pus. The walls of the appendix are thickened. The mucosa is much infiltrated and the specimen is somewhat suggestive of plastic tuberculosis.

On *histological examination* numerous old but very vascular adhesions are seen on the outer surface. They contain quantities of small and several large blood-vessels. The muscular walls show infiltration with small round cells. Scattered throughout the lymphoid tissue are many typical tubercles. The mucosa at numerous points is intact, but in other places has disappeared, the inner surface being represented by caseous material. The lumen of the appendix is practically filled with polymorphonuclear leucocytes.

CASE V.—*The right ovary in the abdominal scar following an operation for appendix abscess.*

Mrs. G. Seen in consultation with Dr. Savage, October 9, 1905. The patient complained of bulging in the scar remaining from a former appendix incision and of a sensation of weight in the lower abdomen. The family history was unimportant. Ten years ago she was operated on by Dr. Kelly at the Johns Hopkins Hospital for a pelvic abscess which was opened into through the vagina. The condition was a very serious one and she was compelled to remain in bed for three months. The second operation was performed shortly after by Dr. J. G. Clark, for an appendix abscess. It was necessary to provide for free drainage and it was between three and four months before the patient regained her strength. Ever since then it has been necessary for her to wear a bandage, and at times there has been an apparent puffiness and tenderness in the abdominal scar. In the right lower quadrant of the abdomen is the scar of the appendix operation. It is about six inches in length. In the middle of the scar there is a small area of tenderness. The tissue here can be pushed in to some extent. In the lower part of the incision is a definite and sensitive thickening. On examination under anæsthesia I found along the appendix scar definite points of thickening and at the lower end a nodule fully 5 cm. long by 2 cm. broad. This was firmly adherent to the skin and felt very much like the thickened omentum. On resecting the old scar and entering the abdomen we found what at first appeared to be an adherent omentum was in reality a large cystic ovary which lay directly beneath the skin. Attached to it was a hydrosalpinx fully 1.5 cm. in diameter. The omentum had come down and had become adherent to the bladder, anterior abdominal wall, and the ovary. We loosened the omental adhesions to the ovary, but in order to avoid leaving fresh raw areas we left the omental adhesions to the bladder and abdominal wall as they were comparatively smooth. After controlling all oozing on the right side we loosened up the left ovary which was embedded in adhesions to the pelvic floor and to minimize the possibility of infection we placed a gauze drain in the pelvis and brought it out through the vagina. The abdomen was closed without drainage. The patient made a very satisfactory recovery.

Path. No. 9184.—The specimen consists of a tube and ovary. The ovary is practically normal in size and is covered everywhere by adhesions and contains several small Graafian follicles, and a partially organized corpus luteum. The tube is also covered by adhesions.

Microscopically, neither tube nor ovary shows anything abnormal.

CASE VI.—*An obscure abdominal tumor in the right upper quadrant consisting of an elongated right hepatic lobe, a prolapsed right kidney, and an appendix adherent to the gall-bladder.*

Gyn. No. 12521.—Mrs. A. D. Age 60. Patient of Dr. Singewald. Admitted to the Johns Hopkins Hospital, November 16, 1905. This patient entered the hospital complaining of pain in her right side. Her family and previous history are negative. Her menses ceased at 44. Married twenty-eight years; has had twelve children. About two years ago

the patient noticed a fullness after eating, and one year ago a swelling in the right side just below the ribs. This has persisted, and she thinks it has become larger and lately has been growing rapidly. The increase in size has been accompanied by some pain and a feeling of pressure. She has been able to walk around the house, but cannot stand much exertion. Pain prevents her from lying down on the right side; she is most comfortable on her back. After eating she has noticed a good deal of discomfort in the right side. Has not lost in weight or in strength. Dr. Rushmore on examination found a cyst-like mass in the right flank which was indistinct; the movements are restricted and the growth does not extend into the pelvis. The vaginal examination yields practically nothing.

Operation, November 18, 1905.—On examining the patient under anæsthesia I readily made out a large firm mass occupying the right upper quadrant of the abdomen. The mass, however, had a rounded contour and extended within 3 cm. of the median line anteriorly, downward it could be traced to a point about 4 cm. below the umbilicus. It was impossible to tell whether we were dealing with a renal tumor, a growth from the bowel, or with some pathological condition implicating the liver or gall-bladder. A small opening was accordingly made through the right rectus to determine the exact condition. On opening the abdomen it was found that a part of this mass was due to a prolapsed and somewhat thickened right lobe of the liver. The posterior portion of the mass was formed by the prolapsed right kidney; and lying in between and extending up along the under surface of the liver for at least 5 cm. was the appendix. This was considerably thickened and adherent to the gall-bladder and cystic duct. The adhesions were gradually liberated, and the appendix was removed without difficulty. The patient stood the operation well.

November 26, 1905.—The patient is in excellent condition.

Path. No. 9229.—The specimen consists of the appendix which apart from a few adhesions appears perfectly normal.

Histological examination.—Attached to the outer surface are several dense and very vascular adhesions. The muscular walls are normal and the mucosa is unaltered.

In this case the symptoms were undoubtedly due entirely to the tugging of the appendix adhesions as evidenced by the fact that the discomfort has entirely disappeared, notwithstanding that the tumor consisting of the right lobe of the liver and the prolapsed right kidney still exists.

CASE VII.—*Abscess between the abdominal peritoneum and omentum four weeks after labor. Involvement of the lower edge of the liver. Opening of abscess; secondary exploration in region of liver with marked tearing of the friable organ. Hemorrhage controlled with blunt liver needles. Complete recovery.*

Gyn. No. 12456.—A. M. Seen in consultation, October 20, 1905, and at once admitted to the hospital. She is 36 years of age, married, white. Her family and previous history are negative. She complains of a good deal of abdominal discomfort and of fever. The patient has been married seventeen years, has had ten children, the oldest 14 years, the youngest born September 19, 1905, just one month before admission. Her labors have all been difficult and instrumental. On several occasions there was tearing. Four years ago her perineum was repaired at this hospital. For several days prior to her labor in September she had been in bed with a fever. The delivery was instrumental. The labor was followed by a most profuse hemorrhage. Fever and chills continned for four days after delivery. Ever since that date she has had chills and fever and a marked pallor has been noted. On admission to the hospital she was extremely anæmic; hæmoglobin 26 per cent, leucocytes 11,200. There were distinct hæmic murmurs, but the heart was otherwise normal; the lung sounds were normal. The right eye was inflamed. A white scar was visible on the cornea and a definite purulent exudate was made out. The abdomen was distended and just to the left and above the umbilicus there was a definite area of bulging. Just to the left of the umbilieus and corresponding to elevations was an indurated area, 2.5 inches in diameter. This was somewhat tender. The lower part of the abdomen was hard, and suggested the existence of a large abdominal tumor. There was no reddening. There was more or less tenderness over the entire abdomen especially over the small tumor elevation noted on the left side. On pelvic examination nothing could be detected. The cervix was high up. The uterus was movable. On both sides the appendages were perfectly free.

Operation, October 21.—An incision was made over the hardened and indurated area on the left side. On passing down to the peritoneum we encountered a large abscess containing foul-smelling whitish pus. On careful exploration the cavity was found to continue upward almost to the free margin of the ribs and downward to within about 8 cm. of the pubes, but apparently lay between the anterior abdominal wall and the omentum. No intestines or abdominal contents were to be seen. The cavity was loosely packed with iodoform gauze and the patient left the table in a precarious condition. Cultures from the pus showed no growth. Anaerobic cultures were not made. For a few days large quantities of pus were discharged. Her temperature kept up and she became delirious and had to be taken to the isolation ward.

On *October 3,* the hæmoglobin was 25 per cent, the leucocytes were 15,200.

November 4, the patient was brought down to the operating room as her condition was not progressing satisfactorily. We could detect an area of induration along the free margin of the ribs on the right side. Artery forceps were introduced in the previous opening and carried up to where the induration was detected on the right side. We then cut down upon the indurated area in the flank. An incision was made on the outer side of the rectus; the peritoneum was found thickened. There was much œdema in the sub-peritoneal tissues. The liver was found lying just beneath the incision and appeared to be necrotic; it broke up very readily under the examining

finger and there was free hemorrhage. The insertion of three or four cat-gut sutures, however, with the blunt needle checked the oozing. We drained down to the edge of the liver and also repacked the large abscess cavity. Apparently the abdominal abscess had its origin from the gall-bladder or had been a primary liver abscess, but in no way involved the pelvic organs and had apparently been almost entirely anterior to the omentum. The patient gradually improved. The temperature dropped from 102 to 100° F. The appetite also improved.

November 20.—She was taken out of doors although her condition was still rather precarious. From this time her mental condition rapidly cleared up and a decided improvement was noted each day and she was discharged on December 21 with the abominal wound completely closed; there was no tenderness at any point, the hæmoglobin was 76 per cent and the mental condition was perfectly satisfactory.

CASE VIII.—*The velvety feel of an unruptured tubal pregnancy.*

E. P., colored, aged 30, married, was admitted to the Johns Hopkins Hospital, September 19, 1905. She has been complaining of uterine bleeding, and pain in the back and right side for seventeen days. Her family and previous history are unimportant. The menses began at fifteen. For two years they were regular without pain, later the periods became painful and lasted longer. Her last period was August 24, the previous one in July. She has been married fourteen years, has had no children but one pregnancy, with an abortion at two months, four years ago. On September 2, she commenced to have considerable pain in the back and on the right side low down; also a bloody discharge. The periods continued without relief. There is continuous aching pain in the lower part of the back and irregular sharp pains in the right side. The abdomen is very sensitive. Examination under anæsthesia disclosed a multinodular myomatous uterus, the organ being about three times the usual size. Several hard nodules could be made out. On the left side was a nodule about 3 cm. in diameter. This differed somewhat from the surrounding ones. The myomatous nodules were uniform, firm in consistency, while the nodule on the left side, although hard in places, gave a sensation of softness. In other words, it gave one the sensation of a firm body with a rather yielding outer covering. I ventured to make a provisional diagnosis of tubal pregnancy, although at that time we had not read the history.

September 23.—On opening the abdomen a small amount of clear fluid was found in the peritoneal cavity. The uterus was multinodular, about three times the natural size. The ovaries were adherent, the right tube was also somewhat adherent. The left tube was swollen and adherent to the uterus. Near the uterus it was 2.5 cm. in diameter, purplish-red in color, and contained an unruptured tubal pregnancy. The uterus and the tubes were removed in the usual way from left to right. The ovaries were not disturbed. On opening the tube, Mr. Broedel found that the fœtus was perfectly preserved and the membranes were still intact. The patient made a very satisfactory recovery.

Our diagnosis was based on a definite and yet apparently undescribed sign, which I think we may designate as the "velvety feel." The examining finger detects a nodule which on gentle pressure seems to be rather soft and yet on firm pressure is found to be hard. The same sensation can be readily obtained by covering a piece of wood with velvet. This "velvety feel" is doubtless due to the soft muscular covering which encircles the pregnant sphere.

CASE IX.—*Pregnancy in one horn of a bicornate uterus, giving symptoms identical with those of tubal pregnancy.*

Mrs. R. C. F. consulted me on November 23, 1905. She has been married about three months. Her period of October 13 was two weeks late, the flow was very scant, dark, and lasted from ten to eleven days. Her period came on again on November 11, and has lasted on and off practically every day since then. For more than a month she has had pain in the lower abdomen, sometimes on the left side, at other times on the right. She has been nauseated, a symptom which she has never had previously. On pelvic examination the cervix was found to be normal, but slightly softened. The uterus was somewhat enlarged; there was no thickening on the right side. On the left there was a sensation of tenderness and in close proximity to the uterus was a mass about half as large again as the ovary.

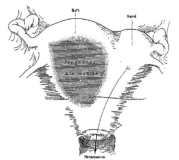

FIGURE 1.

The clinical history and the pelvic examination strongly suggested extra-uterine pregnancy. I accordingly made an ether examination the following morning. I was still able to detect the lump on the left side. After going into the question thoroughly it was decided that an exploratory operation should be performed, although I could not positively exclude intra-uterine pregnancy. On opening the abdomen a 2½ months' pregnancy was found in the right uterus to which were attached the corresponding tube and ovary. The hard mass detected on the left side, apparently plastered up against

the uterus, was the left non-pregnant horn. To the left of this the corresponding appendages were attached. Between the pregnant right horn and the non-pregnant left horn was a depression not more than 1 cm. in depth, a depression that might very readily have been overlooked; in fact when the patient was curetted some three years ago the uterus was apparently normal in size and no unevenness was noted. The abdomen was at once closed. The patient left the hospital in about 12 days. The condition here present is a most interesting one. If we for a moment consider the left uterine horn as a separate uterus, then gestation in the right uterine horn constitutes an extra-uterine pregnancy, consequently we should expect a "sympathic" development of decidua in the left uterine horn. This would naturally for some time be accompanied by a bloody discharge.

CASE X.—*Path. No. 9062.—Adenocarcinoma of the abdominal peritoneum complicating uterine myomata.*

Mrs. R., age 58. Seen in consultation with Dr. Wilmer Brinton, October 4, 1905. Twenty years ago Dr. Brinton saw this patient and found a fibroid about the size of an adult's head. He wisely advised against operation, as at that time the mortality was exceedingly high. He did not see her again until three months ago when she had a definite attack of peritonitis and since then has been forced to sit up all the time. She cannot lie down except with her knees drawn up. The cervix is intact. There is a good deal of offensive discharge. The abdomen is board-like, and is occupied by a tumor which fills the vaginal vault and extends almost to the umbilicus. Although the patient is very anæmic her pulse is of good volume and an exploratory operation seems justifiable.

October 10.—On opening the abdomen we found the omentum greatly thickened and a firm cord running up to the diaphragm just to the left of the median line. Numerous nodules were found scattered throughout the abdomen, and there was a large pelvic tumor. There seemed to be little doubt that we were dealing with a malignant change in a myoma associated with metastases. We removed a small piece of tissue for examination. It was impossible to attempt to completely enucleate the growth.

On histological examination of one of the omental nodules we found that the greater part of adipose tissue had been replaced by fibrous tissue which was very vascular. Scattered throughout this were masses of cells, which showed a tendency toward glandular arrangement. These cells had fairly deeply staining nuclei, in other places isolated cells of the tumor are found lying in the stroma. These were very large, many were multi-nuclear and had deeply staining nuclei. It appeared to be a most rapidly growing form of carcinoma.

In this case we had evidently had a large myoma which had lain dormant for a good many years and then carcinoma, possibly of the body of the uterus, had suddenly developed and gone on to the formation of metastases. With our present perfection in technique early operation in the greater number of myoma cases is clearly indicated as has been so forcibly pointed out by Charles P. Noble, of Philadelphia.

The New Oliver Sphygmomanometer. Dr. Briggs, Washington, D. C.

Since Dr. Cushing brought the first Riva-Rocci apparatus to this hospital I have been much interested in the instrument and its various improvements and modifications in clinical work.

Dr. Erlanger especially has pointed out the errors inherent in earlier appliances and has offered us the only instrument perfectly accurate from the laboratory point of view. Its only practical drawback is that it is too large and bulky for general use.

Lately there has been much interest in the development of a gas manometer as opposed to the ordinary mercury apparatus for measuring pressure; Dr. Oliver, of London, has published in the *Lancet* an account of what, on paper, seems an ideal instrument for the clinical determination of the blood pressure.

The systolic pressure is readily enough determined clinically. By means of the Oliver apparatus the pressure necessary to occlude the artery is determined by the observation of the degree of compression of a volume of gas. A colored fluid—absolute alcohol tinted with "Fettfarben Blau"—is introduced into the open shorter arm of the l-shaped tube until the two surfaces of the fluid register at the two zero levels, one in each arm. The air in the longer arm above the fluid is then considered as the unit volume. All openings are then closed and to the end of the shorter arm, is attached, through a T-piece connected with the compression bulb, the arm band: the broader band (12 cm.) as recommended by Dr. Janeway, of New York, being considered the best. The arm, bag, etc., is then inflated in the usual manner and the diminution in volume of the enclosed air, as registered by the changed level of the fluid, is read off on an empirically calibrated scale in terms of mm. Hg. Readings from this scale and instrument have been found to coincide exactly with readings made with a standard mercury manometer in a series of control tests, at all levels from 50 to 300 mm. Hg., and at all usual air temperatures.

The systolic pressure, however, is not enough even in approximate clinical work, the diastolic being of much importance. I have no intention here of referring to anything beyond the act and means of observation of blood pressure. In the mercury manometer the inertia of the mercury, its high surface tension, and the surprisingly variable error due to its oxidation introduce great sources of uncertainty in diastolic readings. In the Oliver apparatus we use in the determination of the diastolic pressure a column of gas compressed through a bead of liquid, all at an approximately constant or constantly variable temperature. As the gas (air) has practically no inertia and the bead of liquid produces practically no friction within the tube we are enabled to obtain very prompt and ample fluctuations of the bead in response to the rhythmic thrust of the pulse pressure.

The ordinary valve as found in the rubber compression bulbs, found on Riva-Rocci instruments, is not deemed suffi-

ciently positive in closure, and an improved valve is used in this apparatus. It consists of a fine brass tube closed at one end, the side being perforated by two minute holes over which is stretched a tubing of thin rubber membrane. This membrane is forced up and away from the openings by the pressure of the entering air on compressing the rubber bulb, but falls back, closing the apertures directly the pressure of the entering air is diminished, so preventing leakage, and ensuring immobility of the bead in taking readings of systolic pressure.

The principle of this apparatus is an important one and will be far-reaching in its influence on clinical sphygmomanometry. The exactness of a physiological apparatus is at least approached, even if not absolutely attained, in Dr. Oliver's apparatus. Our fortunate—in some senses—brethren of the laboratory must not be too prone to look down upon and patronize the "approximateness" of clinical methods of measurement. The ideal of mathematical precision of determination has often, and justly, to yield the *pas* in the clinic to the practical necessities of sick people. If the physiologists will not admit that the Oliver sphygmomanometer is an appreciable advance in the direction of laboratory accuracy, we can at least feel confident, without their assurance, that it represents a step away from the old attitude of basing clinical judgments of importance in this field wholly on direct sensory palpation impressions of the pulse and vessel wall. This will be perhaps the happier point of view than that which the physiologists would have us assume—it is better to look forward than to gaze back. Dr. Oliver has sensitized the convenience of the finger tip, even if he has not simplified the accuracy of the kymograph.

Discussion.

Dr. Dawson said the large size of the Erlanger instrument was due to the feature which allowed the blood pressures to be recorded. The Oliver instrument admits only of subjective determinations and in so far as objective are superior to subjective methods the Erlanger instrument was necessarily superior. For ordinary purposes the Oliver instrument might be good enough. It was to be regretted that as yet great accuracy had been necessarily accompanied with great bulk in the apparatus.

Dr. Erlanger said he had never used the Oliver apparatus so that any objections he might offer to its principle should perhaps be considered as questions to be answered at the close of the discussion.

(1) The systolic pressure is determined in exactly the same manner as with the Riva-Rocci instrument. The estimation so made is 5 to 15 mm. Hg. below that made by noting the first abrupt increase in the amplitude of oscillations as the pressure on the arm falls at a constant rate from above the systolic pressure.

(2) The method of estimating the diastolic pressure with the Oliver apparatus is essentially the same as with the Hill-Barnard sphygmometer. In the latter instrument the zero is not constant. But even in the physiological laboratory here,

where calibration of a scale is not a serious matter, and in the wards of this hospital, as well as elsewhere, the instrument has been found to be thoroughly unsatisfactory. In many cases it is practically impossible to make a satisfactory reading of the moving needle.

(3) It is difficult to read accurately the levels reached by an object moved by the arterial pulse wave, because the duration of the crest of such waves is too brief and because the form of the crest changes with different pressures on the artery. This objection becomes more serious when, as in the Oliver instrument, equal increments of pressure are associated with diminishing excursions of the indicator.

(4) It must be difficult to read the pressure exerted on the arm when the indicator is constantly oscillating through a range which probably exceeds 10 mm. Hg.

(5) Since there are often two regions of maximum oscillation when the pressure is allowed to fall steadily from a point which exceeds the systolic pressure, and as the first maximum, which does not correspond with the diastolic pressure, may occasionally be higher than the second, it becomes practically impossible to determine with a subjective method which is the proper maximum to choose as the diastolic pressure.

(6) Oliver states that 90 mm. Hg. is the average diastolic pressure and that 10 mm. Hg. is the lowest normal pulse-pressure. The former figure is too high, 75 being the accepted average here; and the latter figure has been seen here in surgical shock and syncope only.

(7) Of the two pressures, sytolic and diastolic, the latter is much the more important since it is much closer to the mean (which is not the arithmetic mean of the systolic and diastolic) and since it follows the variations of the mean pressure much more closely than does the systolic pressure. But a knowledge of both pressures is the most valuable. For example, in orthostatic albuminuria variations in the output of albumin can be predicted from changes in the pulse-pressure only, and during recovery from Stokes-Adams disease the diastolic pressure shows the logical rise of pressure, the systolic pressure falling slightly.

January 22, 1906.

The Toxins and Antitoxins of Poisonous Mushrooms. Dr. W. W. FORD.

The use of mushrooms as a food was known to the ancient Babylonians, and other nations made use of this plant not only as a delicacy, but as the main constituent of meals. The most prized one takes its name from one of the early Roman emperors. The poisonous forms were known and used to kill enemies.

The mushroom has a wide use in European countries, Italy, France, Poland, Russia, and also in China. That its use has not become so general in America is due to a general suspicion of the plant and to its scarcity. Its greatest use in this country is as a condiment.

In the ancient times almost as soon as the mushroom began to come into use cases of fatal poisoning occurred. Up to the last century it was not known to what principle this poisoning was due. Though the actual number of cases is hard to determine, many persons have lost their lives from eating this plant. The best statistics are from France where 100 cases of poisoning were collected in a short time. In another section of the same country 60 cases were reported in a brief period. In Japan during eight years 400 cases were recorded, while from Germany comes a report of 53 cases with 44 deaths. In Italy it is a common cause of death. Near Baltimore two cases were reported last summer neither of which was fatal. Of late there have been a number of scattered cases throughout North America. The number of cases is sufficient to make the study an interesting one and an antitoxin of use.

The nature of the poison involved is important. The French claim that all forms of mushrooms are good if fresh, the Germans claim that all are poisonous. Schmiedeberg isolated muscarine from *Amanita muscaria*, and later prepared this substance synthetically. Its action is on the nerve centers and its antidote is atropine. *A. muscaria*—the ordinary toadstool—is the source of practically all the muscarine in nature.

The most important cause of poisoning with toadstools is *A. phalloides* which differs from *A. muscaria* in color and structure. It is abundant in the woods and grows not only in the shade, but in the sunlight as well. *A. phalloides* is of astonishing toxicity, one-third of the top of a small plant having killed a child. *A. verna* is likewise very toxic, being called the "destroying angel" or deadly amanita.

A 1900 French thesis gives a long list of poisonings by *A. phalloides*, while in other literature 200 cases of poisoning from *A. phalloides* are recorded. *A. phalloides* is the most poisonous and poisoning from *A. muscaria* generally results in slow recovery.

The symptoms of poisoning with *A. phalloides* are very definite and marked pathological changes are found postmortem. In a case where the mushroom was eaten at 6 o'clock in the evening, at 12 midnight the patient complained of severe pain in the abdomen and head, and of intense thirst. There were excessive vomiting, cyanosis, short stertorous breathing, and glazed pupils. Delirium developed, passing on into coma and death, this occurring on the eighth day with typical Hippocratic facies.

Seven postmortem examinations showed lack of postmortem rigidity, widely dilated pupils, ecchymoses in the mucous membranes, and lack of coagulation of the blood. There was fatty degeneration of the liver, kidneys, heart muscle, as in phosphorus poisoning, this occurring to the extent of 53-68% in mushroom poisoning and to 70% from phosphorus.

Kobert, in 1891, and later in 1897, was the first to give definite information as to the poisonous substance, and to him we owe our present knowledge. The active principle phallin is a tox-albumen and possesses a specific action upon the red blood corpuscles being strongly hæmolytic.

Some reference has been made to an antitoxic serum in Italy in 1897, but no account of this can be discovered.

A. phalloides grows abundantly in Maryland, Pennsylvania, and in North Carolina, and possesses a very typical odor and appearance, especially when fresh. Its taste is delicious and this fact leads to the mistakes frequently made in its use. In the preparation of the active principle it is best to extract the fresh plants with distilled water in an ice-box for 24 hours. On pressure this yields a dark brown fluid possessing the characteristic odor of the fungus. This is filtered first through paper and a Berkefeld filter. On concentrating to dryness a sticky residue is obtained, which it is impossible to use because its strength cannot be estimated. It is therefore better to use a certain weight of the fungus and a known unit of water. This substance is a powerful hæmolytic agent, a 1% solution dissolving the red blood corpuscles of many animals and man. This action occurs best at 38° C., more slowly at the room temperature, the corpuscles of the guinea pig being less resistant, those of man and the dog being more so. This dissolving action takes place with very dilute solutions, 1-100 cc. sufficing for 1 cc. of rabbit's blood, laking and dissolving the corpuscles completely.

The hæmolysins are of two classes, normal serum hæmolysins and immune serum hæmolysins. Two substances are required, the amboceptor and the complement, neither of which can act alone. On the other hand different hæmolysins are produced by the bacteria which may act without any complement. Phallin unites directly with susceptible red corpuscles and if the temperature be raised a trifle hæmolysis occurs without the aid of a complement. It is capable of dissolving the corpuscles in the presence of no other substance. Heating phallin to 58° C. causes no diminution in its powers, and only at 65° C. does it begin to lose its hæmolytic action, 70° C. being necessary to render it inactive for certain susceptible forms of cells. If it be inactivated at 70° C., it was thought some substance might be found that would act as a complement. Various sera were tried in many ways, but no such complemental substance apparently exists. Phallin acts therefore directly upon the red blood corpuscles, and, like the bacterial hæmolysins, requires no complement.

Inoculated into animals, the crude extract is very toxic, 1 cc. will kill a rabbit weighing 2000 grains in eight hours. The animals become very weak and lie on their sides with deep, difficult respiratory movements which grow less frequent. The heart continues to beat after the respiratory movements cease. There are no convulsions, as always occur after the administration of muscarine. Inoculations under the skin produce subcutaneous œdema and small hæmorrhages. There is no postmortem stiffness, the bladder is filled with urine, the heart is in diastole with marked bulging of the ventricles, and there are occasionally small hæmorrhages in the pericardium. The stomach may show small ulcers of the mucous membrane and contain blood. With small doses degenerative changes occur in the organs and chronic intoxication.

Graduated doses will determine the lethal dose. The given dose will always kill a given weight of animal in a given time. The ratio between the hæmolytic power and the toxicity varies only within very narrow limits.

With gradually increasing doses it is possible, by using much smaller doses than are toxic and extending the inoculations over a long period of time, to immunize an animal to withstand the inoculation of a rapidly fatal dose, even up to several multiples of that dose. The serum at this point is anti-hæmolytic and stops hæmolysis even if used in dilute solutions. This serum also possesses antitoxic properties and will, if administered to another rabbit, neutralize completely a large amount of phallin so that no poisoning is obtained, not even subcutaneous œdema. Smaller doses of the antitoxin will allow only some of the characteristic features to appear.

We have eventually succeeded in immunizing rabbits to withstand very large doses of phallin. A dose equal in amount to six or seven times the fatal dose has been administered and the rabbit saved by the antitoxin. An amount equal to ten times the fatal dose to be neutralized should be the standard.

Hence phallin seems to be allied to the bacterial hæmolysins and is not only hæmolytic but toxic, and we can accustom small animals to withstand large doses and produce an antitoxin.

It is an open question as to whether this antitoxin will be of any practical use to man. Most cases of mushroom poisoning are due to phallin and the mortality is high. The diagnosis is easy and a physician is generally called at once. As a considerable period (six to eight days in adults and three to five days in children) intervenes before the fatal outcome, the administration of an antitoxin would appear theoretically to be of value.

The " Home Sanatorium " Treatment of Pulmonary Tuberculosis.
Dr. J. H. PRATT, Boston.

As emphasized by Osler, " the vast majority of all tuberculous patients may be treated in their homes." The essential feature of sanatorium treatment must be a careful regulation of the daily life, light, and open air. An outdoor life, if adopted, will in some cases cure. Even in New England's unfavorable climate tuberculosis can be successfully treated. Millet was an early advocate of out-of-door sleeping at night.

Of importance is the regulation of the daily life and this measure has brought good results, as shown by Minor, of Asheville, N. C. We have tried this among the poor in the City of Boston.

In the past the unfavorable results of home and dispensary treatment have arisen from the lack of discipline. The tuberculosis dispensary, although a factor in preventing the spread of the disease, cures few, if any, cases. The difference between the methods of the dispensary and our home treatment is that the dispensary gives a small amount of care to a large number of patients, while we give a large amount of care to a small number of patients.

Every detail of the daily life is supervised. The nurse or friendly visitor is a wise counselor, wise and tactful, and a good disciplinarian. Twenty-five is the largest number of the class at one time. It was organized July 1, 1905, and no one was accepted until the diagnosis of tuberculosis was positive, either by the finding of bacilli or by tuberculin. Not distinctly favorable patients were sought; all were poor, none being able to pay the $4.00 per week demanded by the State Sanatorium, and none were well educated.

The applicant for admission to the class promises that he or she will do no work and will lead the out-of-door life. A clinical history is taken and a complete physical examination made, the latter being repeated once a month. If no available roof, balcony, or porch is at hand the patient must move to where he may live out of doors all the time.

On the first visit the nurse gives the necessary rules to avoid the spread of the disease and the physician is informed. There is a daily visit, many being necessary to impress the important rules on the members of the class. Tents are placed upon roofs and in the yards, if available, and excepting the time for a bath, meals, and exercise, the patient's whole time is spent out of doors in a reclining chair.

The diet consists of milk, bread, butter, fruit, and oil, and the patient must provide it himself. Cottonseed oil is a good and inexpensive substitute for olive oil.

For exercise the patient walks for five minutes in the morning and for the same time in the evening, the temperature being taken before and after. If the patient improves, then the exercise is increased, if he is not so well the exercise is diminished. The exercise is taken watch in hand.

A very important aid is furnished by the individual record books kept by each patient. In them are entered: the food eaten, the hours spent out of doors, the temperature, pulse and weight, and the exercise taken. This system helps the patients to persevere and to keep up courage, and they take great pride in their records.

There is a weekly meeting of the class when there is an inspection of records as to weight, pulse, temperature, food, etc. A payment of two dollars per month is required from each patient.

For the first six months the expenses of the class amounted to $513.

Among nine patients, members of the class for three months or more, one gained 39¼ pounds in weight. In five of these nine the disease was arrested according to the terms of the National Committee, and three of the five are ready to return to work. The bacilli have disappeared from the sputa of the three patients.

Tuberculin was administered to the patient who had gained 39½ pounds and caused a return of cough and of bacilli in the sputum and a great reaction.

In regard to the cottonseed oil one teaspoonful per day is administered at first, some patients taking up to ten tablespoonfuls with no digestive disturbances.

The average gain per patient for the nine who have been in the class the longest is 9¾ pounds per patient.

(The paper is published in full in this issue of the *Bulletin*.)

DISCUSSION.

DR. THAYER.—This is, indeed, an admirable paper, and shows the sort of work that should and might be done here. It is hard to make people do the simplest thing that would do them good, though easy to get them to take medicines of whose composition and action we are ignorant. These simple physical methods should be applied not only to tuberculosis, but to every disease. Rest, for example, the thing worth all the other factors put together, is the hardest thing to get.

DR. JACOBS.—Some maintain the sun is not necessary to the cure of tuberculosis, and in France there are those who will not allow the patient to appear in the direct rays, making the patient carry an umbrella if necessary to walk in the sunlight.

DR. PRATT.—Early diagnosis is important, and our series of cases is perhaps a favorable one. It is important to early recognize the disease and institute a rigid treatment. No case is at too early a stage for the institution of rigid treatment.

February 5, 1906.

A Case of Traumatic Neurosis with Pseudo-Spastic Paraplegia.
DR. BARKER.

The patient, J. F., aged 42, born in Russia, by occupation a merchant, was admitted to Ward F on January 29, complaining of weakness and stiffness of the legs, and pains in various parts of the body. His family history has no bearing upon the case as far as I can learn. Aside from the diseases of childhood the patient has never suffered from any serious illnes. Until eight years ago, he was a strong, healthy man. He denies luetic infection, but admits a gonorrhœal attack some twenty years ago. He has not used alcohol or tobacco to excess.

Eight years ago he slipped and fell on an icy pavement. The injury at the time appeared to be slight, but soon afterwards the patient began to have pain in the right hypochondrium. Soon after his digestion began to be disturbed; various foods disagreed with him, and he suffered from eructations of gas and fluid. Soon after this he noticed increased frequency of micturition, having to rise sometimes as often as five or six times during the night. About five years ago he began to notice that he had occasional swelling and tenderness of the testicles, which lasted only a short time. About three years ago he began to have sharp shooting pains in the frontal region of the head. They were so severe that he stayed in bed for two weeks at one time. The pain in the head sometimes comes on while straining at stool. There is but little disturbance of sexual power. Two years ago the patient began to have shooting pains in the front of the right thigh. These gradually extended further down the leg, and during the past year this leg has been getting weaker. Six months ago the left leg became similarly affected. He states that his calf muscles seem short and that he feels as though he must walk on his toes. The patient complains that his legs are drawn up with pain at times, though the pain can be relieved by rubbing. He thinks the legs are stiffer in the morning, and that they grow weaker just before the bowels move. For several months he suffered very severe pain in the left shoulder. He has also complained of pain over the region of the bladder.

His appetite is good. The bowels are somewhat constipated. On physical examination and careful objective testing of his sensation there is slight hypo-algesia on the back of each leg (over the calves) ; in one or two places he was slow in distinguishing heat from cold. Otherwise the sensory examination was negative.

As far as motion is concerned, he asserts that he is unable to flex or extend the ankles, and that voluntary movement of the toes is impaired. The strength in the knee and the thigh muscles seems good when the individual movements are tested. Power in the muscles of the trunk and of the upper extremities is unimpaired.

The deep reflexes are greatly exaggerated in the lower extremities; almost any touch to the leg will throw the thigh and calf muscles into violent clonus. A tap upon the patellar tendon sets up clonus immediately. The ankle clonus is marked in both legs, but it is interesting that the clonus is irregular; sometimes the movement is very rapid, sometimes much slower. The movements, too, are much influenced by deviation of the attention. The periosteal-radial reflex is active on both sides, as are the triceps reflexes. The cutaneous reflexes are everywhere active, but not changed in quality. Stimulation of the sole of the foot produces plantar flexion of the toes on both sides. In no instance, though the test has been repeated many times, has dorsal flexion of the great toe been obtained. The mechanical excitability of the muscles is markedly increased, especially in the pectorals and biceps.

The patient is decidedly emotional, tears coming to the eyes on slight provocation.

When the patient attempts to walk he has great fear of falling. At first he could walk only with support, but on encouragement he has been able to walk alone. He walks with a broad base and without any marked adduction of the thighs. The feet oscillate as he walks. On the whole, they are dragged forward rather than being swung forward, though he sometimes swings one of the legs.

There are actual organic lesions in the eye-grounds. Dr. Bordley has made a careful examination and finds signs of an old neuritic atrophy and pigmentary changes.

From the history of the case, the state of the reflexes, the gait, the exaggerated mechanical excitability of the muscles and the emotional condition, the case is regarded as, in the main at least, one of traumatic neurosis, resembling spastic paraplegia. We have naturally hesitated in coming to this conclusion on account of the changes in the eye-grounds, and

it is of course possible that further observation may lead to a modification of the view expressed.

The case is being treated by rest, isolation and psychotherapy. He is being encouraged to think that he will recover the use of his legs, and is given systematic exercises in walking at regular intervals. Every effort is being made also to excite in him the desire to get well. As far as has been made out, there is nothing in the way of a damage suit or of invalid insurance to supply a motive for remaining ill. He has, however, been unaccustomed to work for so long that it may be difficult to lead him back to it.

Intention Tremor in a Case of Tertiary Syphilis. Dr. Barker.

This man, 34 years old, a watch-maker, was admitted to the hospital on the 10th of December, 1905, complaining of chills and rheumatism in both legs. At 19 years of age he suffered from gonorrhœa, complicated by orchitis and arthritis in the knees, ankles, elbows, wrists, and hands, which confined him to bed for three months. He recovered, however, entirely from the attack.

Eight years ago he had a hard chancre, followed in five weeks by cutaneous eruption, falling of the hair and sore throat. He was treated by subcutaneous injections of mercury, some forty in all. Salivation occurred during the treatment. He took mercury internally for a month, and received some sixty mercurial inunctions. He followed the mercurial treatment by a course of iodide of potassium in doses increased from 10 to 70 grains three times a day for two months. Two years ago gummata appeared on the head and had to be treated surgically. During the past few years he has developed marked tremor of the hands, and for several years he has suffered from nodes on the tibia. He has used beer and whiskey, sometimes to excess, for many years.

On physical examination the patient is found to have a moderate anæmia of the secondary type. He is fairly well nourished. The glands in places are palpable, but there is no marked general glandular enlargement. The organs of the thorax and abdomen appear to be normal. The urine contains neither albumin nor sugar. There are palpable nodes on both shins, on the right ulna and on the forehead.

The patient has a marked tremor of coarse type, exaggerated on attempts at voluntary movement. It is well marked in the fingers and arms and in the legs. On running the heel down the opposite shin the movement is quite ataxic. There is, however, no objective disturbance of sensation. Touch, pain and temperature sense are normal as far as tested. The sensation of passive movement and the vibration sense are normal.

The deep reflexes are increased, and ankle clonus and patellar clonus can be set up. With Babinski's test the toes nearly always move downward, though sometimes the great toe moves a little upward. The pupillary reflexes are normal. There is no nystagmus, nor is there any disturbance of speech.

As to the nature of this tremor we are in the dark. The history of lues, of alcoholism, and of prolonged mercurial treatment offers clues for etiology.

Gout with Chronic Interstitial Nephritis. Dr. Barker.

This patient, a middle-aged laborer, entered the hospital on January 31, complaining of pain in the left wrist and in both knees and ankles. The joint symptoms have yielded to treatment in the house. The case is one of gout, and I present it on account of the opportunity of emphasizing the frequency of the association of chronic Bright's disease with this affection. The patient's acute paroxysms have been typical, the pains being milder in the day-time and worse in the night. He has tophi in the ears and nose, and crystals removed from them by a needle prick are seen under the microscope to consist of mononatrium urate. The patient is passing from 1500 to 2000 cc. of urine in the twenty-four hours. It is light yellow in color, with a specific gravity varying from 1012 to 1015. It contains from 1.2 to 1.5 grams of albumin to the liter, and microscopically numerous hyaline and granular casts are to be found in the sediment.

Autopsy reports in cases of gout show that it is rare to find an autopsy on acute gouty arthritis unassociated with disease of the kidneys, and that further it is common at autopsies on nephritic patients to find joint deposits which had not been suspected during life. There has been a good deal of dispute as to the nature of this association between gout and chronic nephritis. Some have even gone so far as to assume that the nephritis is primary, and that the gout is due to retention of uric acid owing to faulty elimination by the kidneys. Others maintain that the excess of uric acid in the blood in gout precedes the development of kidney disease, and assert that not a few gouty patients have normal kidneys. The latter believe that the disease of the kidneys so commonly met with in late stages of gout is not the cause, but the effect of the gouty disorder. The question is still more or less open. I have referred to the arguments in some detail in the editorials entitled " Truth and Poetry Concerning Uric Acid " written last year for the *Journal of the American Medical Association.*

I should like to say just one word with regard to the treatment of gout. I need go into no detailed account of this, as Dr. Futcher has so often spoken of it here. The one point I should like to emphasize is the absence of any rational basis for the administration of the so-called uric solvents. Many of the drug manufacturers have made great profits as a result of the theory that uric acid deposits in gouty conditions may be prevented by increasing the solubility of uric acid in the blood and tissue juices. The newer studies in physical chemistry have taught us how futile such attempts are. The researches of the younger His and Paul have demonstrated that the solubility of any urate in the blood is necessarily decreased by the sodium salts of the blood. We cannot increase the solubility of the urates in the blood and tissue juices by attempting to bring into solution along with them bases whose uric acid salts are, outside the body, more soluble than sodium urate. The reason is this. When an acid is brought together with several bases, the first salt to be precipitated is that whose " solubility product " is smallest. Accordingly the administration of lithia, of piperazin and of other bases cannot give rise to the formation of a soluble urate in the blood owing to the excess of sodium ions always present there. It must be concluded, therefore, that the theory of the uric acid solvents no longer has any scientific support. The treatment of gout, aside from the treatment of the acute paroxysm is mainly dietetic and hygienic. Something may be done, it is true, to remove the tophi or the deposits in the joints by the excitation of local phagocytic activity and for this purpose we resort to the application of heat and massage. An out-of-door life, a simple, mixed and rather spare diet, freedom from worry, along with exercise short of fatigue, yield us the best results in the long run in the treatment of gout.

Universal Nævus. Dr. Barker.

This patient is a South American, 39 years old, who came into the hospital on January 21, suffering from certain neurasthenic symptoms which are yielding to treatment. I show him not on account of these, but on account of the peculiar appearance of his skin. All over the body, but most marked on the skin of the arms and trunk, are to be seen innumerable minute brownish red spots, which on superficial examination might make one think of a general secondary luetic eruption, or a generalized receding purpura. On examining the patient closely, however, it is found that the skin affection has nothing to do with either of these diseases. The spots are small, varying in size from that of a pin's head to two or three times that size. They are not elevated above the surface, the skin being smooth and velvety. On pressure the color disappears from the spots and slowly returns after a few seconds. A slight brownish discoloration remains in the spots when the blood is pressed out. The case is an example of the rather rare affection known as universal nævus. It is rather curious that the patient states that he noticed the manifestation for the first time only ten years ago.

A Case of Diabetic Coma With Kussmaul's Air-Hunger in a Boy. Dr. Barker.

This boy was admitted to the ward on December 14, 1905, complaining of extreme thirst and incontinence of urine. No symptoms were manifested until a week before admission. On the ward diet the urine contained from 6½ to 7 per cent of sugar, and he was passing from 150 to 200 grams of sugar per day. Even on a carbohydrate-free diet acetone and diacetic acid remained in the urine. The amount of sugar, however, fell to 2.4 per cent, and he then passed only 16 grams of glucose in the twenty-four hours. Any relaxation of the strict diet, however, has been followed by a rapid rise in the sugar output. This morning as we made the ward visit the onset of diabetic coma was evident. The boy had complained of headache, had gradually become stupid and developed a marked dyspnœa of the mixed type, both inspiration and expiration being prolonged and loud. The condition is a typical instance of the air-hunger in diabetes, so designated by Kussmaul.

The notoriously bad prognosis in the diabetes of children promises to be further substantiated by the progress of this case. The coma is being combatted by the administration of alkalies and by a moderate increase in the administration of the carbohydrates. The boy is brighter by far now than he was this forenoon. I desire to emphasize the danger of persisting in a carbohydrate-free diet when diabetic coma is threatened. The administration of the carbohydrates is often really temporarily life-saving where the excretion of acetone and diacetic acid persists on a rigid diet.

DISCUSSION.

DR. FUTCHER.—In regard to the boy with diabetic coma, I am struck with the difference in his condition now from that at noon to-day. He was then very deeply comatose and oblivious to his surroundings, so much so that an intravenous infusion of a solution of sodium bicarbonate was administered without local anæsthesia. His respirations were also of the characteristic "air-hunger" type. He is now decidedly better and shows well the beneficial effects of the antacid treatment. The patient had previously been getting moderate amounts of sodium bicarbonate, but with the onset of the coma symptoms the alkali had to be pushed, as per mouth and rectum the patient could not take enough to neutralize the beta-oxybutyric acid. As high as a 2 per cent solution of bicarbonate of soda has been given intravenously in these cases, but we prefer to give a 1 per cent solution in normal salt solution, as a too strong solution in our experience has embarrassed the heart's action in some cases.

There is no question as to the ultimate outcome in this case. The patient will no doubt relapse and die in coma within the next few days, although I have seen cases with as deep coma in Naunyn's clinic that did not relapse for three weeks or more.

In regard to the case of gout Dr. Barker has shown, it may be of interest to refer to some very important work that has been done in the Laboratory of Physiological Chemistry here by Dr. Jones and Messrs. Partridge and Winternitz, and by Schittenhelm and Burian in Germany. It has been found that specific ferments play a most important part in the intermediary metabolism of the purin bodies. The purin bodies that play a part in human metabolism are uric acid, xanthin, hypoxanthin, guanin, and adenin, the first having the most and the last the least oxygen in the molecule. Jones and Partridge demonstrated that certain glands of animals contain a specific ferment, guanase, which has the power of hydrolysing guanin into xanthin. Jones and Winternitz showed that some of the glands also contain another specific ferment, adenase, which hydrolyses adenin into hypoxanthin. Schittenhelm found that the liver, lungs, spleen, and muscles possess another ferment, which Burian has called xantho-oxidase, which has the power of oxidizing xanthin into uric acid. Still another ferment, nuclease, has been isolated which possesses the power of splitting off the nuclein portion from the nucleo-proteids taken in the food. After this has been effected the various specific ferments then are able by successive stages to convert the purin bodies one into the other.

A discovery of importance is that the liver and other tissues contain a specific ferment called oxidase, which possesses the power of destroying the formed uric acid and oxidizing it into its end products. This latter discovery has a very important bearing on the effect of alcohol on the uric acid excretion when it is taken with a rich proteid diet. It has been shown in Prof. Chittenden's Laboratory, at New Haven, that when an individual is given a purin-free diet and daily uric acid determinations made and then alcohol added to the diet, there is no increase in the uric acid output. When, however, an individual is given a diet rich in purins (nucleo-proteids) the administration of alcohol causes a marked increase in the uric acid output. In other words, alcohol influences only the excretion of the exogenous uric acid. It is well known that alcohol diminishes oxidation in the liver, and in the light of what has been stated above, Chittenden thinks that it is quite possible that the alcohol interferes with the oxidizing action of the special ferment in the liver whose function normally is to destroy the uric acid already formed. Any interference with this action would naturally lead to a greater excretion of uric acid.

The knowledge thus acquired concerning the action of these specific ferments may lead eventually to a better understanding of the metabolic disturbances at the foundation of gout.

THE JOHNS HOPKINS HISTORICAL CLUB.

January 29, 1906.

The Symposium of the Gold-Headed Cane.

History of the Gold-Headed Cane. DR. McCRAE.

Among the many treasures of the College of Physicians in London not the least interesting is that known as the Gold-Headed Cane. This made its appearance in medical circles probably about the year 1689 and for one hundred and thirty-six years was carried by a leading London practitioner, during this time passing through the hands of Radcliffe, Mead, Askew, the two Pitcairns, and Baillie. The shape of the handle of the cane is rather unusual for the time when it was made, as at that period the head of the physician's cane was generally round and contained a cavity in which aromatic substances were carried, the inhaling of which was thought to prevent contagion. The first owner of the cane, Radcliffe, was a man always impatient of convention, and it is possible that he adopted the unusual shape to be different from the rest of the profession. The cane came into possession of the College as a gift from Mrs. Baillie, the widow of the last of the series who carried it.

The book which is known as "The Gold-Headed Cane" is written in the form of what may be termed an autobiography. The cane is represented as giving an account of the lives of the men who carried it and the more interesting events in which they were concerned. The book was published without the author's name, but was written by Dr. William Macmichael (1784-1839). The first edition was published in 1827 and the second in 1828. The third edition, which was published in 1884, was edited by William Munk, and in it many additions were made. The book is written in a chatty, conversational style, deals with many points in the lives of its possessors and also refers to many of the happenings of the times.

The first possessor of the cane, John Radcliffe (1650-1714), is discussed elsewhere. From him the cane passed to Richard Mead (1673-1754), one of the most interesting figures in British medicine. He studied classics at Utrecht, physic at Leyden, where he was a student with Boerhaave, with whom he kept up an intimate friendship, and graduated at Padua in 1695. He settled in London and was shortly afterwards appointed to the staff of St. Thomas' Hospital. He was a great collector of books, prints, pictures, coins, and gems, as well as Oriental, Greek, and Latin manuscripts. In the chapter of the Gold-Headed Cane dealing with his life we are brought into contact with the interesting people of the time—Sir Hans Sloane, who founded the British Museum, Dr. George Cheyne, who pleaded for a simpler life even at that day, Lady Mary Wortley Montague, and the introduction of the inoculation for small-pox. Accounts are given of meetings at Mead's house in Great Ormond Street, where the Children's Hospital now stands, in which Arbuthnot and Pope figure, and also a description of the last illness of Sir Isaac Newton. Medically, Mead was especially interested in snake venoms and had also much to do with the introduction of inoculation for small-pox. It is interesting to remember that he probably had considerable influence on the founding of Guy's Hospital, as he and Guy were great friends and Mead was consulted as to the best way in which Guy could use his fortune for the establishment of a medical charity. Mead was a great patron of literature and art and has been termed the Mæcenas of his day. It is rather a commentary on what makes for fame that Radcliffe, who did comparatively little during his life, is so well remembered through his bequests, while Mead, who did so much during his life, left little behind him by which he is remembered.

From Mead the cane passed to Anthony Askew (1722-1774), a graduate of Cambridge who studied at Leyden and subsequently spent many years in travelling abroad. He settled in London, was attached to St. Bartholomew's Hospital and became a very intimate friend of Mead. He is perhaps better known as a classical scholar than as a physician. He was a great book collector, and it was even said that it was difficult to get into his house on account of the halls being filled with books. Dr. Cushing will speak more especially of his library. After the death of Askew the cane passed into the possession of Dr. William Pitcairn (1711-1791). He belonged to the same family as Archibald Pitcairn, of Edinburgh, who at one time occupied the chair of physic in Leyden, and was a great exponent of the mechanical school of medicine. William Pitcairn studied at Leyden and took his

degree at Rheims. He was associated with St. Bartholomew's Hospital and was president of the College of Physicians for many years. During the latter part of his life he gave up active practice and transferred the cane to his nephew, Dr. David Pitcairn (1749-1809). He was also attached to St. Bartholomew's and is said to have been the first to recognize the relationship between acute rheumatic fever and endocarditis. He died of œdema of the glottis, and the description of his condition is said to be one of the earliest in which the account of an autopsy was given.

From Pitcairn the cane passed into the hands of Matthew Baillie (1761-1823). About this time the cane ceased to be considered a necessary appendage of the physician, and after the death of Baillie in 1823 the cane was presented by his widow to the college, where it was deposited in 1825. At this point the history of the cane as given in the first and second editions of the work comes to an end, but in the third edition the cane is represented as continuing the history of the college and of some of its most prominent members after 1825. There is also a note regarding many of the portraits and busts in the college.

In this hasty review reference has been made to only a few of the many interesting points in the history of the Gold-Headed Cane. It will probably not be possible for all of you to pick up copies, but those of you who read it will find many facts regarding some of our predecessors which will stimulate interest in the history of the profession, one of the objects of this club.

John Radcliffe. DR. OSLER.

Radcliffe is remembered, first by the Gold-Headed Cane, second by never having written a line, and third by the superb monuments which exist to his memory. He was a Yorkshire man, educated at the school at Wakefield. He took his B. A. at Oxford in 1672, and his M. B. in 1675, when he entered on the "physic line" and secured his M. D. three years later. For some years he practiced in Oxford and laid the foundations for his remarkable success.

Radcliffe was characterized by extraordinary shrewdness and wit. One of his most celebrated sayings shows the opinion in which were held the so-called water-casters of his day. These water-casters made the diagnosis of disease from a specimen of the urine, and they still exist in some parts of England. A woman, hearing how celebrated he was, brought Radcliffe a sample of her husband's urine. He was disgusted at being taken for a water-caster and his reply was that if her husband, who was a shoemaker, would fit him for a pair of shoes from a sample of his (Radcliffe's) urine, then would he give her a diagnosis.

In addition to carrying on an active practice he remained interested in his college and became one of its most munificent benefactors. Proceeding to London, Radcliffe became connected with the court circles, and King William liked him, though at times disgusted at his bluntness, as Radcliffe was not always a user of choice and elegant language. He once said to the king, when the latter was suffering from dropsy, that he would not have his two legs for his three kingdoms. On another occasion he said, " if Your Majesty will forbear making long visits to the Earl of Bradford (where, to tell the truth, the King was wont to drink very hard), I'll engage to make you live three or four years longer." Radcliffe was also called in to see Queen Mary, who died of small-pox. He said he had been called in too late. He had much trouble with his royal patients, offending Queen Anne by telling her her trouble was merely the vapours. In the last illustrious council at the time of her death he was summoned, but sent the blunt answer " that he could not come."

Radcliffe had the reputation of being niggardly and penurious. Later in life he found his money had doubled itself from good investments. He saved money with a specific purpose in view. A remarkable document has lately come out at an auction in Yorkshire. It contains his investments and receipts, entered by his secretary, and shows the great skill exercised in his investments.

Radcliffe's character is well given in the Gold-Headed Cane. It says: " Two years after the death of Prince George, when Radcliffe was in his sixtieth year, I was somewhat surprised, one morning after breakfast, to observe him attired with more than ordinary exactness. His full-bottomed wig was dressed with peculiar care; he had put on his best suit of lilac-colored velvet with yellow basket buttons, and his air upon the whole was very commanding. He reminded me very strongly of his appearance some ten or fifteen years before. He had an elevated forehead, hazel eyes, cheeks telling of the good cheer of former days, if anything a little too ruddy; a double chin, a well-formed nose, and a mouth round which generally played an agreeable smile. When he sat in his easy chair, with his right hand expanded, and placed upon his breast, as if meditating a speech, and clearing his voice for the purpose of giving it utterance; his left wearing his glove, and resting on his side immediately above the hilt of his sword, which was a very usual attitude with him, he certainly had a most comely and well-favored appearance." Kneller's portrait in the library at Oxford gives an admirable presentation of him.

Again here is a little fragment worth reading: " Though my life is, I dare say, pretty well known to you, yet I will mention some of the leading circumstances of it, from which perhaps you may be able to derive some instruction. Since I began the study of medicine, I have devoted myself chiefly to a careful examination of the most valuable modern treatises. In this particular I differ, I know, from you, who are a profound scholar; but my books have always been few, though I hope well chosen. When I was at the university, a few vials, a skeleton, and an herbal, chiefly formed my library. By following the dictates of common sense, while I practiced at Oxford after taking my bachelor of medicine's degree, instead of shutting up my patients who were ill of the small-pox, as was done by the Galenists of those days, I gave them air and cooling emulsions, and thus rescued more than a hundred from the grave. I have always attempted to discountenance the attempts of quacks and intermeddlers in physic, and by the help of Providence I have succeeded most wonderfully. My good Dr. Mead, you must consider this conversation as quite confidential, and if I mention anything that has the air of boasting, you will reflect that I unbosom myself to a friend, and what I am about to say is for your encouragement." The book further goes on to tell of his practice: " My practice rapidly increased, and I was even credibly informed that Dr. Gibbons, who lived in my neighborhood, got more than one thousand pounds a year by patients whom I really had not time to see, and who had therefore recourse to him."

As to the question why Radcliffe never married, the Gold-Headed Cane states: " You will naturally ask me why I never married: it does not become me to speak of my good or ill fortune in that line, especially now when I ought to recall my thoughts from all such vanities, and when the decays of nature tell me that I have only a short time to live. That time is, I am afraid, barely sufficient to repent me of the idle hours which I have spent in riotous living; for I now feel, in the pain which afflicts my nerves, that I am a martyr to excess, and am afraid that I have been an abettor and encourager of intemperance in others."

On his deathbed Radcliffe is said to have made the following statement, that where, when he first started practicing, he had twenty remedies for one disease, when he finished he had twenty diseases for which there was not a single remedy. He died on the first of November, 1714, three months after the Queen; and it was said that that dread of the populace, and the want of company in the country village, where he had retired, shortened his life.

His fortune, by his will, he left wisely and generously. His Yorkshire estate he left to the Masters and Fellows of University College for ever, in trust, for the foundation of two travelling fellowships which still exist. They are conferred upon men who have taken certain degrees at Oxford, the conditions being that six months of the three years during which the fellowship is held must be spent abroad, and any surplus must be turned in and used by University College. In addition, his will provided £5000 for the enlargement of the buildings of University College, where he himself had been educated; £40,000 for the building of a library, and instructions regarding the purchase of books on medicine and natural history. Some years ago this building became so full that the library was moved, and at the cost of the Drapers Company, of London, £60,000 being spent and a new Radcliffe library built. Then in the fourth place he left £500 annually toward mending the diet of St. Bartholomew's Hospital, the balance of his property being handed to his trustees to do as they saw fit. They built the large Radcliffe Observatory and pay all its expenses, and in 1770 built the Radcliffe Infirmary, paying the major part of its cost.

So there are at least four special foundations connected with his name, all are associated with scientific work, and certainly there is no modern physician with so many large and important monuments. Yet he put no line to paper, but saved with a special object in view. One lesson learned from his life is that if you do not write, make money, and, after you finish, leave it to the Johns Hopkins Trust.

Matthew Baillie. Dr. Futcher.

Matthew Baillie was the last possessor of the Gold-Headed Cane, having received it from the younger Pitcairn. He was a Scot, his father being the Rev. James Baillie, who traced his descent from the patriot William Wallace. His mother was Dorothea, the sister of John and William Hunter, the celebrated anatomists. Matthew Baillie was born at Shots, in Lanarkshire, in 1761. Soon after his birth his father moved to Bothwell, thence to Hamilton, and later to Glasgow where he became Professor of Divinity in the University of Glasgow. He received his early education in the grammar school in Hamilton and later in the University of Glasgow. His first leanings were towards divinity or law, but, owing to the exceptional facilities afforded by the influence of his two illustrious uncles, he eventually took up medicine. It was William Hunter's wish that he should receive his medical education under his own immediate direction, but in order that he might obtain an English degree in medicine, his nephew's limited means made it necessary for him to procure an Oxford "exhibition," which the professors of the University of Glasgow have in their power to bestow on deserving merit. The death of his father in straightened circumstances at this juncture rendered the securing of an "exhibition" more urgent, and it was finally granted him. In 1780, armed with a letter of introduction from his mother to William Hunter, he went to London and thence to Balliol College, Oxford, where he eventually was graduated. Between "terms" he spent his vacations in the Anatomical Theatre and Museum of William Hunter in Windmill Street, London, carrying on anatomical dissections.

Two years after the commencement of his anatomical studies Baillie became a teacher in his uncle's Anatomical Theatre. He had not been thus employed more than twelve months when William Hunter died, bequeathing to him for life the use of his museum, which after his death was to go to the University of Glasgow where it is still deposited. His uncle also left him his Anatomical Theatre and house in Windmill Street and Long Calderwood, the old Hunter estate in Scotland, which he had recently purchased. Baillie at once graciously turned over the latter to John Hunter, whom he considered the rightful owner. William Hunter, although wealthy, left his nephew an annuity of only one hundred pounds, stating his reason for this small bequest "that it was his intention to leave him but little money, as he had derived too much pleasure from making his own fortune to deprive him of doing the same."

Two years after William Hunter's death, Baillie, associated with Mr. Cruickshank, gave his first course of anatomical lectures, thus undertaking, in his twenty-second year, the arduous task of filling his uncle's place. It is interesting to note that the number of students did not diminish.

During the years he was particularly interested in normal anatomy and subsequently during his practice as a physician. Baillie lost no opportunity of preserving for a private collection specimens of diseased organs. This museum consisted upwards of 1000 specimens which were nearly all prepared with his own hands. Three years before his death he presented this collection to the Royal College of Physicians with £400 for the purpose of keeping it in a proper state of preservation.

Up to 1787 Baillie devoted almost his entire time to teaching. In this year he took his doctor's degree at Oxford, was elected a Fellow of the Royal College of Physicians and was appointed a physician to St. George's Hospital, the institution in which his uncle was at that time such a shining light. He was elected a Fellow of the Royal Society in 1789. After 1787, Baillie from year to year gradually gave more and more time to practice. His interest in pathology was a marked feature of this period of his life. The museums of the two Hunters afforded him abundant opportunity for the study of morbid lesions and he made admirable use of the specimens they contained. The pathological data derived from these sources as well as from the specimen he himself prepared formed the basis of his work entitled " The Morbid Anatomy of Some of the Most Important Parts of the Human Body," first published in 1795, and constituting his most important contribution to medical literature. This was really an epoch-making work, for, although it was ante-dated by the morbid anatomies of Morgagni and Bonetus, the morbid descriptions in the works of the latter were difficult to get at, owing to their being masked by diffuse clinical descriptions. Baillie was the first to publish, in any language, a work devoted exclusively to the description of morbid processes. He is credited with being the first to describe the simple round ulcer of the stomach and also the morbid appearances of cirrhosis of the liver, although he did not fully recognize their significance in either instance. He is said to have been the first to describe typhoid ulcers, although Thomas Willis has been accorded this honor by some.

In 1799, four years after the appearance of his Morbid Anatomy, he published a volume of engravings for its elucidation. The work is entitled " A Series of Engravings Representing Every Diseased Change of Structure to which the Internal and more Important Parts of the Body are Subject." These superb engravings were made by William Clift, who devoted so much time and care to the preservation of John Hunter's Museum and who was afterwards Conservator of the Museum of the College of Surgeons. It is interesting to note that Baillie's two most important works were published before he was thirty-eight years of age, his Morbid Anatomy appearing when he was thirty-four.

Baillie became so engrossed in private practice that he was forced in 1799 to give up all his teaching. He took a house in fashionable Grosvenor Street and from this time on was the leading consultant in London, and his advice was sought alike by the laity and his fellow practitioners. Some conception of how busy a man he was may be obtained from an account of his daily routine. From 6 a. m. till 8.30 a. m. he was occupied with letters; from 8.30 until 10.30, excepting a short interval for breakfast, he received patients at his own house; and afterwards until 6 p. m., he was out seeing patients chiefly in consultation. From 6 p. m. until 8 p. m. was devoted to dinner and his family, after which, often until a late hour, he returned to outdoor visiting. His practice yielded him £10,000 annually, a fair sum considering that a guinea was the regulation consultation fee. For ten years he was physician extraordinary to King George III and his family and found the visits to Oxford a temporary respite from his arduous daily routine.

Besides the two great works already mentioned, Baillie at intervals published papers on miscellaneous medical subjects in the Transactions of the Royal Society, of the Society for the Improvement of Medical and Surgical Knowledge, and of the College of Physicians, all of which were edited by James Wardrop and published in two volumes in 1825. These contain reports of many interesting cases.

Of the various possessors of the Gold-Headed Cane, Baillie contributed more towards the advancement of the science of medicine than any of the others. His Morbid Anatomy was in many ways an epoch-making work and was a model of conciseness and of accuracy in observation. He belonged to a most talented family. He was the nephew of the two Hunters, and Joanna Baillie, the well-known poetess, was his sister.

Baillie's arduous practice gradually began to tell upon his health. He developed a tracheal affection, for which he visited Tunbridge Wells with some relief. His health seemed permanently undermined, however, and he eventually retired with his family to his country place in Gloucestershire where he died of phthisis on September 23, 1823, at the age of 62.

The Holders of the Gold-Headed Cane as Book Collectors. Dr. Cushing.

Were an uninformed gathering asked, "Which of these five or six men, whose names Dr. McCrae has written upon the board, is most likely to have been a lover of books?" from many the answer doubtless would be, "Radcliffe." But he was, as Dr. Osler has told you, in no sense a scholarly man. The real Radcliffe is well portrayed in Mat Prior's jingle—

> I sent for Dr. Radcliffe: was so ill,
> That other doctors gave me over;
> He felt my pulse, prescribed his pill,
> And I was likely to recover.
>
> But when the wit began to wheeze,
> And wine had warmed the politician,
> Cured yesterday of my disease,
> I died last night of my physician.

He is said to have boasted that a few vials, a skeleton and an herbal constituted his library; and yet in two ways Radcliffe showed the respect that he actually held for the learning to which he himself was a stranger. One was by the magnificent use that he made of his fortune; and though one of the wits of the day said that it would be as appropriate for a eunuch to found a seraglio as for Radcliffe to establish a library, still you have learned from what has already been said how much foresight he showed in the final disposition of his accumulations: the other evidence of his respect for learning was his appreciation of the scholarship shown by his successor, Mead. For it is told that when, early in their acquaintance, he found Mead sitting in his library and reading Hippocrates, he ejaculated, "What, my young friend, do you read Hippocrates in the original language? Well, take my word for it, when I am dead you will occupy the throne of physic in this great town." His vanity must have been tickled by Mead's suave reply that his Empire, like Alexander's, would have to be divided amongst many. And though, in a sense, it did become divided, yet Mead ruled over much of it, and as one of the most remarkable figures in English medicine. He had been educated in Leyden, and, it will be remembered, was Boerhaave's house companion and lifelong friend.

Though it is not my purpose to dwell at any length on his fame as a physician, I wish to show these volumes—Mead's more important contributions to Medicine—as an evidence of his literary activity; for he more than any other of the carriers of the Cane, possibly excepting Baillie, has left us publications of value. The first of these, A Mechanical Account of Poisons, was printed in 1702 while Mead was still a young man. In the first of the four essays that constitute the work he settles the long-disputed point as to whether the viper emits an actual poison with its bite.

De Imperio Solis ac Lunae in Corpora Humana, his second work, appeared soon after, in 1704, and this particular copy was presented by Mead to John, Earl of Orrery, and you may see by the inscription what a careful penman was the author. It is rather a philosophical treatise than a work of medical value, and there seems to be little doubt but that he was led to propound the views herein expressed by the influence of his friend, Sir Isaac Newton, whose deductions regarding the tides had just been brought forth.

The first edition of his Discourse concerning Pestilential Contagion, etc., was published in 1720—this copy is the eighth edition, dated only two years later—and here begin a series of works dealing with infectious diseases and their prevention: and there can be little doubt but that, occupying the position he did, Mead's common-sense attitude toward contagion must have been a power for good. Then, even more than now, people did not take easily to the idea of contagion, and a previous owner has bound up in these covers together with Mead's discourse two other tracts—"The Plague no Contagious Disease" and "The Rise and Fall of Pestilential Contagion"—by anonymous authors, of course.

This paragraph is a sample of Mead's chapter on prevention, and it is upon prevention that he chiefly dwells—"As for *Houses,* the first Care ought to be to keep them *clean;* for as *Nastiness* is a great Source of *Infection,* so *Cleanliness* is the greatest Preservative; which shows us the true Reason, why the *Poor* are most obnoxious to *Contagious Diseases.* It is re-marked of the *Persians,* that though their Country is surrounded every Year with the *Plague,* they seldom or never suffer anything by it themselves; and it is likewise known, that they are the most *cleanly* People of any in the World, and that many among them make it a great part of their religion to remove *Filthiness* and *Nusances* of every Kind from all Places about their Cities and Dwellings."

And, again, when speaking of the necessity of segregating the sick, and of burning their houses after they have been re-moved; " And after this, all possible Care ought still to be taken to remove whatever Causes are found to breed and pro-mote *Contagion.* In order to do this, the *Overseers* of the Poor (who might be assisted herein by other Officers) should visit the Dwellings of all the meaner sort of the Inhabitants, and where they find them *stifled up too close* and *nasty,* should lessen their Number by sending some into better Lodgings, and should take Care, by all manner of Provision and En-couragement, to make them more *cleanly* and *sweet.* No good work carries its own Reward with it so much as this kind of *Charity.*" And this at a time when pestilence was largely regarded as heaven-born.

His Harveian Oration delivered in 1724 shows where his tastes were carrying him, for it deals with the coins which were struck off by the Smyrnæans in honor of physicians.

In 1744 was published this, A Discourse on the Plague, and three years later his work, De Variolis et Morbillis, &c.

A short essay entitled Medica Sacra, a commentary on the diseases mentioned in the Bible and those of biblical heroes, was printed in London, 1749. In it he comments interestingly upon the maladies, among others, of Herod and Job and Saul and "Nabuchodonosor" upon leprosy, paralysis, lunacy, the bloody sweat of Christ, &c., &c.

This final volume, also from Orrery's library, is the author-ized translation of Mead's Monita et Præcepta Medica, his last work, published only a few years before his death, and containing notes and observations from past life upon many diseases, their symptomatology, treatment, &c. There are many excellent chapters: his description of scurvy, for ex-ample, with its prevention and therapy could well supplant that in many a modern text-book.

And so much for his own few writings: but of Mead and the writings of others the story is a far longer one, for there is hardly a more lustrous name in bibliophilic annals. His collections—and not only of books, but of coins, of ceramics, of gems, of pictures, of statuary, of antiquities, and I know not what all—gave him a world-wide reputation that outshone even the repute of his professional attainments. He was everywhere recognized as the Mæcenas of his day, and in this role it is hard to find his peer in history. His house, as Benj. Ward Richardson says, was one great museum and treasury of learning and science. This house stood in Great Ormond Street, the present site of the Hospital for Children, and ow-ing to Mead's express desire that his collections should be dispersed at his death, we now know something of the treas-ures, especially in book form, that it contained. For this

catalogue—Bibliotheca Meadiana—issued by Samuel Baker, the auctioneer, contains the list of the more important vol-umes that passed under the hammer at Covent Gardens be-tween Nov. 18th, 1754, and the following April 7th—a sale extending over 28 days, and bringing in a total sum that would be large even for these extravagant days when million-aires choose to gather in choice volumes unto themselves.

The first day's sale is taken up almost entirely with the disposal of the Bibles and New Testaments. Among these is the Biblia Sacra ex Pagnini translatione, per Mich. Vil-lanovanum (Servetus), bringing only £7—for the prices have all been marked in, on the margin, by the original possessor of this catalogue—and the two-volume Editio Princeps of the Latin Bible, 1462, bringing only £28. Later on, to pick out a few interesting items, we find on the sixth day among eight copies of Pliny's Natural History, which were sold, that the King of France brought the Editio Princeps, Venet op. Spiram, 1469, for something over £16, while Mr. Willock, one of Mead's friends, bought the next item, an illuminated copy of 1472, for £18 18s. Catesby's Natural History of Carolina, " cuts most beautifully coloured by himself " brings £20 19s. 6d.; Winstanley's Prospects of Andley End goes for £50; the rare and first edition of Il Decamerone di Boc-cacio for £16 16s.; Cæsar's Commentaries, Ed. princeps, Rome, 1469, for a song; then there are manuscripts and folios and books of all kinds and descriptions, but mostly rare; Vesalius' Epitome of the Fabrica, Basle, 1543, unobtainable now, brought £8 12s. 6d.; the Aldine Petrarch of 1501 on vellum; Olivet's Cicero, purchased by Askew for £14 14s., to be sold again at the sale of the latter's books for £36 18s.; and on the last day's sale we find a book partly in manuscript sell-ing for £8 18s. 6d., entitled Servetus de Trinitate. It was at some earlier period that "the scarce and perhaps the only copy of Servetus' last book passed from the shelves of one English worthy (Mead) to those of his friend, M. de Boze." The amount of all the sales brought over £16,000; this in-cludes the pictures, antiquities, &c.

In his history of the disease "Bibliomania," Dibdin says that Mead died of the complaint, one of its most splendid victims, and adds in a foot-note:

" It is almost impossible to dwell on the memory of this Great Man without emotions of delight—whether we consider him as an eminent physician, a friend to literature, or a collector of books, pictures, and coins. Benevolence, magnanimity, and erudi-tion were the striking features of his character: his house was the general receptacle of men of genius and talent, and of every-thing beautiful, precious, or rare. His curiosities, whether books, or coins, or pictures, were freely laid open to the public; and the enterprising student, and experienced antiquary, alike found amusement and a courteous reception. He was known to all foreigners of intellectual distinction, and corresponded both with the artisan and the potentate. The great patron of literature, and the leader of his profession (which he practised with a success unknown before), it was hardly possible for unbefriended merit, if properly introduced to him, to depart unrewarded. The clergy, and in general, all men of learning, received his advice *gratui-tously:* and his doors were open every morning to the *most indi-gent,* whom he frequently assisted with money. Although his income, from his professional practise, was very considerable, he died by no means a rich man—so large were the sums which he devoted to the encouragement of literature and the fine arts! "

Anthony Askew was of the same feather with Mead, with like mind, like learning, and the same passion for collecting. Having taken his medical degree at Cambridge and having passed the usual year in study at Leyden, instead of returning to London he travelled widely, and during the three years thus spent, laid the foundation of the library that afterwards became so celebrated. He naturally acquired the warm friendship of Mead, who, we are told, supported him by a sort of paternal zeal; nor did he find in his protege an ungrateful son. Though he never attained to the position in the community held by Mead as a patron of the fine arts in general, his library became perhaps even more widely renowned than that of his predecessor.

Like Mead's, Askew's collection of books was dispersed at auction after his death, and turning the leaves of this catalogue issued by Baker and Leigh—Bibliotheca Askeviana sive Catalogus Librorum Rarissimorum Antonii Askew, M. D.— will enable you to gather some idea of the volumes "rarissimorum" which were knocked down during the nineteen days following February 12, 1775, an occasion memorable in the records of such transactions.

The possessor of this catalogue, too, has carefully marked on the margins the prices bid for the various items, and in many cases the purchaser thereof; and we find "The King," "King of France," "De Bure," "British Museum," and others, including "Wm. Hunter" as purchasers of some of the more notable volumes. We can imagine the many-sided one of the brothers Hunter, the "man mid-wife," rather dandified in person when contrasted with John, sitting at the sale and competing for the possession of books with the royal agents of England and France. And many of the choicer volumes he secured, and they to-day are lying little appreciated and as yet uncatalogued among the treasures that he bequeathed to the University of Glasgow at his death. Mead, Askew, and Wm. Hunter as bibliophiles were cut from the same cloth, and had Hunter been a physician he would have been the natural carrier of the Cane after Askew. Dr. Futcher, however, has told us how the Cane came subsequently into the possession of the Hunter family through Baillie.

Possibly the largest sums offered for any of the items are those under Hunter's name; for example,

817   Anthologia Græca, EDITIO PRINCEPS, IMPRESS. IN MEMBRANA, ET IN LITERIS CAPITALIBUS, compact, in corio turcico, cum foliis deauratis, Florent. ap. Laur. de Alop. 1494, £28-7-0.

1415 Diogenes Laertii Vitæ Philosophorum, Latiné, EDITIO PRINCEPS, exemplar pulcherrimum, compact, in corio turcico, cum foliis deauratis, Venet. ap. Jensen, 1475, £6-6-0.

1876 Homeri Batrachomiomachia, Græcé, EDITIO PRINCIPS, compact, in corio turcico, cum foliis deauratis, Venet, ap. Laonicum Cretensem, 1486, £14-14-0. In this book is this note—This book is so extremely rare that I never saw any other copy of it, except that of

Mons. de Boze, who told me he gave 650 Livres for it. Mr. Smith, our Consul at Venice, wrote me word that he had purchased a copy, but that it was imperfect, &c.

2656 Platonis Opera, Græcé, IMPRESS. IN MEMBRANA, 2 vol. compact in corio turcico, cum foliis deauratis, Ven. ap. Ald., 1513, £55-13-0.

3337 Terentianus Maurus de Litteris, Syllabis & Metris Horatii, EDITIO PRINCEPS, & exemplar pulcherrimum Mediolan per Ulder. Scinzenler, 1497, £12-12-0. In this book is this note—This is judged to be the only copy of this edition in England, if not in the whole world.—If so, it is worth any money.—Dr. Askew could find no copy in his travels over Europe, though he made it his earnest and particular search in every library which he had an opportunity of consulting. —JOHN TAYLOR, Cantabrig.

But I cannot do better than to read again from Dibdin, who sighs with grief of heart over such a victim of the Bibliomania as Askew. He says:

"Dr. Anthony Askew had eminently distinguished himself by a refined taste, a sound knowledge, and an indefatigable research relating to everything connected with Grecian and Roman literature. It was to be expected, even during his life, as he was possessed of sufficient means to gratify himself with what was rare, curious and beautiful in literature and the fine arts, that the public would, one day, be benefited by such pursuits: especially as he had expressed a wish that his treasures might be unreservedly submitted to sale, after his decease. In this wish the Doctor was not singular. Many eminent collectors had indulged it before him: and, to my knowledge, many modern ones still indulge it.

"We are told by the compiler of the catalogue that it was thought unnecessary to say much with respect to this Library of the late Dr. Anthony Askew, as the Collector and Collection were so well known in almost all parts of Europe. Afterwards it is observed that "The books in general are in very fine condition, many of them bound in morocco, and Russia leather, with gilt leaves." "To give a particular account," continues the compiler, "of the many scarce editions of books in this catalogue would be almost endless, therefore the first editions of the Classics, and some extremely rare books are chiefly noticed. The catalogue, without any doubt, contains the best, rarest, and most valuable collection of GREEK and LATIN BOOKS that were ever sold in England." This account is not overcharged. The collection, in regard to Greek and Roman literature, was unique in its day.

The late worthy and learned Mr. M. Cracherode, whose library now forms one of the most splendid acquisitions of the British Museum, and whose bequest of it will immortalize his memory, was also among the "Emptores literarii" at this renowned sale. He had enriched his collection with many Exemplar Askewianum; and, in his latter days, used to elevate his hands and eyes, and exclaim against the prices now offered for EDITIONES PRINCIPES!

The fact is, Dr. Askew's sale has been considered a sort of aera in bibliography. Since that period, rare and curious books in Greek and Latin literature have been greedily sought after, and obtained at most extravagant prices. It is very well for a veteran in bibliography, as was Mr. Cracherode, or as are Mr. Wodhull and Dr. Gosset, whose collections were formed in the days of Gaignat, Askew, Duke de la Valliere, and Lamoignon— it is very well for such gentlemen to declaim against modern prices! But what is to be done? Books grow scarcer every day, and the love of literature, and of possessing rare and interesting works, increases in an equal ratio. Hungry bibliographers meet, at sales, with well furnished purses, and are resolved upon sumptuous fare. Thus the hammer *vibrates*, after a bidding of *Forty pounds*, where formerly it used regularly to *fall* at *Four!*

And with Askew ends Bibliomania so far as it is concerned with the peripatetic life of the Gold-Headed Cane: and perhaps this was none the worse for the patients and certainly it was the better for the purses of the succeeding owners. But for one, I would have wished to see the Cane follow the books and go to William Hunter along with the Aldine Plato for which he paid so dear. Had this happened so, the Cane would probably have ended its active life with Baillie even as it did.

THE DEATH OF JOHN BRUCE MacCALLUM.

A large number of the members of the Medical Faculty of the Johns Hopkins University gathered at the Physiological Building April 11 to take action upon the death of Dr. John Bruce MacCallum, a graduate in medicine of the University, and formerly Assistant in Anatomy, who died on April 6, 1906, at Berkeley, California, while holding the position of Assistant Professor of Physiology in the University of California. The meeting was addressed by Professors Welch and Barker, who gave an account of the career and work of Dr. MacCallum, and expressed their high appreciation of his ability and personal qualities. The following minute, presented by Dr. Lewis, was then adopted:

"John Bruce MacCallum was, to his many friends, an ideal type of man, loved by his associates for his modest, unselfish, and beautiful character, admired by his fellow workers for his ability to solve scientific problems and his talent in presenting them by illustration and description. He possessed the rare combination of artistic tastes and a compelling love for scientific work.

"He entered this Medical School at the age of 20, and pursued with ease his required work for the medical degree. At the same time he began his career as an anatomist by the publication of several scientific papers. His work during the first two years of this period on the histogenesis of heart-muscle and his even more noteworthy contribution to the architecture of the muscular walls of the heart, established at once his position as a productive scientist.

"After his graduation in 1900 he became Assistant in Anatomy, entering a field especially suited to his abilities. He possessed the rare power of attacking problems by the direct method and arriving at their solution with a minimum of labor and time. With the breaking down of his health in the succeeding year and his enforced residence in Colorado and then in California, anatomy lost and ardent disciple in one who would have done much to farther its progress. Undaunted by ill health, he entered the department of Physiology in the University of California, and pursued with credit scientific work in this new field. Most men would have sought health; but MacCallum could not, from his very nature, forego his ideal of a scientific career. His untimely death at the age of 29 is indeed a most grievous loss to his family and friends, and to the science of this country."

NOTES ON NEW BOOKS.

A Text-Book of Pharmacology and Therapeutics, or the Action of Drugs in Health and Disease. By ARTHUR R. CUSHNY, M. A., M. D., Aberd.; Professor of Pharmacology in the University College, London, Eng.; formerly Professor of Materia Medica and Therapeutics in the University of Michigan; Thompson Fellow in the University of Aberdeen, and Assistant in the Pharmacological Institute of the University of Strassburg. Fourth Edition, thoroughly revised. Illustrated with fifty-two engravings. (*Philadelphia and New York: Lea Brothers & Co., 1906.*)

This admirable treatise is prefaced by an introduction of twenty-four pages, in which are discussed a number of questions of practical and theoretical importance. Here are found definitions of such terms as stimulation, depression, irritation, remote, local and general action, elective affinity of drugs, protoplasm poison, pharmacopœial preparations, etc.

A very conservative position is taken in respect to the mode of action of drugs. The great majority of drugs are stated "to act through their *chemical* affinity for certain forms of living matter." "They probably form temporary combinations with some forms of protoplasm and alter the function of all cells which contain these forms." Elective affinity and other points of theoretical importance are well illustrated.

In referring to certain present-day researches, the author says: "A great deal of time and energy has been devoted to an attempt to bring the effects in the organism of certain metals (notably the alkalies) into relation with their atomic weights, their valency, electrical charges, and other properties, but no results are to be expected from these researches, so long as the ordinary chemical reactions of these bodies can only be formulated to a limited extent and imperfectly from such considerations."

That troublesome and complex question—the relation of chemical composition to pharmacological action—is treated with justice. In the body of the work the subject is again taken up in the discussion of narcotics and antiseptics, and the influence of substitution, isomerism, etc., is illustrated. All that is known in this field enables us to say nothing more than that the interaction of drugs with the constituents of protoplasm calls into play the whole range of their *constitutive* properties (not to mention properties that could be classed under other heads). Such a position makes it clear why we have no general theory of toxic or pharmacological action that is worthy of serious consideration. It is the opinion of some chemists that *constitutive* properties can never be completely represented by a general scheme, "for such is contradictory to their nature." Ostwald, for example, declares this to hold particularly for the affinity coefficients, " for in them the whole variety of nature asserts itself within the framework of great and general regularities and produces the finest individualization."

The classification of drugs adopted in this volume is that of Buchheim and Schmiedeberg, with such alterations as are inevitably induced by the personal equation. Part I deals of organic substances which are characterized chiefly by their local action. Here are included such agents as skin irritants, vegetable purgatives and anthelmintics. Part II deals of organic substances characterized chiefly by their action after absorption. Under this heading fall many of the most important classes of drugs used in medicine, as, for example, the anæsthetics, narcotics, antiseptics, the antipyretics, and special alkaloids, such as the mydriatics. Part III treats of combinations of the alkalis, alkaline earths, acids and allied bodies; Part IV, of the heavy metals; Part V, of ferments, secretions and toxalbumins; and Part VI, finally, of menstrua and mechanical remedies.

To undertake the task of writing a comprehensive treatise on pharmacology calls for courage; actually to complete the enterprise, requires also sound judgment, industry and learning. All of the qualities have been manifested by the author of this treatise. No teacher can read the articles on the action of alcohol, ether and chloroform, for example, without a feeling of gratitude toward Professor Cushny for presenting to medical students so good a digest of these topics. There is every evidence throughout the book that its presentations are based on first-hand knowledge of original papers and monographs of importance. More than this, Cushny's activity as an investigator has qualified him in an eminent degree to sift the wheat from the chaff. The field covered is so wide, however, that it is not possible for one man to effect this sifting to the satisfaction of everyone. In the opinion of the reviewer, Part III, which takes up the question of the action of electrolytes (salt action, action of acids, etc.) should be carefully revised in a future edition.

In this section the principles of physical chemistry find their biological applications. Unless an author exercise the greatest care in the presentation of the newer knowledge, the reader is likely to carry away the impression that an ion *as such* is a *free* agent, that, electrically charged though it be, it owes allegiance neither to the molecules of the solvent, nor to the ions, to the atoms, or to the molecules of protoplasm, and that it nevertheless can produce marvellous pharmacological effects. The sentence, "some acids owe their activity in the organism almost entirely to their acidity, *i. e.*, to the hydrogen ion, which is much more powerful than the potassium ion, but otherwise stands on the same plane with it," is a case in point.

It was at one time the custom of physical chemists to single out the hydrogen ion of a given acid as the active agent in the inversion of sugars and in the saponification of esters, and to speak of it as acting "catalytically," but a more careful study of the phenomena has induced later writers to be more guarded in their language. van't Hoff uses such guarded phrases as "if the assumption be made that here the positive hydrogen ion is the essentially active agent, then the process would go as follows." Numerous hypotheses are now on the field. The Traube-Poynting theory of the action of acids as inverting agents makes but little use of the conception of "free" ions in the sense of Arrhenius.

To single out one ion of a compound as the important pharmacological agent is to offer an illusive appearance of explaining the whole matter. The case here is not comparable to that of a series of tartrates, in all of which the rotatory activity is confined to the tartrate ion or to a series of colored salts whose color is due to a common ion. To speak of the hydrogen ion as possessed of proteid precipitating powers (Pauli and others) is to center attention solely on the electrical or dynamical aspect of the reaction and to neglect the concomitant interchanges or linkages of chemical units.

If Professor Cushny believes it to be true (p. 485) that "when KHO comes in contact with a mucous membrane, the molecule does not act as such, but the effects are due to the HO ion, and to a less extent to the K ion," he should also cite cases of caustic action where the same line of argument shows that the undissociated molecules and not the ions are the active agents. Thus, Dreser (1899) in studying the caustic action of aqueous solutions of salicylic acid on the fins of fishes found that equi-molecular (and therefore more strongly dissociated) solutions of hydrochloric acid had no effect, while the salicylic acid caused a white opaque eschar to appear. From this negative result with hydrochloric acid the inference is drawn that hydrogen ions which are present in larger numbers in solutions of this acid cannot be the cause of the etching effect. Similarly, by noting the absence of all caustic action when a highly dissociated solution of sodium salicylate was applied, Dreser concluded that the caustic action of salicylic acid is probably (*vermuthlich*) to be referred to the undissociated molecules and not to the ions.

On page 484 we read: "Cyanide of potassium is said to possess a very poisonous action, but this is due not to the molecule of KCN, as such but to the CN ion which forms from it in solution."

Let us assume for the moment that it can be proved that the toxic action of KCN and of HCN is due to the CN *ion*. Then here also should be cited cases which show that similarly acting and highly poisonous substances act more powerfully in proportion, as they are not dissociated. Thus, hydrazoic acid, HN_3, is intensely poisonous and closely similar in its action to hydrocyanic acid. Like this acid it is feebly dissociated, having only about one-seventieth the avidity of hydrochloric acid. Its sodium

salt is completely dissociated into the ions, $||$ $\substack{N \\ >N-}$ and Na

at the concentrations employed in experimental work. The ions

of the acid are the trinitrogen ion, $||$ $\substack{N \\ >N-}$ and the hydrogen

ion, H. If the toxic action of this deadly acid resides solely or mainly in the *trinitrogen ion* we should expect those of its compounds to be most poisonous which offer the largest percentage of this ion in any given solution. This is not the case. Smith and Wolf have found that three cubic centimeters of a one per cent solution of the acid injected into the marginal vein of a rabbit's ear causes death instantly, while the same quantity of the sodium salt given under like conditions produces only a partial paralysis from which the animal recovers after a few hours. It will be seen then that the intense action of hydrazoic acid as compared with that of the more completely ionized sodium salt cannot be referred solely to the trinitrogen ion. Indeed, its action would appear to be more intense in proportion, as it is not dissociated into its ions. It is at least made evident by such examples that ionization is not the only factor to be considered in explaining the toxic action of electrolytes.

Recent papers on the precipitation of proteids and other colloids by acids and salts of various kinds show that increasingly complicated hypotheses are needed to uphold the notion that one species of ions is inherently endowed by virtue of positive charges, with the power to coagulate proteids while another species has the power to prevent coagulation. It is assumed, but not proved, by these writers that electrical forces alone are concerned in precipitation and in solution. Unless a biological chemical reaction can be followed in all its details, both in a dynamic and in a strictly chemical or stœchiometric way, as for example, in the oxidation of ferrous chloride by chlorine, it gives a misleading impression of accuracy to use terms that are not applicable until all of these conditions have been realized.

The above remarks are made rather to call attention to the difficulties encountered in a new field than to criticise our author. We look forward to a later edition of this treatise in which the divergent views in regard to ionic actions in pharmacology shall all receive due consideration. Take it all in all, there is no treatise on pharmacology in any language that we should prefer to see in the hands of students or other readers of medical works.

JOHN J. ABEL.

Physical Diagnosis. By EGBERT LE FEVRE, M. D., Professor of Clinical Medicine and Associate Professor of Therapeutics in the University and Bellevue Hospital Medical College. Second Edition. (*Philadelphia and New York: Lea Brothers & Co., 1905.*)

In form this is a workmanlike little book, compact in text, well bound, though not without eccentricity in the distribution of its illustrations. In substance it has an unusual virtue in that it lays large emphasis on physical variations which are within the normal. Furthermore the author, realizing in how far physical diagnosis is a craft, does not attempt much description of what needs to be actually heard or seen, but wisely confines himself to a discussion of such findings. He thus makes his book deliberative, as it should be.

Yet one can but feel that the volume is over-classified. It runs constantly to headings and sub-headings, with a resultant lack of proportion. Helped by a table of easy distinctions the student will diagnose many cases as syphilis of the lung; pneumothorax will figure in his records more actively than in those of the wary; and he cannot but be further misled by a neat rule to the effect that the œdema of cardiac disease begins in the feet, whereas that of kidney conditions appears first in the face (p. 248). There are, too, some omissions. Sub-phrenic abscess is not treated, except by a casual word in the discussion of pleurisy with effusion.

Nevertheless, the common physical signs, the important physical signs, are, on the whole, sharply and practically caught. But the work is, like many American text-books, sufficient unto itself, that is to say without references or apparent evidence of their use; and it fails of that more stimulating influence which comes from new facts, or from old facts well put.

F. P. R.

Differential Diagnosis and Treatment of Disease. A Text-Book for Practitioners and Advanced Students. By AUGUSTUS CAILLÉ, M. D. (*New York and London: D. Appleton & Company, 1906.*)

In attempting to include in one volume a complete consideration of the diagnosis and treatment of disease the author has undertaken the impossible. There is no need in medical literature of to-day of a hand-book for the family physician, and yet of necessity, a treatise of such scope in such compass must resolve itself into a work of this character. As such it is a success.

Surgical Diagnosis. A Manual for Students and Practitioners. By ALBERT A. BERG, M. D., Adjunct Attending Surgeon to The Mount Sinai Hospital, New York. (*New York and Philadelphia: Lea Brothers & Co., 1905.*)

This volume is a contribution to the large and constantly increasing class of surgical text-books which aims to present the essential diagnostic points of surgery in a compact form; such books are usually little more than surgical catalogues whose perusal is consequently rather uninteresting. The necessary brevity makes such a book unsatisfactory to students enjoying the advantages of a large clinic while the same quality results in unreliable guidance for practitioners who are dependent on a considerable degree upon text books as a substitute for clinical experience. There is, however, a certain value in such books inasmuch as they present the possibilities briefly; the present volume shares this value alike with other books of the class. The book is full of illustrations, the author having wisely chosen most of them from the standard text-books, and there is the usual number of X-ray pictures whose reproduction is generally unsatisfactory. The author insists frequently upon the use of the more recent methods of diagnosis as tuberculin, X-ray pictures in bone lesions and location of foreign bodies, the cystoscope in disease of the kidney and ureter, etc.; the entire book is devoted to diagnosis and no discussion of surgical therapy is presented. The book is printed clearly, contains few typographical errors and is well bound. There is little to distinguish this volume from its kind; it shares the value and also the faults common to text books of this class.

A System of Physiologic Therapeutics. Edited by SOLOMON SOLIS COHEN, A. M., M. D. Vol. XI.

This volume, which ends the author's " System of Physiologic Therapeutics," deals entirely with the newer methods of therapy.

While this volume deals with subjects which have not been entirely worked out, yet the authors of the various special articles have been conservative in the treatment of their themes.

Serum and Organotherapy are taken up and discussed in detail. The authors, while discussing all important matters, have made no recommendations that have not been substantiated by the test of time.

The section on Radium, Thorium, and Radio-activity is of especial interest. The author has given us a brief but comprehensive outline of the various kinds of radio-activity and their therapeutic effects. The literature on radio-activity has been reviewed and the reader thus gets a good working knowledge of the subject. This section is of especial value in that it has been treated in a conservative way. Radium is not exploited as a universal panacea for all known ills.

Methods of Organic Analysis. By HENRY C. SHERMAN, Ph. D., Adjunct Professor of Analytical Chemistry in Columbia University. (*New York: The MacMillan Co., 1905.*)

The preface states that the purpose of the book is to give a connected introductory training in organic analysis, especially as applied to plant and animal substances and their manufactured products. No attempt is made to touch upon all important branches of his subject but representative topics are treated in considerable detail with reference both to analytical methods and to the interpretation of results. The book is primarily intended for the use of third year students in the School of Chemistry, Columbia University. The author has succeeded in the task which he has outlined for himself. The arrangement of the book and the clear presentation of the subject-matter make us hope that the author may in future editions appeal to the interest of a wider circle of readers. Some of the chapters ought to be treated more in detail. For instance, the space allotted to the proteids seems inadequate and the newer methods of proteid analysis and their results are omitted. It is a valuable feature of the book that the author appends a number of selected references to each chapter.

S. A.

BOOKS RECEIVED.

Progressive Medicine. A Quarterly Digest of Advances, Discoveries, and Improvements in the Medical and Surgical Sciences. Edited by Hobart Amory Hare, M. D., assisted by H. R. M. Landis, M. D. Volume 3. September, 1905. 8vo. 298 pages. Lea Brothers and Company, Philadelphia and New York.

A Text-book of Pharmacology and Therapeutics, or the Action of Drugs in Health and Disease. By Arthur R. Cushny, M. A., M. D., Aberd. Fourth edition, thoroughly revised. Illustrated with fifty-two engravings. 1906. 8vo. 752 pages. Lea Brothers & Co., Philadelphia and New York.

The Surgical Assistant. A Manual for Students, Practitioners, Hospital Internes and Nurses. By Walter M. Brickner, B. S., M. D. With 123 original illustrations. 1905. 8vo. 363 pages. Published by the International Journal of Surgery Co., New York.

The Signs of Internal Disease. With a Brief Consideration of the Principal Symptoms thereof. By Pearce Kintzing, B. Sc., M. D. Illustrated. 1906. 4to. 374 pages. Cleveland Press, Chicago.

Man and His Poisons. A Practical Exposition of the Causes, Symptoms and Treatment of Self-Poisoning. By Albert Abrams, A. M., M.·D. (Heidelberg), F. R. M. S. Illustrated. 1906. 8vo. 268 pages. E. B. Treat & Company, New York.

Progressive Medicine. A Quarterly Digest of Advances, Discoveries, and Improvements in the Medical and Surgical Sciences. Edited by Hobart Amory Hare, M. D., assisted by H. R. M. Landis, M. D. Vol. IV. December, 1905. 8vo. 367 pages. Lea Brothers & Co., Philadelphia and New York.

Nasal Sinus Surgery. With Operations on Nose and Throat. By Beaman Douglass, M. D. Illustrated with 67 full-page halftone and colored plates, including nearly 100 figures. 1906. 8vo. 264 pages. F. A. Davis Company, Philadelphia.

The Physical Examination of Infants and Young Children. By Theron Wendell Kilmer, M. D. Illustrated with 59 half-tone engravings. 1906. 12mo. 86 pages. F. A. Davis Company, Philadelphia.

Second Catalogue of the Library of the Peabody Institute, of the City of Baltimore. Including the additions made since 1882. Part VIII. U-Z. 1905. 4to. Baltimore.

Pathogenic Micro-Organisms. Including Bacteria and Protozoa. A Practical Manual for Students, Physicians and Health Officers. By William Hallock Park, M. D., assisted by Anna W. Williams, M. D. Second edition, enlarged and thoroughly revised. With 165 engravings and 4 full-page plates. 1905. 8vo. 556 pages. Lea Brothers & Co., New York and Philadelphia.

Physical Diagnosis. Including Diseases of the Thoracic and Abdominal Organs. By Egbert Le Fevre, M. D. Second edition, thoroughly revised and enlarged. Illustrated with 102 engravings and 16 plates. 1905. 12mo. 479 pages. Lea Brothers & Co., Philadelphia and New York.

The Era Key to the U. S. P. A Complete List of the Drugs and Preparations of the United States Pharmacopœia. Eighth Decennial Revision. (1905). First edition. Originated and compiled by the Pharmaceutical Era. 1905. 24mo. 83 pages. D. O. Haynes & Co., New York.

Operative Surgery. For Students and Practitioners. By John J. McGrath, M. D. Second edition, thoroughly revised. With 265 illustrations, including many full-page plates in colors and half-tone. 1906. 8vo. 628 pages. F. A. Davis Company, Philadelphia.

A Text-Book of Practical Therapeutics. With Especial Reference to the Application of Remedial Measures to Disease and their Employment Upon a Rational Basis. By Hobart Amory Hare, M. D., B. Sc. Eleventh edition, enlarged, thoroughly revised, and largely re-written. Illustrated with 113 engravings and 4 colored plates. 1905. 8vo. 910 pages. Lea Brothers & Co., Philadelphia and New York.

Genito-Urinary Surgery and Venereal Diseases. By J. William White, M. D., and Edward Martin, M. D. Illustrated with three hundred engravings and fourteen colored plates. Sixth edition. 1905. 8vo. 1092 pages. J. B. Lippincott Company, Philadelphia and London.

Medical and Surgical Reports of the Boston City Hospital. Fifteenth Series. Edited by Herbert L. Burrell, M. D., W. T. Councilman, M. D., and Charles F. Withington, M. D. 1905. 8vo. 242 pages. Published by the trustees, Boston.

Scientific Memoirs. (*New Series*) No. 19. By the Officers of the Medical and Sanitary Departments of the Government of India. On Kala Azar, Malaria and Malarial Cachexia. By Captain S. P. James, M. B., I. M. S. 1905. Fol. 47 pages, and 16 charts. Office of the Superintendent of Government Printing, Calcutta, India.

Saint Thomas's Hospital Reports. New Series. Edited by Dr. H. P. Hawkins and Mr. W. H. Battle. Vol. XXXIII. 1904. 8vo. XIV + 486 pages. 1905. J. and A. Churchill, London.

Baby Incubators. A Clinical Study of the Premature Infant, with Especial Reference to Incubator Institutions Conducted for Show Purposes. By John Zahorsky, A. B., M. D. Reprinted from A Series of Articles in the St. Louis Courier of Medicine. 1905. 8vo. 136 pages. St. Louis, Mo. Courier of Medicine Co.

Minor and Operative Surgery. Including Bandaging. By Henry R. Wharton, M. D. Sixth edition, enlarged and thoroughly revised. With 532 illustrations. 1905. 12mo. 650 pages. Lea Brothers & Co., Philadelphia and New York.

Lectures on Auto-Intoxication in Disease, or Self-Poisoning of the Individual. By Charles Bouchard. Translated, with a preface and new chapters added, by Thomas Oliver, M. A., M. D., F. R. C. P. Second revised edition. 1906. 8vo. 342 pages. F. A. Davis Company, Philadelphia.

Christianity and Sex Problems. By Hugh Northcote, M. A. 1906. 8vo. 257 pages. F. A. Davis Company, Philadelphia.

Organotherapy, or Treatment by Means of Preparations of Various Organs. By H. Batty Shaw, M. D. (London). F. R. P. C. Illustrated. 1905. 12mo. W. T. Keener & Co., Chicago.

Mount Sinai Hospital Reports. Vol. IV, for 1903 and 1904. Edited for the Medical Board by N. E. Brill, A. M., M. D. 1905. 8vo. 418 pages. New York.

A Memoir of Dr. James Jackson. With Sketches of his Father, Hon. Jonathan Jackson, and his Brothers, Robert, Henry, Charles, and Patrick Tracy Jackson; and Some Account of Their Ancestry. By James Jackson Putnam, M. D. 1905. 8vo. 456 pages. Houghton, Mifflin & Company, Boston and New York.

Surgical Diagnosis. A Manual for Students and Practitioners. By Albert A. Berg, M. D. Illustrated with 215 engravings and 21 plates. 1905. 12mo. 543 pages. Lea Brothers & Company, New York and Philadelphia.

The Johns Hopkins Hospital Bulletins are issued monthly. They are printed by the FRIEDENWALD CO., Baltimore. Single copies may be procured from NUNN & CO. and the BALTIMORE NEWS CO., Baltimore. Subscriptions, $2.00 a year, may be addressed to the publishers, THE JOHNS HOPKINS PRESS, BALTIMORE; single copies will be sent by mail for twenty-five cents each.

BULLETIN

OF

THE JOHNS HOPKINS HOSPITAL

Entered as Second-Class Matter at the Baltimore, Maryland, Postoffice.

Vol. XVII.—No. 183.]   BALTIMORE, JUNE, 1906.   [Price, 25 Cents

CONTENTS.

TWO CASES OF STRICTURE OF THE URETER; TWO CASES OF HYDRONEPHROTIC RENAL PELVIS SUCCESSFULLY TREATED BY PLICATION.[1]

By HOWARD A. KELLY, M. D.,

Gynecologist-in-Chief, The Johns Hopkins Hospital.

1. STRICTURE OF THE VESICAL URETERAL ORIFICE AND POUTING URETER.

A number of cases of this extraordinary condition have been reported, but so far as I know, no case has been diagnosed and treated *intra vitam.* The patient of whom I now speak, Mrs. J. W. F. (No. 1787 San.), came to me through the courtesy of Dr. P. M. Hicks, of San Antonio, Texas. She had had one child nine years before, with a difficult instrumental labor associated with a bad laceration. About six months before I saw her, she had suffered with a bad attack of lower abdominal pain, accompanied by a temperature of 102° and much tenderness in the right side. Since that time she continued to complain of backache and much pain in the lower abdomen. Vaginal examination, Dr. Hicks wrote me, revealed a retroflexed uterus and a somewhat fixed tender mass about the size of an egg in the right cul-de-sac.

November, 18, 1904, I made an abdominal incision and found both ovaries small and sclerotic, 2½ by 1 cm. and 2 by 1 cm. and the ureters appeared normal. The appendix was

[1] Read before the Johns Hopkins Hospital Medical Society, February 19, 1906.

removed and the uterus suspended. She made a good recovery from this operation but continued to have more or less discomfort in the lower abdomen. Upon a careful bimanual examination November 23, 1904, I was unable to feel anything upon the left side, while the ureter could be felt on the right through the somewhat senile vaginal wall. Upon making a vesical examination in the knee breast posture the bladder distended well, and the posterior wall dropped 6.5 cm. from the anterior wall. Through a number 10 speculum a curious teat of tissue could now be seen hanging down into the bladder from its base on the right side occupying the position of the ureteral mons. This at first appeared as a short truncate cone about 1.5 cm. in diameter at its base, and 6 mm. from base to apex. From the apex clear urine fell steadily drop by drop. While I was in the act of watching it, a remarkable transformation took place; the cone began to swell and in the act of swelling was forced down into the lumen of the bladder; as it continued to grow larger its walls appeared paler, thinner, and clearer, until at the maximum a few red vessels could be seen coursing over the surface, which looked like a large cyst as big as the end of the thumb, full of water. With this distention the flow of urine increased in amount. Numerous translucent areas were visible scattered over the now hemispherical enlargement, which was from two to three times the size of the eminence originally observed and more rounded in form. Following this distention the cyst collapsed to its former size. I continued to observe it, and noted a periodicity of from 5 to 10 seconds between the intervals of advancement and retraction of expansion and contraction.

The ureteral orifice could fortunately be seen on the anterior inner, or urethral side of this mons, faintly outlined, forming a narrow slit not open at any time.

The left or opposite ureteral orifice lay in a red mucous vesical fold not prominent in its normal position. When the mucous tissues about the right ureteral orifice became distended, the little narrow opening instead of advancing towards the median line of the bladder, remained relatively nearer to the base until the orifice came to lie wholly on one side.

We had here manifestly to do with a stricture of the vesical orifice of the ureter affecting only its mucous surface.

Treatment.—The treatment was very simple. I took a delicate pair of vesical scissors, working on long parallel handles like an alligator forceps, and introduced one of the points into the ureteral slit-like orifice when the sac was fully distended and cut a slit 5 mm. in length. 15 cc. of urine at once gushed out and later 60 cc. escaped, about half of which was estimated to come from the bladder, when the patient assumed a kneeling posture. When examined five days later the right ureteral orifice appeared stellate, widely opened, seated on a red papillary eminence. On introducing a searcher the margins could be readily lifted apart. The opening now looked like a black hole in the bladder wall, instead of a slit situated on the side of a cyst. The patient was discharged well February 9, 1905.

C. Adrian has reported a case of intermittent cystic dilatation of the vesical end of the left ureter (Arch. f. klin. Chir., 1905, Vol. 78, p. 588). The patient had had dull pains in the upper abdomen and in the region of the right kidney, becoming more distressing upon standing or walking; these finally became so intense that she could not sleep. A diagnosis was made when the cystoscope was used; this revealed an intermittent cystic dilatation of the vesical end of the left ureter. The condition was relieved by making a suprapubic opening of the bladder, with an incision into the little mucous tumor, with a suturing of the vesical and ureteral mucosæ with fine catgut.

Adrian calls attention to fifty-two cases of dilatation reported in the literature in twelve of which the diagnosis was made *intra vitam*. See further literature in Th. Cohn (Beiträge z. klin. Chir., 1904, Vol. 41, p. 45).

2. Stricture of the Upper Ureter Treated by Dilatation.

Mr. R. A. W. (San. No. 960), age 42, was under my care for one month from June 10, 1900. He had had repeated attacks of severe pain in the left side seriously interfering with his occupation, which was that of an evangelist. These attacks began January 8, 1879, when he had a long spell of sickness,

associated with a bowel trouble thought to be intussusception. The attacks were clearly renal in their origin and as nothing was found by a physical examination or an examination of the urine, I exposed the left kidney and by rotation brought into view a large hydronephrotic pelvis of about the same size as the kidney itself. It was fusiform in shape and extended down below the lower pole of the kidney a short distance beyond the pelvis. The ureter which began normally, suddenly contracted until it was only about 2 mm. in diameter at a point 2 cm. below the pelvis. There were no signs of any adhesions, or evidence of previous inflammation. The pelvis of the kidney, however, was thick-walled, owing to physiological hypertrophy.

Treatment.—Realizing that it was impossible to do any plastic operation on so delicate a structure, I tried that which seemed to be the only feasible plan. I incised the pelvis of the kidney about a centimetre above the ureter and then through this orifice I introduced metal catheters which I have had made for dilating structures of the lower end of the ureter; with these I gradually dilated the stricture until a catheter about 5 mm. in diameter was passed with some apparent rupture of the inner coats of the ureter. The wound in the pelvis was then closed with fine silk and the kidney returned to its position with a small drain. He made a perfect recovery from the operation and has never had any pain from that day to this.

3. Two Cases of Hydronephrosis Treated with Plication of the Renal Pelvis.

The first case was that of Mrs. G. P. (San. No. 1927), 48 years of age, admitted May 10, and discharged June 13, 1905. She had two children, 26 and 15 years before, with normal labors. For the past six years she had been suffering at irregular intervals with acute lancinating pains in the right lumbar region associated with the development of a tumor the size of an orange and very sensitive to touch. The disappearance of the tumor was followed by an increase in the amount of urine.

After placing the patient in the knee breast position, I catheterized the right ureter and injected 135 cc. of a boracic aniline solution which served to bring on the same pains as those of which she had been complaining. The diagnosis of hydronephrosis was thus made positive and an operation advised. At the operation an oblique incision was made 10 cm. in length from a point over the last rib extending downward and slightly outward. I exposed the kidney through my usual route by opening and bluntly drawing apart the fascia forming the superior lumbar triangle lying just below the rib and bordering upon the upper part of the quadratus muscle. The kidney was found extremely movable, and the pelvis, which had been previously distended, was seen to be the size of an after-dinner coffee cup. The ureter was attached to the side of the pelvis at a point 3 cm. above its lower pole. The fatty capsule was separated from the posterior part of the renal pelvis which was then emptied of 62 cc. of fluid through the renal catheter. I then cut away the fatty capsule from the upper to the lower end of the pelvis and used the remaining portion to sew the capsule together so as to constrict the pelvis, by passing three silk sutures, two mattress and one interrupted, through the margin of the kidney on one side and out into the fibrous tissue of the amputated fatty capsule on the other. When I tied the sutures thus passed, the pelvis was constricted as in lacing up a corset.

One might think that the delicate tissues of the capsule would easily tear and permit a redistension of the pelvis. The tissues proved, however, to be far firmer than I had anticipated, affording a secure snug closure for the pelvis. The ureter was by this means restored to its normal relations, and on pressure on the pelvis, urine was seen to escape downwards without hindrance. The kidney was then suspended by one silk suture around the last rib, and by two others to the quadratus muscle. The patient recovered and was seen by Dr. Hunner six weeks afterwards, who again injected the kidney and found it held only 18 cc.

My next case of plication of the pelvis of the kidney for hydronephrosis, was entrusted to my care by Dr. George Guthrie, of Wilkesbarre, Pa., December, 1905. Mrs. M. J. C. (San. No. 2034), 31 years old, had had one child, after a long, hard labor. During her pregnancy in the fifth month, she was seized with severe pain in the right side followed by the discharge of large amounts of pus in the urine, with albumin which had not been found before. She had suffered from weekly attacks with her kidney from this time until the child was born; after that event the attacks had been monthly. During an attack a tumor would form on the right side which would disappear accompanied with the discharge of pus by the bladder. She had been seen by several other consultants who had found a pyelitis of the right side. Dr. Guthrie had also determined the presence of a right pelvic peritonitis with adhesions, and a chronic appendicitis was suspected.

In my investigation I found that there was no stone in the kidney, and there were no tubercle bacilli. I catheterized both kidneys and discovered a mild pyelonephrosis on the right side, the pelvis of the kidney holding 80 cc. of aniline solution. On the left side I found what had hitherto been unsuspected, a much dilated renal pelvis of a capacity of 35 cc.[2]

[2] I want to call especial attention to this method of determining the presence of hydronephrotic kidney as well as of measuring the degree of the hydronephrosis. The advantages are very manifest. The hydronephrosis is noted in its earliest stages. The exact degree of the hydronephrosis is measured both by injecting

I then did the following operations:

Dilatation and curettage for an excessive menstrual flow.
Restoration of the broken down vaginal outlet.
Removal of the vermiform appendix.
Removal of the inflamed adherent right tube and ovary.
Shortening the round ligaments by attaching them to the posterior surface of the uterus.
Both kidneys were then operated upon, including:
Plication and fixation of the right kidney.
Plication and fixation of the left kidney.

The kidney was exposed through the loin by an incision similar to that used in the last case. The large flaccid pelvis with thickened walls was then reduced in size by plication, by passing three silk sutures so as to gather up the entire pelvis in a V shape, one inside the other and only on the posterior surface. Each suture started by transfixing the margin of the kidney surrounding the pelvis, and was then carried down into the pelvis towards the ureteral orifice, picking up the tissues of the pelvis, without penetrating the mucosa, and catching the strong peripelvic fascia as in the last case, on the extreme edge of the pelvis. The suture then returned and emerged on the margin of the kidney. After passing three sutures in this way, they were drawn up, so as to pucker and draw the pelvis together, when they were tied, each to its own end respectively. After completing this operation the kidney was suspended as described in the preceding case.

A similar procedure was adopted on the left side, except that two sutures were used instead of three for the plication. The patient made a slow but satisfactory convalescence, and left the hospital after 10 weeks, having gained about 8 pounds in weight and feeling well. There were a few leucocytes in the urine. The kidneys could not be felt at all and there was clearly no accumulation of urine in the pelves. By this operation I feel that I have saved a kidney attainted with a mild pyelonephrosis. I realized that there was some risk in treating a much damaged affected kidney in this way, but I felt that it was well worth the effort in view of the condition of the other side.

the kidney to the point of tension distinctly felt at the syringe as well as to the point of bringing on some pain in the pelvis of the kidney. It is also determined by collecting the fluid which escapes from the kidney as soon as the injecting instrument is removed.

THE USE OF QUININE DURING THE CIVIL WAR.[1]

By John W. Churchman, M. D.,
Late Clinical Assistant, Johns Hopkins Hospital.

If coffee, cathartics, and ammunitions were the sinews of the Civil War—arranged in order of importance—quinine was the staple that would have been, after these three and perhaps

[1] Read before the Johns Hopkins Hospital Historical Club, May 8, 1905.

after whiskey, most missed. In the early days of the century, when surgery was still so largely a question of fractures and emergencies, and when medicine was only beginning to know the interest and advance which were to come with applied microscopy and chemistry and physics, quinine was arousing

a lively interest indeed. And it was an interest destined to continue on through its seventh and eighth decades.

From that pride and scandal of medicine—the Surgeon General's catalogue—one may obtain a fair idea of the attention this drug was demanding in the days when the Missouri Compromise and the policy of the Free Soilers, and the Omnibus Bill were the vital things, and Henry Clay and Dred Scott and John Brown the names in the headlines. The literature of the subject rapidly took on dimensions. Articles appeared on almost every conceivable phase of the question. Inaugural theses and ephemeral articles were written on the pharmaceutical preparation of the drug, on the procedure of extraction, on its detection in the urine, on quantitative and qualitative chemical analysis, on the solubility of its salts. Elaborate dissertations appeared labeled, " On the Sulphate of Quinine." Historical studies were published, the beautiful Countess of Chinchon always appearing in one of the early acts. Search for febrifuges to be used as substitutes was instigated, experimental work was carried out as to the action of the drug on this organ and to decide whether it were an oxytocic, an ecbolic, or a partus accelerator—a question which seems to have kept the profession awake nights in the 70's and 80's. Then its dosage was discussed; and methods for disguising its taste invented, and new routes for its administration suggested and accidents following its use reported. Even the surgeons looked to the drug with hope and articles appeared on its antiseptic value and application to surgery. But clinicians were the chief contributors; and the drug was administered in nearly every disease known to man. Convulsions, erysipelas, neuralgia, rheumatism, typhoid, yellow, malarial, and puerperal fevers—these were only a few of its indications. It was used for its effect on the pulse, it was used topically, it was used to reduce an enlarged spleen. It was advised by one observer in " brain disease," and its power in accelerating the action of mercurials was lauded by another. The diseases of childhood seemed to indicate it particularly and " the quinine rub for children " was lauded in a French article.

Even the followers of Hahnemann contributed to the discussion; and it was really little wonder that before long " abuse " began to take the place of " use " in the titles and that a generation of practitioners had sprung up trained to transform their patients' mouths into funnels gaping for quinine.

But for the military interests of the nation an added attention had been given to this drug by the experiences of the strife waging with the Seminoles during the early 40's.

Florida, the scene of this distressing and protracted warfare, was hardly the best State into which to send soldiers unless the supply at home were unlimited. It was the State of hammocks and savannas, of disappearing lakes and streams, of lime-sinks, bay galls, and bad water. From May to August the rain fell in torrents. The humidity was great, the dew-point high, the mean temperature from 80° to 82°. Lake Tuscawilla suddenly disappearing subterraneously in 1838 and leaving a mushy bog behind it, Lake Orange gradually passing from sight throughout several years—these were samples of what not unusually happened. " A dead level," said a medical writer of the time, " and a half drained country alternately drenched with rain and broiled by an almost tropical sun—reeking with the steam from ten thousand swamps, lagoons, bogs, and savannas—would furnish ample materials for vegetable decomposition and miasmatic effluvia." And such material was indeed furnished. " All fevers of malarial origin "—intermittents, remittents, congestive fevers, dysentery—prevailed throughout the State. The first sign, indeed, of residence in Florida—so it was said at the time—was the cutaneo-hepatic sympathy of Dr. James Johnson; an increase of perspiration with an increase and vitiation of bile. Then followed a series of symptoms characterized by increasing malaise, impaired digestion, growing irritability, pallor, languor, and tendency to venous congestion; leading, in the end, to a frank attack of fever—the two never-failing signs of an oncoming attack being peculiar sensations in the right hypochondrium (attributed to hepatic engorgement) and the passage of dark red urine, small in amount. Finally when the attack was over the patient who had brought a vigorous constitution from the north, was left permanently pale, languid, with a poor digestion, torpid liver, muscular debility, and great susceptibility to atmospheric changes. Such was the attraction offered to immigration. And this state of affairs existed not only in the regions of marshes. Malaria was noticeably present in the barren and sandy portions as well—its presence being explained at the time by the geological character of the soil which was studied in great detail. The prevailing northwest winds were also held to account for much of the disease—a pretty distinct relation being established between the occurrence of miasms and the land breezes. Also the drinking of water in the limestone and alluvial regions must, it was thought, have some etiological relation to the diseases; for had not Dr. Rush said, " There can be no doubt of the predisposition to fevers being increased by the use of impure water," and could it be otherwise? So miasma and impure water did valiant scapegoat service while the real sinner went all unrecognized, close at hand. " During the summer season," wrote Dr. Little, describing conditions in middle Florida, "our ears are assailed by the buzzing of myriads of mosquitoes in their murderous attacks. So formidable are their stings that cattle and deer are often compelled to leave the swamps and take up their residence in the pine woods to avoid them." With dead level, then, and a country half drained, with drenching rains and a broiling sun, with marshes and bogs and lagoons, with favorable wind and soil and unfavorable water, with myriads of murderous mosquitoes doing deadly work, it was no wonder that malaria, as Assistant Surgeon Porter put it, was " the great primary and specific cause of most of the diseases of Florida." And so, indeed, the recruits from the North—

sent to this miasmatic morass to undertake for the Government the exceedingly trying and hazardous task of playing at hide and seek with the Seminoles—found the facts to be. But clinical lessons were learned to prove of national value later. Bleeding in malaria, for instance, was found to be injurious —universally and decidedly; and the favorite panacea was generally abandoned. Cathartics, given as a part of routine prophylaxis and as an adjuvant to quinine, were found extremely beneficial; and Porter's statement that they are particularly well borne by soldiers is easily believed when we learn that 8-10 grs. of calomel followed by oleum ricini, or 15-20 grs. of calomel alone were no uncommon dose. Tamarind water was found to be the best nourishing drink, rarely disagreeing with the stomach, always grateful and never causing the gastric pain and vomiting which occurred when limes or lemons were used. The value of capsicum was also amply demonstrated. But the *great* clinical lesson of the war was what it taught of quinine—establishing in part the wisdom of certain methods for its use, in part only corroborating what others had previously suggested. The reports made came chiefly from two United States posts—Fort White and Fort King. At the former, in the very unhealthy summer of 1839 —when fevers were prevailing throughout Florida and yellow fever on the coast—" malarial " diseases occurred in number; but the only fatal cases were two, one from congestive fever and one from cholera infantum: a result to be ascribed, said Surgeon Porter, "almost entirely to the use of quinine in pretty large doses (8-10 grs.) early in the disease." In 1840, the year following, the rainy season was prolonged, 90 inches of rain fell at Tampa Bay and the general health of Florida improved. Yet the troops in the interior suffered severely from fever, diarrhœa, and dysentery. At Fort King an epidemic broke out which involved nearly every man, woman, and child in the post. Two hundred and seventy patients were taken sick in April and May—and this in a garrison four infantry companies strong. Here was an opportunity to study the disease at close range; and Surgeon Porter improved it. He prescribed quinine and he prescribed it in large doses. Chamomile tea, capsicum, and cathartics were used unsparingly but quinine was given and given in confidence. It was ordered at the onset of the disease (grs. xv-xx-xxv) and it was repeated p. r. n.—" quinine sulphate Э ʒʒ " appearing frequently in the medical orders. Here is the way drugs were handed out to these patients—being excerpts from the clinical notes on a Lieutenant of the 2d Infantry:

" 3 p. m.—Slight attempt at perspiration which soon subsided and at retreat the symptoms were the same as at 1 o'clock, with the addition of great restlessness and uneasiness. Ŗ hydrarg. chlor. mit. gr. i, pulv. antimonialis gr. ii, morph. sulph. gr. ¼. *To be continued at intervals during the night.*" (The italics are mine.) The next morning, the clinical clerk who must have had a grim sense of humor, made this note: " Obtained some sleep during the night." Quinine treatment (grs. xv) was instituted. On the 17th the 1 p. m. order was " No medicine ; " and at retreat the significant entry was made,

" Has been in a quiet sleep." The simple life was, however, not to continue and at tattoo this strenuous order was left: " Ŗ hydrarg. chlor. mit. gr. i, pulv. antimon. gr. ii, morph. sulph. gr. ½, a seidlitz powder at 2 a. m. and 10 grs. of quinine at reveillé." The patient recovered. Not only was quinine found to prevent the paroxysms and cure the patient but it seemed, combined with capsicum, to be the best remedy for the distressing gastric irritability—particularly marked among the recruits—which was apparently so important a feature of the disease. " The paroxysms," a medical writer before the Seminole War had written, " continue to recur until either a salutary crisis or death takes place—one or the other of which not infrequently occurs in the third paroxysm." But this was with the ordinary treatment in which quinine was used only as a tonic late in the course of the disease; and the experience of the army physicians with quinine showed that such a fatalistic philosophy was not warranted. The drug was used by them in ten times the usual dose not as a tonic but as " *the certain antidote;* " convalescence was " immediate and invariable; " and " the termination by crisis," to quote Surgeon Porter, " was created rather than awaited."

To the world-wide medical interest, then, in malarial conditions and in quinine manifested in the first decades of the 19th century, the trials and successes of the Florida war had added an interest that was provincial and national; and when Fort Sumter fell, the dreadful diseases for which quinine was to be needed must have loomed large in the medical minds which were planning for a disagreeable and uncertain future and to which the absolute necessity of this staple of war must have been distressingly apparent. For the drug, as was to be expected and as the event proved, was to be the chief reliance in two of the largest groups of disease during the Civil War— the alvine fluxes and the camp fevers.

The alvine fluxes, according to the official nomenclature, included the acute and chronic diarrhœas and the acute and chronic dysenteries; and they were, indeed, the bane of the armies. The statistics are little short of amazing. The fluxes were more frequent and produced a greater mortality than any other disease. They were responsible for about one-half of all the cases of sickness and caused, with scurvy, 831 of every 1000 deaths from disease. They appeared at the beginning of the war and in regiments before organization. It often happened in the hospitals that more were sick from dysentery than from all other causes; and when it is remembered that the proportion of deaths from disease to the deaths from wounds was about as two to one among the whites and as over eight to one among the negroes, the tremendous economic problem this disease presented becomes apparent. In the white and colored troops of the North from the beginning of the war to June 30th, 1863—that is before Gettysburg had been fought, or Vicksburg had fallen, or the draft riots had been quelled in New York—nearly 1,800,000 cases had been recorded under one of the four alvine fluxes; and, at a conservative estimate, almost 60,000 soldiers had died from the disease. The Union had lost, from dysentery, in other words, an army twice the size of the garrison which made Grant famous by surrendering to him, over five times as many men as the killed and wounded at Chancellorsville; troops equal to about three-fourths of the forces which turned the tide of the war by repulsing Lee's invasion of the North. In three Indiana regiments alone, representing a strength of 3000 men, the reports, though exceedingly incomplete and including only a part of the war, list 1567 cases of dysentery. The number of those on sick report for the fluxes was to the total of all diseases as, approximately, one to four. For the single year ending June 30, 1863—the year that began with the Emancipation Proclamation and ended with Lookout Mountain— nearly 522,000 cases of dysentery were reported with 10,554 deaths. Yet Chancellorsville was called a terrible and sanguinary conflict. In the Confederate Army similar conditions were prevailing. From July, 1861, to March, 1862, the Army of the $P_{oto}ma_c$ with a mean strength of about 50,000, reported over 36,000 cases of alvine flux—740 cases, that is, to 1000 of mean strength; and no doubt the medical records, destroyed at the fall of Richmond; would have shown a similar state of affairs throughout the war. The disease, said Surgeon Jones, "destroyed and injured permanently more men than shot and shell." At Capt. Wirtz's notorious Andersonville prison for about 15 months during '64 and '65 nearly 18,000 prisoners were admitted to the hospital. Four hundred and fifty odd of these were wounded and about 16,000 suffered with a specified disease. The results were recorded in about 15,000 cases and the mortality was 73.7 per cent. Over seven thousand cases of diarrhœa were listed; and, excluding cases not followed, 80.3 per cent of them died. In other words in a hospital with 18,000 medical and surgical patients admitted during a short year and a half there were over 5000 known deaths from alvine flux alone.

To combat this wide-spread contagion quinine was, of course, not exclusively or perhaps chiefly used. Ipecac and a whole host of other drugs were the stand-bys. But Peruvian bark and what Dr. Woodward calls its "precious alkaloid," were extensively ordered. The drug had been used with good results by Richard Morton in the London epidemic of 1666 and later by York in 1709. Moreover dysentery was still vaguely thought of as a "malarial" condition and that was indication enough for quinine. And so it was prescribed; prescribed for the prostration accompanying dysentery, for the debility of convalescence and for the cases complicated with malaria; it was even in some cases prescribed to excess; but these errors said Dr. Woodward, were "among the most pardonable and least injurious of the therapeutic errors of the Civil War."

But the chief call for quinine came, of course, from camp fevers; and it was a loud call, and a strong, and a constant. The camp fevers of the war included typhus and typhoid, common continued fevers (after June 30, 1862, reported as "other miasmatic disorders"), remittent fever, quotidian, tertian, and quartan fevers, and congestive intermittent fever. The question of diagnosis was, of course, still somewhat unsettled.

Even typhus and typhoid were not clearly distinguished. The work of Louis had, indeed, appeared in 1829; Gerhard and Pennock had published in 1837, Shattuck in 1839, and Bartlett and Wood in the early 40's. Yet Dickson, of Charleston, as late as 1855 quoted from Campbell with approval, "The necessity which any theory may involve of separating typhus gravior and mitior is enough of itself to declare its absurdity;" and of the three text-books furnished the medical officers during the war (Wood, Watson, and Bennett), two were nonidentist and one monistic. Of course the diagnosis was made entirely from clinical features; and though certain cases of typhus probably got into the typhoid statistics the error was apparently not a large one. As to "typho-malaria," however, there was much confusion. The term was introduced by Woodward in 1862 for those hybrid fevers which he thought due to a combined poison—modified, in some cases, by a "scorbutic taint." He hoped by this innovation to clarify the diagnostic atmosphere; but he succeeded in befogging it. The terms came to be used by the army surgeons to include those febrile remittents which assumed the adynamic form present in enteric fever, and enterics with malarial complications. *True* malaria—remittent and intermittent—was pretty well recognized. But it is, of course, in the statistics of the aggregate camp fevers and not in the statistics of the separate groups, that we are interested; and, as in the case of the alvine fluxes though less notably than in that case, the figures are huge. One quarter of all the cases of disease among the white troops were of a malarial character. This does not include a large number of cases complicated with pneumonia and other diseases and reported under those headings. Nor does it take any account of the great number of recurrent cases which were treated by the men themselves—who recognized and became used to ague fits, took quinine and were simply excused from duty by their company officers without reporting to the surgeons. Yet even so, consider the extensive ravages of the disease. From May, '61, to June, '66, over 1,100,000 cases of pure malaria and nearly 50,000 of typho-malaria were reported among the white troops. Of these 12,199 died. In other words there were 2814 cases of malarial disease and over 26 deaths from malaria per 1000 of mean strength. In three years of service nearly 160,000 cases, with over 3000 deaths, occurred among the colored troops. In the Confederate Army of the Potomac (roughly 50,000 men strong) 1865 cases of malaria occurred between July, 1861, and March, 1862; and at Andersonville in about six months, there were 3000 cases and 119 deaths.

But the camp fevers, so rife throughout the war, made for themselves, a special name and fame in the second twelve-month. The year was 1862, the Bull Run fiasco had been almost forgotten, Scott had retired and McClellan was looming as the most important military figure of the Unionist forces in the East. The giant North, having stood at gaze for some months had taken a few slumbering and blundering steps forward and was now beginning to awake to the true significance of things; but meanwhile the alert David, with a sling and a few smooth stones from the brook, had been doing telling though not fatal work. " On to Richmond " had been the cry at the North during the winter; and in the spring McClellan responded. On account of transportation facilities he chose for his famous campaign that famous strip of land lying between the York and the James. Here it was that the colonies had gone to childbed to be delivered of the nation; and here Lafayette, Cornwallis, and Washington had seen her travail pains, and her rejoicings that a son was born into the world. Through this historic ground McClellan pressed until, by the close of May, he found himself within seven miles of Richmond. Then came the news that expected reinforcements could not be sent and the Army of the Potomac was left to its own resources in the Chickahominy Swamps. Malaria and typho-malaria—familiarly called " Chickahominy fever "—soon became prevalent. Meanwhile Stonewall Jackson had joined Light Horse Harry Lee's son—who was now rapidly forging to the front; and McClellan's thin and fevered army was gradually pushed back by July 1, to Malvern Hill. Richmond was safe and Lee was able to assume the offensive. The Peninsula which had perpetuated the names of Washington and Lafayette and Cornwallis as soldiers, which had tested the mettle of McClellan and had insured the fame of Lee left also its mark in medical history by adding to its nomenclature " Chickahominy fever" and by emphasizing the great disabling power of this disease.

The drug that had to be provided for this second widespread group of diseases was the drug which was being used so extensively in the alvine fluxes; but do not suppose it to have been an entirely settled question, at the outbreak of the war, that quinine was a malarial antidote. Peruvian bark had indeed been so regarded by Lind as early as 1765, and also by Hunter, Clark, and others. But James Johnson, in Calcutta, had re-introduced venesection; and though quinine had been discovered in 1820, Sir J. Martin—writing as late as 1861—said, " Quinine, the great febrifuge acts * * * purely as a nerve tonic to the cerebro-spinal and visceral sympathetic system," and " bleeding * * * is very generally necessary in the severer forms of Bengal remitent fever; then come full doses of calomel and sudorifics short of producing salivation, with saline purgatives, antimonials and refrigerants and quinine in the intervals." At the same time, however, Hare, in India, was using the drug in large doses and as an antidote; and in 1836 Maillot, in France, from a study of many thousand cases spoke of laxatives and purgatives in malaria as obsolete ideas and concluded that quinine should always be used. " All the morbid phenomena," said he, " will disappear as if by enchantment in a few hours." Ten years before this, Perrine, treating the disease in Mississippi, had used and advocated quinine strongly; and it seems probable that he was the first to insist on large doses. Surgeon Harvey, however, in the Florida war had been one of the early extensive users and staunch advocates of the drug; and the result of all this was that, when the war cloud really broke, quinine, though there were still prominent dissenting voices, was regarded as the specific drug

for malaria and became, as a matter of fact, the *sine qua non* throughout the strife, practically no other antiperiodics being used. Even " prophylactic quinine " was recommended in the " Rules for Preserving the Health of the Soldier," published by Van Buren in 1861; so that there can be no doubt as to the fact that the treatment of malaria was then fully understood.

I have said nothing, in calling attention to the terrific dimensions of the camp fevers and the alvine fluxes during the war, of the sub-acute and chronic distress they occasioned; yet, as a matter of history, this feature was quite as marked as the more acute manifestations. For war—the typhoid of nations—resembles its clinical prototype not alone in bringing prostration, depression, and suffering, nor in exacting a high bounty of life. It is like it in this other respect, too, that it collects its usury in long continued instalments, leaves behind, for days after defervescence and convalescence, reminders of itself in the shape of debility, distressing sequelæ, and a motley array of disabilities. One thinks, for instance, of the march of the army of Charles VIII through Europe in 1494, with the conquest of the Italian Peninsula in contemplation and a highly pious ambition to reach Jerusalem; but ending by making the name of Fracastorius' shepherd a household word throughout Europe and starting it on its way toward Persia and Turkey and the Orient. What indeed, for the common weal of Europe, or of the world, were the paltry lives lost on the march? A continent syphilized—here was the real ravage of an army; and that same continent, feeling keenly to-day the distressing and disabling sequels of the acute fever which it has now well-nigh forgotten, illustrates what distress a war can set in motion. Or a few French soldiers buried in Algiers: was *their* loss a national calamity? A calamity, at least, at all comparable to the army's introduction, on its return, of a new febrifuge which turned out to be the baptism—or better—the immersion of French national progress in absinthe? Some day the full story of the late effects of war will be written; and it will be an illuminating chronicle. Of our own intestine upset it is, of course, even yet not uncommon to see the sequelæ in wrecked constitutions and disabilities of every nature; but if we needed any other reminder of the state of affairs than the Pension Budget we would find it in a glance at the statistics of war times. Look, for example, at the facts as to diarrhœa and dysentery. Seventeen thousand three hundred and eighty-nine white soldiers were discharged from the fighting army on certificate for disability due to these two diseases; and a very large number of the 15,000 discharged for " debility " were really dysenteries. So also were a large proportion of those discharged for anæmia, dropsy, etc.; and of the great number of dysenteries mustered out at the end of the war and not entered on the reports we shall never have any accurate conception. So, too, as regards malaria which was the real cause of a large proportion of the, approximately, 102,000 general debilities and miasms, of the 21,872 anæmias, of the nearly 8000 dropsies reported; and when we learn that almost

15,000 white soldiers were discharged for "debility" alone we realize what a tremendous feature the late results of malaria were.

Here then were the elements for a good quinine market when the war came. A widespread medical interest in the drug, a strikingly successful national experimental test of it fresh in the medical mind, a prospect of the wide prevalence of one disease calling loudly and of another calling exclusively for it —these things meant that much quinine would change hands between 1861 and 1865. And much *did* change hands. The Purveyor's Report for the war lists the purchase of about 393,000 dozen quinine sulphate pills; of over 500,000 oz. of fluid extract of cinchona; of 260,000 oz. of powdered calisaya bark; of nearly 600,000 oz. of quinine sulphate; or, briefly, a total of over 19 tons of quinine sulphate, and over 9½ tons of sulphate of cinchona—beside other preparations. Compare this with the 220,000 quarts of castor oil bought; with the 683,000 dozen c.c. pills; with the 515,000 pounds of Rochelle salts, and you will see that quinine was, indeed, as I have already said, playing Romeo to cathartic's Juliet. In the Confederate camp, too, the drug was used in quantity. It was a contraband of war; but it got through. Not, however, in sufficient amount. Nor could it be brought from Europe past the blockade; and Dr. Jones found it necessary to urge a search for an indigenous substitute, which was, strangely enough, to make the South independent of the North not only during the war but afterward, when she had become an established nation. Georgia bark and dogwood were both tried in this extremity; and both proved failures.

So much for the probable needs and the actual demands of the two armies in regard to quinine. To whom was the government to look for the tremendous supply required? On August 29, 1904, William Weightman, popularly known as the richest man in Pennsylvania and certainly one of the largest real estate owners in the country, died in Philadelphia. He was a singularly reserved man, a captain of industry, a practical scientist of rank; a man of sagacity, energy, and thrift, who amassed a fortune of at least $50,000,000 and died in the harness. Eminently fitted to serve the community he had little in common with it, finding his chief interests in the making of a fortune and the raising of chrysanthemums to a variety of which his name became attached. He owned more property in Philadelphia than the Pennsylvania or the Reading Railroads. The Garrick Theatre and the Hale Building— assessed at $2,000,000—were two of his holdings. He made it a point never to sell any of his properties—the only exception to this rule being the sale of the Bingham House, which brought him $1,000,000. The store of Darlington & Co. belonged to him; whole blocks in Philadelphia were his; and his personal property tax return for 1903-1904 was over $5,000,-000. Here we find, then, the resting place of the dollars that went for those 19 odd tons of quinine and of the many thousands of dollars that followed them when the monopoly established during the war lived on and grew fat. At the outbreak of the war there were but two chemical houses in the

country engaged in the manufacture of quinine from Peruvian bark. Powers & Weightman, and Rosengarten & Sons, both of Philadelphia. Previously the properties of the bark had been obtained by a process of suffusion; but these two firms, quickly introducing the method for separating quinine—invented by the French chemists, Pelletier and Coventon in 1820 —were soon without successful rivalry in the American manufacture of the drug. And before long the price of the drug ($2.10 per ounce at the outbreak of the war) was, by reason of this monopoly aided by certain economic conditions, soaring heavenward. Alcohol, the essential solvent of quinine carried a heavy internal revenue tax; so that a duty was placed on imported quinine sulphate in order to allow the American drug to compete with that imported from Germany and other countries where alcohol was free. The duty was 45 per cent; but the government, buying its quinine duty free, was able to avoid the monopoly of the American firms. Not, however, until large bills for the drug had been incurred. In New York alone nearly $591,000 were spent for quinine, $418,000 of this going to J. H. Reed & Co., who were customers of Powers & Weightman; and the payments made to the latter firm themselves for drugs and medicines during the war amounted to over $231,000, of which a large share went for quinine. But, though the records of these transactions are, obviously, not complete in detail, the Confederates, too, were swelling the bank account of the northern Trust. The drug was contraband and had to be shipped South minus all markings. Moreover Powers, the head of one firm, was a loyal and ardent Unionist; while Adolph Rosengarten, a member of the other, was killed at Murfreesboro after having risen to the rank of major in Anderson's Cavalry. Yet the South got its drug—stored on one occasion in mattresses; and it paid for it, at one time as much as $15 an ounce.

After the war, however, the firm, though becoming fabulously wealthy, began to become extremely unpopular as well. The war duty on the bark had been lifted in 1870; in 1872 the duty on the sulphate had been reduced to 20 per cent. Yet the Philadelphia firms became by no means lean kine. The monopoly, it began to be rumored, was being overdone; the tariff-tax on quinine, prohibiting the sick-poor from using the drug, was grimly nicknamed the "tax on blood;" what had been termed business sagacity began to look like scandalous greed; and a popular cry for redress sounded. Even the *New York Tribune*, the most rabid high tariff newspaper in the country, fought valiantly for repeal; and finally the Government yielding to the country's importunity removed the tariff on quinine under the Dingley bill of 1897. Meanwhile the drug has become immeasurably cheaper. Cinchona has been transplanted to Java, Ceylon, and India, where it grows so extensively that the supply exceeds the demand. Improvement in cultivating the bark has resulted in doubling the yield of quinine to the pound of cinchona. Solvents other than alcohol have come into use—fusel-oil and coal-tar chiefly. And the quinine of commerce—which was quoted in 1861 at $2.10 the ounce and brought as high as $15.00 below the line—sells for 21 cents an ounce.

Looking ahead then to our next civil, or perhaps colonial, war, it does not seem likely that the quinine problem will loom large. The question of duty has been settled; and even if this were not so the government would probably settle it in the event of war by passing a general provision, as was done at the time of the Spanish War, to suspend the operation of the tariff law on all materials required by the War Department. There are still only three firms in the country manufacturing the drug—the two already mentioned and the New York Quinine and Chemical Company. Yet the Government might easily elect, if monopoly again threatened to become embarrassing, to establish its own chemical and supply factories—as was done during the Civil War, with a saving to the Gov-

ernment at the Philadelphia laboratory alone of over $766,000 between March, 1863, and September, 1865. As for the supply of the drug to the country—so long as our present coast-line persists a complete blockade seems rather improbable. Yet the quinine problem was a very real one in the struggle between the North and South. If, as Goldwin Smith said in his Manchester speech, the conclusion of the war meant that slavery was dead everywhere and forever this was an achievement worth paying something for. But in estimating the price, do not think only or chiefly of the life lost in the four unfortunate years. Remember as well the disability and debility they left behind them; and in considering the vast financial perplexities which came when reconstruction days began, do not overlook the quinine monopoly which the war had made possible but which a suffering people finally overthrew.

THE IMPORTANCE OF A MICROSCOPICAL EXAMINATION OF ALL GROWTHS REMOVED FROM THE NARES, TOGETHER WITH A REPORT OF EARLY DIAGNOSES OF MALIGNANT GROWTHS.

By Sylvan Rosenheim, M. D.,

Assistant in Laryngology, The Johns Hopkins University.

The use of the microscope as a means of diagnosis has been much neglected by those especially interested in the diseases of the nose and throat. Jonathan Wright has recently called attention to its value as a routine measure. Beaman Douglas points out that the origin and early symptoms of malignant disease of the nose are wanting and reports a case of primary carcinoma of the inferior turbinated body where the diagnosis would not have been made unless the aid of the microscope had been invoked. Trautmann, in a recent long article on carcinoma of the nose concludes that we must be guided in our treatment by the microscopical diagnosis. According to Pasch the views generally held regarding the infrequency of tuberculosis of the nose will have to be revised. This author has found many cases, which would not have been recognized clinically, as neither the ulcerative nor proliferative forms in which this disease occurs have a characteristic appearance. They are usually of long duration and so are readily mistaken.

However, the lack of an early diagnosis of the true nature of a nasal growth is in no class of cases so serious and sure to lead to evil results, as in the malignant growths. Here the usual distinguishing characteristics are apt to be lacking. When these cases ultimately fall into the hands of the general surgeons with the classical symptoms of growths in this region, such as bulging of the nasal wall and upper jaw, protrusion of the hard and soft palate, exophthalmus, and pressure symptoms, they are either inoperable or do not recover after operation. Bloodgood states that none of these cases have been cured at the Johns Hopkins Hospital and that usually the patients are in a worse state after the operation.

By systematically examining all growths from the nose, these growths will be correctly diagnosed while small and at a time when they can as a rule, be readily extirpated by the nasal route. When this route is not feasible a radical operation can be done, at a time when there is the greatest probability of a cure. Moreover, knowing the nature of the growth removed, we are on the watch for recurrences and are prepared to treat them vigorously.

REPORT OF CASES.

The tissues from the growths described below were fixed in 10 per cent formalin. The sections were stained with hæmatoxylin and eosin.

CASE 1. (History lost.)

Diagnosis.—Mixed cell sarcoma. A small round tumor about the size of a pea, made up of a capsule and the tumor proper. The capsule consists of a loose reticular tissue imbedded in which are numerous polynuclear leucocytes. The tumor proper is composed of round, spindle and irregularly shaped cells. It is rich in blood vessels with walls of a single layer of endothelial cells.

CASE 2. Colored man, age 67 years.

Diagnosis.—Giant cell sarcoma. He complained of nosebleed and shortness of breath. He had recently been treated in the hospital for mitral insufficiency.

There is no history of cancer in the family. He gives no history of syphilis. Six months ago he began to get short of breath and four months ago his nose began to bleed, two or three times daily.

On examination of the nose, a tumor mass is seen on the left side blocking up the nares and causing a marked external bulging. From the lower part of the tumor arises a small polypoid mass about the size of a pea. The tumor is of grayish color, firm in consistency, and bleeds profusely on probing. The right nares is atrophic. The post-nasal space is clear. The mucous membrane is pale and atrophic.

Although there was no doubt that here we had to do with a malignant new growth, a small piece was removed for microscopical examination. This patient was seen about six months later and there had been no appreciable increase in the size of the growth.

The tumor is lined by stratified squamous epithelium. Beneath this is a submucosa of connective tissue containing round and spindle shaped cells. The tumor proper has a fibrous capsule which penetrates its substance in places. It consists almost entirely of giant cells each of which contains many nuclei. Between the giant cells are many smaller round cells with small deeply staining nuclei. The tumor is poor in blood vessels which are lined by a single layer of endothelial cells.

CASE 3. A. L., female, white, age 29 years.

Diagnosis.—Mixed-celled sarcoma arising from the middle turbinated bone. It might be said here that in view of the history and appearance of this tumor that it was thought to be a polypoid hypertrophy of the middle turbinate, probably of luetic origin.

The patient complained of something in the nose that moved up and down. Her past history revealed that she had had four miscarriages but no other symptoms suggestive of lues. She had noticed something in the right side of her nose for about one week. It obstructed respiration and moved up and down when she blew her nose. She has no pain in the nose nor headache. There is a slight nasal discharge. The nose has bled frequently for the last month and a half.

On examination a pale polypoid growth is seen on the right middle turbinate and a perforation of the septum. Otherwise the examination is negative.

Microscopical Examination.—The tumor is one centimeter long by one-half centimeter broad. It is covered for the most part by stratified columnar epithelium but in one small area there has been a metaplasia to stratified squamous epithelium. The tumor proper is a sarcoma consisting of a mixture of spindle-shaped and round cells, the former predominating. It is very rich in blood vessels, which consist of large spaces with a lining of endothelial cells. Some are empty, some filled with blood corpuscles.

CASE 4. H. C., female, colored, age 31.

Diagnosis.—Papilloma on anterior part of septum nasi, showing epithelial ingrowths.

The patient complained of matter falling back into her throat.

No history of any new growth in the family. She has had four miscarriages. Her hair came out in spots last year; no other luetic symptoms.

Her present trouble began about two months ago. The right nostril bleeds when she blows it. When she lies down she has cough and difficulty in breathing.

On examination a papilloma the size of a pea is seen attached by a broad pedicle to the anterior part of the nasal septum of the right side. Removed with the cold snare. The left inferior turbinate is chronically inflamed.

Microscopical Examination.—The tumor is lined by stratified squamous epithelium, cornified in places. It is increased in places to at least a dozen times the normal thickness of mucous membrane in this region. In these areas there are irregular ingrowths into the underlying parts and sections of these ingrowths appear as little epithelial islands. However, the epithelial cells of these ingrowths do not show any irregularities in shape or staining properties. There is no infiltration with young round cells in their neighborhood. The rest of the tumor consists of connective tissue, for the most part rich in cells of an embryonal type closely packed together; in other places these cells are not so closely packed together and here there are many blood spaces.

While one would hesitate to call this tumor malignant, it belongs to a class of cases which should be carefully watched.

The stroma of the tumor is a vascular œdematous connective tissue with few cells and blood vessels.

CASE 5.—R. R., male, age 62 years, white.

Diagnosis.—Polypoid tumor in right nares. Microscopical Diagnosis: Nasal polypus of epithelial type with tendency to become malignant.

The patient complained of something growing in his nose. His family history is negative for any new growth. His past history is unimportant. He has felt the growth in his nose four or five months. It bleeds at times when touched with the finger. For two months the patient has breathed through the mouth at night. He has no pain in the nose or head; has not lost in weight or strength.

On examination a grayish colored firm growth is seen in the right nares, occluding it and apparently coming from the region of the middle turbinate. Otherwise the examination is negative.

After thorough cocainization, preparatory to operation, the growth is seen to come from the bulla ethmoidalis. It was removed in one piece with the cold snare (see photograph). The bulla ethmoidalis was removed with Grunwald's cutting forceps exposing the anterior ethmoidal cells, which appeared normal. The patient was seen a number of times and was finally discharged cured. He was, however, warned of the danger of a recurrence and told to report every few months for examination.

The photograph shows very well the shape of the tumor.

Microscopical Examination. (See photographs.)—The tumor is covered with thick stratified columnar epithelium, the base line of which is thrown into scalloped curves. In places there are downgrowths of epithelium forming alveoli composed of the same type of cells. Some of these alveoli have holes in the centre. The epithelial cells are regular in shape and staining; between the cells are seen many polynuclear cells. There is no infiltration of young round cells about the epithelium.

CASE 6.—A. S., female, white, age 27.

Diagnosis.—Nasal polypi, one of which shows beginning epithelioma. Complained of constant spitting and cough.

Her husband died of consumption 7 years ago. She has been a healthy woman, suffering occasionally from colds and headaches.

Her present trouble began about one year ago. She hawks a great deals and coughs all day long. No pain about the head. Has not lost in weight or strength.

On examination polypi are seen on both sides of the nose in the region of the middle turbinate. The left tonsil contains a small abscess. The larynx is normal. The polypi were removed with the cold snare and one was kept for microscopical study. This is the one showing beginning epithelioma. Seven months later the patient was seen again, when she still complained of hawking and spitting a great deal. On examination of the nares two small polypi were seen, arising from the anterior end of the right middle turbinate. These were removed together with the anterior end of the turbinate with the cold snare, and preserved for examination. A small polypus was also removed from the right nares. These polypi were of a translucent grayish-white color.

Microscopical Examination.—The growth removed at the first operation is of irregular shape, about the size of a large pea. The accompanying photograph gives a very good idea of its structure.

The investing epithelium is of the stratified squamous variety, varying greatly in thickness. As seen in the photograph, it dips deeply into the underlying structure, where it is cut off in places as small epithelial islands. The nuclei of the cells forming these ingrowths vary much in their staining properties, an indication of division. Between the lowermost cells are seen many polynuclear leucocytes.

Just beneath the epithelium is a dense infiltration with small round cells, which is more marked where the ingrowths occur. Deeper down are the acini of numerous mucous glands, imbedded in a fibrous matrix, rich in spindle-shaped cells.

The growth removed at the second operation is about the same size as the first growth. Its epithelial covering varies in variety and thickness. In some places it is of the stratified columnar, in others of the stratified squamous variety. There are no ingrowths of the epithelium but the epithelium shows great variations in thickness, being in places but three layers of cells. In one place where the epithelium is slightly

thickened and of the stratified squamous variety there is an infiltration with numerous young round cells.

The tumor proper consists of a loose connective tisue rich in young cells of round and spindle shape. It contains many mucous glands, some of which are dilated (one to a cavity the size of a pin point filled with pink staining material).

In all of the text books on diseases of the nose and throat, the infrequency of malignant growths is noted. Dreyfuss notes 19 cases among 9,554 cases of malignant tumors in various parts of the body. Of these 15 were sarcoma and 4 carcinoma. Among 28,000 patients in Frankel's clinic, Finder found 10 cases of sarcoma and 2 cases of carcinoma of the nose. Darnall mentions having found but 76 cases of carcinoma described in the literature. In an analysis of the literature, Cordes was able to find but eight cases of adenocarcinoma of the nose. Watson states that there are records of about 200 cases of sarcoma of the nose since the middle of the last century and gives a summary of 150 of these cases.

The form of carcinoma most often found is the squamous-celled variety. Next in frequency are the cylindrical-celled, the medullary form and the adeno-carcinoma. Of the sarcomas, the small-celled, mixed-celled and fibro-sarcoma are most common. According to Watson melano-carcinoma forms 7 per cent of all cases, its occurrence here being next in frequency to melano-carcinoma of the skin and choroid. Moritz Schmidt says, however, that it occurs here very infrequently and that one must not mistake hemorrhages into ordinary sarcoma for it.

The origin of both carcinoma and sarcoma is most frequently on the septum, middle turbinate body and ethmoid bone. Carcinoma originates very frequently in the antrum of Highmore (Bloodgood, Schmidt, Majutin) and gives rise to symptoms of an empyema. Sarcoma rarely arises in the antrum.

Nasal obstruction is the earliest symptom that these growths give rise to. Hemorrhage is often an early symptom, especially in sarcoma. There is usually some nasal discharge. Pain is usually a late symptom and is of a deep boring character. Glandular enlargement and metastases are rarely noted and only when the disease is very far advanced.

In the nose, as elsewhere, sarcoma occurs equally at all ages, whereas carcinoma is usually found after the fourth decade. Sarcoma of the nose pursues a milder course, as a rule, than carcinoma. It is also more amenable to treatment, even when discovered late. Watson reports 39 per cent cured after a radical operation and 54 per cent cured by intranasal treatment. However, it must be noted that in only 28 of the 62 cases reported cured were the histories followed longer than six months. Histories of these cases showed that incomplete operations did not tend to hasten the growth of the tumor (sarcoma) but prolonged life.

Regarding the transformation of benign into malignant growths, Moritz Schmidt is of the opinion that it is possible but that it does not occur frequently. Cobb says that as yet no case has been published that proves this hypothesis.

Sir Felix Semon also holds this view. He has not seen this transformation in over 10,000 cases. Zuckerkandl has not observed this form of degeneration. In his monographs on polypi of the nose, Hopman states that he has observed the combination of polypi and carcinoma but is not prepared to state the relationship. Heymann found that polypi constituted about 10 per cent of all his nasal cases and Zuckerkandl found polypi of the nose in one out of every ten autopsies. Kümmel mentions that as nasal polypi form 2 per cent of all cases of disease of the upper respiratory tract it is not surprising that we frequently find the combination.

However, much is to be said in favor of this hypothesis. In a recent address, von Hansemann states that none of the usually mentioned factors, namely heredity, infection or trauma, can be proved as the cause of cancer. He points out that we must still search for a definite cause. The careful study of this class of cases should aid us in this search. Very few cases, if any, can be adduced that prove this point conclusively. Still there is much evidence to show its probability. As Watson remarks, we know that fibrous and myxomatous tissue become converted into bone, fat and cartilage. Why should they not revert to embryonic connective tissue? In many of the intranasal growths the epithelium is of the squamous-celled variety. This transformation from the cylindrical cell type normally in this region is called epithelial metaplasia and is usually thought due to irritation of the tissue. It is only a step farther for this epithelium to take on malignant tendencies. Heyman regards fibroma, angioma, adenoma, lipoma and epithelioma as modifications of the hyperthrophied nasal mucous membrane.

In Watson's series of 150 cases of sarcoma of the nasal passages, there were 24 cases in which there was a previous history of polypi, that is in 16 per cent. Bloodgood records 18 cases of carcinoma of the antrum, of which five arose in the antrum. Thirteen cases arose from the nasal fossae, and in 9 of them there was a history of polypi lasting from one to twelve years. Bayer reports a case which strongly supports this form of degeneration. In a man aged 50 years, who had previously been treated for nasal polypi, examination showed a large growth in the upper part of the right nares, the lower part being ulcerated and the upper part having the appearance of an œdematous fibroma. Examination of the excised growth showed the structure of the usual mucous polypus in the upper part, while the lower part was carcinomatous. In Case 6 of our series, it seems most probable that the tumor represents a polypus that has undergone carcinomatous degeneration. No note was made as to which nostril the growth came from. The polypi subsequently removed from this patient were ordinary œdematous fibromata, the epithelium of which, however, had undergone metaplasia and was thickened in places. Heyman described six cases similar to this, which he says might be called benign epitheliomata. He could find no mention of this class of cases in the literature. These growths either arose from the middle turbinated body or in its neighborhood. After removal there was no return in two of these cases after two and three years; one recurred in three years,

after which the patient remained well for fourteen years; another case had five recurrences after operation within three years; the fifth also had numerous recurrences during four years, when death intervened from heart failure; the sixth was seen but once. None of these patients had accessory sinus trouble.

In our study of these cases, we must remember that the reverse of this transformation may take place. Hermann reports a case of carcinoma of the antrum, in which a number of typical œdematous fibromata were found in the middle meatus of the nose.

BIBLIOGRAPHY.

Bayer, L.: Ueber die Transformation von Schleimpolypen in bösartigen (krebsige oder sarkomatose) Tumoren; Deutsche med. Wochenschr. 1887, S. 174.

Bloodgood, Jos. C.: Tumors and Inflammations of the Jaws; April, 1903.

Burnett, Ingalls and Newcomb: Diseases of the Ear, Nose and Throat.

Cobb, F. C.: Proceedings of Tenth Annual Meeting of American Laryngological, Rhinological and Otological Society; Abstract in Journal of Laryngology, Rhinology and Otology, Jan. '05·

Cordes, H.: Das Adenocarcinom der Nase; Berliner klin. Wochenschr., 1903, S. 164.

Douglas, B.: Primary Carcinoma of Inferior Turbinated Body; N. Y. Med. Record, Aug. 1896, p. 210.

Felix, E.: Die Schleimpolypen der Nase; Sammlung zwangloser Abhandlungen aus dem Gebiete der Nasen-, Ohren-, Mund- und Halskrankheiten, 1901, No. 9, S. 263.

Von Hansemann: Was wissen wir über die Aetiologie der Krebse? Münchener med. Wochenschr., 1905, No. II, S. 531.

Herrmann, Carl: Ueber die Combination von Carcinom und Polypen der Nasenhöhle; Inaug. Dissertation, Würzburg, 1898.

Kummel, W.: Die bösartigen Geschwülste der Nase; Heymann's Handbuch der Laryngologie und Rhinologie, 3. Band, 2. Hälfte, S. 874.

Kyle, B.: Diseases of the Nose and Throat, 1904.

Mayer, Emil: Adenoma of the Nose, with Incipient Sarcomatous Metamorphosis; American Medicine, 1902, August, page 179.

Packard, Francis R.: The Etiology of Nasal Polypi, with Especial Reference to their Association with Other Pathological Conditions; Amer. Jour. Med. Sc., 1903, p. 824.

Schmidt, Moritz: Die Krankheiten der oberen Luftwege; Berlin, 1903

Wyatt, Wingrave: Proceedings of the Laryngological Society of London; Journal of Laryngology, Rhinology and Otology, Feb. 1905.

Trautmann, G.: Carcinoma des Naseninneren; Archiv für Laryngologie und Rhinologie, Band XVII, Heft 3, 1905, S. 386.

Watson, J. A.: Sarcoma of the Nasal Passages; Amer. Med. April, 1904, p. 553.

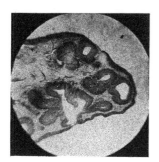

CASE 5.

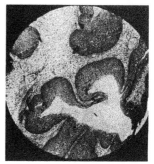

CASE 5.

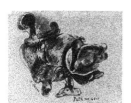

CASE 5.

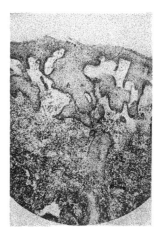

CASE 6.

AN EXPERIMENTAL STUDY ON THE RECURRENCE OF LYMPHATIC GLANDS AND THE REGENERATION OF LYMPHATIC VESSELS IN THE DOG.

By ARTHUR W. MEYER, M. D.,

Assistant in Anatomy, The Johns Hopkins University.

(*From the Anatomical Laboratory of the Johns Hopkins University.*)

The careful anatomical studies (1 and 2) on the axillary lymphatic glands; on the tracheal and bronchial glands (3), and on those adjacent to the common and external and internal iliac arteries (4) show conclusively that we have not the necessary data for a thorough description of the lymphatic glands in man, at the present time. These painstaking studies show that there is a great variation in the size, number and location of the lymphatic glands in a given region, that they are but poorly developed in infancy and tend to disappear with old age. They have also confirmed the belief that the lymphatic glands reach a maximum of development in adult life and that they undergo fatty degeneration and involution at a later age.

Unfortunately, in these studies sufficient account of the modifying influences of disease was not taken. This omission necessarily detracts greatly from their value, for it is manifestly inaccurate to regard as normal what may be abnormal. When we recall how rapidly disease may permanently affect the lymphatic glands it is evident that a statistical study of the size and number of glands is apt to be especially misleading. The influence of either local or general disease makes the whole problem a complicated one. A histological study of every gland seems quite impossible; yet only in this way can we decide to what extent a given gland has in years past been affected by disease. The question as to what is normal is further complicated by the reported fatty involution of glands and by the difficulty of distinguishing between mere accumulations of lymphocytes and true lymphatic glands. In a histological examination of the fat of the axilla of normal individuals Zehnder (2 and 5) found lymph nodules of follicular structure, streaks of lymphadenoid tissue with and without lymph passages, and isolated follicles outside of the true capsule of the gland. Bartel and Stein (6) also speak of lymphadenoid formations in adults, which consist of a collection of lymphocytes with a marginal sinus. These they regard as embryonic stages in which follicles, medullary cords and trabeculæ are not to be found. Glands of microscopical size have also been described in adults by Kling (7). They are found in the walls of the stomach and are known to occur in great numbers in the mesentery.

Aside from microscopical examinations it is not an easy matter to determine what is and what is not a lymphatic gland by ordinary dissecting-room methods. The number of glands found in any region will depend largely upon the acuteness of the observer, the care with which he works, and the age and past history of the subject. In order to locate small glands, special methods of treating the adjacent fat are required. The studies above referred to and some personal observations lead me to believe that in any given region, glands of such varying sizes exist that the smaller ones are recognized only with difficulty by the unaided eye. Only a microscopical examination can reveal the smallest glands and enable us to distinguish between a minute gland which has undergone fatty degeneration and a small fat lobule. That these involuted and small glands and irregular accumulations of lymphocytes have been concerned in the reported recurrence of glands after extirpation and the observed increase in the number of the lymphatic glands in disease, pregnancy and lactation is highly probable.

I. REGENERATION OF LYMPHATIC GLANDS.

A review of the literature on regeneration, recurrence and formation of lymphatic glands in adult life reveals three forms of evidence: clinical, pathological and experimental. In this discussion only the experimental evidence will be considered in detail. The clinically observed recurrence of lymphatic glands after extirpation and their increase in number in such diseases as tuberculosis, malignant tumors, and in such conditions as pregnancy and lactation, naturally led to a series of experiments on animals. These experiments have up to the present, been performed upon dogs and rabbits and consisted in the removal of a part or of the whole of a gland or, *presumably* of all the glands in a given region. Consequently both the question of regeneration and that of the recurrence of glands after resection have been experimentally investigated. The results of these experiments have been very conflicting. To what extent this disagreement is due to the fact that different species of animals of varying ages have been used and that no account was taken of the existence of lymphatic glands of microscopical size, involuted glands and accumulations of lymphocytes it is impossible to say.

Although Bayer (8) published a paper entitled "Ueber Regeneration und Neubildung der Lymphdrüsen" in 1885, the first experiments on regeneration *per se*, were done by Delius (9) in 1888. Delius experimented upon dogs and rabbits lymphaticæ cervicales superficialis of rabbits. In some cases the glands were perforated by a small knife which was rotated after piercing the gland. In others a wedge-shaped portion of the gland was removed. A piece of catgut was then placed in the defect to mark the seat of the operation. A series of nine experiments was made, but we are not told how old the animals were, and whether or not account was taken of the catgut, or of hairs from the animals operated on which were accidentally introduced during the operation, and which must have given rise to infection.

From an examination of tissue removed from seven hours to eight days after operation, Delius concluded that regeneration took place by proliferation of elements like those in normal lymphatic glands. Leucocytes appeared in enormous numbers by seven hours, but decreased after the third day. Degeneration of the leucocytes which began by the seventeenth hour reached a maximum by forty-eight hours. After five days leucocytes were found near the catgut only. In every case after seventeen hours mitoses appeared in the fixed tissue elements. Daughter cells of the fixed tissue elements were present by forty-eight hours. These were the only kind of cells which underwent mitoses in the whole process of regeneration. Later the fixed cells of the gland grew into the defect from the periphery, and formed a network which contained mitotic cells and after forty-eight hours, also lymphocytes. Delius conceived the lymphocytes to be pushed forward from the older areas or more probably, to have arisen from the daughter cells of the fixed tissue elements. He reports giant cells near the foreign bodies—hair and catgut.

In 1899 Ribbert (10) repeated these experiments of Delius on rabbits, but chose the submaxillary instead of the superficial cervical lymphatic glands. The operation consisted in the removal of wedge-shaped pieces including one-fifth to one-sixth of the gland. Instead of catgut Ribbert interposed silk thread, pieces of sponge, or pieces of injected lung which had been preserved in alcohol. The age of the animals is again not given, but the histological report is a very complete one. The rabbits were killed from seventy-four hours to five to eight days after operation, when sponge was introduced into the defect; and from twenty-four hours to ten to thirty-six days, when alcoholic specimens of injected lung were so used. The results showed only partial regeneration of the glands with encapsulation of the foreign bodies and the formation of a lymphatic network in small areas of the foreign body. This regeneration Ribbert ascribed to the fixed tissue elements, the endothelium of the lymph-vessels, the fixed cells of the reticulum, to the corresponding cells of the medullary cords and follicles and to the elements of the walls of the vessels. These various elements are said to grow into the foreign body accompanied by blood vessels, where they divide mitotically and form free round cells which transform themselves into lymphocytes. Lymph cells do not take part in the regenerative processes save as some of them wander in later and help to increase the number of lymph cells found in the newly formed tissue. Ribbert adds that he does not attribute much significance to infiltration by lymphocytes!

The only other experimental study of the question of regeneration is that of Heuter (11). Heuter's experiments were done on the cervical lymphatic glands of dogs with examination of tissues from two to fourteen days after operation.

After removal of part of a gland no regeneration, but scar tissue formation was found. Heuter did not interpose a foreign body to mark the defect and for examination used tissue from cases in which healing took place by first intention. He points out that areas of adenoid tissue become isolated by the development of connective tissue into the adenoid tissue surrounding the defect at the expense of the adenoid tissue, in such a manner as to suggest the development of lymphatic tissue. He objects to Ribbert's experiments because a foreign body was introduced, because Ribbert's conception of reticulum was faulty and says that since Ribbert saw the beginning of regenerative changes as early as the fourth day, the picture must have been obscured by the inflammatory reaction following the operation. Heuter also points out that the process of encapsulation of the foreign body, the removal of the pigment from the pieces of injected lung and the presence of giant cells must all have influenced the regenerative processes.

My own observations on the regeneration of lymphatic glands were incidental and quite unimportant; but since they have some bearing upon the question under discussion, I feel justified in reporting them. In my series of experiments on dogs there were two cases of partial excision of a popliteal gland. In these cases from one-half to two-thirds of the gland was removed, in dogs three and four months old respectively. After the skin incision had been made the gland with the fat over it was caused to protrude from the incision by lateral pressure. The incision was then extended to the upper surface of the gland and the latter freed from the surrounding fat by blunt dissection, special care being taken not to injure the afferent and efferent vessels. After from one-half to two-thirds of the gland had been excised what remained was replaced into the wound which was closed by a subcutaneous silver-wire suture. Healing promptly followed and in five days there was little evidence of the operation. By the seventh day in one case and by the tenth day in the other, a deep abscess had begun to form and finally discharged about one centimeter laterally from the line of incision. There was no further trouble and in a few weeks granulation was complete. In the one case in which a histological examination of tissue taken one hundred and sixty-one days after the operation was made, there was no sign of regeneration. Apparently suppuration had destroyed all glandular tissue and healing by granulation may have prevented regeneration from taking place. It is evident that in both of these cases the infection must have been secondary. It seems probable to me that this arose through infection of the lymph which had exuded from the cut surface of the gland for no such result as this followed any of the other operations. When infection occurred in these it was always in the skin incision itself, never in the depth of the wound, and followed promptly after operation.

So far as regeneration in the cervical and submaxillary lymphatic glands of *rabbits* is concerned we must conclude from these experiments of Delius and Ribbert that the question is still an open one. Delius and Ribbert observed regenerative processes as early as the fourth day after operation, without taking any account of the inflammatory reaction following an operation which included the introduction of catgut, and hairs from the animals operated on in Delius's cases. Besides, the histological report is not convincing and does not agree at all with that of Heuter. Ribbert, who reported only partial regeneration by thirty-six days, also failed to lay sufficient stress on infiltration and the presence of a foreign body. Besides, as Heuter has pointed out his conception of reticulum was faulty and we may add that his opinion as to the origin of lymphocytes has not been confirmed.

In dogs we can, I think, accept Heuter's experiments as conclusive for the dogs operated on. No foreign body was introduced and the histological report is very satisfactory. It must be remembered that regenerative activities might be present in young dogs but absent in older ones and even if regeneration does not occur in the dog it may do so in the rabbit. In any study on regeneration it is of great importance to consider the age of the animal operated on and its place in the animal kingdom. Studies in regeneration although conflicting, have shown quite clearly that these powers are more active in the lower orders and the earlier in embryonic or postembryonic life that the experiment is performed. They may indeed be present in early life and absent later, and that regeneration may be present in principle even when its capabilities are insignificant, seems to be indicated by the studies on regeneration of the epithelia of the larger gall ducts and by the regenerative activity observed in ruptured human livers by Orth and Heile.

II. RECURRENCE OF LYMPHATIC GLANDS.

Bayer (8) (in 1885), undertook the first experiments on the recurrence of extirpated lymphatic glands in the axilla of the dog. The age of the dogs varied from two weeks to several years and the interval between operation and death from several weeks to four months. Bayer removed all the axillary lymphatic glands after the injection of India ink. Before killing the animals cinnabar was injected in order to distinguish the newly formed glands from those left after operation. In the first dog which was one and a half years old, changes in the fat were noticed six weeks after operation around the places stained by India ink, at the seat of operation. From these changes Bayer says we must assume a change from fat to connective tissue cells and further asserts that the sheaths of the vessels give off the material for the formation of new lobules of fatty tissue. The fact that more cinnabar than India ink is found in the glands is taken as an evidence of the young stage of the glands.

In the second dog the result was a negative one. This Bayer attributes to healing per secundam and to the enlargement of the collateral lymphatics by which means stasis, the main impulse to regeneration was prevented. From these two contradictory experiments the following conclusion is reached. After removal of lymphatic glands recurrence takes place in a comparatively short time from the surrounding fat

unless a collateral lymphatic circulation develops or healing takes place by granulation.

In 1886 Bayer (12) elaborated his views from a study of diseased glands which he conceives to impede the flow of lymph, cause dilatation of lymphatic vessels, saturation of the surrounding tissues, secondary emigration of lymph cells and proliferation of cells in circumscribed areas near blood and lymph vessels. These latter areas are later transformed into follicular structures through cell activity.

In 1891, Bayer (13) developed his theory of the formation of lymphatic glands from fat still further from a study of the phenomena observed in adjacent fat after extirpation of tumors. At the outset of the paper the author states that the opinion of Klein (15) that adipose tissue really belongs to the lymphatic system and is to be considered as changed lymphatic tissue, won more and more truth with him. From the examination of an extensive cavernous lymphangioma Bayer says he is able to confirm and to extend his former observations. He traces transitions from fat to endothelium of lymph spaces and says that the capillaries are in some places surrounded by accumulations of cells which are formed not only by proliferation of cells of the adventitia but by proliferation of fat cells as well. These accumulations he further considers as having a possible origin in the cells of the sarcolemma and he regards it a proven fact that adventitia cells can give rise to fat cells at one time and furnish material for new blood vessels at another time.

In 1895 (14) Bayer says that since *experimentation introduces unavoidable obstacles to a good observation of the facts,* he has confined himself to the examination of glandular tumors such as lymph-angiomata and angiose-lymphomata. The following reasons are given for the recurrence of lymphatic glands: (1) lymphatic glands lie in fat; (2) glands and fat lie as a separate whole; (3) disease of the glands is accompanied by striking macroscopical and microscopical changes in the surrounding fat; (4) total destruction of lymphatic glands by disease leads to a decrease of fat; (5) the number of glands increases pari passu with the decrease of fat; (6) unmistakable pictures of newly formed glands in all stages of development can be found; (7) the surrounding fat contains separate lymph channels which are in communication with those formed pathologically and with the lymph channels of glands; (8) changes occur in the fat surrounding lymphatic glands, which must be considered regenerative. Bayer also reports a direct communication between lymph clefts lined only by fat cells and the lymph channels and says he has traced the transition from fat cells bounding these clefts to perfect lymphatic glands. He adds, however, that the complete process only occurs under propitious circumstances.

I have reported Bayer's work at some length in order to show that his main evidence is not experimental but pathological. While fully aware that pathological and physiological regeneration have been shown to be practically identical and that pathological regeneration is thought to be only an enhanced and modified physiological regeneration following either mechanical injury or disease, yet, it seems to me, granting that Bayer's observations are correct, his error lies in the assumption that regenerative processes which may be present in pathological states, are also present normally. That this is not the case Bizzozero (16) has well expressed in the following words: " Wenn sich die Verhältnisse ändern und gewisse pathologische Zustände eintreten ändert sich auch die Regenerationsthätigkeit und kann auch an solchen Orten sehr lebhaft werden wo sie normal nicht zu finden ist."

Number of the dog	Age	Interval in days	Nature of the healing	Region operated upon	Side operated upon	Nature of operation
I.	2-3 yr.	7	Per primam	Mesentery	Both	One gland 3.5x6x5 mm removed.
II.	3-4 yr.	91	Per primam	Mesentery	Both	Two glands removed on each side. R. S.—48x12x8 and 6x8x5 mm. L. S.—40x8x 8 and 32x10x8 mm.
IV.	6 mo.	25	Per secundam	Popliteal	Right	One gland and one third of surrounding fat removed.
			Per primam	Popliteal	Left	Two glands and no fat were excised.
V.	3 mo.	161	Per primam	Popliteal	Right	One gland and most of the fat was removed.
			Per primam	Popliteal	Left	Two-thirds of the gland only was removed—abscess after seven days.
VI.	2-½ mo.	89	Per secundam	Popliteal	Right	All (?) the fat and glands were removed.
			Per primam	Popliteal	Left	Gland only was removed. A piece of the capsule remained.
VII.	4 mo.	53	Per primam	Popliteal	Right	Gland only was removed. Animal lost.
			Per primam	Popliteal	Left	One-half of gland removed—abscess after ten days.
VIII.	3-½ mo.	85	Per primam	Popliteal	Right	Gland and fat removed.
			Per primam	Popliteal	Left	Gland only removed.

The table above gives a summary of the experiments on the popliteal and mesenteric glands.

Through the suggestion of Prof. Sabin, a number of experiments on the lymphatics were undertaken in order to obtain, if possible, additional evidence on these questions. These experiments included the extirpation of lymphatic glands and the resection of lymphatic trunks in dogs from two months to several years old. In two cases the large glands lying at the root of the mesentery near the spinal column were removed and in seven instances the popliteal glands were extirpated. Although the lymphatic system of the dog (17) is not highly developed, one and occasionally two, palpable glands are found in the popliteal region.

The difficulties necessarily associated with abdominal operations caused me to choose the popliteal region as especially adapted to my purpose. The operation here was less severe, the seat of operation was not hidden from view by adhesions between coils of intestine after operation, a more complete extirpation was possible, the area drained by the removed glands could easily be ascertained, the progress of healing could be better observed and the nutrition of the animal was not disturbed. In these operations the ordinary surgical technique was adopted and every care was exercised to prevent infection. Where infection did occur a special note was made and account was taken of this fact in the histological examination of the tissue. Daily notes were made on the condition of the wounds and the state of health of the animals.

In four cases the popliteal glands and all the fat in the popliteal region were removed as thoroughly as possible. This could easily be done as deep down as the popliteal vessels. In three cases the gland with the overlying fat was caused to protrude by pressure from the skin incision and the gland freed by blunt dissection from the surrounding fat after the necessary superficial incision into the overlying fat. In these operations especial care was exercised not to disturb the adjacent fat because Bayer laid considerable stress upon this fact. The skin incision was closed by a subcutaneous catgut, silk or silver suture and a sterile dressing was applied. The afferent and efferent lymphatic vessels were not ligated.

From the table opposite it will be seen that the intervals varied from seven to ninety-one days in the two abdominal operations, and from twenty-five to one hundred and sixty-one days in those on the popliteal glands. So that for all practical purposes we have an interval of experimentation varying from twenty-five to one hundred and sixty-one days. An earlier examination of tissue than twenty-five days seemed unnecessary to me since it hardly seems possible that the evidences of attempted regeneration would not be visible after three and a half weeks if present at an earlier day. If regeneration had occurred a later examination would have revealed this as well as an earlier one, while it would not have had to reckon with the inflammatory reaction following injury. The nature of the operations varied from partial excision of fat and glands to as complete an excision as possible. If we exclude those cases in which healing took place by granulation and the two instances in which a part of the gland was left in situ, there remain five operations on the popliteal glands and two on the mesenteric glands against which no objection can be urged. In three out of five operations on the popliteal glands the gland or glands and no fat were removed. In two cases the gland or glands and all the fat possible, were removed. In the abdominal operations the glands only were removed by blunt dissection.

Before killing the animals they were etherized and the lymphatics of the extremity injected from the pad of the foot with India ink, as far as the inguinal and lumbar glands. In several cases the animals were bled to death after injection of the lymphatics and half a litre of one per cent formaline injected into the aorta. These animals were then skinned and the bodies placed in five per cent formaline for two days, after which they were transferred to alcohol. In other cases the fat with the contained lymphatics was removed *en masse* from the popliteal region, spread on wax and fixed in formaline. In every case the fresh tissue was carefully examined macroscopically as to the condition of the injected lymphatic trunks and the presence of small glands. After fixing and hardening, the tissue was cut into blocks of convenient size, imbedded in celloidin and cut 10-30 microns thick, each tenth section being stained and mounted. All sections were preserved, however, and more were stained as required. In some cases every fifth section was examined.

Such an examination of the tissue in three out of the five experiments on the popliteal glands showed no evidences whatever of the presence of lymphatic glands or of lymphatic nodules. In those cases in which total excision of the fat had been done the amount of fat found post mortem was much smaller but the histological picture was exactly the same as in those in which only part or none of it had been removed. In two of the five cases of extirpation a small gland was found. In one of these operations the gland only, while in the other case, both gland and fat had been removed. One of these specimens was from a dog two and a half months old at the time of operation. Healing was by first intention, the interval was eighty-nine days, and a piece of the capsule of the gland was left *in situ*. This remnant was plainly visible in the sections, but there was no lymphatic tissue in the neighborhood of it. The gland which was found, lay in a distant part of the section; it had the appearance of a mature gland and was surrounded by a definite capsule of connective tissue. This gland was about 3x2½ mm. in size, and the fat around it showed no infiltration or other changes indicative of active regenerative processes of any kind.

The small gland found in the other case looked also like an adult gland, or rather follicle. There were evidences of degeneration in the center and the gland lay in a mass of connective tissue which showed no signs of cellular proliferation. This gland which was only one millimeter in size also lay distant from the seat of operation. On referring back to my memoranda I found the following note made on the fifth day after operation: "On the left hind leg a nodule about seven millimeters in size is felt in the depth of the popliteal region. It is hard and shot-like and suggests an enlarged, unremoved gland." Aside from the value of this note the fact that no regenerative changes were found in the regions from which the glands had been removed seems to indicate that we have to deal with unremoved glands. The existence of glands of microscopical size and of irregular masses of lymphatic tissue in man has already been referred to. There seems to be no good reason why these may not exist in the case of dogs, and especially in young dogs. In order to determine whether or not small glands are commonly present in the popliteal region of dogs, the popliteal fat was removed in eight dogs, from two to four years of age. This

fat was pinned on wax, all blood was removed by washing, and fixed in formaline. After hardening in alcohol the specimens were cleared in creosote and xylol and some in oil of bergamot. An examination by means of the dissecting microscope revealed five small lymphatic glands from 3-6 mm. in size, in these sixteen specimens. From these facts it cannot be doubted that still smaller glands are equally common. It may be recalled that Arnold (18) has shown that accumulations of round cells which look like small follicles, are found normally in rabbits and dogs in the interacinous bands of connective tissue about the gall ducts. If such be the case it is evident that complete extirpation of the lymphatic glands of any region is quite impossible and that the small glands found in the above cases were most likely unremoved mature glands and not newly formed ones. Since also none of the specimens in which healing took place by granulation showed any signs of regeneration or recurrence, I feel justified in concluding from this and from the above facts that in these seven instances of extirpation of the popliteal glands there was no recurrence.

In the two cases of abdominal operation in which the large lymphatic glands lying in the root of the mesentery of the small intestine were removed by blunt dissection, the condition of the intestine was a very interesting one. The glands removed were approximately 3x1x1.5 cms. and drained all of the small intestine save the duodenum and all of the large intestine save the rectum. In neither of these cases was there any ascites or sufficient disturbance of nutrition to cause an unusual loss of weight in the animals. Indeed, in one of the dogs there was a steady weekly gain in weight of one-half to two pounds after the first week.

Upon opening the abdomen of the first dog seven days after operation, the folds of the mesentery of the small intestine were matted together and the omentum was adherent to the small intestine and mesentery. On gently breaking the adhesions little pockets of chyle were found. The omental adhesions had sealed off the cut ends of the peripheral lymphatic ducts and evidently prevented the escape of chyle into the peritoneal cavity. The wall of the intestine was œdematous along the mesenteric border. Injections of Prussian blue into the walls of the small intestine could be followed to the seat of operation but never went into the receptaculum. The latter could be injected from the duodenum, however. The thoracic duct was distended with lymph and not with chyle. These injections seem to show that the central ends of the lymphatic ducts had not been regenerated. Tissue taken from the seat of operation showed a typical picture of a granulating wound. There were no evidences of regeneration of the removed lymphatic glands but there was an intense infiltration.

The other dog on which a similar operation was made was killed eighty-four days after operation. In this case, too, there was no ascites and no loss of weight beyond that following any abdominal operation. The omentum was found adherent to the parietal peritoneum along the linea alba and the adjacent coils of small intestine were firmly adherent to each other in numerous places near the seat of operation.

No pockets of chyle were found though the dog had been fed milk before the killing, as a result of which the intestinal lymphatics and the receptaculum were well filled with chyle. Owing to the manipulations made necessary by the adhesions these naturally injected lymphatics could not be traced to the seat of operation. However, injections of Prussian blue made from various parts of the small intestine under ether, seemed to show a direct connection with the receptaculum. In some cases the injection seemed to run across the seat of operation and in one case an injected duct was traced from the ileum to the duodenum. After all the injections had been made the viscera were fixed *in situ* by the intra-arterial injection of a one per cent solution of formaline.

The histological examination of the tissue from the seat of operation showed small lymphatic glands present in some of the sections. These glands were always enclosed in a definite capsule which was sharply delimited from the surrounding fat. They did not lie at the places where the granulation tissue was found and had all the appearances of mature glands. There were no signs of cellular proliferation. Consequently it seems probable that these are also small glands which existed previously to operation and which are so numerous in the mesentery; or small lymphatic nodules which lay outside of the capsules of the removed glands. Although, in my opinion, all these experiments on dogs were negative so far as recurrence of lymphatic glands is concerned, such recurrence may take place in younger dogs or in case of disease. As pointed out above, the only *experimental* evidence of such recurrence is the one case in a dog one and a half years old, reported by Bayer. Bayer's second case was negative and against his first case serious objections can be urged. Besides, although Bayer reports having operated on a series of dogs whose ages varied from two weeks to several years, the rest of the series are not reported.

It does not seem probable to me that recurrence is likely to occur after years, unless in disease, if there be no signs of recurrence in five or six months. Regenerative processes, when they do occur, have been shown to take place *pari passu* with the repair of the injury. Both the blood supply and cellular activity are greatest at this time, obstacles to growth are absent, a collateral circulation has not developed, and other organs have not assumed a vicarious activity. When granulation is complete the granulation tissue would seem to interpose an obstacle to regenerative processes and in the case under consideration both injury and stasis are absent as stimuli.

III. Regeneration of Lymphatic Vessels.

The injections of Prussian blue into the intestine in one case of resection of the mesenteric glands already referred to, seemed to indicate that the severed lymphatic trunks had after eighty-four days or previously, re-established central connections with the receptaculum. I say seemed to indicate, because it is impossible to say whether or not some lymphatic vessels remained uninjured on the outside of the gland when the latter

was removed by blunt dissection. It is also probable that small blood vessels were injected, for the study of the sections from the seat of operation show many blood vessels containing injection material.

In order to test the question of regeneration of the larger lymphatic vessels by actual experiment a series of sections and resections were done on the large lymphatic trunks lying on either side of the saphenous vein, near the knee of the hind leg of the dog. Preparatory to operation the lymphatics of the hind leg of the dog were studied by means of injections of Prussian blue, methylene blue and India ink. By these methods it was found that twenty-five minims of a one per cent solution of methylene blue when injected into the pad would make the main lymphatic trunks plainly visible.

Before making the skin incision at the time of operation, a sterile normal salt solution containing one per cent methylene blue was injected into the pad of the foot. One and sometimes two, of the largest lymphatic trunks lying just anterior to the saphenous vein in the region of the knee were then ligated with black silk thread and cut between ligatures, in four cases. In four other cases from 3-5 mm. of the trunk was resected between the seat of the ligatures. The skin incision was closed by a subcutaneous catgut or silk suture and a sterile dressing applied. There was never any œdema of the leg below the seat of operation save when the dressings had been applied too snugly. The following table summarizes the operations with results, as found by injections after killing the animals and by microscopical examination of the tissue.

Dog	Age	Interval in days	Healing	Region	Operation	Result
III.	4 yr.	91	Per primam	Left hind leg	Resection of largest trunk	No regeneration
....	....	91	Per secundam	Right hind leg	Section of largest trunk	No regeneration
....	....	14	Per primam	Left front leg	Resection of largest trunk	No regeneration
....	....	14	Per primam	Right front leg	Section of largest trunk	No regeneration
VI.	2-½ mo.	84	Per secundam	Left hind leg	Resection of two trunks	No regeneration
....	....	..	Per primam	Right hind leg	Section of two trunks	No regeneration
VII.	3-½ mo.	27	Per primam	Left hind leg	Resection of largest trunk	No regeneration
....	....	27	Per primam	Right hind leg	Section of largest trunk	No regeneration

In these experiments the intervals between the time of operation and the death of the animals varied from fourteen to ninety-one days, and the age of the animals from two and a half months to four years. In two out of the eight cases healing was by granulation, in six by first intention. After etherizing the animals preparatory to killing, 10-20 cc. of Prussian blue or India ink were injected into the pad and the leg alternately flexed and extended while the pad of the foot was massaged, in order to assure a thorough injection. In some cases the dog was then bled and a solution of formaline injected intravascularly. After fixation the skin of the leg was removed and the condition of the lymphatic trunks especially noted. In all cases the ligated and resected lymphatic trunks were distended with the injection fluid up to the seat of operation, but never across the same. The injection of the resected trunks above the seat of operation was always accomplished through the collateral subcutaneous and anastomosing vessels. The accompanying lymphatic trunks were usually found considerably larger near the seat of resection than at the time of operation even when only the same amount of injection fluid was used as at the time of operation.

The tissue including the saphenous vein and the three large accompanying lymphatic trunks, at the seat of operation, was excised and after the usual procedures cut 10-30 microns thick, in celloidin. Four specimens were examined in series and four by staining every fifth or tenth section. All unstained sections were preserved, however. The presence of the black silk ligature made it easy to recognize the exact seat of the operation in the sections. The resected or sected lymphatic trunks could never be traced across these regions and were often found with thickened walls in an obliterative condition. The results of the histological examination agreed entirely with those of injection and were exactly the same whether section or resection had been done. Around the ligatures there was an intense accumulation of lymphocytes and leucocytes such as is characteristic about encapsulation of a foreign body in granulation tissue. Regeneration of lymphatic trunks was found in no instance. It may be urged that the silk ligature being a foreign body may have interfered with the process of regeneration. This may be so; yet in all the operations on the popliteal glands the afferent and efferent trunks which were always cut close to the hilum of the gland were never ligated and still it was never possible to inject these large trunks across the seat of operation. The large afferent lymphatic trunk could always be traced into the fat in the popliteal region, but the injection never extended across the gap left by the removal of the glands, to the efferent part of the same trunk. Since there were such operations it seems quite probable that if the silk ligature had been the only obstacle to regeneration, connection between the cut ends of the lymphatic trunk in the popliteal region would have been re-established in some cases at least.

If stasis be the main stimulus to regeneration it is quite probable that resection and ligation of one or two principal trunks in the region of the knee and elbow did not interpose sufficient obstruction to the flow of lymph. This can hardly have been the case in the operations on the popliteal glands, however, for here all the large trunks of the hind leg converge to form a single trunk. Consequently, all the superficial

lymph from the lower extremity must have been carried past this point of obstruction by the numerous small lymphatics of the skin. Further experiments in which all the superficial lymphatics of an extremity are divided have been undertaken, and it is hoped that some evidence bearing on the question of regeneration of the larger lymphatic trunks and of the formation of lymphatic channels in granulation tissue may be obtained.

The fact that in these experiments the large lymphatic trunks have, in all respects, acted like blood vessels under similar conditions makes it probable that the capillary lymphatics act similarly also in the case of a granulating wound. Talke (19) found epithelial tubes which he recognized as lymphatic vessels, in the adhesions about the ascending colon in a case of perityphlitis and in a case of thickened pleura. In the latter Talke could trace branches from the visceral subpleural lymphatics into the pleural thickening. These newly-formed lymphatic capillaries joined the old lymphatic vessels and extended in the general direction of the blood vessels. They were composed of epithelial tubes from 6-10 microns in diameter, which in some cases contained lymph, coal dust and pigmented leucocytes. Although Talke was not able to see the mode of formation of these lymphatic sprouts because of the absence of sufficient granulation tissue in his specimens, he thinks that the new formation of lymphatics proceeds as in case of the blood vessels, from the pre-existing lymphatic vessels. Further evidence of a similar nature is offered by Behre (20) in a case of tuberculosis in which coal pigment *seems* to have been carried across a much thickened and densely adherent pleura. However, these pathological evidences, though valuable and suggestive need verification, before we can accept the formation of lymphatic vessels in granulation tissue as a fact. As far as I am able to learn, such experiments have not yet been done nor can I find any reference in the literature to experiments on the question of regeneration of lymphatic trunks such as reported here.

It is a pleasant duty to acknowledge my indebtedness to Prof. Mall for his interest and many suggestions.

REFERENCES.

1. Stiles, H. J.: Edinburgh Medical Journal, Vol. XXXVIII, 1893.

2. Zehnder: Virchow's Archiv. Vol. CXX.

3. Sukienikow: Berl. kiln. Wochenschrift, Vol. XL, 1903.

4. Rept. of Com. of Collective Investigation of the Anat. Soc. of G. B., Jr. of Anat. & Phys., Vol. XXXII, 1898.

5. Sanderson: Edinburgh Medical Journal, Vol. XV, 1870.

6. Bartel u. Stein: Arch f. Anat. u. Phys.; Hft. II u. III; Anat. Abt., 1905.

7. Kling: Arch. f. mikr. Anat., Bd. LXIII, 1904.

8. Bayer, K.: Zeitschrift f. Heilkunde. Bd. VI, 1885.

9. Delius: Ueber die Regeneration der Lymphdrüsen. Dissert. Bonn, 1888.

10. Ribbert: Beiträge z. path. Anat. u. allg. Path., Bd. VI, 1889.

11. Heuter: Verh. d. Deutsch. Path. Gesellsch., Heft I, 1904.

12. Bayer, K.: Archiv f. Heilkunde, Bd. VII, 1886.

13. Bayer, K.: Zeitsch. f. Heilk. (Berl.), Bd. XII, 1891.

14. Bayer, K.: Arch. f. Chir., Bd. XLIX, 1895.

15. Klein and Smith: Atlas of Histology, Phila., 1880.

16. Bizzozero: Virchow's Archiv, Bd. CX, 1887.

17. Richter, Johannes: Archiv f. mikr. Anat., Bd. LX, 1902.

18. Arnold: Virchow's Archiv, Bd. LXXXII, 1880.

19. Talke, Ludwig: Beitr. z. path. Anat. u. allg. Path., XXXII, 1902.

20. Behre, K.: Zur Frage der Lymphgefäss-Neubildung. Kiel, 1898.

NOTES ON NEW BOOKS.

Distribution of the Cells in the Intermedio-lateral Tract of the Spinal Cord. By ALEXANDER BRUCE, M. D. XLV, 105-131, 1 pl. *(Reprinted from the Transactions of the Royal Society of Edinburgh, 1906.)*

Professor Bruce has increased the debt of neurologists to him by adding to his well-known atlases of the medulla and spinal cord the present study, which deals with the exact distribution of the cells in the intermedio-lateral tract of the spinal cord. This intermedio-lateral tract, first so designated by Lockhart Clarke, and the adjacent cell-groups have long interested investigators of neural anatomy. The studies of Waldeyer and of Argutinsky will be especially recalled. No one had, however, worked out carefully, by modern methods, the exact distribution of the cells in the tract.

Bruce has examined serial sections from the upper part of the cervical enlargement to the lower extremity of the spinal cord, studying in all some 7000 sections, of which more than 5000 contained cells of the intermedio-lateral tract. These cells, as found on both sides of the cord, were carefully counted independently by four different observers. The study illustrates the topography in the various segments. It proves that the intermedio-lateral tract is present in the upper cervical region, in the lower cervical, thoracic and upper lumbar regions and in the lower sacral region, though it is absent in the cervical enlargement from C.5 to C.7 and in the lumbo-sacral region from L.3 to the upper part of S.3 inclusive. It is interesting that the middle cells described by Waldeyer do not form any part of the intermedio-lateral tract. Bruce's counts show some 89,000 cells in the tract on each side. The cells do not form a continuous column, but occur in groups or clusters. The distribution on the two sides may be asymmetrical. There appears to be a remarkable increase in the number of cells of the tract in the third thoracic segment. The vascular supply to the tract is said to be largely independent of that of the motor cells of the anterior horn.

Though Bruce's study is anatomical, he comments upon the physiological function of the cells, and points out that where there is the greatest outflow of sympathetic fibres from the cord, there the number of cells in the intermedio-lateral tract is greatest. He mentions the suggestions of Anderson and Herring and of Onuf and Collins that the intermedio-lateral tract is the source of the sympathetic fibers, but he feels that further researches are necessary before anything definite can be said on the subject.

There is as yet scarcely any pathology of the intermedio-lateral tract. It escapes entirely in cases of chronic degeneration of the anterior horns, such as occurs in progressive muscular atrophy and in amyotrophic lateral sclerosis. In one case it has been found to be degenerated in connection with erythromelalgia. Bruce expresses the hope that future research will succeed in explaining symptoms of visceral and vascular diseases hitherto imperfectly understood. L. F. B.

Lectures on Auto-intoxication in Disease, or Self-Poisoning of the Individual. By CH. BOUCHARD, Professor of Pathology and Therapeutics, with a preface and new chapters added. Translated by THOMAS OLIVER, M. A., M. D., F. R. C. P. Second Revised Edition. *(Philadelphia: F. A. Davis Company, Publishers, 1906.)*

The publication of a second, revised translation of Professor Bouchard's book shows that there has been a demand for it, which may be regarded as a testimonial of its value. The reviewer does not feel, however, that this demand is justified by the character of the book. Its success simply proves that the medical profession has not completely outgrown a love for the metaphysical and theoretical. It is because it is so much easier to think than to try, and so much more simple to accept elaborate reasons ready made than to scrutinize proofs carefully that this book appeals to so many. The terms uric acid diathesis and auto-intoxication have furnished so many with material to glibly cover what they don't know that it may seem cruel to try to deprive still others of this comfort. So much semi-scientific work of this sort has come from American sources and this has been so often held up against us that it is a true pleasure to know that this book has been written by a professor in the University of Paris and that he has permitted its republication after ten years.

The main experimental work from which the broad and far-reaching conclusions are drawn is the writer's well-known work on the toxicity of the urine as tested by injection into animals. It is to the credit of the translator that he has introduced some of the criticisms which have been uttered against Bouchard's work. Interesting and valuable as it has been because stimulating to further and more accurate work, it by no means possesses the importance or justifies the conclusions given to it by Bouchard.

A great many allusions are made to the scientific work of others, but as no accurate references are given, the book has no value as a reference book on abnormalities of metabolism. It would be useless to quote many of the absurd theories which the book contains, such as the series of ills which are believed to follow in the train of dilatation of the stomach. "Chlorosis in young girls and pulmonary phthisis are often induced by dilatation of the stomach." There is even thought to be a close relationship between "nodosites on the second articulations, dilatation of the stomach and typhoid fever."

"The healthy man is both a receptacle and a laboratory of poisons. In fact, he receives them in his food, he creates them by dissimilation, and he forms them in his secretions."

Truly, one may say with Sir Thomas Browne, that "men . . . quarrel with their constitutions for being sick; but I . . . do wonder that we are not always so."

No one can deny the grains of truth upon which this book is built, and we recognize the important rôle which organic poisons play in disease, but this book does not approach these problems in any scientific or national spirit.

It will only aid in keeping alive and spreading the *theory* of auto-intoxication, about which we have already heard too much in internal medicine.

Christianity and Sex Problems. By HUGH NORTHCOTE, M. A. (*Philadelphia: F. A. Davis Company, 1914-16 Cherry Street, Publishers, 1906.*)

The author deserves much credit for approaching a difficult subject with delicacy and dignity. His aim throughout is to benefit the young and his standpoint is of the highest, in refreshing contrast to much of the pornographic literature of the past two decades. It is to be feared, however, that he underestimates the degree to which the comparatively young become informed upon these forbidden topics through the traditions of school-mates and servants. If the book is designed for the young it should be simpler in style and less ambitious in treatment. When persons have reached an age to appreciate and profit by a semi-religious and philosophical treatise upon sex relations their habits and views are generally well-fixed. The book, however, will be useful to teachers and helpful to those who have the responsibility of the moral training of aggregations of young people. It contains many valuable chapters.

The National Standard Dispensatory. Containing the natural history, chemistry, pharmacy, pharmacopœias of the United States, Great Britain and Germany, with numerous references to other foreign pharmacopœias. In accordance with the United States Pharmacopœia, 8th decennial revision of 1905 by authorization of the Convention. By HOBART AMORY HARE, Jefferson Medical College; CHARLES CASPARI, JR., Maryland College of Pharmacy; and HENRY H. RUSBY, College of Pharmacy of the City of New York. Imperial octavo. (*Philadelphia: Lea Brothers & Co., 1905.*)

This ponderous volume of 1860 pages arrayed in magnificent calf, high tribute to the bookbinders' art and a distinct credit to its publishers in paper, type and editing, supersedes the "National Dispensatory" of Stillé & Maisch, which for a quarter of a century held sway as a standard work on the botany, chemistry and therapeutics of drugs and medicines. None of the original editors are now alive, and while in its previous edition Professor Charles Caspari, of Baltimore, was associated with Messrs. Stillé & Maisch, the present work is the product of the efforts of Professors H. A. Hare of Philadelphia, who edits the therapeutical portion, Charles Caspari, Jr., of Baltimore, who edits the pharmaceutical and chemical portions, and H. H. Rusby, of New York, who edits the botanical portion. These are assisted by Messrs. Edward Kremers, of the University of Wisconsin, Daniel Base, of the University of Maryland, and Joseph Geisler, of the New York State Department of Agriculture.

As the U. S. Pharmacopœia, 1900, is a decided improvement upon and change in its predecessor, the Pharmacopœia of 1890, so this Dispensatory, based as it is upon the new Pharmacopœia, is a distinct advance and improvement upon its predecessor, the National Dispensatory. The most marked feature of difference is practically the entire elimination of the old part of the former edition. It had been the custom of former editions to let the old views it contained remain and merely add modern views, so that the book throughout was a symposium of views upon the chemistry, therapeutics, etc., of drugs from time immemorial almost down to the present day. As the present views of scientists of half a century ago upon therapeutics in the past interest us little except in an historical way, it seems wise of the present editors

to eliminate the antique from their work. The prime purpose of a Dispensatory is to serve as a commentary upon the Pharmacopœia, inasmuch as the latter gives no why's and wherefore's, and the raison d'être of many of its statements and methods and conclusions is not clear to the average practitioner of medicine and pharmacy. Our first Pharmacopœias were hence not used to any great extent and it was not until the Dispensatory was born that the Pharmacopœia became as it should be a vade-mecum to doctor and druggist.

The Dispensatory contains all that the Pharmacopœia contains, but explains each step of the latter in a readily intelligible form, and besides volunteers information upon all kindred subjects not contained in the Pharmacopœia. While for instance the Pharmacopœia contains only a small portion of all the plants, animal products and chemicals that are used in medicine, the Dispensatory attempts to, and in the main succeeds in bringing to our attention all drugs that are used anywhere in the civilized world, certainly all that are used in this country. As old drugs are continually becoming new and popular in use while new ones are dropping by the wayside, it is apparent how important it is to have at hand a work which will supply us with desired information upon any drug we may be looking for or intending to use. The general arrangement of the book is alphabetical and a perfect index makes finding the subject sought a very easy task. The Latin title prevails in all cases as the heading, followed by the English title and then the French and German title. Then follows a description or formula of the article, and thereafter its preparations, then its properties, then tests for its purity or assay methods for determining its strength and finally its therapeutical action and uses and its dose. Under any given drug all of the preparations which contain it are also given. Besides this substitutes and adulterants are also treated of in each case as a warning to the uninitiated in the all-too-much practiced arts to-day of the "just as good" and of the sophisticator.

While all the assay processes for the standardized drugs of the Pharmacopœia are given in full it would have been desirable to add in some instances explanatory remarks as to the reasons for certain steps and processes, which to the unskilled practitioner must be more or less mysterious. The idea of arranging various members of one plant family under the head of that family is an acceptable innovation and will meet with deserved approbation no doubt. The illustrations throughout the work appear to be new and specially drawn and are very creditable. The microscopical drawings of cross sections of leading drugs also add to the value of the book as a means of determining the genuine from possible adulterations or spurious drugs. The chemical and pharmacognostical part of the book is well written and thoroughly up-to-date, while the botanical part reflects a close study on the part of the editor of the most modern research on botany. A special chapter is devoted to physiological testing as an innovation in this book, and while it cannot be claimed that standards of drugs can be definitely established by animal experiments, still in cases of those drugs whose chemistry is insufficiently developed to warrant a chemical standard of strength, such as ergot and cannabis, it may be said that such a physiological test standard is better than none at all. The appendix like that of the Pharmacopœia is very extensive and follows the latter pretty closely, embracing reagents, test solutions, volumetric solutions of all kinds, and how to use them, saturation and solubility tables, molecular weights, equivalents of weights and measures in the avoirdupois, apothecaries and metric systems, alcohol and specific gravity tables, weight and volume relations and thermometric equivalents. In fine, the National Standard Dispensatory unquestionably presents the best work of its kind that has yet been published, combining fully the accuracy and thoroughness of the best German works with American completeness.   A. R. L. DOHME.

THE JOHNS HOPKINS HOSPITAL REPORTS.

VOLUME I. 423 pages, 99 plates.

VOLUME II. 570 pages, with 28 plates and figures.

VOLUME III. 766 pages, with 69 plates and figures.

VOLUME IV. 504 pages, 33 charts and illustrations.

VOLUME V. 480 pages, with 32 charts and illustrations.

CONTENTS:

The Malarial Fevers of Baltimore. By W. S. THAYER, M. D., and J. HEWETSON, M. D.

A Study of some Fatal Cases of Malaria. By LEWELLYS F. BARKER, M. B.

Studies in Typhoid Fever.

By WILLIAM OSLER, M. D., with additional papers by G. BLUMER, M. D., SIMON FLEXNER, M. D., WALTER REED, M. D., and H. C. PARSONS, M. D.

VOLUME VI. 414 pages, with 79 plates and figures.

Report in Neurology.

Studies on the Lesions Produced by the Action of Certain Poisons on the Cortical Nerve Cell (Studies Nos. I to V). By HENRY J. BERKLEY, M. D.

Introductory.—Recent Literature on the Pathology of Diseases of the Brain by the Chromate of Silver Methods; Part I.—Alcohol Poisoning.—Experimental Lesions produced by Chronic Alcoholic Poisoning (Ethyl Alcohol). 2. Experimental Lesions produced by Acute Alcoholic Poisoning (Ethyl Alcohol); Part II.—Serum Poisoning.—Experimental Lesions induced by the Action of the Dog's Serum on the Cortical Nerve Cell; Part III.—Ricin Poisoning.—Experimental Lesions induced by Acute Ricin Poisoning. 2. Experimental Lesions induced by Chronic Ricin Poisoning; Part IV.—Hydrophobic Toxæmia.—Lesions of the Cortical Nerve Cell produced by the Toxine of Experimental Rabies; Part V.—Pathological Alterations in the Nuclei and Nucleoli of Nerve Cells from the Effects of Alcohol and Ricin Intoxication; Nerve Fibre Terminal Apparatus; Asthenic Bulbar Paralysis. By HENRY J. BERKLEY.

Report in Pathology.

Fatal Puerperal Sepsis due to the Introduction of an Elm Tent. By THOMAS S. CULLEN, M. B.

Pregnancy in a Rudimentary Uterine Horn. Rupture, Death, Probable Migration of Ovum and Spermatozoa. By THOMAS S. CULLEN, M. B., and G. L. WILKINS, M. D.

Adeno-Myoma Uteri Diffusum Benignum. By THOMAS S. CULLEN, M. B.

A Bacteriological and Anatomical Study of the Summer Diarrhœas of Infants. By WILLIAM D. BOOKER, M. D.

The Pathology of Toxalbumin Intoxications. By SIMON FLEXNER, M. D.

VOLUME VII. 537 pages with illustrations.

I. A Critical Review of Seventeen Hundred Cases of Abdominal Section from the standpoint of Intra-peritoneal Drainage. By J. G. CLARK, M. D.

II. The Etiology and Structure of true Vaginal Cysts. By JAMES ERNEST STOKES, M. D.

III. A Review of the Pathology of Superficial Burns, with a Contribution to our Knowledge of the Pathological Changes in the Organs in cases of rapidly fatal burns. By CHARLES RUSSELL BARDEEN, M. D.

IV. The Origin, Growth and Fate of the Corpus Luteum. By J. G. CLARK, M. D.

V. The Results of Operations for the Cure of Inguinal Hernia. By JOSEPH C. BLOODGOOD, M. D.

VOLUME VIII. 552 pages with illustrations.

On the role of Insects, Arachnids, and Myriapods as carriers in the spread of Bacterial and Parasitic Diseases of Man and Animals. By GEORGE H. F. NUTTALL, M. D., PH. D.

Studies in Typhoid Fever.

By WILLIAM OSLER, M. D., with additional papers by J. M. T. FINNEY, M. D., S. FLEXNER, M. D., I. P. LYON, M. D., L. P. HAMBURGER, M. D., H. W. CUSHING, M. D., J. F. MITCHELL, M. D., C. N. B. CAMAC, M. D., N. B. GWYN, M. D., CHARLES P. EMERSON, M. D., H. H. YOUNG, M. D., and W. S. THAYER, M. D.

VOLUME IX. 1060 pages, 66 plates and 210 other illustrations.

Contributions to the Science of Medicine.

Dedicated by his Pupils to WILLIAM HENRY WELCH, on the twenty-fifth anniversary of his Doctorate. This volume contains 38 separate papers.

VOLUME X. 516 pages, 12 plates and 25 charts.

Structure of the Malarial Parasites. Plate I. By JESSE W. LAZEAR, M. D.

The Bacteriology of Cystitis, Pyelitis and Pyelonephritis in Women, with a Consideration of the Accessory Etiological Factors in these Conditions, and of the Various Chemical and Microscopical Questions involved. By THOMAS R. BROWN, M. D.

Cases of Infection with Strongyloides Intestinalis. (First Reported Occurrence in North America.) Plates II and III. By RICHARD P. STRONG, M. D.

On the Pathological Changes in Hodgkin's Disease, with Especial Reference to its Relation to Tuberculosis. Plates IV-VII. By DOROTHY M. REED, M. D.

Diabetes Insipidus, with a Report of Five Cases. By THOMAS B. FUTCHER, M. D.

Observations on the Origin and Occurrence of Cells with Eosinophile Granulations in Normal and Pathological Tissues. Plate VIII. By W. T. HOWARD, M. D., and R. G. PERKINS, M. D.

Placental Transmissions, with Report of a Case during Typhoid Fever. By FRANK W. LYNCH, M. D.

Metabolism in Albuminuria. By CHAS. P. EMERSON, A. B., M. D.

Regenerative Changes in the Liver after Acute Yellow Atrophy. Plates IX-XII. By W. G. MACCALLUM, M. D.

Surgical Features of Typhoid Fever. By THOS. MCCRAE, M. B., M. R. C. P. (Lond.), and JAMES F. MITCHELL, M. D.

The Symptoms, Diagnosis and Surgical Treatment of Ureteral Calculus. By BENJAMIN R. SCHENCK, M. D.

VOLUME XI. 555 pages, with 38 charts and illustrations.

Pneumothorax: A historical, clinical and experimental study. By CHARLES P. EMERSON, M. D.

Clinical Observations on Blood Pressure. By HENRY W. COOK, M. D., and JOHN B. BRIGGS, M. D.

The value of Tuberculin in Surgical Diagnosis. By MARTIN B. TINKER, M. D.

VOLUME XII. 548 pages, 12 plates and other illustrations.

The Connective Tissue of the Salivary Glands and Pancreas with Its Development in the Glandula Submaxillaris. Plates I-III. By JOSEPH MARSHALL FLINT, M. D.

A New Instrument for Determining the Minimum and Maximum Blood-Pressures in Man. Plates IV-X. By JOSEPH ERLANGER, M. D.

Metabolism in Pregnancy, Labor, and the Puerperium. By J. MORRIS SLEMONS, M. D.

An Experimental Study of Blood-Pressure and of Pulse-Pressure in Man. Plates XI and XII. By JOSEPH ERLANGER, M. D., and DONALD R. HOOKER, A. B., M. S.

Typhoid Meningitis. By RUFUS I. COLE, M. D.

The Pathological Anatomy of Meningitis due to Bacillus Typhosus. By WILLIAM G. MACCALLUM, M. D.

A Comparative Study of White and Negro Pelves, with a Consideration of the Size of the Child and Its Relation to Presentation and Character of Labor in the Two Races. By THEODORE E. RIGGS, M. D.

Renal Tuberculosis. By GEORGE WALKER, M. D.

VOLUME XIII. (In press).

The Johns Hopkins Hospital Bulletins are issued monthly. They are printed by the FRIEDENWALD CO., Baltimore. Single copies may be procured from NUNN & CO. and the BALTIMORE NEWS CO., Baltimore. Subscriptions, $2.00 a year, may be addressed to the publishers, THE JOHNS HOPKINS PRESS, BALTIMORE; single copies will be sent by mail for twenty-five cents each.

BULLETIN

OF

THE JOHNS HOPKINS HOSPITAL

Entered as Second-Class Matter at the Baltimore, Maryland, Postoffice.

Vol. XVII.—No. 184.]　　　　　　BALTIMORE, JULY, 1906.　　　　　　[Price, 25 Cents

CONTENTS.

BARON LARREY: A SKETCH.[1]

BY J. CHALMERS DA COSTA, M. D.[2]

Among the many remarkable men that stood with the greatest captain of modern times in his Titanic combats was one whose career attracts the particular interest of surgeons. He was a military surgeon for over half a century, and he participated in twenty-six campaigns, from Syria to Portugal, and from Moscow to Madrid. He followed Napoleon with love that never failed, with constancy that never faltered; and gave all his best skill to friend and foe alike, as duty called. He was brave on the battlefield and in the plague-hospital, but he was braver in the Tuilleries and in the imperial tent; for he always dared to tell his master the truth. That master loved and trusted him; ennobled him; decorated him before the army; when at St. Helena, referred to him in his will as

" the most virtuous man I have ever known ; " and bequeathed to him ten thousand francs as a souvenir of enduring affection.

It is needless to say that I refer to the greatest military surgeon that ever lived,[3] to Dominique Jean Larrey, Baron of the Empire, Commander of the Legion of Honor, Inspector General of the Medical Staff of the French Armies, Chief Surgeon of the Grand Army and First Surgeon of the Imperial Guard. He was born in 1766, in the romantic region of the High Pyrenees. His birthplace was the little village of Beaudeau, which is distant about a mile from Bigore, a well-known watering-place, celebrated since Roman days for the medicinal virtues of its mineral springs.

At the period of Larrey's birth, centuries of misrule were

---

[1] Read at a meeting of the Johns Hopkins Historical Club, February 12, 1906.

[2] The chief sources of information for this article are the Surgical Memoirs of Baron Larrey. (The first two volumes have been translated by Richard Willmott Hall; the third volume, by John C. Mercer); Sloane's Life of Napoleon, Taine's Ancient Régime, Levy's Private Life of Napoleon. The Memoirs of Baron Marbot, The Memoirs of Marshal MacDonald, The Hospitals and Surgeons of Paris, by F. C. Stewart, and A Memoir of J. Mason

Warren, M. D., edited by Howard Payson Arnold. The Life of Larrey, by Paul Triaire, I was not familiar with when writing this sketch and I did not see it until Dr. Harvey Cushing showed it to me in Baltimore. Had I been able to use this excellent and complete work errors would have been corrected which doubtless exist in this article, and the subject would have been treated more accurately.

[3] Mitchell Banks calls him so and I think justly. See " The Surgeon of Old in War."—*Medical News*. September 4, 1897.

about to culminate in a mighty catastrophe. All faith and loyalty had gone out of life; there were no real leaders; the nobles devoted their time to debauchery, intrigue and the chase; love was dead, and gallantry reigned instead. The ambitions of the Bull's Eye were directed purely to getting influence, so that this influence might bring power and gold. Everything went by favor, and nothing by merit; and harlots wheedled from the king every appointment, from Archbishop to Gamekeeper. The nobles thronged Versailles, leaving their estates in utter neglect and ruin, and permitting their peasants to starve and rot. The people, in the words of Macaulay, were beasts of burden and were soon to become beasts of prey. They were ignorant beyond conception, were brutal as pigs or oxen, and were regarded by the authorities as mere material for the tax-gatherers. Famine stalked through every district; and lust, anger, ferocity, and brutal hatred brooded in every workshop and hovel. The best that could happen to a son of the people was to become the steward of an estate and oppress his brothers; the best that could happen to a daughter of the people was to become the bed-room slave of a well-to-do captor. The people could truly say, as the Corn Law Rhymer was to say many years later:

"Our sons are the serfs of the rich by day,
"And our daughters their slaves by night."

It was thirteen years before Larrey's birth that Lord Chesterfield, traveling in France, wrote: "All the symptoms which I have ever met with in history previous to great changes and revolutions in government exist and daily increase in France"; but the rulers were blind and could not see. In 1766, the old Satyr, Louis XV, in spite of the dreadful poverty of the people, still kept four thousand horses in his stables, and still spent every year sixty-eight million francs for his household expenses, the equivalent of at least twice that sum to-day. Pompadour, who had cost him directly thirty-six million francs, and indirectly had cost him wars, famines, pestilences, and his immortal soul, had been dead but two years; and the beautiful and brazen DuBarry reigned in her stead. The easy view among the rich and powerful was that what had been would continue to be; but even Louis was a little wiser and said: "After me, the Deluge,"—and after him the Deluge came. As has been said: "At this time there were trees growing in the forest out of which the frame of the guillotine was to be made." The educated world had become skeptical, philosophical, utterly cynical, and prated and canted continually of philanthropy and the rights of man. A young fellow named Charles Henri Sanson was taking from his father the lessons that were to fit him to be the great M. de Paris, the public executioner of the time of the Terror. Voltaire was living at Ferney in Switzerland, was attacking with searing sarcasm and almost Satanic mockery the most cherished traditions of the court and of the church, and was placing in a pillory before all the world every hideous instance of public wrong and injustice. Diderot, with some great contemporaries,—notable among whom were Grim, D'Holbach, and d'Alembert—was editing the Encyclopédie, and was helping

to lay broad and deep the foundations of modern thought. Rousseau was in England, just preparing to return to France, where he was to hide in a garret, and in that garret brood out the dread retribution of the French Revolution. Marat, the future editor of the Ami de Peuple, the future advocate of a sacrifice of two hundred and seventy thousand lives, the future victim of Charlotte Corday, was a poor, unknown doctor, and was leading a wandering existence. Robespierre, the future creator of the Terror, the sentimentalist who dearly loved dogs, the man who was to move the abolition of capital punishment, and was to resign a judgeship rather than impose a death-sentence, the man who came to make slaughter a creed and to kill friend and foe alike, was a school-boy at Arras, living with his father, the advocate. Danton, the lion-hearted Danton of later days, the one that was to defy the threats of united Europe and was to "cast down as a gage of battle the head of a king," was but seven years old and was living at Arcis-sur-Aube. Napoleon Bonaparte, whose loving follower Larrey was destined to become, had not yet been born. This illustrious man was born on the fifteenth of August, 1769. It must have been evident to all thoughtful minds in 1766 that the world was on the threshold of great events, that the future was pregnant with portentous happenings, and that Jean Jaques spoke the truth when he said: "This is an age of revolutions."

Larrey, like most great men, was born poor. His parents were too poverty-stricken to pay for his education; and what instruction he got was obtained gratuitously from the Abbé de Grasset, a good and kindly churchman, who had originally become interested in the boy because he possessed a good voice and sang in the choir. When Larrey was thirteen years of age, his father died; and the son went to Toulouse to live with his uncle, Alexis Larrey, a successful surgeon of that city, and the chief surgeon to a large hospital. The city of Toulouse had recently rung in the ears of men; for it was there, in 1762, that probably the most infamous verdict ever given by a judicial tribunal had been rendered by the Parliament of Toulouse against the Calas family. This verdict excited Voltaire to frantic rage, and is dealt with in his book "Sur la Tolerance."

While in Toulouse and under the guidance of his uncle, Larrey finished his education in the College of Esquile, and then studied medicine and surgery. He left Toulouse in 1787, when he was twenty-one years of age, and went direct to Paris. This was two years before the convocation of the States General. Soon after reaching Paris, he took a public examination and obtained an appointment as auxiliary surgeon in the navy. He went to the great naval station at Brest, underwent another examination, was appointed chief surgeon of a war-vessel, and was assigned to the Vigilante.

As the boat was not to sail for some months, Larrey passed the time in lecturing to students on surgery and anatomy, an instance of that fiery activity that possessed him all his life. He was also interested in visiting the prison of the galley-slaves. Ten years later, the notorious Vidocq, who afterwards became chief of the French police, was a convict in this same dreadful Bagne of Brest, from which he made a remarkable escape. We learn of its terrors in his Autobiography, and the conditions were probably much the same at the time of Larrey's visit. In the Bagne, Larrey saw a man seventy years of age, who was totally blind during the daytime, but could see at night. This condition of day-blindness had resulted from a confinement of over thirty years in a dark, underground cell. Larrey believed that the blindness was the result of the long exclusion of light, which, of course, is one of the known causes of this interesting condition. In a postmortem examination made upon a galley-slave at this time, Larrey found transposition of the viscera.

The newly-appointed naval surgeon sailed from Brest for Newfoundland in April, 1788, and was gone six months on his trip. He made many interesting observations, which are recorded in his Memoirs. For instance, he discusses sea-sickness, a condition from which he suffered himself, and which he justly calls "the most painful disease with which a mariner can be affected." He studied its development and theorized on its cause, and came to the conclusion that it results from oscillation of the brain, saying that when the brain is large and soft it is more liable to be affected. Hence, young persons, whose brains are voluminous, are most usually the subjects of sea-sickness; while persons of advanced ages, with firm brains, are less liable to the disease. He says graphically that the first effects are "sadness and panic, which seizes the individual. The face becomes pale, the eyes are suffused with tears, and the appetite for food is entirely removed. The patient is silenced; seeks solitude and repose; reels like one intoxicated; is affected with vertigo, tinnitus aurium, and unpleasant weight of the head. Nausea succeeds and, soon after vomiting, which becomes frequent and painful, and continues almost without intermission until the cause ceases." It, therefore, becomes evident to us not only that Larrey was sea-sick, but that he was most extremely sea-sick.

He also discusses frost-gangrene; the catching, cleaning and salting of cod-fish; and the tastes and habits of the Newfoundland caribou, which in some respects were extraordinary; as one of them broke into fold, and as the result of this forcible entry, a cow became pregnant. Larrey always wondered what the product of this ill-assorted love affair could have been.

He was very much interested in the change of plumage of the birds in Arctic climates, and noted that the black-birds are red-brown in the summer and white in the winter. He also presents a dissertation on the habits of the Esquimaux. It had always been my impression that the Esquimaux, almost alone among races, use no intoxicants; but Larrey found the Newfoundland Esquimaux using a fermented liquor made of the buds of the fir-tree. He speaks, likewise, of the insect-pests in Newfoundland during the summer; says particularly that "a species of gnat called the mosquito is very troublesome, and produces by its sting local inflammation and fever, which are but ephemeral. The effects of these stings were removed by washing with salt-water and by rest and refreshment. By my advice, our men protected their skin from them by anointing themselves with camphorated oil and by wearing a piece of gauze over the face." The phenomenon of phosphorescence also interested him greatly. This he believed to be the result of the presence of numerous animalcules "and putrid animalmatter. The situations where these lights appear most brilliantly is consequently unwholesome, if persons continue in it."

Larrey reached Brest on his return voyage in October, 1788; and early in the winter of 1789, he went to Paris. The winter of 1789 he justly calls "the memorable winter," and says that between the time of his return to Paris and of his departure for the campaign of the Rhine "many remarkable events transpired in this capital to which I was a witness"; but, unfortunately, he does not tell the events, but confines himself to speaking purely of surgical matters. He departed for the Army of the Rhine in April, 1792, just thirteen months before the beginning of the Terror, and the very month in which the guillotine was adopted as the official instrument of execution. It had been invented by Dr. Guillotin and had been improved by Sanson, the executioner. A musician that boarded with Sanson suggested the obliquely set knife; and, irony of fate, Louis XVI suggested the neat little basket to catch the separated head.[1]

It was in the winter of 1789 that the people awoke to their wrongs and their power, and that the earthquake-tread of red Democracy began to echo through the land. Tumult and disorder became common in the capital. We read in history of the attack of the mob of the St. Antoine Quarter upon the paper-warehouse of Réveillon, who was falsely charged with saying: "A workman can live well on fifteen sous a day." In this attack on the paper-warehouse, five hundred were killed and very many were wounded; and Réveillon himself took refuge in the Bastille. Larrey saw many of those wounded in this affair. They were brought to the Hotel Dieu in the service of the celebrated Desault.

Desault demonstrated these cases, and used them to emphasize his views upon the treatment of gun-shot wounds. He strongly opposed the popular alcohol-dressing, and used lead-water, as recommended by Paré. He opposed the attempt to alter the nature of the wound by excision and suture, except in wounds of the face and mouth, when he advocated it. He opposed immediate amputation, a view from which Larrey subsequently positively dissented.

Desault must have had many harrowing experiences during the Revolution. He was physician to several of the chief jails; he did not attend the Dauphin—Peleton having been the surgeon that had him in charge; but he saw most of the prisoners that went to execution from the Conciergerie. Desault must have freely moved among the prisoners, jailers, and revolutionists, just as did Dr. Manette in Dickens's Tale of Two Cities; and he seems to have been almost universally loved and respected. He was a man of violent temper, as we learn from the following account of him, given by Sir Astley Cooper (A Book about Doctors, by J. Cordy Jeaffreson, Vol. I, p. 8):

It was in the winter of 1792 that Sir Astley Cooper was a student under Desault and Chopart. A boy, sixteen years of age, was brought to Desault's clinic. He was said to have paralysis of the right arm; but the surgeon suspected that he was malingering. Desault spoke to the boy by name and calmly said: "Take off your hat." The boy thoughtlessly took the supposedly paralyzed hand and removed the hat. "Hand me a stick," called Desault; and then, he attacked the boy before everybody and soundly beat him. This remedy he called "club cordial."

Once during the Revolution Desault was arrested, and was confined in the Luxembourg Prison for three days. This was in many respects the least terrible of all the Revolutionary jails. It was considered the aristocratic prison. It was a palace that had been made into a prison, and the first noble suspects in the beginning of the Revolution were sent there. Later,

however, the ordinary, every-day citizen occasionally found his way there; and finally, on a certain notable night, Danton, Camille Desmoulins, and their friends were brought in, at the order of their one-time friend, Robespierre. Desault was quickly liberated: returned to his work as a teacher of surgery in the Hotel Dieu; and was not arrested again.

At the height of his fame. six hundred pupils attended his clinics. The horrors of the Revolution depressed him greatly and embittered his final years. At his death, he was attended by two friends, both of them celebrated, and both remembered to-day; Bichat, the founder of histology, and Corvisart, subsequently the physician to Napoleon and a great authority on the heart. At the present day, we remember Desault particularly by his circular amputation of three incisions, a cone being thus made, the apex of which is the divided bone; by his long extension-splint for fracture of the thigh; and by his operation for one form of salivary fistula. Chopart, Desault's hospital colleague. is still remembered in this age for his amputation through the middle tarsal joint, this articulation being yet called in anatomy the line of Chopart. The writings of neither of these men endure, but we may say with Longfellow:

> "Happy those whose written pages
> Perish with their lives,
> If among the crumbling ages
> Still their name survives."

Some writers have stated that none of the crowd was killed at the taking of the Bastille; but there must have been some of them injured, for Larrey says that he saw the wounded of the tumult of that day. The day that martial law was declared in the Champs de Mars, many wounded persons were brought into the Invalides; and our surgeon saw them being treated by Sabatier, whom we remember to-day as the surgeon that advocated suturing a divided intestine over a cylinder made of a playing-card smeared with turpentine. This method of Sabatier was a modification of the method of Four Masters of the Thirteenth Century, who used the trachea of an animal; of the method of William of Salicet, who employed the dried and hardened bowel of an animal; and of the method of Watson, who used a cylinder of isinglass.

On May 13, 1789, Larrey seems to have seen a genuine case of anthrax. He tells us in his Memoirs that an ox having a carbuncle was purchased at a market by a butcher; and that the butcher killed the animal in haste, because he was afraid that the carbuncle would be fatal and that he would lose the sale of the meat. One of the boys that had killed the ox developed a black pustule of the face and stiffness of the left jaw. This tumor grew purple-red around its margins, and was black and depressed in the center; and the patient died within a few days, by which time the lesion had spread over half the face. Another boy in the family had the same fate, the tumor having arisen on the neck. The wife of the butcher also developed a similar condition; and when Larrey saw her, she seemed on the point of death. He ordered what he called "cordial antiseptic drinks," aromatic cataplasms, and min-

[1] Memoirs of the Sansons.

eral lemonade; and had vinegar evaporated in the chamber. He then held a consultation with M. Boyer, a celebrated surgeon of La Charité. Boyer is remembered as the author of a noted book which was supposed to embody all the surgical knowledge of his time, in which he makes the statement that any further progress in the art or science of medicine is impossible. The surgeons agreed that the pustules should be extirpated, and the raw surfaces cauterized. The patient so treated recovered.

During the winter that Larrey stayed in Paris, he passed a competitive examination for the position of interne of the Hôtel Dieu; but the appointment was given to someone else having more influence. He also passed an examination for Second Surgeon of the Invalides, and this place was given him. A short time afterwards, war was declared; and Larrey was sent as a surgeon of the first class to the Army of the Rhine, then commanded by Marshal Luckner, but soon afterwards put under the charge of Lieutenant-General Kellermann. Marshal Luckner, a fine old soldier, came to the guillotine during the Terror. Lieutenant-General Kellermann soon afterward won the great conflict of Valmy; and when Napoleon became Emperor, Kellermann was created a Marshal of France and Duke of Valmy. He was soon displaced from the command of the Army of the Rhine by General Biron, who was quickly succeeded by General Custine. The latter occupied Frankfort, and was then obliged to retire to the Rhine. In the fall of this year, Dumouriez won the great battle of Jennappes, and thus secured possession of a large portion of the Austrian Netherlands.

It was in the Campaign of the Rhine that Larrey first became impressed with the "inconvenience to which we were subjected in moving the ambulances and military hospitals. The military regulations required that they should always be one league distant from the army. The wounded were left on the field until after the engagement, and were then collected at a convenient spot, to which the ambulances repaired as speedily as possible; but the number of wagons interposed between them and the army, and many other difficulties, so retarded their progress that they never arrived in less than twenty-four or thirty-six hours; so that most of the wounded died for want of assistance." Larrey saw that it was absolutely necessary to construct vehicles that would readily convey the wounded actually during the battle. He was unable to perfect the plan at this period, but did so soon afterwards; and the principle of actively treating men on the battlefield and quickly transferring them to a field-hospital seems to have originated in the mind of this distinguished surgeon.

When he was at Mentz, or Mayence, a town in Hesse that the army occupied for some time, he attended the anatomical demonstration of the celebrated Dr. Sömmering, whose method of numbering the cranial nerves is the one that we follow to-day; and he also repeated with Dr. Straak some of the very earliest experiments in galvanism. He was able to carry out on a recently-amputated leg some experiments that had previously been made only upon animals. The contraction of the muscles that followed the galvanization of the popliteal nerve led Larrey to believe that galvanism might restore paralyzed limbs; but he says that the very slight benefit that had since been derived from galvanism and electricity in the cure of such conditions led him to give up this idea.

It was at this period of his career that he invented the needle that was long known by his name. These needles were made of fine and highly-tempered steel and were of different sizes. The needle was curved into a semi-circle, the extremities being parallel. The point was a small curve with sharp edges, and the edges terminated toward the body in obtuse angles. The edges were rounded and slightly thinner than the middle of the needle.. There was a square, transverse opening through the eye, and a groove; so that a cord or ribbon could lie in it. The advantages that he claimed for these needles were the readiness with which they would pass through the skin and the fact that the ligature would lie free and keep its flattened form, thus supporting the wound-edges.

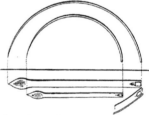

Fig. 1.—Larrey's Needles (Larrey's Memoirs).

Larrey was in several actions during this campaign, and became very seriously impressed with the difficulties of handling the wounded; through the fact that at Limbourg the French were obliged to leave them on the field, and they fell into the hands of the enemy. He applied for permission to construct a flying ambulance. He at first thought of having the wounded carried on horses in panniers, but he soon gave this idea up; and he was led to devise a carriage that united "swiftness to solidity and ease." He began to use his ambulance in this campaign with great success.

He was in some very serious battles, in which he made some extremely interesting observations on gun-shot wounds. His experience led him to advocate immediate amputation in certain grave injuries of the extremities—a view that he never abandoned. He became convinced that people were sometimes killed by what was known as "windage" of bullets; there being no external wound, but a postmortem examination showing grave internal injury. Surgeons then believed that such injuries were caused by the wind from a cannon-ball or a shell-fragment that had passed close to the body, but had not struck it. Larrey thought there must have been a blow by the projectile, in spite of the absence of surface-contusions. Military surgeons have entirely abandoned the idea that injury by the wind of a ball is possible, and attribute the so-called wind-contusion to a projectile that has lightly passed across the surface and in doing so has left no surface bruise.

The health of the soldiers in this campaign was excellent, although thousands of them were new recruits that had been hurriedly gathered; but they received good food and had plenty of exercise. It was in this campaign that Larrey first met General de Beauharnais, a native of Martinique, of whom he became extremely fond. The general addressed to the Convention a letter highly commending the surgeon for his services and speaking in flattering terms of the ambulances that he had recently invented. This unfortunate gentleman likewise fell a victim to the guillotine, and left a widow to become Empress of the French.

After the Army of the Rhine had lost several combats, General Pichegru took command. In a few days the army joined the Army of the Moselle; and the chief command was given to that brilliant young man, General Hoche. We remember Pichegru as the able but unfortunate soldier who conquered Belgium and the Netherlands; suppressed the Parisian insurrection in April, 1795; became, later, involved in the conspiracy of Georges Cadoudal; and, after being captured by the police of Fouché in 1804, committed suicide. Hoche was one of the most promising and brilliant soldiers of the Revolution. He suppressed the Vendean revolt in 1795-96; and, when only twenty-nine years of age, died at Wetzler. Had he lived, he would unquestionably have been one of the greatest of Napoleon's marshals.

During the campaign, Larrey amputated a foot between the tarsal and the metatarsal bones, doing what we now call the amputation of Lisfranc. He also extirpated the head of the humerus, saving the arm—an operation of which he afterward became a warm advocate. When the troops went into cantonments, an adynamic fever, which was probably typhoid, broke out. Larrey was then sent for to go to Paris and complete the organization of an ambulance-service, and to establish it in the different armies of the Republic; as the value of these ambulances had been most conspicuously demonstrated in the campaign of the Rhine.

In 1794, Larrey was appointed Chief Surgeon to the army that was intended for Corsica, and was ordered to report at Toulon. This city had been captured from the English the previous year. At the siege, a certain Napoleon Bonaparte had been a captain of artillery; and in the same company of which he had been captain, Marmont and Suchet had been junior officers, and Junot had been a sergeant. In the army destined for Corsica, Bonaparte was a general of brigade.

During the few days that Larrey remained in Paris, he married a lady to whom he had long been engaged, a daughter of M. Leroux, who had been for a time Finance Minister under Louis XVI. On reaching Toulon, Larrey met General Bonaparte for the first time. Bonaparte was then twenty-five years of age, and commanded the artillery. He was beginning to be known, and the command of Paris had been of-

fered him by Robespierre; but he had had the good sense to decline to take Henriot's position. The uncertainty of official life, however, was well manifested; for about this time he was put in prison for thirteen days as a suspect, and not long afterward he lost his commission altogether.

The squadron was to repair to Nice and take on soldiers; and Larrey went there by land, traveling with the Inspector of Hospitals, M. Heurteloup, a man remembered by us as the inventor of the artificial leech.

The presence of the English fleet prevented the French expedition from reaching Corsica, so Larrey spent some time with the Army of the Maritime Alps. At this time, he formulated his views on the treatment of the apparently drowned, advocating a form of artificial respiration that consisted in blowing into the mouth of the person to distend his lungs, and pressing on his chest to empty them.

He then went to Spain as Chief Surgeon of the Army of the Pyrenees, and was present at the taking of Figuières and the sack of Roses. He speaks in his journal of individuals of whom he had amputated more than one extremity, and says that they had afterwards become very fat; and, because their circle of nutrition was so much lessened in extent, their alvine evacuations became much more frequent.

At this time, he became very much interested in the treatment of burns, and insisted that a person that has been burned requires a generous diet; although this view is entirely contrary to the opinion of Hippocrates, who restricted them to a low diet. This solemn quotation of Hippocrates suggests that the latter must still have been regarded as an authority. In fact, in the age of which we speak, surgery was in a chrysalis-state and was barely emerging from its cocoon; and the first few hesitating words of truth had, as yet, but scarce been lisped by the baby lips of science. Another of Larrey's views regarding burns was that opium should not be given in their treatment.

He notes that the Spanish love of beauty and good taste appeared even in the preparation of their linen for dressings, which was like cambric; and of their lint, which was as fine as silk, and was tied up in small packages, tastefully arranged in different colors by the Queen of Spain and the ladies of the court.

In 1796, Larrey's health broke down, and he obtained permission to go to Paris. The city was at times somewhat turbulent, but there were no actual outbreaks; for young General Bonaparte had discouraged anarchy by filling several commodious grave-yards with the bodies of enterprising revolutionists. Larrey soon went to Toulon, where he learned that the Corsican expedition had been postponed without date; so he stayed a while at Toulon, and began to teach military and naval surgeons, giving courses in anatomy and theoretical and clinical surgery. He pursued this custom wherever he went. We find that whenever the army remained for a few weeks or months in one place, this indefatigable man organized a school and caused all the surgeons of the army to attend it. In this school they would perform operations on the cadaver, study anatomy, and question one another about important topics of military surgery. It seems to have been an infinitely valuable method, and it probably affords one of the reasons why the French army-surgeons of that day were the best in the world.

In May, 1787, Larrey set out as Chief Surgeon of the Army of Italy, which had been recently placed under the command of General Bonaparte. Since Napoleon and Larrey had met for the first time at Toulon, the former had gone through many trials, and had achieved some notable triumphs. He had lost his commission; had been harassed by poverty; had walked along the streets of Paris contemplating suicide; had thought of going to Turkey to fight under the Sultan; had, in a critical moment, when all others were afraid, accepted the command of the city from Barras; and had defeated the National Guard, which, at the behest of the Sections, had come thirty thousand strong, to attack the Convention. As a reward for

ury, and its indolence. The contrast between the voluptuous, luxurious Venetians and the rough and hardy French soldiers is shown in the well-known pictures by Georges Clairin. The French are encamped in front of the Ducal Palace. Some soldiers and a woman are preparing dinner, and some men are resting on a great pile of straw. A grim, white-moustached, red-vested revolutionary soldier, with a gun in his hand, is looking with unspeakable disgust at the dandies of Venice, who, arrayed in laces and silks of many colors, are gazing at him with languid surprise and supercilious disgust.

Larrey tells us in his Memoirs that the Winged Lion, which he then saw in the Square of St. Mark, now adorns the Esplanade of the Invalides at Paris. It did adorn this for a while, but it went back again after the fall of Napoleon. Our traveler was very much struck with the Cathedral and the four gilded bronze Corinthian horses that surmount the front

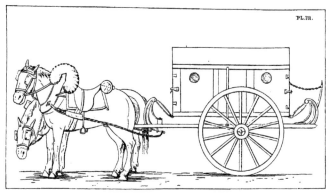

PL. III.

FIG. 2.—AMBULANCE (LARREY'S MEMOIRS).

this achievement—in fact, probably as the price of it—the command of the Army of Italy had been given him; and he had married Josephine de Beauharnais, whom he had met at Madame Tallien's. At the age of twenty-eight years, this remarkable man had won a coveted object of his ambition, the command of an active army about to enter a campaign.

While Larrey was proceeding to Italy, he saw, among the Alps, the victims of goiter and the cretins. They interested him a great deal; and he believed that the drinking of snow-water was responsible for the conditions. The difference between travel then and now is well exemplified by the fact that the surgeon had to wait forty-eight days at the foot of Mt. Cenis, owing to the snow-drifts and the avalanches.

He visited most of the important towns of northern Italy, establishing schools of military surgery. He was particularly interested in Venice, a city then noted for its gaiety, its lux-

piece. These horses had been found, centuries before, on the Island of Chios; had been taken to Alexandria; removed to Rome by Augustus Cæsar; taken to Constantinople by Constantine; and to Venice by the Doge Dandalus, who captured Constantinople in 1204. Larrey says that these horses have also been transported to Paris, and are now on the Triumphal Arch of the Tuilleries. This arch is what we, at the present day, call the Arch of the Carrousel; and it has horses on it, but they are not the genuine horses from Venice. They were taken home again, as was the Winged Lion—a commentary, both these circumstances, on the mutability of human affairs.

The gondolas interested Larrey greatly, and he describes them in his journal. We cannot help but think of Byron's description in a few words, when he says that a gondola is like "a coffin clapt in a canoe."

We gather from Larrey's account that the well-to-do inhabitants of Venice had a reasonably comfortable life. The custom of a fashionable Venetian was to rise from bed between two and three o'clock in the afternoon; to pass the remainder of the daylight in his apartment, clad only in a morning robe; to take a light meal, array himself in his finest, and walk to the Square of St. Mark or some adjacent island; to idle about for a time; to go to dinner, and then to the theatre, which did not begin until nine o'clock and did not let out until about one in the morning. After leaving the theatre, he would pay any ceremonial calls he had to make, going from place to place in a gondola; keeping on making visits until five o'clock—or perhaps six—in the morning; and then going home to bed. The law forced the workingmen whose occupations produced noise to live in a remote section of the town, so that the day-slumbers of illustrious personages might not be disturbed.

While traveling to Trieste, Larrey met Desaix, already a well-known general, who was soon to go with Napoleon to Egypt and to return with him, only to be killed at Marengo. The surgeon became very fond of Desaix and regarded him as a most lovable character. We remember Desaix at Marengo. Bonaparte said: "The battle is lost." Desaix looked at his watch, found the hour was four o'clock, and said: "Yes, this battle is lost; but there is time to win another." The other battle was won. Desaix was killed; and long years afterward Napoleon said that had Desaix lived, he would have made him a king.

When at Pavia, the surgeon called on Spalanzi and Scarpa. The latter gave him a copy of his recent treatise on the nerves of the heart. Scarpa's dissections of the nerves of the heart were studied by Larrey with the utmost interest. He greatly preferred them to the wax models of all the different portions of the human system copied from those in Florence; because he loved reality more than imitation, however accurate the latter might be.

Larrey was ordered to Toulon, with directions to prepare to assume the position of Surgeon in Chief to the expedition that was to go to Egypt and Syria under General Bonaparte. The Chief Surgeon wrote a letter to the medical schools of Montpelier and Toulouse, requesting them to send him at once a number of intelligent young surgeons whose health justified the belief that they could stand the fatigues of a most laborious campaign. This request met with an ample response, and Larrey appointed those that suited him. How differently it would have been done in this country! It would not have been possible for the Surgeon General of our army to write to any non-political bodies to send him capable men; for these capable men could not have been appointed, unless they had had political endorsements; and most medical men with high political endorsements are not capable men. In this country, United States Senators, Congressmen, and other outcasts, would have sent peremptory orders to the War Department as to who was to be appointed; and most of them would have been appointed, irrespective of their fitness. I am not, of course, speaking of the regular army-surgeons, who

enter by examination; but of the volunteer-surgeons, who go out in time of war.

This expedition had a Chief Physician, as well as a Chief Surgeon. The Chief Physician was Desgenettes, a most humane and able man. The expedition embarked on the 13th of May, 1793; and its leader was filled with enthusiasm as to its destiny. The idea of conquering Egypt was not a new one to the French mind. Four centuries before, Philip le Bel had thought of it. Sixty years before, D'Argenson had suggested the cutting of the Suez Canal; and Choiseul had advocated the conquest of Egypt, because it was the highroad between the East and the West. This remarkable expedition carried the name of Bonaparte into the remotest parts of Asia, and led the Mamelukes and the Arabs to think that he was invincible and to call him El Kebir, the Exalted One; and through all these countries, his fame still lingers in stories and traditions.

Ever since, as a boy, he had read Plutarch and of the achievements of Alexander the Great, Napoleon had dreamed of and longed for the East. When in Paris without an occupation, his thoughts had turned to the East for a career. He went there as a poet goes to the source of his inspiration; and while there, he acted a veritable epic. During all the rest of his life, and particularly near its close, when at St. Helena, he regretted that he had failed to found an Empire of the East.

In this Eastern Campaign, we see some of the most impressive and some of the most dramatic events in the marvelous career of Napoleon. At Alexandria; near Cairo at the Pyramids, when he called upon forty centuries to look upon their deeds; at the bombardment of Jaffa; at the bloody, desperate, and unfortunate siege of Acre; at Mt. Tabor; and at Aboukir. Traveling the fiery deserts on a camel, sharing all the hardships of his soldiers, he was the great, forceful, inscrutable figure that ever since has entranced the imaginations of men.

He took with him on this expedition some of the best soldiers of France. He took Desaix, who afterwards won the battle of Marengo and was killed there, and whom he said he would have made a king. He took Kleber, who was assassinated in the East. He took Berthier, who was so long his close companion; Menou, who turned Mohammedan; Davout, who afterward won Auerstadt and became one of the most celebrated marshals of France; Murat, the cavalry-leader who surprised the very Mamelukes by the splendor of his horsemanship, and who later became King of Naples; and his close friend, Lannes, who afterward became Marshal of France and Duke of Montebello, who lost his life at Essling, and of whom Napoleon said: "He was the most distinguished soldier in my army."

Three of the colonels in this expedition came later to great celebrity: Marmont, who became a marshal and a duke; Junot, who became one of the best known of the generals and a duke; and Bessières, who became Marshal, Duke of Istria, and Commander of the Imperial Guard, and who lost his life at Lützen. One hundred scientists skilled in various sciences, many of them students of the East, were taken along to study the country, the people, the inscriptions, etc. One find of these learned men was the Rosetta Stone, the key by which the hieroglyphics were deciphered by Young and Champollion.

The expedition visited Malta, which was still ruled by that curious Order, the Knights of Malta, and had been so ruled since 1530. Napoleon broke up the Order and placed the Island under the flag of France; but, three months after he had left, it was captured by Lord Nelson; and it has been an English possession ever since.

Larrey participated in all the dangers and troubles of this most harassing campaign. At Acre, he was wounded; and Napoleon complimented him in public for his gallantry and usefulness. It was at this battle that the general saw that the surgeon was dismounted, gave him his own horse, and directed that the horses of the staff be placed at the disposal of the Surgeon General to assist in removing the wounded soldiers. He had the satisfaction, he tells us, of bringing all the

midst of the plague, but he never took the disease. In the course of eight weeks, in one plague-hospital, every nurse that had started in died of the disease; as well as three physicians, fourteen surgeons, and eleven apothecaries (see the Memoirs).

The journal of Larrey's campaign in Egypt and Syria is rich in striking incidents. He shows us how afraid the soldiers were of being bitten by scorpions, and yet that the bites were not dangerous; that severe home-sickness compelled certain persons to return to France; and that the Commander-in-Chief was kicked by a horse, contusing his right leg severely, and threatening dangerous consequences. Larrey succeeded in curing this injury, in spite of the marches and the great activity of the general, which prevented him from giving the hurt member rest. Larrey also tells us of a hernia that became strangulated and gangrenous, and killed a man in the space of two hours. He speaks of the wounds inflicted by the

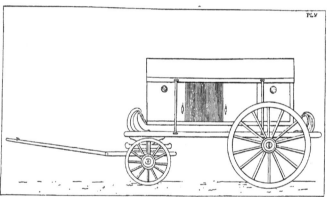

FIG. 3.—AMBULANCE (LARREY'S MEMOIRS).

wounded off, and thus saving them from the Arabs. After the battle, Bonaparte presented Larrey with a sword of honor; on account of his having operated, in the very midst of a conflict, upon one of the best generals, General Fougières. This operation was an amputation at the shoulder-joint, and was done by the method that we still call Larrey's amputation. This sword was engraved, by the order of Napoleon after he became Emperor, with the words, "Aboukir and Larrey"; and Larrey wore it nearly all the rest of his active military life. When he was captured at Waterloo, it was stolen from him by the Prussians.

On one occasion during this campaign, the men were obliged to kill their horses to make soup of them. Larrey, in speaking of a later campaign, tells of flavoring soup with gunpowder, as a substitute for salt. He was constantly in the very

swords of the Mamelukes. One chief of brigade had seven severe wounds; two on the shoulders, cutting through the muscles and some of the bones, and one on the back, cutting through the muscles and through the spinous processes of the dorsal vertebræ. He also had a bullet in the chest, producing a copious effusion of blood in the pleural sac, and followed by empyema; but he recovered.

Larrey trephined a number of cases, and warmly advocated operation for meningeal hemorrhage, recording successful cases. He describes cases in which leeches lodged in the nose and naso-pharynx, and remained there for weeks before the condition was understood, producing exhausting hemorrhage. He blames bad water for liver-abscess; and also for nervous putrid fever with bloody fluxes, which was probably typhoid. He points out that the inhabitants protect themselves from plague by inserting setons; that pannier-bearing camels were used to carry wounded men; and that maggots in wounds hastened the processes of nature and rapidly removed dead material. He tells us of the establishing of a school of practical surgery at Cairo; and discusses that dreadful disease, the Egyptian ophthalmia, which caused much blindness. We learn that many amputations were necessary, owing to the character of the missiles used by the enemy. He describes the bas-reliefs in the ruins of Luxor, representing surgical instruments similar to those used at the present time for amputating.

Tetanus seems to have been a veritable scourge among the French, killing many men; and it must have been a haunting nightmare to the surgeon. Larrey believed that when the body bent back into opisthotonos, the prognosis was much worse than when it bent forward into emprosthotonos. He insisted on the causative influence of a wound in this disease, and believed that cold and wet helped tetanus to develop. He advocates incision and cauterization in tetanus, if the wound is on the face or the body; and amputation, if it is on an extremity. He gives some notable examples of recovery from tetanus. One is the case of the celebrated General Lannes, who was wounded at Aboukir, and whom Larrey treated merely with internal remedies, emollient applications, and bleeding. General d'Estaing developed this disease after a wound through the right arm, and Larrey says that he cured him by amputation.

He tells us that at the Siege of Acre there were two thousand wounded; and that seventy amputations were performed, two of them being hip-joint amputations. One of these patients seemed on the high-road to recovery, when he took the plague and died of it. The other one died of shock. At the time, it was considered useless to attempt hip-joint amputation. Larrey advocated it, in spite of Pott's view "that it is a bloody, dreadful, and unjustifiable procedure." Larrey was seven years ahead of Brashear of Kentucky in advocacy. In his later campaigns, he twice performed this operation with success, although Brashear's success in 1806 antedated Larrey's by several years. Larrey did six amputations at the shoulder-joint, and four of them were successful. He trephined seven cases, and five were cured. General Caffarelli received a compound gun-shot fracture of the elbow-joint. The arm was amputated; but he developed " a nervous fever," and died of it. Undoubtedly, however, this fever was pyemia; for the postmortem examination disclosed an abscess of the liver and an abscess of the lung. General Murat, afterwards Marshal of France and King of Naples, received a serious gunshot wound. A bullet entered the neck, below the angle of the jaw, on the right side; and emerged on the left side, passing in front of the jugulars, injuring the ninth pair of nerves, and traversing the mouth. He was cured. M. Duroc, afterwards Grand Marshal of the Palace, received an enormous wound of the right thigh by the bursting of a bomb. Eugene de Beauharnais, Bonaparte's stepson, received a grave wound of the orbit. Both these gentlemen recovered. General Lannes was wounded again, by a bullet striking him in the face and pass-

ing behind the ear. M. Arrighi, afterwards Duke of Padua, received a wound that divided the external carotid artery. One of the soldiers put his finger into the wound, to arrest the bleeding temporarily by pressure; and Larrey was obliged to go to his assistance "in the midst of a shower of bullets." He arrested the bleeding, strange to say, by the use of a compress and a bandage.

He tells us that the wounds often became full of maggots, the larvæ of the blue flies of Syria. He gives full accounts of the plague, in all its horrors; speaks of the marvelous endurance and great bravery of Bonaparte; tells the story of the sacking of Jaffa, and of the martial deeds of Kleber; and mentions men that swallowed leeches in their drinking-water, in spite of the efforts to keep them from drinking from the pools. He speaks of abscess of the liver, and says that there were many cures. His rule was to open it when it had become glued to the surface. He writes of atrophy of the testis; of leprosy; of elephantiasis; of the death of Kleber, and of the military brilliancy of Desaix; of scurvy, syphilis, Arabian horses, Syrian midwives, abortionists, slaves, women, baths, seraglios, embalming, mummies, camels, sarcocele, wounds of the head and incubators—truly a wide variety of subjects exhibiting enormous intellectual activity. He was very much interested in the bathing-habits of the women, and engaged in the questionable proceeding of getting a female physician who was matron and proprietor of a bath at Cairo, to allow him to witness ladies bathing. He saw them through a small opening that commanded a complete view and also enabled him to hear. He describes the scene in an entertaining manner, and it evidently afforded him considerable personal satisfaction. He says that they " relate the adventures of the scraglio, dispute with each other of their charms and of the favors that they have received from the sultans."

Napoleon, it will be remembered, returned home on account of the critical state of public affairs and the peculiar conduct of Josephine. The army had been left under the command of Kleber. Kleber was assassinated by a fanatic, and Menou took command. The entire absence of re-enforcements and supplies finally necessitated surrender. Alexandria was given up, and the army received all the honors of war. The officers and soldiers were returned to France in British vessels. In 1801, Larrey came back to Toulon. Thus ended the famous expedition to the East.

After his return, on the 24th of December, 1801, the following letters were issued by the War Department: The first was one stating that the Commander-in-Chief had notified the Government of the devotion and success of Larrey and his colleagues in preserving the army. The next letter, dated January 8th, and signed by Berthier, tells Larrey that he has rendered most important service and has received the particular attention of the First Consul. The third is dated the 28th of January, and states that the Government has lost no chance to let the French Nation know of the services rendered by Larrey in Egypt, and tells him that his name will henceforth be regarded as that of a benefactor of his country. It also says that fifteen thousand francs had been sent to his wife, as a very small testimonial of gratitude; and that, to the personal knowledge of the writer, Larrey, with his brave associates, had attended the wounded under the fiercest fire, and even in the trenches.

The Revolution of the 18th Brumaire had cast the imbecile Directory out of power. The new Constitution, which was largely the work of the Abbé Sieyes, had established the Consular Government; and Napoleon had become First Consul. He was practically a king, without the title. He moved into the Tuilleries in the beginning of the year 1800, and was soon afterward made First Consul for life.

It will be remembered that Larrey had remained in the East for a long time after Napoleon's return; and the Second Italian War, with its magnificent triumphs—the war in which the Battle of Marengo occurred—was fought before the surgeon

ceasing and marvelous. He had conquered Italy; had made peace with England; had adjusted matters with the Papacy; had built roads and canals, improved the drainage and the water-supply of Paris, created numerous industries; had stimulated ship-building, science, and art; had become President of the Cisalpine Republic; had encouraged education—particularly the higher education, and had, with Cambaceres and others, drawn up the Code Napoleon, which is the basis of the criminal law of France to-day.

The peace with England was broken in 1803; and Napoleon gathered a large army in the neighborhood of Boulogne, with the intention of invading England. He had been beset by the Chouan Conspiracy, headed by Georges Cadoudal, General Pichegru, and probably Moreau. He had instigated—or, at least, accepted—the execution of the Duc d'Enghien. Soon after having been made Emperor, he also became King of

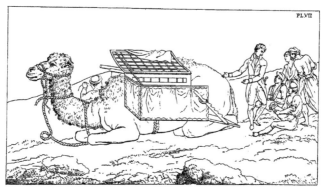

Fig. 4.—Pannier-bearing Camel for the Wounded (Larrey's Memoirs).

returned. On his arrival, he was received most affectionately by the First Consul; and was made the Chief Surgeon to the Consular Guards a few days before the signing of the Treaty of Amiens, which made peace between France and England. It was just about this time that the famous Concordat was drawn up, the agreement or understanding between France and the Papacy that has been under active discussion in the newspapers within recent months. Soon after Larrey arrived at Paris, he commenced a course of lectures to a very large number of students; and it is extremely interesting to find that at that early day in surgery, he was lecturing on Experimental Surgery, a branch that is still rarely taught and too rarely thought about.

In March, 1804, Napoleon became Emperor of the French. In the interval between his assumption of the office of First Consul and his becoming Emperor, his labors had been un-

Italy, and appointed his step-son, Eugene de Beauharnais, as Viceroy.

Larrey tells us in his Memoirs that the Emperor made mighty preparations for the invasion of England, and gathered vessels in every harbor and soldiers at every port. Larrey, who was now Chief Surgeon of the Imperial Guard, went with his master to Boulogne. At this time, as never before, the Emperor felt the need of a great admiral. The Channel was practically open, and all he required was the convoy; but the convoy did not come. At the most, there were probably but a few thousand regular troops in England; and could his army of veterans have crossed what Gladstone called the silver streak of the Channel, it seems as though London would have fallen. But the splendid activity of the English navy, in contrast to the supine imbecility of the French navy, together with the violent storms that beset the coast, hindered the passage. Just at this time, too, the European Coalition against the French power was formed, having been instigated by Austria.

Without a moment's hesitation, Napoleon turned this gigantic army, marched it through France, crossed the Rhine, and was in Germany almost before the enemy knew that a single man had started. It was just then that Lord Nelson defeated the combined French and Spanish fleets in the memorable Battle of Trafalgar. Napoleon, as we have said, always wanted an admiral and never found one. It is an interesting speculation what might have happened had Paul Jones lived but a few years longer. It seems more than probable that he would have been the admiral that the Emperor was seeking. Had this daring sailor and most capable seaman been in command of the French forces at Trafalgar, perhaps history might have had a different story to tell.

Larrey, as Chief Surgeon of the Imperial Guard, was under the direct orders of Marshal Bessières, the soldier in command of the Guard. The surgeon went to Strasburg and organized his ambulances, and the army marched rapidly toward the Danube. The Austrians were quickly cooped up in Ulm, where almost their whole army was lost. This was done by a masterly piece of strategy. They were unable to sustain a siege, because there were no stores in the city. The remainder of the Austrians retreated toward Vienna, and the French followed them. While passing a few days in Munich, Larrey again visited Sömmering; and, although in the midst of the fierce excitement of war, he made a study of the anatomical museum. The Emperor soon established his headquarters at Schönbrunn, and the Marshal Prince Murat occupied Vienna.

This campaign throughout had been one of exposure, with almost constant snow or rain. The marches had been hard and harassing. The haste had been so great that there had been difficulty in transporting baggage, and even necessary articles had been left behind; yet there were very few sick. Larrey says, in his Memoirs, that as he watched the development of the army at this time, he was satisfied that the French soldiers were becoming more robust; and he insists that a soldier will stand almost any fatigue, if he gets sufficient food. This view confirms the axiom of Frederick the Great, that " an army, like a serpent, travels on its belly."

The portion of the Austrian army that had escaped from Vienna retired into Moravia, to effect a junction with the Russian army; and the Emperor Napoleon set out to meet them. He found them in a little town in Moravia, in the neighborhood of Brunn. The name of this town will always be remembered. It is Austerlitz.

The Battle of Austerlitz was the greatest victory that Napoleon ever won. It is often called the Battle of the Three Emperors; the Emperors of Austria and Russia being on the one side, and the Emperor of the French on the other. Napoleon had about eighty thousand men; the allies, in the neighborhood of one hundred thousand.

The direction of the Medical Corps of the army was in the hands of Larrey, Baron Percy having remained in Vienna.

The night before the battle, the Emperor, without warning, rode along the French line. Larrey tells us that the army "was electrified by his presence. By a unanimous and spontaneous motion, the whole army grasped wisps of straw and set them on fire; and in a moment, you beheld a new kind of illumination, symmetrical and brilliant, by more than forty-five thousand men."

The rain stopped during the night. Napoleon watched the sun rise through the mists on the morning of the battle; and his mystical nature was impressed with it as a favorable omen. He always referred to it subsequently as the " sun of Austerlitz." At seven o'clock in the morning, the battle began; and the Russians and Austrians were completely destroyed. A portion of the allied army tried to escape by crossing a frozen lake; but the French artillery fired at the ice with cannon and broke it up, and thousands drowned. Marshal Soult, the Duke of Dalmatia, was the hero of the combat, and bore the brunt of it on the French side.

In this battle, Larrey tells us, the enemy lost forty stands of colors, five hundred pieces of cannon, twenty generals, thirty thousand prisoners, and twelve thousand killed; besides thousands of wounded, who were transported to Brunn. Almost all the wounded of the French army were dressed on the field of battle. Inspector General Percy returned during the height of the engagement, and took charge of the General Medical Staff; and Larrey returned to his own position with the Imperial Guard. He had established a field-hospital in a granary, and the French wounded were quickly removed there and satisfactorily cared for. He says that no battlefield ever presented such a fearful picture of destruction as did Austerlitz. The day afterward, the French wounded were taken into Brunn, to quarters that had previously been prepared for their reception. Colonel Morlan, of the Chasseurs, had been killed in the combat. The Emperor was very fond of him and desired Larrey to embalm the body, which he did most successfully by methods he had learned in Egypt. Soon after the battle, the Treaty of Presburg was signed, which forced Austria to give up Venice, the Austrian Tyrol, and Suabia.

Larrey describes the appearance of an epidemic disease in Brunn, among the French and the Russians. He speaks of it as a " malignant, nervous, and putrid hospital-fever (adynamico-ataxick)." It was characterized by severe headache, chills, and fever. The wounds that existed tended to become putrid and gangrenous. There was a quick and irregular pulse, turbid urine, and usually diarrhœa. There were also tremor of the limbs, subsultus tendinum, delirium, pain in the belly, sweating, bleeding from the nose, and discharges from the bowel of black blood. The tongue was black in the center, and dry and red at the edges; and there were sordes on the gums and teeth. The patient was heavy and drowsy, and tended to become insensible. There was a most remarkable change in the features of the face; and when this facial condition, which was surely the Hippocratic face, was noticed early, it was always regarded as of fatal augury. The sick person passed into very great debility, and often sank and died.

Some patients died on the ninth, and some even on the seventh day of the disease. In this account, Larrey unquestionably describes typhoid fever, confusing it, perhaps, in some instances, with hospital-gangrene.

Soon after this period, Larrey returned to Paris and again took up teaching. His Memoirs contain at this point an essay on aneurysm, in which he maintains that this condition arises only in a diseased artery, and that very frequently the artery has been diseased by syphilis. He also discusses the effect of rheumatism on the fibrous and osseous structures, and considers movable and preternatural cartilages of the joints. He tells us that the first instance of movable cartilage of the knee was reported by Ambroise Paré in 1558. This surgeon opened a suppurating knee-joint, and a concretion about the size of an almond emerged. Larrey gives the other reported cases, and shows how many had been operated upon with success—particularly by his own masters, Sabatier and Desault. It is rather horrifying to us to-day to think of opening knee-joints without asepsis, for the purpose of removing these movable bodies; and yet, Larrey seems to have operated with very great success. He also considers the subject of epilepsy, as met with among the soldiers; and says that in many instances mercurial treatment was curative; thus agreeing with our modern view that epilepsy that begins late in life,—that is, after youth,—if not alcoholic or due to organic brain-disease, is usually syphilitic.

His memoir on amputations is a very important one, and somewhat lengthy. In it, he strongly advocates immediate amputation for certain serious injuries. In amputating in continuity, he employed the circular method, using several cuts. He did not sew up his flaps, but retained the edges together merely by applying a roller-bandage with a piece of lint over the wound. His operations were remarkably successful, probably because he had the freest kind of drainage and did not cover the wounds with foul and nasty greases, which would retain discharges. In confirmation of his views as to the value of early amputation, he quotes what he had heard of the experience of surgeons in the War of the American Revolution. He says that at this period the French surgeons would not amputate until late in the case, but that the American had the courage to amputate at once or within twenty-four hours. The mortality among the French was large, and among the Americans very small; yet the French hospitals were infinitely superior to the American. We thus see that even at this early day, American surgeons had independent convictions and the courage to carry them out.

Not a great while after the battle of Austerlitz, Prussia, undeterred by the lesson just administered to Austria and Russia, made a league with Saxony and began war. The Emperor immediately took the field, and very soon the great Battle of Jena was won. There was some difficulty here about the ambulances. They were too far back of the line of battle, and there was considerable delay in dressing the gravely wounded. Larrey insists upon the necessity of placing the ambulances near the line of battle, and of establishing a headquarters to which the wounded requiring serious operations can be rapidly taken. He says that those dangerously wounded must be attended to first, entirely without regard to their rank or distinction; and that those less severely injured must wait until the gravely hurt have been operated upon and dressed. The slightly wounded can go to the hospital of the first or second line, especially officers; because officers have horses to transport them, and these merely trivial wounds do not immediately endanger life. The Emperor marched his army into Berlin, and took back with him to Paris the keys of the city. He also took back with him to Paris the sword of Frederick the Great. Prussia had to wait a great many years; but she frightfully punished her old conquerors in the fearful war of '70-'71; and now again France bends all her energies to keep up her army to the highest level, in the hope that she may take vengeance upon Germany and march her soldiers beneath the linden trees.

While in Berlin, Larrey visited the distinguished physicians and scientists; and his relations with them seem to have been agreeable. He was particularly indebted to Humboldt, the great explorer; and to the elder and younger Walther, the eminent surgeons. A great many French soldiers, while in Berlin, became asphyxiated through having slept in rooms containing the stoves used by the inhabitants, after having closed the doors and windows. It was in Berlin that the ravages of syphilis were particularly noticeable in the army.

The next campaign participated in by Larrey was that in Poland, where he saw for the first time that remarkable disease, plica polonica. He noted that it was most common among the Jews, and regarded it as a result of syphilis—especially of hereditary syphilis. He took part in the fearful battles of Eylau and Friedland. Eylau is in East Prussia, twenty-two miles from Königsberg; Friedland is in East Prussia, twenty-six miles from Königsberg. After the Battle of Eylau, both Larrey and Percy were made Commanders of the Legion of Honor. At this point in the Memoirs, there is a treatise on dry gangrene produced by frost, which he calls gangrene from congelation. In Poland, he saw a number of cases of anthrax, which he thought came from eating the meat of animals that had the disease. In this campaign, for the second time, Larrey made a counter-opening in the cranium to reach a bullet. He introduced a gum-elastic catheter as a probe, and trephined over the point of it. He found a flattened bullet on the inside of the bone. The patient died five days afterwards, of hospital-fever.

At Tilsit, peace was made, the monarchs meeting on a pontoon anchored in the middle of the river. Königsberg interested Larrey greatly. Here he saw the point of a javelin that had been within the cranium of the Chevalier Erasmus for fourteen years without impairing his faculties. An abscess formed in the frontal region. It was opened, and this piece of javelin was removed. Larrey thinks that the javelin had probably been in the frontal sinus. He recalls that he himself saw a French soldier that, a little while after the Polish campaign, had had his head pierced with an iron-ramrod from a gun accidentally discharged. He had no bad symptoms at all, although it seems that the ramrod must have penetrated the brain. In Königsberg, the surgeon also saw a knife that a man had swallowed in 1613. Dr. Gruger, a Polish surgeon, had performed gastrotomy successfully; and the man had lived for ten years afterward. Larrey recalls that once, while he was a pupil, he had seen M. Frizac, Professor of Surgery at Toulouse, make an incision into the abdomen parallel with the linea alba, and discovered the point of a knife sticking through the wall of the stomach. He removed this fragment of knife-blade, which was about two inches in length; sutured the stomach with two sutures; and sewed up the integument. The man recovered. The sutures used were not inversion sutures, as the Lembert suture was not introduced until the third decade of the nineteenth century. Larrey then gives an account of a soldier of the guard who was wounded in the left extremity of the stomach by the point of a saber, which penetrated the thorax between the seventh and eighth ribs; injured the lung; split the diaphragm; and entered the stomach. The man vomited blood, and fluids that he had swallowed escaped from the wound. He was very ill for several days. Cooling medicine and emollient enemata were given, and venesection was performed. He was made to lie continuously on the right side. The wound healed without trouble. He got entirely well, and became one of the veterans of the Old Guard. The only difficulty left as a legacy was a hernia of the lung, which he kept in place by wearing a bandage.

After this campaign, Larrey again returned to Paris, where he received from the Emperor the title of Knight of the Iron Crown and was decorated with the insignia of that order. His Memoirs set forth next the stories of the campaigns in Spain. On his way to Spain, he visited Toulouse and demonstrated to the students of the College the views of Dr. Gall, which have been perverted of recent years, and have been utilized by the quack and the imposter; yet Gall sems to have been the first man that ever really indicated the localization of cerebral functions. Larrey also visited his own birth-place, and became much interested in studying goiter in the Pyrenees. He disliked the bull-fights of Spain very much, and thought that they should be disapproved by all that love tranquility and by all that are humane.

In Spain, as elsewhere, Larrey founded his military school and lectured on clinical surgery. He was in many fierce battles, and had numerous striking experiences. At one time, a hospital was attacked by Spaniards; and he, and the surgeons and the convalescents, were obliged to take up guns and defend it.

He reports interesting cases of wounds of the brain; of penetrating wounds of the thorax; and of abdominal wounds with protrusion of the intestines, followed by recovery. He considers traumatic gangrene and the Madrid colic, which he thinks was due to some deleterious properties in the wine sold by the people, but which some of the French surgeons thought was due to the wine having been actually poisoned. In order

to reach a conclusion as to the action of poisons and the way to treat cases of poisoning, he says that experiments should be made on living animals, in order to find remedies to counteract the poisonous effects. He was much impressed with the virtue of calisaya bark in treating intermittants.

He gives the following interesting case, which happened to Marshal Lannes, Duke of Montebello: The Marshal's horse fell down on a mountain covered with frozen snow; and, as a consequence, Lannes was severely bruised about the thorax and abdomen, and seemed to be gravely injured. He was completely covered with bruises. His abdomen was distended and very tender. He had violent pain and dyspnea, and could not voluntarily move. His pulse was small and tense. His face was deadly pale. His voice was weak, and his extremities were cold. The very slightest touch of the abdomen produced agonizing pain.

Larrey recalled a wonderful cure that he had seen made by the Esquimaux on some sailors of the Vigilante, whose boat had been cast against the rocks. These sailors had been dreadfully bruised. Larrey tried the same treatment, and afterwards used it on others besides the Marshal with success. He got a large sheep and had it stunned by a sudden blow on the neck, and two excellent butchers quickly flayed it. While this was being done, the Duke was greased all over with camphorated oil of camomile. His body was then completely wrapped in the skin of the sheep, which had been taken warm from its back. This reeking skin was still covered with serous fluid, and it was fastened together at the edges so as completely to surround the injured man's body. His extremities were wrapped in warm flannel, and the Marshal was allowed to take internally a light tea with lemon-juice and sugar.

His pain was very quickly relieved, although the sheep-skin pricked and irritated the skin of his body for a little while. Ten minutes after its application, he went to sleep and slept for two hours. When he awoke, the sheep skin was taken off; and it was found that he had been sweating tremendously. The sweat was wiped off, and an embrocation of warm, camphorated brandy was applied to the injured regions. Camphorated enemata and mucilaginous drinks, with milk of sweet almonds, were given him. The next morning the swelling of the abdomen had abated, and the Marshal felt very much more comfortable. It was found that his urine contained quantities of blood. He was then put into a warm bath. The aromatic embrocations were continued, and he went on duty on the fifth day, being able to ride a horse.

In the wounds inflicted in the Battle of Benevento, Larrey did not think it proper to remove the dressings that had been applied until the third day; because they had been put in place by skilful surgeons, and he was evidently opposed to the meddling interference that is so often productive of harm. One of the Mamelukes, Ibrahim, received a pistol-shot wound of the knee-joint that fractured the patella. Larrey removed the separated bone-fragments, and this man recovered completely.

Larrey lays down the rule that in any severe wound of a

hinge joint, the surgeon should always take amputation into consideration; and before the days of antiseptic surgery, this must unquestionably have been sound practice.

We learn from the Memoirs that a Dragoon of the Guard received a saber-cut in the right inguinal region. The abdomen was opened, and the epigastric artery was cut. A large mass of the great omentum stuck out of the wound. The plug of omentum stopped the hemorrhage from the divided epigastric artery. The protruded part became cold, without tenderness, and of livid hue. Larrey cut away the part that exhibited these phenomena. He then tied the bleeding arteries, and restored the healthy portion of omentum to the abdominal cavity. The man was entirely well in six weeks.

We find the record of another remarkable case: The patient was a Chasseur of very vigorous constitution, and of a strongly amorous nature. A saber-cut received in the Battle of Benevento chopped off a large piece of the occipital bone, with a portion of the dura mater, and exposed the right cerebellar lobe. Pressure upon this lobe did not cause any pain; but produced immediate vertigo, convulsions, and then syncope. Larrey removed the loose portion of the occipital bone, which was stuck to the flap, and placed the skin-flap directly in contact with the cerebellum, having retained an opening at the lower end for drainage. Quantities of fluid, which must have been cerebro-spinal fluid, were discharged at each dressing. The day after the injury, the man lost the sight of his right eye and the hearing of his right ear, and developed severe pains in the dorsal region and severe prickling, like the stinging of ants, in the testicles. These organs atrophied; and, in the space of fifteen days, reached the size of Windsor beans. The man was taken from Benevento to Valladolid, and stood the journey very well; but inflammation appeared, and the pains in the head and back became agonizing. He had convulsions; and, on attempts at swallowing, had attacks of syncope. Tetanus developed; and the patient died of it, thirty-nine days after the injury. Postmortem examination showed that there was no suppuration in the wound. There was a great contraction of the right lobe of the cerebellum. The medulla oblongata and the spinal cord were dull white, indurated and greatly shrunken; and the nerves that emerged from them were obviously atrophied. The cranium of this remarkable case was placed in Larrey's anatomical collection. The surgeon regarded this case as confirmatory of Gall's view that the cerebellum is the seat of the sexual instinct, a view long since abandoned. Larrey was aware that critical injuries impair the intellect, and states that basal and ventricular injuries produce paralysis; and that in severe injury of one hemisphere, the limbs of the opposite side are paralyzed. He also knew that even when such conditions of the limbs are old, relief may follow the performing of an operation to relieve brain-pressure on the side of the head opposite to the paralysis. He reports a case that Mumford [2] regards as undoubtedly a fracture of the base, in which there was coma and bleeding from the ears and mouth. A day after the injury, there was ecchymosis behind each mastoid, which we now call Battle's sign.

The health of the surgeon broke down in this campaign, and he consequently handed over his duties to M. Percy and returned to France. He was so ill that he was in great danger of dying. While he was still far from well, the Austrian campaign opened; and without waiting to recover his strength completely, he set out to join the army in Bavaria. On reaching Strasburg, he found that the French had beaten the Austrians at Ratisbon.

Baron Marbot, in his Memoirs, gives a most interesting account of the fight at Ratisbon. It was in this engagement that the greatest difficulty arose in surmounting the walls in making an assault. Each party that went to take the scaling ladders was destroyed by the well-directed fire of the Austrians. Fifty volunteers were called for twice to place ladders, and twice every volunteer was killed or wounded. Marbot says that every man in the army would have gone, if ordered to do so; but when volunteers were called for a third time, no one responded. Marshal Lannes, who was in command, became extremely angry. He said that he had been a grenadier before he was a marshal, and would show them that he was a grenadier yet; and he grasped a ladder and started forward with it alone. The officers were ashamed to think of his making the movement personally, so they struggled with him for the possession of the ladder. When the soldiers saw a marshal of France and his staff fighting desperately to have the honor of an enterprise, hundreds jumped forward to participate. Among those that did so were Marbot and Labédoyère, who were the first two men up the ladders. They ascended side by side and hand in hand, steadying each other as they mounted. They got over; a swarm of grenadiers followed; and the city was taken. A fine aquarelle of these two men mounting the ladders may be seen in Sloane's Life of Napoleon.

It was in the fight at Ratisbon that Napoleon was wounded for the second and last time in his life. Some rifleman from the Tyrol succeeded in just grazing him with a shot. The Emperor and Marshal Lannes were talking together when the Emperor was struck. The injury was of the right ankle. Marbot makes a mistake in one point: he says that the pain was so sharp that the Emperor leaned upon the Marshal, and that Dr. Larrey quickly arrived and said that the wound was a trifle: but Larrey did not arrive, as we learn from his Memoirs. He was then at Strasburg. It was a young surgeon that took charge of the case. He felt extremely the responsibility of his position. This was obvious to the Emperor, who counseled him to proceed just as though he were dealing with the most unimportant man in the army—which was unquestionably the best of good advice.

The army marched forward and occupied the Island of Lobau, and soon afterward fought the desperate Battle of Aspern, from the field of which the French had to fall back,

[2] "Teachings of the Old Surgeons," by J. G. Mumford.—*Boston Med. and Surg. Jour.*, October 3 and 10, 1895.

and in which Marshal Lannes was killed. There is a graphic account of this in Marbot's Memoirs.

Marbot tells us that the Marshal, tired out with his exertions, had got off his horse and was walking about with Major General Pouset. At this moment, the General was struck in the head and instantly killed. Lannes was warmly attached to the General; had, all through his life, advanced the latter's interests; and was grief-stricken at his death. The Marshal was almost overcome with grief. He walked about one hundred paces away, sat down on the side of a ditch, and seemed buried in deep thought. About fifteen minutes later, some soldiers were carrying the dead body of an officer covered with a cloak, and they stopped to rest directly in front of the Marshal. The cloak fell aside, and Lannes recognized Pouset. He cried out: "Is this terrible sight going to follow me everywhere?" He then got up; walked a little distance away; and sat down again on the edge of a ditch, with his legs crossed and his hands held over his eyes. In a moment, a three-pound shot ricochetted and struck him just where his legs were crossed. He was dreadfully injured, and Marbot rushed toward him. The Marshal said: "I am wounded, but it is nothing. Give me your hand and help me up." He tried to rise, but could not. He was suffering fearfully, and the soldiers started to carry him away. As they began to lift him, it was observed that he was not wrapped up. Some one ran and took the cloak from General Pouset's dead body, and laid it upon Launes; but the Marshal recognized the cloak and said: "This was my poor friend's. It is covered with his blood. I will not use it. Drag me along, rather, as you can." So the grenadiers made a stretcher out of some boughs from an adjacent clump of trees, and carried the Marshal to the dressing-station, where Larrey took charge of him.

Larrey, in his Memoirs, says that a bullet of large size had struck the left knee, passed through the joint, grazed the right thigh, and lacerated the integument, and a part of the vastus internus muscle, just above the left knee-joint; and that the Marshal also suffered from concussion of the brain and general prostration—by which, of course, Larrey means shock. He says that the face was livid, the lips pale, the eyes dull and watery, the voice extremely weak, the pulse almost absent, and the intellect deranged; and that the sufferer did not at all realize his danger. The surgeon was almost overcome at the sight of this devoted old-time friend, whom he had attended in Syria, Egypt, and Spain, and whose life he had saved on several previous occasions.

Larrey at once called some of his colleagues into consultation. The wound of the right knee was of the gravest description, there being a comminuted fracture of the bones, laceration of the ligaments and tendons, and destruction of the popliteal vessels. Marbot says that Larrey was in favor of amputating the right leg; another surgeon wanted to cut off both legs; but Dr. Yvan believed the Marshal's firm character would give him a chance of cure without any amputation at all, and that the operation performed in the hot weather would kill him. Larrey says that all of them were in favor

of immediate amputation; but that each of the other surgeons hesitated to perform it, because he was so sure that the result in any case would be fatal, and he hesitated to do it because his duty to the army called him elsewhere. Finally Larrey himself performed it, the operation requiring less than two minutes, and apparently causing but little pain.

The Marshal was then taken to the Island of Lobau, where the Emperor saw him, and where Larrey left him in the care of M. Paulet. He says that he left the Duke with great regret, and continues: "But I was the only inspector on the field of battle; and a great number of wounded on the island, whither they had been transported, still required our assistance. We never rested from our labor until all the wounded had been operated on and dressed."

The interview between Marshal Lannes and Napoleon has been told in many histories and memoirs, and a celebrated picture of it has been painted by Boutigny. It shows the Marshal, after his leg has been amputated and dressed, lying down, with the Emperor on his knees beside him, grasping the Marshal's hands. Larrey, with his apron still in place, stands back of them, looking upon the scene. Marbot tells us in his Memoirs that the interview between the Emperor and the Marshal was extremely touching; that Napoleon shed tears as he embraced the Marshal; and that the latter's blood stained the Emperor's white waistcoat. Marbot should have known; for he was at that minute supporting the Marshal's head and shoulders; although he is not put in the painting. Lannes was very much touched by the Emperor's grief. When Napoleon was obliged to leave, in order to provide for the safety of the army, he said: "You will live, my friend, you will live." The Marshal pressed the Emperor's hand and replied: "I trust I may, if I can still be of use to France and to Your Majesty." [*]

Marbot goes on to tell us that every moment Lannes asked the position of the troops, and exhibited pleasure when he learned that the enemy had not ventured to pursue. He asked how his wounded aides-de-camp were doing, and requested Dr. Larrey to examine Marbot's wound. Marbot says that they had to keep the Marshal all night on the island, lying on a bed of cavalry-cloaks; and that there was not even good water to give him to quench his thirst. The water of the Danube was filled with mud, and Lannes would not drink it; so Marbot devised a filter, which he made of one of the Marshal's fine shirts. This water was eagerly taken. The next day, the Emperor sent a boat to bring the Marshal to the right bank; and he was taken to a house in Ebersdorf, Marbot remaining with him.

We now return to Larrey's account in his Memoirs. On reaching Ebersdorf, he found the Marshal extremely weak, pale, and incoherent. He was very restless, suffered with dyspnœa, and sighed frequently. The next day the wounds were found to be purulent; but the stump looked well; and Larrey had some hopes of recovery. On the evening of the

_____

[*] Marbot's Memoirs.

sixth day after the injury, a dangerous fever arose. Two hours after the first attack of fever, there was another attack; and in the course of the day, another, with delirium and gangrene. The Marshal died in the ninth day after the accident—in all probability of pyemia. Larrey had the unpleasant task of embalming the body of his old friend, so that he might be sent back to France.

After this battle, there was a dreadful mortality in the army from lock-jaw and hospital-fever. The next great battle participated in by the surgeon was the tremendous conflict of Wagram, upon which the fate of the Empire was staked. It was this fight that made Larrey a Baron of the Empire; and Macdonald, a Marshal of France. The latter had been regarded as one of the ablest soldiers of the Republic; but he was a personal friend of Moreau's, and, although he had not joined in the conspiracy with Pichegru, the Emperor was suspicious of him. Furthermore, he was a man blunt of speech, truthful to a fault, and as courageous in counsel as on the battlefield. He had come from a family noted for courage; for his father, Macdonald of Glencoe, had agreed to go with Prince Charles Edward Stuart when all the other Scottish chiefs had held back, and after the Battle of Culloden had gone to France and remained there.

The original list of Marshals was as follows: Augereau, Bernadotte, Berthier, Bessières, Brune, Davout, Jourdan, Kellermann, Lannes, Lefebvre, Masséna, Moncey, Mortier, Murat, Ney, Perignon, Sérurier, and Soult. It had caused universal comment that Macdonald had been left out of this illustrious list. The Marshals afterward appointed by Napoleon were Grouchy, Marmont, Oudinot, Poniatowski, St. Cyr, Suchet, Victor, and Macdonald. The latter said himself that, in the long run, it was worth being left out; because his achievement at Wagram caused him to have the baton of a Marshal given him on the battlefield, and to have the honor of being made a duke there—honors that had never come to anyone else on the field of battle.

Macdonald made at Wagram the charge upon which the whole battle hinged. It was his duty to break the center of the Austrian army. He had but fifteen thousand men to do it with, and one hundred cannon were playing upon them in a semi-circle. He accomplished the task; but when it was done, only fifteen hundred men were left around him. The Emperor rode up to him and said: "No more trouble between us, Macdonald. You have been reserved for a higher honor than your brothers-in-arms. I make you a Marshal here, on the field of your glory."

In contemplating the names of the illustrious soldiers that were selected as Marshals of France, one is struck by the curious fact that all but three of them seem to have begun life in humble circumstances, with very few advantages. Of these three Poniatowski, the Polish Prince, was not made a Marshal until October, 1813; and he was drowned in the Elster six days later. He was a gallant soldier and an aide to Napoleon. The stories of the other two of better origin were different. One was Marmont. and the other Grouchy; and

these two men ruined the man that had made them. Marmont surrendered Paris when the Emperor had almost reached there. If it had been held but a few days longer, far different terms could have been made. Grouchy, by indecision that is simply incredible, lost the Battle of Waterloo, which should have been won.

After Wagram, a great many amputations had to be done, on account of the severity of the gun-shot wounds. In two of the Guard, amputation at the hip-joint was performed. In telling the story of one of these cases, Larrey says that he ligated the femoral artery; and then amputated at the hip-joint in fifteen seconds, without any loss of blood. One of these two patients died of shock within three hours; the other died at six o'clock the next morning.

One remarkable case was that of an artilleryman struck by a ball that had rebounded before hitting him. It buried itself behind the bone and lodged near the groin. The patient said that the ball had glanced from him and killed another artillerist. Larrey says: "On seizing the limb to amputate it, I found it unusually heavy; and I decided that there was a ball in it, as I had often seen while making incisions and during operations. Under this impression, and supposing that the thigh was injured high up, I wished to amputate with the flaps. I then made an incision parallel with the skin of the thigh, and discovered a five-pound ball, which was extracted." The surgeon then completed the amputation.

With this campaign, the second volume of the Memoirs of the surgeon is terminated. The third volume shows us that Larrey continued with Napoleon until the last. He went through all the horrors of the Russian Campaign—the cold; the exposure; and the dreadful conflict at the Borodino, in which thirty thousand Frenchmen lost their lives. He was at the desolation of Moscow, and at the passage of the Beresina, where he got safely over; but, finding that important hospital-supplies had been left behind, he took his life in his hands and went back for them. The men cried: "Let us save the man that saved us." The frantic mob gave way, and the soldiers brought him in their arms safe to the army again. He was in the hideous tramp in midwinter, from Moscow back to France; and in all the actions of the winter of 1813-14, in which Napoleon fought united Europe and contested, step by step, the road to Paris.

The genius of the great captain never shone brighter than in this period; for he won battle after battle against vastly superior numbers; but, as he had no re-enforcements and few supplies, he was compelled, slowly and gradually, but surely, to fall back. On one occasion during this campaign, he captured a whole German army corps; but the faces of the French had to turn to Paris, no matter what the result of the battles might be. We all remember that picture by Meissonier in which the Emperor and his staff, gloomy and depressed, but resolute, are going on their way back to the capital, through the desolate country, over a road cut to pieces with wagons and artillery.

When the order to send the Emperor to Elba was given,

Larrey begged to be taken along; but Napoleon would not let him go, telling him that the army needed his services, and that it was his duty to stay with it. Bonaparte returned from Elba in 1815, and the old surgeon was one of the first to welcome his Emperor. The latter, after speaking of the joy that it gave him to be thus received, expressed regret that he had left Larrey so long without a fortune, and said that he hoped soon to be able to recompense him for his services. Soon after coming back from Elba, when the colors were being distributed to the different departments, the Emperor handed the flag of the High Pyrenees to Larrey and asked him to give it to the President of that Department; saying, as he did so, that he was glad that this color should be presented by their countryman, Larrey, a man that was an honor to humanity on account of his courage and his disinterested conduct—a man that had saved great numbers from death in the deserts of the East, had given water reserved for himself to suffering soldiers in Egypt and Syria, and had always loyally and faithfully served his Emperor.

On the eve of the Battle of Waterloo, Larrey was long with Napoleon in confidential conversation, seeking to rouse him from his depression; for this great man seemed to have dipped into the future, and to have had a glimpse of what was coming.

At Waterloo, when the news of the defeat arrived, Larrey, who was involved in the rout, endeavored to reach the French frontier. He had to fight his way with sword and pistol through a party endeavoring to take him. He succeeded in getting through this party, but his horse was shot under him; and before he could get up, he was struck on the head and the left shoulder with sabers. He was left for dead where he fell; but he regained consciousness, got on a horse, and proceeded on his road. He was, however, captured afterwards. Nearly all his clothing was taken away, and the sword given him by the Emperor was also taken. He was a short man, somewhat stout, and wore a gray great-coat. He thus somewhat resembled the Emperor in appearance, and was at first taken for him. His hands were tied together, and he was brought before a Prussian officer, who saw that he was not Napoleon and ordered that he be shot. Just as the soldiers were about to fire at him, the Prussian regimental surgeon recognized Larrey and succeeded in stopping the contemplated execution. He then took the French surgeon before General Bulow, who also recognized him. The general was grieved to see this distinguished man without shoes to his feet, almost without clothing to his back, wounded, hungry, and suffering. His hands were untied, and he was taken before Marshal Blucher, who knew of him; because in the Austrian campaign Blucher's own son had been wounded and taken prisoner, and Larrey had cared for him and saved his life. The Marshal at once liberated Larrey, gave him clothing and money, and had him sent forward into France; and he soon afterward reached Paris.

When the Bourbons mounted the throne, Larrey lost his position and fell into a state of absolute poverty. His mother and one of his brothers died, and he almost made up his mind

to go to the United States to practice surgery. The Emperor of Russia endeavored to secure his services in a high position with the Russian army, and Dom Pedro of Brazil made every effort to have him come to that country: but he refused both these offers.

Napoleon died in 1821, and Larrey was plunged into grief at the death of his old chief. He was greatly touched to learn that the Emperor had spoken of him in his will; had referred to him as "the most virtuous man that I have ever known"; and had left him some money, as an evidence of his continued affection.

Soon afterwards, Larrey was restored to the army. In 1826, he took a trip to England, and was received with the greatest distinction by the English surgeons. He then returned to Paris, and continued to practice and teach his profession; and he was again made Surgeon-in-Chief of the army, and Chief Surgeon of the Invalides. In the Revolution of July, 1830, which overthrew Charles X, he directed personally the care of the wounded. A year later, at the invitation of the King of Belgium, he visited all the army hospitals of that country and suggested regulations and improvements.

In 1834, he made a tour through southern France, visiting his birth-place. He was received with the greatest honor by all the citizens, and members of the Imperial Guard flocked from long distances to see him. At his birth-place, he found the Abbé de Crasset, his old instructor, still living.

In 1842, he was sent to visit the army in Algeria. He inspected it carefully, and then returned toward home; but when at Lyons, he was taken ill; and he died there on the 25th of July, 1842.

We find an interesting picture of Larrey in his old age at Paris in "A Memoir of J. Mason Warren," the father of the present distinguished Professor of Surgery in Harvard College. This interesting volume is edited by Howard Payson Arnold. Dr. Warren was a student in Paris during the reign of Louis Philippe, that greatest day of French medicine and surgery, which I have discussed in another paper;[1] the day of Dupuytren, Lisfranc, Roux, Marjolin, Civiale, Velpeau, Ricord, Falret, Trelat, Calmeil, Fauville, Dubois, Baudelocque, Guerin, Vidal-de-Cassis, Cazenave, Jobert, Lugol, Rostand, the younger Larrey, Boyer, Maisonneuve, Richerand, Blandin, Chassaignac, Hugier, Sanson, Denonvilliers, Cloquet, Amussat, Nélaton, Cullerier, Breschet, Sappey, Magendie, Andral, Gay-Lussac, Broussais, Malgaigne, and others. On November 5, 1832, Dr. Warren wrote as follows:

My dear Father.—I made a very pleasant and instructive visit, a few days since, to the Hotel des Invalides, where I attended Larrey in his wards. He is a short, corpulent man, with a very agreeable face. His hair, which is gray, falls in curls over the straight, ornamented collar of the military coat that he wears during his visits. He was very polite to Dr. Pierson, who was introduced to him by an Italian gentleman, and took great pains to show us all the remarkable cases, many of which he referred to as being described in his books. He also showed a case of

---

[1] "Medical Paris During the Reign of Louis Philippe," by J. Chalmers DaCosta, M. D., *University of Pa. Med. Bul.*, March, 1904.

amputating-instruments that he had had with him in Egypt. He spoke much of his inventions of different kinds, particularly of an amputating-knife with a curved blade, which, he said, cuts off the leg more expeditiously from its embracing a greater surface. I think I have heard you state in your lectures that, no matter how much a blade was curved, nothing was added to the celerity of the operation; as it cut only on one point at the same time. Larrey, however, if he has anything he thinks his own, will not give it up for anybody. The most remarkable cases were:

"1. Lower jaw shot off, the tongue hanging down upon the front of the neck. To remedy this, a curved plate was tied to the head, having a silver lip. When this was on, the man was able to articulate distinctly. He had been nourished with broth for ten or fifteen years.

"2. Three cases of disarticulation at the shoulder-joint, with a beautiful union. One of the cases had been operated on two days previously, and was doing well.

"3. Baron Larrey showed us a case of neuralgia of the arm from amputation's having been performed too low down. The flap is not sufficient, and the cicatrix presses on the bone. He says he has seen a number of cases like this, and the best remedy is to amputate again.

"He is very fond of the hot iron.[*] He says he applies it to large ulcers of the leg, forming an eschar over the whole. He stated that he had wrought some wonderful cures in erysipelas of the face by passing an iron over the whole surface. The patients were cured in twenty-four hours, but he did not say how their faces looked after the operation.

"4. He showed us a case of cataract in which the man had been totally blind, but had been restored to sight by applying moxas to the back of the neck. From this he infers that cataract always depends on inflammation of the capsule. I did not see him operate, but intend to go there again for the purpose."

We have said more than once in these pages that Larrey was noted for his truthful and decisive character, and never hesitated to tell the Emperor what he thought, even though it irritated his master. As an illustration of this, we may mention the disagreement between the Emperor and Larrey after the Battle of Bautzen. This is related in the sketch of Larrey in F. C. Stewart's book on the Hospitals and Surgeons of Paris, and is briefly referred to in Larrey's own Memoirs.

There were a very large number of wounded in the Battle of Bautzen, which misfortune Larrey attributed to the very large percentage of recent recruits present; the fierce nature of the combat; and the positions occupied by the armies. Some of the officers, who wished the war to end and wanted to get home, said that the army could not be depended on; that the troops were dissatisfied; and that the soldiers, in order to make the army go home, had in many instances wounded each other, or had pretended to have injuries that they had not sustained. The Emperor ordered Larrey and some other surgeons to examine all the wounded, so that he might signally punish anyone guilty of such a lack of patriotism.

Larrey went to the Emperor for the purpose of insisting that these statements were untrue. Napoleon was extremely angry, and told the surgeon that any observation he might make must be official, and not personal; and that he should at once go on with the duty he had been ordered to perform.

Larrey, with quiet dignity, went about this duty; and he refused to be hastened, although the Emperor was in a passion of impatience. The surgeon obtained, with the utmost care, every particular about each wounded man. He was told by his companions in arms that he had better not be so careful, and should hurry for his own good, or the Emperor would punish him; but he took the time that he knew was necessary to do this duty thoroughly and well.

When he had finished, the Emperor asked him whether he still retained his former opinion. Larrey said: "More than that, Your Majesty. I come to prove to you that our brave soldiers have been subjected to calumny. I have not discovered a single one that is guilty. There is not a wounded man that has not been examined. I have here a wagon-load of manuscripts; and I shall be pleased, if Your Majesty has them all read." Napoleon snatched the report out of Larrey's hands, and said sternly: "I will have it attended to." He then paced uneasily up and down the room; but, after a few moments, his frown broke away. He stopped before Larrey; shook him warmly by the hand; and, with every evidence of affection, said: "Good-bye, M. Larrey. A monarch is extremely lucky who is served by such men as you; and my further orders shall be conveyed to you." That same evening, the Emperor sent Larrey his portrait set with diamonds, six thousand francs in money, and a pension of three thousand francs a year. This story is creditable to both these distinguished men.

The surgeon's decision of character and willingness to assume responsibility are shown by the following anecdote: After a battle, many officers complained that their horses had been shot by Larrey's order. The Emperor sent for him and said: "Why have you dared to have these horses shot? Was it to feed the wounded?" Larrey answered simply: "Yes, Your Majesty"; and Napoleon thanked him for it.

In summing up the achievements of Baron Larrey, we should mention the following:[*]

1. The avoidance of meddlesome surgery, leaving a simple healing wound practically to take care of itself.

2. The use of warm salt-solution to wash wounds with; and the use of Labaraque's solution, a powerful antiseptic, to wash putrid and sloughing wounds.

3. The demonstration that the union of two granulating surfaces may take place, if one surface is laid against the other and the wound is cleansed frequently with an antiseptic. We call this to-day union by third intention.

4. The belief in the necessity of supporting treatment after severe injuries, stimulants and nourishing food being given the patient, instead of fierce purgatives and copious bleedings. In certain cases, Larrey fed persons with the stom-

---

[*] Larrey, in his Memoirs, says he used the hot iron around an area of erysipelas to prevent its spread.

[*] In this connection, see the admirable article on "Teachings of the Old Surgeons," by J. G. Mumford, in the *Boston Med. and Surg. Jour.*, October 3 and 10, 1905.

ach-tube; in others, by means of a catheter passed through the nostril, as is often done in lunatic asylums to-day."

5. The demonstration of the very great value of heat in suppurating areas. We now know why heat is of such value; as it relieves circulatory stasis, and brings millions of leukocytes to encompass the area of infection. Napoleon's Surgeon General knew clinically its usefulness.

6. The view that granulating wounds require no special dressing, some ordinary non-irritating ointment being sufficient; Larrey's rule was to abandon poultices as soon as the pain abated, the inflammation disappeared, and the temperature became normal.

7. The employment of rest in the treatment of wounds. Larrey believed rest to be imperatively necessary, in order to permit nature to do her work; and he would allow a first dressing, if properly put on, to remain undisturbed for several or many days. He associated rest with judicious compression, made by bandages—particularly flannel-bandages.

8. The belief in the imperative necessity of drainage for large wounds, for certain injuries of the skull, and for some injuries in the pleural cavity.

9. The use of the conservative operation of the resection of joints. The view regarding the usefulness of this had been put forth, but three or four years before, by Mr. Park, of Liverpool; and had been originally suggested by Bilgner, the Surgeon General of Frederick the Great.[10] Larrey showed that resections save a large number of amputations.

10. The insistence upon the necessity of enlarging, by incision and drainage, all punctured wounds—a point of view not yet accepted by all practitioners.

11. Trephining for hemorrhage of the middle meningeal artery; although, strange to say, after thus having reached the bleeding vessel, Larrey arrested the bleeding with the actual cautery.

12. Trephining for depressed fracture, comminuted fracture, or any condition that causes compression of the brain.

13. The value of drainage in preventing pressure in intra-cranial hemorrhage.

14. The recognition of discoloration over the mastoid process as a result of fracture of the base—the condition we now call Battle's sign, after Mr. Battle, of St. George's Hospital, London.

15. A knowledge in advance of his time regarding the symptoms of cerebral injuries. He said that injuries of the cortex of the brain impair the intellect; that injuries of the ventricles and the base produce paralysis; and that the paralysis is on the side of the body opposite to the brain-injury. Further, he stated that even in old cases of such paralysis, good results sometimes follow trephining the opposite side of the head, to relieve pressure.

16. The view that a fungus cerebri should not be cut off, and that no effort should be made to reduce it; because the

cause is actual swelling of the brain, and the only treatment that promises good results is equable compression.

17. In hemorrhage of the lung into the pleural cavity, he made a large incision. Le Cuite has recently showed us that a large incision arrests bleeding by producing pneumothorax. Larrey stated that when drainage was thus inserted, bleeding stopped and the person was safe from subsequent dangerous empyema.

18. The belief that empyemata should be operated on, and that this is a very successful operation.

19. On several occasions, in gun-shot wounds of the head, he explored the track of the bullet with a soft catheter; and, finding that the missile was on the opposite side of the cranium, he trephined on the side opposite the wound and extracted the bullet.

20. The belief in the great superiority of immediate amputation over the secondary operation so long in vogue.

21. The introduction of the flying ambulances into warfare. This method was soon imitated by every nation. It has saved countless thousands from death and from horrible agony, and may be regarded as one of the greatest of Larrey's achievements.

22. A description of adynamic ataxic fever, the typhoid of our own time; and the fact that gangrene may occur during its existence.

23. The inauguration of the custom of carefully attending to the wounded men, as well as to the wounded officers; the prisoners, as well as his own people.

24. Finally, his ideas as to reaching, removing, and caring for the wounded after the battle constitute the foundation-stones of military surgery to-day.

The name of this eminent man is on the Arch of Triumph. His statue is at the Val de Grace. His body lies in the Cemetery of Père-la-Chaise, where his monument can be seen at the present time. Near him are a number of scientists; and about him are many of those soldier-comrades with whom he marched into most of the capitals of Europe. Near him is Saint Hilaire, the naturalist; Arago, the physicist; Monge, the mathematician; Laplace, the astronomer; and Gay-Lussac, the chemist. Around him we note a group of soldiers; Marshal Masséna, who held Genoa in the great siege, who fought Wellington, and who was one of the best strategists and grimmest fighters in the army; Marshal Lefebvre, who was the first man made a noble by Napoleon, and who commanded in his will that he be buried near Masséna, adding: "We lived together in camps and combats; our ashes ought to have the same asylum;" Marshall Kellermann, one of the first generals under whom Larrey served, and the man that won Valmy; Marshal Grouchy, who had had a great reputation as a strategist, and whose inexplicable hesitation lost Waterloo; Marshal Ney, "the bravest of the brave," who commanded the rear-guard in the retreat from Russia and who was shot as a traitor by the treacherous and wretched Bourbon king; Colonel Labédoyère, who, with Baron Marbot, was the first over the walls

[10] J. G. Mumford.
[11] J. G. Mumford.

of Ratisbon; Marshal Macdonald, who won Wagram, and was made a Marshal on the field of battle, a man who was a gallant and loyal gentleman all his days: Marshal Suchet, who had been a junior officer in Napoleon's company, when the latter was a captain; Marshal Davout, the hero of Auerstadt; General Junot, whose wife Napoleon wished to marry, when she was a young girl—Junot, reckless to gallantry, who resembled Mad Anthony Wayne of our Revolutionary struggle; and General Foy, who was sent to Turkey to fight the Russians and the English, and was wounded fifteen times in his various arduous campaigns. It seems a pity that Larrey's old friend and patient, Lannes, is not near him. This celebrated Marshal's body lies in the Cemetery of Montmartre.

Those of us that go to Paris and look at the tomb of Baron Larrey can feel with justice that there is buried a soldier, a patriot; a great, learned, and brilliant surgeon; a brave, truthful, and loyal man; a gentleman; and a benefactor of the human race.

ON SOME EXPERIENCES WITH BLOOD-CULTURES IN THE STUDY OF BACTERIAL INFECTIONS.[1]

By E. Libman, M. D.,

Adjunct Visiting Physician and Assistant Pathologist Mt. Sinai Hospital, New York.

When, a few months ago, you honored me by asking me to present something here, I was much concerned. I felt unequal to the task of addressing you, and I was at a loss as to the choice of my subject. After a few days' thought I decided that the subject which has been announced to you would be an advantageous one in a number of ways.

In the first place, I could combine the paper with a demonstration. This I was anxious to do because Professor Welch, when he was kind enough to visit our hospital last spring, expressed a wish that some of our material be presented here. In the second place, I thought that it would be of value to speak of blood-cultures here because you have been engaged in such work; therefore, the paper would, be of particular interest to you, and I could have the benefit of your opinions for our later work. And finally, the subject is one of direct interest to men engaged in nearly all the branches of medical work.

Since the fall of 1897, when I found streptococci in the blood of a child suffering from streptococcic intestinal infection (1), in the clinic of my friend and teacher, Professor Escherich, I have been much interested in systemic bacterial infections, and, during the past eight years I have attempted from time to time to study especially the general infections by the pyogenic cocci. The number of cases which we have studied by means of cultures is between 700 and 750. Not all are of value. Many were made at request in cases which proved to be examples of fever due to tuberculosis, or cases not bacterial in origin. Some were unsuccessful for one reason or another. I shall not attempt to cover the entire material—that would be impossible. Only certain points will be taken up and digressions will be made here and there so as to mention observations that are unusual or particularly interesting. The literature (2) will not be discussed as I prefer to speak at this time of our own experiences. The subject of infections by the typhoid bacillus will be omitted and only such pneumococcus infections as occurred independently of pneumonia will be included.

While the paper will not be a connected one,—the breadth of the subject prevents that—I shall take up the following main points:

1. The terminology to be used in the paper.
2. Technical considerations.
3. Organisms found, their frequency, and the types of diseases in which they were encountered.
4. Notes on osteomyelitis, secondary parotitis, intra-abdominal infections, infections of otitic origin and those arising in the genito-urinary tracts of the male and the female.
5. Notes on certain groups of cases belonging to the domain of internal medicine.
6. Endocarditis; embolic aneurysms.
7. Discussion of negative blood-cultures.
8. Discussion of positive blood-cultures.
9. Diagnostic points.
10. The prognosis in cases in which bacteria have been found in the blood.

1. Terminology.

The terminology (3) that I shall use is one based on the work itself and will, I hope, be justified by the observations I shall record. When bacteria attack any part of the body we call the resultant lesion a local infection. There may or may not be evident toxemia; usually there is. If such a local infection is so situated that it is not diagnosed we can call the lesion a cryptic infection. If there is toxemia we have a cryptogenetic toxemia.

If bacteria are present in the blood we have a bacteriemia, or systemic infection. Such a bacteriemia may or may not be accompanied by the establishment of secondary foci (metas-

[1] Read before the Medical Society of the Johns Hopkins Hospital, February 5, 1906.

tatic infections or so-called pyemia). If, when bacteria are in the blood, the point of infection is overlooked, or has healed or is so situated that it is not diagnosed, we are dealing with a cryptogenetic bacteriemia.

In the use of the word bacteriemia I wish to agree with those who use the term to signify the presence of bacteria in the blood without implying anything concerning the question of whether they are multiplying or not. Canon (4) uses the word bacteriemia to indicate the cases in which bacteria are discharged from a local focus and do not multiply in the blood, whereas by septicemia he refers to their multiplication in the blood. The word septicemia, if used at all, should, I believe, be used only to designate the presence of bacteria in the blood. The reasons for this will be made apparent later.

The term secondary infection is best reserved for those cases in which one bacterial infection follows another. For the occurrence of a bacterial infection in the course of a disease not bacterial in origin, the term intercurrent infection .is better. By a mixed infection we mean the co-existence of infections by two or more organisms. The two infections may have occurred simultaneously, or one may be secondary. The first infection at times disappears. For secondary and mixed invasions of the blood-current we can use the terms secondary bacteriemia and mixed bacteriemia.

The term agonal invasion needs no explanation; it is not yet known how often it really occurs. The expression terminal infection (5) needs a commentary. I believe it should really be used to indicate an infection that comes when the patient is about to die of his original disease. Often, however, it is used to indicate the infection that terminates the life of a patient with a chronic disease. Not infrequently a patient in a hospital ward with a chronic nephritis or endocarditis, whose condition is supposed to be hopeless, spontaneously or as the result of treatment rallies and leaves the hospital in quite good condition for a shorter or longer time. If such a patient has the misfortune to acquire a fatal infection in the ward, he is sometimes put down as having died of a terminal infection, when in reality it was a terminating infection. It would be better, I believe, to restrict the use of the expression terminal infection and use at times the expressions secondary fatal infection and intercurrent fatal infection. This would lead to greater stress being laid on preventing such infections.

2. Technical Considerations.

In the remarks which I shall make on the technical side, I shall not go into the question of how the blood is to be obtained or the difficulties which we may meet. It is generally agreed that the amount should be large, 25 cc. if possible. We do not rely on microscopic examinations.

The question of the media to be used we must touch upon, even if briefly. For several years we have used a variety of media for each culture, so as to study their relative value, and so as to be able to state, when results were negative, that optimum methods had been used. The routine, except in cases of typhoid fever, was to use plates of agar, serum-agar, glucose-agar and serum-glucose-agar and flasks of bouillon and glucose bouillon with and without serum. When we expected to find streptococci, staphylococci or pneumococci the blood was used more concentrated. If there was no clue to the organism that was possibly present, the blood was used in varying dilutions. In obscure cases, more than one culture was necessary when all the variations in media were to be tried.

It is hardly possible to state briefly and definitely the relative value of each of these media. In cases in which only a few organisms are present it may be more difficult to decide this question than when they are numerous, as the occurrence of the organisms on one particular plate may be due to chance. At times the fluid media were better, at times the plates. Glucose-agar rarely proved to be of any greater value than ordinary agar; generally it was less favorable. Possibly at another titre it might have been better. Serum-agar often gave a better result than ordinary agar. Glucose-serum media (6) which I suggested some years ago as simple optimum media for bacterial growth, often gave an earlier result, and in some instances were the only media to show growth even when the bacteria were abundant. (This refers especially to the cocci found in certain cases of subacute endocarditis).[1] We have found these media often of advantage in routine work for cultivating the meningococcus and the gonococcus. It would be wise to use them in blood-cultures in cases in which these organisms are looked for. Staphylococci usually grow well on all media.

At times streptococci would grow in glucose-bouillon when they would not grow in ordinary bouillon, and occasionally the opposite was found. At times they seemed to grow better when the blood was well diluted, but as a rule concentrated blood was more favorable. At times streptococci and staphylococci were found in the flasks growing only in the clot at the bottom.

Media in tubes have been used very little in the past six years, but there is no doubt that in cases in which bacteria are present in very large numbers an earlier result can be obtained by pouring some blood over the surface of slanted media. In obscure cases it is wise to use one or two plates of serum-glucose-agar on the surface of which the blood is poured. This gives the possibility of using pure blood and avoids the overheating of the organisms which may occur during plating.

Glycerine-agar was found to be of no particular advantage. The Wassermann medium (7) (made of 2% Chapoteaut peptone and pork infusion with a markedly alkaline reaction) in a

---

[1] Although glucose-agar is not particularly advantageous we continue to use it because it serves as a control on the glucose-serum-agar. If on the serum-glucose-agar plates bacteria are found that grow easily on all media and there is no growth on the glucose-agar plates we can suspect a contamination of the serum.

couple of instances gave very good results.[a] I believe, however, that similar results are obtained by using agar made up of beef infusion with 2% Witte's or Merck's peptone with a reaction neutral to phenolphthalein.

In certain cases anaërobic work was done. Either the Novy jars or Buchner tubes were used, or the blood was mixed with glucose-agar in deep tubes according to the Veillon method.(8) This last method was used especially in case of abdominal disease. Tissier (9) has pointed out that the intestinal tract contains anaërobes that can be isolated only by the Veillon method, and we have encountered such organisms either by staining methods or in cultures in a number of intra-abdominal infections. They are also to be found in necrotic foci in the mastoid, lungs and other organs. The difficulty in using this method for blood cultures lies in the fact that a small quantity of blood makes the medium opaque and colònies cannot be seen. To carry out the method properly very many tubes would have to be used. . One could think of attempting in some way to rid the blood of red corpuscles.

Before considering the findings in the positive cases, it is necessary to refer to the question of contaminations and to the methods of identifying certain organisms.

In the hands of beginners contaminations are frequent, but with experience they can be almost entirely avoided. It is advisable to study carefully all. contaminating organisms, so that if one of them is found in the blood of an obscure case, it be not looked upon as the cause of the disease. Not infrequently one encounters publications in which organisms are described as being the cause of certain diseases, which organisms accurately correspond to those often met with as contaminations.

The contaminations most frequently met are *Micrococcus epidermidis albus*, Gram-positive bacilli with and without spores, Gram-negative bacilli of different kinds, organisms of the psuedo-diphtheria group and *Micrococcus tetragenus*.[b] An interesting organism occasionally met is a short Gram-negative bacillus which it is difficult to cultivate on other than blood media.

Several years ago one of the laboratory workers found a remarkable contaminating organism in two cases. It was a streptococcus growing like the ordinary streptococcus on media without glucose, but growing in large mucoid masses on glucose media. It was Gram-negative. If the Gram test had not been applied and if glucose media had not been used a serious blunder would have been made. Cultures made the next day in both cases proved negative, a result more in accordance with the clinical picture.

The organisms concerning the identification of which I

wish to speak are the pneumococci, streptococci, staphylococci, gonococci and meningococci.

Much of the earlier work of other observers and myself is unreliable as the methods for identifying pneumococci were not sufficiently definite in all instances. From what I have seen during the last year I believe that a few of the so-called streptococci[c] which I found in earlier cases may have been pneumococci and vice versa. This is a question into which I enter gladly because Dr. Buerger worked on that subject in our laboratory. Dr. Epstein, the present pathological interne, has been working along the same lines and so far has corroborated Dr. Buerger's results. We have, therefore, adopted them for routine work.

If the organism (Gram positive) has the typical capsule described by Dr. Buerger (10) it is a pneumococcus. This capsule or rather the capsular membrane is situated at a fair distance from the organism, stains sharply and the capsular substance (between the membrane and the organism) shows little tendency to stain. The capsule often shows indentations; these occur at the intervals between the organisms in the diplococcus-form; in chains, the indentations occur between each pair of cocci. (*Streptococcus mucosus capsulatus*[c] is almost never lancet-shaped; its capsule is at a fair distance; it is mucoid and the capsular substance tends to take the stain. There are no indentations). Other streptococci do not usually have capsules; when they do, the capsule is very close to the organism, and has deep indentations between each of the cocci in the chains.

When the typical capsule of the pneumococcus (or *Streptococcus mucosus capsulatus*) is present, the identification can at once be made. If the organism has the streptococcus type capsule, or no capsule, it must be studied, for the organisms just mentioned may lose the type capsule after successive inoculations or under adverse circumstances.

To determine whether such an organism is a streptococcus or a pneumococcus one can use the inulin test and the precipitation test. Dr. Hiss (11) of New York, made the very valuable discovery that pneumococci ferment inulin and streptococci do not. He uses the inulin in his well-known serum-water mixture. The reaction is shown by acidification or coagulation of the medium. We found that all the pneumococci fermented inulin (12, 13)[e] and a very few streptococci.

As a control, we have used the precipitation test (15). Some years ago I noted that streptococci regularly precipitated (whitened) serum-glucose-agar within 48 hours and pneu-

---

[a] Wassermann in his article states that the medium should be very alkaline, using litmus as an indicator. I found the most advantageous titre was neutrality to phenolphthalein.

[b] There are some cases reported in which this organism is supposed to have caused a systemic infection (53). We have not encountered such a case.

[c] All the organisms recognized as streptococci precipitated serum-glucose-agar (see below):

[d] This organism will doubtless be soon identified in the blood-current, now that local infections produced by it are more often recognized.

[e] But not in all generations. Sometimes it was necessary to use Dr. Buerger's modification (14) (addition of peptone). All the organisms identified as pneumococci by the type capsule fermented inulin.

mococci very rarely did. Dr. Buerger (12) found that this held true in a large series of tests.*

We have, therefore, followed this scheme. If when the type capsule is absent the organism ferments inulin and does not precipitate, it is a pneumococcus, and vice versa it is a streptococcus. If it does both, animal inoculations should be made to try to restore the type capsule.*

The differentiation of the organisms by the characters of their growth in plates of blood-agar (16), though useful, cannot be entirely relied upon. I show you a plate made by Dr. Epstein from the blood of a case of pneumonia (17). Whereas the pneumococcus colonies are supposed not to be surrounded by clear areas (hemolysis) this pneumococcus not only produces a large clear ring, but at some distance away there is a second ring of hemolysis.¹⁰ Otherwise the organism has the typical pneumococcus characteristics. The pneumococcus in the sputum caused no hemolysis.

We have had a specimen of a pneumococcus from the blood of a case of infection of the foot, which, when first isolated, had no capsule, grew in chains, fermented inulin and precipitated. After animal inoculation the organism was coccoid, often bacillary, and groups were found surrounded by single capsules. Later animal inoculations resulted in the production of the type pneumococcus capsule.

I cannot enter more fully into this question now, but have said enough to indicate the great care that is necessary in identifying these organisms.

The literature shows that not sufficient care has been taken in distinguishing staphylococci. Professor Welch (19), already in 1891, pointed out that the pigment of *Micrococcus aureus* often requires several days for its development and that potato is a favorable medium for its production. Glucose media, we have found, often temporarily cause a loss of the color. We are in the custom of inoculating all white staphylococci on agar, potato and serum-agar, leaving them in the thermostat for 24 hours, and then allowing them to stand outside in diffuse daylight for seven days. We have made no studies on the differentiation of staphylococci by means of hemolysis production or agglutination tests. (20) ¹¹

The Gram-negative cocci found in future will need careful study, and their exact status may, in some instances, remain in doubt (particularly if there is no meningitis or gonorrhea present), for we now know that there is a group of organisms

---

* In my original experiments I used ½ per cent glucose medium. Dr. Buerger, through a suggestion of mine used 2 per cent. We have been using the ½ per cent medium for the last few months and find that it is more advantageous.

Only when a streptococcus grows so sparsely that there is little evident growth, is precipitation absent, so that a good growth without precipitation seems to exclude a streptococcus.

* *Streptococcus mucosus capsulatus* ferments inulin and does not precipitate.

¹⁰ We have seen concentric (intermittent) hemolysis once before (18). The organism was a streptococcus.

¹¹ A possible influence of icteric serum will be discussed later.

---

closely allied to the gonococcus and meningococcus. (21) ¹² It will not be enough to identify an organism as a gonococcus because it is Gram-negative and cannot be grown on media. It must be cultivated and studied. We have met with a Gram-negative contaminating diplococcus which was found to have been derived from the ascitic serum used. In another case we found in a post-mortem culture in a case of osteomyelitis (due to *Micrococcus aureus*) a Gram-negative organism which was neither the gonococcus nor the meningococcus.

The blood-cultures were usually observed for 5 to 7 days, hanging-drops from the flasks being made daily, as well as inoculations on serum media and into glucose-bouillon. The time in which the cultures became positive varied. The earliest two periods were six and eight hours. Often results were obtained in 12 to 16 hours; at times 48 hours or more elapsed. If the organism was a staphylococcus that was slow in its pigment production, 5 days might elapse before a definite report could be given, but this was very exceptional.

The number of organisms varied from one in 15 cc. up to 2676 to the cubic centimeter, or up to such a number that the colonies could not be counted. At times the growth was so marked that the separate colonies were indistinguishable and the medium looked simply discolored. The variation in the number of colonies in a given case will be discussed later.

In every instance in which the culture was positive we attempted to confirm the result by cultures made from the primary focus or secondary foci, or by means of later cultures of the blood, before or after death.

In only eight cases were we unable to obtain confirmatory cultures. Either there were no evident lesions, or cultures were not sent in from them when present. In some instances the patient died and a further culture could not be obtained. But in each of the eight instances the clinical picture was in accord. In seven, the diagnosis was acute endocarditis; the eighth was a terminal infection. All of the cases showed pneumococci or streptococci. All staphylococcus findings were confirmed.

Comparatively few cultures were taken just prior to death, because we were interested in the problems mainly from a diagnostic standpoint. Had more been taken we might have met with more positive findings; a greater variety of organisms might have been found.

We laid no stress on cultures made after death, except as a means of confirming those made during life. A little experience was sufficient to show how cautious we must be in interpreting post-mortem findings.¹³ (Of course, the presence of such organisms as the anthrax or glanders bacillus is

---

¹² We encountered one such organism (in the pus in a case of otitis media) which produced a disagreeable odor in all media. And Dr. Boggs (22) has described one as occurring in bronchiectasis, which grew in blood only, and produced an odor.

¹³ I shall not discuss the question of whether some positive postmortem findings may not be due to agonal invasion and postmortem multiplication.

diagnostic.) Whether cultures made from the arm veins would give more reliable results than the heart-blood, as Canon (23) and Gradwohl (24) claim, our experience is too small to permit us to state.

3. ORGANISMS FOUND: FREQUENCY: SHORT LIST OF CONDITIONS IN WHICH THEY WERE ISOLATED: MIXED AND SECONDARY INFECTIONS.

Before giving the facts of interest in this connection I want to state that I shall give no percentages as to the frequency of positive findings in various forms of diseases. Such figures are misleading, the results depending on the type of cases studied and the stage of the disease at which they were studied. This will be made more evident by the general remarks on negative blood-cultures.

The organisms found were: streptococci, the pneumococcus, *Micrococcus aureus, Micrococcus citreus, Micrococcus albus, Bacillus pyocyaneus,* paracolon bacillus, *Bacillus coli, Bacillus proteus vulgaris* and the gonococcus.

Streptococci were isolated in 58 cases. Some were instances of terminal infections, or infections arising from the tonsils, the ears and mastoid processes, or the genito-urinary tract. In some cases there were infected wounds; in others the source of infection could not be found. Some were characterized by joint or bone lesions. Endocarditis was frequent. One was a case of erythema nodosum. In one case the source of infection was an abscess at the root of the lung secondary to esophageal carcinoma; in another it was a suppurating tabetic joint of the great toe. In one case there resulted a hemorrhagic myositis of both forearms. Metastatic bone lesions were not uncommon; once there resulted an extensive osteomyelitis of the vertebral column.

Micrococcus aureus was found 28 times (25). Many of the cases were instances of osteomyelitis; some were secondary to furuncles or cellulitis; some were cryptogenetic bacteriemias. Two were post-partum infections; bacteriemia due to staphylococci is rare under such conditions.

In a number of cases endocarditis was present. In one case a cystitis was the primary focus, and in two cases abscesses of the prostate occurred secondarily. Of particular interest were two cases with metastases in the muscles and one with a small abscess of the sclera.

The only staphylococcus albus findings confirmed by subsequent cultures were made (with one exception to be discussed later) within two days ante-mortem and were confirmed by heart-cultures. These were looked upon as agonal invasions. We have not met with a single case in which the finding of the albus in the blood was followed by the establishment of a metastatic depot. On the whole we look upon the organism as playing little rôle in systemic infections. This is in keeping with the infrequency of our finding it in local lesions of any importance, a point long ago emphasized by Professor Welch (19).

There are two observations in this connection which I wish to mention. One refers to a case of acute endocarditis of the

aortic valve with an inflammatory swelling in the septum. The staphylococcus albus was cultivated in the blood 12 and 10 days ante-mortem, and also at the autopsy. The spreads made from the swelling in the septum showed many staphylococci. Although there is no doubt of the validity of the cultures, the organisms at the time were not observed as we now observe them, and, therefore, we cannot exclude the possibility that we were dealing with a staphylococcus aureus.

The other observation was made in the case of an infant two weeks old, suffering from hemorrhages of the new-born with jaundice and fever, supposedly due to an infection. The blood which we were fortunate enough to obtain from a vein in front of the ankle showed *Micrococcus albus.* A culture made 40 hours post-mortem showed a pure aureus in the first colonies. As I had never observed a *Micrococcus albus* invasion followed by one by the aureus, I suspected that the icterus may have temporarily inhibited the pigment production.

A short time later a specimen of bile from a case of cholecystitis was sent to us. The first culture showed an albus that could not be changed to an aureus. A culture made the next day showed an albus that became aureus after 3 days; the third culture gave an aureus in two days, and all subsequent cultures showed the aureus at once.

We made a few experiments trying to prove that bile might temporarily inhibit the pigment production, but were unsuccessful. We hope to repeat the experiments with icteric serum (or bile from inflamed gall-bladders), because it is known that they act differently from normal bile itself. This is shown by the work on the agglutination of typhoid bacilli by icteric serum. Whereas icteric serum has more or less agglutinating power, bile itself has practically none (26).

For the present, *Micrococcus albus* found in a case with icterus should be particularly studied, and carefully considered.

Pneumococci, apart from pneumonia cases, were found 4 times. Twice there was an acute endocarditis,[14] source unknown. Once there was an infection between two toes, and once there was a suppurative ethmoiditis and frontal sinusitis with brain abscess.

Micrococcus citreus was isolated once in a case of osteomyelitis; the bone showed the same organism. The patient recovered.

Bacillus pyocyaneus was found once (in a case published by Dr. Brill and myself) (27) secondary to *Micrococcus aureus* bacteriemia. The case was fatal.

A paracolon bacillus was isolated once in a case clinically resembling cholecystitis (published in extenso by Dr. A. A. Berg and myself) (28).

The gonococcus was believed to have been found once, antemortem, with a streptococcus, in a case of post-abortive infection. The Gram negative coccus could, however, not be further cultivated, and to-day I would not be willing to say that

---

[14] In one of these two cases, in the service of Dr. Alfred Meyer, there was an embolism of the abdominal aorta.

it was definitely a gonococcus (see above under Technical Considerations)."

Bacillus proteus was found by Dr. J. Gerster one day antemortem with streptococci in a case of uremia." *Bacillus coli* was found in the blood of a patient upon whom the operation of internal urethrotomy had been performed. The case was fatal.

In a case of infection of the gall-bladder by the gas bacillus (Welch) an attempt was made to cultivate the organism from the blood. Cultures were made and also direct animal inoculations, but the result was negative. The organism has been found several times in the blood by other observers.

Mixed and secondary infections were uncommon. All such cases were fatal. Those encountered were:

(a) A streptococcus with a possible gonococcus.

(b) A streptococcus and the proteus bacterium.

(c) In the paracolon case, a culture made one day antemortem showed also streptococci and *micrococcus albus*. This was confirmed at the autopsy.

(d) In a child dying of an umbilical infection, a streptococcus was found with *Micrococcus aureus.*

(e) A pyocyaneus infection secondary to one by the aureus.

(f) In a case recently under the observation of Dr. Rudisch and Dr. Sachs, with the clinical picture of a hemichorea, *Micrococcus aureus* was found; the second culture showed mainly the same but also a streptococcus; in the third culture the streptococcus predominated. The post-mortem cultures showed no aureus in the blood. This was a striking example of a secondary infection crowding out the primary."

When a primary focus shows two or more organisms, the blood sometimes shows only one. Recently, in a case of phlegmon of the arm, due to a streptococcus and the *Micrococcus aureus*, only the former was found in the blood.

4. NOTES ON THE FINDINGS IN SOME SURGICAL CONDITIONS.

In most of the cases of acute osteomyelitis," particularly those due to the *Micrococcus aureus*, organisms were found in the blood. There is a peculiar difference between the cases due to staphylococci and those due to streptococci. In the staphylococcus cases the bone disease is apt to stand out in the clinical picture, whereas in the streptococcus cases we look upon it more often as the result of a bacteriemia. Of course, we know that all the osteomyelitic lesions are secondary, due to a recent invasion by bacteria or old deposit. But the staphylococcus bone lesion once established seems to cause a more marked bacteriemia than the streptococcus cases.

Most of the acute staphylococcus cases occurred in children. As Jordan (29) well says, "Osteomyelitis is the septicemia of adolescence." That is to say, in children bacterial invasion

of the blood is apt to set up bone lesions because the growing bones are points of diminished resistance. In adults metastatic bone infections are less common.

In some of the staphylococcus bone infections in children, when the bacteriemia was marked, interesting cutaneous lesions were found. These consisted of pustules in the scalp and slightly purulent miliaria or pustules scattered over the entire body or part of the body. The lesion usually first appeared on the scalp or over the shins. The lesions, including the miliaria, all gave cultures of the *Micrococcus aureus* (ordinary miliaria alba show the *Micrococcus epidermidis albus.*) All the cases in which these lesions were found were fatal. Skin lesions have been often described in cases of bacterial infections, but I do not know that attention has been called particularly to the scalp lesions. I believe the lesions which I have described are due to infections of sweat glands. The question of whether this is due to an attempt at elimination is left open."

The few cases of osteomyelitis of the jaw which were studied showed no bacteriemia even when accompanied by cavernous sinus thrombosis.

A remarkable case was that of a man who died of a fulminating osteomyelitis of the femur after he had suffered for eight years from recurrent staphylococcic bone and joint infections (31). The original infection followed an operation for the relief of hemorrhoids. On the day before death no bacteria were found in the blood. It would look as if the blood had developed marked bacterial power, and as if the infection of the femur were due to cocci deposited long before. This was the only case of severe staphylococcus osteomyelitis, in which bacteria were not found in the blood.

In many cases of secondary parotitis no bacteria were present in the blood. In only one case of streptococcemia did we find a streptococcus infection of the parotid. In other cases of local or general streptococcus infection, or intra-abdominal infections, a secondary parotitis was due to the *Micrococcus aureus*. These observations strengthen the view that most cases of secondary parotitis are not metastatic infections, but are mouth infections (32).

In intra-abdominal infections the results were quite unexpected. I shall cite a few. In cholecystitis the results were negative. Even in some cases with secondary pulmonary metastatic infections there was no bacteriemia."

In a series of 25 cases of appendicitis, the results were negative, even anaerobically. Here also in some very severe cases the ante-mortem cultures were negative (in a few, the post-mortem also). Occasionally systemic infection must occur, as shown by a case with a negative blood-culture which died a few weeks later and showed an acute endocarditis and

---

" Post-mortem the gonococcus was found twice. (See under "Endocarditis.")

" I am indebted to Dr. Goldenberg for this case.

" This case was studied by Dr. Epstein and Dr. A. Cohn.

" These cases occurred in the services of Dr. A. Gerster and Dr. Lilienthal.

" Werther (30) describes a case of streptococcus osteomyelitis with papules in the skin having a central vesicle; in one excised lesion he found a necrotic inflammation of a sweat gland.

" In making blood cultures in cases of cholecystitis, the methods should be adapted to the finding of the typhoid bacillus, as the latter occurs fairly often in cholecystitis.

purulent infarcts in the kidney. A later culture would probably have been positive.

In one of the series of cases there was a chronic endocarditis with erythema nodosum. In another, the pus showed *B. proteus fluorescens*, the cause of certain cases of acute toxic febrile icterus (33)—(so-called Weil's disease).[n]

In about 25 cases of peritonitis (mainly of intestinal origin), the blood was sterile; in some just before death. In the series are a few of the cases of streptococcus and pneumococcus peritonitis occurring in the course of chronic parenchymatous nephritis. These cases have a peculiar clinical picture which I hope to describe at a later time. Bertelsmann (34) has also had negative results in peritonitis.

In 7 cases of pylephlebitis[n] and 3 supposed cases (no autopsy in 2, recovery[n] in one) most of which were suppurative, the results were negative. There are positive cases in the literature. I have not yet gone over all of them to see in how many cases cultures were made early in the disease (35) (36).

In infections arising from the female pelvic organs[n] (especially after abortion or delivery at term) the findings were of particular interest. The organisms found were streptococci and the *Micrococcus aureus*. (The latter occurred twice; such cases are rare). There was quite a large number of positive results. ·But in some of the cases with extensive thrombosis in the veins, with or without parametritis, the blood-cultures remained sterile. In one of these cases the cava was completely thrombosed; in another there was parietal purulent thrombosis of the cava with metastatic abscesses of the lungs and pyopneumothorax. In a third case, there was an abscess of the clitoris, with abscess in the broad ligament due to thrombo-phlebitis and pulmonary abscesses. In a fourth there was a parametritic abscess with thrombosis of the cava and metastatic abscesses of the lung, all the lesions showing streptococci, a pseudo-tubercle bacillus and some other organisms.

In infections of otitic origin[n] there were similar results. There were severe cases without bacteriemia. There were cases with bacteriemia and recovery. At times the disappearance of the bacteriemia was due to operation on the sinus or jugular vein. And there were cases of sinus thrombosis with secondary pulmonary lesions without bacteriemia. In all the cases a streptococcus was found.

In bladder and kidney infections there were few instances of systemic infection (the material studied was small). In one fatal case of suppurative thrombosis of the iliac vein

---

[n] We had no opportunity of investigating any case in which the appendicitis appeared to be the result of a systemic infection.

[n] Included among surgical conditions because most often occurring in connection with surgical diseases.

[n] For the privilege of investigating this private case I am indebted to Dr. Manges.

[n] These cases were in the services of Dr. Brettauer and Dr. Krug.

[n] In Dr. Gruening's service.

after urethrotomy, the first culture was positive and the later one negative. The organisms found were the streptococcus, *Micrococcus aureus* and *B. coli*. In these organs, metastatic lesions were common.

NOTE.—The frequency of negative results in the types of intra-abdominal disease discussed are particularly interesting when one remembers that the causative organisms are, except for the anaërobes, capable of easy cultivation. I would like to repeat that if more cultures had been made within a few days before death, there might have been more positive results. Clinically, the results are in harmony.

5. NOTES ON FINDINGS IN CERTAIN MEDICAL CONDITIONS.

I should now like to direct your attention to the results obtained in some selected types of disease usually regarded as belonging to the domain of internal medicine. In some of the conditions which I shall mention there is no evidence that they need be associated with a bacteriemia. Positive results have been obtained in some of the diseases grouped here by other writers.

In several cases of pseudo-leukemia the results were negative, even when the temperature was of the intermittent type described by Ebstein.

In tuberculosis we met with no secondary systemic infections.

In two cases of multiple obliterating endophlebitis (one fatal),[n] two cases of acute ascending paralysis (Landry's) and in one of febrile neuro-myositis, there were also negative results.

In the group of cases described by Dr. Brill (37), which resemble typhoid fever somewhat, and which have been considered to have been possibly cases of paratyphoid fever, we could not succeed in isolating any organisms from the blood. There is no proof yet that they are cases of paratyphoid, and should, therefore, be classed for the present as a separate group.

Of a large number of cases of acute leukemia, cultures were made in six. All gave negative results except two in which there was an agonal invasion by *Micrococcus albus*. A positive finding in a case of acute leukemia would have to be carefully analyzed. Besides the possibility of a terminal infection there might be a bacteriemia arising from one of the infections often found in these cases (particularly about the mouth). Apart from this I can imagine that a case might arise in which it would appear probable that the disease was due to a bacterial infection. For, a study of a large number of cases certainly gives one the impression that the disease is due to changes in the blood-forming organs (particularly the marrow) which could be due to a variety of causes, just as has long ago been found to be the case with pseudo-leukemia infantum. In children, in infections, one occasionally meets with blood-pictures that resemble those found in some cases of acute leukemia.

In cases of " visceral lesions of the erythema group " (Osler) (38) and in various forms of purpura, the results were nega-

---

[n] In these cases anaërobic cultures were also used.

tive. In a series of remarkable cases of erythematous lesions with fever, lasting a number of weeks, with secondary renal or pulmonary lesions, there were negative results, except in one. This was a case in Dr. Brill's service of erythema multiforme (particularly erythema nodosum) with joint inflammations and high fever running several weeks, and ending in recovery with stiff joints. In one culture out of five a few colonies of an attenuated streptococcus were found, possessed of feeble pathogenic power (transient joint symptoms in rabbits). This shows the necessity of repeated cultures in such types of disease.

Of five fatal cases of acute degeneration of the liver (acute yellow atrophy) cultures were made in two, with negative results.[37]

In rheumatism, arthritis deformans and gonorrheal rheumatism, no bacteria were found in the blood. (In two cases of rheumatism the fluid aspirated from the joints showed no bacteria. These cells were mainly polynuclear).

NOTE.—In this section we have discussed a number of medical diseases, most of which are probably due to different causes in different cases. Dr. Epstein, will, I hope, later report in cases of typhoid fever, pneumonia and meningitis.

6. ENDOCARDITIS: EMBOLIC ANEURISMS.

The most interesting condition connected with the subject of bacteriemias is endocarditis (39). The study of these cases by means of blood-cultures makes very definite Leube's (40) view that the acute endocarditis in these cases is a secondary infection. As is well known, such a bacteriemia may affect normal valves, but more often diseased valves (41). A primary focus may or may not be evident. Some of the cases are examples of terminal infections.

There is often a marked disproportion between the number of bacteria in the blood and the extent of the lesion. There may be an almost countless number of bacteria in the blood and only very small deposits on the valves, or there may be large vegetations with hardly any bacteria in the blood. As a rule, they are present in fair numbers.

Again, in a case of chronic endocarditis there may be a marked bacteriemia and at the autopsy we may find only a little deposit of fibrin on the wall of the heart or no lesion whatsoever. I show you some hearts to illustrate this. One is of particular interest. The patient, who was admitted into Dr. Brettauer's service because of a post-partum infection, had a marked bacteriemia, heart-murmurs and all the symptoms of so-called " ulcerative endocarditis " (petechiæ, high temperatures, chills, etc.). And still, as you see, the heart shows only an old mitral stenosis and no recent lesion. The case was one of bacteriemia in a patient with chronic endocarditis. There is no reason why such a case (with a less marked bacteriemia) should not get well. It might then wrongly go on record as an " ulcerative endocarditis " with recovery.

[37] I believe that it would be better to include in this group only cases for which no cause is found.

I believe it is best to call all the cases, acute, subacute or chronic endocarditis, according to the clinical course, then attach the name of the infecting organism when it is found (thus, " acute streptococcus endocarditis "), and attach an adjective—vegetative, polypoid, ulcerative, etc., descriptive of the type of lesion, when it is seen. The hearts which I demonstrate to you to-night show how difficult it often is to diagnose beforehand the type of lesion.

The organisms found by us in these cases have been streptococci, pneumococci, Micrococcus aureus and gonococcus.

Of the last there were two cases. In the first, the cultures were made when we started the work and favorable media were not used. The result was negative, the gonococci being found post-mortem. The second case was diagnosed post-mortem: no cultures were requested during life. In a third case of endocarditis following gonorrhea, streptococci were found in the blood during life and at the autopsy. When the patient entered the hospital there were no longer gonococci in the urine, but there were streptococci.[38]

In some of the cases of endocarditis the number of bacteria varied from time to time. In some, they increased up to the time of death; in one, they decreased. There seem to be two types of cases: one in which a bacteriemia which in itself would not necessarily be fatal, sets up an endocarditis which keeps up the bacteriemia and dominates the clinical picture. In the second type the original bacteriemia plays the main role.

In some cases of acute endocarditis with marked lesions we have looked for and found acute enlargement of the nodes at the bifurcation of the trachea. In cases in which there were no acute pulmonary lesions present we have attributed the enlargement to the endocardial lesions, as the lymphatics which drain the heart enter these nodes (intertracheo-bronchial group of Poirier) (42). I might mention here that in cases of marked bacteriemia one finds at times the lymphnodes all over the body somewhat enlarged, pink or red in color.

In two cases of acute staphylococcus endocarditis with marked cerebral symptoms, the cerebro-spinal fluid presented interesting changes. In both, leucocytes and cocci were present, the latter being mainly intra-cellular. In one of the cases the cocci were numerous but it was very difficult to cultivate them. The cultures from the blood gave profuse growths (2,200 colonies to the c.c.).[39] There was but slight increase in the leucocytes.

There are many cases of chronic endocarditis with fever without any demonstrable bacteriemia. In some cases causes for the fever may be found elsewhere in the body. If no cause can be found, the acute symptoms may be due, at least

[38] Since writing the above we have encountered two cases of general gonococcus infection, one with negative result and one with two positive cultures. At the autopsy in the former, the gonococci were found in an abscess of the mitral valve. The surrounding thrombus mass showed no gonococci.

[39] A study of the relative opsonic contents of the blood and cerebro-spinal fluids in such cases might give results of interest.

at times, to organisms not to be cultivated by our present methods. I have suspected that in some cases with irregular fever, at times quite high, recurring from time to time, the temperature may be due to discharge into the blood-current of bits of thrombotic masses or old vegetations (43).

There is another group of febrile cases lasting a number of weeks or months, in which bacteria are repeatedly demonstrable in the blood (44). In such cases we have never found staphylococci but always attenuated streptococci or diplococci. In some cases the organisms are fairly abundant; in some very sparse. In one case, a week before death, they were very numerous and grew on serum-glucose-agar plates only. Later they grew on other media but were kept alive with great difficulty. In one case we found only two colonies in 25 cc. of blood. In five instances they were short, small streptococci and in three a lancet-shaped diplococcus which did not appear to be a pneumococcus.* The last case in which the diplococcus was found occurred during the past year, and we made a careful study which showed that the organism had no capsule, did not ferment inulin and did precipitate serum-glucose-agar. It was, therefore, definitely not a pneumococcus.

Several of the organisms correspond to those described by Lenhartz (39) and Schottmueller (45), but the others seemed to be even more attenuated (they grew at first only on serum-glucose-agar or the Wassermann medium). I wish I could give an accurate differential description of these organisms from ordinary streptococci by means of their fermentative reactions (in carbo-hydrates) but careful studies made by Dr. Buerger (to be published soon) show that it is not wise at present to depend upon differentiation by such means. The organisms were hardly pathogenic—at most they would produce peritonitis in mice, and then at times by repeated transfers only. Direct inoculations of blood into mice, rabbits, and guinea-pigs were tried in two cases with negative results.

In all these cases there was a history of joint manifestations at the apparent onset of the symptoms or months or years previously. In all which we could examine post-mortem, there was present an old, chronic endocarditis on which recent lesions were grafted. I show you hearts from four such cases. You will notice that the vegetations are very friable (in one less so), and in each instance there is a mural endocarditis of the left auricle (in one also of the anterior flap of the mitral and the wall of the left ventricle over the septum membranaceum).

Some of these patients are able to walk about the wards although there are cocci in the blood. But although the symptoms are generally mild, and though the temperature may be quite low for a long time, it may rise sharply from time to time, and toward the end of the disease there may be chills and high temperatures.

All of the cases of this type which we could follow were

fatal. One of them left our hospital feeling quite well after an illness lasting some months, and died four months later at another hospital. Streptococci had been found three times in her blood.

One patient who was in Dr. Manges' service developed an aneurism in the right popliteal artery with subsequent thrombosis in the sac. He left the hospital after a prolonged stay; the subsequent history is unknown. Lenhartz describes two recoveries but does not state how long the cases were observed. What the portal of entry in these cases was, I do not know. It may have been the tonsils. The possibility of acute exacerbations due to bacteria which have remained dormant and become attenuated in old endocardial lesions, must be thought of (analogous to what is known to occur in osteo-myelitis).

At this time I do not wish to discuss in detail the question of the etiology of rheumatism (46), but will say that I believe it would be wiser for the present to call all these cases subacute or chronic streptococcus or diplococcus endocarditis, and not to call them rheumatic endocarditis because of the rheumatic history. According to the terminology that I would suggest, cases of endocarditis occurring in what we call rheumatism should be called acute, subacute, or chronic endocarditis, and the fact that no organism was indicated in the name would at once show that the cause of the endocarditis in the particular case had not been found.

I have indicated the importance and frequency of acute and subacute endocarditis associated with bacteriemia, and, without attempting to discuss the diagnosis of such conditions, I would like to refer to a point which has been of great value. It is well known that petechiæ occur in these cases. The particular value of the occurrence of conjunctival petechiæ and " the small hemorrhages in the palms and soles with slightly nodular character " I learned from Dr. Janeway when I had the privilege of serving under him.* Very occasionally conjunctival petechiæ are found in cases of chronic endocarditis in which no bacteria are demonstrable in the blood, and occasionally they occur when there is a bacteriemia without any acute endocarditis. Further, in some of the cases of acute endocarditis with bacteriemia the petechiæ may appear late or not at all. Nevertheless, a sharp lookout for them will often direct attention to an acute endocarditis to which there was no other clue.*

One of the most striking features of some cases of endocarditis is the establishment of aneurisms. We have seen five cases (48). In two no cultures could be obtained during life; in one, streptococci were found post-mortem, and in the other streptococci and *Micrococcus aureus*. Twice the lesion occurred in the cases in which streptococci had been repeatedly found in the blood. In one, streptococci were found in the walls of the aneurisms (of the hepatic, mesenteric, and a branch of the femoral arteries) post-mortem. The other case

---

* I am indebted to Dr. A. Mayer and Dr. H. Herman, of New York, for the privilege of investigating two of these cases.

* The observation was later published by Dr. Janeway (47).
* I have, of course, made no attempt to discuss causes of conjunctival petechiæ other than endocarditis and bacteriemia.

was the patient with the aneurisms of the popliteal artery mentioned above.

In a fifth case, recently observed in Dr. Rudisch's service, there developed embolic aneurisms of the left iliac artery and a branch of the renal artery. Repeated blood-cultures were negative. At the autopsy there were none of the usual lesions of acute endocarditis, but there was a large mass of calcareous vegetations, and a piece of lime was found in the aneurism of the iliac artery. (There was also an aneurism of the mitral valve). This case shows that it is probable that embolic aneurisms are not always bacterial in nature.

In some cases of acute bacterial endocarditis one finds occasionally a small, tender swelling on a superficial vessel, which persists or disappears. I have not been able to determine yet whether these may be very small aneurisms or inflammatory deposits.

7. REMARKS ON NEGATIVE BLOOD-CULTURES.

It is necessary to discuss, even if briefly, the significance of negative and positive results, particularly with reference to the cases of infection by the ordinary pyogenic cocci. The first and most important question is, do bacteria enter the blood-current in every case of local infection? This question is a difficult one to answer because we cannot examine the blood every day for bacteria. We can obtain a general idea, however, from the results in a large series of cases. And from these we cannot deny the possibility that in every case of local infection bacteria may enter the blood-current at one time or another. Even very small foci may be the starting-point of a bacteriemia. How often all the bacteria which enter the blood are gotten rid of by the bacterial powers [m] of the body and can, therefore, not be cultivated, even on optimum media, one can only surmise. Practically these are cases without bacteriemia.

From a study of all the cases in our series, I am inclined to the following beliefs as to negative findings: [n]

1. The case may not be one of infection by one of the ordinary bacteria. It may be a case of tuberculosis, actinomycosis or syphilis; it may be due to an infection by protozoa; it may be due to parasites of any kind which have not been isolated.

2. The case is due to one of the ordinary organisms, but there are no bacteria in the blood-current. This may occur in any type of infection. I have indicated how it can occur, at least at times, in certain cases of intra-abdominal infections, and in cases with even extensive thromboses of the cerebral sinuses, or of the intra-abdominal veins with or without

secondary foci in the liver or lungs. For such cases as the last I am in the habit of using the term incomplete or partial bacteriemia. (In all these cases the bacteria are, of course, usually carried into the liver or lungs by pieces of thrombi). [m] When the diagnosis is not made this is a cryptic bacteriemia. The cases involving the portal system can be called portal bacteriemias.

3. Bacteria may have been present in the blood and have disappeared from it with or without the disappearance of the primary focus and with or without the establishment of secondary foci. They may, of course, remain after metastatic foci are established. We have never seen them disappear completely when the endocardium was involved.

4. In the cases in which we can take for granted that a secondary (and possibly a fatal focus) is established by the passage through the blood of a bit of infected clot, it is easy to see how there need be no bacteria demonstrable in the blood (example: A brain abscess due to embolism from a thrombosed branch of the pulmonary vein in empyema). At times without evident thrombosis a secondary focus is set up by a very short invasion of the blood-stream (para-nephritic abscess due to a small focus in the kidney after a furuncle of the face).

The last two types of formation of metastases are sometimes called infection by transport (50).

8. REMARKS ON POSITIVE BLOOD-CULTURES.

Concerning positive results I wish to make the following remarks: I group the cases of infection into two groups: A. With a primary focus of some extent. B. With a minute (e. g. a small furuncle) or no demonstrable primary focus.

I shall refer to endocarditis separately from other metastatic foci, for reasons which will be very evident from my remarks.

A. 1. If the bacteria are present in the blood and the primary infection is successfully treated, the bacteria in the blood may slowly or rapidly disappear. At times one finds what one may consider the end of the bacteriemia (e. g. one colony of pneumococci in 12 c. c. of blood in a case of infection of the foot, when the patient was apparently recovering). Occasionally the bacteria disappear from the blood even though the primary focus is not eradicated.

2. Whether the primary focus has been successfully treated or not, the bacteria may remain in the blood and the metastatic foci may or may not develop, the endocardium may or may not be involved. If the primary focus has healed and no endocarditis has resulted and no metastatic infections, we can presume that the bacteria have multiplied. Whether they mul-

---

[m] As you are aware, it is not definitely settled how large a role the bactericidal power of the blood plays; some believe other agencies play a much greater role in ridding the body of bacteria. When I use the term "bactericidal power," I use it to indicate briefly all the defensive powers of the body.

[n] The remarks on negative and positive blood-cultures are made on the basis of clinical observation, the blood-cultures and the post-mortem examinations.

---

[m] I believe, although I have had no proof of such a condition, that it is possible that blood-cultures might at times be negative when metastatic foci were set up in the lungs by way of the thoracic duct. Dr. MacCallum (49) has drawn attention to processes in the lung set up by emboli of cells by way of the thoracic duct in typhoid fever. In a personal interview he has told me that he believes that in agreement with what I had suspected bacteria are carried along with the cells and are responsible for many of the local phenomena.

tiply in the large vessels or only in the capillaries, or, as some maintain, in the endothelium of certain organs, it is not necessary to discuss now.

3. When secondary foci develop (excepting endocarditis) the bacteria may not persist in the blood-current (as mentioned under "negative results.")

4. There is a possibility that bacteriemia may result from surgical intervention or an infected focus, when much manipulation has to be done or from extensive handling during dressings. We have seen a possible instance of the former and Mœller describes an example of the latter. Both cases recovered. How often such a bacteriemia might be harmful future studies may show. Such studies would have to include cultures before and after operations, and would have to be very carefully interpreted.[38]

B. When the original focus is very small or none can be found and there is a bacteriemia, conditions are the same as discussed under heading A-2.

If an acute endocarditis develops the number of bacteria found may be small or large. If there is no endocarditis and no other secondary foci, the number is large.

In general it seems that the bacteriemia is often due mainly to the invasion of bacteria from a local focus, and many organisms may be found in the blood under such conditions. In one case of osteomyelitis of the humerus there were found 500 colonies of *Micrococcus aureus* to the cubic centimeter of blood. A blood-culture made four days after operation was sterile, the patient recovering.

Multiplication of the bacteria is probably not as common as it was supposed to be, and it is only when there are large numbers present without the presence of a focus from which they could be discharged, that we can presume that they have multiplied.

It is very tempting to enter into a discussion of the problems concerning the elimination of the bacteria from the body (by the bile, sweat, milk, and urine). Much has been written concerning the question whether the presence of the bacteria in the urine is due to an active eliminative process or whether it is simply an accident due to the fact that the lesions set up by the bacteria and their poisons make the renal filter less perfect. It would exceed the limits of this paper to discuss this problem alone (51). But I would like to draw attention to a few of our findings in the urine of the cases with bacteriemia. The difficulties in this work, and points to be regarded for a careful interpretation of the findings I shall not now detail.

When the bacteria were present in fairly large numbers in the blood they were usually found in the urine, and in cases in which they disappeared from the blood, the bacteria in the urine disappeared first. In a couple of cases, however, they persisted in the urine after none were

demonstrable in the blood. In one such case we found metastatic abscesses in the kidneys. Whether the bladder lesions found in seven cases of invasion of the blood by streptococci or staphylococci cause a persistent bacteriemia, I do not know. (In all cases in which marked secondary bladder lesions were present at autopsy, the bacteriemia had persisted.)

10. DIAGNOSTIC CONSIDERATIONS.

Much might be said in a tentative way concerning the diagnostic uses of blood-cultures, but I shall refer to a few points only, basing my remarks on some of the observations embodied in the paper.

1. In some cases a blood-culture is the only means of recognizing that the patient is suffering from a bacterial infection. This is so well known that it need not be further referred to. It is important to remember, however, that the bacteriemia which is found may be secondary to a previous local or general infection by another organism (e. g. secondary bacteriemia), or it may represent an intercurrent or terminal bacteriemia in some non-bacterial disease. As an example of the former I might mention a case with streptococci in the blood in whom a subphrenic abscess was diagnosed. The autopsy showed that the original disease was typhoid fever, with splenic infarction.

2. The fact that bacteria are not demonstrable in the blood-current in some cases of pylephlebitis may be made use of in a diagnostic way. In some cases of this condition when there is no evidence of a primary focus, it is necessary to differentiate it from acute endocarditis. In the cases of acute endocarditis which would be simulated, however, we have always found bacteria in the blood if two cultures were made (very rarely were two cultures necessary). A year ago we made use of this point in a case in which we suspected the existence of a suppurative thrombosis of the splenic and portal veins. Two negative blood-cultures spoke against an acute endocarditis. The autopsy corroborated the diagnosis.

3. Similarly, negative results may be of use in the differential diagnosis between endocarditis and thromboses of the pelvic veins or vena cava due to infection through the genitourinary tract (especially post-partum infections). In some of these cases, even when the inferior cava is partially or entirely closed, there are no local symptoms, not even edema of the legs or distension of the veins.[38]

The main point to be emphasized is that in fevers of obscure origin, especially if the temperature is intermittent and there are chills, and the blood cultures are negative, one must keep in mind the possibility of the existence of venous thromboses acting as a form of cryptic focus.

4. In two cases of sinus thrombosis of otitic origin, the

---

[38] If the Bier treatment of acute local infections by hyperemia should continue to be as favorably looked upon as it is now, it would be a great advantage from the standpoint under discussion. Canon has also drawn attention to this in his book.

[38] Professor Welch (52) states that this may be due to the fact that the deep veins dilate. We had come to the same conclusion as we often observed that in cases of severe bacterial infection there was a collapse of the superficial veins all over the body; at times this was so marked that it was impossible to obtain any blood when it was attempted to make a culture.

finding of some streptococci in the blood induced the surgeon (Dr. Gruening) to operate, although the local signs were apparently insufficient to account for all the symptoms. In both cases extensive thromboses were found; both patients recovered."

In the one case the clinical picture looked like typhoid; in the other like malaria. The local signs were such that it was possible that the patients were suffering from the otitic disease plus the other conditions, but the finding of streptococci in the blood was considered to signify that the local disease could be the cause of all the symptoms.

5. When a local infection has been operated upon and the symptoms persist for a number of days, and there is a bacteriemia, the primary focus should be carefully examined. If it is in good condition careful search should be made for metastases so that they can be attended to promptly. Only if an acute endocarditis develops, or if the bacteria are present in large numbers, should one be satisfied with not finding metastases. In some infections there may be a secondary purulent phlebitis which gives no local symptoms. This is one of the difficulties. At times it is difficult to diagnosticate metastases in the internal organs (especially the lungs, kidneys, and spleen).

6. If the primary focus is healed or healing and there is no bacteriemia and the symptoms persist, metastases must be carefully looked for. (In the case of a colleague who had had a cellulitis of the arm, which had been incised, but in whom the fever persisted, the diagnosis of "sepsis" and "pleurisy" had been made, but the blood-culture being negative a careful search was instituted. A paranephritic abscess was located after a few days. An operation upon this focus was followed by recovery).

The metastases may be very difficult to locate, as mentioned above. In one case, there were found multiple abscesses of the kidney due to *Micrococcus aureus;* the blood-culture had been negative and there were no local symptoms. I believe that careful studies of the urine may in the future help us to locate such lesions. The data which we have thus far collected on this point are insufficient for publication.

7. Under the same conditions as described under heading 6, the symptoms may be due to the onset of some other condition. (Example: A child with empyema; local focus apparently doing well; fever re-appears; blood-culture negative; condition proves to be tubercular meningitis).

The conditions that hold good (under heading 6) when no bacteriemia is evident could also be stated to hold true when very few bacteria are found, except that in a few cases endocarditis may occur with only a few bacteria in the blood.

It becomes clear that although blood-cultures are of great service, they do not lessen the necessity for careful clinical observation, diagnosis and judgment.

"The bacteriemia disappeared shortly after operation. The jugular vein was tied in only one. A third case has recently been observed.

10. PROGNOSIS.

What is the prognosis in the cases in which a bacteriemia can be demonstrated?

To consider this question fully would necessitate entering into a discussion of the problems concerning how the bacteria are disposed of in the body—problems which have not yet been definitely solved, and the exposition of which it is best to leave to others better equipped for the purpose. But we can say this much—that we must allow that even a moderate number of bacteria in the blood does harm by the demands made upon the protective agencies of the body and by means of the toxins liberated by the bacteria (before and after destruction) and that the character and location of the primary focus and the secondary foci play a great role in the prognosis.

Acute endocarditis plays a very important role. In all the cases in which we have made the clinical diagnosis, the case has been fatal. Others have reported recoveries. And it cannot be stated how often the valves of the heart are implicated in such a way that the lesion is not recognized (and how often such a lesion could become the origin of chronic disease).

In our series of cases the results have been as follows: In 58 cases of streptococcemia, there were 6 recoveries, or almost 11 per cent. Of 28 cases of staphylococcemia, 8 recovered, or nearly 29 per cent. Taking both sets together we have 86 cases with 16 per cent recoveries. (Of pneumococcus cases there were 4 with one recovery; the cases are too few in number to be included in the calculations).

The lower percentage of recoveries in the streptococcus cases does not necessarily mean that they are the more serious, for our observations cover medical as well as surgical cases; they therefore, include many cases of terminal infections and of endocarditis.

Bertelsmann, who studied surgical cases only, found 48 instances of bacteriemia in 154 cases; 21 cases recovered or 43 per cent. Of 28 streptococcus cases, 19 recovered, or 68 per cent; and of 13 staphylococcus aureus cases 4, or 30 per cent.

Lenhartz, who studied mainly medical cases (there were included a number of cases of post-partum infections) found 17 per cent recoveries in 77 cases. Of 47 streptococcus cases, 8 recovered or 17 per cent; and of 13 staphylococcus cases, one recovered (7½ per cent).

Canon reports 38 cases of bacteriemia with 5 recoveries (13 per cent).

While I do not think the number in any of the series is large enough, and while I do not believe in comparing the results obtained by different investigators in work of this kind, I think we can draw two conclusions:

1. That the number of recoveries reported depends to a great extent on the type of cases studied.

2. That the bacteriemia met with often does not prevent a favorable outcome.

Concluding Notes.

The statements which I have made, especially regarding the significance of negative and positive results, I present to you as theses. It is not possible for any one investigator to establish in a reasonable period their validity. They embody our experience up to the present time and we shall be glad to publish any observations that may be contradictory.

There are many points on which I might have touched, especially of a more direct therapeutic nature, which might have been of greater interest than those which I have presented to you. But I have said enough to indicate how many and how varied are the problems connected with the subject of bacteriemia, and if I have succeeded in throwing any new light on any of these problems or in suggesting some new lines of thought, I shall feel that I have in some small way earned your kind attention.

It is a pleasure and a duty to express my thanks to numerous former and present members of the house staff of the hospital for much help in making many of the observations, and to them and the visiting staff for many suggestions and much kind co-operation and encouragement.

To Dr. J. C. A. Gerster I am indebted for the beautiful mounting of the specimens and to him and Dr. Epstein for the preparation of the demonstration.

Addendum: April 29, 1906.

Since reading the paper, we have investigated many additional cases, some of which present unusual points of interest. Some of these I hope to publish with Dr. Epstein, who has carried on most of the recent work. I wish to make only two short notes now:

1. A concentric intermittent hemolysis produced by pneumococci on blood plates has been observed twice more. It cannot therefore be a rare phenomenon.

2. The streptococcus mucosus has been reported as being found in the blood current by Otten (D. Arch. f. Klin. Med., Bd. 86, p. 434).

References.

1. Libman: Centralblatt fuer Bakteriologie, Bd. XXII, 1897, p. 376.
2. The literature will be found in Bertelsmann: Deutsche Zeitschrift fuer Chirurgie, Bd. LXVII, 1902.
3. Canon: Die Bakteriologie des Blutes bei Infektionskrankheiten, 1902.
   Lenhartz: Die septischen Erkrankungen, 1903, Nothnagel Handbuch.
   Full accounts are given by these authors of the work of v. Eiselsberg, Kraus, Garré, Rosenbach, Czernowsky, Brunner, Petruschky, Kuehnau, Sittmann, Moeller, and Jochmann.
   Compare.
   Gussenbauer: Septhæmie u. Pyhæmie: Deutsche Chirurgie, 1882.
   Kocher and Tavel: Vorlesungen ueber Chirurgische Infektionskrankheiten, 1895.
   Kretz: Zeitschrift fuer Heilkunde, Bd. XXIII, Heft 1.
   v. Kahlden: Centralbl. Allgm. Pathologic, Bd. XIII, p. 784.
4. Canon: Mitth. aus den Grenzgeb., Bd. X, Heft 3 and 4.
5. Flexner: Journal of Experimental Medicine, Vol. I. 1896, p. 559.
6. Journal of Medical Research, Vol. I, 1901, p. 94.
7. Westphal, Wassermann and Malkoff: Berliner Klin. Wochenschrift, 1899, No. 29.
8. Veillon: Soc. de Biologie, 1893, Juillet.
   Rist: Centralblatt fuer Bakteriologie, 1901, Bd. XXX, p. 287.
9. Tissier: La Flore Intestinale, Paris, 1900.
10. Buerger: Centralblatt fuer Bakteriologie: Originale: Band XXXIX, pp. 20 and 216.
11. Hiss: Jour. Exp. Med., 1905, VI: 317 and VII, p. 556.
12. Buerger: L. c. p. 346.
13. Journal of Exp. Med., 1905, VII, p. 524.
14. Ibidem.
15. Libman: Journ. Med. Research, VI, 1901, p. 89.
16. Schottmueller: Muenchener Med. Woch., Bd. L. No. 20, May 19, 1903.
17. Trans. New York Path. Soc., December, 1905.
18. Trans. New York Path. Soc., April, 1905.
19. Welch: Amer. Jour. Med. Sci., Vol. CII, 1891, p. 439.
20. See, Neisser and Wechsberg: Zeitsch. f. Hygiene, etc., Bd. XXXVI, 1901.
   Klopstock and Bockenheimer: Arch. Kl. Chirurgie, Bd. LXXII, p. 324.
   Kolle and Otto: Zeitsch. f. Hyg., Bd. XLI, Heft 3.
   Kutscher and Konrich: Zeitsch. f. Hyg., Bd. XLVIII, Heft. 1 and 2.
   Otto: Centralbl. f. Bakt., Bd. XXXIV, Orig. p. 44.
21. Ghon and Albrecht: Zeitschr. fuer Klin. Med., Bd. XLIV.
   Libman and Celler: Trans. N. Y. Path. Soc., December, 1902.
22. Boggs: Am. Jour. Med. Sci., V. CXXX, p. 911.
23. Canon: Centralbl. fuer Pathologic, Bd. XV, No. 4, p. 143.
24. Gradwohl: Annales de l'Institut Pasteur, Vol. 18, 1904, p. 767.
   See also Simminds. Muench. Med. Woch., December 22, 1903; and Gioyn and Harris: Journ. of Infect. Diseases, Vol. II, p. 514.
25. Libman: Medical News, 1903, Vol. 82, p. 733.
   Trans. N. Y. Path. Soc., February-March, 1903.
26. Libman: Medical News, January 30, 1904.
   Mt. Sinai Hospital Reports, Vol. IV.
27. American Journal of Med. Sci., August, 1899.
28. Journal of Med. Research, Vol III, 1902, p. 168.
29. Beitraege z. Klin. Chir., Bd. X, 1893, p. 587.

30. Deutsch. Archiv. f. Klin. Med., Bd. LXXXV, Heft. 1 and 2.
31. Cf. Kocher and Tavel, L. c.
    Jordan: Muench. Med. Woch., No. 21, 1904.
32. First suggested by Hanau and Piliet: in 1889. See Bucknall: Lancet, 1905, II, pp. 1158-1164.
33. Libman: Philadelphia Med. Journal, V. III, 1899, p. 620.
34. Bertelsmann: L. c.
35. Cf. Rolleston: Diseases of the Liver, 1905, p. 77.
    Dr. Rolleston has kindly written to me that the remarks made in his book were based on the literature. The main cases of pylephlebitis with negative cultures are contained in Dr. A. Gerster's paper, which cases were studied by me. Langdon Brown (Brit. Med. Journal, November 25, 1905, p. 1393) cites one case with negative culture, but does not state what media were used.
36. Gerster: A Medical Record (N. Y.), June 27. 1903.
37. Brill: New York Med. Journ., 1898, January 15, "A Study of 17 Cases of a Disease Resembling Typhoid Fever, but Without the Widal Reaction."
38. Osler: Jacobi Festschrift, 1900.
    Amer. Journ. Med. Sci., V. CXXVII, 1904, p. 1.
39. See Lenhartz: l. c., also Muenchen. Med. Woch., 1901, Nos. 28 and 29.
    In these places will be found the literature and many original observations. Of particular interest are Litten's studies:
    Zeitschrift fuer Klin. Medizin, Bd. II, 1881; Berlin. Klin. Woch., 1899, No. 28, and Verhandl. Congr. inn. Mediz., 1900.
40. Leube: Spez. Diagnose der inneren Krankheiten, Bd. II, 6th Edition, p. 577.
41. A full discussion of pathology and clinical aspects is given by

42. Osler: Gulstonian Lectures: British Med. Journal, March 7, 1885, and Practitioner: Vol. 50, March, 1893.
42. Poirier and Cunéo: The Lymphatics, 1904, p. 229.
43. Thacher: American Journ. Med. Sci., January, 1906, p. 33, suggests the possibility of passive congestion of the viscera as a cause for the fever.
44. The first findings in such cases in our laboratory were made by Dr. Gershel, a former assistant, without any knowledge of Lenhartz's paper. The latter contains an admirable account of the clinical picture in these cases.
45. Schottmueller: l. c.
46. Cole: Journ. Inf. Diseases, V, 1905, p. 714.
    Harris: Trans. Chicago Path. Soc., June 12, 1905, p. 303.
    Beattie: Journ. of Med. Research, Vol. XIV, 1906, p. 399.
47. Janeway, E. G.: Med. News, August 26, 1899.
48. These have been published in detail by the writer in the Transactions of the N. Y. Path. Soc. for April and October, 1905. The literature is given in these papers.
49. MacCallum, W. G.: American Medicine, 1903, p. 452.
    See also Risel: Virch. Arch., Bd. CLXXXII, p. 258, and Loehlein: Virch. Arch., Bd. CLXXVII, p. 269.
50. v. Kahlden; l. c.
51. A good review of the literature is given by Churchman: Amer. Med., Vol. XI, 1906, p. 111; see also
    Noetzel: Wiener Klin. Woch., Bd. XVI, 1903, p. 1036.
    Schwarz: Zeitschr. f. Heilk., Neue Folge, Bd. VI, 1905, p. 295.
52. Welch: "Thrombosis," Allbutt's System, 1899, Vol. VII, p. 217.
53. Fornaca: Rev. in Centralbl. f. innere Med., 1903, p. 1056. See also Muench. Med. Woch., 1905, p. 2385.

PROCEEDINGS OF SOCIETIES.

THE JOHNS HOPKINS HOSPITAL MEDICAL SOCIETY.

February 19, 1906.

A Case of Cerebral Lues with Anæsthesia of the Face, with Remarks on the Epicritic Sense and Protopathic Sense of Head. DR. THOMAS.

This patient, A. C., a very light colored woman, is interesting in several particulars. She came to the dispensary in February, 1905, was at that time 31 years old, married. She complained of inability to raise her eyebrows and of pain in the left side of her face. Her family and personal history are negative and unimportant, except that two years before coming to the dispensary she had a miscarriage. No definite history of syphilis could be obtained.

July 4, eight months before coming to us, she noted, while eating that the left side of her face became stiff and two days later there was intense pain all over the left side of her face. This pain was very severe and persisted until her admission. In September, 1904, she had some difficulty in reading which was helped by glasses. On December 4, there was some drooping of the lids and the eyes closed. At this time she went to the Presbyterian Eye and Ear Hospital where she was given iodide of potassium, and there was some improvement.

The examination when we first saw her showed a remarkable picture. Her head was held back and her forehead wrinkled, the eyelids covering the iris almost completely.

She could see only by holding the head far back. Her sense of smell was unaffected, and the eyes were normal as regards the optic nerves and vision. The left eye was fixed in the mid-position, and the right eye was deflected outwards and could be moved only a little outwards and up and down. The pupils were inactive to light and to accommodation. There was therefore on the left side a complete paralysis of the 3d, 4th, and 6th nerves, and on the right of the 3d, and 4th, the 6th only functioning. Further there was paralysis with atrophy of the muscles of mastication, the mouth being deflected to the left when opened. There was anæsthesia of practically the whole side of the face as is seen after the operation for trifacial neuralgia. This area was anæsthetic to all qualities tested. All the other cerebral nerves acted normally.

The patient was given mercurial inunctions and potassium iodide was continued and she began to improve immediately. The eye movements returned markedly in a few weeks. An ulcer developed on the cornea of the left (anæsthetic) eye. The patient was referred to the eye department and in spite of all treatment the condition became worse, and the eye was lost and removed one month after the ulcer appeared. Since that time the specific treatment has been continued and the improvement has been good though somewhat slow of late.

As you see, the movements of the remaining eye are perfect and the pupil reacts to light and accommodation. When the mouth is opened the jaw is deflected to the left, showing that the pterygoids are still weak, but the masseter begins to show some action. In testing for sensation an interesting condition is found. There is present an area over the left forehead absolutely insensitive to all forms of sensation. This area extends down on the side of the face somewhat, but beyond this there is a band which borders the completely anæsthetic area, extending from the level of the tragus downward to the chin in which the patient feels some abnormal sensation. In this band the patient cannot appreciate a delicate touch, but will feel the prick of a pin. In this area the patient cannot distinguish between one and two points of the compass, nor can any but the extremes of temperature be appreciated—ice being felt as cold and a very hot tube as warm. Any stimulation within this area, causes a peculiar, unpleasant tingling sensation, which is poorly localized and radiates throughout the area.

There are then these two distinct areas, the first, anæsthetic to all forms of stimulation, and the second this band-like area in which only certain forms of stimuli are appreciated, and in which they are not localized but give rise to a diffuse radiation.

It was on account of these sensory changes that the case was shown to the Society, for they exemplify conditions to which Dr. Henry Head, of London, has recently called attention. Dr. Thomas had a number of the plates from Head's article thrown on the screen. He said that Head's work was of the first importance, and had apparently been done with the greatest care and thoroughness. Head and his associates had examined very many surgical injuries to peripheral nerves, and Head had had the radial and external cutaneous nerves cut on his own arm, and had made a most careful study of the sensory disturbances. He believes that it was this personal experiment that gave him the clue to the explanation of the condition found in the cases of injury. When a peripheral nerve is cut, there are, as in the patient before the Society, two areas of cutaneous sensory disturbance. One in which no sensory stimuli are perceived, and the other, beyond this area, in which peculiar sensory disturbance is present. In this border area, light touch is not perceived, the patient cannot distinguish between one and two points of the compass, even when widely separated, nor can he distinguish between a cool and a warm test-tube. He can, however, appreciate the prick of a pin, can distinguish between the extremes of temperature, and the responses are all associated with a widespread tingling, disagreeable sensation. This is what he calls his "protopathic sensation," and he believes it depends upon peculiar nerves. The power of appreciating light touches, as with a cotton wool, of distinguishing between the intermediate grades of temperature, and between one and two points, and in accurately localizing the stimuli, he groups together under the term "epicritic sensation," and believes that this depends also upon special nerves. These two kinds of nerves run together in the peripheral nerves. There seems to be very little overlapping of the epicritic nerves, for, as Head's figures show, when the ulnar nerve is cut, the loss of epicritic sense extends almost exactly to the same line. The overlapping of the protopathic nerves, however, is great and variable and this is the explanation why the area of total anæsthesia varies so much and is always so much less than the anatomical distribution of the nerve would lead one to expect. The rapidity with which these two kinds of nerves recover after injury varies considerably. The protopathic nerves recover first and more certainly. As they recover, the area of complete anæsthesia diminishes and at a certain stage we have the whole area of disturbed sensation occupied by protopathic sensibilities. Head's arm was a beautiful example of this, and gave him a unique opportunity for the study of this peculiar sensory condition. He has promised to present a future article which will deal with this part of the subject more fully.

Head also believes that deep sensation depends upon the sensory nerves which run with the muscular nerves, and he places these nerves in a third category.

DISCUSSION.

Dr. Barker said that the case interested him much, especially on account of Dr. Thomas' reference to the epicritic and protopathic sense of Head and to the nature of the sensory disturbance present in the case. He stated that he had described a very similar dissociation of sensation in an article entitled " A Case of Circumscribed Unilateral and Elective Sensory Paralysis," published in the Journal of Experimental Medicine in 1896 and simultaneously in the Deutsche Zeitschrift fur Nervenheilkunde (1895). The anæsthesia in the case reported affected the author's own arm and was supposedly due to pressure from a cervical rib. The area of anæsthesia extended in the form of a strip from the axilla down the medial side of the left arm to the little finger. It had been examined by Dr. Thomas in 1894, and during the summer of 1895, while in the physiological laboratory at Leipzig, at the suggestion of Prof. von Frey, the sensory disturbance was exactly worked out by most accurate physiological methods. The pressure points, warm points and cold points were localized one by one at the margins of the anæsthetic area. The great interest of the dissociation of sensation lay in the fact that whereas there was complete absence of certain nervous functions in the anæsthetic area, namely, heat sensation, cold sensation and pressure sensation, the pain sense was preserved. Pricks with a fine needle excited only a feeling of pain without calling forth previous touch or pressure sensations, and were answered by lively reflexes. Ice and heat when first applied called forth no sensation of cold or warmth, but after the lapse of a very short time excited a diffuse sensation of pain. Dr. Barker regarded the findings as strongly supporting von Frey's doctrine of the existence of pain nerves separate from touch and temperature nerves. The reactions to ice and heat he regarded as examples of " temperature pain " wholly independent of the temperature sensation which on the normal skin accompanies or precedes it. In the course of the work exact values for threshold stimuli were made out, for an account of which Dr. Barker referred to his paper. At the time these studies were made it was pointed out that the capacity to localize was very incomplete within an area where pain exclusively is felt. The situation of compass points was appreciated only very inaccurately. Pin points separated from one another by as much as 10 cm. could not be distinguished when care was taken in the application of the test. There are some discrepancies between Head's description of his protopathic sense and the pain sense which was preserved in the arm studied, but Dr. Barker thinks it very likely that Head's protopathic sense may turn out to be identical with the form of sensation he has described under the designation of von Frey's pain sense in the article above referred to.

Head has made a most important contribution in his recent articles, and has had the good fortune to work with an abundant material. He has also resorted, as Dr. Thomas has pointed out, to experiment on himself, a procedure of the greatest help if one desires to be sure of his findings when very delicate matters of skin sensation are in question. Head's theories regarding the nature of what he calls protopathic sensation and its relation to the sympathetic nervous system are of the highest interest and will doubtless stimulate much further study. .

March 19.

An Analytical Study of Acute Lobar Pneumonia in the Johns Hopkins Hospital from May 15, 1889, to May 15, 1905. Dr. Chatard.

The following statistics were gathered from the records of the hospital for the sixteen years, during which time 658 patients were treated for pneumonia, excluding ether pneumonias. Of this number 200 died, a percentage of 30.39, though if terminal pneumonias are excluded the number of deaths is 165, or 25.07 per cent.

The number of patients increased steadily up to 1899, but in 1900 and 1901 there was a sharp rise in the number, followed by a large drop during 1902 and 1903, followed again by a rise in the number during 1904 and 1905. During 1900 there was a general increase in the number of patients as ascertained by comparing other records.

Age.—The greatest number of cases of pneumonia occurred in young adults, 20-40 years old, 55 per cent. In patients from 20-30 years old 32 per cent occurred, and 16.5 per cent occurred in patients younger than 20 years. A comparison of the mortality with the age table is interesting. In early adolescence the mortality may be as low as 4 per cent; during the period of greatest frequency, 20-30 years, it is about 20 per cent; and after that period we find a steady rise to 80 per cent of deaths.

Sex.—The male patients far outnumber the female patients, 533 with 154 deaths, compared with 125 females, with 46 deaths. The death rate in the females, 36.8 per cent, far outnumbered that in the males, 28.8 per cent.

Race.—White, 238 patients, with a mortality of 30.6 per cent; foreign, 170 patients, with a mortality of 29.4 per cent; black, 250 patients, with a mortality of 31.2 per cent.

Male mortality, 29.2 per cent; female mortality, 40.4 per cent.

Seasonal Variation.—From January to March there is a rise in the number of patients when the greatest morbidity occurs; while during the summer months there is a great diminution in the number of patients, although the mortality is increased. In March the total number was 116 with a mortality of 28.4 per cent. In July, 19 patients, mortality 52.6 per cent. September, 24 patients, with a mortality of 45.8 per cent.

Occupation.—Greatest number of patients were laborers, or 203, with a mortality of 35.9 per cent; other outdoor occupations gave a total of 347, with a mortality of 34 per cent. Patients with indoor occupations 274 or 26.6 per cent. Alcohol was admitted by 426 patients or 64.7 per cent; mortality 30.9 per cent.

Previous Attacks of Pneumonia.—One previous attack was claimed by 88 patients, two previous by 8, three previous attacks by 3 patients, and 1 patient claimed to have had four previous attacks.

Condition of Patients.—One hundred and twenty-one of

the patients were exposed to bad weather, 19.9 per cent; eight to extremes of temperature; there were eight cases in nurses and orderlies, and three cases among doctors. As regards family history there was a history of tuberculosis in 11.3 per cent of the patients.

Symptoms.—The most frequent symptoms were cough, pain in the side, 79.7 per cent; chill, 49.3 per cent, and dyspnœa, 66.4 per cent. Abdominal pain was present in 51 of the cases or 7.7 per cent. The pulse was considered slow when it registered below 90 beats per minute, and of the patients 3.3 per cent exhibiting this pulse rate, 13.6 per cent died. Patients with a medium pulse rate, up to 125 per minute, showed a death rate of 14.9 per cent, this medium pulse rate occurring in 50.7 per cent. Patients with a rapid pulse, 125 or over per minute, showed a death rate of 49.4 per cent. Of these the number was 289 or 43.9 per cent.

Temperature.—This was subnormal, below 98.5 degrees in five cases with two deaths, 40 per cent mortality; between 98.5-102 in thirty-nine cases, with thirteen deaths, 33.3 per cent mortality; between 102-104 degrees, in 181 patients, with 49 deaths or 27.07 per cent mortality, and between 104-106 in three hundred and eighty-four patients, with 106 deaths, or 27.6 per cent. The temperature was above 106 degrees in forty-nine patients, with 55 per cent of deaths. The admission temperature was generally between 102 and 104, though in one-sixth of the patients it was below 100 degrees.

The respiratory rate was rapid in the majority of the patients; when over 50 respirations per minute the mortality was 54.8 per cent; those patients exhibiting labored respiration and cyanosis gave nearly 50 per cent mortality.

The sputum in the majority of the patients was mucopurulent, tenacious and rusty. In ninety-three patients the pneumococci were found in the sputum, though doubtless present in many more.

Involvement.—In 354 patients the right side alone was involved, with a mortality of 26.5 per cent; the right lower lobe 139 times, being the most frequent. The left side was involved alone 168 times, with a mortality of 20.2 per cent. In double pneumonia, which occurred in one-fifth of our patients, the mortality was about 54.07 per cent.

Pneumococci were isolated from the blood in 25.2 per cent of the patients, and of these 69.1 per cent died. The joints were aspirated in a number of patients and the pneumococci obtained in one. Lumbar puncture was done 9 times, the pneumococcus being found 6 times in cultures and once by smears alone.

Complications.—There were 338 patients with pleurisy, and 11 patients with effusion, a total of 52.8 per cent; mortality about 40 per cent; empyema occurring in 27 patients, 22.2 per cent mortality. Pericarditis was present in 35 patients, mortality 82.8 per cent; endocarditis in 13 patients, 76.9 per cent mortality, and jaundice in 76 patients, with 21 deaths, 27.6 per cent mortality. This latter complication varied in frequency with the years; in 1901 there were 20

patients with jaundice, 13 in 1902, and only 6 in 1900, though there were the greatest number of patients during the latter year. There were 13 cases of meningitis, all fatal. Abscess of lung 5 times, 3 were fatal.

The greatest number of patients showed a leucocyte count of between 25- and 30,000, with the lowest mortality, 19 per cent. The highest mortality occurred among the patients with the lower (below 10,000) leucocyte count, and also in the very high ones, 70,000-80,000. Albumen was present in the urine of 511 patients, 77.6 per cent; casts in 166 patients, 25.2 per cent, and the Diazo reaction in 16.8 per cent. Bile was present in 34.3 per cent of the urinary examinations made for it. The chlorides were diminished and below 1 gm. per liter in over 50 per cent.

Otitis media occurred 9 times, all recovered; parotitis 4 times; conjunctivitis 4 times; thrombosis, peritonitis, tonsillitis, and arthritis occurred each three times. There were eight cases of septicæmia, one hundred and forty-nine patients with delirium, mortality 44.9 per cent; twelve being admitted with delirium, 58.3 per cent mortality. Herpes was noted in one hundred and eighty patients, and not noted in two hundred and sixty-five. Where a note was made herpes occurred on the lips in eighty-seven patients, on the nose in forty-three, on the ears in three. In 47 patients the special spot was not noted.

Among the special features delayed resolution was noted in thirty-five patients; relapses occurred in five patients. The average blood pressure was between 125 and 150 mm. of mercury. Terminal pneumonia occurred thirty-five times, or 5.3 per cent.

Defervescence.—Crisis was considered as "true" when occurring in twelve hours or less; "protracted" when occurring in from twelve to twenty-four hours. It was "true" in 99 patients or 15 per cent, and "protracted" in seventy-one patients, 10.8 per cent, and there were seventeen cases of pseudo-crisis. Temperature fell by lysis in 288 patients, or 43.7 per cent. The crisis was usually associated with a fall in the number of leucocytes. The crisis usually occurred from the seventh to the ninth day, though in one patient occurring as early as the third and in two as late as the fifteenth day.

For treatment, stimulants were used in five hundred and thirty-six patients, and symptomatic treatment was employed in four hundred and sixty patients. Measures employed were the ice bag, poultices, sponges, oxygen, and in a few cases the anti-pneumococcus serum. The anti-pneumococcus serum gave little, if any, good results.

Typhoid fever occurred in twenty-one patients as an associated condition, nephritis eighteen times, and heart lesions occurred next in order of frequency.

Note.—The above is a brief report of an article on the "General Statistics" to appear later with a series of collected papers entitled, "Studies in Pneumonia."—J. A. C.

DISCUSSION.

DR. McCRAE.—Complications are of little value in the prognosis of pneumonia as Dr. Chatard's paper shows, while in typhoid fever there are a tremendous number of complications, and yet the mortality is low compared with pneumonia. In this series there have been a comparatively small number of empyemata, and the small number (35) of delayed resolutions is surprising. Another point is the heavy death rate with delirium, this symptom speaking for a severe toxæmia. The low death rate with jaundice is surprising.

DR. MARSHALL spoke of the difficulty in diagnosing pneumonia in young children early in the disease. There was a house epidemic of twelve cases in which the young children would for two or two and a half days have a marked rise of temperature, with a high leucocytosis, without physical signs. The ratio between the rate of the pulse and the respiration, emphasized in the text books, proved to be a fallacy. In these cases an early diagnosis was aided by the suppressed breath sounds, and a slight diminution in the expansion of the affected side, followed later by a few râles and some dullness.

Clinical and Experimental Observations on Cheyne-Stokes Respiration. DR. EYSTER.

This communication is based upon the results obtained from ten cases in which continuous tracings were taken as records of the blood pressure in its relation to the respiratory changes.

There were found two groups of cases: first, cases with a rise of blood pressure and an increase in pulse rate during the period of dyspnœa, and a fall during the period of apnœa, and second, cases with a fall during dyspnœa and a rise during apnœa.

In the first group there were two cases of increased intracranial tension, the first of which was admitted to the hospital with a history of left-sided clonic spasms, intense headaches, and a choked disc of the left eye. The Cheyne-Stokes breathing was marked, with periods of apnœa of one minute or longer, the dyspnœic periods being relatively short. The blood pressure tracings were made by means of the Erlanger sphygmomanometer. The systolic and diastolic pressures were first determined and the instrument set midway between these points and a continuous record taken. With a fall of the blood pressure the pulse waves decreased in size owing to the diastolic pressure being removed from the point at which the instrument was set. A rise of pressure produces the opposite effect.

The following points were observed: first, the Traube-Hering waves of blood pressure disappeared with the disappearance of the periodic respiration; second, the relative lengths of the periods of apnœa and dyspnœa varied with the extent of the rise and the fall of the blood pressure.

Increased intracranial tension was produced experimentally in dogs by trephining the skull and screwing into this opening a canula connected to a pressure bottle filled with salt solution that could be elevated and lowered at will, thus securing various degrees of tension. Periodic respiration was obtained and was always accompanied by changes in the blood pressure. The simple rise and fall in the blood pressure is not sufficient to produce periodic respiration, but the rise must be above and the fall below the line of intracranial pressure. With these conditions it was found in the periods of dyspnœa there was a rise of blood pressure, and during apnœa a fall of the pressure, the rise and fall being above and below the intracranial pressure.

Tracings from the cases of increased intracranial tension, showed a rise in the blood pressure associated with each group of respirations, and an increase in pulse rate accompanying the increased blood pressure. Cheyne-Stokes respiration in these increased intracranial tension cases is not by any means always the typical text-book type, small groups being common, groups of two or three respirations. After the disappearance of the periodic respiration there was disappearance of the blood pressure changes.

The second case of this series, one of cerebral hæmorrhage, shows the same changes described above.

In a second group of eight cases of Cheyne-Stokes respiration associated with cardiac and arterial disease, tracings were shown from a case of aortic insufficiency and myocarditis. The tracings from this case showed a fall of blood pressure leading up to about the first third of the period of dyspnœa with a decrease of the pulse rate, then up to the middle of the following period of apnœa there is a rise of blood pressure and an increase in the pulse rate. A curve was also shown demonstrating that the blood pressure changes are not due to the effects of the periodic respiratory activity itself. This tracing was taken from a normal individual who breathed periodically and simulated Cheyne-Stokes respiration. In this tracing an entirely different series of blood pressure changes is observed. The periodic respiration obtained in a dog after section of both vagi was accompanied by no difference in the pulse rate during the periods of apnœa and dyspnœa.

The underlying condition of periodic respiration in cases of increased intracranial tension is evidently an alternate anæmia and period of blood supply to the brain and medullary centers. The former is associated with apnœa and occurs when the blood pressure is below the line of intracranial pressure. The period of respiratory activity is associated with the period of blood supply to the brain, and occurs with the rise of the blood pressure above that of the intracranial pressure. These changes in blood supply should cause the opposite effect upon the respiratory center to those observed, if the stimulus to the center were all that need be considered, as this stimulus (increase in carbon dioxide and decrease of oxygen) is certainly greatest when the anæmia is greatest. Another factor has to be considered, however, a loss of irritability of the respiratory center with a much decreased blood supply. This irritability is periodically much reduced or lost when the blood pressure is below the line of the intracranial pressure, and hence such periods are associated with apnœa. This loss of irritability of the respiratory center is also shown in experiments upon brain anæmia following the ligation of the cerebral arteries. Entirely different conditions are present under these circumstances from those in asphyxia of the center following ligation of the trachea. Here the carbon dioxide increases and the oxygen decreases to an enormous extent, but the blood supply to the brain and centers is normal or increased and the respiratory center responds almost until the death of the animal.

The explanation of the second group of cases is not at all clear at present. Mosso has recently obtained continuous records of the blood pressure in periodic respiration occurring in normal persons at high altitudes, and he separates apparently a third group. This group shows a rise of the blood pressure accompanied by a slowing of the pulse rate with each respiratory period.

DISCUSSION.

DR. ERLANGER emphasized two points. First that Cheyne-Stokes respiration was described as early as 1816 and again in 1850, and that since that time it had been investigated by scores of physiologists, but no clear cause had been given until Dr. Eyster had taken up the problem. Secondly the reasons for this were no doubt due to two causes: first; to improved methods of investigation, and second, to the assistance from clinicians and the members of the staff of the hospital. This offspring was the first to result from the union of the wards and the laboratory.

The Toxic Constitution of Amanita Phalloides. DR. W. W. FORD.

This paper deals with a toxic principle found in the fungus and not noted by Kobert. The phallin of Kobert is strongly hæmolytic and to it may be attributed all the lesions found in man due to destruction of red blood cells. Experimentally lesions referable to hæmolysis may be produced, such as hæmoglobinuria and pigmentation of the spleen, but in addition, subcutaneous œdema, hæmorrhages, and necrosis of various organs are found. Are these the result of intracorporeal hæmolysis?

In animals the amount of blood destruction produced by fatal doses is too small, by itself to account for the profound intoxication. We may explain the lesions by first, the liberation of poisonous substances by the breaking down of red blood cells; second, the action of phallin on other cells of the body; third, the presence of others poisons in *Amanita phalloides* in addition to phallin.

The last hypothesis is shown to be correct by the following experiments:

(a) Extracts of the fungus when heated to 65 degrees C. for one-half hour, the temperature at which the hæmolysin is completely destroyed, are still strongly toxic to animals, in which they produce hæmorrhage and necrosis, but no subcutaneous œdema, no pigmentation of the spleen, and no hæmoglobinuria.

(b) Pepsin and pancreatin digest the hæmolysin but leave unimpaired the heat-resistant body.

· (c) Extracts of the fungus cannot be neutralized by blood, as tetanus toxin and the neuro-toxic constituent of cobra venom are by brain tissue. There are present in *Amanita phalloides*, therefore, thermolobile (hæmolytic) substances and thermostabile (necrotising substances). In ricin Jacoby has shown that, whereas the first believed there were separate poisonous substances present each with its own haptophoric and toxophoric group, in all probability there is but one substance composed of two toxophoric groups attached to one haptophoric group. In *Amanita phalloides* we may imagine two different toxic constitutions.

1st. A single haptophoric group united with two toxophoric groups, one hæmolytic and one necrotising.

2d. Separate haptophoric groups each united to its own toxophoric group. The true conception may be determined experimentally.

If we destroy the hæmolysin and immunize animals to the heated material, if the anti-serum is merely anti-toxic and not anti-hæmolytic then there must be different haptophoric groups in the extracts. On the other hand if the anti-serum be anti-hæmolytic as well as anti-toxic then but a single haptophoric group is present. Animals immunized to extracts heated to 65 degrees C. and to 80 degrees C. one-half hour, develop anti-sera, which are anti-toxic to the heated material only, no anti-hæmolytic principles being found. We have present in the fungus therefore, toxic and hæmolytic principles, each with its own separate and distinct toxophoric and haptophoric groups.

In short *Amanita phalloides* contains in addition to phallin another distinct toxin.

April 2, 1906.

Report of Five Cases of Pneumonia Occurring in One Family. DR. FABYAN.

Dr. Fabyan reported a series of five cases of pneumonia which entered the colored wards during the March of this year. There were two girls and three boys, all from one family. A careful study of these cases and the home conditions was made.

Among the etiological factors might be mentioned the house where the family lived. This is a dilapidated old wooden structure near which is running dirty water. A privy is situated about 50 feet away. On the first floor of the house the two older girls of the family occupied one room until about three weeks before the outbreak of the disease, when they moved to the garret. There was great crowding in one of the rooms on the first floor, four persons occupying one bed, and two and three others, cots. Some of the children had suffered from whooping cough a short time previous to the pneumonia outbreak.

The father stopped work March 8 complaining of a cold and misery in the stomach. There was no pain in the side, dyspnœa, cough or fever. On March 11, one child was taken ill, three days later, March 14, a second child became ill, three days after this another child became sick, still another one day later, and still another two days later. The eldest daughter returned home at this time to assist the mother in nursing the sick members of the family but up to the present time they have both remained well.

There are no animal pets in the house, nor is there any illness in the neighboring factory. Second-hand blankets had been purchased and after cleaning, had been used on the beds of the family. The nursing was all done by the mother, father, and eldest daughter.

In the earlier cases the onset was sudden, with headache, epigastric pain, and cough. Diarrhœa was a constant feature in all but one of the cases. The first patient entered the hospital with the typical signs and symptoms of pneumonia, the pneumococcus being isolated from the blood in pure cultures. This patient died. At autopsy there was found a yellowish pleural exudate, the lungs contained firm areas, especially the upper lobes. There was a similar yellowish exudate in the abdominal cavity, with a general involvement and reddening of the abdominal and pelvic viscera.

The second patient entered the hospital with consolidation of the left lower lobe. The third patient presented signs of an involvement of the right upper lobe, the fourth patient signs of involvement of the right upper lobe—this patient is now up and about the ward. The fifth patient was the only one to have herpes, and had indefinite signs of consolidation. There was no diazo reaction present in any of the cases.

The occurrence of these cases suggests contagion, though this is not absolutely necessary. In 1885 Blyth called attention to the probable infectious nature of pneumonia. Epidemics have been reported at different times, epidemics of many hundred cases occurring in communities and having high mortalities. Dr. Osler has reported 10 cases in one family, cases of a very severe type of the disease.

Under the head of house infections there are records of as many as 32 cases occurring in one house in 4 years, and 8 cases in another house in 9 years.

Still another group of cases reported are those in which house pets, especially parrots, played an important part in spreading the disease. Also certain articles from the sick room have been known to carry infection. In one instance the bedding from the deathbed of a pneumonia patient after being carried two miles, was 3 weeks later placed on the bed of a child who immediately developed the disease.

To summarize this series of cases, there were nine persons living in one house, five of whom developed the disease. In four cases it was a frank pneumonia. One case died and showed typical pneumococcus pneumonia and clinically the disease is supposed to be the same in the other cases. The rooms in the house where the infections occurred were generally neat, and the sputum was well taken care of. All but one of the patients were predisposed by previous attacks of whooping cough. As a possible means of infection the blankets must be thought of.

Metaplastic Bone Formation. DR. BUNTING.

The ossification of calcified cartilages in the aged is so frequently seen that it excites no comment, but the presence of foci of bone in organs where there is no pre-existing perichondrium or periosteum arouses one's interest and at first seems difficult of explanation. The specimen submitted is from the calcified aorta of a man aged 72 years, who died of broncho-pneumonia. The bone masses lie in the thickened intima and adjacent to a deposit of calcium salts in the hyaline media, at a point where the media is penetrated by an artery accompanied by granulation tissue.

Such a picture is unusual but not unparalleled, as a search of medical literature shows five cases of bone formation in the aorta and more numerous cases where the foci have been found in smaller vessels and in heart valves. One cannot resort to the Cohnheim displacement theory in explanation of these foci because of the frequency of their occurrence in calcified vessels, and in fact in practically every organ where calcium deposits are found, surrounded by granulation tissue, and finally because of the experimental production of such foci about calcium-containing foreign bodies in the peritoneal cavity—and in necrotic and calcified kidneys following ligature of the renal vessels. The process is a metaplasia of cells of the young granulation tissue and appears as a result of the chemical stimulation of the calcium salts. The bone may be formed apparently either by the formation of a callus or ostoid tissue with its subsequent conversion into bone or by erosion of the calcified material and deposit of bone by osteoblasts as in the normal development at the epiphysis.

This specimen is interesting further in the presence adjacent to the bone of a focus of cellular marrow containing all the elements usually found in the red marrow of cancellous bone. Here too one probably has the result of metaplasia of cells of the granulation tissue, and it seems most likely of cells of the mononuclear type, hæmatogenous in origin, such as are always found in granulation tissue, rather than of the fixed connective-tissue cells. This seems more probable than the assumption that one has here the emigration of a parent cell for each of the types found in the focus of marrow. Such being true the case is strong evidence for the presence in the hæmoporetic organs of a cell of indifferent type which retains throughout life the capability of differentiating into the various types of blood cells.

April 23, 1906.

Experimental Heart Block. DR. CULLEN AND DR. ERLANGER.

The main object of this communication was to show to the society a dog in which heart block had been produced by crushing the auriculo-ventricular bundle of His, but unfortunately the animal died a few days ago.

The series of experiments which included this case was undertaken at the suggestion of Dr. Welch with the object of attempting to produce Stokes-Adams disease in the dog by destroying the auriculo-ventricular bundle of His. The operations to destroy the bundle were performed as follows: Under artificial respiration through a tracheal cannula, two ribs were resected, the pericardium was opened, and, by means of an instrument attached to the aorta, the heart was drawn well up into the wound in the chest wall. After heart block had been produced the pericardium was sutured and the wounds in the chest wall and trachea closed.

In the first series of experiments the attempt was made to destroy the auriculo-ventricular bundle by injecting into it with a hypodermic syringe a solution of iodin in alcohol. On account of the small size of the bundle and its hidden position this procedure is a difficult one, but in each case the operation was successfully completed not, however, until several attempts had been made.

Case 1. After the completion of the operation this animal had heart block but the block was gradually passing off when the animal died 18 hours after the operation.

Case 2. This animal also presumably had a partial block from which it was recovering when it died of secondary hæmorrhage two hours after the completion of the operation.

Case 3. After recovery from the operation this animal had a partial block with a two or three to one rhythm, but the auriculo-ventricular sequence became normal one month later. A second operation was then performed at which it was found that the return of the heart to normal was due to the resumption of conduction by the auriculo-ventricular bundle.

Case 4. This animal became normal after one day of very slight heart block.

The recovery of the heart from the block produced in this first series of experiments was probably due to the fact that the method did not suffice to destroy completely the auriculo-ventricular bundle. Therefore in the second series of experiments another method was employed; the bundle of His was crushed with a specially devised clamp.

Case 1. This dog died from hæmorrhage.

Case 2. This dog died on the table from some unknown cause.

Case 3. In this case the operation was entirely successful and the animal forms the most important case in the entire series. The date of the operation, which was thoroughly successful, was March 17, 1906, and the dog lived until April 13, 1906. Before the operation the rate of the animal's heart had been 150 per minute. After the destruction of the auriculo-ventricular bundle the heart block was permanently complete. The rate of the auricles, when the first observations could be made, was 140 per minute while that of the ventricles was about 60 per minute. The rate of both the auricles and the ventricles decreased more or less progressively up to the time of death, the rate of the ventricles decreasing to about 40, and that of the auricles to about 70. The animal fed well, was playful, and seemed normal in almost every way till the day of its death, which was sudden and unexpected. At the autopsy the only cause of death found was pulmonary œdema.

This dog had no symptoms of syncopal attacks but never-theless it occasionally had the cardiac signs sometimes seen in human beings during these attacks. In simultaneous tracings of the respirations and heart beat made at such times the following phenomena may be seen: The respirations are of the Cheyne-Stokes type. Simultaneously with the beginning of the periods of hyperpnœa the auricular rate increases and the ventricular rate decreases. The auricular rate decreases and the ventricular rate increases usually somewhat before the onset of the period of apnœa. These changes in rate are very marked. In one instance, for example, one ventricular period lasts 1.6 seconds during the apnœic period while during the subsequent hyperpnœic period the longest ventricular period is 4.4 seconds. Similar changes in heart beat and respirations have been seen in man in association with syncopal attacks.

Since there is every reason for believing that in the case of this dog the heart block was absolute, it becomes necessary to abandon the explanation, suggested in another place, of the syncopal attacks seen in man in association with Cheyne-Stokes respiration. In the absence of experimental data it might now be suggested that the variations in the auricular and ventricular rates, as well as that of the respiratory rate, are associated with rhythmic variations in the activity of the nerve centers in the medulla. It has been demonstrated that the vagus nerve exerts but a minimal influence over the ventricles in complete block, whereas the accelerators in such a case preserve their normal influence over auricles and ventricles. Therefore, in heart block, simultaneous stimulation of the medullary centers would probably slow the auricles and accelerate the ventricles, and simultaneous depressions of the centers would have the opposite effects.

Physiologically these experiments are significant in that they demonstrate beyond doubt that the auriculo-ventricular bundle of His constitutes the only path of conduction from auricles to ventricles. The objection might previously have been raised that the results obtained in experiments of comparatively brief duration do not suffice to prove that the auriculo-ventricular bundle is the sole physiological connection. Thus it might have been objected that in the limited time of an experiment other connections which perhaps exist did not have time to become functional. However this objection loses its force in the light of the fact that heart block may remain complete 27 days after crushing the auriculo-ventricular bundle. Furthermore, this fact indicates, although it does not prove, that the conducting tissue of the auriculo-ventricular bundle is muscular and not nervous.

That in man the auriculo-ventricular bundle is the only physiological connection between auricles and ventricles is proved by the autopsy findings in at least three cases of Stokes-Adams disease. Perhaps the clearest of these instances is the one reported by Jellick, Cooper, and Ophuls. In this case the block was caused by anæmic necrosis of the auriculo-ventricular bundle.

The results of histological examinations of the material obtained in these experiments will be reported to the Society at a later date.

Surgery of the Blood-Vessels and its Application to the Changes of Circulation and Transplantation of Organs. DR. A. CARREL, OF CHICAGO.

The work along this line was begun in 1891 at Lyons, in France, and it may be divided into a number of groups or divisions.

I. Operations acting directly on the blood-vessels, of which there are the following subdivisions.

(a) Partial stenosis, an operation to produce a diminution in the lumen of a vessel.

(b) Longitudinal exclusion of a vessel by means of longitudinally placed purse-string suture to lessen the circumference of the vessel.

(c) Patching, by sewing patches into the walls of a vessel. We have used many substances, among them the peritoneum, which latter substance functioned perfectly, the animal—a cat—living for seven months after the operation. To anastomose small vessels with big ones we use the patch method, flaring out the end of the small vessel by means of a longitudinal incision and applying this as a patch to the side of the large one.

(d) Anastomoses. These may be termino-terminal, termino-lateral, the important part of the operation being anchor threads which divide the circumference of the vessels into quadrants, and which allow of good approximation and suturing. There are some slight modifications of the technic as when arterio-venous or arterio-arterial anastomoses are made. In all work of this kind the most perfect technic and asepsis are necessary to obtain any results at all.

(e) Transplantation of veins and arteries. We may dissect out the vessels and transplant either the vein to the artery or the artery to the vein. The main purpose of such experiments is to judge the effect on the veins when an artery is transplanted into them and the venous walls subjected to the arterial pressure. By this method it is also possible to increase the pressure in the veins and diminish it in the arteries. When the pressure in an artery is increased by transferring all its pressure into a closed venous system like the thyroid veins for example, the arterial walls undergo a sclerosis. This results from increased pressure alone and is assisted by no toxic factor. On the other hand by transferring the arterial pressure into an open system of veins we get a diminution of the arterial pressure with a weakening of the walls. This might be used as a possible cure for sclerosis.

Accompanying these changes in the arterial walls the veins thicken enormously from the increased pressure, becoming from two to three times their normal thickness and exceeding that of the arterial wall. The nutrition of the wall of the transplanted piece is perfect and an interruption of this nutrition for from twenty minutes to two hours appears to have no evil effect.

In the experiment of transplanting a piece of artery into another artery there is no change in the walls of the transplanted piece, but in the walls of a piece of vein transplanted into an artery there is the same great hypertrophy. We may conclude that vessels adapt themselves very quickly to changes in pressure and circulation.

II. Operations on the blood-vessels indirectly through their nerves. a. temporary denervation, by (1) elongation, and (2) by crushing. This series of experiments and their results is still in a crude state as fibers of nerves of different functions are cut at the same time, e. g., constrictor and dilator fibers.

The experimental application of these operations is very broad. The following experiments are described to show the effects of many of these methods:

a. Artificial modification of the circulation through (1) the limbs, (2) the head, and (3) other organs. First in the limbs. The lateral anastamosis between the femoral artery and vein showed three hours after the operation that the valves in the vein were still competent and there was no effect noted. However four hours after an end anastamosis the red blood flowed through the vein and the artery contained the dark blood. A complete reversal of the circulation in its major portion caused death, due to the accumulation of red blood in the veins.

Secondly, the arterial modification of the circulation to the head is easily accomplished, as the veins in this area are without valves. In one case where the arterial circulation was turned into the superficial veins of the neck, eight months later the superficial veins were like arteries and the skin was much thickened. The circulation to the head may be modified (a) by the transformation of the superficial veins of the neck into arteries, (b) by the attempt to supply arterial blood to the brain through venous channels, and (c) operations regulating or diminishing intracranial blood pressure.

Thirdly, in regard to organs we may (a) change the kind of blood to an organ. This was accomplished in the case of the thyroid gland in a goitre case in a dog. By this reversal of the circulation the thyroid became smaller and smaller and the symptoms of the disease disappeared. Or (b) the circulation may be modified to produce an active hyperæmia by means of a temporary denervation or by an elongation.

Under still another head will be considered replantations and transplantations of organs and limbs. First, replantations of the thyroid are readily performed. The gland is extirpated and replaced by making careful anastomoses of the blood-vessels and eight months later the glands have been examined and found perfectly normal. Second, the transplantations and replantations of the kidney have been successful. Third, limb replantations have been done. The thigh of a dog was amputated with a circular incision and the vessels cut in the region of Scarpa's triangle. After one and one-half hours disturbance of the circulation the bone, muscles, aponeuroses, vessels and skin were carefully sutured. Of course there was a complete paralysis of the limb and some elevation of temperature resulted from the operation.

In the first case tried there was considerable œdema of the limb below the amputation but this was found to be due to the dressings. The main difficulties of this operation are asepsis and a suitable means of dressing the limb.

Transplantations of organs are of two types, (a) simple, and (b) *en masse,* and have been successfully performed on the thyroid, ovary, thigh, lungs, and the suprarenal bodies. First, the simple form has the great drawback of cutting all the nerves to the transplanted organ and therefore the second form of the operation, *en masse,* is the best. By this method all the connective tissue, nerves, and large segments of the main vessels are preserved. A portion of the small bowel in this manner was transplanted into the space left by removing a portion of the œsophagus with a perfect result, also was the heart transplanted in various manners, and, twenty minutes later the auricles began to beat, and one hour later the ventricles, the experiment being terminated two hours later. Lungs have been successfully transplanted but become œdematous.

The kidney and suprarenal have been successfully transplanted, both homo- and auto-transplantations, normal urine having been obtained from kidneys thus implanted. Likewise in a case of homo-transplantation of both kidneys to another dog, the animal remained perfectly normal for eight days, the urine showing variations within perfectly normal limits.

From the above experiments I believe it is improper to draw definite conclusions. I do not say we will get as good results in man, as the conditions of the circulation and the red blood corpuscles are no doubt different. However this new technic may be of some use in the course of time, and some of the experiments may lead to the establishment of therapeutic methods, especially in the treatment of wounds of the large arteries and veins.

The methods are very simple, the fine silk, fine needle, vaseline for the coating of the suture, accurate approximation without invagination, and perfect technic being the only requirements.

The present surgical treatment of disease is either cutting or extirpating; now why not influence the circulation to the diseased part or organ and thus its nutrition, or extirpate it and replace it with a sound one. It is reasonable to suppose that by increasing the red circulation to a diseased organ or part that it will aid its attaining a more normal function.

The clinical application of these methods may be divided as follows: a. to present vascular surgery, (1) treatment of aneurysms, (2) to the treatment of artery wounds; b. to surgery of organs and limbs, (1) operations changing the metabolism of diseased organs by acting through the circulation, (2) transplantations of organs, (3) through the nerves instead of by the vessels directly, though caution must be observed here as, while a partial denervation of the kidney is not to be feared, a complete one will cause degenerative changes in the cells of the tubules.

The question of the transplantation of organs in man is a very serious one and difficult, for will the transplanted organ remain and function normally after a long period of time? Another difficulty would be that of finding organs suitable for transplantation into man. A process of immunization would no doubt be necessary before organs of animals would be suitable for transplantation into man. Organs from a person killed by accident would no doubt be suitable.

In closing I wish to say that this work is still very incomplete as it has been carried out under not the best circumstances. I hope others will continue with the research.

DISCUSSION.

DR. HALSTED said he had been especially interested in the paper and that there was work here for an army of investigators. It seems but reasonable to expect that in a short time there will be great revelations resulting from such work.

This work has another side of especial interest to surgeons—for the first time it seems necessary for surgeons to develop great manual dexterity, it not being possible for every one to employ these methods. This work also emphasizes the great importance that the surgery of the arteries bears to surgery in general, and even those who do not expect to make contributions would do well to familiarize themselves with this work in order to gain facility in the handling of large vessels.

DR. WATTS said he wished to emphasize what Dr. Carrell had said in regard to perfect technic. Dr. Watts had done ten operations upon the jugular vein and the carotid artery, all of which had been successful, though a number of cases on the femoral vessels had failed, as absolute cleanliness is harder to obtain in this latter region.

DR. WELCH said this paper had been a most startling presentation of a field suggesting an entirely new line of work. In regard to one point made by Dr. Carrell, that increase of blood supply alone could produce an increase of growth as shown by increased karyokinetic figures, Dr. Welch thought other factors were necessary besides the mere increase in the blood supply.

Common Yeast (Saccharomyces cerevisiæ) in the Treatment of Rheumatic Affections. DR. PENROSE.

The common yeast, Sáccharomyces cerevisiæ, is a sprouting fungus producing spores, and causing an alcoholic fermentation with the liberation of carbon dioxide. This yeast can split up albumen, and its powerful germicidal action, both inside and without the body, is due to its great vitality and powers of propagation, and to its power of stimulating the formation of lymphocytes. Yeast also has a laxative effect which is an aid to its other effects.

Salicylic acid is of benefit to the rheumatic patient and it is reasonable to suppose it is because it favors the growth of the yeast present in the stomach. Yeasts added to the salicylic acid treatment greatly aid the action of the former.

In one case of severe acute inflammatory rheumatism the yeast treatment was tried and the man was up and about the ward free from pain in two weeks. The yeast is given often during the day and does not interfere with the liquid food. Several other cases have been markedly aided by this form of treatment.

May 7, 1906.

Loco Disease in the West. DR. H. T. MARSHALL.

(To be published later.)

Exhibition of Medical Cases. DR. EMERSON.

Unilateral paroxysmal hæmoglobinuria.—The first patient is a man aged twenty-eight years, who has been in this hospital four times, the first admission five years ago. His personal history is negative except for the fact that six years ago he made a voyage to the West Indies as a sailor. For five years the patient has been suffering from a severe anæmia, with an oligocythemia of about one million red cells and a color index of about one. The leucocyte count is normal; there have been few nucleated red cells.

At no time have the blood counts been over one and a half million cells. This case is of interest as illustrating on his previous admission the independence of the blood count and the subjective symptoms so common in pernicious anæmia, although the count was no higher on his discharge than on admission, the patient felt well enough to go home. In other cases the count rises during their stay, then falls, and the death comes when the count is that on admission. This independence of the blood count to the symptoms has been a striking feature of our series of cases in this hospital.

The first symptom for which this patient was admitted was bloody urine, which turned out to be pure hæmoglobinuria. This has continued for a few weeks, then clears up entirely, later to reappear. The hæmoglobinuria in this case is of particular interest in that for a time it was present from one until nine o'clock in the morning, while during the rest of the day the urine was clear. Examination with the cystoscope showed red urine coming from the right kidney only. The condition is therefore one of *unilateral paroxysmal hæmoglobinuria.* The diagnosis has not been made in this case. He has tuberculosis of the lungs, a large spleen and liver and a pulsating mass in the left renal region.

A Case of Combined Morbus Errorum and Addison's Disease.—The second case is a man aged fifty years, who has worked as a tobacco seller. He came in complaining of weakness. His personal history is negative, his habits good. The patient led an active life up to one month ago. Associated with the weakness there has been shortness of breath and pigmentation of the skin.

On admission there was found a marked condition of vagabond's disease, the pigmentation being general over the body, but most marked on neck, shoulders, waist line, genitals,

and proximal segments of both extremities. However, in addition to this body pigmentation there is considerable pigmenting of the mucous membranes of the mouth. The blood pressure is low—60 to 80 mm. of mercury.

The question arises, is the pigmentation due entirely to the body louse or to Addison's disease also. In favor of the latter view is a positive tuberculin reaction, the low blood pressure and the weakness, all of which point rather strongly to Addison's disease, though there has been no gastric or muscular irritability.

Tetany.—Case three is that of a colored woman aged thirty-five, who came in complaining of "drawing up of the hands"—a case of tetany. The family history is interesting since one brother died at thirty-four years of age with spasms of the same nature as those complained of by this patient. The patient's personal history is negative as regards gastro-intestinal symptoms, positive as regards pelvic troubles.

The present illness began four months ago, at which time the patient was ill in bed for one week. Two months later she had her first attack of tetany in the wrists and fingers. Since her admission the spasms have been limited to the hands and the fingers.

The patient has no enlargement of the stomach but there is almost total anacidity. There is definite chronic nephritis.

DISCUSSION.

DR. MACCALLUM mentioned a case of tetany in a woman sixty-five years old, with anacidity and without dilatation of the stomach in which case the parathyroid glands showed abundant mitotic figures demonstrating that these glands were trying to overcome the poison of tetany.

The Relation of Various Strains of Dysentery Bacilli to the Diarrhœas of Infancy. DR. KNOX.

The following results of investigations on infant diarrhœa were carried out by Mr. Schorer and myself and I regret that he is unable to be present this evening to communicate his portion of the subject.

The association of some variety of the dysentery bacillus with a large number of the cases of epidemic diarrhœa in infancy has been definitely shown, through investigations carried on under the direction of the Rockefeller Institute for Medical Research. In the present series of cases an effort was made to isolate all organisms which could be supposed to be casually related to the disease, i. e., all pathogenic organisms, all bacteria which agglutinated with the patient's blood and all dysentery bacilli. Seventy-four cases in all were studied. They were not selected but were taken *seriatim*, according to the admissions, at The Thomas Wilson Sanitarium. The series comprised several clinical varieties of the disease: (a) toxic forms with fever and an acute onset (dyspeptic diarrhœa); (b) cases with evidence (either clinical or post mortem) of definite inflammatory changes in the intestine in addition to the symptoms of group a (ilio colitis). Of the first variety there were thirty-six cases out of the total seventy-four, and of the second, or inflammatory type, there were twenty-nine cases. A third and smaller group (c) of cases were termed cases of intestinal indigestion.

The methods of obtaining cultures were two: from the stools, by selecting bits of mucus and washing these in salt solution before making cultures, and secondly by scraping the intestine at autopsy. In our series the cases showing blood were thirty, and thirty-one had purulent material in the stools. The dysentery organism was found more readily when there was pus present—in 93 per cent of the cases with pus and in but 63 per cent of the cases when the stools contained only mucus with or without blood, while in 22 per cent of the cases studied the organism was found only at autopsy and had not been demonstrated during life. Altogether there were three hundred isolations made.

The organisms isolated were as follows: In six cases, streptococci in pure cultures; streptococci were present in eleven other cases; in two cases colon bacilli were present alone; in two cases, pyocyaneus alone, both of which organisms agglutinated with the blood of the patients. There were two cases with more or less extensive pseudo-membrane, one of which yielded a pure culture of the dysentery bacillus immediately while the other did not. All the cultures fell into one or another of the four groups of dysentery bacilli described by Hiss. The commonest strain found was the " Y " bacillus of Hiss and Russell, then the Flexner-Harris, and then the original Shiga. The agglutination reactions were tested as a routine with anti-dysentery serum and with the patient's blood, though with varying success. The serum reaction does not play as important a part in the diagnosis of this disease as it does in the case of typhoid fever. Absorption with the various sera—experiments showed that the Flexner-Harris serum had the largest amount of common agglutinins, the other forms possessing less, though all forms possessed some agglutinins in common.

The largest number of cases associated with any one form of bacillus was fourteen in which the " Y " form was found. Many infants belonging to this group were very ill; five were admitted in partial collapse. Several were very young (under one month old) on admission. Six cases were found infected with the Flexner-Harris organisms, the cases presenting widely different symptoms. Of these latter six cases, four recovered and two died. There were thirteen cases with mixed dysentery bacilli infection and all of these were severe cases, including eleven cases of definite ulcerative ilio-colitis, and one of tuberculous colitis, a double infection. These cases were usually admitted late in the summer. The stools were for the most part muco-purulent and blood stained. Nine died and seven at autopsy showed an ulcerative ilio-colitis.

The dysentery bacillus was associated with the streptococcus eleven times, of which cases seven resulted fatally, a mor-

tality of 67 per cent, and of the seven two had dyspeptic diarrhœa and five ilio-colitis. Streptococci were found alone in six instances, one case with ilio-colitis, three mild cases with dyspeptic diarrhœa, one with a mild diarrhœa after prolonged malnutrition, and one with an intestinal indigestion.

In five cases were other organisms found: two cases of colon bacillus infection, two of pyocyaneus, and one of a non-pathogenic organism.

In ten cases no organism was found at all, but several of these cases came in late at the end of the season and no autopsies were obtained.

The summary of the seventy-four cases studied is as follows: Forty-two, or 58 per cent, showed the presence of some of the four varieties of bacilli studied: streptococci were found in fifteen cases or 22.9 per cent; in ten cases no pathological organism at all was found. These were the late cases mentioned above. The organisms were found twice in other places than the alimentary canal, once in the liver and once in the mesenteric glands.

Differences in the severity of the illness can be noted in the several groups into which the cases have been divided according to the bacterial findings. Thus the largest proportion of instances of ilio-colitis and the highest mortality in any one group was noted in the series associated with more than one type of the dysentery organism. Here twelve out of the thirteen cases were ilio-colitis and nine died, a mortality of 69 per cent. Next in order of the severity of the infection is the group in which streptococci were found together with dysentery bacilli. Of these cases, eleven in number, seven were ilio-colitis and seven or 63.6 per cent died.

Of the fourteen cases associated with but one type of dysentery organism those with group II or Hiss " Y " bacilli seemed most severe. Six of them were instances of ilio-colitis and seven of them, or 50 per cent, ended fatally.

There were no extremely ill patients among those in whose dejecta unclassified dysentery bacilli, or pathogenic micro-organisms other than dysentery bacilli, or streptococci, were present.

NOTES ON NEW BOOKS.

Lectures on Tropical Diseases. Being the Lane lectures for 1905, delivered at the Cooper Medical College, San Francisco, U. S. A., August, 1905. By Sir PATRICK MANSON. 230 pp. [86 figs.] 8°. (*Chicago: W. T. Keener & Co.*)

An interesting, rather than a profound discussion of tropical medicine, illustrated with figures, most of which contribute but little to an exact understanding of the subject.

The Surgical Assistant. A Manual for Students, Practioners, Hospital Internes and Nurses. By WALTER M. BRICKNER, B. S., M. D., Chief Surgeon of Mt. Sinai Hospital Dispensary. (*Published by International Journal of Surgery Co., New York, 1905.*)

An interesting book to one who is making his debut in the operating room, giving some idea of what one's attitude should be and what a high potentiality of usefulness one may carry; a book indeed which may be even of more value to the hospital resident or operator who needs to instruct new assistants from time to time, inasmuch as by referring them to it he can expect them to be wise when they come into the operating room to the things which under usual circumstances he may find himself telling them at the end of the first month. The "dont's" alone, especially the shorter ones, if kept in mind will aid much in maintaining the proper relation of the new man on the staff.

The advice on cleaning up is good and quite thorough. It is to be regretted that the limited size of the book and extreme abundance of material treated prevents a consideration of those bacteriological findings which demonstrate experimentally the relative value of the different methods. One rather objects to the statement "for additional disinfection desirable if the asistant has recently been in contact with pus or other infectious material . . . . hands may be immersed in potassium permanganate . . . . ." Every person who uses rubber gloves must feel as did Dr. Halsted on introducing them in 1890, and as recently expressed by Sarwey, " dass die Hand niemals, der Handshuh stets keimfrei gemacht werden kann." (Bakteriologische untersuchungen über Handedisinfektion. Sarwey, Tubingen.) The "surgical assistant" with his various ward examinations, laboratory work, and even the exposure in daily life must feel that the most thorough is the only way and that the so-called " surgical habit," which licenses any one connected with operative work to think that cleaning up should be done less thoroughly on account of his not coming into contact with infectious material, is greatly to be deplored.

Were not anæsthetization such a large part of the duties of the surgical assistant, the chapter relating to this subject could well be omitted. It contains many valuable hints but the subject is so important that one who has any of it to do should necessarily be familiar with some more complete work which would make this chapter unnecessary. One is shocked to read, both in text and in illustration, " The index finger is on the facial artery, the thumb is testing the conjunctival reflexes." No one, we are certain, would touch the delicate conjunctiva of a person who is awake to ascertain what his general condition might be, much less while he is anæsthetized and unable to resist such dangerous and uncalled-for insult. Better to cover the eyes with rubber protective and do without any of the eye reflexes, even the much more important ones, than subject the patient to a possible unnecessary traumatic conjunctivitis.

It is truly remarkable that a man in writing a book could think of so many important and minute details which really give the book its chief value. We all know that no operator would be able to write down his exact procedure for an immediate operation, and this makes us feel that the part of the book devoted to the description of the various operations and what is expected of the assistant is chiefly of value in that it points out that an assistant after some experience with certain operations can be expected to be clever enough to outline a theoretical procedure, though he cannot reasonably hope to see it carried out in any subsequent identical operation. The illustrations are uniformly poor. The book contains formulæ for the preparation of surgical material to which, for personal use, it would have been well if a number of blank pages had been left so that methods could be added from time to time as the owner of the copy might see fit.   F.

Materia Medica. Pharmacy, and Therapeutics. By S. O. L. POTTER, M. D. (*Philadelphia: P. Blakiston's Son & Co., 1906.*)

The recent revision of the pharmacopeia has brought out new editions of almost all the works on materia medica and therapeutics. The present is the tenth edition of Dr. Potter's work and many additions have been made in it. The book opens with an introduction which contains some general statements regarding the subject and the various constituents of organic drugs. Following this is a section on the classification of medicines which is clear and satisfactory; the methods of administration and dosage are also described. Then follows a large section on materia medica and therapeutics in which the drugs are taken up alphabetically, and after a description of their preparation, the action and therapeutic use are described. Dr. Potter gives a great deal of information and it is interesting to see that he has devoted some attention to the historical side where this is possible. This section as a whole seems exceedingly well done and it is a pleasure to express appreciation of it. In this and the following sections on prescriptions and some methods of pharmaceutical preparations, there are many excellent practical points given.

The third part of the book deals with special therapeutics and it is regarding this that the reviewer feels regret that Dr. Potter has not used his materials in a better way. Diseases and symptoms are given alphabetically and under each one is a long list of remedies that may be used, so that for instance under albuminuria we have " aconite in incipient albuminuria with high body temperature. Lead diminishes the albumen. . . . Cannabis indica is indicated when bloody urine." Surely no one would hold that this is a satisfactory way to set out treatment and it cannot be regarded as either rational or scientific. Many other examples of this might be given, but it would seem that to-day we should be past this nickel-in-the-slot method of teaching therapeutics. Thus under diphtheria we find proper reference to the use of antitoxin but in addition twenty-one drugs mentioned as useful for their internal action, among which we find myrrh, cubeb, and sanguinaria. Does any one to-day consider that these drugs are indicated as internal remedies in diphtheria? There are many excellent recommendations for treatment, but this method of presenting them we believe to be bad and unlikely to tend to rational treatment.

It is surprising in this section on special therapeutics to find five and a half pages devoted to the clinical examination of the urine. This doubtless gives some excellent information, but a work on therapeutics is not the place for it and the space might have been put to better use. In the appendix with a list of contractions and Latin phrases, certain formulæ for hypodermic administration and of some patent medicines, we find six pages given to differential diagnosis. It is difficult to understand what possible excuse there is for putting this in a work on therapeutics.

And when we find the differential diagnosis given between yellow fever and bilious remittent fever one feels like making the humble query as to what is meant by bilious remittent fever? The best text-books of medicine do not mention it.

It is a pleasure to commend the good features of this work, as shown especially in the section on materia medica, but we consider it as much our duty to speak out plainly regarding the section on special therapeutics. It seems too bad that an author to-day would put out such an arrangement. There are of course excellent therapeutic directions given, but it is the irrational and unscientific arrangement which should be so strongly condemned. The work as a whole fails to give anything like a proper discussion of therapeutic measures other than the giving of drugs, which after all is but a small part of the subject of treatment.

Atlas and Epitome of Operative Gynecology. By DR. OSKAR SCHAEFFER, Privatdocent of Obstetrics and Gynecology in the University of Heidelberg. Edited by J. CLARENCE WEBSTER, M. D. (Edin.), F. R. C. P. E., F. R. S. E.; with 42 colored lithographic plates and many text illustrations, some of them in color. (*Philadelphia: W. B. Saunders & Co., 1904.*)

The author of this volume prefaces it by saying that it seems to him appropriate, in an atlas designed to represent technic as it appears to the eye, to classify operations, not according to the parts or organs on which they are performed, but according to the methods of gaining access to them for purposes of operation. He divides his subject, therefore, into " Operations that are performed without the speculum," " Operations requiring for their performance exposure of the vagina," and other divisions of the same character, the whole number being ten. This idea is certainly a new departure in gynecology, but there does not seem to be anything sufficiently advantageous in the results to justify so great a departure from accepted methods.

Apart from the matter of division there does not appear to be anything new or striking in the book, the text of which is written in accordance with principles and methods which are certainly conventional if not antiquated. For example, in discussing perineal operations, the writer adheres to the restricted classification of some time ago, by which lacerations were divided into three classes, namely, those extending to the thicker part of the perineum; those extending to the sphincter; and those extending through the sphincter. In other words, lacerations of the first, second, and third degrees. All the various modifications of these great divisions, upon which modern gynecology has developed such a variety of plastic work, are not alluded to, except for a passing mention of the class of cases in which the integument remains intact though the tissues underneath have given way. The treatment of other subjects is similar to this and the book as a whole, while it is clear in expression and reliable in methods, cannot be regarded as fruitful in new ideas or expedients.

The text, however, as in all books of this kind, is subordinate to the illustrations, with which it is liberally provided. Every variety of operation is depicted with most conscientious attention to detail, but it is impossible not to regret the crudity of the means employed. As a means of designating the position of nerves and blood-vessels, of reproducing the stains employed in the preparation of pathological specimens, and of demonstrating the details of surgical operations, such as the lines of incisions, areas of denudation, and the like, color has its use and purpose; but when the most florid tints and the highest possible glaze are employed solely for the purpose of making the whole illustration as striking as possible to the eye, we can only recall the gaudy picture books of our infancy and wonder at what age the public outgrows its childish tastes. Another matter for regret is the want of accuracy in the proportion of different objects and of

judgment in the selection of tints; as for instance, in the representations of surgical procedures where the needles, scissors, and sutures are all of the same shade of gray (which belongs by nature to none of them), and all three objects are of nearly the same size.

The translator has done his work well, and the editorial comments, which show a marked tendency to enlarge the ideas presented, add greatly to the value of the book.

Man and his Poisons. A practical exposition of the causes, symptoms, and treatment of self-poisoning. By ALBERT ABRAMS, M. D. (Heidelberg), F. R. M. S. Illustrated. (*New York: E. B. Treat & Co., 1906.*)

This little volume is a step in the right direction. The whole trend of modern medical knowledge goes to show that man carries within himself the causes of disease, and that a long train of morbid conditions, hitherto misunderstood, are occasioned either by poisons generated within his own system or by the impairment of the processes known as internal secretion, the importance of which to our well-being we are now beginning to estimate. The question of self-poisoning, as the writer truly remarks, ' Has advanced from a plausible and fascinating theory to a verity."

We took up the book with strong hopes of finding the subject of self-poisoning greatly illuminated by it, but we must confess to considerable disappointment at finding it to consist largely of discursive reviews of the speculations hitherto rife upon the subject when we had expected (not unreasonably, we think,) some practical contribution to our present knowledge. The chapter treating of the influence of mind upon body contains some interesting instances of results obtained by suggestion in persons of susceptible temperament, but we cannot help feeling a greater share of interest in the side of the question which is left untouched, namely, the extent to which such influences can be exercised upon persons whose temperament does not lend itself to them. Dr. Abrams tells a story of a French scientist who gave one hundred hospital patients some water, telling them that it was for purposes of experiment. Shortly afterwards he informed them, in a state of great apparent alarm, that he had given them an emetic by mistake. The result was that four-fifths were taken violently sick. No attention, however, is given to the one-fifth who remained unaffected, and this to our thinking really begs the question, for it leaves the most interesting side of it untouched. We have already abundant evidence that the effect of suggestion upon impressionable persons is very strong, and we are, moreover, fully satisfied that the majority of people are impressionable. It is the minority who are not affected by influences to which their fellows succumb upon whom our interest is centered; and to ascertain how far they also can be affected by the same processes of a stronger degree, or by other processes of a different character is a problem which would well repay investigation.

The whole book is characterized by this same excess of discussion and speculation and while it is, as we have said, a step in the right direction it cannot be said to lead us far along it.

The Four Epochs of a Woman's Life. A study in hygiene. By ANNA M. GALBRAITH, M. D.; with an introductory note by JOHN H. MUSSER, M. D., Professor of Clinical Medicine, University of Pennsylvania. Second edition, revised and enlarged. (*Philadelphia, New York, and London: W. B. Saunders & Co.*)

There is a good deal of sound common sense in this little book, which should recommend it to those who wish to understand the best means of preserving the health and strength of women, either in their own case or in that of others committed to their care. The literary style is clear and simple, and the writer has been successful in what is often a matter of some difficulty, namely, the use of technical terms without confusion to the uninitiated. She has, however, foreseen the possibility of difficulty in this respect, for she has added a glossary in which the meaning of any word not familiar to the reader is at once at his command.

The chief defect is one common to all books of the class to which it belongs, and that is an unconscious assumption that all claims and obligations should and will yield to the requirements of an ideal hygienic life, as depicted in its pages. From one point of view this is, of course, the proper attitude, for a medical or quasi-medical book is nothing if not didactic; nevertheless, we must believe that a certain amount of adaptation to the difficulties and hindrances with which all women, and especially all self-supporting women, have to contend would be both possible and advisable. The book, as a whole, however, is useful and wholesome; and the fact that it has reached a second edition shows that a niche was ready for it to fill.

Obstetrical and Gynecological Nursing. By EDWARD P. DAVIS. A. M., M. D., Professor of Obstetrics in the Jefferson Medical College, etc. Illustrated. (*Philadelphia, New York, and London: W. B. Saunders & Co.*)

The obstetrical part of this work is full and interesting. All the various peculiarities of obstetrical nursing as compared with nursing of the ordinary character are judiciously pointed out and clearly discussed. Some of the statements strike us as a little behind the times, as, for example, the recommendation of the obstetrical binder, which the best authorities now regard as injurious and a potent factor in the causation of retro-displacements.

The gynecological division of the book occupies much less space than the obstetrical, and the subject is insufficiently treated. It would, however, be impossible to treat both subjects adequately in a volume the size of this one. The importance and scope of gynecological nursing and the many variations of pathological conditions with which it has to deal, cause it to require a much greater space than obstetrical nursing, which in the majority of cases does not deal with any pathological condition at all. It is only a matter of surprise that the two subjects should be treated together at all.

Baby Incubators. A clinical study of the premature infant with especial reference to incubator institutes conducted for show purposes. By JOHN ZAHORSKY, A. B., M. D., Clinical Professor of Pediatrics, Medical Department Washington University, St. Louis. Reprinted from a series of articles in the St. Louis Courier of Medicine, 1905. (*St. Louis: Courier of Medicine Co., 1905.*)

There is a great deal in this little book to render it of unusual interest. It is, in all probability, the first comprehensive account of the work accomplished by the so-called show incubators, and although the detailed descriptions of the various kinds of incubators and their comparative merits are acceptable to only a few, there is much in the nature and results of the work accomplished that is full of general interest.

The writer of the little volume was in charge of the institute where infants were reared in incubators at the St. Louis Exposition of 1904, and he shows plainly that he entered heartily into the good which such an establishment accomplishes, even though it owes its origin to the gratification of the public curiosity. The display of incubators at the Exposition was, of course, purely a business affair, but it was none the less well managed, under the charge of competent physicians and well-trained nurses. Its results show plainly that much good can be accomplished by such means among the poorer classes. In private practice and among well-to-do people, the writer thinks the method is not to be rec-

ommended, for, as he points out, the sole function of the incubator is to lessen heat loss, and any methods which serve the purpose for the individual case do all that an incubator can accomplish. The supply of artificial heat, however, is only one, and that not the greatest benefit which public incubators bestow upon premature children. Their value is really much greater in what they effect indirectly than in what they accomplish through the exercise of their own proper function, for, as Dr. Zahorsky shows, the greatest difficulty in the rearing of premature children is not the prevention of heat loss, but the maintenance of a proper nutrition, and this is an end which the public incubators achieve incidentally, but none the less efficiently. The attendance which is essential to their success is really the source of greatest benefit to the infant, for by means of it he obtains the care which the homes of the poorer classes cannot afford.

There can be no doubt from the results shown here that public incubators in our large cities would be a source of great good, not only through the exercise of their proper functions, but on account of the attendant nursing, which of course includes suitable nutrition and all the minor hygienic accessories, such as cleanliness and ventilation. If some of our generous benefactors would find the wherewithal to establish free institutions for the raising of premature infants by means of incubation, there is no doubt that many little lives which are otherwise doomed would be saved.

The book is one which will repay reading. It is full of interesting detail and its attraction is increased by the impression it creates of personal interest on the part of the writer. He admits frankly that the elimination of what he calls "hospital atmosphere" is an important factor in the success of the work, and it is the absence of a certain coldness and indifference that is often associated with accounts of institutional work together with the presence of an indefinable sensation of heartiness and kindly feeling which render the book so attractive.

The Signs of Internal Disease. With a brief consideration of the principal symptoms thereof. By PEARCE KINTZING, B. Sc., M. D., Professor of Physical Diagnosis and Diseases of the Heart, Maryland Medical College. Illustrated. (*Chicago: Cleveland Press, 1906.*)

The book is divided broadly into diseases of the chest and of the abdomen, together with a general outline of the examination of the urine and fæces.

In the chapters devoted to the diseases of the chest the various methods of examination are discussed. A brief review follows of the more important anatomical points from a clinical standpoint, elucidated by many diagrams and plates, not all original, which should clear away any uncertainties in the student mind. The various physical signs are then considered and their significance noted. Finally the more common signs of such diseases of the lungs, as bronchitis, pleurisy, pneumonia, and tuberculosis, are passed hastily in review. This same general scheme is carried out in regard to the heart and the various abdominal conditions. There is also a short chapter on the Roentgen ray in diagnosis.

In order to cover so much ground in 355 pages it has been necessary to be brief and to treat many subjects in a more or less superficial manner. Indeed in one or two instances there have been important omissions, as a consideration of empyema and fibroid phthisis in the diseases of the lungs.

In order to be concise, many of the statements appear rather dogmatic and in some of the diseases, notably pericarditis, exceptions are taken to them. On the whole, however, the writer has given a brief outline of internal medicine, which should prove of value to the beginner in this subject.

The Diseases of Infancy and Childhood. By HENRY KOPLIK, M. D. Second edition. (*New York: Lea Brothers & Co., 1906.*)

A second edition of this text-book on The Diseases of Infancy and Childhood by Dr. Koplik has recently appeared. The writer's large clinical experience and thorough laboratory training render this work peculiarly valuable. The arrangement of chapters in the first edition has been somewhat altered in this one and considerable new material has been added.

A fairly complete introductory chapter on the anatomy in infancy and childhood would improve the book for the general reader, who could then easily turn to facts concerning the structure and relationship of the important organs at several important age periods before taking up the systematic study of the diseased conditions. A very good account of the urine in infancy appears in the introductory chapter, page 31, but little is said of the character of the feces and the description of the blood in normal children is reserved until Chapter IX.

In the directions for history-taking, more emphasis could properly be laid upon the character of the diet before the onset of the illness; and in the methods of procedure in the physical examination of infants, the desirability of proceeding with auscultation of the chest after inspection and before palpation and percussion is not impressed upon the reader, and there are some situations in which the phonendescope is of great service.

Dr. Koplik's description of the management and hygiene of the normal infant and of the various methods of therapy is concise and accurate. Fortunately gavage or forced alimentation is rarely necessary, but in our experience, the introduction of food through a nasal catheter is often more satisfactory than by means of a stomach tube.

Section II of the book is devoted to the much-discussed question of infant feeding. The section has been completely recast and much new matter added. The chemistry of human milk and cow's milk is carefully presented but with sufficient fulness to enable the student to understand the nature of the infant's natural food and the important differences which exist in the milk of animals.

The writer lays more stress, very properly, on the necessity of clean milk and less on the minute modification of the ingredients except for a few cases. The value of the so-called American System of Milk Modification is not that there is any special advantage to be gained in changing the baby's proteid from 1% to 1.1% or the fat from 2% to 2.2%, but that largely through the introduction of the percentage feeding the physician has it in his power to change the particular ingredient of the diet that seems to be at fault without altering the remainder of the formula.

Dr. Koplik details his method of milk modification, using as a rule 12% top milk, upper 9 oz., of a quart of milk allowed to stand several hours. It is probable that the ratio of fat and proteid is nearer 4:1 than 3:1 as calculated by Dr. Koplik, and that he has used the method so successfully only illustrates that minute variations in percentages are not as important as pure milk. Probably in another edition less stress will be laid on treating milk either by Pasteurizing or sterilizing, even in hot weather, and more on the bacterial count of the milk on delivery and on its proper refrigeration. At present some form of treating seems necessary among the poorer classes. The discussion of the proprietary foods is fair. Their use in exceptional cases and with full knowledge of their composition is permissible.

Koplik's experience with plain barley water versus dextrinized gruel for very young infants is difficult to explain. It is well to have the admirable method of Keller for making cereal gruels, described in an American text-book, page 149.

All the ills the newly-born baby can be heir to are discussed in the following section. Fortunately many of these are exceedingly rare and others are more often seen by the Obstetrician than by the Pediatrician. The care necessary for the successful raising of premature babies is well described. Possibly in this connection a little too much emphasis is laid on the importance of the incubator, which even in its simplest form requires constant and skilled attention, and moreover brilliant results can often be obtained at room temperature and with properly applied external heat.

The chief addition which Dr. Koplik has made to the section on infectious diseases is in the chapter on meningitis which has been admirably rewritten and the writer's unusual large experience during the recent epidemic in New York has been freely drawn upon. The bedside distinctions between the epidemic and the tuberculous forms of the disease are clearly stated. Lumbar puncture is advised in all cases of meningitis. A precise description of the best method of carrying out the procedure in children is given and there is a sufficiently full account for clinical purposes of the cytology of the spinal fluid. Considerable new material has been added to the account of typhoid fever in infancy and childhood and the probability that the disease is more frequent during early life than was formerly supposed is properly suggested. The disinfection of the urine as well as the stools should be specifically insisted upon. Various psychoses should be included among the complications and sequelæ. The discussion of the other infectious diseases has been little altered in this edition and few of the more recent references to the literature have been added.

The serum treatment of scarlet fever which seems helpful in the hands of Escherich and his assistants deserves mention, as does the Dock method of vaccination.

The section on Diseases of the Digestive System has been rearranged; no notable additions have been made. Added experience has shown the prognosis in surgical interference in cases of pyloric stenosis to be better than Dr. Koplik leads one to hope, and the cause of the stricture is now known to be a hypertrophy of the circular muscular layer.

In the discussion of the etiology of Summer Diarrhoeas of infancy it is to be regretted that Dr. Koplik has apparently given no credence to the recent investigations conducted by many workers under the direction of the Rockefeller Institute for Medical Research. These have shown conclusively that the dysentery bacillus is associated with a considerable number of even the milder forms of epidemic summer diarrhœa as well as with many cases of ulcerative ileocolitis and is not confined to those forms of diarrhœa resembling adult bacillary dysentery. The term dysentery of infants if etiologically employed must include intestinal affections of varied nature and intensity.

The excellent research of Wentworth should be mentioned in any recent description of infantile atrophy.

There are many useful suggestions in the chapter on constipation in infants and children.

Congenital dilatation of the colon, acute intestinal obstruction, and appendicitis are all fully considered (there are no references for the student appended later than 1901). In the discussion of the diseases of the throat, bronchi, and lungs and heart the extensive bedside experience of the writer is used to good purpose.

Following the chapter on rickets, in which the important contributions of Kassowitz and his students are given full credit, there is a brief discussion of the more unusual diseases of the skeleton, Chondrody's trophia fœtalis and osteogenesis imperfecta.

As Dr. Koplik says, diabetic mellitus is of rare occurrence in infancy and childhood, and hardly sufficient attention is called to the very grave prognosis from this disease in early life.

The blood diseases are fully treated. The author accepts the pseudoleukemia anæmia of Von Jaksch as a clinical entity, a position which is denied by some of the latest writers. Concerning the relationship between the lymphatic apparatus and the number and nature of the lymphocytes few positive statements of fact can be made at present.

The section on diseases of the ear is timely. It would have been well to follow it with a brief consideration of the diseases of the external eye, as simple affections of the lids and conjunctiva must often be treated by the pediatrician and the subject is omitted in most of the American text-books.

In the discussion of the diseases of the kidney Dr. Koplik has adopted the somewhat disputed classification of nephritis advanced by Delafield. In the treatment of nephritis the recent suggestions of Dr. Morse deserve mention, by which the proteid metabolism is decreased and yet the calorific value of the diet maintained by increasing the proportion of cream in the milk mixtures. One misses also any allusion to the regional anatomy of the kidney.

The discussion of the infections of the urethra, bladder, and external genitalia is excellent.

The affections of the nervous system are considered rather briefly in Section XIII. In the treatment of convulsions Dr. Koplik places the patient's head low to relieve the cerebral anæmia which he asserts is present through the attack. It has usually been taught that the brain is in a state of venous congestion during the eclamptic seizure, in which case this postural treatment would be contraindicated.

The outlook in congenital internal hydrocephalus, absolutely grave under the older methods, has been made somewhat better than Dr. Koplik indicates, by surgical interference and the establishment of permanent drainage from the spinal canal to the cavity.

The first section of Book IX is devoted to the more important diseases of the skin in infancy and childhood.

The book is carefully edited and well printed. It is especially valuable among other American text-books on pediatrics on account of the distinction of the author and because it perhaps more than any text-book on the subject in this country reflects the influence of the fundamental contributions that have been made to our knowledge in this field from the German laboratories and clinics.　　　　　　　　　　　　　　　　　　　J. H. M. K. Jr.

Burdett's Hospital and Charities, 1906. Being the Year-Book of Philanthropy and the Hospital Annual, containing a review of the position and requirements, and chapters on the Management, Revenue, and Cost of the Charities. An exhaustive record of Hospital Work for the year. It will also be found to be the most useful and reliable guide to British, American, and Colonial Hospitals and Asylums, Medical Schools and Colleges, Nursing and Convalescent Institutions, Consumption Sanatoria, Religious and Benevolent Institutions and Dispensaries. By Sir Henry Burdett, K. C. B. (*London: The Scientific Press Limited, 28 and 29 Southampton Street, Strand, W. C.*)

The Annual for 1906 contains its usual valuable and instructive figures. The book, in fact, is interesting to an American from cover to cover as indicating the condition of hospital administration abroad as well as in America. The advertisements even convey much food for reflection; as, for example, where Guy's Hospital makes an appeal for £43,000 to pay debts and an annual fund of £25,000 for running expenses. There is a degree of comfort in reading these appeals, because hospital men in America have been led to think that they were extravagant and foolhardy in projecting improvements beyond the income of the hospital. We know of no hospital, however, in this country which has upwards of $200,000 of debt and which requires an annual subscrip-

tion of $125,000 for running expenses. It is interesting to see that nowhere else can we get as reliable statistics concerning the hospitals in America as are contained in this Annual. The labor incident to the analysis of the figures presented in this volume is colossal, and a master-mind is required to make the proper deductions from them.

A chapter from Dr. Goldwater, of the Mt. Sinai Hospital in New York, on American hospitals is of interest, however reluctant we may be to accept his conclusions. We would commend the chapter on the "League of Mercy" to charitable workers in America. The book should be in the hands of every hospital worker and might be consulted with advantage by every board of trustees.

The World's Anatomists. By G. W. H. Kemper, M. D. (*Philadelphia: P. Blakiston's Son & Co., 1905.*)

This little book of seventy-nine pages is a compilation of a series of papers originally published in the Medical Book News during 1904. A number of names have been added so that in the present form there are treated two hundred and twenty-nine names. There is a brief description of the life of each anatomist, mention of his most important writings, and of his principal anatomical discoveries, making a very convenient reference book to those who wish to refresh or add to their knowledge of medical history. The criticism might be made that the notes are too brief, but perhaps were they longer they would be referred to less often. The book is a most convenient and valuable one and every physician and student should have one on his work table.
　　　　　　　　　　　　　　　　　　　　　　　　　　W. R. D.

Chirurgie Oto-Rhino-Laryngologique. Par George Laurens. (*Paris: G. Steinheil, Editeur.*)

This monumental work represents, in our opinion, the best exposition of the surgery of the affections of the nose, throat, and ear in any language. As the title indicates, this work deals solely with the surgical treatment of diseases of these organs.

The operations on the various parts are preceded by a short but thorough anatomical description. The treatment before, during, and after the operation is given with minute detail. The various complications that may arise are carefully considered. The various operations devised for a particular disease are described in detail, their rationale as well as their advantages and disadvantages.

This work of one thousand pages indicates in a way the tremendous progress that has been made in these special branches. One cannot understand how any surgeon untrained in special technique, can attempt this class of surgery.　　　　　S. R.

Genito-Urinary Surgery and Venereal Diseases. By J. William White, M. D., and Edward Martin, M. D. Sixth Edition. (*Philadelphia and London: J. B. Lippincott Company, 1905.*)

The general value of this work and its high standing among English text-books on genito-urinary diseases are well recognized by the medical profession. It is desirable now merely to note the innovations and additions in this recent edition. The arrangement of presentation is improved. The general features of disorders of the urinary tract are taken up in a separate chapter and not appended to the article on the bladder as heretofore. Urethritis is considered broadly, its etiology systematically stated, and gonorrhea is made a sub-head, yet of course is given the minute attention its etiological importance demands. In the section on gonorrhea we note the condensation or elimination of many paragraphs, a refining process which might advantageously be pushed further throughout the book. Cystoscopy and ureteral catheterization are considered at greater length. However, the value of cystoscopy in prostatic hypertrophy is not brought out—scarcely mentioned. In the section on enlarged prostate is given a good brief résumé of the operative treatment of benign hypertrophy, although the authors still insist that castration is indicated in some cases. The chapters on syphilis are placed at the end of the book, and a newly arranged index completes the volume.

In general, the subject matter has been brought up to date, and with the many improvements in arrangement, this edition promises to be of great value to both the student and practitioner.

Die Placentation Beim Menschen. Von J. Clarence Webster. Translation into German by Dr. Gustav Kolischer. (*Berlin: Oscar Coblentz.*)

The present monograph is a translation of the volume published in English in 1901, and already made the subject of review in the Bulletin. Profesor Webster is to be congratulated on the demand to render his work more accessible to German readers.

Two notable changes from the former edition are to be found: First, there is a most striking improvement in the illustrations. These remain the same in subject-matter with the addition of two or three new cuts, but the reproduction is invariably larger. The result is a much clearer and more detailed picture than formerly. Again, the more diagrammatic drawings now given do away with the indistinctness which diminished so much the value of the earlier ones.

The second change lies in extending the text so as to include a chapter on placenta prævia. A review of the various theories regarding the causation of the condition is given. The author regards the formation of the placenta from the decidua reflexa as the more common factor in the etiology of the condition. However, these cases most frequently eventuate in early abortion. Those instances in which pregnancy advances to term are more likely explained by an originally low implantation of the ovum in the uterine cavity.

The work of translation has been very well done.

Scientific Memoirs. By Officers of the Medical and Sanitary Departments of the Government of India. Serum-Therapy of Plague in India. Reports by Mr. W. M. Haffkine, C. I. E., and Various Officers of the Plague Research Laboratory, Bombay. Edited with an introduction by Lieut.-Col. W. B. Bannerman, M. D., B. Sc., F. R. S. E., I. M. S., Calcutta. (New Series) No. 20. *Office of the Superintendent of Government Printing, India, 1905.*

The conclusions reached by careful observers of the effect of different anti-plague sera are that the remedy is far less effective than the serum used in the treatment of diphtheria, that to be most effective, injections of any sera are those which pass directly into the blood stream and overwhelm the bacilli at once by mass action, as it is believed, and finally that the use of sera does not affect the case-mortality in the slightest degree. It is believed, however, that sera do prolong life. They also lower the temperature, lessen the pulse and respiration rate, diminish delirium and restlessness, cause a disappearance of buboes and lessen pain in them. This gives encouragement to a further trial of serum-therapy.

The Physical Examination of Infants and Young Children. By Theron Wendell Kilmer, M. D. (*Philadelphia: F. A. Davis Co., 1906.*)

In the preface the author states that nearly all the text-books on pediatrics are deficient in their treatment of the subject of the physical examination of infants. " We must forget and unlearn all the things we ever knew about adults when we come to the examination of children." He also states " that he makes no pretense as to outlining physical diagnosis nor pathological conditions of any kind whatsoever; his only aim is to instruct the student and physician how to examine a baby."

In spite of the author's statement in the preface the book contains little else than a rather crude review of the technique of physical examination, including history-taking, inspection, palpation, auscultation, percussion and the examination of the special organs, excretions, etc. The book contains 84 pages and 59 illustrations. The only illustrations which might be of value to a student are four indicating the outlines of organs at the ages of 11 months and 5 years, and two indicating the technique of lumbar puncture.

Nursing: Its Principles and Practice. For hospital and private use. By Isabel Hampton Robb, late Superintendent of Nurses and Principal of the Training School for Nurses, Johns Hopkins Hospital; late Superintendent of Nurses, Illinois Training School for Nurses. Third edition, revised and enlarged. Illustrated. (*Cleveland: E. C. Koeckert, Publisher, 715 Rose Building, 1906.*)

Notices of previous editions of this book have appeared in the Bulletin. The important changes which have been made in the third edition indicate in a striking manner how much the training of nurses has developed during the past twelve years. The book has been practically rewritten and brought up to date. It is unquestionably the best manual for teaching the principles and practice of nursing which we possess. The specific directions given for nursing the sick, the hygiene of the sick room, sterilization and disinfection, the care of patients, methods of taking temperature, giving baths, making external applications, giving medicines, observing and recording symptoms, feeding the sick, and the like, are clear, explicit, and well stated. The special chapters also on the operating room, gynecological operations, the administration of anesthetics, and the nursing and care of infectious diseases are to be especially commended. All things considered, the book has profited greatly by its careful revision and can be commended for use in all training schools.

A Laboratory Manual of Physiological Chemistry.. By E. W. Lockwood, M. D., Ph. D. Second edition. (*Philadelphia: F. A. Davis Company, 1906.*)

The first edition of this elementary manual was reviewed in this journal in February, 1900. The work has been somewhat enlarged, the number of experiments described being increased from 340 to 425. The author has failed to correct some obvious errors which occurred in the first edition. Thus on page 142 he still maintains that the reaction of milk " may be amphoteric to litmus; that is, it turns red paper blue and blue paper red." However, the manual is fairly satisfactory and deserves to be recommended.

Nasal Sinus Surgery with Operations on Nose and Throat. By Beaman Douglas, M. D. (*Philadelphia: F. A. Davis Co., 1906.*)

This small excellent work briefly summarizes the operative treatment of the diseases of the nose and throat. We recommend it to those interested in the surgery of these affections. Well illustrated anatomical descriptions are given of the affected parts, previous to the description of the operations.

The book is nicely printed and is an agreeable addition to the various works in this field.   S. R.

THE JOHNS HOPKINS HOSPITAL REPORTS.

VOLUME I. 423 pages, 99 plates.

VOLUME II. 570 pages, with 28 plates and figures.

VOLUME III. 766 pages, with 69 plates and figures.

VOLUME IV. 504 pages, 33 charts and illustrations.

VOLUME V. 480 pages, with 32 charts and illustrations.

CONTENTS :

The Malarial Fevers of Baltimore. By W. S. THAYER, M. D., and J. HEWETSON, M. D.

A Study of some Fatal Cases of Malaria. By LEWELLYS F. BARKER, M. B.

Studies in Typhoid Fever.

By WILLIAM OSLER, M. D., with additional papers by G. BLUMER, M. D., SIMON FLEXNER, M. D., WALTER REED, M. D., and H. C. PARSONS, M. D.

VOLUME VI. 414 pages, with 79 plates and figures.

Report in Neurology.

Studies on the Lesions Produced by the Action of Certain Poisons on the Cortical Nerve Cell (Studies Nos. I to V). By HENRY J. BERKLEY, M. D.

Introductory.—Recent Literature on the Pathology of Diseases of the Brain by the Chromate of Silver Methods; Part I.—Alcohol Poisoning.— Experimental Lesions produced by Chronic Alcoholic Poisoning (Ethyl Alcohol). 2. Experimental Lesions produced by Acute Alcoholic Poisoning (Ethyl Alcohol) ; Part II.—Serum Poisoning.—Experimental Lesions induced by the Action of the Dog's Serum on the Cortical Nerve Cell ; Part III.—Ricin Poisoning.—Experimental Lesions induced by Acute Ricin Poisoning. 2. Experimental Lesions induced by Chronic Ricin Poisoning ; Part IV.—Hydrophobic Toxæmia.—Lesions of the Cortical Nerve Cell produced by the Toxine of Experimental Rabies ; Part V.—Pathological Alterations in the Nuclei and Nucleoli of Nerve Cells from the Effects of Alcohol and Ricin Intoxication ; Nerve Fibre Terminal Apparatus ; Asthenic Bulbar Paralysis. By HENRY J. BERKLEY, M. D.

Report in Pathology.

Fatal Puerperal Sepsis due to the Introduction of an Elm Tent. By THOMAS S. CULLEN, M. B.

Pregnancy in a Rudimentary Uterine Horn. Rupture, Death, Probable Migration of Ovum and Spermatozoa. By THOMAS S. CULLEN, M. B., and G. L. WILKINS, M. D.

Adeno-Myoma Uteri Diffusum Benignum. By THOMAS S. CULLEN, M. B.

A Bacteriological and Anatomical Study of the Summer Diarrhœas of Infants. By WILLIAM D. BOOKER, M. D.

The Pathology of Toxalbumin Intoxications. By SIMON FLEXNER, M. D.

VOLUME VII. 537 pages with illustrations.

I. A Critical Review of Seventeen Hundred Cases of Abdominal Section from the standpoint of Intra-peritoneal Drainage. By J. G. CLARK, M. D.

II. The Etiology and Structure of true Vaginal Cysts. By JAMES ERNEST STOKES, M. D.

III. A Review of the Pathology of Superficial Burns, with a Contribution to our Knowledge of the Pathological Changes in the Organs in cases of rapidly fatal burns. By CHARLES RUSSELL BARDEEN, M. D.

IV. The Origin, Growth and Fate of the Corpus Luteum. By J. G. CLARK, M. D.

V. The Results of Operations for the Cure of Inguinal Hernia. By JOSEPH C. BLOODGOOD, M. D.

VOLUME VIII. 552 pages with illustrations.

On the rôle of Insects, Arachnids, and Myriapods as carriers in the spread of Bacterial and Parasitic Diseases of Man and Animals. By GEORGE H. F. NUTTALL, M. D., PH. D.

Studies in Typhoid Fever.

By WILLIAM OSLER, M. D., with additional papers by J. M. T. FINNEY, M. D., S. FLEXNER, M. D., I. P. LYON, M. D., L. F. HAMBURGER, M. D., H. W. CUSHING, M. D., J. F. MITCHELL, M. D., C. N. B. CAMAC, M. D., N. B. GWYN, M. D., CHARLES P. EMERSON, M. D., H. H. YOUNG, M. D., and W. S. THAYER, M. D.

VOLUME IX. 1060 pages, 66 plates and 210 other illustrations.

Contributions to the Science of Medicine.

Dedicated by his Pupils to WILLIAM HENRY WELCH, on the twenty-fifth anniversary of his Doctorate. This volume contains 38 separate papers.

VOLUME X. 516 pages, 12 plates and 25 charts.

Structure of the Malarial Parasites. Plate I. By JESSE W. LAZEAR, M. D.

The Bacteriology of Cystitis, Pyelitis and Pyelonephritis in Women, with a Consideration of the Accessory Etiological Factors in these Conditions, and of the Various Chemical and Microscopical Questions involved. By THOMAS R. BROWN, M. D.

Cases of Infection with Strongyloides Intestinalis. (First Reported Occurrence in North America.) Plates II and III. By RICHARD P. STRONG, M. D.

On the Pathological Changes in Hodgkin's Disease, with Especial Reference to its Relation to Tuberculosis. Plates IV-VII. By DOROTHY M. REED, M. D.

Diabetes Insip dus, with a Report of Five Cases. By THOMAS B. FUTCHER, M. B. (Tor.).

Observations on the Origin and Occurrence of Cells with Eosinophile Granulations in Normal and Pathological Tissues. Plate VIII. By W. T. HOWARD, M. D., and R. G. PERKINS, M. D.

Placental Transmissions, with Report of a Case during Typhoid Fever. By FRANK W. LYNCH, M. D.

Metabolism in Albuminuria. By CHAS. P. EMERSON, A. B., M. D.

Regenerative Changes in the Liver after Acute Yellow Atrophy. Plates IX-XII. By W. G. MACCALLUM, M. D.

Surgical Features of Typhoid Fever. By THOS. MCCRAE, M. B., M. R. C. P. (Lond.), and JAMES F. MITCHELL, M. D.

The Symptoms, Diagnosis and Surgical Treatment of Ureteral Calculus. By BENJAMIN R. SCHENCK, M. D.

VOLUME XI. .555 pages, with 38 charts and illustrations.

Pneumothorax: A historical, clinical and experimental study. By CHARLES P. EMERSON, M. D.

Clinical Observations on Blood Pressure. By HENRY W. COOK, M. D., and JOHN B. BRIGGS, M. D.

The value of Tuberculin in Surgical Diagnosis. By MARTIN B. TINKER, M. D.

VOLUME XII. 548 pages, 12 plates and other illustrations.

The Connective Tissue of the Salivary Glands and Pancreas with its Development in the Glandula Submaxillaris. Plates I-III. By JOSEPH MARSHALL FLINT, M. D.

A New Instrument for Determining the Minimum and Maximum Blood-Pressures in Man. Plates IV-X. By JOSEPH ERLANGER, M. D.

Metabolism in Pregnancy, Labor, and the Puerperium. By J. MORRIS SLEMONS, M. D.

An Experimental Study of Blood-Pressure and of Pulse-Pressure in Man. Plates XI and XII. By JOSEPH ERLANGER, M. D., and DONALD R. HOOKER, A. B., M. S.

Typhoid Meningitis. By RUFUS I. COLE, M. D.

The Pathological Anatomy of Meningitis due to Bacillus Typhosus. By WILLIAM G. MACCALLUM, M. D.

A Comparative Study of White and Negro Pelves, with a Consideration of the Size of the Child and its Relation to Presentation and Character of Labor in the Two Races. By THEODORE F. RIGGS, M. D.

Renal Tuberculosis. By GEORGE WALKER, M. D.

VOLUME XIII. (In press.)

The Johns Hopkins Hospital Bulletins are issued monthly. They are printed by the FRIEDENWALD CO., Baltimore. Single copies may be procured from NUNN & CO. and the BALTIMORE NEWS CO., Baltimore. Subscriptions, $2.00 a year, may be addressed to the publishers, THE JOHNS HOPKINS PRESS, BALTIMORE; single copies will be sent by mail for twenty-five cents each.

BULLETIN

OF

THE JOHNS HOPKINS HOSPITAL

Entered as Second-Class Matter at the Baltimore, Maryland, Postoffice.

Vol. XVII.—No. 185.]   BALTIMORE, AUGUST, 1906.   [Price, 25 Cents

CONTENTS.

AN ADDRESS AT THE FORMAL OPENING OF THE LABORATORIES OF THE ROCKEFELLER INSTITUTE FOR MEDICAL RESEARCH ON MAY 11, 1906.

By WILLIAM H. WELCH, M. D.

The support of hospitals has always made a strong appeal to the philanthropy of the State and of individual citizens, and the importance to the community of educated physicians has been appreciated, although in this country until recent years most inadequately, but the recognition of medical science as a rewarding object of public and private endowment is almost wholly the result of discoveries in this department of knowledge made during the last quarter of a century. An eloquent witness to the awakening of this enlightened and beneficent sentiment, is the establishment, in 1901, of the Rockefeller Institute for Medical Research with its laboratories formally opened to-day.

While the scientific study of infectious diseases is, of course, not of recent origin and had been pursued as a part of the functions of health departments and of university laboratories of hygiene and of pathology, the first provision of a special laboratory for this purpose was made by the German Government in 1880 in the Imperial Health Office in Berlin, and to the directorship of this laboratory was called from his country practice Robert Koch, who four years before had startled the scientific world by his memorable investigations of anthrax. The supremacy of Germany in science is due above all to its laboratories, and no more fruitful record of scientific discoveries within the same space of time can be found than that afforded by this laboratory during Koch's connection with it from 1880 to 1885. Thence issued in rapid succession the description of those technical procedures which constitute the foundation of practical bacteriology and have been the chief instruments of all subsequent discoveries in this field, the determination of correct principles and methods of disinfection, and the announcement of such epochal discoveries as the causative germs of tuberculosis—doubtless the greatest discovery in this domain—of typhoid fever, diphtheria, cholera, with careful study of their properties.

The leading representative, however, of the independent laboratory devoted to medical science is the Pasteur Institute in Paris founded in 1886 and opened in 1888. The circumstances which led to the foundation of this Institute made probably a stronger appeal to popular sympathy and support than any others which have ever occurred in the history of medicine.

There stood in the first place the personality and the work of that great genius, Louis Pasteur, of noble and lovable character, one of the greatest benefactors of his kind the world has known, who for forty years had been engaged, often under adverse conditions, in investigations which combined the highest scientific interest with important industrial and humanitarian applications. Pasteur's revelation of the world of microscopic organisms in our environment—the air, the water and the soil—and his demonstration of their relation to the processes of fermentation and putrefaction had led Lister in the late sixties, even before anything was definitely known of the causative agency of bacteria in human diseases, to make the first and most important application of bacteriology to the prevention of disease by the introduction of the principles of antiseptic surgery, whereby untold thousands of human lives have been saved.

In 1880 came the most momentous of Pasteur's contributions to medical science and art in the introduction of the method of active immunization by the use of the living parasites of the disease attenuated in virulence, a method which until this date had remained without further application since its employment by Edward Jenner in 1796 in vaccinating against smallpox. Pasteur's researches in this field of immunity, marvelous in their originality, ingenuity and fertility of resource, culminated in 1885 in the announcement of his successful method of protective inoculation against that dread disease, rabies, and most of those here present will recall the enthusiasm with which this great triumph of experimental medicine was hailed throughout the civilized world.

It was under the immediate impression and the incentive of this discovery and as a mark of gratitude to Pasteur that over two and one-half million francs were raised within a short time by international subscription for the construction and endowment of an institute to bear his name, where the Pasteur treatment was to be carried out and ample facilities afforded for investigations of microorganisms and the problems of infectious diseases. This model Institute, much enlarged since its foundation and after the death of Pasteur under the directorship of Duclaux and now of Roux and, in one of its most important divisions, of Metchnikoff, has been a fruitful center of productive research and through its contributions to knowledge affords a signal illustration of the benefits to science and to humanity of the endowment of laboratories for the advancement of medical science.

It was under much the same influences that the important Imperial Institute for Experimental Medicine in St. Petersburg, with even wider scope than the Pasteur Institute, was founded and munificently endowed by Prince Alexander of Oldenburg in 1890.

In the following year the Prussian government established in Berlin under the directorship of Professor Koch the admirably organized and equipped Institute for Infectious Diseases, to which is attached, as to the Pasteur Institute, a hospital for infectious diseases. This and the excellent Institute for Experimental Therapeutics in Frankfort, under Professor Ehrlich's direction, founded also by the Prussian government in 1896, are unsurpassed in their scientific activities and in the number and value of their contributions to our knowledge of infection and immunity.

In 1891 was founded in London the British, later the Jenner, and now the Lister Institute of Preventive Medicine designed to be a national institute similar in character and purpose to the Institut Pasteur in Paris. The funds were contributed by the public and subsequently increased by Lord Iveagh's generous gift of two hundred and fifty thousand pounds.

Within less than a year after the foundation of the Rockefeller Institute for Medical Research the Memorial Institute for Infectious Diseases was founded in Chicago by Mr. and Mrs. Harold F. McCormick, and placed under the capable direction of Professor Hektoen.

The Institute for the Study, Treatment, and Prevention of Tuberculosis which bears the name of its beneficent founder, Henry Phipps, was incorporated in Philadelphia in 1903, and, while devoted to a single disease, it must be ranked among those of wide scope, when we consider the magnitude and surpassing importance of the problems pertaining to this disease.

It may also be noted that the Carnegie Institution in Washington, with its unequalled endowment of ten million dollars, includes within its scope the support of biological and chemical investigations of great importance to medical science, so that our country now stands in line with Germany, France and Great Britain in the opportunities afforded for research in medical and other sciences.

These various institutions have been mentioned as typifying the general aims and character of the Rockefeller Institute for Medical Research rather than to afford any complete picture of the material aid now available for the advancement of scientific medicine. If the latter were the purpose it would be necessary to travel far afield so as to include independent medical laboratories of more restricted scope, such as those for the study of cancer, the laboratories connected with departments of health, so well exemplified in our own country by those of the State Board of Health of Massachusetts and of the Department of Health of the City of New York, hospitals and the laboratories connected with them, the medical laboratories of universities and medical schools, such as the Thompson Yates and Johnston laboratories in Liverpool and the splendid new laboratories of the Harvard Medical School, laboratories established in recent years for the study of tropical diseases, such as our government laboratories in Manila, and funds available for special grants to investigators.

Impressive and encouraging as is this remarkable growth within recent years of laboratories devoted to the medical sciences no one who has any knowledge of the vast field to be covered, of the difficulty·and complexity of the problems, of the expenditure of money required, and of the returns in increased knowledge and benefits to mankind which have been attained and which may be expected in increasing measure, can for a moment suppose that the existing opportunities, considerable as they are, are adequate to meet the present and the future needs of scientific medicine.

As I have already stated, the wider recognition of medical science as a rewarding object of endowment is a result of discoveries made during the last quarter of a century, and it is of interest to inquire why this increased knowledge should have borne such abundant fruit. The result is not due to any change in the ultimate aims of medicine, which have always been what they are to-day and will remain—the prevention and the cure of disease, nor to the application to the solution of medical problems of any higher intellectual ability and skill than were possessed by physicians of past generations, nor to the growth of the scientific spirit, nor to the mere fact of a great scientific advance in medicine, for the most important contribution ever made to our understanding of the processes of disease was the discovery by Virchow in the middle of the last century of the principles and facts of cellular pathology, the foundation of modern pathology.

The awakening of this wider public interest in scientific medicine is attributable mainly to the opening of new paths of investigation which have led to a deeper and more helpful insight into the nature and the modes of prevention of a group of diseases—the infectious diseases—which stand in a more definite and intimate relation to the social, moral and physical well-being of mankind than any other class of diseases. The problems of infection which have been solved and kindred ones which give promise of solution are among the most important relating to human society. The dangers arising from the spread of contagious and other infectious diseases threaten not the individual only but industrial life and the whole fabric of modern society. Not medicine only but all the forces of society are needed to combat these dangers, and the agencies which furnish the knowledge and the weapons for this warfare are among the most powerful for the improvement of human society.

Great as was the material, intellectual and social progress of the world during the past century there is no advance which compares in its influence upon the happiness of mankind with the increased power to lessen physical suffering from disease and accident and to control the spread of pestilential diseases. Were we to-day as helpless as the physicians of past centuries in the face of plague, smallpox, typhus fever, cholera, yellow fever and other epidemic diseases, even if the existence of our modern crowded cities were possible, which may be doubted, the people would sit continually in the shadow of death. Great industrial activities of modern times, efforts to colonize and to reclaim for civilization vast tropical regions, the immense undertaking to construct the Panama canal, are all in the first instance dependent upon the successful application to sanitary problems of knowledge, much

of it gained in recent years, concerning the causation and propagation of epidemic and endemic diseases.

And yet probably a fair measure of the general realization of these facts is the provision by Congress that of the seven members of the Isthmian Canal Commission four shall be engineers, without a word concerning a sanitarian on the commission. There could hardly be a more impressive opportunity to demonstrate to the world the practical value of our new knowledge concerning the mode of conveyance of malaria and yellow fever, the two great scourges of Panama, than that afforded by the digging of the Isthmian canal. The sanitary problem is not surpassed in difficulty by the engineering problem, but we may feel reasonable assurance that with the sanitary control in hands as trained and capable as those of Colonel Gorgas the ghastly experiences of the old French Panama Canal Company and in the construction of the railway will not be repeated.

To comprehend fully the degree and the character of the progress of modern medicine requires a kind of knowledge and a breadth of vision not possessed by the average man. He is concerned mainly with the prompt relief of his own ailments or those of his family. Of the triumphs of preventive medicine he knows little or nothing. With such dull matters as the decline in the death rate by one-half and the increase in the expectation of life by ten or twelve years during the last century he does not concern himself. He takes no account of the many perils which have been removed from his pathway since his birth, and indeed at the time of his birth, nor does he know that had he lived a little over a century ago and survived these perils he would probably be marked with smallpox.

While it is true that in the relief of physical suffering and in the treatment of disease and accident the progress has been great and the physician and the surgeon can do more, far more to-day than was possible to his predecessors, and while improvement in this direction must always be a chief aim of medicine, still it is in the prevention of disease that the most brilliant advances have been made. The one line of progress, that with which the daily work of the physician is concerned, affects the individual, the unit, the other, like all the greater movements in evolution, affects the race. It has been argued with a certain measure of plausibility that the interference with the law of the survival of the fittest assumed to be a result of the success of preventive medicine will bring about deterioration of the race. I believe the argument to be fallacious and that we already have sufficient experience to show that there need be no serious apprehension of such a result.

Before some accurate knowledge of the causation of infectious diseases was secured preventive medicine was a blundering science, not, however, without its one great victory of vaccination against smallpox, whereby one of the greatest scourges of mankind can be controlled and could be eradicated, if the measure were universally and efficiently applied. The establishment upon a firm foundation of the germ doctrine of infectious diseases, the discovery of the parasitic organisms of many of these diseases, the determination by experiment of the mode of spread of certain others, and the experimental studies of infection and immunity have transformed the face of modern medicine.

The recognition, the forecasting, the comprehension of the symptoms and lesions, the treatment of a large number of infectious diseases have all been illuminated and furthered, but the boon of supreme import to the human race has been the lesson that these diseases are preventable.

Typhus fever, once widespread and of all diseases the most dependent upon filth and overcrowding, has fled to obscure, unsanitary corners of the world before the face of modern sanitation.

In consequence of the knowledge gained by Robert Koch and his co-workers Asiatic cholera, to the modern world the great representative of a devastating epidemic, will never again pursue its periodical, pandemic journeys around the world, even should it make the start.

Of bubonic plague, the most dreaded of all pestilences, which disappeared mysteriously from the civilized world over two centuries ago, we know the germ and the manner of propagation, and, although it has ravaged India for the last ten years with appalling severity, it can be and has been arrested in its spread when suitable measures of prevention are promptly applied.

Typhoid fever, the most important index of the general sanitary conditions of towns and cities, has been made practically to disappear from a number of cities where it formerly prevailed. That this disease is still so prevalent in many rural and urban districts of this country is due to a disgraceful neglect of well-known measures of sanitation.

To Major Walter Reed and his colleagues of the Army Commission this country and our neighbors to the south owe an inestimable debt of gratitude for the discovery of the mode of conveyance of yellow fever by a species of mosquito. On the basis of this knowledge the disease, which had been long such a menace to lives and commercial interests in our Southern States, has been eradicated from Cuba and can be controlled elsewhere.

Another army surgeon, Major Ross, acting upon the suggestion of Sir Patrick Manson, had previously demonstrated a similar mode of inoculation and transportation of the parasite of malaria, discovered by Laveran, and it is now possible to attack intelligently and in many localities, as has already been proven, with good promise of success, the serious problem of checking or even eradicating a disease which renders many parts of the world almost uninhabitable by the Caucasian race and, even where less severe, hinders, as does no other disease, intellectual and industrial activities of the inhabitants. It is gratifying that one of our countrymen and a member of the Board of Directors of this Institute, Dr. Theobald Smith, by his investigations of Texas Cattle Fever, led the way in the discovery of the propagation of this class of disease through an insect host.

The deepest impress which has been made upon the average death rate of cities has been in the reduction of infant mor-

tality through a better understanding of its causes. The Rockefeller Institute by the investigations which it has supported of the question of clean milk and of the causes of the summer diarrhoeas of infants is already made important contributions to this subject, which have borne good fruit in this city and elsewhere.

No outcome of the modern science of bacteriology has made a more profound impression upon the medical profession and the public, or comes into closer relation to medical practice than Behring's discovery of the treatment of diphtheria by antitoxic serum, whereby in the last twelve years the mortality from this disease has been reduced to nearly one-fifth of the former rate.

The most stupendous task to which the medical profession has ever put its hands is the crusade against tuberculosis, whose preeminence as the leading cause of death in all communities is already threatened. Sufficient knowledge of the causation and mode of spread of this disease has been gained within the last quarter of a century to bring within the possible bounds of realization the hope of even the most enthusiastic, but it will require a long time, much patience and a combination of all the forces of society, medical, legislative, educational, philanthropic, sociological, to attain this goal.

Time forbids further rehearsal even in this meagre and fragmentary fashion of the victories of preventive medicine. Enough has been said to make clear that man's power over disease has been greatly increased in these latter days. But great and rapid as the progress is been, it is small in comparison with what remains to be done. The new fields which have been opened have been explored only in relatively small part. There still remain important infectious diseases whose secrets have not been unlocked. Even with some whose causative agents are known, notably pneumonia and other acute respiratory affections and epidemic meningitis, very little has yet been achieved by way of prevention. The domain of artificial immunity and of the treatment of infections by specific sera and vaccines, so auspiciously opened by Pasteur and by Behring, is still full of difficult problems the solution of which may be of immense service in the warfare against disease. Of the cause of cancer and other malignant tumors nothing is known, although many workers with considerable resources at their disposal are engaged in its study. With the change in the incidence of disease due at least in large part to the repression of the infections of early life, increased importance attaches to the study of the circulatory, renal and nervous diseases of later life, of those underlying causes we are very imperfectly informed. There are and will arise medical problems enough of supreme importance to inspire workers for generations to come and so make demands upon all available resources.

In directing attention, as I have done, to some of the practical results of scientific discovery in medicine and in indicating certain of the important problems awaiting solution there is always the danger of giving to those unfamiliar with the methods and history of such discovery a false impression of the way in which progress in scientific knowledge has been secured and is o be expected. The final victory is rarely the result of an immediate and direct onslaught upon the position ultimately scored. The advance has been by many and devious and gradual steps, leading often, it might appear, in quite differentlirections, and mounted more frequently than not to secure avider prospect, but without any thought of the final goal. Th army contains a multitude of recruits drawn from the mos various fields, the biologist, the chemist, the physiologist cctributing their share to medical triumphs just as truly as th pathologist, the bacteriologist, the hygienist, the clinician. The inspiration has been the search for truth and joy in th search far more than any utilitarian motive. In the fullns of time comes the great achievement; the leader is haile, but he stands upon the shoulders of a multitude of predecessors whose contributions to the result are often lost from view.

In full recoition of the dependence of success in the warfare with disese upon increase of knowledge the Rockefeller Institute for Medical Research was founded by the enlightened munificence of Mr. John D. Rockefeller, to whom we make grateful acknowledgment. Likewise to the broad sympathies and active interest of his son, Mr. John D. Rockefeller, Jr., the origin and development of this institute are largely indebted.

What has already been accomplished, as well as the general scope and aims of the Institute have been concisely indicated to you by Dr. Holt. My purpose has been to show, although of necessity most inadequately, that these aims relate to matters of the highest significance to human society, that the present state of medical science and art requires large resources for its advancement, and that the returns in benefits to mankind have been and will continue to be great out of all proportion to the money expended. May the hopes of the founder and of those who have planned this Institute be abundantly fulfilled! May it contribute largely to the advancement of knowledge, and may the streams of knowledge which flow from it be " for the healing of the nations."

(N THE TEACHING OF PATHOLOGICAL PHYSIOLOGY.

BY W. G. MacCallum, M. D.,

Associate Professor of Pathology, The Johns Hopkins University, Baltimore, Md.

The following outline of the course in pathological physiology recently begun at the Johns Hopkins University is intended to show the plan and aims of this work and to argue its importane in the general scheme of medical education. Heretofore, curses in pathology have concerned themselves chiefly if not exclusively with the study of pathological anatomy, practicl demonstrations of the lesions met with at autopsy being varied here and there, by didactic lectures upon the underlyig principles involved and the nature of the mechanical ad chemical processes at work. As far as the practical wor—that is the intimate contact of the student with real objets, is concerned, such courses are purely morphological and cal with the end results of the processes mentioned in th lectures. With these processes in action the student gair no direct acquaintance until he reaches the later years o his medical course when he is introduced into the wards an allowed to study the patients clinically. Then, it is true, h directly observes the altered functions of diseased organsout, as it were, at a distance. He may not apply other than cnical methods to these patients, such as auscultation and pcussion, although it is clear that of recent years the perfectio of the methods of clinical investigation approaches me and more closely that of the physiological laboratory. Che fact, however, that he is dealing with a fellow huma being, and that a suffering one, will necessarily limit greatlyin many if not in all instances, the thoroughness and coipleteness of his application of these methods. Many of themost instructive of the precise methods at the command of the physiologist are not applicable to human beings at all, or if so, only indirectly, and by means of apparatus much less delicate and exact than that commonly used in the laboratory.

Further, it is well known that unless special care is taken to avoid such a thing the student is likely to complete his study of pathological anatomy before he begins his clinical work, and he is in the position then of trying in each clinical case to correlate sometimes faintly remembered anatomical changes with the signs and symptoms which he now finds before him. It was for these reasons that it seemed desirable to teach pathology, not merely from the morphological standpoint, but more particularly to bring clearly before the student the alterations in function which result from disease, by applying to the organs in the course of their reaction to experimentally produced lesions, all of the exact methods of the physiologist. By this means, always in association with anatomical studies, it is possible to correlate in the mind of the student much more closely than otherwise the changes in function and the anatomical alteration.

In this study of disturbed function it was planned to produce experimentally such lesions of the various organs as are commonly met with in the wards, and any available methods were used to this end. It may be remarked in passing that ideal uncomplicated lesions may be produced in this way which will illustrate the principle involved often in a way seldom seen in clinical cases.

Facilities for the prosecution of this work were afforded in

the new Hunterian Laboratory for Experimental Medicine which the trustees of the University have generously erected for such purposes. Of this building, Dr. Cushing has already written a description in which he details the arrangements for the accommodation of animals in the whole basement, and the operative work which is carried on for and by the students in one-half of the upper floor. The other half of that floor is devoted to experimental pathology and is divided into several small rooms provided with the necessary apparatus. Fig. 1 shows the general arrangement of one of these rooms, in which a skylight furnishes a particularly advantageous illumination.

In planning a course in pathological physiology it immediately became obvious that the whole field could not be covered even in the most superficial way within the portion of the academic year at our disposal, and it was therefore decided to subdivide the course, taking up the diseases of a different set of organs each year. Thus the course already given, which lasted about two months with the three afternoon exercises a week, was devoted entirely to the circulatory system, while next year it is proposed to study in a similar way the diseases of the organs of internal secretion and so on.

In a general way the lectures of Cohnheim formed a model for this course, the experiments described there being actually carried out. It was not thought desirable, however, to limit the course to experimental work, but certain days were devoted to the study of the gross and microscopical anatomy of the lesions to be studied experimentally, as exemplified by specimens in the museum, etc. Thus the course was actually a course in the general pathology of the circulatory system.

Diseases of the pericardium were first taken up and studied anatomically, especially with regard to the nature and quantity of the exudate and its position with reference to the heart. These being the factors of especial importance in affecting the function of the heart, the experimental study was designed as described by Cohnheim, to render clear the effects upon the circulation produced by such an exudate imitated by the introduction of fluid under pressure into the pericardium. The apparatus was so arranged that fluid might be introduced or withdrawn at will and the pressure correspondingly changed. The effect of rather rapid distension of the pericardium with fluid is shown in Curve 1, in which it is seen that the arterial pressure rapidly sinks to a minimum, the pulsation disappearing in time. The pressure in the pulmonary artery (green) is also lowered and the pulsation obliterated, while in the innominate vein (blue) the pressure is elevated slightly. The death of the animal would rapidly ensue if this distension of the pericardium thus suddenly produced were maintained, but the pressures return to normal and pulsation reappears when it is withdrawn. When the exudate appears gradually, as it usually does, the heart is able to tolerate the pressure of much larger amounts. Evidently its power of dilating actively is called into play there.

Anatomical study of various acute and chronic lesions of the endocardium and especially of the heart valves with the resulting changes in the heart and circulation was followed by the experimental study of these lesions, nearly all of which can be reproduced by various methods. Exact records of pulsation and pressure could then be taken from any portion of the circulatory system, such as the pulmonary arteries and veins, or the chambers of the heart, although these are entirely inaccessible to the clinician. Such records have been produced systematically by von Basch, Moritz, and others by the aid of ingeniously constructed models of the circulation made of glass and rubber, and fitted with valves to imitate the actual conditions, but nervous and muscular control is lacking in these models and one feels sure that the reaction of such a model to the production of an obstruction or insufficiency of one of its valves must differ frequently in unsuspected ways from the reaction of the living animal with its wonderful adaptive mechanisms. Nevertheless, they are able to produce curves which show fairly well the mechanism of the various alterations. Rosenbach, Kornfeld, Bettelheim, Kauders, and several others have studied quite extensively, some of these lesions experimentally produced in animals with their results, and Klebs and others have constructed special instruments to produce tears in the more inaccessible valves.

During this course we were able to study various degrees of insufficiency and stenosis of each of the valves recording before and after the production of the lesion the pulsation and pressures in different parts of the circulation. By methods which will be described elsewhere similar valvular lesions were produced without exposing the heart, and the animals kept for a time to determine the effect upon the heart, but in the experiments of the course it was found desirable to expose the circulatory apparatus so that students might directly observe the changes in the size of the heart and in the character of its contractions and further might listen to the murmurs by applying the bell of the stethoscope directly to the wall of the heart and to the large blood-vessels. For this purpose a stethoscope was constructed with a very small bell, by the aid of which murmurs could be traced along the vessels and localized on various points over the heart wall as will be described in a separate paper.

The nature of the alterations in the pulse could also be recorded by the use of a tambour attached to the leaden tube leading from the canula in an artery, this being necessary from the fact that the ordinary mercury manometer does not record exactly slight variations in the character of the pulse.

The lesions were produced in various ways. Insufficiency of the valves was brought about by tearing them, either in the case of the aortic valves by the method of Rosenbach, which consists in inserting a blunt probe through the carotid and rupturing the valve, or in the case of the mitral or tricuspid by the insertion of a blunt hook with inner cutting edge (Fig. 2) through the vein, or preferably through the auricular appendage, which could then be tied off after removal of the hook. It was found that such a hook was also very serviceable instead of the probe in tearing the aortic valves, for after being pushed through the base of a segment it could then be

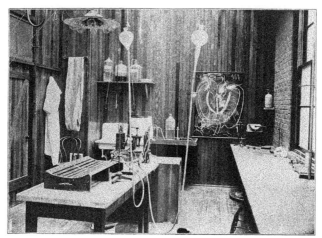

Fig. 1.

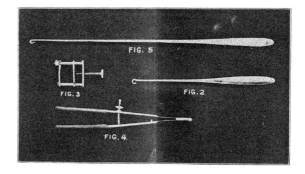

Femoral artery.

Pulmonary artery.

Jugular vein.

Femoral artery.

Curve 1. Pericardial effusion.

Femoral artery.

Femoral artery.
Pulmonary artery.

Innominate vein.

Curve 2. Aortic insufficiency.

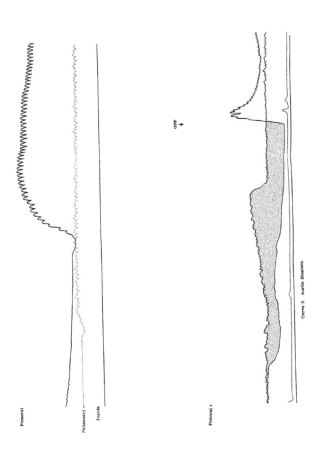

Femoral

Pulmonary

Jugular

480

Femoral :

Curve 3. Aortic Stenosis.

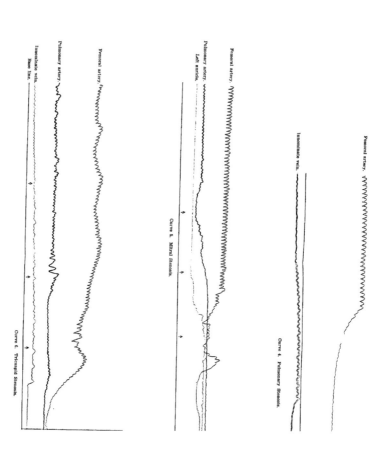

Femoral artery.

Innominate vein.

Curve 4. Pulmonary Stenosis.

Femoral artery.

Pulmonary artery.

Left auricle.

Curve 5. Mitral Stenosis.

Pulmonary artery.

Femoral artery.

Innominate vein.

Base line.

Curve 6. Tricuspid Stenosis.

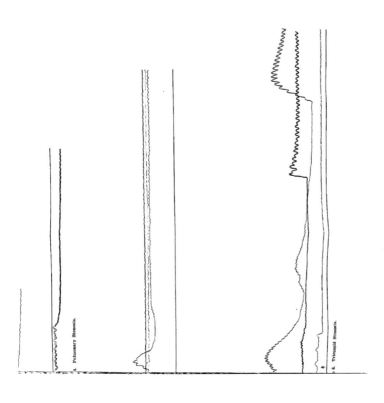

Pulmonary Stenosis.

6. Tricuspid Stenosis.

turned toward the lumen and would cut the valve cleanly on its return. Stenosis of the arterial orifices was easily produced by the application of a screw clamp with one movable limb (Fig. 3) by means of which any degree of constriction could be brought about. In the case of the mitral and tricuspid orifices a clamp of the form shown in Fig. 4, with the ends guarded with rubber tubes, could be applied and constriction produced by means of the screw in the center. It was also found possible to attain almost the same result by passing a suture with a long curved needle through the heart about the mitral ring and drawing it tight, but this method is less easy.

Aortic insufficiency was first studied and the remarkable maintenance of arterial blood pressure with peculiar collapsing pulse shown in a curve (Curve 2). A loud diastolic murmur could be heard over the heart and to some extent along the vessels. Even in the smaller arteries far from the heart a pistol-shot clap could be heard with the stethoscope.

Aortic stenosis produced the effects upon arterial and venous pressure, shown in Curve 3, the line recording venous pressure showing but little change, while that from the pulmonary artery shows the gradual rise in pressure in the pulmonary circulation. A harsh thrill could be felt beyond the clamp by placing the finger upon the arch of the aorta and this was associated with a loud murmur best heard along the aortic arch.

Stenosis of the pulmonary artery similarly produced (Curve 4) has a somewhat similar effect but brings about a much greater elevation of the general venous pressure.

Mitral insufficiency was studied in detail and the phenomena associated with it are described in a separate paper. It was found easy to reach through the left auricular appendage and cut the valve with the knife hook figured above, while manometers were connected with several parts of the circulation. Briefly it was found in these rapidly produced and excessive lesions that the arterial pressure sinks at once, while the pressure in the pulmonary circulation is affected by the addition of the regurgitant amount, by the diminution in blood supply owing to the incomplete expulsion from the left ventricle, and by the communication of a more or less violent backward pulsation to the pulmonary stream of blood. It is necessary to take into account all of these factors in explaining the hypertrophy of the right ventricle. Since it is so rare to find an entirely uncomplicated mitral insufficiency in human beings and to observe its exact and unaided influence in producing cardiac hypertrophies it has been thought interesting to tear the valves by a long knife hook (Fig. 5) introduced along the carotid and between the aortic valves; on its return the hook catches and cuts the free edge of the mitral curtain, and a loud systolic murmur appears over the apex of the heart. The results of such experiments when the dogs are kept alive will be detailed in another paper. In most instances in which an extensive lesion is produced the effects offer too great a strain for the heart, and dilatation with fibrillary twitchings and cessation of the heart beat result.

In one case, however, while a curve was taken from innominate vein and femoral artery a mitral insufficiency was produced which proved to be so extensive that a break in compensation occurred, the arterial pressure sank to almost nothing, the heart became dilated, and with each beat there was seen a high pulsation in the innominate, due doubtless to relative insufficiency of the tricuspid. After stimulation the heart gathered strength, brought the arterial pressure back to normal, and withdrew from the distended veins the abnormal amount of blood gathered there. The excessive pulsation communicated to the veins disappeared with the contraction of the right heart to its normal dimensions. In this experiment the condition of broken compensation with recovery seemed well imitated.

Mitral stenosis was studied after its production by one of the methods mentioned above; the most satisfactory being the application of the screw clamp, which narrows the orifice without also producing insufficiency as the suture is apt to do.

When canulas are inserted into left auricle, pulmonary artery, systemic vein, and systemic artery great elevation in pressure is recorded by those in the left auricle and pulmonary artery, while within the time occupied by these experiments at least no great change appeared in the systemic veins. The arterial pressure, however, drops markedly. The diminished circulation is in the systemic vessels while the overloaded circulation with stagnation of blood is found in the pulmonary vessels (Curve 5).

In *tricuspid stenosis* on the other hand, produced in the same way, a very sharp elevation of venous pressure is at once evident, the obstructed circulation being now the systemic one (Curve 6). When *tricuspid insufficiency* was produced the effects of various lesions of the other valves, particularly of the pulmonary, upon the venous pressure became much more evident.

Every valvular lesion or experimentally produced limitation of the activity of the ventricle tends to diminish the amount of blood in actual circulation, and to allow of the stagnation of the rest in the part of the stream bed behind the incompetent portion.

In addition to the functional disturbances of the myocardium, such as were mentioned above, it was sought to imitate the effects of anatomical lesions by the actual destruction of portions of the myocardium. This could easily be done by the injection of alcohol or some similar substance into the heart muscle by means of a hypodermic syringe, the extraordinary power of the heart to maintain the blood pressure in spite of extensive injuries being demonstrated.

The experiments of Porter with the ligation of the branches of the coronary arteries were repeated, and it happened that in the experiment watched by the class, the ligature of the anterior descending branch of the left coronary vessel produced only a temporary irregularity of the heart and lowering of the pressure, while the subsequent additional ligature of the circumflex branch gradually brought the pressure and pulsation to zero.

Coincidentally with these experiments or on alternate days the anatomical study of museum preparations was carried out, the anatomical results of the experiments being compared with those of the actual disease in man. There were of course changes in the heart which could not be imitated experimentally, and the results of the prolonged existence of cardiac lesions were also for the most part impossible to attain by experiments but could be well studied in the museum.

Some time was spent in the study of congenital malformations of the heart, in which the museum is rather rich, and the effects upon the circulation of these distortions was considered.

The time did not allow of the experimental study of arteriosclerosis or of aneurysms. Such experiments, however, as well as the production of collateral tracts of circulation, etc., could be prepared beforehand, if the course were given again, but long-prepared experimental imitations of disease do not seem to present any special advantage over clinical or autopsy material, unless it be in the readiness with which they may be investigated. On that account these things were studied chiefly from their anatomical results. More immediate interest could be found in the observation of the effects upon blood pressure of the ligation or clamping of various arteries and arterial systems, it being easily shown that the ligature of both renal arteries caused a slight rise in pressure; even the aorta below the splanchnic vessels may be ligated without changing the pressure very markedly while the ligature of the splanchnics themselves causes an extraordinary rise. The effects of hæmorrhage and infusion were also studied, manometers being connected with both the general arterial and pulmonary circulation, and it is remarkable that while the systemic pressure suffers great changes, the pressure in the pulmonary circulation is but slightly altered.

The effects of various drugs, such as adrenalin, nitroglycerin, amyl-nitrite, etc., were demonstrated and it was shown that neither these nor any electric stimulation of nerves had any effect except indirectly upon the blood pressure in the pulmonary circulation (best tested by connecting a manometer with the pulmonary vein, in which the pulsation from the right ventricle is almost unchanged by the pulmonary capillaries).

Thrombosis and embolism were studied anatomically, thrombosis being especially adapted to experimental production and study while the effects of emboli in producing infarctions were demonstrated by injecting into an artery against the stream a quantity of poppy seeds. These produced extensive hæmorrhagic infarctions of the intestine and anæmic infarctions of the kidney, the white seeds being readily found where they occluded the supplying vessels.

Such in brief is an outline of the portion of this experimental course already carried out, a course experimental in two senses and definitely settled only in so far as the conviction is firm in our minds that the study and teaching by experimental methods of the pathology of function is a broad and promising field as yet by no means exhausted. Already in this new laboratory the detailed study of one or two of the conditions has been carried out with a view to the better comprehension of the resultant changes in function, and these will shortly be published. The aim of the course will be accomplished if it helps to stimulate the more minute study of the behavior of living pathological organs, in addition to the long-accustomed anatomical study of the dead organ.

PHLEGMONOUS ENTERITIS.

By W. G. MacCallum, M. D.,

Assoc. Prof. of Pathology, The Johns Hopkins University, Baltimore, Md.

Nearly all text-books make some mention of phlegmonous enteritis, but the actual material upon which this description is based is very small. Seven cases have been described as far as can be ascertained and of these five were affections of the upper part of the small intestine while in one there was a lesion of the colon, and in another the whole digestive tract was involved. The condition is, however, so analogous to the phlegmonous gastritis that one may construct the pathological picture from that similarity. The first case reported was that of Belfrage and Hedenius [1] whose patient was a man aged 52, who was suddenly taken sick with symptoms of peritonitis. Belfrage being called in on the third day found an incarcerated hernia in the right crural region. Operation revealed an omental mass strangulated there, and the patient died.

At autopsy there was found a generalized peritonitis. At a point 40 cm. below the pylorus the jejunum became greatly widened and thickened measuring 18 cm. in circumference throughout a stretch of about 18 cm. The mucosa was grayish yellow and on the broad valvulae conniventes were seen a number of bright yellow flecks sometimes coalescing into streaks running across the intestines. Here the mucosa was occasionally ulcerated and the ulcers showed at their base a loose tissue infiltrated with pus. On incision it was found that the thickening arose chiefly from swelling of the submucosa and muscularis. The first was especially swollen and was 8 mm. thick in places, being quite loose in texture and of light yellow color. The musculature, too, was infiltrated with pus. Hedenius considered this phlegmonous infiltration to be of infectious nature and similar in that respect to the phlegmons of the subcutaneous tissue.

Goldschmidt [2] saw a similar condition in the colon of a

---

[1] Belfrage och Hedenius, Upsala Läkaref. Förhandl., XI, p. 132, 1876. Ref. Virchow Hirsch Jahresber. 1876, II, 210.

[2] Goldschmidt, Dtsch. Arch. f. klin. Med., 1886-7, Bd. 40, p. 400.

woman aged 41, who after an indiscretion in diet had a chill, pain in abdomen, cough and pain in her chest. Obstipation and meteorism were continuous with severe pain in the abdomen until her death on the tenth day.

At the autopsy the peritoneum over the transverse colon and small intestine was dulled by fibrin and by an exudate of thick yellow pus. The transverse colon was widened to a circumference of 30 cm. the mucosa covered with thick mucus. It appeared mottled with pale and bloody suffused areas and on section was found to be extensively infiltrated with pus. In places the serosa alone persisted, the remainder of the wall being ulcerated away and this in one place was perforated.

Goldschmidt explains the condition as being analogous to gastritis phlegmonosa, the infection occurring primarily in the mucosa and extending later to the submucosa. Atony of the intestinal musculature allows of coprostasis which is soon followed by ulceration of the mucosa and extended infection. It is questionable whether there is any relation between this infection and the pneumonia which was also found.

Hofman[3] reports a case of phlegmonous enteritis in a Russian journal. The anatomical diagnosis reads as follows: Hypertrophia ventriculi sinistr. cordis. Atrophia fusca musculi cordis, dilatatio et sclerosis aortæ, Pleuritis adhæsiva chr. duplex partialis, emphysema et œdema pulmonum. Peritonitis acuta purulenta; hyperplasia acuta lienis. Degeneratio parenchymatosa hepatis. Gastritis chronica polyposa. Tumor (adeno carcinoma) curvaturæ minoris ventriculi cum exulceratione. Enteritis phlegmonosa circumscripta intestini jejuni. Enteritis acuta hæmorrhagica intestini ilei. Colitis chronica. Nephritis interstitialis chronica et acuta parenchymatosa.

The remainder of the paper being in Russian, I cannot read it.

Askanazy[4] reports a similar case. It was that of a man aged 51, who fell into a hole and injured his knee. This disabled him for several days, during which time he suffered from severe pain in the abdomen. After making an indiscreet attempt to walk, he became worse and died sixteen days after the injury. At autopsy 50 cc. of thing purulent fluid was found in the peritoneum. The intestinal folds and especially the duodenum and jejunum were greatly enlarged, the jejunum measuring 12½ cm. in circumference. The mucosa beginning at a sharp line was greatly swollen, rather transparent and gray, the valvulae conniventes being 1 cm. high. The crests of the folds were in places brown and necrotic with small defects through which the infiltrated yellowish tissue below appeared. At many points pus welled out. Section showed a purulent infiltration of the entire wall, the submucosa being converted into a broad layer of purulent tissue. The affected part of the jejunum was 20 cm. long. Cultures showed the streptococcus and staplylococcus albus, which were also found in sections.

Microscopically the infiltration is chiefly in the submucosa

[3] Hofman, Bolnitschnaja Gazeta Botkina, 1896.
[4] Askanazy, Centralbl. f. Allg. Pathologie, Bd. 6.

and muscularis, the mucosa itself being relatively unaffected. Askanazy thinks that trauma is important in producing this and that as the jejunum is fixed, it is most of all likely to suffer rupture in such a fall as this patient had. To support this he refers to several cases of traumatic rupture of the jejunum. Further he regards the streptococcus infection as coming directly from the intestine.

P. Matthes[5] describes a case observed in Dresden in which the whole intestinal tract including the stomach and colon was affected. The case was that of a woman aged 53 years who had suffered no traumatism, but in whom the abdomen gradually became distended. Great œdema of the legs ensued but throughout the temperature was normal. Three days before death erysipelas appeared in right leg.

At the autopsy there was found a widespread fibrinous peritonitis. The liver was in a state of advanced cirrhosis, the spleen greatly swollen, the intestine throughout thickened and rigid, the thickening of the wall being due especially to purulent infiltration of the submucosa, which was most marked in the jejunum, about the cæcum and in the stomach. Streptococci were found in smears, and in cultures from the walls. The author attempts to explain the mode of infection by the possibility that the ascites produces slight injuries of the mucosa of the jejunum, which is tightly bound down, which allow of the entrance of organisms from the intestine. More probable, however, in his opinion, is the injury and infection of the intestine by the needle used to evacuate the ascitic fluid. A third possibility is the metastatic infection from the erysipelatous patch.

Deutelmoser[6] describes the case of a farmer aged twenty-one years, who was well up to 14 days before his entrance into the hospital. At that time he took to his bed with vomiting, pain in the abdomen and jaundice. On admission the abdomen was distended, tender in epigastrium and mesogastrium where there was a definite resistance which could be outlined. Vomiting frequent, but the vomitus was not blood stained, and gave an acid reaction. Icterus was quite deep. Several days later the abdominal tumor was still readily palpahle and gastric succussion was to be heard over it. Vomiting frequent. Temperature normal or subnormal. Death occurred 25 days after admission to hospital with sudden elevation of temperature.

Autopsy: Most of the intestine appeared normal, the duodenum much thickened, the region of the bile papilla being especially affected, and causing great dilatation of the bile ducts. The wall of the intestine was 10 mm. thick, the mucosa intensely yellow and œdematous. There was no peritonitis. Deutelmoser inclines to the idea that this infection was due to some slight lesion of the mucosa of the duodenum, which allowed of the invasion of the streptococci from the intestine.

[5] P. Matthes. Ein seltener fall von phlegmonöser Darmentzündung. Inaug. Diss. Leipzig, 1905.
[6] Deutelmoser, Ueber enteritis phlegmonosa idiopathica. Inaug. Diss. Greifswald, 1905.

In addition to the cases already cited, he quotes another Russian paper by Moissejew,[1] who described the case of a peasant aged 67 years, who died after a brief illness characterized by pain in the abdomen but no fever. There was peritonitis and swelling of the jejunum throughout 40 cm. The mucosa was grayish yellow, opaque and swollen. The folds of the mucosa broad and flat; no visible injuries were present. The submucosa was in places 5 mm. thick, grayish white and exuded a milky fluid. These changes reached their maximum 20 cm. from the end of the duodenum, after which they faded gradually away. The rest of the ileum and the colon were unaltered. Microscopically and culturally the streptococcus pyogenes was found.

The case which we have observed was as follows:

John Chase, aged 75, a negro laborer was brought into the hospital complaining of pain in the abdomen and vomiting. He himself was unable to answer questions as to his past history, but it was ascertained that about three weeks before he had been struck by a street car, and carried unconscious to the Maryland General Hospital. The only injury seemed to be a scalp wound, but during the week that he remained in the hospital he complained of considerable pain in the "stomach." After coming home he seemed to be quite well up to the beginning of the present illness.

Present illness: 4 p. m., November 4, 1905. Patient awoke at 5 a. m. yesterday (November 3) with pain in the abdomen, which, however, he is unable to locate very definitely. In a general way he places his hand over the lower right ribs, and across the epigastrium and left flank as the site of the pain. Pain was apparently quite severe, although no definite history of cramps can be obtained. Shortly after the onset of pain the patient began to vomit and has vomited at short intervals ever since. At present he regurgitates every few minutes, without effort, a mouthful of yellowish bile-stained fluid of a foul, faintly fæcal odor. Patient states that bowels moved very slightly yesterday morning.

Note by Dr. Sowers:

Patient looks ill, tongue moist, lips dry, no very marked expression of pain. Abdomen. Symmetrical, rather full, but not distended. There is slight bulging in each flank, but it is everywhere soft. There is some general tenderness on deep palpation, but no muscle spasm. Apparently the tenderness is slightly greater below the umbilicus. There is relative dullness in the left flank. Liver dullness extends to costal margin, but neither liver nor spleen can be felt. On pressure in the epigastrium a great deal of gurgling and succussion can be made out, although there is no marked distension in this region. There is suggestive peristalsis visible over the abdomen, but no definite cramps; soreness is sufficient to make the patient lie on his side. Temperature 100°F. Leucocytes 24000, urine contains albumen and numerous granular casts.

Operation. Because of the signs of high obstruction ex-

ploratory laparotomy was decided upon, although the patient's condition was very bad.

No general peritonitis was found, but in the left side of the abdomen there was found a slight excess of turbid fluid. Cæcum and appendix, pelvis, gall bladder and liver, and stomach were explored and found normal. Nothing abnormal was found in the large intestine nor in the small intestine up to a point about 25 cm. below the duodenum. At the beginning of the jejunum, just beyond the point where the duodenum crosses the spinal column, the bowel wall was very markedly thickened, and had a brawny appearance. This distended loop was situated low down beneath the spleen, below the splenic flexure of the colon, and when it was drawn out a small amount of turbid fluid was found about it in this corner of the abdominal cavity. This was wiped out. The distended loop seemed not to have been kinked, and at no point was there an evident obstruction. The color of the bowel was a little darker than that of the surrounding bowel, but there was no evidence of any local pressure or strangulation, and the circulation in the mesentery seemed normal. The increased size of the bowel, which was perhaps 5 cm. in diameter, whereas the bowel below this loop was only about 2½ cm. seemed to be due to the thickening of the walls rather than to the distension of the loop. On palpation the much enlarged rugæ could be felt. There was no sign of ulceration or perforation. The serous coat was, however, slightly injected and there were a few fine flakes of fibrin upon its surface, which had lost in part its gloss.

Nothing further was found to account for the condition, although there was felt a hard mass in the region of the left kidney, which was thought to be either a calcified retroperitoneal gland or a renal calculus.

The patient's condition did not permit of any further operative interference even had there been any clear indication for such procedure, and he gradually grew weaker and died about 1 a. m. November 5th.

Autopsy was performed a few hours later. From the protocol those portions are copied which are of interest in this connection.

The body is that of a small man 165 cm. in length. There is a wound about 20 cm. in length in the median line closed with silver sutures. A smaller wound in the left flank has been made to receive a protective gauze drain. In the peritoneum there is a little blood-stained fluid, but the purulent fluid found at the operation is no longer present. The omentum, duodenum and adjacent tissues are somewhat reddened, but there is no distinct fibrinous exudate on their surface. The appearance is practically what might be expected after handling the abdominal organs. The greater part of the intestine is collapsed and lies in the pelvis. The appendix is quite free and normal looking. Mesenteric glands are not especially enlarged, except one that lies opposite a high point of the intestine. This one is not caseous but opaque and indurated and on section swollen-looking. The thoracic viscera show no abnormality.

[1] A. J. Moissejew, Bolnitschnaja Gazeta, 1900, No. 33.

Spleen and liver are practically normal, the gall-bladder containing clear green bile, which passes easily through the ducts, although there is in the duodenum a small concretion resembling a gallstone. The gall duct and bile papilla appear entirely normal.

The stomach is not dilated. It contains a greenish fluid. The mucosa is everywhere thickened and studded with prominent mushroom-like polypoid masses, about thirty in number. The largest of these is no more than 1 or 2 cm. in height and 1.5 cm. in diameter. The mucosa is covered with thick mucus, and shows abundant ecchymoses. Just below the pyloric ring there are one or two small, irregular, punched-out ulcers in the mucosa. The intestine viewed from the outside is greatly enlarged from a point about 5 cm. below the pylorus for a distance of about 30 to 35 cm. It is not only distended but its walls are greatly thickened so that it stands out as a stout rigid tube, which gives place abruptly, lower down, to the normal collapsed intestine. The abrupt transition between the thickened and the normal part can be plainly felt by the palpating finger, as was observed at the operation. No kink is found at this point nor any narrowing to explain the symptoms of obstruction. The serosa covering the rigid portion is somewhat dulled but there is no conspicuous deposit of fibrin upon it.

On cutting open the intestine its lumen is found to be perfectly open and filled with a soft, yellowish white, pasty, granular material. On removing this the mucosa is seen to be remarkably altered. It is very pale, grayish white in color, and there are no visible ulcerations or defects in its surface, a few minute hemorrhages only being seen. The lining of the intestine differs from the normal, however, in that the transverse plicæ instead of being thin, soft flaps of mucosa stand up as thick, opaque, swollen, and rigid folds, sometimes reaching a height of 1 cm. or more and returning to their erect position when bent over. This change is most intense at a point about 15 cm. from the pylorus, but it extends throughout a length of about 30 cm., that is from a point about 5 cm. below the pylorus to a point 35 cm. below, where the folds again suddenly resume the normal aspect.

On making an incision across one of these swollen, firm, valvulæ conniventes it is seen that the swelling is not in the mucosa itself, which appears on the cut edge as a thin, opaque, grayish white line forming the surface. The submucosa, however, is very greatly thickened and is gray and translucent and moist. On squeezing it a slightly turbid fluid oozes out, and the tissue collapses into a soft spongy mass. No such infiltration can be definitely seen macroscopically in the musculature.

The mesentery of this part of intestine is not thickened or grossly altered in any way. The blood vessels are perfectly patent and contain fluid blood. The left kidney is much contracted about some calcified masses of mortar-like material; its ureter is obliterated.

The other organs show nothing of special interest.

Numerous cultures were made from the tissues in this case, but through some misfortune they were lost and the organism concerned can only be described morphologically.

Sections of the intestine in the affected area show a remarkable condition. The mucosa is everywhere practically normal. It is true there is a considerable desquamation of epithelial cells, but those which line the crypts and in large part those which cover the villi are intact. The stroma of the mucosa shows practically only its normal cells, there being little if any infiltration with leucocytes. The muscularis mucosæ, however, is spread apart and immediately upon passing through it into the submucosa the most extensive infiltration is met with. The tissue elements of the submucosa are widely separated and isolated by an accumulation of fluid and cells with a delicate network of fibrin, which extends everywhere among them. The cells are so abundant as to form a homogeneous mass which occupies the whole area of the section of the fold and everywhere separates the mucosa widely from the underlying musculature.

Not only is the submucosa so infiltrated, but the musculature shows the same condition, the muscle fibers are spread apart and isolated in bundles of various sizes, by quantities of cells with fluid and fibrin. Even the subserous tissue is densely infiltrated, and along the edge of the section its surface is seen to be covered with a thin layer of fibrin. The cells are chiefly of the polymorphonuclear neutrophile type, but there are mononuclear cells scattered among them in limited numbers. These are larger than the more abundant leucocytes, and possess a large vesicular nucleus. They vary a good deal in size, however, some being smaller and resembling the lymphocyte more closely while others are very large and are evidently very actively phagocytic since they often contain the bodies of other cells. The lymphatic channels are sometimes seen stuffed with these various types of cells, and the same cells are recognized on closer examination of the infiltrated muscularis. Section of the adjacent mesentery also shows an acute inflammatory infiltration, the lymphatic channels there also being filled with cells. Weigert's fibrin stain brings out very clearly the delicate network of fibrin which stretches among the cells and also demonstrates the presence of myriads of bacteria, most of which are enclosed in the polymorphonuclears, although a certain number are free. These are micrococci in chains, and there seems little doubt that the organism is the *streptococcus pyogenes*. The cocci are rather elongated however at time and occur in pairs, but in general they form short chains, which may be entirely engulfed by the leucocytes.

It is interesting to note that the neutrophile leucocytes exhibit an extraordinary avidity for these organisms, while they seem but little attracted by fragments of other cells. On the other hand the mononuclear polyblastic elements apparently do not ingest bacteria, but do eagerly engulf other cells and fragments of cells, and only when these had contained cocci are the organism to be found within the body of the large cell. Evidently the two types of cells respond almost specifically to certain chemiotactic stimuli, a fact which is of course well enough known.

There is, therefore, a close resemblance betwen this case and the others which have been described. Askanazy's case is especially similar not only in that there was a history of traumatism, but also in its clinical and anatomical features. It seems plausible, as Askanazy suggests, that traumatism to the abdomen may affect the upper part of the intestine most readily on account of its relatively fixed position and thus give rise to a chance for infection. It is of course possible that the bacteria invade directly from the intestine, but in the light of the recent work upon the relative freedom from bacteria of the uppermost part of intestine, it seems also possible that the trauma may have produced a point of lowered resistance into which streptococci are carried by the blood from elsewhere. The mucosa in this instance was so completely intact over the affected area that some support is lent to this latter view.

Little else can be said in general about a condition which has been so rarely observed. Diagnosis must remain very difficult unless aided by an exploratory laparotomy, but the symptoms of obstruction which in this case were doubtless due to the paralysis of peristalsis throughout the affected part of the intestine, together with the pain and high leucocytosis may perhaps offer some suggestion as to the nature of the condition. On exploring the abdomen the rigidity of the bowel once seen could hardly be mistaken for anything else, especially when a definite obstruction cannot be found and when there is also evidence of peritonitis.

Suggestions as to treatment are not backed by experience of good results since all reported cases have quickly died, but enterostomy below the paralyzed area might at least relieve the symptoms of obstruction. With such an extensive focus of infection within the abdomen and involving generally the duodenum and jejunum, the outlook seems very grave under the best of circumstances.

MULTIPLE CAVERNOUS HÆMANGIOMATA OF THE INTESTINE.

By W. G. MacCallum, M. D.

Associate Professor of Pathology, The Johns Hopkins University.

A case has recently come under observation in this laboratory which shows throughout the small intestine many small cavernous venous tumors, a condition which seems to have been observed by few, if any, other writers. There is so little in the literature bearing upon the subject that it is possible for me to give in abstract all that has been found after fairly careful search.

Laboulbéne[1] described an erectile tumor of the intestine, which gave rise to a fatal hæmorrhage. The case was that of a man aged 64, who had suffered from slight constipation which was however easily relieved by mild purgatives. One morning he passed blood in the stools. This lasted for several days after which the stools were normal. One month later this was repeated and he vomited black coagulated blood, but after two or three days his condition seemed normal. Physical examination was negative and the physician regarded the case as one of ulcer of the duodenum. A few days later there was an extensive hæmorrhage from the bowel and the patient died. At autopsy the intestine was found full of blood; in the duodenum above the bile papilla there was a tumor of about the size of an almond, elevated and covered by mucosa except for a ragged ulceration which lay bare the tumor tissue. This was composed of widened capillaries dilated regularly or laterally into saccular dilatations. Laboulbéne considered the tumor to be an angioma developing in the mucosa and emphasized the danger of hæmorrhage in such cases.

Boyer[2] describes a case in a man aet. 62, who on dying of pneumonia, showed at autopsy numerous small varices in the

jejunum and the upper part of the ileum. There were rounded blackish nodules visible by transmitted light, the largest being of the size of a pea, while most of them were much smaller. They were very closely set throughout the tissue. No alteration of the larger arteries or veins could be found, but when examined with a lens, these nodules appeared to be situated upon arterial loops and to be themselves formed of vascular loops like a renal glomerulus. They were fairly sharply outlined and the walls of the vessels which were twisted together to form them were parallel and in continuity with those of the arterioles. There were no aneurysmal dilatations or ruptures, and a connective tissue envelope surrounded them at least in part so that they could hardly be entirely emptied of blood.

Paci[3] reported the case of a woman who, having suffered for a short time from obstruction of the intestine, suddenly passed together with fæces, a mass of tissue which Paci recognized as a pedunculated cavernous tumor. The central portion was composed of a cavernous tissue with large lacunæ filled with clotted blood. Capillaries were numerous in the trabeculæ and the whole was covered with mucosa. Apparently hæmorrhage had occurred into the substance of this tumor, enlarging it to such an extent as to cause obstruction after which it was torn from its peduncle and passed out, the obstruction being thus relieved at once.

Hektoen[4] describes in a case of aortic and mitral endocarditis, many large veins running transversely under the mucosa like varicose veins, occasionally anastomosing and sometimes overlapping. These occupied a limited area of the

[1] Laboulbéne, Bull. de l'Acad. de Méd., 2 ser., t. I., 1872.
[2] Boyer, Bull. de la Soc. Anatomique de Paris, t. 52, 1877.
[3] Paci, Lo Sperimentale, 1882, p. 149.
[4] Hektoen, Trans. Chicago Path. Soc., 1897-9. 1900, iii., p. 192.

small intestine and sometimes presented globular dilatations full of blood. Microscopically they proved to be irregularly dilated venules, and Hektoen speaks of the condition as a simple hæmangioma.

Our case differs from all of these in certain respects. It was as follows: C. Y., white male aged 54 years, a salesman who had had no infectious diseases except pneumonia, complained only of digestive disturbances which had lasted for months. He vomited before breakfast and once two years ago vomited a quantity of blood. In the present illness he has had headache and dizziness and frequent micturition. Had always been an excessive whiskey drinker, and on entering the hospital had drunken to great excess and was in a condition of acute alcoholism. Death occurred April 10.

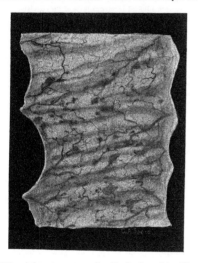

1905, and the autopsy was performed a few hours later (No. 2513).

Anatomical diagnosis.—Arteriosclerosis; atrophy of cerebral convolutions. Chronic diffuse pancreatitis; beginning cirrhosis of liver; œdema of brain. Broncho-pneumonia; multiple cavernous angiomata of intestine.

There was nothing in the other lesions which seemed to bear directly upon the appearance of the angiomata, so that they will not be described in detail. The small intestine seemed practically normal throughout as far as the mucosa was concerned, but throughout its length and especially in the upper portions there could be felt either from the inside or from the peritoneal side small fairly firm areas which shone through the mucosa as blackish purple patches, the

largest of which reached a diameter of not more than 7 or 8 mm. By transmitted light these were plainly seen as dark red thick nodules situated in the course of the veins and connected by abundant branches with the larger veins.

They were thought at first to be hæmorrhages since they seemed in many cases to be clotted drops of blood under the mucosa. On cutting through them, however, it was found possible to squeeze out liquid blood which left a spongy tissue mass. Sometimes the clots were visible, adhering in this spongy tissue.

The mucosa was in no way altered over these nodules, and there appeared to have been no hæmorrhages from them at any time. They were quite numerous, perhaps forty, to be found throughout the whole affected portion of the ileum, a portion of which is shown by transmitted light in the drawing which was kindly made for me by Mr. Shore. It can be seen that they are irregular in outline and in density as if composed of a plicated mass of vessels. Sections show that these nodules are in reality not hæmorrhages but vascular tumors of cavernous structure composed of wide sinus-like spaces lined by endothelium and full of blood. They lie chiefly in the submucosa, not invading the mucosa itself nor extending to any degree into the musculature, although in places portions of these dilated channels may be found among the muscle bundles.

On approaching such a nodule it is found that the veins of the submucosa in the neighborhood are very numerous, large, and tortuous and at the margins of the nodule suddenly become widened and pass over into widely anastomosing blood channels, the walls of which consist of little more than the endothelium and one or two layers of fibrous tissue. The arteries are easily distinguished wherever they occur, from these sinuses which rapidly coalesce as one approaches the centre of the nodule and form large, irregular sacs. Some of these are partly thrombosed and contain masses of leucocytes, the thrombi sometimes showing a definite architecture, sometimes being granular or hyaline. Toward the center of the nodule the mucosa is separated very widely from the musculature by the tangled mass of blood sinuses, which open so widely into one another, that the cavernous character becomes very evident even from a single section, in which the partitions between the large blood spaces are seen to end abruptly in the centre of a space. No hæmorrhage seems to have taken place from these angiomata, although it is possible that the vomiting of blood which occurred two years before the man's death may have been due to the rupture of one of them.

Since this paper was finished there has appeared a short paper by H. Bennecke in the last number of Virchow's Archiv. Bd. 184, Heft 1 "Ueber kavernöse Phlebektasien des Verdauungstraktus," in which the author describes a case practically identical with the one described here except in that the cavernous "phlebectasies" existed throughout the œsophagus and stomach, as well as the intestine, and concludes that they resemble in their general nature the cavernous angiomata of the liver.

ON THE MECHANICAL EFFECTS OF EXPERIMENTAL MITRAL STENOSIS AND INSUFFICIENCY.

By W. G. MacCallum, M. D.,

Associate Professor of Pathology,

AND

R. D. McClure,

Johns Hopkins Medical School.

The pressure relations in mitral stenosis are quite simple and easily understood, even when, as is so often the case, it is complicated by the existence of mitral insufficiency. It differs from a pure mitral insufficiency essentially in that the right ventricle and left auricle are unable to force the blood into the left ventricle which assumes no part of the responsibility, while in mitral insufficiency the stagnation of blood in the lesser circulation may be, in some degree, at least, favorably influenced by the increased activity of the left ventricle. In the one case the obstruction is obviously at the valvular ring; in the other it consists in the ineffectual mechanism of the left ventricle, part of the work of which is wasted.

Curves illustrating the change in pressure in the various parts of the circulation in experimental mitral stenosis may be introduced to illustrate the condition. Experimental stenosis is readily produced by one of several methods, either by applying a screw clamp with arms guarded by rubber tubes, or by passing a suture about the auriculo-ventricular ring or by introducing a distensible balloon through the auricular appendage. The immediate result is the lowering of the general arterial pressure and the great elevation of the pressure in the pulmonary arteries and in the pulmonary veins and left auricle. The pressure in the systemic veins is little if at all elevated, unless there arise an insufficiency of the right ventricle or. with the dilatation of the right ventricle, relative insufficiency of the tricuspid valve. The essential feature of the process, as indeed of all the changes of blood pressure due to any obstruction of the blood stream from alterations of the heart, lies in the fact that the amount of blood in actual circulation is diminished while the rest of the blood stagnates behind the obstruction, and therefore in this case in the pulmonary circulation. (Curve 1.)

In mitral insufficiency we find again precisely the same principle; the incompetency of the mitral valve to maintain the direction of the stream for all the blood, renders a part of the work of the left ventricle useless, and the result is that the general arterial and systemic pressure falls while that in the pulmonary veins tends to rise. In other words the quantity of blood kept in circulation is decreased, the remainder stagnating behind the incompetent valve.

Insufficiency of the mitral valve may be easily produced experimentally by means of a hook with blunt point and inner cutting edge such as is shown in Figure 1. This we had made in such a way that the outer surface is very smooth and round so that only thin structures such as the chordæ tendineæ and

valves are reached by the knife edge. This hook is introduced through the left auricular appendage into the left ventricle where the valves and chordæ tendineæ may be cut to the desired extent. Canulas connected with mercury manometers having been adjusted in various parts of the circulatory system, the one designed to record the pressure in the left auricle, is quickly tied into the aperture in the auricular appendix on the removal of the hook.

It is now found by comparing the curve with that recorded before the insufficiency was produced, that great alterations have immediately taken place. The arterial pressure always sinks; the degree of lowering depending upon the extent of the insufficiency. Its pulsation is not greatly altered. The pressure in the pulmonary artery is relatively little altered; with extreme insufficiency it usually sinks with the general arterial pressure; with slight insufficiency it rises but not very high.

The systemic venous pressure is also not greatly altered. The most striking change is seen in the curve from the left auricle in which before the injury to the valve there is low pressure and only the slightest waving pulse. Now the blood is ejected from the left ventricle not only into the aorta, but also directly into the auricle and with extreme insufficiency, the auricle may be regarded as forming part of one chamber with the left ventricle. It is therefore not surprising that it is seen to become distended with blood and to beat violently and synchronously with the ventricle. The manometer connected with it shows that the pressure becomes markedly elevated and the curve shows great excursions which are due to the contractions of the left ventricle. This was clearly described by von Basch[1] from his experiments with his model and he states that the results of animal experiments are the same.

In all these experiments the heart was carefully examined at autopsy, and it was found that in each instance the hook had cut some of the chordæ tendineæ and had made a more or less extensive rent in one or both curtains of the valve.

It is evident that the disturbance produced consists in placing the left ventricle at a disadvantage in that an orifice is made in its wall so that in its contraction the blood escapes not only in the normal direction, but backward also. Unless therefore it pumps more actively and controls a larger amount

---

[1] v. Basch. Allg. Physiologie und Pathologie des Kreislaufs. Wien, 1892.

Femoral arter
le = Pulmonary
a = Left auricle.

Red = Femoral artery.
Blue = Pulmonary artery. Canula receiving pressure from right heart.
Purple = Pulmonary artery. Canula receiving pressure from lung.
Green = Left auricle.
Black = Base line.

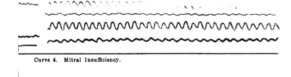

Curve 4. Mitral Insufficiency.

Red =
Purpl
Green

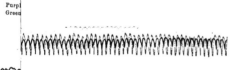

the quantity of

may be thought
arily selected to
this is of course
ay of describing
andled by any
right ventricle,
ive 10 and the
he mitral valve
e left ventricle
orta. With the
and meets the
eft auricle now
oon the activity
more than the
is thrown into
ne 6 is thrown
ead of 10 and
p 14 of which
culating blood
pulmonary cir-
orces 6 into a
nd into which

e under such
force in the
ived, we may
to receive the
it is probable
reater than 4,
out if we sup-
r 10 into the
at ventricle to
t sent on into
t which there
maintained in
ount of blood
at instead of
orta they are
only the nor-
and in order
of contraction
m the tissue.
quantities of
y must be, if
tained.

epresented as
6 into the
cle dilates at
at sufficiently
ta while 4 is
now with 6
nd from the
the ventricle

Curve 1. Mitral Stenosis.

Red.=Femoral artery.
Purple.=Pulmonary artery.
Green.=Left auricle.
Black.=Base line.

Curve 2. Mitral Insufficiency

Red.=Femoral artery.
Blue.=Pulmonary artery.   Canula receiving
Purple.=Pulmonary artery.   Canula receivin
Green.=Left auricle.
Black.=Base line.

Curve 4. Mitral Insufficiency.

Red.=Femoral artery.
Purple.=Pulmonary artery.
Green.=Left aortic appendage.

of blood, the amount ejected into the aorta will be diminished. Whether in the case of mitral regurgitation the amount thrown into the aorta can ever reach the normal is one of the questions which first presents itself. It is of course obvious that in order that the circulation may continue, precisely the same amount must be thrown out by the right and left ventricles, for one ventricle could not eject more than the other for any length of time without finally forcing the greater part of the blood into the vessels which lie in front of it. Further it seems clear that although the amount of blood handled by the heart in one beat is a very small portion of the whole mass of the blood, and although the position of the greater part of the blood may be changed by vascular contraction and dilatation, all of the blood is moving at all times and under ordinary conditions its actual amount does not change. Hence one may reason that if for any cause the left ventricle fails to perform its normal work and throws out a smaller quantity of blood the amount furnished to the right auricle and ventricle will also decrease. By active contraction of the vessels the normal amount might be kept up for a few heart beats, but this reserve would soon be exhausted and the systemic organs left anæmic while the blood is crowded into the pulmonary circulation. This has been pointed out by Kornfeld, who finds that the venous pressure falls with a fall in the arterial pressure.

From this it is seen that when regurgitation occurs at the mitral valve the amount of blood thrown into the aorta must be constantly less than normal as long as the cavity of the ventricle retains its normal dimensions and the wall its normal force of contraction. This may be modified by the power which the ventricle possesses of dilating to receive more blood and expelling it with great force; but in order to throw the normal quantity of blood into the aorta the left ventricle must receive that amount plus the amount regurgitated. This is possible, however, in only one of two ways, either there must be an actual addition of fluid to the blood from somewhere to make up to normal the smaller amount thrown into the aorta, or there must be such a vascular contraction that when the diminished amount thrown out by the left ventricle reaches the venous side of the heart the amount is made up to normal by the narrowing of the vessels, and thus while the circulating amount is maintained at the normal, the actual amount in the tissues and larger vessels is diminished by so much as has accumulated in the lungs. Probably there would in such a case be a rapid addition of fluid to the blood from the ingested fluid, and the total amount of blood would be increased by as much as accumulates in the lungs. Indeed one receives the impression from observing the amount of blood in the vessels at autopsy in cases of long standing chronic passive congestion from cardiac lesions, that there is a great increase in its quantity.

In our experiments we have not attempted to measure the quantity of blood thrown out by a beat of the heart, but merely the pressure which is of course very different and since it also depends upon the resistance and degree of contraction

of the vessels gives only a rough clue as to the quantity of blood concerned.

The changes in the distribution of the blood may be thought of perhaps in terms of numbers quite arbitrarily selected to represent the amounts of blood concerned. This is of course entirely schematic but it serves as a concise way of describing the probable changes. Thus if the amount handled by any one part of the heart in one systole, say the right ventricle, be represented by 10, the left auricle will receive 10 and the left ventricle also 10. If now insufficiency of the mitral valve arises a portion, say 4, is driven back from the left ventricle into the left auricle and 6 goes on into the aorta. With the same systole 10 again reaches the left auricle and meets the 4 regurgitated from the ventricle so that the left auricle now contains 14. That which follows will depend upon the activity of the left ventricle. If it will not receive more than the usual 10, 4 remains stagnant in the auricle, 6 is thrown into the aorta and 4 more regurgitates. By this time 6 is thrown into the auricle from the right ventricle instead of 10 and meets with 8 of regurgitated blood making up 14 of which 10 again goes into the ventricle. Thus the circulating blood amounts to 6 while the stagnant blood in the pulmonary circulation amounts to 4. The right ventricle forces 6 into a pulmonary circulation already containing 4 and into which the left ventricle simultaneously forces 4.

It is usual, however, for the left ventricle under such circumstances to dilate and to exert greater force in the expulsion of the greater amount of blood received, we may imagine then that the left ventricle dilates to receive the whole 14 of blood from the auricle. Even so it is probable that the amount regurgitated would now be greater than 4, and that thrown into the aorta less than 10, but if we suppose the ventricle to regurgitate 4 and throw 10 into the aorta, we now find only 6 furnished by the right ventricle to meet the 4 regurgitated, while 10 is by this beat sent on into the veins. This is the point mentioned above at which there must be, in order that the normal amount be maintained in circulation, either an actual addition to the amount of blood in the body or the veins must contract so that instead of giving up only the 6 sent to them by the aorta they are drained of 10, with the next beat they receive only the normal 10 and not the extra 4 which was removed and in order that they may return to their normal degree of contraction there must be more fluid brought to them from the tissue. All this seems possible and indeed even greater quantities of blood may be handled by the heart, and probably must be, if the normal amount in circulation is to be maintained.

A more probable state of affairs may be represented as follows: when the left ventricle has thrown 6 into the aorta and there is 14 in the auricle the ventricle dilates at the next diastole, not to receive the whole 14, but sufficiently to receive 12. Of this it expels 8 into the aorta while 4 is again regurgitated. The regurgitated 4 meets now with 6 driven in by the right ventricle and 2 left behind from the 14, making in all 12. With the next diastole the ventricle receives the whole 12, regurgitates 4, and throws 8 into the aorta. By this time the amount 8 thrown out by the ventricle into the aorta reaches the auricle and meets the 4 regurgitated. The whole 12 passes into the ventricle and thus a circulation is established in which 8 circulates while 4 is regurgitated with each systole.

Still another case may be mentioned. The left auricle receives 10 and regurgitates 6, throwing 4 into the aorta. At the second diastole 16 being in the auricle, the ventricle dilates to accommodate the excess of blood, but can receive only 12, 4 remains stagnant. Of the 12, 6 is regurgitated and 6 thrown into the aorta. Four remaining in the auricle plus 4 received from the right ventricle makes up 14. Of this the ventricle receives again 12, leaving 2 regurgitating 6 and expelling 6. The condition established is a circulation of 6, with a regurgitating of 6 and a constant residue in the pulmonary circulation of 2. This probably represents a common condition in which as in the first example there is some blood constantly stagnant in the pulmonary circulation while with each systole more is introduced.

Let it be repeated that it is of course not intended to convey the idea that these figures really represent the condition or the changes in them the actual character of the changes in distribution of the blood. They may only stand as symbols to illustrate the general principles involved and are far too rough when we consider the various ways in which the different parts of the circulatory system adapt themselves to the conditions forced upon them. It is especially evident that no allowance is made for the different proportions of regurgitated and ejected blood which would arise with changes in the quantity received by the ventricle and the force exerted.

From this discussion it is, however, clear that unless the ventricle is capable of receiving and handling all the blood which fills the auricle at each systole there will be some constant obstruction to the outflow of blood from the auricle, and this is important, since Gerhardt in a recent paper (Verhandl. des Kongresses für innere Medicin, 1905), states that in the diastole of the ventricle there is no obstruction to the emptying of the overfilled auricle—that the obstruction really occupies only the portion of systole during which blood is being driven back into the auricle.

In each of our experiments there has finally arisen a dilatation of the heart, especially marked in the left ventricle, with diminished vigor and lowering of the pressure in all the curves. This may be expressed as follows: Take for example the condition in which 8 is circulating, while 4 is regurgitated at each systole. The left ventricle receives 12; with the weakening of its beat, it regurgitates 4 but drives only 6 into the aorta; at the next beat since the ventricle retains 2, it receives 12 and is distended to hold 14, again it drives out 6 into the aorta and 4 into the auricle. By this time 6 only reaches the auricle from the right heart and the left ventricle which retained 4 from the last systole receives 10 from the auricle, thus maintaining a circulation in which only 6 is circulated, 4 is regurgitated and the left ventricle is constantly

receiving 14. Or the left ventricle may regurgitate only 2 and drive out into the aorta only 6. There is a residual amount of 4 to which is added in the next diastole the 2 regurgitated and the 8 previously forming the amount circulated. Of the 14, 2 is again regurgitated and 6 thrown out into the aorta. The diastole brings to the ventricle only 6 from the systemic circulation and the regurgitated 2 which with the residual 6 restores the 14 in the ventricle. The circulating blood is now only 6, the regurgitating only 2. It is easy to see that under such circumstances the pressure in the pulmonary artery must be lowered as well as that in the aorta.

From all this it is evident that when insufficiency of the mitral valves appears there is either a constant stagnation of a certain amount of blood in the pulmonary circulation together with the systolic regurgitation of an additional quantity, or when the ventricle accommodates itself to the reception of the increased amount of blood from the auricle merely a systolic regurgitation of a certain amount of blood. At the systole both right and left ventricles force blood into the pulmonary circulation from opposite ends and at the end of the systole the blood is under some tension, a sufficient tension to distend the elastic wall to accommodate the amount of blood in excess of normal. It is seen that as was clearly pointed out by von Basch, the situation is dependent upon the activity of the left ventricle, the right ventricle being powerless to do more than furnish its quota of blood to keep pace with the left ventricle. It has the task of forcing a quantity of blood never in excess of the normal into the pulmonary artery. In those instances in which there is a constant stagnation of blood there, it does this against a constantly increased tension. In case the conditions are such that in diastole the left auricle is able to empty itself, there will be no excessive resistance to the entrance of blood into the pulmonary circulation until that moment when (both ventricles simultaneously pouring blood into those vessels) the amount of blood exceeds the amount normally accommodated there. Then both right and left ventricle would feel the increased resistance simultaneously were the walls of the pulmonary vessels rigid. In the elastic vessels, however, the elevation of pressure is transmitted from each end in the form of a pulse wave and the resistance is felt when this wave reaches the opposite end.

In the human being insufficiency of the mitral valve with regurgitation is generally associated with other changes in the heart, which complicate the effects produced, but the results of uncomplicated mitral insufficiency are as a rule dilatation and hypertrophy of the left ventricle, chronic passive congestion of the lungs, hypertrophy of the right ventricle and if muscular insufficiency of the heart wall ensues a chronic passive congestion of the systemic veins. The problem which offers most difficulty lies in the explanation of the hypertrophy of the right ventricle and as to this there has recently been some discussion.

From any or all of the conditions indicated above it is readily seen that no matter what the character of the mitral insufficiency, any approach to a normal circulation is only to be maintained by the increased activity of the left ventricle which receives an increased amount of blood and ejects it against a pressure which is not diminished. Sufficient explanation of its hypertrophy and dilatation is given in this statement.

As to the hypertrophy of the right ventricle the explanation is less simple. It has been said that the right ventricle throws into the pulmonary artery an amount of blood which in most instances of mitral insufficiency is less than normal and cannot exceed the normal unless by a great increase in the total amount of blood, and by great activity on the part of the left ventricle. In order to produce hypertrophy of the ventricle therefore the resistance opposed to the ejection of this amount of blood must be increased and the cause for this increased resistance we must seek in the stagnation of blood in the pulmonary circulation and in the systolic regurgitation of blood from the left ventricle.

The presence of the stagnant blood offers resistance to the entrance of more blood when the sum of the two exceeds the bulk of the blood normally received by the pulmonary circulation. To these there is always added, however, the regurgitated blood and in every instance the sum of the three is sufficient to overdistend the pulmonary vessels. As Volhard has pointed out, therefore the elasticity of the wall of the auricle and of the pulmonary vessels has a direct bearing upon the extent of the resistance opposed to the right ventricle.

If now just before systole the pulmonary circulation contains no more blood than normally present there, the hypertension will appear at that point in the systole when the distension becomes greater than that normally present at the end of systole. The same thing is true if there is already an excess of blood there, but the condition of hypertension will begin sooner and occupy more of the period of systole. We can imagine a condition in which the amount of blood in the pulmonary circulation might be so great that even at the outset of systole the normal maximum tension is overreached. Such a condition is, however, far more probable in mitral stenosis than in mitral insufficiency. The cause for hypertrophy of the right ventricle exists therefore in different cases for different lengths of time during the systole, the duration of the hypertension being longer when there is a constant excess of blood in the pulmonary circulation than in the case in which only the normal amount remains there after diastole and hypertension begins only when nearly all of the blood forced in by the right ventricle and regurgitated by the left is added to it. All this would be strictly true were the pulmonary circulation composed of a rigid tube in which equalization of pressure would occur at once.

It is seen that the condition of maximum tension is reached only toward the end of systole and since we are dealing with an elastic tube and not with a rigid one the question arises as to the rapidity of equalization of the pressure throughout, for we may imagine a condition in which the length and great elasticity of the tube connecting the two ventricles is such that the effect of the synchronous systole of both is to send waves of heightened pressure from each end which require a considerable time to reach the opposite end. Further the size of the capillaries of the lung and the friction of the passage through them might be supposed to affect the passage of the waves of pressure. We may even imagine a condition in which the length and elasticity of the tube are such, and the modification produced by the resistant capillaries in the center such that the task of the right ventricle during its systole consists practically in the distension of the pulmonary artery while the regurgitation of the blood from the left ventricle distends during systole the pulmonary veins, the equalization of the pressure occurring only after the pulmonary valves are closed and the systole over, so that the effect of the regurgitation in elevating the pressure is never felt by the right ventricle.

It will be shown, however, that the pulmonary capillaries are so wide that they may be practically neglected and the pulmonary circulation regarded as one elastic tube and it is then only necessary to determine its length and time occupied in the equalization of pressure throughout it.

Jürgensen and Sahli and more recently Gerhardt have expressed the opinion that the hypertrophy of the right ventricle may be largely due to the direct shock from the systole of the strong left ventricle. Jürgensen makes the statement that the normal blood stream which is thrown into the left auricle from the pulmonary artery and the reflux wave from the left ventricle must, since the systole is synchronous, interfere with one another. The two ventricles work directly against one another and part of their force is spent uselessly. This does not seem to be a precise way of expressing the condition of things, for the work of the right ventricle consists not exactly in moving the blood into the left ventricle but in injecting it into the elastic pulmonary vessels where it begins its motion into the left ventricle at the beginning of diastole—a motion produced essentially by the right ventricle but in part maintained by the elastic contraction of the vessel walls and the muscular contraction of the left auricle. The pause is so short that the pressure has not time to become equalized throughout the distended pulmonary tract, but a wave travels along distending the tube as it passes. Such a wave represents the force imparted to the particles of blood by the right ventricle which are in turn communicated to those in front of them and on all sides. The particles pushed laterally stretch the vessel wall which again contracts and returns part, at least, of the energy to be transmitted again to the particles in the center and added to the impulse to go forward; thus continually losing by the energy needed to distend the elastic wall the impulse travels on, the particles moving only in a certain orbit as far as the effect of the wave is concerned. At the end of the tube the impulse is exerted in distending the wall and is returned in such a way that the wave starts back again. If such a wave meets another wave coming in the opposite direction, the energy at the point where they meet will be applied to the elastic walls and since the particles move easily upon one another there will be little effect other than the dispersion of these particles and the great distension of the elastic walls. The elevation of pressure produced by the systole is not an instantaneous one, and the reflux wave on meeting the advancing one unites with it in its effect in distending the vessel, the maximum distension being produced at the point where the crests of the waves meet. If now these waves reach the opposite ends while the ventricles are still contracting, it is plain that the tension of the wall against which they discharge the last of their content of blood is greater than normal. If any work is wasted, it is in the unnecessarily great distension of the pulmonary vessels and not in opposing the shock from the left ventricle. This presupposes that the tube is so short that the wave from the right ventricle is still being formed when the van of the other reaches the right ventricle. If the tube were much longer there might be a lower pressure in the artery after the departure of the wave from the right ventricle when the wave from the left ventricle arrives, so that at each end of the tube there would be felt at the moment of its arrival only the distension produced by that wave. Jürgensen and Gerhardt made no experimental study of the conditions of which they speak, but it is possible to record the pressures so that the actual happenings may be studied. One may study the pressure relations by the aid of mercury manometers, but the character of the pulsations and the time relations are of course best studied by means of the Hürthle manometer or small tambours connected with the canulas by lead pipes and each moving a lever.

If now one adjust canulas suitably arranged in the carotid or femoral artery, in a branch of the pulmonary artery, and in the left auricular appendage and record a curve of the normal relations, the canula in the left auricle may then be removed for a moment, the hook introduced and mitral insufficiency produced and the canula replaced and tied in. The results as compared with normal may be seen in the curves appended. The pressure rises in the left auricle slightly and there is a great pulsation, the waves being synchronous with the contractions of the left ventricle. In different cases the effect upon the pulmonary artery may vary slightly, but when the insufficiency is great and the pulsation of the auricle consequently great, the pulsation in the pulmonary artery assumes the same character (Curve 2). The pressure in the femoral artery in extreme insufficiency is greatly lowered and in these cases that of the pulmonary artery is also lowered. If, however, the left ventricle is stirred up to extreme effort, the arterial pressure may be brought up and with it that of the pulmonary (Curve 3). Now in order to explain the effect upon the pulsation in the pulmonary artery of the mitral insufficiency a canula from a fourth manometer was inserted into the severed end of a branch of the pulmonary artery toward the lung so as to receive any possible reflux wave which may have passed through its capillaries. The result is shown in Curve 4, in which it is seen that while before the insufficiency this manometer registers

zero pressure and no pulsation, the pressure rises at once on the production of the insufficiency and pulsations of the character of those in the left auricle are seen. It is obviously therefore the addition of these pulse waves to those from the right ventricle in the pulmonary artery which produces the peculiar pulsation seen in that vessel. This shows further that the pulmonary capillaries offer practically no resistance to the passage of a pulse wave, a fact which is sufficiently evident to anyone who will inspect a pulmonary vein which pulsates actively, and is shown clearly by merely inserting a canula into a pulmonary vein when the pulsation from the right ventricle is recorded practically unchanged. In such curves, however, it is difficult to determine more than the gross effect of the reflux pulse on account of the inertia of the mercury, and from what was said above it is necessary to decide whether this reflux wave merely increases the height of the normal pulmonary pulse wave or is added to it as a shoulder or separate wave, in other words to observe the length of time it requires to traverse the length of the pulmonary vessels.

Canulas attached to tambours were therefore inserted into the left auricle and the pulmonary artery as near the heart as possible and the pens adjusted to write precisely in one vertical line. Curve 5 shows the result of this. It is seen that while the crest of the wave in the auricle is precisely synchronous with that of the higher wave in the pulmonary there is a second small wave following these higher elevations, and evidently the effect of the reflux wave which requires a little time to reach that end of the pulmonary vessel. To make this clearer the canulas were put side by side pointing in opposite directions in the cut ends of a branch of the pulmonary artery, so that one would receive the reflux wave only while the other recorded the combined wave. Curves 6, 7, and 8 show the result of this experiment in which it is seen that while in Curve 6 in the normal animal the pulmonary beats have a sharp rise and fall, after the mitral insufficiency is produced and the reflux wave appears, the fall in the pulmonary wave is not so rapid, but is delayed by a sort of shoulder which is seen to be exactly synchronous with the apex of the reflux wave taken as it will be remembered at practically the same spot (Curves 7 and 8). The exact representation of the interval in this curve required by the reflux wave to travel from the left ventricle to the arterial end of the pulmonary tract is shown in Curve 9, in which the upper curve is drawn by the pen from the left auricle while the lower is from the distal portion of the cut pulmonary artery, from the same case and with the drum running at the same speed as in the Curves 6, 7, and 8. The question still remains as to whether it can be said from these curves that the elevation of pressure from the reflux wave is felt at the root of the pulmonary artery, i. e., by the right ventricle before the pulmonary valves close. It is fairly clear that this may be answered in the affirmative since it is seen that the reflux wave begins to arise before the pulmonary wave has quite

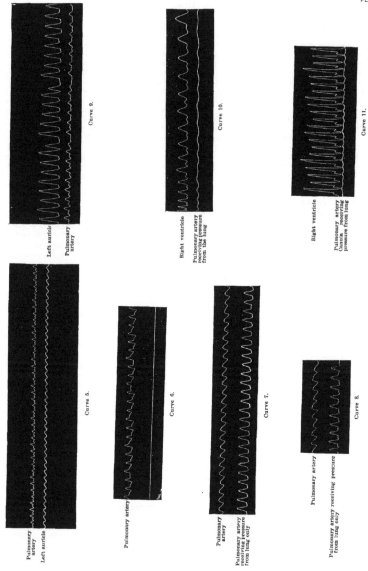

elastic walls and since the particles move easily upon one another there will be little effect other than the dispersion of these particles and the great distension of the elastic walls. The elevation of pressure produced by the systole is not an instantaneous one, and the reflux wave on meeting the advancing one unites with it in its effect in distending the vessel, the maximum distension being produced at the point where the crests of the waves meet. If now these waves reach the opposite ends while the ventricles are still contracting, it is plain that the tension of the wall against which they discharge the last of their content of blood is greater than normal. If any work is wasted, it is in the unnecessarily great distension of the pulmonary vessels and not in opposing the shock from the left ventricle. This presupposes that the tube is so short that the wave from the right ventricle is still being formed when the van of the other reaches the right ventricle. If the tube were much longer there might be a lower pressure in the artery after the departure of the wave from the right ventricle when the wave from the left ventricle arrives, so that at each end of the tube there would be felt at the moment of its arrival only the distension produced by that wave. Jürgensen and Gerhardt made no experimental study of the conditions of which they speak, but it is possible to record the pressures so that the actual happenings may be studied. One may study the pressure relations by the aid of mercury manometers, but the character of the pulsations and the time relations are of course best studied by means of the Hürthle manometer or small tambours connected with the canulas by lead pipes and each moving a lever.

If now one adjust canulas suitably arranged in the carotid or femoral artery, in a branch of the pulmonary artery, and in the left auricular appendage and record a curve of the normal relations, the canula in the left auricle may then be removed for a moment, the hook introduced and mitral insufficiency produced and the canula replaced and tied in. The results as compared with normal may be seen in the curves appended. The pressure rises in the left auricle slightly and there is a great pulsation, the waves being synchronous with the contractions of the left ventricle. In different cases the effect upon the pulmonary artery may vary slightly, but when the insufficiency is great and the pulsation of the auricle consequently great, the pulsation in the pulmonary artery assumes the same character (Curve 2). The pressure in the femoral artery in extreme insufficiency is greatly lowered and in these cases that of the pulmonary artery is also lowered. If, however, the left ventricle is stirred up to extreme effort, the arterial pressure may be brought up and with it that of the pulmonary (Curve 3). Now in order to explain the effect upon the pulsation in the pulmonary artery of the mitral insufficiency a canula from a fourth manometer was inserted into the severed end of a branch of the pulmonary artery toward the lung so as to receive any possible reflux wave which may have passed through its capillaries. The result is shown in Curve 4, in which it is seen that while before the insufficiency this manometer registers

zero pressure and no pulsation, the pressure rises at once on the production of the insufficiency and pulsations of the character of those in the left auricle are seen. It is obviously therefore the addition of these pulse waves to those from the right ventricle in the pulmonary artery which produces the peculiar pulsation seen in that vessel. This shows further that the pulmonary capillaries offer practically no resistance to the passage of a pulse wave, a fact which is sufficiently evident to anyone who will inspect a pulmonary vein which pulsates actively, and is shown clearly by merely inserting a canula into a pulmonary vein when the pulsation from the right ventricle is recorded practically unchanged. In such curves, however, it is difficult to determine more than the gross effect of the reflux pulse on account of the inertia of the mercury, and from what was said above it is necessary to decide whether this reflux wave merely increases the height of the normal pulmonary pulse wave or is added to it as a shoulder or separate wave, in other words to observe the length of time it requires to traverse the length of the pulmonary vessels.

Canulas attached to tambours were therefore inserted into the left auricle and the pulmonary artery as near the heart as possible and the pens adjusted to write precisely in one vertical line. Curve 5 shows the result of this. It is seen that while the crest of the wave in the auricle is precisely synchronous with that of the higher wave in the pulmonary there is a second small wave following these higher elevations, and evidently the effect of the reflux wave which requires a little time to reach that end of the pulmonary vessel. To make this clearer the canulas were put side by side pointing in opposite directions in the cut ends of a branch of the pulmonary artery, so that one would receive the reflux wave only while the other recorded the combined wave. Curves 6, 7, and 8 show the result of this experiment in which it is seen that while in Curve 6 in the normal animal the pulmonary beats have a sharp rise and fall, after the mitral insufficiency is produced and the reflux wave appears, the fall in the pulmonary wave is not so rapid, but is delayed by a sort of shoulder which is seen to be exactly synchronous with the apex of the reflux wave taken as it will be remembered at practically the same spot (Curves 7 and 8). The exact representation of the interval in this curve required by the reflux wave to travel from the left ventricle to the arterial end of the pulmonary tract is shown in Curve 9, in which the upper curve is drawn by the pen from the left auricle while the lower is from the distal portion of the cut pulmonary artery, from the same case and with the drum running at the same speed as in the Curves 6, 7, and 8. The question still remains as to whether it can be said from these curves that the elevation of pressure from the reflux wave is felt at the root of the pulmonary artery, i. e., by the right ventricle before the pulmonary valves close. It is fairly clear that this may be answered in the affirmative since it is seen that the reflux wave begins to arise before the pulmonary wave has quite

PLATE XV

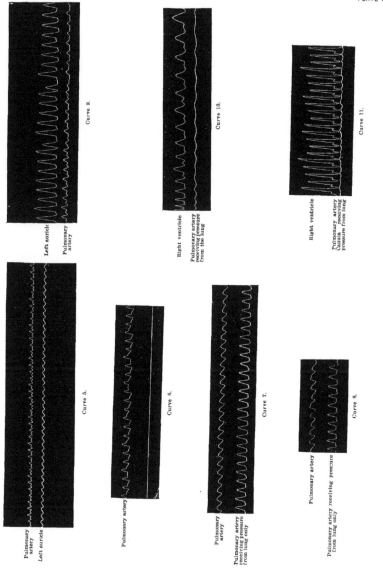

reached its climax, but it was thought that it would be clearer if it were possible to trace a curve from the cavity of the right ventricle simultaneously with one from the distal portion of the cut pulmonary branch, i. e., one showing the reflux wave alone. For some reason we had great difficulties with this, but the curves finally obtained are fairly clear and show (Curves 10, 11) that the elevation from the reflux wave begins before the ventricle has finished its systole and therefore before the pulmonary valves close.

From all of this it is seen that there is less cause for hypertrophy of the right ventricle in pure uncomplicated mitral insufficiency than in mitral stenosis or in mitral insufficiency associated with myocarditis or other causes for inadequate work of the left ventricle. The cause in those cases in which the regurgitation and the activity of the left ventricle are such that there is a constant residuum of blood in the pulmonary vessels greater than normal, consists in the rapid rise in tension during systole to a point above the maximum normal tension such that an excessive effort is required on the part of the right ventricle. In this case there is the additional influence toward the end of systole of the increased tension produced by the reflux of blood from the left ventricle, the effect of which is felt by the right ventricle before the end of its systole. Even when there is no constant residuum of blood in the pulmonary circulation this hypertension due to regurgitation is felt toward the end of systole.

ACUTE HÆMORRHAGIC PANCREATITIS FOLLOWING OBSTRUCTION OF THE BILE PAPILLA.

By C. H. Bunting, M. D.,

Associate in Pathology, Johns Hopkins University; Pathologist to Bay View Hospital.

In his monograph on "Diseases of the Pancreas," Opie has emphasized the importance of cholelithiasis as a factor in the causation of acute hæmorrhagic pancreatitis and has clearly demonstrated the mechanism by which a gall stone may bring about this lesion of the pancreas. There are several conditions which must be fulfilled before this may occur. The anatomical arrangement must be such that the duct of Wirsung is the main duct of the pancreas and it must join the common duct so as to form an ampulla of Vater whose length is greater than the diameter of its orifice at the papilla—a condition which is present in about three out of ten individuals. The stone must be of such size that it may close the orifice of the ampulla and not at the same time that of the pancreatic duct, thus converting the bile duct and pancreatic duct into a single closed channel. With a greater pressure in the common duct, bile may then be forced into the pancreatic duct and by its irritative action set up an acute inflammatory reaction.

This mechanico-chemical theory of acute pancreatitis, Opie bases upon the autopsy findings in which the above conditions were fulfilled—a stone 3 mm. in diameter blocking the orifice of an ampulla which measured 10 mm. in length—and in which bile was found in the pancreatic duct; also upon the experimental proof that bile injected into the pancreatic duct of animals under sterile precautions will produce the lesion of acute pancreatitis; and upon the frequency with which cases of acute pancreatitis occur in people who give a history of biliary colic or are found to have gall stones in the gall bladder or common duct at operation or autopsy. In the reference cited Opie quotes in addition to two cases of his own 39 others in which cholelithiasis was present, in eight stones being found in the common duct, in one in the duodenum, and in the others in the gall bladder, though in ten of these jaundice suggested the recent passage of a stone with temporary obstruction of the duct. In a more recent paper [1] in summarizing the evidence for this view he expresses the opinion that cholelithiasis is the usual if not the only cause of acute hæmorrhagic pancreatitis; and concludes that "whenever a biliary calculus passes through the diverticulum of Vater into the duodenum the pancreas is subjected to the danger of injury, the character and extent of which are dependent on the size of the calculus and the duration of its impaction."

Little of value has been added by subsequent work save the important demonstration by Flexner [2] that the bile salts are the constituents of the bile which produce the inflammatory reaction in the pancreas while the colloid constituents have a protective action. Acute pancreatitis was produced in dogs by the injection of a sterile solution of sodium taurocholate.

In view of the clinical and especially the experimental evidence it is difficult not to accept the theory of pathogenesis of the disease proposed by Opie and quite impossible to concur in the opinion of Robson,[3] who, though recognizing the importance of cholelithiasis in the production of the lesion, says, "For my own part I believe that infection is the important factor and that the bile is simply the conveyor of infection."

Although numerous cases of pancreatitis in which the connection with cholelithiasis has been established have been published since the work of Opie, I have been unable to find any in which at operation or postmortem a stone was found blocking the orifice of the ampulla and in consequence desire to record the following case in which there was definite obstruction of the orifice of the papilla and, though through an error in technique, the obstructing mass was lost, there is little doubt but that it was a biliary calculus.

The patient was a well nourished white man, 51 years of

[1] Journal of the Am. Med. Association, 1904, xliii, 1102.

[2] Journal of Experimental Medicine, 1906, viii, 167.

[3] Lancet, 1904, i, 845. Montreal Med. Journal, 1904, xxxiii, 741.

age, an inmate of the Bay View Almshouse, who had had not infrequent attacks of epigastric pain with some constipation usually easily relieved. On January 25, 1906, he was seized with intense pain in the epigastrium, became collapsed and showed considerable abdominal distension. On a diagnosis of intestinal obstruction he was explored; some peritoneal adhesions were freed, and the wound closed. There was no generalized fat necrosis to attract attention to the pancreas and the condition of that organ was not determined at operation. The patient died at six o'clock the following morning and the postmortem examination was made five hours after death.

The examination showed beside numerous chronic lesions, as may be seen from the appended anatomical diagnosis an acute hæmorrhagic inflammation of the pancreas, which was large, swollen and mottled with red areas of hæmorrhage and opaque yellowish areas of fat necrosis. The gall bladder was large, distended and tense with bile, and the bile ducts were also dilated and firm to the touch, clearly showing that there was an obstruction to the outflow of bile. With gentle pressure there was no escape of bile from the papilla but with increased pressure there was a sudden spurt of bile carrying before it a small yellowish white mass which was distinctly seen in transit but was not recovered from the material in the abdominal cavity in which it fell. On opening the bile duct a small stone about 2 mm. in diameter was found in the apex of the ampulla close to the orifice and in the gall bladder and cystic duct there were about 400 soft, light colored cholestrin stones, varying in size from 0.5 to 6 mm., so there seems little doubt that the escaped mass was another stone, or a stone with mucus and desquamated epithelium. Whether or not the mass was a stone there was definite obstruction and the anatomical relations of the ampulla and ducts were such that the obstruction of the orifice set in progress the mechanism described by Opie, and resulted in retro-injection of bile into the pancreatic duct. The duct of Wirsung joined the common duct 11 mm. from the tip of the papilla and on dissection was found dilated and bile stained for 4 cm. from its orifice. The duct of Santorini was obliterated at the duodenal wall and opened into the duct of Wirsung. The common duct was dilated and somewhat hypertrophied and this in connection with an induration of the pancreas seemed to indicate that the previous attacks of pain of the patient were referable to the passage of other gall stones, some of which may have been of sufficient size to block the pancreatic duct in transit and thus cause atrophy of the parenchyma and the chronic interstitial process.

The anatomical diagnosis and that portion of the protocol which is of interest from the standpoint of this paper follow:

AUTOPSY 2664. *Anatomical diagnosis.*—Cholelithiasis, with stone in the ampulla of Vater; chronic interstitial pancreatitis; acute hæmorrhagic pancreatitis; peri-pancreatic fat necrosis; exploratory operation; acute fibrinous peritonitis; cloudy swelling of viscera; emphysema; chronic bronchitis; broncho-pneumonia; arteriosclerosis; chronic fibrous myocarditis; cardiac hypertrophy and dilatation; chronic passive congestion of viscera; atrophic scars in kidney cortex; hypertrophy of prostate; hydronephrosis; chronic interstitial orchitis; chronic gastritis; round ulcer of the pylorus.

The body is that of a well nourished white man 173 cm. in length. The left leg has been amputated through the lower third of the thigh and shows old pale fibrous scars on the stump. Rigor mortis is well marked; pupils are equal and moderately dilated. The face shows marked suffusion. The abdomen is prominent and shows in the mid-line a surgical incision extending for about 10 cm. below the umbilicus and closed by through and through silver sutures. The panniculus adiposus is well developed. On opening the peritoneal cavity there is found a small amount of blood-stained fluid in the neighborhood of the operation wound, the parietal peritoneum is injected and shows numerous small ecchymoses and the intestines are lightly adherent to each other by a slight fibrinous exudate.

Pancreas.—The pancreas is large, swollen, firm and mottled in color. Across the middle of the body it measures 45 mm. in width and 23 mm. in thickness. Over its surface in the peripancreatic fat there are numerous small irregularly shaped opaque yellowish areas, evidently areas of fat necrosis. Similar areas are found in the fat at the base of the mesentery. Several small dark red areas of hæmorrhage are also found in the peri-pancreatic fat. On section of the pancreas it is found infiltrated with adipose tissue separating the parenchymatous lobules somewhat. The latter in general are more homogeneous than normal and are firmer to the touch save in some small dark grayish areas which are softened. The parenchyma of the tail of the organ appears more indurated than that toward the head. Throughout the organ but especially marked toward the head there are numerous small irregular areas of hæmorrhage, and opaque yellowish areas of necrosis similar to those seen upon the surface. Toward the middle of the body there is one grayish black area about 1 cm. in diameter which is softened.

Bile passages.—The gall bladder and bile ducts are found tense and much distended; on gentle pressure bile does not flow through the papilla into the duodenum, on increased pressure, however, there is a sudden spurt of bile carrying before it a small yellowish white mass. (This mass was unfortunately lost in the body cavity). On opening the common duct it is found filled with thick greenish bile, and at the tapered summit of the ampulla of Vater is a small gall stone between 2-3 mm. in diameter and a small amount of mucoid material. On opening the duct fully it is found to measure 17 mm. in width, in its lower portion and 19 mm. just below the junction of the cystic and hepatic duct. Eleven mm. from the papilla the pancreatic duct enters. On dissecting out the duct of Wirsung it is found to be somewhat dilated, measuring 12 mm. across when opened; and is bilestained for 4 cm. above its junction with the common duct. It is joined by the duct of Santorini which tapers toward the periphery of the gland and is obliterated at the duodenum. The gallbladder and cystic duct contain many small calculi which are on section white, crystalline, quite soft and evidently composed almost entirely of cholestrin. They vary in size from 0.5 mm. to 6 mm. and are about 400 in number.

Microscopical Examination of the Pancreas. Sections made at various portions show islands of parenchyma separated by fat cells. In these islands the lobules show an increase in fibrous stroma about them, with some invasion of the lobules. The acini are in most places well preserved. The most striking features in the microscopical sections are the extensive necroses of the fat and interstitial tissue in some areas including also areas of the parenchyma. In these areas nuclear stain is entirely lost and the architecture of the tissue can just be made out. Small extravasations of red blood cells are also present in the sections both in the interstitial and fatty tissue, normal and necrotic, and between almost normal acini. In many places there is exudation of leucocytes, especially on the edges of the areas of hæmorrhage and necrosis, and many of them show fragmentation of their nuclei.

SO-CALLED SPONTANEOUS FOCAL MYOCARDITIS AND THE OCCURRENCE OF CALCIFICATION OF THE DEGENERATE MUSCLE FIBRES.

By Ernest K. Cullen, M. B.,

Fellow in Pathology, Johns Hopkins University.

(*From the Pathological Laboratory of the Johns Hopkins University and Hospital.*)

Focal changes affecting the muscle fibres of the heart are usually secondary to sclerosis of the coronary arteries but may occur in association with various infectious diseases, notably diphtheria, typhoid fever, and scarlet fever. The lesion in the infectious diseases is usually characterized by a fatty or albuminous degeneration of the fibres, hyaline degeneration being occasionally present, together with a variable increase of cellular elements in the interstitial tissue. In rapidly fatal cases the lesion, if present, is prone to be diffuse in type, while in those of longer duration the focal character is prominent. This has been confirmed experimentally by Mollard and Régaud.

In the early discussion of myocarditis in the infections diseases, considerable controversy arose as to the nature of the degenerative process. Romberg maintained that the changes in the interstitial tissue were primary, the muscle fibre being secondarily affected. Ribbert took the opposite view, considering the muscle fibre the seat of primary change, with subsequent inflammatory alterations in the connective tissue. He based his contention on the fact that in the earliest stages of diphtheria the muscle fibre was alone affected. Subsequent observations have favored Ribbert's view.

The experiments of Babes, of Welch and Flexner, and of Mollard and Régaud, have shown conclusively that the ætiological factor in the production of myocarditis in diphtheria is the toxin and not necessarily the bacillus itself. This was determined by the injection into animals of the sterile filtrate of diphtheria cultures. Similar myocardial changes have been experimentally produced with several toxic substances of organic origin.

Ziegler has expressed the view that fibrous patches in the myocardium are not always due to arterio-sclerosis, but in some instances are the result of intoxication, with consequent replacement of the degenerative fibres by scar tissue. Romberg adheres to this view. Basing his opinion upon a case following typhoid fever, in which the vessels were unaffected, he maintained that definite sclerotic changes may be produced in the myocardium, thus concluding that arterio-sclerosis is not the sole cause of fibrous myocarditis.

CALCIFICATION: The occurrence of calcification in certain pathological conditions, especially in arterio-sclerosis and myoma uteri is comparatively common. Calcareous deposits are also found occasionally in the skeletal muscles of animals, but involuntary muscles, except of the arteries, appear to be rarely affected.

Weigert has conclusively shown that calcium salts are never deposited in living tissues. In recent studies on the microchemistry of calcification Klotz has observed that in pathological processes the deposit of calcium salts is preceded by fatty degeneration of the affected tissues. The ætiology and pathogenesis of calcification have been summarized in the paper of Aschoff and the recent experiments of Klotz have shed much new light upon the process.

Two cases of calcification occurring in the cardiac muscle fibres have been reported by Coats, and single cases by Jacobsthal, Heschl, Roth, Köster, and ·Langerhans. Liebscher has reported a case of multiple disseminated calcification co-incident in the myocardium, liver, and spleen, but no reference is made to the microscopical picture.

The interesting feature of the case to be presented is the focal distribution of the calcium deposits in groups of muscle fibres, the fibres in most instances being still recognizable. The changes in the interstitial tissue form an inconspicuous part of the microscopical picture.

CASE I. Gynecological No. 77. Pathological No. 69.

Clinical history.—Jane Johnson, colored, single, age 28, admitted into the service of Dr. Kelly on January 6, 1890. The following is an abstract of the clinical history.

No satisfactory history can be obtained from the patient, who exhibits much hebetude. She first noticed a tumor in the abdomen about four years ago. This tumor has gradually increased in size.

Physical Examination.—Pulse is 100 and regular, the radial artery seems atheromatous. The abdominal wall is uniformly rounded out by a large tumor mass which on palpation presents two small nodules in the lower abdominal zone. The vagina is large and the cervix is high up, being on a line with the superior strait. The mass is entirely out of the pelvis. A slight, exceedingly fetid, discharge is present in the vagina.

The patient was examined by Dr. Osler, who found nothing abnormal, other than symptoms resulting from upward pressure upon the thoracic organs.

From January 6, the date of admission, until January 18 the patient's condition showed comparatively little change, the pulse beat ranging from 84 to 124 per minute, and the temperature from 98° F to 99° F. On admission the urine contained a small amount of albumin. Two weeks later pus cells were found and the albumin was increased in amount. From this time on the temperature ranged between 102.3° F and 100.5° F. The patient became gradually weaker and died on January 31.

The autopsy was performed by Professor Welch on February 1, 1890.

Anatomical Diagnosis.—Myoma of the uterus with central necrosis, pyonephrosis due to pressure on the ureters, chronic passive congestion of lungs, displacement of diaphragm and abdominal viscera by pressure of the tumor, marasmus, hypertrophy and hyaline degeneration of the heart.

The body is emaciated. The abdomen is distended by a large tumor which is quite smooth except for two nodular masses in its lower portion. The diaphragm on the left side is on a level with the second inter-space and on the right side reaches to the third rib.

The pericardial cavity contains a few cubic centimetres of clear fluid.

Heart: The heart is slightly enlarged and weighs 245 grammes. The pericardial surfaces are smooth. Fluid and coagulated blood are present in both sides of the heart. With the exception of a very slight contraction of the mitral orifice, the valves appear competent and normal. A few pale patches are seen scattered throughout the endocardium. The wall of the left ventricle measures 17 mm. and that of the right 4 mm. in thickness. The heart muscle is tolerably firm and dark brown in color. On tangential section of the left ventricular wall small yellowish foci are visible immediately beneath the endocardium. The orifices of the coronary arteries are dilated.

Lungs: The anterior borders of both lungs are emphysematous. The remaining parts of both lungs show the picture of chronic passive congestion.

Liver: The liver is rather small, the surface is smooth and shows a mottling of dark brown and yellowish colored areas. The same appearance is seen on section. The gallbladder is normal in appearance.

Stomach: Intestines and pancreas appear normal.

Kidneys: The left kidney measures 17x7x5.5 cm. The pelvis is enormously dilated and turned towards the front. The capsule is adherent and the surface irregular and lobulated. Beneath the capsule are numerous small white colored foci. Throughout the kidney are purulent foci, the pus following lines running from pelvis to cortex. The pyramids are flattened. The pelvis is generally smooth, but here and there is covered with a fibrino-purulent exudate. The ureters are dilated and closely adherent to the posterior surface of the tumor. The dilatation extends to the point of attachment to the tumor.

The right kidney is about the same size as the left and presents essentially the same features.

The adrenals are apparently normal.

Uterus.—The uterus is 19 cm. in length, is antiflexed and occupies the anterior portion of the tumor. The ovaries are flattened. The tubes are both patent till lost in the tumor mass.

Tumor.—The tumor is nodulated and divided into two distinct lobes corresponding to either side of the vertebral column. It is quite firm in consistence. On section it presents towards the center a triangular cavity which at its base measures 11 cm. This cavity is filled with a slightly blood-stained fluid and dense masses of firm white elastic tissue. Sections from these masses show perfectly preserved muscle fibres more refractive and clearer than those in other parts of the tumor. Sections from the tumor itself show a large amount of fibrillar connective tissue between the bands of muscle fibres.

Lymphatics.—The lymphatics in the lower part of the abdomen are greatly dilated and contain a faint yellow colored fluid. The lymph glands are small.

Bladder.—The mucous membrane shows ecchymoses, is deeply injected and contains a small amount of turbid urine.

Apart from the microscopical appearance of fresh specimens of the tumor and both fresh and hardened sections from the heart, we unfortunately have no microscopical picture of the other organs as specimens were not preserved.

Microscopical Appearance of the Heart Muscle.—Scattered throughout the wall of the left ventricle, especially, near the endocardium are numerous isolated groups of opaque, deeply staining fibers which appear to have undergone calcification. (Fig. 1.) These areas are composed of adjacent fibres ranging in number usually from three to twelve. Such fibres in most instances are well defined but occasionally appear irregular in outline, as if disintegrating. They have lost both their cross and longitudinal striations and appear quite homogeneous and opaque, staining deeply blue with both methylene blue and hæmotoxylin. No nucleus of the fibre is discernible, but often small, oval or rounded nuclei are situated about the fibre. In the interventricular septum the process appears to be much less extensive. Here single fibers are observed, which present a homogeneous granular appearance and with hæmotoxylin and eosin stain differently from the surrounding fibres. Fig. 2.) Such fibres are stained faintly brown in color. The nucleus is absent. Definite calcification is, however, observed in this situation in small groups of fibres which in general appearance resemble those found in the wall of the left ventricle. In sections taken from other parts of the heart no alteration of the fibres was visible.

At the time of autopsy Professor Welch studied the microchemical reaction of those altered fibres in the fresh specimens and found on the addition of glacial acetic acid to those fibres which contained a highly refractive substance, a slow dissolution of this material without the evolution of gas. This refractive material dissolved rapidly in hydrochloric and nitric acids also without the evolution of gas. As it dissolved the fibres swelled, lost their refractive property and appeared hyaline. This substance was insoluble in strong caustic potash and ammonia. In frozen sections left over night in an aqueous solution of bichromate of potash the refractive material dissolved slowly. The most interesting reaction was observed in specimens treated with strong sulphuric acid. The refractive material changed without the evolution of gas into beautiful clumps and rosettes of narrow rhombic crystals of calcium sulphate. Similar crystals, usually single, appeared in the fluid close by. No such reactions were obtained in specimens from other parts of the heart.

Professor Welch also observed that the refractive material appeared in the form of little coarse blocks or granules, with a suggestion often of an arrangement in the line of normal longitudinal and cross striation. Fatty degeneration of the fibres close to these areas of calcifications was observed.

The connective tissue immediately in relation to these altered fibres presents a variable amount of cellluar increase. In areas where only one or two fibres are involved, as in the interventricular septum, there is a very slight increase of cells while in those situations, in which the process is extensive, the number of cells is considerably larger than normal. The nuclei of these cells are oval or rounded in outline and appear slightly larger than those of the connective tissue in other parts of the section. The greater number of these resemble most closely young connective tissue cells, but a few appear

PLATE XVI

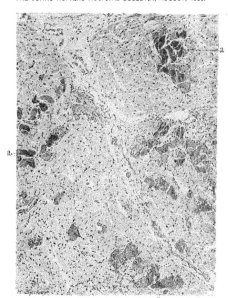

Fig. 1.

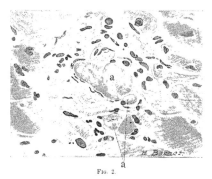

Fig. 2.

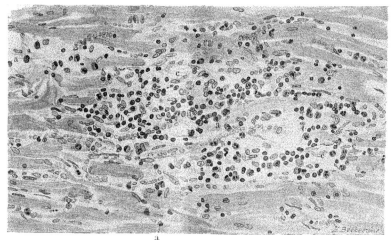

Fig. 3.

to be small lymphocytes. There is some slight increase of nuclear elements in the connective tissue not immediately in apposition to the degenerate areas. The vessels close to these foci of calcification contain a few red blood cells and some small round cells in their lumina, but there is no appreciable increase in the number of cells in the perivascular connective tissue, nor is there any evidence of alteration in the vessel walls.

The ætiology of the cell necrosis in this case cannot be definitely determined, but it is possible that the same ætiological factor concerned in the production of the existing pyonephrosis, may also be responsible for the lesion in the myocardium. The pressure exerted upon the thoracic organs by the large abdominal tumor may also have entered into the causation. This case appears to be no exception to the rule, that death of the cells precedes the deposit of calcium salts. In a study of the fresh specimens, as was mentioned in the microscopical report, Professor Welch observed the presence of fat granules in the fibres adjacent to the calcareous deposits. In hardened specimens such fibres presented a granular appearance and in some instances the typical ground glass picture was present.

From these observations it appears that a fatty degeneration of the fibres most probably preceded the deposit of calcium salts.

Acute myocarditis occasionally occurs unassociated with any other lesion, the ætiology being quite obscure. Two such cases have been reported by Freund and Rindfleisch. The patient of Freund was a man forty-eight years of age, who first complained of pain, reddening and swelling of the extremities. Symptoms of failing cardiac compensation developed and death followed in the fifth week. Microscopically the myocardium was the seat of degenerative changes in the muscle fibres with prominent cellular increase in the interstitial tissue. Freund was inclined to regard this case as belonging to the interstitial type of myocarditis.

The case reported by Rindfleisch was that of a man thirty-five years of age who fell from a height, striking on his left breast. A week later he complained of pain in the epigastrium. Cardiac distress and prostration gradually developed and the patient died at the end of the fifth week. At autopsy the heart was found to be hypertrophied and both ventricles dilated. Microscopically the muscle fibre was the seat of extensive fragmentation and the interstitial tissue was diffusely infiltrated with polymorphonuclear leucocytes, many eosinophilic cells being present.

Our second case to be presented belongs to this type of obscure origin, the so-called " primary myocarditis." Unlike the cases of Freund and Rindfleisch, the lesion is essentially focal in type. It is characterized by extensive degeneration of the fibres, accompanied by inflammatory changes in the interstitial tissue. The lesion is in no way referable to pre-existing alterations in the blood vessels, nor is there any history of existing infectious disease.

Gen. Med. No. 12,851. Pathological No. 1726. John G., age

47, German, unmarried. Admitted into the service of Dr. Osler on May 4, 1901.

Family history.—Negative.

Personal history.—Patient has been a bartender for the past four years and has used alcohol rather freely.

Previous illness.—The patient had typhoid fever several years ago.

Present illness.—For the past four months the patient has complained of a gradually progressive weakness, but until four days ago remained at his work. He has suffered considerably from cough and for some days past has complained of severe soreness down the middle of the chest. His appetite has been poor and he has suffered much from thirst. The bowels have moved quite regularly. There is no history of chills.

Physical Examination.—The patient is very weak and the face appears ashen. The radial pulse is feeble, twenty-six to the quarter and regular; the volume is small and the tension is low. Owing to his dyspnœa the patient has difficulty in answering questions.

The percussion note over the thorax is apparently everywhere resonant. Respiration is harsh and rather vesicular in character. A few moist râles are heard in the lower part of the axillae and posteriorily over both bases. The abdomen is soft and is free from distension. The liver and spleen are not palpable.

Immediately on admission to the ward stimulants were administered. There was temporary improvement of the pulse, but it soon became very feeble. Dyspnœa and cyanosis developed rapidly. Examination of the lungs showed a rapidly increasing oedema. The patient died two hours after admission. The chart on admission showed a temperature of 97.5° F, pulse 112, respiration per minute 30. No urine was obtained.

The autopsy was performed at 9.30 A. M. on May 5, by Dr. Opie.

Anatomical Diagnosis.—Hypertrophy of the heart with slight effusion into pericardial and both pleural cavities, oedema of lungs.

On opening the abdomen the stomach and intestines are found to be moderately distended. There is no excess of fluid in the peritoneal cavity. The left pleural cavity contains about 50 cc. of a clear straw colored fluid. The right pleural cavity contains a slightly greater quantity. Light fibrous adhesions are present over both lungs.

The pericardial cavity contains 125 cubic centimeters of a clear straw colored fluid. The pericardial surfaces are quite smooth.

Heart.—The heart weighs 445 grammes. The surface is smooth and covered by a moderate amount of fat. The endocardium is smooth. The heart muscle is pale in color and loose in texture. The wall of the left ventricle is 16 mm. in thickness and that of the right ventricle measures 3 mm. in thickness. The mitral segments show no thickening but are large and the papillary muscles are hypertrophied. There is slight thickening of the aortic segments about their bases and corpora aurantii, their free edges, however, being thin. The tricuspid and pulmonary valves are normal in appearance. The coronary arteries contain a few very slightly raised opaque patches, but the intima is otherwise smooth. The lumina are not obstructed. The aorta is smooth with the exception of an occasional raised yellow patch.

Lungs.—Both lungs are very oedematous and a few fibrous adhesions are present on their surfaces. The bronchial glands are deeply pigmented.

Apart from some slight hyperplasia of the lymphoid elements in the small intestine the other organs present a practically normal appearance both macroscopically and microscopically.

Microscopical Appearance of the Heart Muscle.—The heart muscle shows a decided change. Patches are observed in which the muscle cells have partially or completely disappeared, having been replaced by loose fibrous connective tissue, which in many instances shows an extensive infiltration with leucocytes. (Fig. 3.) The small round cell predominates, but a striking feature is the large number of eosinophilic leucocytes, which in some instances constitute the only type of polymorphonuclear leucocyte present. The septa of pre-existing connective tissue close to these areas appear œdematous and show a varying amount of infiltration with leucocytes. Coursing across the areas above mentioned may be seen capillaries containing single rows of red blood cells. The areas seem to bear no definite relation to the vessels, which themselves show no evidence of degeneration.

Adjacent to these areas of connective tissue the muscle fibres present a distinctly hyaline appearance. They stain deeply with eosin, are atrophied, very irregular in outline and often broken. The cross striation has in most instances completely disappeared, but the longitudinal is often indicated. The nuclei of the degenerative fibres vary to some extent, in size and shape, but are usually shrivelled and deeply stained. In many of these fibres occur ridges, which stain more deeply than the rest of the fibre. In several sections degenerate muscle fibres are found wholly isolated from the patches of connective tissue. About the larger of these foci there is an extensive accumulation of nucleated cells which is much less abundant about the smaller foci. The nuclei are usually oval or rounded in outline and appear larger than those of the connective tissue in other parts of the section. In some foci are found definite fibroblastic cells. Many of the cells resemble this type, but a few are observed which appear to be lymphocytes. The connective tissue not immediately in apposition to these foci shows some slight infiltration. The vessels in the neighborhood are free from any alteration. Specimens stained both for bacteria and fibrin were negative.

The lesion described above was found only in the wall of the left ventricle. Other parts of the myocardium appeared normal. The similarity of the lesion in this case to the type found in those cases associated with infectious diseases of longer duration, leads us to regard it as one of toxic origin. The lesion is limited to the wall of the left ventricle. The wall shows slight hypertrophy. As factors in the causation of this hypertrophy, valvular lesion, arterio-sclerosis and Bright's disease may be excluded. The patient was a beer drinker and possibly this hypertrophy may be similar in origin to that found in the lesion termed by the Germans "beer drinker's heart." In such hearts the hypertrophy is attributed to the increased work, consequent upon the excessive amount of fluid in the circulation.

The lesion in these two cases reported is essentially focal in character, and although. the onset of fatal symptoms in each instance was rather acute, it seems justifiable to regard them as belonging to the subacute rather than the acute type of myocarditis.

BIBLIOGRAPHY.

Aschoff: Laubarsch Ostertag. Ergenbnisse, 1904, VIII, 561.

Babes: Virchow's Archiv. 1890, CXIX, 460-488.

Coats: Manual of Pathology, 1883, p. 318.

Freund: Berl. Klin. Wochenschr., 1898, No. 49, 1077-1079.

Heschl: Cited by Jacobsthal.

Jacobsthal: Vidchow's Archiv., 1900. CLIX, 361-364.

Klotz: Journal of Experimental Medicine, 1905, VII, No. 6, 633-674.

Koester: Cited by Coats.

Langerhans: Cited by Jacobsthal.

Liebscher: Prag. Med. Wochenschr., 1902, No. 17, 195-197.

Mollard and Régaud: Annal. de L'Institute de Pasteur, 1897, XI, 97-133.

Ribbert: Mitteil. a. d. Grenzgeb. d. Medizin. u. Chirurgie, 1900, V. 1-14.

Rindfleisch: Ein Fahl von diffuser akuter myokarditis. Diss Königsberg, 1898.

Romberg: Deutsches Archiv. f. Klin. Med., 1891, XLVIII, 369-413, XLIX, 413-441.

Roth: Cited by Jacobsthal.

Welch and Flexner: Johns Hopkins Hosp. Bull.; Balt.; 1892, III, No. 20.

Flexner: Johns Hopkins Hosp. Reports; 1897, VI, 259-409.

Ziegler: Centralbl. f. Allgemein. Pathol., 1890, s. 883; 1891, s. 583.

DISSEMINATED TUBERCULOSIS IN RELATION TO THE THORACIC DUCT AND VASCULAR TUBERCLES.[1]

By G. H. WHIPPLE, M. D.,

Instructor in Pathology.

Since Weigert's work on the relation of tuberculosis of the blood vessels to acute miliary tuberculosis it has been generally believed that the disseminated tubercles found in various organs in cases of acute tuberculosis, were due to leakage of the tubercle bacilli into the blood stream from small vascular tubercles. Benda (1) and others have emphasized the pathology of the thoracic duct, which has been found packed with

[1] Read before The American Association of Pathologists and Bacteriologists, May 18, 1906.

tubercles or caseous material in some cases of acute miliary tuberculosis. Longcope (2) reports several such cases and mentions the fact that smears from 2 ducts which were apparently normal showed a number of tubercle bacilli. Ravenel (3) has reported interesting experiments on dogs. He fed the fasting animals with a mixture of tubercle bacilli and butter, 3½ hours later examined the thoracic duct and mesenteric glands by inoculation and demonstrated the presence of bacilli in these structures.

During the past winter the thoracic ducts in all cases of tuberculosis have been studied with regard to the presence of the tubercle bacillus. In all, smears have been made from 27 cases, including nearly every type of the disease. The method is very simple. The duct is dissected out and a small opening made in its upper portion. A slender pipette is introduced and pressure is made over the receptaculum, fluid accumulating to the amount of 1-5 drops. Smears of this fluid are stained with carbol fuchsin and methylene blue.

One may subdivide these cases for comparison into three groups.

(1) Acute miliary tuberculosis, 2 cases: Both showed ulcers in the intestines and caseation of the mesenteric glands. The smears contained many tubercle bacilli. The main vascular focus in one was a tuberculous thrombus of a pulmonary vein; in the other, a large caseating aortic tubercle.

(2) Subacute tuberculosis usually with the most extensive lesions in the lungs and numbers of disseminated tubercles in the organs. There were 19 cases in this group, of which 14 showed tubercle bacilli in smears, some only 2 or 3, others 40 or 50 on a single slide. Of these 14 positive cases, caseation of the mesenteric glands was present in all, intestinal ulcers in 11. It is of interest to note that one of these cases was at first placed in the third group, as no disseminated tubercles were seen with the naked eye, but examination of the smear showed 20 or 30 tubercle bacilli. A series of sections from the lungs, liver, and spleen showed the presence of very many minute tubercles in the very earliest stage of development.

(3) Chronic tuberculosis (usually of the lungs) with no disseminated tubercles. There was 6 cases in this group—none of which showed any bacilli in smears, 4 with tuberculous mesenteric glands, and 2 with intestinal ulcers.

From this analysis it would seem that the tubercle bacilli which are swallowed can pass through the intestinal mucosa, in some cases causing no visible lesion. The majority of these cases however showed intestinal ulceration. In their passage through the mesenteric lymph glands, in every instance, the bacilli left traces in the form of more or less extensive cascation, but the most interesting feature is that they seem able to traverse the thoracic duct with no damage to its intima.

The ducts in these series with one exception showed a smooth normal intima and delicate vessel wall. Some of the ducts appeared somewhat dilated and occasionally a little thickened, but the valves and intima were always smooth and glistening.

The one exception showed a slight constriction in its upper thoracic portion, just at the site of three of its delicate similunar valves.

A small nodule of an opaque gray color (2-2½ mm.) was situated in the duct wall just below the smooth intima and showing through it. Microscopic sections showed this nodule to be a tuberculous focus in some lymphatic tissue just outside the duct wall with extension through the adventitia. A lymphatic radicle at the margin of this area showed a small tubercle just rupturing into its lumen and the subintimal tissue of the main duct showed an infiltration with large and small round cells.

One may imagine this small lymphatic intimal tubercle as the type of many similar ones in the radicles of the mesenteric lymphatics, which are in relation to the caseating glands and from which the duct collects the bacilli which it pours directly into the blood stream.

These cases would indicate that in adults the bacilli do not pass through the lymphatic glands without causing more or less pathological change, that the bacilli can easily pass through the mucosa and lymphatic channels, but are blocked by the glands which may encapsulate them and prevent further damage (as is usually the case). On the other hand, the glands may liberate bacilli into their efferent lymphatic channels, which finally end in the thoracic duct.

Since Weigert's first description, recent methods have shown an increasing number of small vascular or intimal tubercles in cases of acute or subacute miliary tuberculosis. Ribbert (4) in a recent communication lays great stress on these small vascular tubercles as foci of distribution of tubercle bacilli. He believes that the great majority of disseminated tubercles, even in cases of acute miliary tuberculosis, are derived from these small intimal tubercles which he demonstrates by serial sections, oftenest in the lungs. In this connection a study of the development of young, rapidly growing vascular tubercles in the liver showed such tubercles of the portal vein. Microscopical sections show that the tubercle bacilli are oftenest deposited at the margin of the lobule, being carried there by the hepatic artery or portal vein. In their growth such tubercles naturally invade the portal veins more frequently and it is quite rare to see an invasion of the larger central veins.

The growth of such a tubercle may be outlined as follows: It soon begins to invade the wall of the adjacent portal vein, causing some accumulation of wandering cells in the middle coat and subintimal tissue. There may be some necrosis of the adventitia and infiltration of the media with the slender epithelioid cells, but the most interesting feature of this stage is the heaping up of polyblasts and small round cells below the intima, thus elevating it to some distance from the elastica interna. It is remarkable how many of these cells can accumulate below this thin layer of intimal cells before it ruptures or degenerates. A thrombus forms at once on this damaged area and closes the vessel if it is of small size, but in any case seems to wall off the young tubercle effectively from the blood stream. If the tubercle has grown into a larger vessel one may see this thrombus form and become smoothed over by the blood current, as Benda has pointed out. The next step is most interesting and consists in a rapid overgrowth of the fresh thrombus mass, by a delicate layer of endothelial cells, and in some instances one can see an intact layer of these cells roofing over a fresh thrombus in which can be made out the lines of Zahn and fresh fibrin with no signs of organization. It is difficult to believe that these small vascular tubercles, walled off as they are by a layer of endothelial cells, can take an active part in the dissemination of the bacilli, as is held by Ribbert. It is possible that they contribute a few tubercle bacilli to the blood stream, but proof one way or the other would be very difficult, while it can be shown conclusively that in many cases the thoracic duct takes an active part in such dissemination of bacilli.

Two other types of vascular tubercle were encountered in this series and may be briefly alluded to.

(1) Intimal or implantation tubercles—may be found in any vessel—for example portal, renal, and pulmonary veins, and the aorta as well as the conus of the right ventricle. There seems to be no doubt that in the larger vessels at least, such tubercles begin by the adhesion of one or more bacilli to some part of the intima which may have been previously damaged. The subintimal tissue is invaded immediately and here the growth takes place below an intima, which usually has repaired the primary damage and presents an intact roof of thin cells covering the young tubercle. Such a tubercle may grow to a large size by the formation of a large thrombus mass, its partial organization, and then caseation. In one case there was formed in the aorta such a tubercle the

size of a small pea. Even in these large tubercles there is a tendency for the endothelium to cover over part at least of the nodule by an upgrowth from its edge. (2) Medial tubercles—are not frequent but in the early stage of their development are quite definite. The bacilli are undoubtedly carried by the vasa vasorum into the middle coat; in their growth such tubercles tend to invade the lumen of the vessel, so that in an advanced case it may be very difficult to decide whether one is dealing with a tubercle which was primary in the intima with some invasion of the media, or vice versa.

Summary.—Cases of acute miliary tuberculosis usually show a vascular focus from which most of the bacilli are derived, but in the more common subacute cases with a variable number of disseminated tubercles, the thoracic duct may be the channel of infection.

Small vascular tubercles would seem not to take an active part in the dissemination of bacilli because during a greater part of their development they are covered by an intact endothelium which, if it ruptures or degenerates, is rapidly coated by a thrombus mass. This either occludes the vessel or is smoothed over, then roofed in by a rapid overgrowth of endothelium. In these cases the bacilli are usually derived from the intestine, which may or may not show ulcers. The organisms in their passage through the lymphatic apparatus give rise to caseation or tubercle formation in the glands, but usually have no effect on the lining of the thoracic duct.

REFERENCES.

1. BENDA: Lubarsch-Ostertag Ergebnisse, 1898, Bd. V.
2. LONGCOPE: Ayer Clin. Bul., 1906, No. 3.
3. RAVENEL: Jr. Med. Research, 1903-4, X, 460.
4. RIBBERT: Deutsch. Med. Wchnschr., 1906, No. 1.

NECROSIS OF EPITHELIUM IN THE KIDNEY IN INFECTIONS AND INTOXICATIONS.

By J. H. HEWITT, M. D.

Johns Hopkins Medical School, Baltimore.

(From the Pathological Laboratory.)

Several cases which have been observed at autopsy in the Pathological Department of the Johns Hopkins Hospital, in which widespread necrosis of the kidney cortex was found, roused interest in this phenomenon and its relation to other lesions and the search for descriptions of similar lesions and the study of all such cases as had occurred here was undertaken under the direction of Dr. MacCallum.

The literature contains very little direct reference to any such change. What could be found more or less closely related to the process to be described was as follows:

Orth[1] mentions necrosis of the epithelium of the tubules as the result of anæmia of the tissue from various causes, obstruction of the blood-vessels by thrombi, amyloid degeneration, hydronephrosis, etc., further necroses of toxic nature

in gout, diabetes, icterus, hæmoglobinuria, and poisoning with cantharidin, chlorates, chromates, petroleum, etc., and finally necroses which follow infectious diseases such as pyæmia, septicæmia, typhoid fever, diphtheria, acute atrophy of the liver, acute tuberculosis, etc.

Nearly all writers in speaking of acute and chronic forms of nephritis, mention in addition to the ordinary degenerative changes in the epithelium of the tubules the necrosis of some, at least, of the cells which may occur.

Aufrecht,[2] Israel,[3] Kossa,[4] Schmaus,[5] and others have studied

---

[1] Orth, Lehrb. Spec. Path. Anat., II; 1893.

[2] Aufrecht, Ctbl. f. inn. med., 1895, XVI, 241.
[3] Israel, Virch. Arch., Bd. 123, 1891, p. 310.
[4] Kossa, Ziegler's Beitr., Bd. 29.
[5] Schmaus, Atti. di. XI Kongr. med. internaz. Roma, 1894, II, 215.

experimentally the histological changes leading to necrosis of the kidney substance after ligation of the vessels, the nature of the change, its relation to coagulation, the occurrence of calcification and the processes of karyorrhexis being the points of interest.

Leutert,[4] Gebhardt,[7] Ebstein, Nicolaier[8] and others have described the severe injuries to the epithelial cells, which result from poisoning with sublimate and oxalic acid and show that calcification appears most extensively before complete necrosis is reached.

Ebstein[9] gives in his paper on diabetes with cirrhosis a plate illustrating the change in the kidneys, which consists in a general necrosis of the epithelium of the convoluted tubules.

Lorenz[10] also finds in erysipelas necrosis of the epithelium of the convoluted tubules while the straight tubules and the descending portion of Henle's loop as well as the glomeruli are preserved. So also in septic processes, while in diphtheria the necrosis, although sometimes occurring, is less intense.

Recently a few cases have been described in which extensive necrosis of the renal epithelium occurred and which have been explained on mechanical grounds.

Bradford and Lawrence[11] observed the case of a young woman who immediately after confinement developed anuria; death followed without uræmic symptoms. Thrombosis and obliterative endarteritis were found to have occluded all the smaller cortical arteries, complete necrosis of the cortical epithelium resulting.

Griffith and Herringham[12] have quite recently described a case similar in all details to this.

Zaaijer[13] describes a similar case in which anuria and death followed confinement. There was necrosis of the whole cortex of the kidney which the author thought to be due to increased intrarenal pressure compressing the vessels which were not otherwise obstructed. The anæmia resulting from this is described as the cause of the necrosis.

Practically nothing else except vague statements that necrosis may occur in the course of nephritis due to various causes could be found in the literature, and it was consequently thought advisable to collect the cases which have occurred here and attempt to determine their underlying cause. Among 2500 autopsies ten cases of this character were found and will be described briefly as follows:

CASE 1.—White woman, aged 50 (Med. No. 12,577, autopsy 659). Family and personal history unimportant. For 8 to 10 years has had periods of dull pain in right hypochondrium, never any jaundice. During last two months has had several attacks of severe pain in that region and since the last one,

[4] Leutert, Fortschr. d. med., Bd. 13, 1895.
[7] Gebhardt, Inaug. Diss. Freiburg. Bd., 1897.
[8] Ebstein and Nicolaier, Virch. Arch., Bd. 148.
[9] Ebstein, Deutsches Arch. f. klin. med., Bd. 28, p. 143, 1880.
[10] Lorenz, Ztsch. f. klin. med. XV, 416, 1889.
[11] Bradford and Lawrence, I. Path. and Bacteriology.
[12] Griffith and Herringham, Brit. Med. Journ., 1905, 2, 1182.
[13] Zaaijer, Mitth. a. d. grenz. d. med. u. chir., Bd. XII, 1900.

has gradually become jaundiced. Vomiting is frequent. Stools decolorized. Died ten days after admission to hospital. *Urine* on admission showed a specific gravity of 1015, deep brown color, traces of albumen and bile stained casts.

Later the urine showed leucin and tyrosin crystals, while in the hospital it varied from 200-300 cc. per diem. Temperature was subnormal for the greater part of the time.

The patient died ten days after admission. Only the essentials from the autopsy are given.

Anatomical diagnosis.—General infection with *B. coli.* Anatomical occlusion of the cystic duct and narrowing of the common bile duct. Acute yellow atrophy (?) of the liver. Jaundice. Chronic adhesive peritonitis. Ecchymoses in intestine and stomach.

Body strongly built; deep jaundice of the skin and all tissues; hæmorrhages here and there beneath the peritoneum.

Liver.—Capsule is smooth and free from adhesions. Its surface is dark in color. The whole organ is diminished in size, weighing about 1400 gms. It is soft and when placed on the table tends to flatten out. The edges are thin. On section it is of a greenish black color, with numerous lighter areas scattered through it. The bile ducts within the liver are dilated. The gall bladder is collapsed, its coats are much thickened and it contains glutinous mucus with little or no bile stain. The cystic duct is thickened and its lumen reduced. There is a considerable dilatation of the hepatic duct. This forms a pouch the size of the thumb, which contains greenish bile, and from which bile may be expressed into the duodenum. The liver shows central areas of complete necrosis and obliteration of the structures in the center of the lobule. The peripheral liver chords are not so seriously affected but the cells are filled with numerous granules and fatty globules.

Kidneys.—Combined weight 370 grammes. Capsule strips off with ease. On section the cortex is bile stained, the striations plainly seen, the glomeruli visible as bright red points. There are ecchymoses in the pelvis. The cortex is almost entirely necrotic; the medullary portion has been fairly well preserved. The glomeruli are fairly well preserved although their epithelium seems to have suffered somewhat. The epithelial cells of the convoluted tubules are for the most part completely necrotic; at the best, they contain only deeply staining shrunken nuclei or merely a dust of black nuclear fragments. In many places the cells are broken to fragments and form a mass of granules in the lumen of the tubule. The conducting tubules are better preserved, although their cells in many places are swollen and contain deeply stained shrunken nuclei. There is no evidence of inflammatory exudate, and no new growth of fibrous tissue. In the medullary portion there are some casts.

CASE II.—Colored man, aged 22, Med. No. 32,784. Autopsy 1621. Family and personal history negative. Always well up to 10 days before death. when jaundice appeared with general malaise. Four days later he began to vomit at first a greenish material, but later a material containing altered blood. The day before his death he became delirious, passed urine involuntarily and was seized with convulsions which persisted until an hour before death, when he passed into coma in which he died.

Urine was red in color, sp. gr. 1018, reaction acid and contained some bile pigment. Much albumen present. Microscopically red blood cells, hyaline casts, epithelial cells all deeply bile stained.

The amount excreted could not be determined as the patient died a few hours after admission.

Leucocytes 25,000 on admission, red corpuscles 5,200,000. Hæmoglobin, 90 per cent.

*Autopsy.—Anatomical diagnosis.—*Acute yellow atrophy of the liver, jaundice, submucous and subserous hæmorrhages. Parenchymatous degeneration of the kidneys. Adhesive perisplenitis. Tuberculosis of the bronchial lymph nodes.

Body sparely nourished; skin and tissues deeply tinged with yellow. Ecchymoses over epicardium, peritoneum, etc.

Liver weighs 770 gms., flaccid in consistence. The surface is reddened, roughened by areas about 4 mm. in diameter which are reddish yellow in color and slightly raised above the surrounding deep red surface. On section the cut surface is bright yellow with a greenish tinge with alternating red and yellow patches. Gall bladder contains viscid greenish bile. Very extensive necrosis involves the whole central part of the lobule extending from one lobule to another, so that only portions of tissue about the portal veins lie isolated in a mass of collapsed necrotic material. There is a new growth of bile ducts about the original bile ducts, and the connective tissue seems increased in amount. About these portal vessels extremely little liver tissue remains preserved.

*Kidneys.—*About normal in size. The capsule strips off readily leaving a smooth red surface. On section the cortex averages 7 mm. in thickness and is brownish red with a greenish tint. Striations well marked. Glomeruli visible as bright red dots. Ecchymoses are present in the pelvis. Combined weight, 420 gms.

The blood-vessels are quite clear. The medullary part shows some degenerative changes in the epithelial cells. On passing into the cortex it is found that almost all the convoluted tubules while still sharply outlined are completely filled with a homogeneous granular pink staining mass, in which the epithelial cells are merged. No nuclei are to be seen, except those of the intertubular tissue. The glomeruli are quite well preserved, except that their epithelium seems to have been destroyed in many cases, while in others it is for the most part intact. The conducting tubules are still better preserved, and in their lumen, but not in those of the necrotic tubules, there are abundant accumulations of a small rounded mass of calcium salts, which take a blue stain. (This supports the results of Leutert and Gebhardt, who find that the calcium deposit takes place rather in the injured than in the already dead cells.)

The *Streptococcus pyogenes* and *B. coli* were found in the blood and in the organs.

CASE III.—Colored man, aged 49. Surgical No. 38,604. Autopsy 1913. The patient complained of symptoms which led to the diagnosis of carcinoma of the stomach and an exploratory laparotomy was performed which revealed an inoperable carcinoma. After the operation the temperature became elevated and the pulse rapid and he died four days later.

*Autopsy.—Anatomical diagnosis.—*Adeno-carcinoma of the stomach with metastases, acute splenic tumor. Cloudy swelling of the kidneys. Stomach presents a large tumor mass involving the omentum and adjacent glands and extending beyond the pylorus into the wall of the duodenum.

*Liver.—*Weighs 2200 gms., measures 32 x 18 x 9 cm. On section the lobules are distinctly outlined, the periphery being gray, the centers more reddish. Gall bladder and ducts normal. The liver shows some disarrangement of the epithelial cells, some of which are shrunken. There are no definite areas of necrosis.

*Kidneys.—*Combined weight, 320 gms. Each meaures 11 x 7.5 x 4.5 cm. The cortex is 8 mm. in thickness. Capsule strips off with some difficulty but does not tear the surface. On section the cortex is pale and yellowish, the striations indistinct, but the glomeruli are plainly visible. The blood-vessels are clear. The cells in the pyramidal part of the kidney are for the most part preserved. In the cortex, there is most extensive necrosis of the epithelium particularly of the convoluted tubules, but this is not so advanced as in the previous cases, many tubules showing a few nuclei, while the remaining cells have none. The glomeruli and conducting tubules are much better preserved, but the epithelium of the glomeruli is much disintegrated, and at times necrotic. There is no inflammatory exudate, and no new-formed fibrous tissue. The *Streptococcus pyogenes* was found in the heart's blood; spleen and abdominal incision together with the *B. coli.*

CASE IV.—White woman, aged 24. Surgical No. 48,840. Autopsy 2413. Patient was admitted suffering from extreme dyspnœa and symptoms of a severe toxæmia. The tonsils were greatly swollen and were evidently the site of an abscess. The patient was quite cyanotic and became unconscious. Tracheotomy was performed and the respiratory distress somewhat relieved, but she died without ever regaining consciousness.

*Autopsy.—Anatomical Diagnosis.—*Abscess of tonsils with generalized infection; Cirrhosis of liver; acute bronchitis; acute splenic tumor.

*Liver.—*Distinctly smaller than normal, soft and flabby with many ecchymoses. The surface is covered with projecting masses of liver substance between which there are depressions in which lie injected veins. There are old scars with regenerative changes indicating long past injuries to the liver substance. There are some hæmorrhages in the substance of these scars. There is marked hypertrophy of the remaining liver substance, but there are no fresh injuries to the liver, unless the hæmorrhages form an index to such injury.

Kidneys.—Are quite soft and enlarged, weighing 400 gms. The capsule is slightly adherent and tears the surface on removal. The surface is, however, fairly smooth and the lobulations are very distinct. On section the cortex is of about normal thickness, striations are fairly regular, the blood-vessels are injected and the glomeruli appear as bright red spots. The pelvis contains some greenish opaque fluid. Its walls are injected and there are some ecchymoses.

The tubules in the pyramidal portion show marked degenerative change, the epithelial cells containing much fat, and being disintegrated in places in the cortex. The epithelial cells of all of the convoluted tubules are quite necrotic and converted into shapeless masses of red staining material, without nuclei which have fallen off from the basement membrane. The glomeruli have lost their epithelium, but otherwise are fairly well preserved. The conducting tubules are still lined with nucleated cells. There is no inflammatory reaction. The blood-vessels are clear throughout and show no thrombi. *Streptococcus pyogenes* and *Micrococcus aureus* were found in the form of a general infection.

CASE V.—White man, aged 50. Med. No. 40,387. Autopsy 2021. Entered the hospital twenty-four hours after receiving a severe blow on the side which was followed by intense pain and dyspnœa.

Evidences of pleural inflammation soon appeared with with dyspnœa and cyanosis. Leucocytosis of 11,400, marked delirium cordis with loud systolic murmur at apex. Dulness and tubular breathing developed over the bases of the lungs and the Cheyne-Stokes type of respiration appeared. Death occurred 24 days after admission with elevation of temperature.

Urine.—Spec. gravity, 1017; color, dark yellow; acetone present; urea averaged 12 gms. daily. Patient excreted 350 cc. on admission, which diminished to 120 cc. before his death.

Autopsy.—Anatomical Diagnosis.—Fracture of 6th, 7th and 8th ribs. Sero-fibrinous pleuritis. Atelectasis of lower lobe of right lung. Acute bronchitis. Subacute fibrinous adhesive pericarditis. Chronic mitral endocarditis with insufficiency. Chronic passive congestion of viscera.

Thorax contains about 1500 cc. of turbid fluid, in the left pleural cavity. Right lung bound to the chest wall by old adhesions.

The layers of the pericardium are bound together by recent adhesions, the mitral valve thickened and shortened. Heart is enlarged, the right ventricle being especially hypertrophied.

Liver.—Weighs 1500 gms., consistence firm. Surface is smooth and on section the lobules are indistinct. There is apparently some induration of the tissue. The epithelial cells are very much swollen; capillaries are seen with difficulty between them. They are granular, contain pigment and fat lobules, but there are no areas of necrosis.

Kidneys.—About normal in size, capsule firmly adherent and strips off with some difficulty, leaving a rough surface. Stellate veins are injected. On section the cortex is of a general purplish color, the vessels are quite prominent and

the glomeruli may be seen as dark red points. The cortex measures 7 mm. in thickness.

The kidney is much congested. Blood-vessesl are patent throughout. In the cortex practically all of the convoluted tubules are filled with necrotic masses of epithelium; their lining cells having lost their nuclei, and having become coalescent into a formless mass. There are patches here and there in which the cells are preserved. The conducting tubules show a lining of nucleated cells. The glomeruli are fairly well preserved, but seem to have lost their epithelium. Cultures were unfortunately contaminated.

CASE VI.—White man, aged 75. Surgical No. 48,704. Autopsy 2439. Entered complaining of shortness of breath and cough. Had recently indulged heavily in drink. Mental derangement. On November 30, the temperature rose from subnormal to 101°, and next day constipation and retention of urine began. Afterwards until his death urine was obtained only on catheterization. Leucocytes, 8500.

Cheyne-Stokes respiration, rapid and irregular pulse. During the last few days temperature steadily rose until his death, when it was 108°.

Urine.—Spec. gravity, 1030-1034, otherwise negative.

Autopsy.—Anatomical Diagnosis.—Arterio-sclerosis; cardiac hypertrophy and dilatation with myocardial degeneration. Chronic passive congestion of the viscera; œdema of lungs; fatty degeneration of the liver. Hypertrophy of prostate.

Liver.—Slightly increased in size and weight. Its surface is slightly irregular, there being numerous depressed reddish areas separating elevated areas of light yellow. There are well marked furrows due to the pressure of the ribs. The edge is rounded and the whole organ is soft. On section the central veins are injected. The parenchyma is extremely light in color and has a greasy feel. There appears to be no increase in the connective tissue. The gall bladder is very large and distended with dark greenish bile. It contains no concretions and the bile ducts are all open. The liver shows a slight cirrhosis. The liver tissue which remains, is extremely fatty, almost all the cells being occupied by large fat globules. There are no areas of necrosis, but the scars are quite extensive throughout the liver substance.

Kidneys.—Are surrounded by a thick, fatty capsule, and weigh together, 450 gms. They are slightly enlarged; the capsule strips easily, leaving a smooth surface, which is somewhat injected. Striations are regular, parenchyma is somewhat pale and cloudy with a yellowish color toward the boundary zone. The pelvis appears normal.

The blood-vessels are patent. Some of them are greatly distended with blood. The pyramids are fairly well preserved, but some of the tubules show marked degeneration of epithelium. In the cortex all the epithelial cells of nearly all the convoluted tubules are necrotic. There are a few which still show nucleated cells. The glomeruli are congested. The epithelial cells much disintegrated. There is no evidence of inflammatory reaction; no scarring of the kidney.

Culture from the spleen, shows the *Bacillus coli* and *B. acidi lactici.*

CASE VII.—Colored woman, aged 35. Gynæcol. No. 26,172. Autopsy 1353. Entered hospital April 13, complaining of hæmorrhoids and pain in abdomen. On April 20, and again on April 26, she was examined under an anæsthetic, chloroform being used on April 26. After that she grew weak and passed into coma April 29, in which she died. Temperature was much elevated before death. Urine on admission showed sp. gr. 1024, acid; no sugar; no albumen. Heavy pinkish sediment. There was no further examination of urine.

Autopsy.—Anatomical Diagnosis.—Ulcerative colitis; disseminated fat necroses. Acute atrophy of the liver.

Heart, lungs, spleen, etc., show no abnormality.

Opaque white areas were found in the fat of the omentum and mesentery about the pancreas.

Intestine shows extensive shallow ulcerations with remaining islands of mucosa.

Liver.—In general is smooth. There are a few tags of old adhesions. It is about normal in size and weight. On section it is not homogeneous. In the superficial portion the lobules are plainly marked out, the anterior being congested. In the more central portion of the liver the lobules are even more sharply marked out and present a net-work of white and yellow lines, surrounding opaque yellowish areas. The center of the lobule is pale and whitish, but toward the periphery it becomes ocher yellow. Gall ducts and gall bladder normal.

The liver shows a distinct midzonal necrosis, which causes the disappearance and coalescence of all the cells of the lobule, except those quite near the portal vessels, and those quite near the efferent vein. The remaining cells contain a good deal of fat, and show here and there mitotic figures. There is no scarring of the liver.

Kidneys.—Are normal in size and weight, the capsule strips off readily, leaving a smooth surface. On section the cortex is 6 mm. in thickness. Striations well defined and the glomeruli apparent as red dots. The cortex is rather pale. The blood-vessels are patent. The pyramidal portion of the kidney shows hæmorrhages and necrotic fragments in the conducting tubules, but the lining cells are for the most part preserved in the cortex. Many of the convoluted tubules have a well preserved lining, but many show complete necrosis of the epithelial cells. The injury is not so intense as in the preceding cases; and shadows of the nuclei at least may be seen in almost all of the cells. The conducting tubules and glomeruli are better preserved, but the glomeruli show frequently a loss of epithelium. There is no inflammatory reaction. Heart's blood, liver and kidney showed *Streptococcus pyogenes* and *Bacillus coli*.

CASE VIII.—Colored woman, aged 21, Gynæcol. No. 9380. Autopsy 1879. Confinement 8 months ago, uncomplicated. Abscess developed in pelvis, which was punctured and drained, 200 cc. of pus being evacuated. February 23, the peritoneum became infected. Symptoms of general peritonitis ensued

and continued in spite of operation and cleansing of abdominal cavity. Intestinal obstruction ensued and amount of urine secreted diminished greatly in amount. Continual vomiting; death on April 2. Temperature rose to 105° before death; urine examined only on admission, and on February 27, at latter date, just after operation, it showed albumen and many leucocytes and squamous cells.

Autopsy.—Anatomical Diagnosis.—Operation wounds in vagina and abdomen. General fibrino-purulent peritonitis; purulent endometritis. Bilateral salpingectomy. Sero-fibrinous pleurisy. Fatty degeneration of heart and liver.

The abundant exudate in the peritoneum and pleura need not be further described.

Liver.—Slightly enlarged, very pale and yellowish, mottled with yellowish opaque and red foci, which are also seen on the cut surface. In some areas the center of the lobule is red, the periphery yellow. Gall bladder contains dark bile. The lobules are sharply marked out by lines, throughout which the liver cells are loaded with fat. These occupy the periphery of the lobule extending from portal space to portal space. There are no actual necroses in the liver.

Kidneys.—Slightly enlarged. Capsule strips off easily, leaving a smooth surface with injected stellate veins. Cortex is 7 mm. in thickness and slightly injected. The striations are indistinct, but the glomeruli are quite prominent. The pyramidal portion is somewhat congested. The epithelial cells fairly well preserved. In the cortex all the convoluted tubules have become necrotic with the exception of a few epithelial cells, which still show faded nuclei. There is an extensive desquamation of the epithelial cells of the conducting tubules, as also of the epithelial lining of Bowman's capsule. There is no inflammatory reaction. There are some hæmorrhages throughout the cortex of the kidney. *Streptococcus pyogenes* with *B. coli* was found in all the exudates.

CASE IX.—Tissue from miscellaneous collection (No. 569) probably from New York. The jar is labelled a case of acute yellow atrophy of the liver, duration of the disease one week; acute symptoms two days; mania and delirium.

Liver.—Weighed two and one-half pounds, and showed reddish brown and yellowish lobular markings. There was no liver tissue to examine.

Kidney.—The blood-vessels are patent. All the convoluted tubules show complete necrosis of the epithelium, which lies in a formless mass without any nuclei staining in the tubules. The epithelium of the conducting tubules is better preserved and contains nuclei; that of the glomeruli as well as the glomerulus itself, seems but slightly injured. The tubules are everywhere swollen and tightly packed together. There is no inflammatory reaction and no new growth of connective tissue.

CASE X.—White woman in private practice of Dr. Williams. Autopsy 2110. This case which is described by Dr. Williams in his paper on "Pernicious Vomiting of Pregnancy" (J. H. H. BULLETIN, March, 1906), was seen in the third month of pregnancy; all efforts to check the continual vomiting being in vain, an abortion was performed in the hope of saving the patient's life; but she grew weaker and died a few days later.

Examination of urine a few days before death showed nothing of importance.

*Autopsy.—Anatomical Diagnosis.—*Laceration of vagina and cervix uteri. Adherent placenta in uterus of early pregnancy. Focal necrosis and bile staining of liver. Fatty degeneration and bile staining of kidneys. No cultures were taken. There was no peritonitis or other fresh inflammatory process.

Liver.—Decreased in size, weighs 1000 gms. It is bright yellow in color, and is quite soft. Its surfaces are everywhere smooth. On section it is bile-stained and fatty. Areas and lines of degeneration and necrosis are evident by their opacity to the naked eye. Between these areas the capillaries stand out very plainly. Gall bladder normal. The liver shows a midzonal necrosis frequently affecting also the central zone. Throughout the necrotic area, the nuclei have disappeared, or are represented by fine dust of nuclear fragments. The more peripheral liver cells are very full of fat and show very abundant mitotic figures.

Kidneys.—Increased in size. The capsule strips off readily leaving an opaque yellow surface. No vessels are to be seen. On section the cortex measures 7-8 mm. and is very yellow and opaque. No structures, vessels, or glomeruli can be distinguished in the cortex. It has a granular appearance and is slightly raised above the level of the pyramids. The pyramids are pale and their peripheries show lines of opacity.

The blood-vessels are clear. The pyramidal portion of the kidney is a little altered. The cortical portion shows complete necrosis of the epithelium of all the convoluted tubules which are still packed with the coalescent mass of pink staining granular material, in which the cell outlines and nuclear shadows are only faintly visible. The glomeruli and convoluted tubules are better preserved, and show nuclei in all their cells, even the epithelium of the glomeruli being pretty well preserved.

SUMMARY.

The cases may be summarized as follows in a table:

No.	Age.	Sex.	General condition.	Duration of illness.	Bacteriological report.
1	50	F.	Jaundice, acute yellow atrophy of liver	2 weeks	B. coli, general infection
2	22	M.	Acute yellow atrophy of liver	10 days	Streptococcus pyogenes, B. coli
3	49	M.	Carcinoma of stomach; streptococcus infection following operation	4 days	Streptococcus, B. coli
4	24	F.	Suppurative tonsillitis; generalized infection	2 days	Streptococcus, micrococcus aureus
5	50	M.	Fracture of ribs; pleuritis and pericarditis	3 weeks	Cultures contaminated
6	75	M.	Chronic alcoholism, delirium, hyperpyrexia	18 days	B. coli and B. acidi lactici
7	35	F.	Acute yellow atrophy of liver, acute enteritis	16 days	Streptococcus and B. coli
8	21	F.	Pelvic abscess; general peritonitis, pleuritis	5 days	Streptococcus and micrococcus aureus
9	21	F.	Acute yellow atrophy of liver	7 days	Streptococcus and micrococcus aureus
10	21	F.	Pernicious vomiting of pregnancy; acute yellow atrophy of liver	3 weeks	Streptococcus and micrococcus aureus

This summary makes it clear that the kidney in these cases has been affected by some poison circulating in the body whether bacterial or not, which quickly destroys all the highly specialized and sensitive epithelial cells, so quickly indeed that there has been no time for reaction of any sort. This injury to the kidney is quite analogous to those necroses of the liver which are usually classed under the name of acute yellow atrophy and indeed of the 10 cases, 5 showed also the lesions of acute yellow atrophy of the liver. Nevertheless just as in the cases of hepatic necrosis there is not always complete necrosis of the renal epithelium so herein the remaining cases in which bacterial or other toxins destroyed the renal epithelium, the liver escaped.

The changes differ obviously from those seen in acute nephritis in the completeness and suddenness of the destruction and in the lack of reaction.

ON THE GROWTH OF LYMPHATICS IN GRANULATION TISSUE.

By T. Homer Coffin, M. D.

(From the Pathological Laboratory, Johns Hopkins University, Baltimore.)

The mode of growth of the lymphatics in the development of the embryo has been fairly satisfactorily worked out by Ranvier, MacCallum, Sabin and others, but there seems to be but little in the literature referring to the new formation of these channels in the course of regeneration of tissue in the adult animal. The following work was therefore carried out under the direction of Dr. MacCallum in the attempt to clear up their mode of growth in granulation tissue.

It has been shown by MacCallum in a study of the relation of the lymphatics to connective tissue that in the embryo,

growth takes place by an active proliferation of the endothelial cells which constitute the complete walls of the channels and which may extend in the form of elongated rows of cells sometimes branching, sometimes sending out long lash-like processes for a considerable distance in advance of the lumen.[1] Later it was shown by Dr. Sabin that this process of growth begins in the form of buds from the endothelium of

[1] Johns Hopkins Hospital Bulletin, XIV, No. 142, January, 1903, Figs. 5, 6, and 7.

the veins which push their way radiately far and wide into the tissues of the animal, finally meeting and anastomosing with ramifications from the opposite side.[2] It seemed entirely probable that this method of growth which is in most respects similar to that of the blood vessels would be carried out in the formation of granulation tissue or indeed in the furnishing with lymphatics of any new-formed tissue, and it was determined to put it to a test in a position where such tissue formation could be easily controlled.

It is well known that it is very easy to inject the lymphatics of the wall of the intestine by inserting a hypodermic needle into the subserous tissue, and on that account the granulation tissue to be investigated was made to grow upon the serous

was experienced in recognizing the injected vessels as lymphatics, but in some cases to make quite sure the blood vessels were first injected from the larger arteries with a mass of another color. Serial sections were then made through the intestinal walls and overlying granulation tissue.

Microscopically it was found in these sections that the original lymphatics of the intestinal wall are distended with the injection mass and that from them there spring up sprouts into the granulation tissue which resemble closely sprouting blood vessels except perhaps in that their walls are quite thin. The tips of these sprouts are represented in Figures 1-2, in which it is seen that the injection mass proceeds toward the surface between endothelial cells until the

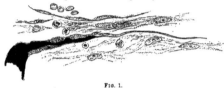

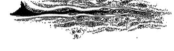

Fig. 1.   Fig. 2.

surface of the intestine. For this purpose a loop of intestine was drawn out and sewed into a wound in the skin, only a portion of the circumference of the gut being allowed to project. In the course of a week or ten days the loop was usually found to be well covered with granulation tissue, which rendered it inconspicuous in the bottom of the wound. The animal was then killed and an injection of the lymphatics of the wall of this loop of intestine was made by plunging the needle of the syringe into the quite smooth intra-abdominal part of the loop near the line along which it adhered to the inner surface of the body wall. It was found that it is quite easy to make an injection of the intestinal lymphatics in this way and that the injection will run for a certain distance into the granulation tissue which grows upon the exposed portion of its surface. It is thus evident at once that lymphatic channels spring from those present in the original tissue and advance into the overlying granulation tissue. No difficulty

lumen of the channel narrows to a point where the injection stops. Beyond this there are continued for a short way the endothelial cells in a single or partly double row. These cells are quite plump and their nuclei are large and vesicular. Nuclei and cell bodies are seen sometimes to diverge from the line and to send forth protoplasmic processes into the adjacent tissue and the terminal cell of the advancing strand is frequently seen, as in Figure 1, to be continued into a long lash of protoplasm which reaches far forward into the tissue crevices. In this advance portion there is no lumen and it is difficult to understand exactly by what mechanism the lumen is produced unless it be by the lateral growth of the cells which may lead to their separation. It is seen here as always that the lymphatic channels are perfectly sharply outlined independent structures completely formed of endothelial cells and standing in no more intimate relationship with the crevices of the connective tissue than do the capillary blood vessels.

[2] Am. Journal of Anatomy, Vol. 1, 1901-2.

OBSERVATIONS ON THE GROWTH OF CARCINOMA CELLS WITHIN THE MUSCLE FIBRES IN CARCINOMATOUS METASTASES TO VOLUNTARY MUSCLE.

By G. Howard White, M. D.

(From the Ayer Clinical Laboratory of the Pennsylvania Hospital, Philadelphia.)

In the histological examination of a carcinoma of the mammary gland, it was noted that about the margins of a metastatic nodule situated in the pectoralis major muscle the carcinoma cells appeared to be within the muscle fibres, surrounded by sarcolemma and replacing the sarcoplasma. To

determine the frequency of this condition and the method by which the cells entered the muscle fibres, a study was made of all the carcinomatous metastases to voluntary muscle which could be obtained; and the present paper embodies the results of this study.

The early observations on carcinoma of muscle are closely connected with the question of the specificity of tissues, and one finds in the literature many discussions as to whether muscle cells can give rise to carcinoma, either as a primary or secondary growth; and whether the sarcolemma or the connective tissue of the muscle can be considered as the point of origin of the growth.

The earliest article found was one by Chevalier in 1826, who said that carcinoma invaded muscle by insinuating its gristly sprouts between the muscle fasciculi—retracted these into its substance—and caused them by pressure or by absorption to lose their fibrous or muscular character; while sarcoma, he said, engulfed the muscle but the muscle fasciculi preserved their character better and could be traced through the tumor pulp. Walshe considered that the cancer was primary in "the cellular membrane separating the fasciculi of muscle fibres" and stated that the muscle was transformed into an "encephaloid structure" though the form of the fibres was retained. Bennett made microscopic examinations of carcinoma of muscle but had not apparently in 1849 discovered carcinoma cells lying inside the sarcolemma.

In 1848 Lebert saw, in a case of carcinoma of the tongue, carcinoma cells in some of the muscle bundles. Little notice was taken of this observation and after the publication of Schroeder van der Kolk's article [1] describing the same condition, the latter author was usually regarded as the first to have made this observation. Van der Kolk and Lebert both believed the cells to be transformed muscle cells. Following these communications, much interest was shown in the matter. Billroth thought that possibly the muscle cells were changed to carcinoma cells but later decided that the carcinoma arose from the myolemma which he considered as evidence of connective-tissue origin. Böttcher believed that the cells arose from the sarcolemma, and though Weber believed that most of the cells arose in this manner he also contended that some arose from the muscle nuclei. Kölliker adopted the view of the origin from muscle tissue.

Virchow stated that the cells arose not in the muscle fibres or the sarcolemma, but in the connective tissue, and later penetrated the sarcolemma. Neumann a year later repeated this view, and said that he had seen sections which showed that the growth spread from only one point in the sarcoplasma, a fact which he considered was in favor of the view that the process was an invasion of the mucle fibres and not a transformation of muscle cells into tumor cells.

Förster's opinion seems to have varied. In 1863 he upheld the theory of origin from connective tissue, but believed that "secondary carcinoma" could sometimes arise from the muscle cells. Sick considered that the origin of the cells was in the capillaries of the muscle. Popper said that carcinoma could arise both from connective tissue and from muscular tissue interchangeably.

Waldeyer's article in 1867 was the first on carcinoma of

muscle which advocated his now universally accepted view that the growth must arise from epithelial cells elsewhere. He admitted that there was a proliferation of the nuclei of the muscle but insisted that these nuclei could not produce carcinoma cells. At this time he believed that the tumors were metastases carried to the muscle by way either of lymph- or blood-vessels.

Volkmann described sections showing the openings through which the carcinoma cells entered the sarcolemma but thought that the primary point of origin was the connective tissue.

The only statement which could be found from America concerning this question is an incidental sentence in a lecture by Woodward, where he emphasizes the presence of a small round cell infiltration and suggests that it may have given rise to the idea that the proliferation of the muscle nuclei may produce carcinoma cells.

The later articles of Schaeffer and Christiani treat the subject from a modern point of view, and Cornil and Ranvier have an excellent article in the last edition of their "Manuel d'Histologie Pathologuique," in which they desribe the occasioual occurrence of carcinoma cells within the muscle fibres of voluntary muscle, the seat of carcinomatous metastases.

A search of the literature for any definite information concerning the lymph vessels of muscle was unfruitful. The usual statement is that they exist only in the connective tissue and accompany the blood-vessels. Sappey says that the main trunks in the muscle itself run parallel to the muscle bundles, and give off many branches forming anastomoses with the neighboring trunks. An attempt made in the laboratory to inject and demonstrate lymph vessels in muscle was unsuccessful. The material which was studied consisted of tissue from six cases of carcinoma of the breast with involvement of the pectoral muscles. Zenker's fluid was used as a fixative. Sections were cut in paraffin and stained with hæmatoxylin and eosin. One serial set of 115 sections was obtained through a small metastasis in the pectoral muscle. These were cut transversely to the muscle fibres. Much the same mode of growth was seen in all the cases.

Sections through an area of advanced tumor growth show nests of carcinoma cells usually with a large proportion of fibrous tissue between; and no vestige of the original muscle can be found. Sections of a less advanced stage show, however, a striking persistence of the arrangement of muscle fibres. In sections cut transversely to the muscle bundles and studied under the low power one finds rounded masses of cells corresponding to the muscle bundles and giving at first glance an appearance much like that of a gland; while on longitudinal section one sees elongated cellular masses stretching across the field.

The reaction on the part of the muscle is shown by a small round-cell infiltration which may be intense or almost entirely lacking, and by a marked degree of interstitial myositis. The cross striation is preserved until the muscle is markedly involved in the tumor growth. The nuclei are almost always increased in number, often forming lines in longitudinal

---

[1] Content known only through references in the literature.

sections. The sarcoplasma appears granular, and takes the stain irregularly, giving the impression of rifts in the protoplasm. In some bundles, especially in the portion nearest the epithelial cells, the sarcoplasma shows a hyaline degeneration and stains very deeply in eosin.

On closer examination of the cross-sections under the high power, one finds, particularly about the margins of the metastases, small masses of carcinoma cells lying in the muscle bundles among the muscle fibres. Some are quite round and are seen to be surrounded by a delicate membrane. These do not lie between the muscle fibres but are in a position which corresponds exactly to a muscle fibre itself (see Fig. 1, C). Often it can be made out that this delicate membrane is really the sarcolemma of a muscle fibre, for in some cases a little sarcoplasma is present beneath the apparently intact sarcolemma (Fig. 1, A), separating it from the collection of carcinoma cells. This sarcoplasma may form a crescent or a half-moon on one side of the carcinoma cells (Fig. 1, D and E), or sometimes a ring surrounding one or more cells; occasionally one sees a single cell lying just beneath the sarcolemma in an indentation in the sarcoplasma. Between the fasciculi of muscle bundles one sees carcinoma cells lying in the lymphatics which surround the blood-vessels in these situations (Fig. 1, B).

Longitudinal sections show a corresponding picture (Fig. 3). The carcinomatous tissue occupies the sarcolemmata with some or no sarcoplasma along its edge. One can occasionally find bundles showing how the carcinomatous and muscular tissue dovetail into one another inside the sarcolemma, giving the picture in the cross-section of a fibre half filled with carcinoma cells. Here, too, there are strands of cells which cannot be shown to be within the sarcolemma but which lie in the perivascular lymphatics of the connective tissue.

Serial Sections.—One end of the series is in a dense tumor growth, and at the other end, in certain parts of the sections, the epithelial cells have almost entirely disappeared. Starting from the portion where the growth is most developed and following the sections toward the advancing edge of the metastasis, one finds that the masses of cells grow smaller and more discrete until they come to occupy only the spaces within the sarcolemmata with no free tumor cells near them. One can trace very clearly all the stages of transition from the round nests of epithelial cells to the perfect muscle fibre (Fig. 2). Following up any one muscle bundle the epithelial cells will be found to show first a thin border of sarcoplasma, at one side or perhaps surrounding them; then the area of the epithelial cells gradually decreases with a proportional increase in the area of the sarcoplasma. This decrease in the number of epithelial cells is not always steady, but may cease for a few sections or there may even be a slight and transitory increase. Further on one finds only one or two epithelial cells lying either in the central or peripheral part of the sarcoplasma (Fig. 2, A), and finally the carcinoma cells disappear entirely, leaving a perfect muscle bundle.

No bundles were found containing epithelial cells in which it was not possible to trace these cells to a point where the bundles were lost in dense carcinomatous growth. That is to say, no islands of carcinoma cells were found isolated from the main growth.

The deep red hyaline appearance of the muscle fibres in the neighborhood of the tumor cells is very well marked in these sections, and on tracing the sections toward the carcinoma one can tell by the change in appearance of a bundle that epithelial cells are present within its sarcolemma before one sees the cells themselves, and can foretell that they will appear a few sections further on.

From a study particularly of serial sections it seems possible to explain the method by which the carcinomatous growth penetrates the muscle fibres. The carcinoma cells evidently reach the muscle through the lymph vessels supplying the muscle; since the lymph vessels so involved are usually located in the connective tissue between the muscle fasciculi, the original metastasis first starts its growth from this situation. The possibility of a similar involvement of the lymph vessels lying between the muscle bundles—if such exist—cannot so far be excluded.

The carcinoma cells which proliferate in the lymph vessels secondarily involve the fasciculi of the neighboring muscle bundles, destroying in their growth many fibres. In this way it is possible that tumor cells may extend into the broken ends of muscle fibres and develop along the course of the muscle bundle, the sarcolemma acting as a sheath. The sarcoplasma seems to offer a comparatively weak resistance to the carcinoma and permits its rapid advance in a longitudinal direction, whereas the sarcolemma offers a comparatively high resistance to the carcinoma and prevents the lateral spread of carcinoma which exists within it.

The interaction of the low resistance of the sarcoplasma and the high resistance of the sarcolemma, causes the presence of carcinoma cells within the sarcolemma, as can be followed in serial sections, far removed from the point at which the carcinoma entered the muscle bundle; giving an appearance in section of carcinoma cells lying within an apparently intact sarcolemma.

No evidence could be found to support the view that carcinoma cells are carried directly to the sarcoplasma through openings normally present in the sarcolemma, and communicating with the lymph vessels; or through openings which they themselves have made by destruction of the sarcolemma at one point.

REFERENCES.

Bennett: On Cancerous and Cancroid Growths, p. 85, Edinburgh, 1849.

Billroth: Virchow's Arch., Vol. IX, p. 172, 1856.

——— Beiträge zur path. Histologie, p. 67, Berlin, 1858.

——— Virchow's Arch., Vol. XVIII, p. 74, 1860.

Böttcher: Virchow's Arch., Vol. XIII, p. 237, 1858.

Chevalier: London Med. and Phys. Journal, LV, p. 95, 1826.

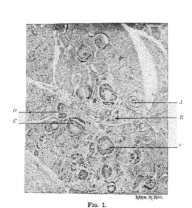

Fig. 1.

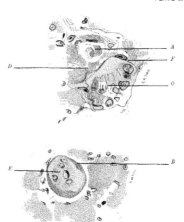

Fig. 2.

Fig. 1.—Cross-section through margin of a carcinomatous metastasis to the pectoral muscles, showing varying grades of replacement of sarcoplasma by carcinoma cells. (Zeiss, oc. No. 4; obj. AA.)

A. Carcinoma cells completely within muscle fibres.
B. Carcinoma cells within perivascular lymphatic.
C. Round mass of carcinoma cells about which no muscle fibres are visible.
D and E. Carcinoma cells partially surrounded by muscle fibres.

Fig. 2.—Tranverse section of muscle fibres, showing varying grades of replacement of sarcoplasma by carcinoma cells. (Zeiss, oc. No. 4; Bausch & Lomb, obj. No. 1/6.)

A O and E. Carcinoma cells.
B and D. Sarcoplasma. In B, the hyaline appearance of the sarcoplasma is well seen.
F. Delicate membrane surrounding mass of carcinoma cells.

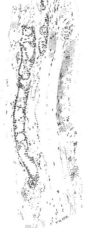

Fig. 3.

Fig. 3.—Longitudinal section through carcinomatous metastasis to pectoral muscle. (Zeiss, oc. No. 4; obj. AA.)

Christiani: Arch. de Physiologie, Vo. X, p. 107, 1887.

Cornil and Ranvier: Manuel d'Histologie Path., Paris, 1902.

Förster: Allg. path. Anat., Leipzig, 1863.

*Korpovitsch: Ke vopruso o razoitii raka ve mishtsache ve patologo-gistolog otnoschenii, St. Petersburg, 1868.

Lebert: Abhandlungen aus den Gebiete der prakt. Chirurgie, p. 256, Berlin, 1848.

Neumann: Virchow's Arch., Vol. XX, p. 152, 1861.

Popper: Med. Jahrbücher, Wien., Vol. XXXI, p. 37, 1865.

Rosenbach: Der Epithelial Krebs im quergestreifte Muskel, Göttingen, 1873.

Sappey: Traite d'Anatomie, p. 775, Paris, 1888.

Schaeffer: Virchow's Arch., Vol. CX, p. 443, 1887.

----

* Not read.

* Schroeder van der Kolk: Nederlandsch Lancet, September, p. 129, 1853.

Sick: Virchow's Arch., Vol. XXXI, p. 331, 1865.

Virchow: Virchow's Arch., Vol. XVIII, p. 15, 1860.

Volkmann: Virchow's Arch., Vol. L, p. 543, 1870.

Waldeyer: Virchow's Arch., Vol. XLI, p. 512, 1867.

Walshe: Nature and Treatment of Cancer, p. 133, London, 1848.

Weber: Virchow's Arch., Vol. XV, p. 526, 1858.

—— Virchow's Arch., Vol. XXIV, p. 182, 1864.

—— Virchow's Arch., Vol. XXXIX, p. 254, 1867.

Weil: Med. Jahrbücher, Wien., p. 285, 1873.

v. Wittich: Virchow's Arch., Vol. VII, p. 324, 1854.

Woodward: Toner Lecture, No. 1, p. 20, Smithsonian Institute.

TYPHOID NODULAR COLITIS.

By G. H. Whipple, M. D.,

Assistant in Pathology, The Johns Hopkins University, Baltimore.

The following case seems to be of interest from several points of view; first, in that it is a case of typhoid fever clinically unsuspected, the symptoms being overshadowed by those arising from the disease of the heart valves; secondly, because the intestinal lesions were confined to the colon, and in the third place, because these lesions closely correspond with the description given by Orth and others for the so-called nodular colitis. The following is a very brief outline of the clinical history of this case:

Otto Kast, aged thirty-seven years, German.

Family history, negative.

Past history.—The patient had rheumatism and chorea in his youth; no lues; no typhoid fever. His habits were good. He ran the course of a heart case with mitral stenosis and insufficiently showing frequent breaks in compensation, which caused him to enter the hospital at various times. His last admission was on August 25, 1905, with a bad break in cardiac compensation; he showed marked dyspnœa, edema and cyanosis. There was considerable improvement under treatment. His temperature was constantly subnormal until October 6, when it gradually rose to 101.5° on October 9, where it remained steadily for the greater part of this last illness.

His leucocytes numbered 7,800 on October 8; 9,500 on October 16. During this febrile period he developed signs of pulmonary infarction. He was very restless and uncomfortable, and gradually grew weaker, the weakness being apparently due to his cardiac lesion; was finally delirious the day before death, which took place on October 20. No record was made of any signs pointing to an abdominal complication. The case came to autopsy in the service of Dr. Welch from the medical service of Dr. Barker at the Johns Hopkins Hospital.

Anatomical Diagnosis.—Chronic mitral endocarditis with stenosis; cardiac dilatation and hypertrophy; sclerosis of pulmonary artery; chronic passive congestion of the viscera; localized subcutaneous edema; anæmic infarctions of spleen; hemorrhagic infarctions of lungs; acute bronchitis; bronchopneumonia; nodular colitis (typhoid); lymphadenitis; old tuberculous foci in lymph glands and lungs; chronic adhesive pleuritis; chronic adhesive peritonitis.

The following is an abstract of the autopsy report: Lower limbs show considerable subcutaneous edema. Abdominal and pleural cavities are clear except for a few old fibrous adhesions. The spleen is adherent to the diaphragm.

Heart weighs 620 grams; there is great distension and hypertrophy of its right side. The pulmonary artery shows several large, opaque, yellow areas of sclerosis, some of which stand fully 1 mm. above the surface. The left auricle is dilated and shows a few sclerotic areas. The mitral orifice shows a typical "button hole" opening which just admits the tip of one's little finger. Aortic and pulmonary valves are delicate. Aorta shows little sclerosis. The coronaries show only an occasional patch of moderate thickening.

Lungs show some old pleural adhesions and one apical scar with a small caseous central focus. Some of the bronchial lymph glands show caseous encapsulated foci.

The bronchi show a deeply injected mucosa of a purplish color. Cut sections show areas of broncho-pneumonia and wedge-shaped infarctions scattered over the elastic, tough, salmon-red-colored lung tissues.

Spleen weighs 450 grams; there is some thickening of the

capsule and tags of old adhesions over it. It is firm and the cut surface is sharp. The trabeculæ are not distinct. The pulp scrapes off on the edge of the knife with difficulty and is of a pale purplish color. The malpaghian bodies are clearly visible as small gray dots. There are several pale, cream-colored infarcts with their bases at the surface, extending some distance into the parenchyma and surrounded by a zone of injection.

Pancreas is normal.

Liver weighs 1,750 grams. It is adherent to the diahpragm by old adhesions, and to the duodenum by pericystic fibrous adhesions. The cut surface is fairly typical of chronic passive congestion.

Kidneys weigh 530 grams. Their capsules come off readily and both are fairly typical examples of the kidneys of chronic passive congestion, with some cloudy swelling of the cortex.

Pelvic organs are normal. The mesenteric glands are slightly enlarged, the change being most marked in those glands situated along the transverse and ascending colon.

cular outline; some are quite deep extending down through the thickness of the nodule, but in no instance do they invade the muscularis. The deep ulcers may show some undermining of their edges, and their bases are covered with an adherent, grayish-yellow slough. The solitary follicles are visible in this area and were described as the earliest stage in the formation of the nodules.

The ascending and transverse colon show much the same appearance, except for the fact that the nodules are more thickly placed, and in some areas as many as ten or twelve can be made out in a space measuring 3x3 cm. The transverse colon shows some enlargement of the solitary follicles up to 1 mm. in diameter, these being evenly distributed over the mucosa between the larger ulcerated nodules. The descending colon and sigmoid show fewer of the larger ulcerated nodules as one approaches the rectum, but the smaller nodules are quite numerous in this region.

Rectum shows intense injection, giving its mucosa a deep, purplish color, but no nodules.

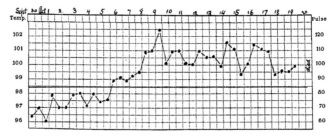

Some of the larger ones measure 1.5 cm. in diameter, and cut section shows scattered areas of focal necrosis on a translucent background.

Digestive Tract.—Stomach is normal. The upper part of the duodenum shows some injection and a pinkish smooth mucosa. The jejunum and ileum are normal, showing a pale, pinkish mucosa. The lower portion of the ileum was preserved in formalin together with the cæcum, appendix and ascending colon. This specimen shows not the slightest swelling of the Peyer's patches, or solitary follicles in the ileum.

The appendix is thick and short, but free from adhesions. Its lumen is patent for only 2 cm. from its junction with the cæcum, but there is no evidence of any ulceration or swelling of its lymphatic tissue. The ileo-cæcal valve is normal.

The mucous surface of the cæcum is thickly sown with small sessile nodules from 2 to 10 mm. in diameter, in some instances projecting 4 mm. above the surface. The larger nodules show small round ulcers on their crests, but elsewhere the mucosa is intact and of a pale purplish color. The ulcers vary from very minute dots to areas 5 mm. in diameter. The majority of them are superficial with a clean cut edge and cir-

At the time of autopsy there was not the slightest suspicion that the lesion was due to the typhoid bacillus, and it is very unfortunate that no cultures were made from the intestinal lesions, spleen and glands. The culture from the heart's blood was sterile.

MICROSCOPICAL SPECIMENS.

The Intestinal Lesions.—Small intestine shows a perfectly normal mucosa. The Peyer's patches and solitary follicles do not show any hyperplasia, and the submucosa is normal except for a marked degree of chronic passive congestion. The appendix is negative.

Large Intestine.—The mucosa except over the larger nodules is normal. The solitary follicles, which were quite conspicuous in the transverse colon, show little, if any, hyperplasia but in some instances seem raised above the surface and rendered prominent by an infiltration of the submucous stroma with wandering cells of various types, some of which are phagocytic. In such areas too there is a certain amount of edema of the stroma and injection of the capillaries. Several of the nodules from different parts of the intestines, measuring 2 to 5 mm. in diameter and showing no superficial ulceration, were cut in serial sections and stained with polychrome methylene blue and eosin or haematoxylin and eosin. Such nodules usually contained one or two solitary follicles which might be located at the summit of the nodule or on one side, never in the centre of the nodule. These solitary follicles showed no hyperplasia as a rule, but one or two which occurred in the stroma of a nodule showed a little edema and infiltration with epithelioid cells, maintaining sharply their independence however from the main bulk of the nodule. Some follicles in the mucosa near the nodules are perfectly normal and show absolutely no evidence of any hyperplasia. The nodules themselves appear to be made up of an edematous stroma infiltrated uniformly with numbers of lymphoid cells and a few leucocytes. The predominating cells, however, are large, oval, "epithelioid" cells with eccentric nuclei, often phagocytic and showing a variety of granules. There are many cells which correspond to the "polyblasts" of Maximow. The capillaries in the nodules are always dilated and some of the smaller ones as well as many sinuses are packed with phagocytic epithelioid cells. These nodules all show scattered focal areas of necrosis with fragmented nuclei, usually of small size but sometimes conglomerate and containing clumps of pale-staining, slender bacilli. The larger ulcerated nodules, averaging from 5 to 10 mm., show a typical picture of typhoid hyperplasia in the submucosa round the ulceration, the loose edematous stroma being packed with large, oval, flat epithelioid cells which are actively phagocytic. There are many round cells and polyblasts of all kinds but few leucocytes. Solitary follicles are seen in these areas, sometimes on the shoulder of a large nodule, maintaining its normal appearance and showing absolutely no change, and again at the edge of a nodule but unchanged as a rule and taking no active part in the reaction. A few follicles are found which show a little edema and invasion with epithelioid cells, but only to a limited degree.

The ulceration in some cases seems to extend from the surface, due to anæmia of the mucosa consequent on its stretching over a large nodule. More commonly the ulceration merely connects a large area of focal necrosis in the middle of the nodule with the lumen of the bowel, in many such cases the ulcer being very small with extension of the necrosis under the overlying intact edges of mucosa. Gram-staining micrococci are found in the edges of the ulcers, but no gram-staining organisms in any other tissues. No acid fast bacilli were demonstrated in any sections. Large areas of focal necrosis are usually present and appear to be formed by fusion of the smaller foci seen in the smaller nodules. Strands of fibrin are interwoven with these focal areas and connect them to each other, interlacing with strands of fibrous tissue (as is sharply brought out by Mallory's connective tissue stain). The meshes of fibrin are full of the wandering cells, described above, with many fragments of nuclei and leucocytes in the more central portions of the necrotic areas and in the bases of the ulcers. Some of the smaller vessels in and near such

areas are thrombosed. Beneath some of the larger nodules the internal muscular coat shows some injection of its capillaries, edema and separation of the muscle cells with slight infiltration of round cells and a delicate tracery of fibrin.

The mesenteric glands near the cæcum and transverse colon were cut in serial sections and stained with polychrome methylene blue and eosin. They all show a typical picture of typhoid lymphadenitis with numerous small scattered areas of focal necrosis and infiltration of the lymph sinuses with phagocytic epithelioid cells. Numerous large clumps of bacilli are found. The capillaries are congested.

Liver sections show advanced chronic passive congestion of the lobules and some fatty degeneration. Scattered areas of focal necrosis are found similar to those seen in typhoid fever.

Spleen sections show chronic passive congestion and a few scattered phagocytic cells like those described in the lymph glands. The most characteristic thing is the finding of large clumps of bacilli in the pulp. These organisms decolorized by Gram and stained clearly but not deeply by polychrome methylene blue and eosin. They always occurred in large clumps as is so characteristic of the typhoid bacillus in this organ. Studied with a one-twelfth objective the organisms appear as slender bacilli and correspond exactly in morphology to the typhoid bacillus. Exactly similar organisms are found in large clumps in the base of the intestinal nodules, mesenteric lymph glands and liver. The spleen also shows several fresh anæmic infarcts with a halo of leucocytes and hemorrhage. Some sections show focal necroses in the malpighian bodies.

Kidneys show congestion of the capillaries everywhere, especially in the glomeruli, and marked cloudy swelling of the secreting structures of the cortex.

Lungs show advanced chronic passive congestion with scattered areas of red infarction and bronchopneumonia. There is an old tuberculous focus with a thick fibrous capsule.

The other organs are negative.

Lesions in the large intestine, which give a similar picture, are not infrequently found in typhoid fever cases, but associated with swelling and ulceration of the lymphatic apparatus of the ileum. Woodward reports a case (No. 882, Med. History of the War of the Rebellion, Part II, page 360). A man dead of a severe attack of typhoid fever showed at autopsy a colon which presented a remarkable picture of nodular swelling with superficial ulceration. The illustration of this case is almost an exact duplicate of a portion of the colon in this case. He says that the nodules are due to hyperplasia and ulceration of the solitary follicles, but gives no microscopic report. The small intestines showed a remarkable hyperplasia of Peyer's patches and follicles. In a previous case of typhoid fever in this hospital (autopsy 1435) the mucosa of the colon was dotted over with nodules of various sizes up to 10 mm. in diameter, showing in places slight superficial ulceration. The small intestine showed extreme hyperplasia of the lymphatic tissue. Microscopic examination of these nodules showed a picture corresponding fairly closely with the lesion in the nodules described above. The bulk of the nodules was made up of an edematous stroma packed with large flat, epithelioid cells, which were very actively phagocytic. Several lymphoid follicles occurred in all the large nodules and preserved their integrity, although a little swollen and infiltrated by many of the large wandering cells. It was quite evident that the nodules were not due to hyperplasia of any one or of several lymphoid follicles, which formed only a small fraction of these nodules. Focal necroses were seen, but widely scattered and of small size. Ulceration was slight and very superficial, extending scarcely beyond the muscularis mucosæ. Clumps of bacilli were seen in the stroma of the nodules which coresponded in morphology to the typhoid organism. Cultures from various organs showed growth of B. typhosus.

Typhoid ulceration confined to the large intestine, the colo-typhus of the French writers, was not thought to be exceptionally rare before the literature was looked over in pursuit of such cases. Many of the larger text books of Pathology make no mention of such cases. Nothnagel as well as Brouardel and Thoinot (La Fièvre Typhoide) state that "colotyphus" is extremely rare. Hoffmann[1] in a study of 250 cases at Basel only reports one case, as follows:

Male twenty-five years old.

The patient came in with high fever and soon became delirious. He later developed a purulent discharge from both ears. Shortly before death on the forty-second day of his illness the sputum became purulent and foul-smelling with other signs of pulmonary complications.

Autopsy: Chest.—The left pleural cavity contained 200 cc. of thin, clear, yellow fluid. Heart was normal. Lungs showed acute bronchitis and perhaps bronchiectasis or gangrene.

Abdomen.—The stomach was enlarged and showed a few submucous ecchymoses near the fundus. The intestines were distended with gas. The small intestine showed no swelling or ulceration throughout its course. There were a few ecchymoses near the ileocæcal valve. In the cæcum, ascending and transverse colon the follicles were swollen, and some of them show ulceration of slight extent but yet extending to some depth, even to the muscularis in some instances. Some of the ulcers were covered by a thin delicate membrane whose margins are pigmented and of a grayish color. The mesenteric lymph glands were scarcely enlarged and of a dark, grayish-red color. The liver was very large and cut section of a pale, grayish-yellow color. The spleen measured 16.5 cm. in length, capsule wrinkled, parenchyma soft, pulpy and of a purplish color. The kidneys showed a "horseshoe" malformation with firmly adherent capsule and cloudy cortex. Brain was negative, middle ear findings not relative.

[1] Untersuchungen über die pathologisch anatomischen Veränderungen der Organe beim Abdominaltyphus, 1869, Von C. E. E. Hoffmann.

Marchand[2] reports a case of a young man clinically one of severe Typhoid Fever. Autopsy showed intestinal lesions limited to swelling and superficial ulceration of the solitary follicles of the large intestine. The spleen was greatly enlarged and the cut section studied with grayish-red enlarged malpighian bodies, which at first sight suggested tubercles. He considered this appearance to be due to active hyperplasia of the malpighian bodies with comparative escape of the spleen pulp. The mesenteric glands were enlarged and showed on section little pale dots in the parenchyma which microscopically were small areas of necrosis. Most of his paper was devoted to a discussion of the method of formation of the sloughs in typhoid ulceration.

Hodenpyl[1] reports a case at the Roosevelt Hospital of a man thirty-one years old, who ran a typical course of typhoid fever. Autopsy showed a small intestine which was entirely normal. The colon, except the sigmoid and rectum, was studded with ulcers from 2 to 15 mm. in diameter, having sharp edges and a circular outline. Cultures from the spleen showed B. typhosus. Microscopical sections showed hyperplasia at the margins of the intestinal lesions and focal necroses in the liver. The small intestine showed no hyperplasia of the lymphoid elements. The spleen and mesenteric glands were not examined.

In looking over the available literature on the subject these three cases were the only ones found which were satisfactorily reported. Doubtless cases have been mentioned in reports on other lesions, as in Marchand's case, which have escaped our notice, but it may be stated with some certainty that typhoid intestinal lesions limited to the large bowel are very rare. The case reported from this laboratory is the only one in a series of 217. It is unfortunate that in this case no cultures were taken from the spleen and other organs, but the microscopic picture of the intestinal lesions and mesenteric lymph glands, together with the finding of typical clumps of bacilli in the spleen and mesenteric glands seems to leave no doubt that this was a case of typhoid fever. A review of the clinical history shows a temperature curve and leucocyte count which support this conclusion.

The term "nodular colitis" was used in this instance because it seemed to fit exactly and accurately describe the lesion. The terms "enteritis nodularis" or "enteritis nodularis hyperplastica" seem to have been introduced by Orth, who described these lesions in cholera, diphtheria, typhus and typhoid fevers. The illustration which is found in his book was taken from a case of cholera and resembles this case very closely, but he describes the lesion as due to a hyperplasia of the solitary follicles with central softening and ulceration. He classifies the lesion under Infectious Granulomata.

Rokitansky seems to have confused several kinds of ulcers of the large intestine. He describes an increase in size of the

[1] Centralblatt für Allgemeine Path. u. Path. Anatomie, 1890, I—121.

[2] Brit. Med. Journal, 1897, II, pp. 1850.

solitary follicles going on to central softening with ulcer formation, but says that these ulcers may undermine the mucosa, coalesce with one another and finally lay bare large areas of the muscular coat. The last part of his description is suggestive of amebic ulceration.

Ziegler describes enteritis follicularis as consisting of marked swelling of the lymph nodules and Peyer's patches, which may go on to central softening and ulceration. There may be any type of associated enteritis. He does not use the term "enteritis nodularis," nor does Nothnagel refer to it. The latter uses the term "follicular ulceration" and says that it is more common in the large than in the small intestine; further, that the ulcers are commonly of small diameter but may extend through the muscular coats and even perforate. Histologically the lesion consists of a great accummulation of wandering cells in the submucosa and solitary follicles. The mucosa on the summit of the nodule undergoes a pressure necrosis and the ulcer grows from the surface.

Bamberger[4] confused follicular ulceration and chronic cystic colitis in that he considered the small cysts, full of mucus and formed from dilated glands, to be small abscesses in the solitary follicles.

Virchow[5] calls attention to this error and states that this type of follicular ulceration can be confused with colotyphus as there are many points of similarity.. However, the follicular ulceration is preceded by abscesses in the follicles which rupture through a *small* opening, thus forming a tiny ulcer. On the other hand, the typhoid ulceration of the swollen follicles is not cavernous and undermined with a punctate opening, but superficial and having more of a ring shape with no evidence of abscess formation, or suppuration.

Woodward described the specimen from the case cited above as "Transverse Colon with Enlarged Glands Ulcerated at their Apices." He states that he places this case, not in the typhoid section where it would seem to belong logically, but in the section on ulcerations of the colon, because it differs only in *degree* from similar enlargements of the solitary glands found in cases of simple acute diarrhœa. He pictures numerous types of such enlargement of the follicles in diarrhœa and describes a "follicular ulceration." He says the first step consists of an enlargement of the solitary follicles by accumulation of cells from the blood or by proliferation of the fixed cells. Ulceration may take place in quite small as well as large follicles by two methods, either by central softening and surface rupture or by a superficial loss of mucosa and extension downward. These ulcers are described as circular in outline, with undermined, overhanging edges. More or less inflammatory reaction is always present in such areas, giving a cellular infiltration of the submucosa as well as the underlying muscular coats. According to Woodward the process always begins in a follicle and results in its des-

truction, if ulceration occurs. Once started the ulceration may involve the infiltrated submucosa and even the underlying coats.

This short review of the subject of enteritis nodularis, follicularis, etc., shows how varied is the nomenclature regarding the inflammation or hyperplasia affecting the lymphatic tissue of the large intestine. It would seem that no writer has called attention to the difference existing between the cases of follicular or lymphatic hyperplasia of the intestine, which are so commonly seen in children dead from any acute intoxication (for example diphtheria) and the class of cases described in this paper and pictured by Orth, Woodward and others.

The term lymphatic hyperplasia is used in this laboratory to designate cases showing swelling of the lymphatic tissue of large or small intestines. This lesion is most common in children dying from some acute infection when the large intestine may show nodules up to 2 mm. in diameter sometimes with superficial ulceration. These nodules, however, are evenly distributed over the mucosa and correspond in number and distribution to the solitary follicles. Histologically each nodule consists of a solitary follicle, which may show some edema and infiltration with wandering cells, but chiefly a simple hyperplasia. The submucosa is usually quite normal, but may show a moderate degree of congestion of its capillaries.

The term nodular colitis should not be confused with that of lymphatic hyperplasia, for in the former case the solitary follicles would seem to play only an unimportant role and form a small fraction of the nodules which, as described above, are made up of an edematous stroma infiltrated with various types of polyblasts or wandering cells. The nodules are dotted over the colon in a haphazard fashion with no fixed relation to the follicles and are as a rule larger than those seen in lymphatic hyperplasia. This lesion appears to be found most frequently in cases of typhoid fever, but at best is quite rare, whereas lymphatic hyperplasia is common in children and not infrequent in adults. Probably the lesion can be produced by a variety of organisms, for example, those of cholera and typhoid, and may be classed (Orth) under the infectious granulomata.

SUMMARY.

1. Typhoid intestinal lesions limited to the colon are very rare.

2. The term "nodular colitis" should be restricted to such cases as show a marked infiltration of the submucosa with wandering cells, giving rise to prominent isolated nodules having no relation to the solitary follicles which are comparatively unaffected. These cases are of rare occurrence.

3. The term "lymphatic hyperplasia" may be used to describe the cases showing a simple hyperplasia of the solitary follicles of the intestines and a relatively normal submucosa. These cases are commonly found at autopsy.

[4] Virch. Handbuch der Spec. Path. und Ther., 1864, VI, 1—356.
[5] Virch. Archiv., 52, p. 22, "Kriegstyphus und Ruhr."

PROCEEDINGS OF SOCIETIES.

THE JOHNS HOPKINS HOSPITAL MEDICAL SOCIETY,

May 21, 1906.

A Simple Method for the Quantitative Determination of Proteid in Milk. DR. Boggs.

Dr. Boggs presented a new, simple method for the quantitative determination of proteids in milk. This will be published in full in a future number of the BULLETIN.

He also exhibited two unusual malarial specimens obtained from the blood of a patient. These specimens represent the parthenogenetic division or development of the organism as described by Schaudinn in explanation of the recrudescence. The female form persists after the others have died out and throws out a polar body-like structure followed by a division of the nucleus unequally, which is in turn followed by a division of the protoplasm. Eventually a number of spore bodies are formed similar to the merozoites of the asexual cycle.

The Blood in Pernicious Anæmia. DR. EMERSON.

I wish to call attention to certain points in the blood of patients with pernicious anæmia which we have noted in the cases admitted to the wards during the past five years.

First, the blood on admission shows a higher average count (about 1,500,000) than in other clinics, and I believe this is due to the fact that cases are admitted for other than the condition of the blood itself—the nervous manifestations of the disease for example.

Secondly, there is quite frequently a non-parallelism between the blood count and the patient's condition. The patient will enter with a certain count, feeling badly, and will leave later with exactly the same count though he feels well. In another group illustrating this same fact the count will rise steadily though the patient dies. In still another group there is a rise, then a fall to about the first count and the death of the patient then occurs. This rise and fall is of interest. With a 50,000 variation in the count per day this is often not due to the new formation or destruction of the red blood corpuscles but to changes in the concentration of the plasma, changes which are greater in this disease than in any other. A rise, however, of from 15,000 to 20,000 cells per day may mean a new production of corpuscles as these rises are often accompanied by an increase in the leucocytes and eosinophiles which shows bone marrow activity.

In a certain number of cases with a count of from 300,000 to 700,000 cells at the time of death, death appeared to have resulted from the anæmia alone as there were no complications. This seems to be the average count at the time of death from the anæmia alone.

Megaloblasts—and by this term I mean a large nucleated red blood cell the nucleus of which is about the size of a normal erythrocyte, all with smaller nuclei being considered as intermediate forms—are of considerable interest. The reason for the line of division given is as follows. The marrow of an infant or of a case operated on for empyema shows two groups of cells, one with a large nucleus, the megaloblast described above, and secondly a red cell with a smaller nucleus. We suppose the larger cells represent the centers of the islands for proliferation of the red blood cells and after the outer zone of normoblasts is stripped off in this disease, pernicious anæmia, these float out, and are the megoblasts.

The line drawn here in this clinic for a crisis is the finding of 50 nucleated red blood cells per 1000 leucocytes, and fully one-half of the crises do not result in a gain in the red cells. There are two kinds of crises, normoblastic and megaloblastic, and the latter seem the last efforts of the marrow, often unavailing.

A color index of over 1½ is open to criticism. The color index in this disease is high for, (a) the large size of the cells, though the color of the cells at times seems to indicate an increase in iron content, though this is probably not any higher than normal, (b) large numbers of microcytes, (c) the most important factor is the poor instrument used, and our high indices are due to the v. Fleischl instrument.

The leucocytes in pernicious anæmia are interesting. As a rule they vary directly with the red corpuscles, rising and falling with them. In many of these variations the percentage of the leucocytes remains the same. Cases with a leucocytosis usually have some complication.

In considering the percentages of the leucocytes a thing to be emphasized is the finding of say 60 per cent of small mononuclears. This does not mean a lymphocytosis as the absolute, rather than the relative count, must always be considered. In only 17 per cent of all our cases has there been a true lymphocytosis.

The last point I wish to emphasize is the count of the eosinophiles, not the percentage, as this cannot amount to much, but the absolute count. If these cells are rising the case is improving, and if they are decreasing the opposite is true. This is well shown by a case with a count of 2,700,000 cells right along during the stay in the hospital. During this time the eosinophiles were steadily dropping and reached zero at the time of the patient's death. Even with a rising red blood count the falling eosinophiles tells of the approach of death.

INDEX TO VOLUMES 1-16 OF BULLETIN.

A subject and author index of the first sixteen volumes of the Johns Hopkins Hospital Bulletin is now ready. As the edition will be limited, it is desirable that orders be sent in as promptly as possible.

Price bound in cloth is fifty cents.

Orders should be addressed to the Johns Hopkins Press, Baltimore, Md.

NOTES ON NEW BOOKS.

Materia Medica and Therapeutics. By J. MITCHELL BRUCE, M. A., LL.D. (Hon.), Aberd., M. D. Lond. (*Chicago: W. T. Keener & Co., 1906.*)
A Manual of Medical Treatment or Clinical Therapeutics. By I. BURNEY YEO, M. D., F. R. C. P. (*Chicago: W. T. Keener & Co.*)

In these recent editions of English works on Therapeutics the formulæ has been adapted to the American Pharmacopeia by Oscar Oldberg of Chicago. In both the apothecary weights and measures only are used, which seems unfortunate, as tne metric might well be added. These works differ widely in scope and perhaps that of Dr. Bruce's may be regarded as more adapted for the student who has his materia medica to learn and finds it easy to pick up some therapeutics with it, while that of Dr. Yeo is more for the final student or graduate.

The arrangement of Bruce's work is excellent. After the introduction dealing with preparations, weights and measures, etc,. comes the discussion of the inorganic and organic materia medica. The arrangement here is good and may well be commended. The various preparations are given, with concise notes as to their preparation, solubility and dosage. These are complete and put in very concise form. Following this is a section on their action and uses, first the external and then the internal action being given. The drug is followed through the body and its action in excretion, if there be any, is noted. Then there is a brief summing up of the uses of the various preparations of the drug. By this method we think Bruce has ⸺rhaps the best section in the action of drugs of any text-book, certainly there is none in which the student can get such a clear idea of the action of a drug and its preparations. The work which enables the student to learn something of the use and purpose of drugs at the same time as the details of preparation and dosage are being gained, has certainly a great advantage.

The latter part of the book deals with general therapeutics and this is necessarily much condensed. In each section the general physiology, the pharmacodynamics, the pathological relations, natural prevention, and recovery, and lastly therapeutics are discussed. We are glad to see that Dr. Bruce does not consider drug giving to be the sole aim of therapeutics. Throughout this section the treatment advised is rational and sound. The work as a whole is excellent and compact. One criticism might be made on the character of the printing. This is poor and the type is not an easy one to read. It is to be hoped that this will be improved in later editions.

Turning to Yeo's book, the reviewer finds it much more difficult to express an opinion. It deals with treatment solely: there is no materia medica. It contains more than therapeutics, for many times the author wanders from the field of treatment into that of general medicine. Much space is given to the discussion of symptoms which doubtless in some ways is a help to the later discussion of treatment. The book is well written and one has no special objection to reviewing symptoms again, but it is doubtful if this is quite the province of a work on treatment. Certainly the discussion of methods of diagnosis—*e. g.*, in stomach diseases—must be regarded as out of place in this work. There are sections given to the treatment of symptoms which are valuable, if they do not lead the student to be too content with the handling of these and so less likely to strive for the solution of the essential causal condition. Yet we are likely to have to continue to treat symptoms.

In the matter of treatment there are many minds and there may be various methods of aiding a patient to get well, but it seems in some things Dr. Yeo hardly holds what may be considered the best modern views. Take the treatment of pleurisy with effusion for example. That early and repeated tapping is the best treatment seems well established, and yet Dr. Yeo advises against this except in the case of large effusions. In moderate effusions he says " we should, however, be in no haste to advise paracentesis." Leave out the *no* and we should agree with him. In the treatment of typhoid fever, Dr. Yeo of course advocates his chlorine water. As a young house officer, the reviewer, full of therapeutic hopefulness, tried it with a number of patients, but the expected results as given by Dr. Yeo were conspicuously absent. To those of us who know the Brand treatment, the reference to it here must be irritating. If many of those who write on it would take the pains to inform themselves accurately on the method and what is hoped for by its use, there would be fewer such comments as we see here. Dr. Yeo is right when he says it involves trouble, but is that not a cheap price to pay for six to eight patients saved in every hundred? To suggest that the bath treatment is especially to reduce pyrexia shows that the author does not understand it. It seems to be a Britannic idea that the bath treatment must be used only for desperate conditions which is fair neither to the patient nor to the method. The administration of gallic acid for intestinal hæmorrhage cannot be commended.

While comment has been made on some points which might be improved, yet the greater part of the work is excellent. It has the advantage of making one think of the reasons for given procedures and that is a desirable feature. Measures, other than drugs, receive proper consideration, in which particular many of the works on therapeutics are conspicuously lacking.

Refraction, Including Muscular Imbalance and the Adjustment of Glasses. By ROYAL S. COPELAND, A. M., M. D., Professor in the University of Michigan, and ADOLPH E. IBERSHOFF, M. D., Instructor in the University of Michigan. (*Philadelphia: Boericke & Tafel, 1906.*)

We believe that this treatise on refraction will be found especially useful to those who are about to take up the practice of ophthalmology. The word practice is used advisedly, for the work is thoroughly practical, as any treatise on this subject to be a real help to an ophthalmologist should be. It is free of technicalities and consequently does not demand that we refresh our minds with the significance of mathematical formulæ and terms. The illustrations of the myopic, hyperopic, and astigmatic eye and of the effect of the correcting lens upon each of these conditions are excellent. The experience of the authors, however, is certainly at variance with that of the reviewer in that they " succeed in coaxing out the most obstinate accommodation and accurately measuring the degree of eye-strain without the use of a cycloplegic, the latter being necessary in exceptional cases only." The longer we treat this class of cases the more we are convinced of the importance of knowing what the eye shows with a paralyzed accommodation. There is nothing more uncertain than the behavior of a ciliary muscle and we are surprised to find how often this is true after thirty-five, from which age on, according to the authors, cycloplegics are rarely necessary because spasm of the accommodation is very rare. We cannot help thinking that the sentiments which bear upon the value of cycloplegics, will be differently expressed in the next edition of the work. The instructions as to the correction of myopia are too meager to be of much help. But what is useful in the book outweighs its shortcomings and we recommend it as a reliable and interesting introduction to the applied principles of refraction.

International Clinics. A Quarterly of Illustrated Clinical Lectures and Especially Prepared Original Articles. By leading members of the medical profession throughout the world. Edited by A. O. J. KELLY, M. D., Philadelphia, U. S. A., assisted by a corps of collaborators. Vol. IV. Fifteenth Series, 1906. (*Philadelphia and London: J. B. Lippincott Company, 1906.*)

These papers are all interesting, but of unequal value. The best are those which relate to practical topics or present the results of actual clinical experience. Among these in the present volume are Gwyn's "Treatment of Some Common Gastric Disorders," Deaver's "Results of Operations Such as Gastroenterostomy, Pyloroplasty, etc., in the treatment of Diseases of the Stomach," Freiberg's "Study of the Clinical Course of Joint Tuberculosis by Means of the X-Rays." Of the remaining papers some are sketchy and others are profound; while several of them seem to have been written to bring forward a single special feature of a disease or a feature in operative technique. Occasionally the impression is left upon the mind of the reader that the article was written perfunctorily in response to an urgent request for a paper, without special preparation or investigation. And yet there are many excellent monographs upon special topics which give evidence of careful painstaking preparation and subsequent elaboration, such as Brown's "Thyroid Gland," Craig's "Symptomatology and Diagnosis of Malta Fever," and Warthin's "Experimental Study of the Effects of Röntgen Rays Upon the Blood-forming Organs." The book as a whole is valuable and can be commended to the medical profession. The clinical lecture form which characterizes most of the papers renders the style easy and readable. The volume is fully equal to its predecessors.

THE JOHNS HOPKINS HOSPITAL REPORTS.

VOLS. XIII AND XIV,

OF ABOUT 600 PAGES EACH, WITH NUMEROUS ILLUSTRATIONS.

(NOW IN PRESS.)

STUDIES IN GENITO-URINARY SURGERY. By HUGH H. YOUNG, M. D., Associate Professor of Genito-Urinary Surgery, The Johns Hopkins University, and Associate in Genito-Urinary Surgery, The Johns Hopkins Hospital, and F. H. BAETJER, M. D., of Baltimore; HENRY A. FOWLER, M. D., of Washington, D. C.; STEPHEN H. WATTS, M. D., of Baltimore; JOHN W. CHURCHMAN, M. D., of Breslau; LOUIS C. LEHR, M. D., of Washington, D. C.; J. T. GERAGHTY, M. D., of Baltimore, and A. R. STEVENS, M. D., of Baltimore.

CONTENTS.

1. The Seven Glass Test. By Hugh H. Young, M. D.
2. The Possibility of Avoiding Confusion by Bacillus Smegmatis (Smegma bacillus) in the Diagnosis of Urinary and Genital Tuberculosis. An Experimental Study. By Hugh H. Young, M. D., and John W. Churchman, M. D.
3. Urethral Diverticulum. By Stephen H. Watts, M. D.
4. Case of Urethrorrhagia. By H. A. Fowler, M. D.
5. Paraurethritis. By John W. Churchman, M. D.
6. Use of Ointments in the Urethra. By Hugh H. Young, M. D.
7. Treatment of Stricture of the Urethra. By Hugh H. Young, M. D., and John T. Geraghty, M. D.
8. The Treatment of Impermeable Stricture of the Urethra. By Hugh H. Young, M. D.
9. The Treatment of Bacteriuria by Medication. By John W. Churchman, M. D.
10. Use of the Cystoscope in the Diagnosis of Diseases of the Prostate. By Hugh H. Young, M. D.
11. Chronic Prostatitis. An Analysis of 358 Cases. By Hugh H. Young, M. D., John T. Geraghty, M. D., and A. R. Stevens, M. D.
12. The Treatment of Prostatic Hypertrophy. By Hugh H. Young, M. D.
13. Recto-Urethral Fistulæ. By Hugh H. Young, M. D.
14. Modern Method of Performing Perineal Lithotomy. By Hugh H. Young, M. D.
15. Early Diagnosis and Radical Cure of Carcinoma of the Prostate. By Hugh H. Young, M. D.
16. Operative Treatment of Vesical Diverticula. By Hugh H. Young, M. D.
17. Case of Double Renal Pelvis and Bifid Ureter. By Hugh H. Young, M. D.
18. Pyonephrosis Due to B. Typhosus. By Hugh H. Young, M. D., and Louis C. Lehr, M. D.
19. The Use of the X-ray in the Diagnosis of Renal and Ureteral Calculi. By F. H. Baetjer, M. D.
20. Nephritis and Hematuria. By H. A. Fowler, M. D.
21. Microscopic Study of Urinary Calculi of Oxalate of Lime. By H. A. Fowler, M. D.
22. Cystinuria and the Formation of Calculi. By H. A. Fowler, M. D.
23. Post-Traumatic Atrophy of the Testicle. By John W. Churchman, M. D.

Price per volume in paper, $5.00; in cloth, $5.50.

Orders should be addressed to

THE JOHNS HOPKINS PRESS, BALTIMORE, MD.

The Johns Hopkins Hospital Bulletins are issued monthly. They are printed by the FRIEDENWALD CO., Baltimore. Single copies may be procured from NUNN & CO. and the BALTIMORE NEWS CO., Baltimore. Subscriptions, $2.00 a year, may be addressed to the publishers, THE JOHNS HOPKINS PRESS, BALTIMORE; single copies will be sent by mail for twenty-five cents each.

BULLETIN

OF

THE JOHNS HOPKINS HOSPITAL

Entered as Second-Class Matter at the Baltimore, Maryland, Postoffice.

Vol. XVII.—No. 186.]   BALTIMORE, SEPTEMBER, 1906.   [Price, 25 Cents

CONTENTS.

THE RESULTS OF OPERATIVE TREATMENT OF VARICOSE VEINS OF THE LEG BY THE METHODS OF TRENDELENBURG AND SCHEDE.

By Robert T. Miller, Jr., M. D.,

Assistant Resident Surgeon, Johns Hopkins Hospital.

Many methods are employed in the treatment of varicose veins of the legs, no one of them being generally accepted or satisfactory. The aim of almost all operative procedures is to block the saphenous vein in order to do away with abnormal circulatory conditions existing in the leg as a result of valvular incompetency of the superficial venous system. The particular method employed is perhaps one of arbitrary choice since it is unusual to find any procedure recommended because its results, ultimate as well as immediate, are known to be good.

Schede, in 1877, published the method which goes by his name, consisting of a more or less extensive division between ligatures of the superficial veins a short distance above an ulcer. In 1884 Madelung published the method with which his name has become associated; this consists of excision of the varicose saphenous vein and its branches, the extent of operation varying with cases. This procedure had been employed by others before Madelung's paper appeared. In 1891 Trendelenburg published a paper in which was embodied the

first accurate statement of the hydrostatics of the condition together with a description of his operation consisting of division between ligatures of the long saphenous vein. The point of division elected by him was in the lower third of the thigh but the tendency has been to divide at a higher and higher point until today the attempt is made to block the venous stream just at the saphenous opening in the deep fascia of the thigh. In general, the present operative therapy consists of the employment of some one of these classical methods or a combination of them; the choice of method, however, is often blind, being influenced by little else than the immediate future simply because late results are unknown.

Attempt is made to present in this paper the results of treatment of varicose veins of the leg as practiced in the Surgical Clinic of the Johns Hopkins Hospital. Inasmuch as it has been possible to follow some of the cases for 10 years or more, we are perhaps able to place a comparative value upon the various operative methods.

ANALYSIS OF CASES.

There have been 128 cases of varicose veins of the leg and associated disorders treated in this clinic up to July 1, 1905.

Race.—107 or 84% are white and 21 or 16% colored, a fact which is of no relative significance.

Sex.—73 cases are male, 57%; 56 or 43% female.

Age of Onset.—

Years.	Number of cases.
At birth	1
10-19	10
20-29	41=32%
30-39	29
	81 cases=69%
40-49	19
50-59	13
60-69	5
	37 cases=31%
Unrecorded	10

It was usually possible to learn when the patient first noted enlargement of the veins. Inasmuch as noticeable enlargement is probably preceded for an uncertain time by actual disease, the date of onset fixed by the patient is probably late rather than early. However, dating its onset at the appearance of visible enlargement it is seen that the disease becomes evident in one-third of the cases between the 20th and 30th year. Over two-thirds of all cases appear before the 40th year. This is rather striking; the usual and natural view that venous varicosity is a senile change appears erroneous.

Etiology.—In general, there are two great groups which can be sharply defined, viz.: inflammatory and non-inflammatory.

1. Inflammatory. This is by far the smaller group; in 128 cases there are but 40 with a definite history of phlebitis.

a. Pregnancy: There are 25 cases showing initial symptoms during pregnancy; of these 7 have a history of thrombosis.

b. Typhoid fever: 9 cases have a history of phlebitis in connection with typhoid, in 3 of which there was thrombosis of uncertain extent and location. Six of these cases occurred during convalescence.

c. Erysipelas: 2 cases have a history of preceding erysipelas.

d. Pneumonia: 1 case occurred during convalescence. The patient was a male aged 20; phlebitis occurred in the right leg.

e. Acute enteritis: There are 2 cases; one suffered a left phlebitis during an attack of "bloody flux," and one had a double phlebitis during severe dysentery.

f. Post-operative: 1 case had a double phlebitis 40 days after operation for strangulated hernia, the wound healing per primam.

The long saphenous vein was probably involved in all these cases of phlebitis. It seems reasonable that inflammation of the vein might, through resultant fibrosis of the valves, lead to valvular incompetency; this etiological relation seems fairly definite.

2. Non-inflammatory. In 128 cases, 88 are grouped here. Various causes are mentioned; constipation and excessive walking about or standing while at work are, as usual, the most frequent. Pelvic tumor is noted once. There is no case in which a heart lesion or cirrhosis of the liver was thought to have any bearing on the condition although routine physical examination was made in every case. The etiology of this group of cases is obscure since it is by no means certain that the mechanical conditions usually mentioned in this connection hold anything more than an incidental relation to the disease.

Location.—The right leg was noted as alone involved in 21 instances, the left alone in 25 instances and 74 cases had bilateral clinical signs among which those with most marked signs in the left leg were slightly in the majority. The lower leg was noted as alone showing clinical signs in 94 cases; the lower leg and thigh were involved together in 25 cases and the thigh alone in 1 case. These figures are probably not entirely reliable since the vein in the thigh has not been noted except when it was the site of visible or palpable enlargement or actual varix formation; manifestly many diseased veins have thus escaped detection. The presence or absence of Trendelenburg's sign has not been noted as a routine.

OPERATIVE METHODS.

In this clinic the three classical methods have been followed almost exclusively; occasionally the Schede and Trendelenburg operations have been combined but usually only one method has been applied in any given case. The operations are carried out in the following manner:

1. *Trendelenburg.*—The long saphenous vein is approached through a short incision at right angles to its course and divided between ligatures near the saphenous opening. The point of division is probably within 10 cm. of the saphenous opening in every case and usually considerably nearer. Each end of the divided vein is doubly ligated with silk; occasionally a small portion of the vein, never more than 2 or 3 cms., is resected. The operation is usually done with local anæsthesia. Ninety-eight legs have been treated in this manner, the operation being bilateral in 30 cases. In addition to the high section of the vein in 16 cases a varicose mass below the ligation was excised; a partial Schede operation was done in one case; in one case extensive excision of varicose veins in the leg and thigh was practiced, and in 13 instances excision of an ulcer and skin graft.

2. *Schede.*—A partial or complete circumcision is done in the upper third of the leg dividing between ligatures all the superficial veins encountered; if the circumcision is partial it, at least, divides the veins of the anterior, internal and posterior aspects. There have been 19 legs so treated, the operation being bilateral in only one instance, while combined with 3 of these cases there was excision of an ulcer and skin graft and with 3 others scarification of an ulcer.

3. *Madelung.*—In 5 cases a more or less complete excision of the varicose saphenous vein was made.

Results of Trendelenburg's Operation.

In 11 instances a personal examination was possible, and 30 results were reported by letter. The majority of these cases were rather severe, extensive varicose veins of the internal saphenous system being present at or below the knee; well marked varicose clumps were present in 10 thighs and ulcer was present in 22 of the 41 legs. Nine of these cases had, in addition, excision of a varicose clump below the ligation and in 8 cases an ulcer was excised and skin grafting was done.

Of these 41 cases, 32 legs or 78% have been cured or greatly improved. Approximately this result has been obtained rather generally; Goerlich, in a recent report from von Bruns' Clinic, found 84% cured or improved subjectively in a series of 69 observed results, while after an exhaustive review of the literature since 1892 he found that the cures varied from 85% to 56%, averaging about 75%.

The post-operative interval in this series varies from 6 months to 10 years, 4 months. If the cases are grouped by the following method,

Years since operation.	Cases.	Cure.	Percentage.
1-4	19	17	89%
5-8	19	12	63%
9-11	3	3	100%

there is seen a higher percentage of cures in the first four years than is found in the general average of the series, while the percentage of cures for the second quandrennium is considerably below the general average. Between the fourth and eighth year the percentage of cures drops from 89% to 63%.

The same tendency to recurrence of symptoms is shown, though in not quite so striking a form, by the following groupings:

Years since operation.	Cases	Cure.	Percentage.
1-4	19	17	89%
5-11	22	15	68%
1-3	12	10	83%
4-6	14	10	71%
7-9	12	9	75%
10-11	3	3	100%
1-5	22	18	82%
6-11	19	14	74%

Of the 9 instances of failure, there was recurrent ulceration in 7, and in 2 swelling and pain were very severe; obliteration of the saphenous vein in these cases afforded only temporary relief and the tendency to recurrence of symptoms was more marked as the post-operative time lengthened. Among the 17 cases examined it was possible to demonstrate in 8 a return of intact venous stream in the saphenous bed after division of that vein.

Return of venous circulation after division of the vein may take place in three ways, adopting the classification of Goerlich, viz.:

1. Anastomosis around the scar.

2. Formation of varices in the scar.

3. Union of the ligated stumps with formation of an intact vein.

Examples of all these types were found, of the first and second following Trendelenburg operations, and of the third following Schede operations. Anastomosis around the scar was found in one case. A man, aged 30 years, suffering with extreme varicosity of both legs and thighs was submitted to a bilateral Trendelenburg operation which relieved his pain entirely. For 6 weeks the veins of the lower legs were much smaller and then there was progressive increase in venous dilatation. Examination of the right leg 6 months after operation showed, internally to the scar, an anastomosing system of small superficial veins which could be distinctly traced from the dilated proximal saphenous stump into the distal stump of the divided saphenous vein. There was a somewhat similar finding on the left leg where the distal saphenous stump gave rise to a superficial set of small anastomosing veins which was situated internally to the scar and ran upward to become lost slightly above the level of Poupart's ligament; although this superficial anastomosing set could not be traced definitely to the proximal saphenous stump yet there can scarcely be a doubt that such was its ultimate destination. Trendelenburg's sign was not present in either leg, however, the saphenous vein filling visibly from the periphery in about 3 minutes; evidently the anastomosing system was still possessed of competent valves.

There are three instances of formation of varices in the scar. The first instance is in a woman, 57 years of age, upon whom a bilateral Trendelenburg operation was practiced 6 years ago. She suffered recurrence of ulceration, pain and swelling in both legs and experienced from the operation no relief whatever. Upon examination there was found to be extreme venous dilatation and varicosity in both feet and lower legs, while small ulcers were present near each ankle; the vein in the thigh was visible and palpable and in each scar there was a clump of varices whose individual vessels were 1-2 cm. in diameter. With pressure over the proximal stump Trendelenburg's sign was suggested but was not prompt.

The other case is a man, 37 years old, who was submitted to a Trendelenburg operation and division between ligatures of the external saphenous vein in the popliteal region 3 years and 3 months previously. The result was perfect subjectively, but there developed in the lower scar a varicose bunch of veins and below this point dilated, tortuous veins were moderately prominent.

It is of interest to note in this connection that in 69 cases examined from 1 to 12 years after Trendelenburg operations, Goerlich found 21 instances of anastomosis around the scar and 24 examples of varix formation in the scar. Recurrence of intact venous column does not necessarily mean recurrence of symptoms; this is a curious fact whose explanation is difficult. Goerlich distinguishes sharply between subjective and objective results; while he found 84% cured or greatly improved subjectively, he also found in the same series but 27% cured objectively and there were in the series of 69 cases 47 instances of functional restoration of the saphenous vein.

RESULTS OF SCHEDE'S OPERATION.

There have been 19 legs treated in this manner; of these we have the results in 9, 6 by examination and 3 by letter. Complete circumcision has been made in 4 cases and partial circumcision in 5, an ulcer being excised and a graft applied in one of the latter group. The conditions were well marked in these cases, œdema and decided varicose veins being present in the lower legs in all. Ulceration was present in 6 legs, scars in one other, and no note was made in 2 cases. From a clinical standpoint, the cases eventually submitted to Schede operations have not differed essentially from those submitted to Trendelenburg operations; the decision between these two operations has been a matter of personal choice by the operator and usually an arbitrary one, inasmuch as no knowledge of late results could be brought to bear upon the subject.

There are but 33% cured or greatly improved in the series of 9 Schede cases when grouped as a whole. The results arranged according to the post-operative interval, which varies between 1 and 10 years, follow:

Years since operation.	Cases.	Cure.	Percentage.
1	1	1	100%
2	1	1	100%
3	1	0	0
4	1	0	0
9	2	0	0
10	3	1	33%

The series, though a small one, is suggestive. The 2 cases of two years' standing or less are cured, while the older ones are almost uniformly failures. In each of the six unsuccessful cases, ulceration has recurred since operation. As in the series of Trendelenburg operations, there is again seen the tendency to recurrence of symptoms which becomes more pronounced as the post-operative interval lengthens, while the evidence of regeneration of an intact saphenous vein is much more striking in this series than in the previous one.

There returned for examination 6 cases, of which 4 were operative failures. In 3 of these cases were found one or more dilated veins running directly through the scar to unite the veins divided and ligated at operation; there was functional, if not actual anatomical, regeneration of the saphenous vein. In two of these three cases, Trendelenburg's sign was positive showing beyond a doubt that the hydrostatic conditions existing before operation had become fully re-established. The curious phenomenon of subjective cure and objective failure coexisting was well illustrated by the following case, in which 10 years previously a partial Schede operation had completely and permanently relieved the pain consequent upon a moderate varicosity of the veins of the right lower thigh and leg. This was a complete subjective cure; however, upon examination, there was found an intact saphenous vein running directly through the scar and below the knee many large tortuous veins. Trendelenburg's sign was positive in this case. These three cases may be grouped as examples of the third type of reestablishment of the venous stream, viz.: union of the ligated stumps with the formation of an intact vein. The

possibility of dilatation of an anastomosis is excluded by the fact that in each instance regeneration took place at about the mid point of a circumferential incision.

In one of these cases the regenerated vein was obtained at a second operation; inasmuch as it is a case of unusual interest the history is given in some detail.

Surgical Number, 5062. J. J., colored, male, aged 41. Admitted Jan. 3, 1896, complaining of ulcers on his leg. The patient had suffered for 15 years with enlarged veins and chronic ulceration of his right lower leg. Upon examination there was found a varicose long saphenous vein in the thigh and general varicosity of the veins between the knee and the junction of the middle and lower thirds of the leg where there was a small superficial ulcer. Œdema and induration of the skin were slight.

Operation, Feb. 4, 1896.—Under ether anæsthesia a partial Schede operation was done in the upper third of the leg, leaving intact only a small bridge of skin on the outer side of the leg. Many small veins were divided between ligatures of fine black silk. Convalescence was without event; the ulcers healed and the patient was discharged on the 27th day.

In November, 1905, at the end of 9 years and 10 months the patient returned with the following interesting story: the operation was followed by increased œdema of his foot and recurrent ulceration within a year. Six months ago he noticed "a big vein cross the scar"; almost immediately one of the ulcers increased about 4 times in size and became much more painful. Upon examination the internal saphenous vein was found functionally intact from ankle to thigh, passing directly through the Schede scar. The vein was considerably enlarged, being about the size of the index finger at the knee, and there were numerous dilated varicose veins upon the posterior and internal aspects of the calf. Upon the anterior surface of the lower third of the leg were four superficial ulcers, three about 2 cm. in diameter and one about 6 cm. in diameter. Trendelenburg's sign was positive. There was complete regeneration of the divided saphenous vein and the condition was virtually that presented 10 years previously upon his first admission; it was decided to do a modified Trendelenburg operation which procedure had afforded him complete relief from a more aggravated condition in his other leg.

Operation, November 20, 1905.—Under ether anæsthesia 12 cm. of the vein were excised just beneath the saphenous opening, 6 cm. opposite the internal condyle and the recurrence through the scar was taken. Convalescence was uneventful except for extensive thrombosis in the remaining sections of the vein, although healing was per primam; the patient was discharged in the 5th week with marked decrease in size of the veins of the lower leg and no ulcers. This case is of especial interest, inasmuch as it illustrates graphically the relationship between ulceration and excessive venous pressure at the base of a valvularly incompetent saphenous vein.

The accompanying illustration of the hardened specimen shows the condition found. At A is the saphenous vein whose walls are greatly thickened, but retain roughly their normal architecture. Between the ends of the relatively normal vein and uniting their lumina is a venous sinus (E) which is crossed transversely at about its mid point by the Schede scar (B). A white cord marks the intact lumen within which it has been placed; a probe was passed along this course before the specimen was cut and met no resistance whatever. No trace of the black silk ligatures was found. Arising from the main vessels are the cords C, which on microscopic examination proved to be veins obliterated by irregularly arranged fibrous tissue. The wall of the sinus is very fibrous, adherent to the adjacent structures and less than one-half the thickness of the adjoining vein wall. The lumen of the sinus measures 3.5 cm. by 1.5 cm. in greatest dimensions, is smooth and glistening throughout and receives numerous minute tributary venules. The transition from actual vein wall to sinus wall is gradual. The wall of the sinus consists chiefly of connective tissue, though there is a considerable amount of smooth muscle present; there is no definite arrangement of the muscle cells to be recognized. The lumen is lined by a layer of endothelial cells. It is impossible to say whether there was anastomosis between the ligated stumps of the saphenous vein itself or between some of its branches; the site of ligation is not accurately marked, and it is possible that the cords C represent the obliterated saphenous stumps while the anastomosis was between branches. The important point, however, is the anastomosis between veins, which had been ligated and divided, restoring the function of the saphenous vein and its pathological consequence of ulceration.

The question of regeneration of a vein divided between ligatures is an old one; cases have been reported by Langenbeck in 1860, Velpeau in 1862, Perthes in 1895, Grzes in 1900, and more recently Ledderhose in 1904. Trendelenburg denied the possibility and regarded supposed regeneration as dilatation of the second stem of a double vein; this position was supported by the fact that in many animal experiments Minkiewitsch had not seen regeneration after division between ligatures. Minkiewitsch regarded supposed regeneration as dilatation of one of the many minute collaterals around the point of division; inasmuch as the anastomosing vessels to which he refers are so small as to escape detection during operation, it is difficult to deny this possibility in certain cases, nor is it unlikely that many recurrences are of this type. However, in the case reported above, the possibility of dilatation of preexisting anastomoses is probably excluded by the fact that regeneration took place at the mid-point of an almost circumferential incision which divided everything external to the deep fascia. In the two cases reported by Ledderhose recurrence of symptoms occurred 7 and 9 years after division between ligatures in the thigh. In each instance there was found a thin sinuous sac uniting the vein stumps whose limits were not sharply defined; the sac wall consisted of connective tissue and did not show the architecture of a vein. No trace of the ligatures was found. Goerlich found two cases which clinically presented the appearance of regeneration after ligation and division in the thigh, but was unable to obtain the specimen for examination.

There are two additional objections to the Schede operation that have been observed in our cases. There usually develops after operation a more or less marked œdema of the leg below the incision. This is possibly caused by too extensive division of the veins but in many cases it cannot be avoided without running the chance of doing too little. The second objection lies in the fact that the incision necessarily divides many cutaneous nerves and patients often complain considerably of anæsthesia below the scar while a certain number suffer from hyperæsthesia or even pain in the scar itself.

MADELUNG'S OPERATION.

It is impossible to obtain reports from any of the five cases in which Madelung's operation was practised; they were among the early admissions to the hospital and all trace of them has been lost. This is unfortunate since excision of the saphenous vein is followed probably less frequently by recurrence of symptoms than either a Trendelenburg or Schede operation. Symptoms may recur, however, even after complete excision. Madelung described his method and reported eleven cases before the Deutsche Gesellschaft für Chirurgie in 1884; v. Langenbeck, in discussing the paper, described a case in which there was recurrence of a varicose clump above the knee and of numerous varicose veins in the lower leg 3 years after excision of the saphenous vein. Whether probable freedom from recurrence of symptoms is enough to offset the additional risk incurred by a much longer and bodier operation is open to question. Attempts to simplify and shorten the operation have been made. In 1899 Casati of Ferrara described a method of tearing out the vein through multiple short incisions, and the same operation, together with a special instrument, has recently been described by C. H. Mayo. Both of these operators disregard the lateral branches and control hæmorrhage by elevation and pressure, resorting only occasionally to ligation. Complete removal of the varicose internal saphenous vein is, of course, the most radical therapy, but it is doubtful whether it will ever be practised as generally as Trendelenburg's operation.

COMPARISON OF TRENDELENBURG AND SCHEDE OPERATIONS.

The operative cases reported in this paper are of approximately the same clinical severity and the post-operative interval in each series extends over 10 years; we may, therefore, justly compare the results. Trendelenburg's operation resulted in 78% cured in 41 cases; Schede's operation resulted in 33% cured in 9 cases. Absolute conclusions concerning the relative therapeutic value of these two operations would perhaps be unsafe if based upon the results of no more than 50 cases; however, in the present series the Trendelenburg operation has given a percentage of cure more than twice as great as the Schede operation. There are several minor points of comparison which may be mentioned. Trendelenburg's operation does not necessitate division of any large cutaneous nerve trunks, while Schede's operation results in extensive anæsthesia and often in a hyperæsthetic or painful scar.

Schede's operation is often followed by persistent œdema of the leg. From a technical standpoint, though there is no difficulty in either procedure, ligation of a single vein in the thigh is somewhat easier than multiple ligations in the calf. Local anæsthesia is satisfactory in practically every instance for Trendelenburg's operation and, though it doubtless suffices in circumcision of the leg, the tendency is to resort to general anæsthesia, a procedure which limits the practice of any operation.

It has been shown that division between ligatures does not ensure permanent obliteration of the saphenous vein and that its function may be restored by varix formation in the scar, by dilatation of small anastomotic loops not injured at operation and, infrequently, by union of the ligated stumps. Resection of 8 cm. or more of the vein will probably maintain a hiatus between the stumps sufficient to prevent subsequent formation of varices bridging the defect as well as occurrence of union of the ligated stumps. Recovery of function through dilatation of uninjured anastomoses is best avoided by dividing the vein just at the saphenous opening before it has received any branches and by using a generous transverse incision in the skin and subcutaneous tissue, thereby ensuring ligation of adjacent anastomosing loops such as that described above. Although objective failure and subjective cure seem to coexist in certain cases, yet objective failure is often accompanied by return of subjective symptoms and, therefore, an attempt should be made to prevent recovery of function by the saphenous vein. For these reasons resection of 8 cm. or more of the vein just at the saphenous opening, made through a generous transverse skin incision is to be preferred to a simple division between ligatures. This procedure has been suggested before and is practised by many surgeons. After a careful comparative review of results, Goerlich found that it resulted in a greater percentage of cured cases than any other of the many modifications of Trendelenburg's operation.

COMPLICATIONS.

There are few complications of these three operations. The most interesting, and luckily a rare one, is embolism. Reports are infrequent not only because fatal cases are unlikely to find their way into print, but also because symptoms of embolism may be so slight as to escape notice. Of 125 operations for varicose veins at the Johns Hopkins Hospital in which either excision or division between ligatures was practiced the following is the only case of possible pulmonary embolism.

Surgical Number 12463. L. J., colored, female, aged 32. Admitted October 11, 1901, complaining of ulcer on the left leg. The patient had suffered for 5 years with enlarged veins of the legs and for 1 year with chronic ulceration of the left leg. Routine physical examination revealed a functional heart murmur in the pulmonic area but was otherwise negative. There was decided general varicosity in the distribution of both internal saphenous veins, phleboliths being palpable in the right leg. A superficial ulcer 3 x 5 cm. was present upon the left leg. Trendelenburg's sign was positive in both legs.

Operation, October 15, 1901.—Under ether anæsthesia the left long saphenous vein was divided between ligatures high in the thigh and a mass of varices extending from the knee to the ankle excised, thrombi being encountered at each point of section of the vein. The duration of anæsthesia was one hour and 15 minutes, the pulse varying between 110 and 140 to the minute.

Convalescence was uneventful till the 5th day (Oct. 19) when the patient was suddenly stricken with dyspnœa and tachycardia; she "seemed to be suffocating." Her pulse was weak and beating 140 to the minute, while respirations were labored and ranging 55 to the minute. Strychnia and morphia were administered and within a few minutes her extreme distress disappeared. The respiratory and pulse rate gradually dropped and she was "in good condition" by the 10th day, apparently having sustained no permanent injury. Healing was per primam except for the presence of a small hæmatoma in the lower womb; there was no infection. Unfortunately no examination of the chest was recorded at the time, and, therefore, a positive diagnosis is not possible; however, the clinical picture of abrupt transient dyspnœa five days after ligation of a large thrombosed vein is very suggestive and similar, in its essential points, to that of the most frequent form of postoperative pulmonary embolism seen in these cases.

Goerlich found two cases of embolism in a series of 147 Trendelenburg operations and collected four others. The first case was that of a woman, 47 years old, in whom 2 cm. of the saphenous vein were resected in the upper third of the right thigh. The wound healed per primam, no note of thrombosis being made, and upon the 5th day the patient, arising from bed to urinate, was suddenly stricken with dyspnœa, cyanosis and pain in the right side. Absolute flatness and bronchial breathing were present over the right lower lobe and her temperature was 38° centigrade. During the next few days the signs subsided and an uneventful recovery ensued.

The second case was that of a woman, 47 years of age, in whom division between ligatures in the left upper thigh was made, the wound healing per primam. On the 10th day the patient complained of pain in the left side accompanied by cough and bloody sputum. There was flatness and tubular breathing in the left back and a temperature of 39° centigrade. The physical signs subsided slowly, and the patient was discharged on the 25th day.

Franz reports the case of a woman, 35 years of age, in whom, following ligation in the mid-thigh and curettage of an ulcer, there was thrombosis from the ligation to the mid-calf, although healing was per primam. Pulmonary embolism followed, resulting in infarct and effusion; the physical signs slowly subsided and the patient was discharged in 1½ months.

In the case of Nauwerk double resection of the saphenous vein was made in a woman 64 years old, the wound healing per primam. Ten days after operation the patient suffered sudden dyspnœa, and death followed within half an hour. At

PLATE XVIII

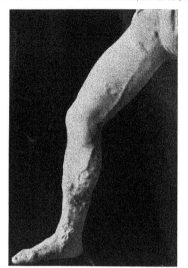

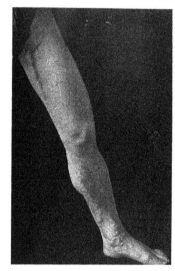

FIG. 1.

FIG. 2.

FIGS. 1 and 2.—Venous anastomosis around the scar; 6 months after a bilateral Trendelenburg operation.

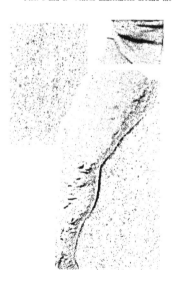

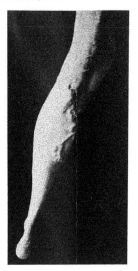

Fig. 5.—Varices in scar uniting stumps of external saphenous vein which was divided between ligatures 3 years previously.

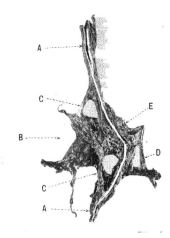

Fig. 6.—Regeneration of internal saphenous vein by anastomosis of ligated stumps; 10 years after a Schede operation.
Alcohol specimen.

autopsy there was found occlusion of both pulmonary arteries by clots and a finger-sized thrombus in the proximal stump of the right saphenous vein. Thrombosis was attributed by the author to microscopic necrosis of the ligated stump.

Perthes reports sudden transient dyspnœa of but a few hours duration in a case which had slight fascia-necrosis in the wound and thrombosis near the point of ligation.

In Studsgaard's case embolism with transient symptoms followed per primam healing.

In addition to these cases there is one other reported by G. H. Sylvester. In the case of a man, aged 34, suffering with varicose veins in both legs, six clumps of dilated veins were excised, including three inches of the left saphenous vein in the thigh. Dressing was made on the twelfth day, finding per primam healing throughout; splints were worn up to this time and then discarded. "That night he suddenly sat up in bed, complained of feeling faint, fell back and died almost immediately." At autopsy there was found occlusion of the pulmonary artery at its bifurcation by a clot; no thrombi were found in the iliac veins, but the veins of the legs were unfortunately not examined.

There are thus on record eight cases of pulmonary embolism following operations upon varicose veins of the legs, viz.: Franz, Nauwerk, Perthes, Studsgaard, Goerlich 2, Sylvester and one case in this report. Four cases occurred after division between ligatures in the thigh, two cases after multiple partial excisions with ligation and division, and one case after bilateral complete excision of the saphenous veins. In three cases there was a slight wound complication, but in no instance was infection thought to be present. Embolism occurred after the simplest as well as the most extensive procedure.

Symptoms appeared on the 5th day twice, on the 10th day twice, and on the 12th day in one instance.

In four cases the symptoms were transient, subsiding within a few days; of these four, two cases followed division between ligatures and one followed division with resection of a varicose mass. In two cases there were definite physical signs of pulmonary infarct, the symptoms persisting for three and six weeks respectively; both followed division between ligatures and in one of them there was extensive post-operative thrombosis below the ligation. In two cases sudden death resulted; both of these followed extensive procedures, viz., bilateral resection and multiple excisions. There seem to be three fairly distinct types of post-operative pulmonary embolism which may be recognized; the mildest is transient and comparatively harmless, causing more or less marked respiratory distress for a few hours. The more severe results in definite infarct which may cause symptoms for four to six weeks and probably leaves a definite pulmonary lesion, while the most severe causes immediate death by occlusion of the pulmonary arteries. Although it is, perhaps, a suggestive fact that the two fatal cases of pulmonary embolism have followed extensive operative procedures, it is unsafe, as yet, to draw definite conclusions in regard to such a possible relationship.

CONCLUSIONS.

1. Varicose veins of the leg are not an incident of senility; the condition is rather a disease of young and middle-aged individuals, over one-third of the cases appearing before the 30th year and two-thirds before the 40th year.

2. From an etiological standpoint, there are two classes, viz., inflammatory and non-inflammatory. The inflammatory group includes about one-third of all cases, phlebitis occurring as a complication or sequel of pregnancy, post-operative convalescence or an acute infection, among which typhoid fever is the most frequent. The pathology of the non-inflammatory group is obscure.

3. In 128 cases the right and left legs are affected in about equal proportion; over one-half of the cases are bilateral.

4. Trendelenburg's operation cured 78% in a series of 41 cases; this is about the result generally reported. In the first four post-operative years 89% were cured, in the 5th-8th post-operative years but 63% were cured; the tendency to recurrence of symptoms increases as the post-operative interval lengthens.

5. Schede's operation cured 33% in a series of 9 cases. Of two cases, 2 years or less since operation, both were cured; of seven cases, more than 2 years since operation, but one was cured. The tendency to recurrence of symptoms as the post-operative interval lengthens is much greater after a Schede than after a Trendelenburg operation.

6. Division between ligatures of the saphenous vein does not ensure permanent occlusion. The venous stream may be reestablished in three ways, viz., dilatation of anastomoses around the point of division (two cases), formation of varices in the scar (three cases), or end-to-end anastomosis of the ligated stumps (three cases). The Schede operation is followed particularly by anastomosis of ligated stumps; of six cases examined three showed an intact saphenous vein running directly through the scar.

7. Functional restoration of the saphenous vein may be, but is not always, accompanied by recurrence of symptoms.

8. Resection of 8 cm. or more of the saphenous vein at the saphenous opening made through a generous transverse skin incision is to be preferred to simple division of the vein.

9. Post-operative pulmonary embolism is rare, but has occurred between the 4th and 13th days. The onset is marked by sudden dyspnœa, cyanosis, tachycardia and signs of collapse accompanied by rise in temperature; the symptoms may subside rapidly, may persist with the physical signs of pulmonary infarct, or may be followed immediately by sudden exitus.

I wish, here, to express my thanks to Professor Halsted for the opportunity of reporting this material from his clinic; and to Dr. Bloodgood for the privilege of the laboratory.

REFERENCES.

1. Schede: Berliner klin. Wochenschrift, 1877, No. 7.
2. Madelung: ⎰ Verhandlungen der Deutschen Gesell-
3. Langenbeck: ⎱　　schaft für Chirurgie, 1884, p. 114.

.4. Trendelenburg: Beiträge zur klinischen Chirurgie, Band 7, p. 194.

5. Goerlich: Beiträge zur klinischen Chirurgie, Band 44, p. 278.

6. Velpeau: Manuel d'anat. chirurg génér. Bruxelles, 1837, S. 51, and Bull. de la soc. de chir. de Paris, 1862, T. III, p. 137. (Reference from Goerlich.)

7. Grzes: Beiträge zur klinischen Chirurgie, Bd. 28, p. 501. (Reference from Goerlich.)

8. Perthes: Deutsche med. Wochenschrift, 1895, p. 253. (Reference from Goerlich.)

9. Ledderhose: Deutsche Zeitschrift für Chirurgie, Bd. 71, p. 401.

10. Minkiewitsch: Virchow's Archiv. Bd. 25 and 48.

11. Casati, E: Ferrara. 1899. Reference: Centralblatt für Chirurgie, Bd. 26, p. 807.

12. Mayo, C. H.: St Paul Medical Journal, Sept. 1904.

13. Franz: Deutsche Zeitschr. für Chirurgie, B. 47, p. 295.

14. Nauwerk: Sitzungsbericht für wissenschaftl. Heilkunde, Nov. 22, 1897. (Reference from Goerlich.)

15. Studsgaard: Reference: Hildebrand's Jahresber., 1895, p. 1149.

16. Sylvester, G. H.: Journal of the Royal Army Medical Corps, Vol. 4, p. 215.

17. Viannay: Revue de Chirurgie, Vol. 31, p. 78.

18. Carothers: Transactions of the Southern Surgical and Gynæcological Association, December, 1905. Abstract in Surgery, Gynæcology and Obstetrics, Vol. 2, p. 226.

BLOOD PRESSURE CHANGES IN CHEYNE-STOKES RESPIRATION.

By J. A. E. EYSTER, M D.,

Assistant in Physiology.

(From the Physiological Laboratory of the Johns Hopkins University.)

In ten clinical cases of Cheyne-Stokes respiration, the periodic alternation of dyspnœa and apnœa was associated with Traube-Herring waves of blood pressure. These cases may be separated into two groups. In the first, the period of respiratory activity was accompanied by a rise of blood pressure, the period of apnœa by a fall. In the second group, the inverse relations were present. In both groups there was a change in the pulse rate. The slower pulse was associated always with the fall in blood pressure. In the first group therefore it was present during the apnœa, in the second during the dyspnœa.

Historical Note.—Murri,[1] by the use of the plethysmograph, observed a decrease in the blood contents of the arm during the first part of dyspnoea. Hill,[2] by the same means, in a single case, the nature of which he does not state, observed a constriction of the vessels during dyspnœa and a dilatation during apnœa. Cushing,[3] by the employment of the Riva Rocci sphygmomanometer, found a rise of blood pressure with each group of respirations in two cases of cerebral hæmorrhage. Mosso,[4] by means of the sphygmomanometer devised by himself, found in the periodic respiration occurring in normal men at high altitudes, a rise of blood pressure associated with each group of respirations.

Methods.—The blood pressure was obtained by means of

the Erlanger sphygmomanometer.[5] The recording pen of this instrument shows the largest pulsations when the pressure exerted upon the arm by the cuff is equal to diastolic blood pressure, and these pulsations decrease as the pressure is raised or lowered. The systolic and diastolic pressures were first obtained by the method of increasing the pressure until the pulse at the wrist disappears, and then allowing it to slowly fall. The pressure upon the arm was then adjusted so that it was permanently at a point midway between systolic and diastolic pressures, and a continuous tracing of the pulse was recorded. Any change in blood pressure produced an effect upon the size of the pulsations of the recording pen. A rise of blood pressure increased the size of the pulsations, because such a rise brought the diastolic pressure nearer to the point at which the instrument was set. A fall in blood pressure had the opposite effect by making more distant the diastolic pressure from this point. The respirations were registered upon the same record by means of a Marey double tambour.

Group I. Cheyne-Stokes respiration in which there is a rise of blood pressure and an increase in the pulse rate with each respiratory group.—Two of the series of ten cases belong in this group. The condition with which it was associated was in both cases increased intracranial tension. The first was a case of solitary tubercle of cerebrum with tuberculous meningitis. The patient was admitted to the hospital in Dec. 1905 (Surg. No. 18,531). The increase in the intracranial tension was indicated by the symptoms and confirmed at a subsequent exploratory craniotomy and decompression. This

---

[1] "Sulla genesi del Fenomeno di Cheyne-Stokes," Rivista Clinica, Fasc 10, 2-11, 1883. Also "Scritta Medici di Augusto Murri, Bologna," 1902. Tome II.

[2] "Cerebral Circulation." London, 1896.

[3] American Journ. of the Med. Sci., September 1902, and June, 1903.

[4] Fisiologia dell'uomo Sulli Alpi. Also Archiv. ial. de Biol. T. XLIII. Fasc 1, 1905.

[5] Johns Hop. Hosp. Reports, 1904, XII.

patient had well marked Cheyne-Stokes respiration for the first five days after admittance to the hospital. The respiratory groups varied greatly in character. Atypical groups, such as descending groups of a few respirations and groups of irregular respirations, were unusually frequent. The true Cheyne-Stokes type with an ascending and descending phase to each group was however common. Numerous tracings obtained during the course of observation of this patient showed well the blood pressure changes associated with the respiratory periods. The rise in blood pressure which was constantly associated with the periods of dyspnoea, in some cases preceded, in others was coincident with, and in others followed slightly the beginning of respiratory activity. There was marked slowing of the pulse during apnoea, and the tracings showed the greatest slowing to be present with the most marked fall of blood pressure. A gradual rise of blood pressure occurring during the first five days of observation, was associated with a decrease in the periodicity of the respirations; an increase in the length of the dyspnœic periods at the expense of the apnœas. On the fifth day, a complete disappearance of periodic respiration was accompanied by a rise of 12 mm. in systolic pressure occurring in the course of five hours. Following this there was no return of Cheyne-Stokes respiration. The blood pressure continued to rise until the operation, on the seventh day after admittance. One and one-half hours after the operation the systolic pressure had fallen 35 mm. Tracings taken after the disappearance of the Cheyne-Stokes respiration showed an entire absence of the blood pressure changes previously observed.

The second case occurred in the service of Dr. Arthur Hebb, and to him and to Dr. Cushing, who was called in consultation, I am indebted for the privilege of obtaining tracings from this patient. The case was one of cerebral hæmorrhage of two weeks duration. Cheyne-Stokes respiration had been present at intervals, interspersed with periods of normal respiration. The records showed a similar relation of blood pressure to the respiratory variations as in the previous case.

Tracing No. 1 is from the case first described. The upper line is the tracing of the sphygmomanometer pen, obtained by the method above described. The middle tracing is the respiratory curve. The lowermost line records the time in one second intervals.

Group II. Cheyne-Stokes respiration in which there is a fall of blood pressure and a slowing of the pulse rate with each group of respirations.—This group includes eight cases of Cheyne-Stokes respiration occurring in association with cardiac and arterial disease. The blood pressure changes in relation to the groups of respirations are shown in Tracing No. 2. Commencing usually at the first half of apnœa, there is a fall of blood pressure which continues to about the third or fourth respiration of the following group. The slowing of the pulse is associated with the most marked fall of blood pressure. It is usually to be observed several seconds before respirations begin and reaches its maximum during the first

few respirations. A rise of blood pressure and a gradual increase of pulse rate occur from this point and reach a maximum in the first half of the following apnœa. This rise is at first slow; toward the end of dyspnœa and the first part of the following apnœa it is more rapid.

Discussion and Comparison of the Two Clinical Groups of Cheyne-Stokes Respiration.—Disappearance of the periodic respiration in both groups of cases is accompanied by a disappearance of the blood pressure waves. The intensity of the respiratory variations furthermore corresponds to the intensity of the blood pressure changes. In one of the cases of Group II, the gradual disappearance of the Cheyne-Stokes respiration over a period of three hours showed well the gradual decrease and finally the disappearance of the blood pressure changes. The same has been observed in several cases in records taken during sleeping and waking in the same patient. The Cheyne-Stokes respiration was frequently more marked in the former case and was accompanied by more marked blood pressure changes. The blood pressure changes cannot be regarded as a mechanical result of periodic respiratory activity, because in normal individuals the latter gives an entirely different series of blood pressure changes. Numerous records were obtained in which a normal man respired periodically and endeavored to simulate Cheyne-Stokes respiration, and the blood pressure changes that were associated differed entirely from those that occurred in either of the groups of true Cheyne-Stokes respiration. Tracing No. 3 is the record of such an experiment. Besides the difference in the blood pressure changes in the two groups described, and the different conditions under which they occur, certain other characteristics serve to distinguish them. The regular alternation of apnœa and dyspnœa was more constant in Group II and the respiratory groups, were much more uniform and nearly always of the typical Cheyne-Stokes type, with an ascending and descending phase to each group. Groups of irregular respirations and especially groups of a gradually decreasing scale in which the first respiration is the largest, were common in the intracranial cases. The periods of apnœa in Group I were associated with deep unconsciousness. In Group II· there was usually mental dullness and quiet at that time, but the impairment of consciousness was not nearly so marked and in several cases was not noticeable. The periods of respiratory activity in the second group were much more dyspnœic in character than those in Group I.

Experimental Cheyne-Stokes Respiration.—Cheyne-Stokes respiration was produced in dogs by means of cerebral compression. A full description of these experiments will appear shortly in the "Journal of Experimental Medicine." The method used for increasing the intracranial tension was that employed by Cushing.[1] An isotonic solution of sodium chloride was run into the closed cranial cavity through a

---

[1] Loc. cit.

trephine opening, into which was screwed an accurately fitting brass canula. The pressure of the entering fluid was measured by a mercury manometer. The blood pressure from the carotid or femoral was recorded by another mercury manometer, the pen of which wrote upon the same record and as nearly as possible in the same vertical line. The zero pressure of each system was represented by the same base line. Periodic respiration was obtained when the blood pressure rose and fell in the form of waves above and below the line of intracranial tension, the periods of respiratory activity accompanying the rise, the periods of apnœa the fall. When this relation between the intracranial and blood pressure was lost, periodic respiration disappeared. The periodic respiration thus produced varied in character. Groups of two to twenty respirations of equal size, groups of an ascending scale and groups of a descending scale, and finally groups which presented both an ascending and a descending phase (true Cheyne-Stokes type). The occurrence of the respiratory groups was associated with an increase in pulse rate. After section of both vagi, the pulse rate was the same in dyspnœa and apnœa.

A series of experiments upon brain anæmia consequent upon ligation of the cerebral arteries was performed. The results of these may be briefly summarized as follows: (a) The irritability of the respiratory centre is markedly susceptible to a considerable reduction in its blood supply, and if this reduction is sufficiently great the centre soon becomes incapable of response, even to the strongest stimulation. The irritability is rapidly regained upon the occurrence of a renewed blood supply if the preceding anæmia has not lasted too long. (b) The irritability of the other medullary centres is much less susceptible to a reduced blood supply. The vasomotor centre may respond to stimuli many seconds after the occurrence of absolute anæmia. (c) The effects of increased intracranial tension upon the medullary centres are due to the anæmia that results and not to any pressure effects directly.

Discussion of the Experiments in Relation to Group I.— In experimental Cheyne-Stokes respiration occurring in increased intracranial tension, the dyspnœic periods are accompanied by a rise of blood pressure above the line of intracranial tension, the periods of apnœa by a fall below this line. When the intracranial pressure is greater than the blood pressure, the brain and medullary centres must be in a condition of anæmia, for the pressure without the capillaries being greater than that within, these vessels must fall into a state of collapse. A rise of blood pressure above the line of intracranial pressure is associated with a renewed supply of blood to the centers and brain. The changes in blood supply may be observed directly by observation of the cortex through a glass window screwed into a trephine opening in the skull. The periods of respiratory activity were therefore associated with the periods of blood supply to the medullary centres, the periods of apnœa with anæmia. Anæmia in-

creases the stimulus to the respiratory centre by diminishing the rate of diffusion of the CO_2 from the cells of the centre and at the same time decreasing their oxygen supply. In a condition in which blood pressure waves vary through a considerable degree, and hence cause periodic variations of the blood supply to the respiratory centre, we should expect the response of this centre to be greatest when the stimulus is greatest, i. e., during the fall of the blood pressure wave. Apnœa, if such were present, we should expect to occur when the rise of the blood pressure wave sufficiently decreased the stimulus. In periodic respiration occurring in increased intracranial tension, the opposite condition prevails. This is most probably due to periodic variations in the irritability of the respiratory centre as a result of the marked periodic variations in its blood supply. During the apnœa, the blood supply is so reduced that the irritability of the centre suffers greatly, and it is not capable of responding until the irritability is regained as a result of a renewed blood supply, or the stimulus, as a result of the long apnœa, is greatly increased.

Summary and Conclusions.—In ten cases of Cheyne-Stokes respiration occurring in man, the periodic alternation of dyspnœa and apnœa was accompanied by long Traube-Herring waves of blood pressure. These cases may be separated into two groups as regards the relation between the respiratory periods and the blood pressure wave. In Group I, each dyspnœic period was associated with a rise of blood pressure; in Group II, the opposite relations existed. In the former, the pulse rate was slowed during the apnœa, in the latter during the dyspnœa.[1]

Periodic respiration may be produced in animals by an increase of intracranial tension, and blood pressure changes are observed which bear the same relations to the respiratory periods as occur in clinical cases of periodic respiration associated with increased intracranial tension. In the former case, the waves of blood pressure rise and fall above and below the line of intracranial tension, and the underlying cause of the periodic respiration is a periodic alternation of anæmia and blood supply to the brain and medullary centres.

From the clinical standpoint, in the opinion of the author, the following conception is important. Cheyne-Stokes respiration occurring clinically in cases of increased intracranial tension, in all probability represents similar conditions to that observed in the animal experiments, namely blood pressure waves rising and falling *above and below the line of intracranial tension*. According to this conception, the appearance of this condition in a patient indicates one of two things, either a still further increase in the intracranial tension, or

---

[1] Mosso, in a recent publication, separates what is apparently a third group of Cheyne-Stokes respiration. In the periodic respiration occurring in normal men at high altitudes, he has observed a rise of blood pressure and a decrease in the pulse rate with each group of respirations (Fisiologia dell'uomo sulli Alpi. Fig. 31 and 32, and Archiv. ial. de Biol. T. XLIII, Fasc 1, 1905. Fig. 21). This differs from both of the groups described by me.

a beginning loss of the blood pressure reaction to the increased intracranial tension.[*] In either case the prognosis is bad. A disappearance of Cheyne-Stokes respiration in a case of increased intracranial tension means on the other hand either a decrease in the tension or a rise of blood pressure, and hence is of good prognosis. Cheyne-Stokes respira-

tion that is accompanied by a rise of blood pressure and increase of pulse rate during the dyspnœic periods is probably always associated with increased intracranial tension.

The cause of the second group of cases is not as yet clear. The author is engaged upon a special research in this subject, and a subsequent report will be made.

---

[*] Cushing has shown in a most striking way, both experimentally and clinically, the rise of blood pressure that follows an increase of intracranial tension. (Physiol. u. anat. Beobacht. u. d. Einfluss v. Hirnkompression u. s. w. Mitteil. a. den grenzgebieten d. Medizin u. Chirurgie, Bd. 9, Hft. IV & V, 1902.) Amer. Jour. Med. Sciences, September, 1902, and June, 1903. Johns Hop. Hosp. Bul-

letin, Vol. XII, No. 126, September, 1901. He states as a general law that "an increase in intracranial tension occasions a rise of blood pressure which tends to find a level slightly above that of the pressure exerted against the medulla." The results of my experiments have confirmed his conclusions in all essential details.

OBSERVATIONS ON A CASE OF PALPITATION OF THE HEART.

BY ARTHUR D. HIRSCHFELDER, M. D.

(From The Medical Service of the Johns Hopkins Hospital.)

The sensation of palpitation of the heart is so distressing, and its causation so obscure, that the following observations may not be without interest. It is not uncommon for persons, especially for neurasthenics, to be conscious of each individual heart beat and to be greatly distressed by it, partly from fear of "heart disease" and partly from the nature of the sensation itself—although the exact character of the sensation seems to vary in both its nature and the region to which it is referred. In some, the sensation is referred to the region of the apex and is slightly painful in character. In the present case each systole was accompanied by a feeling of pressure or almost of traction referred to a point within the thorax about the level of the Angle of Ludwig. No symptoms were felt during diastole. The patient being a physician, was thoroughly conscious of its trivial nature, and not at all disturbed mentally by the occurrence, being interested in the symptom only from the scientific standpoint.

The main interest in the case lay in determining whether or not the symptom of palpitation was associated with any irregularity or disturbance in rhythm or force of contraction, in irritability, or in conductivity in the heart, or whether it was in any way associated with characteristic changes in pulse rate or blood pressure. For this purpose blood pressure records of maximum and minimum pressure were taken with the Erlanger apparatus. Tracings of the brachial pulse and other pulsations were taken with the author's modification of this apparatus.

Patient L. N. is a physician, 26 years old, married, of more or less nervous temperament. Has had measles, chicken-pox, whooping cough, but no other diseases except an annual tonsillitis. Has had no other phases of rheumatic cycle. No venereal diseases. Does not smoke. Takes very little wine and beer, no whiskey; drinks coffee in moderation. No drug habits.

Heart has always been normal; blood pressure, which has

been taken at intervals during the past three years, has been maximum 110 to 120 mm.; minimum, 80 to 90 mm. Pulse rate when patient is quiet 64 per min. Palpitation was first felt during extreme excitement in April, 1905, being then accompanied by slight but definite irregularity of pulse rate lasting but 5 to 10 minutes; palpitation ceased with the subsidence of the irregularity, and the latter has never returned. Since then palpitation has occasionally been felt after excitement, but never enough to keep patient awake. It is associated with a slight smothering sensation, and sense of fulness and traction referred to about the bifurcation of the trachea—never precordial; the sensation being always of distress rather respiratory than cardiac, although it is always exactly synchronous with cardiac systole and can be used to count the pulse rate.

On Feburary 23, after mental excitement such an attack of palpitation set in, lasted throughout day and night and was present next day, when observations were made with a view to determine the presence or absence of irregularities of contractility (as found by Mackenzie[1] in some cases, with precordial pain or palpitation), or of any other cardiac complications.

Note on Physical Examination Made by Dr. Cole, February 24.—With patient standing, point of maximal impulse is not well seen nor felt. In recumbent posture, P. M. I. also not well seen and felt. No visible impulse at the base. Fairly well marked throbbing in the neck and epigastrium. Very slight diffuse heave over the precordium.

The area of deep cardiac dulness extends 9.5 cm. to left at the 5th rib, 7.5 cm. in 3d interspace parasternal line; above to upper margin of 3d rib. To right 3 cm. in 3 i.s., 5 cm. in 4 i.s. On auscultation, heart sounds are best heard in 5th i.s.

---

[1] James Mackenzie, An Inquiry Into the Cause of Angina Pectoris, British Medical Journal, Vol. 2, 1905, p. 845; New Methods of Studying Heart Affections, ibid. Vol. 1, 1905, p. 815.

9 cm. from mid-sternal line. Sounds are a little distant, slightly muffled though well heard. Both sounds quite clear at apex, second sound a little snapping, both of almost equal intensity. Second sound becomes more ringing as one approaches base and over sternal articulation of 3d rib second sound is snapping, more so than to right of sternum. Heart sounds are quite clear.

First sound is faint and just audible. No murmurs can be heard anywhere. Heart action is quite regular.

Pulse is quite regular with patient lying 15 to ¼ m. There is a definite dicrotic wave felt and a well marked capillary pulse is visible. Patient on standing suddenly pulse rate jumps to 22 to ¼ m.

The palpitation gradually disappeared after four days—and with it the throbbing of the vessels, and the visible capillary pulse—but there were no changes in objective findings otherwise.

The blood pressure maximum 110, minimum 80-85 (Fig. 1-I), and pulse rate 64 to 76 (reclining position) are normal for the individual upon whom these observations had frequently been made when he was in normal condition. Tracings taken from cuff on arm at different pressures (Fig. 2) show normal and uniform form of beats—showing no abnormality in contractility. The same may be said of the changes in blood pressure and pulse rate observed after five minutes chest-weight exercises (Fig. 1-IIa), and upon suddenly rising from the reclining to the standing position.

The same relation of pulse rate and blood pressure to respiration (inspiration 72.7 per min.; expiration 69.0 per min., with rise of blood pressure in inspiration and fall during expiration), is also quite normal and not exaggerated. In other words, during the period when palpitation was noted, the heart was responding to stimuli in the same degree as when no palpitation was felt.

Comparison of the tracings obtained from the carotid artery, jugular vein, and apex show that each ventricular systole (Fig. 6, s-d) is preceded by a normal auricular systole (Fig. 5, a-c) the period of conduction (a-c=0.16 sec.) being normal. The time (s-c=0.04 sec.) from the beginning of systole to the beginning of the carotid wave is also normal, as is the period of systolic output from the heart (Fig. 4, c-d=0.26 sec.). There is no sign of irregular or aborted systoles nor of abnormal auricular contractions. The only objective abnormality observed was that there was marked throbbing in the vessels of the neck, marked capillary and dicrotic pulse.

None of these factors, however, throw any light upon the causation of the symptom of palpitation, as each and all may be present to a much more marked degree without bringing it about. Moreover, the palpitation was not felt for a few minutes after the chest-weight exercises when the heart was being subjected to the greatest strain; but on the other hand, it was always the most intense when patient had been lying down for a few minutes. It may be stated that the patient's attention was directed toward the palpitation quite as much

after exercise as at other times, so that the psychical factor, as the sole cause, may here be excluded.

Several other possibilities may also be considered.

1. The maintenance of the normal blood pressure (maximal and minimal) with normal pulse rate in spite of the presence of a marked capillary pulsation and throbbing carotids showing an abnormal peripheral vasodilation would indicate an increased total blood flow (although the product of pulse pressure by pulse rate is normal), which, according to the work of Erlanger,[3] would be possible only if there were an increased amount of blood put out at each systole. However, even if this is present in the case under discussion, increased systolic output has no relation to palpitation in other cases with pulse irregularities, in which the weaker beat can be noticed by the patient quite as well as the stronger ones. On the other hand, in many tachycardias with imperfect systolic emptying of the heart the patient is nevertheless not conscious of the individual beats. Palpitation is therefore quite independent of the degree of contractile power, or effort.

In the case under consideration it was more marked with slower rhythm than with rapid rhythm, and had no relation to the work done by the heart.

2. The nature of the sensation described above and its reference by the patient suggested the possibility of traction from adhesions, etc. But the absence of pulsus paradoxus, tracheal tug, Broadbent's sign, and of signs of enlarged bronchial glands, rather excludes this interpretation. In order to determine the presence, if any, of abnormality in the intra-tracheal pressure, tracings were made of the pressure in the air passages, with glottis closed (Fig. 8), and with glottis open (Fig. 9). These, however, are normal,[4] showing the carotid wave when glottis is closed, and the negative wave in systole when glottis is open—no abnormal waves.

3. Considered from the standpoint of a purely functional neurosis, it may be stated that there were no signs of abnormality in the reflex action of vagus or accelerator, nor of increased cardiac response, nor were there at any time any psychic disturbance such as Henry Head (Brain, Part 95, page 345, 1901) found to be frequently associated with "visceral pain" from the heart.

4. Since the above observations were made, the patient has several times experienced marked throbbing of the vessels of forearms and hands—of which he was made conscious by the shock felt in these parts throughout the whole systolic period—corresponding closely to the duration and occurrence of the palpitation felt in the chest on February 23 and 24. Blood pressure determinations could never be made during the short periods (fifteen to twenty minutes) when this symptom prevailed; but at these times there was marked reddening of

[3] Erlanger, J., Johns Hopkins Hospital Reports, Vol. 12, p. 53, 1904.

[4] Cf. Mosso, Sul Pulso negativo.—Arch. per. le. Sc. Med., Torino, Vol. III, 1878, cit. from E. J. Marey, La Circulation du Sang, Paris, 1882, p. 434.

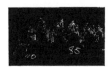 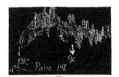

Fig. 1—I. 1:40 p. m. Blood pressure maximum 110 mm. hg., minimum 85 mm. Pulse rate, 72 per min. II. 1.52 p. m. After exercise. Maximum 138 mm., minimum 90 mm. Pulse rate 132 per min.

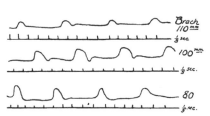

Fig. 2.—Pulse tracings from cuff on upper arm at 110, 100, 80 mm. hg., respectively, showing regularity in force and rhythm.

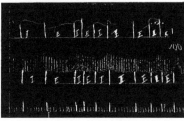

Fig. 3.—Tracing of respiration and brachial pulse. Average pulse rate: inspiration, 72.7 per min.; expiration, 69.0 per min.

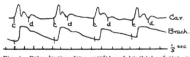

Fig. 4.—Pulse tracing from carotid and brachial arteries simultaneously.

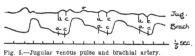

Fig. 5.—Jugular venous pulse and brachial artery.

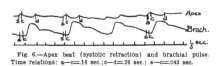

Fig. 6.—Apex beat (systolic retraction) and brachial pulse. Time relations: a—c=.16 sec.; c—d=.26 sec.; s—c=.043 sec.

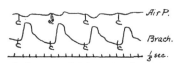

Fig. 8.—Pressure of air in mouth—glottis closed.

DESCRIPTION OF THE FIGURES.

Car. = Pulse tracing over carotid artery.
Jug. = Pulse tracing over jugular vein.
Brach. = Pulse tracing from cuff applied to upper arm at 100 mm. hg. pressure.
Air P. = Tracing of pressure in air passages.
Resp. = Respiration I=Inspiration, E=Expiration.
  c = time of carotid wave.
  d = time of dicrotic notch on carotid pulse tracing.
  a = time of wave due to auricular systole.
  s = time of beginning of ventricular systole.

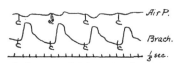

Fig. 9.—Same—glottis open.

the hands, and a very definite capillary pulse in the finger nails, not present at other times. Moreover, extreme throbbing of the abdominal aorta is not uncommonly associated with palpitation of the heart, although not in the case described above. It seems, therefore, not improbable that the symptom of palpitation of the heart in the above-mentioned case, and perhaps in many others, may have been due entirely to the throbbing of the aorta and may be quite independent of the heart itself, since the latter showed no other signs of abnormal spontaneous or reflex action.

THE IRISH SCHOOL OF MEDICINE.[1]

By JAMES J. WALSH, M. D., PH. D.,

Professor of the History of Medicine and of Nervous Diseases, Fordham University Medical School, New York City; Adjunct Professor of Medicine at the New York Polyclinic Hospital and School for Graduates in Medicine, and Professor of Physiological Psychology at St. Francis Xavier's College, New York.

[The main reason for my choice of the subject of the Irish School of Medicine is my own interest in it. A secondary though very important reason for the choice, is that Professor Osler, who is responsible, I suppose, for a great deal more of the medical thoughts that this generation thinks in America than either the generation itself gives him credit for or he himself might care to acknowledge, met me one day in New York, and finding that I was to be in Dublin, offered to give me letters of introduction that facilitated some study on the spot of the conditions in which the Irish School of Medicine developed. To his kind introduction to Sir John Moore and Sir Christopher Nixon, and Sir John Moore's recommendation to Sir Charles Cameron, whatever I may have to say owes any of value that it has. Sir Charles Cameron, especially, who is the historian of the Royal College of Surgeons in Ireland, proved an invaluable source of suggestions, hints, precious bits of information and references, that made further study easy and fruitful.]

It is with no idea of impressing the value of any narrow, national type of medical investigation or development in medicine that I have come to Johns Hopkins this evening. There are not many things in life that I deprecate more than scientific Chauvinism. I sincerely hope that the medical science of the future will be above and beyond all such limitations. Personally, I consider that one of the most interesting features of the Congress of Arts and Sciences at the Exposition at St. Louis was the fact that Russian and Japanese scientists cooperated in certain work for the Congress, though their countrymen on the other side of the globe were engaged in a bitter struggle over political matters. It is perhaps the most encouraging outlook for humanity at the present time that true science may raise men above the narrow national feeling that now drives them to war, and so help to usher in an era of universal peace that has been so long waited for but is surely coming.

I select "The Irish School of Medicine" as a topic for historical treatment because in the second quarter of the nineteenth century a trio of young men, physicians in Dublin, revolutionized the practice and the teaching of medicine by devoting themselves to the clinical investigation of disease, to the study of patients rather than to the elaboration of medical

theories, and to the training of students to look to the condition of their individual patients rather than to any preconceived notions if they would make correct and helpful diagnosis and at the same time promote what is the dream of every young medical man, I hope, the development of this science of medicine of ours which is destined to accomplish so much for humanity.

Any single nationality has had very little to do with the development of our modern clinical medicine, and it is interesting to realize how medical progress has skipped from one country to another, quite contrary to what might have been expected from the influence of association and environment, and has received its best advances at the hands of genius wherever it might be and in spite of the discouraging influences that surrounded originality. Perhaps the most precious lesson in the history of clinical medicine is the fact that most of our discoveries came from young men, men under thirty-five, men as a rule somewhat out of the busiest current of medical thought in which the greatest progress might be expected, men whose initiative and genius for original investigation had not been smothered by the ineffectual attempt to master all the details of previously acquired medical information and technical methods.

The beginning of our modern clinical medicine came when Morgagni, at Bologna, began to keep notes of the cases that he saw clinically and compare them with the notes of the autopsies which he had the opportunity to see. This confrontation of bedside and autopsy room details seems so obvious to us now that we can scarcely think of it as a great discovery, yet great discovery it was, and the man who did it is the father of modern pathology, if we shall adopt Virchow's expression, and who was better able to judge? Morgagni began his note-taking when he was scarcely twenty, in a series of little books called Adversaria, the Latin name for note book, and these contained the foundations of modern medicine.

It might surely have been expected then that the next great step in medicine would come in Italy from some of the young men closely associated with Morgagni and with his practical methods of observation and pathological comparison. It did not, however, but came nearly a thousand miles away

[1] Read before the Johns Hopkins Hospital Historical Club. December 11, 1905.

in Vienna, where a young man named Auenbrugger, not yet 25 years old, began to realize that if he tapped with his finger on the chests of people suffering from various thoracic diseases he could tell something about the condition of the organs beneath his fingers from the sounds elicited by this tapping or percussion. For ten years he studied his patients carefully and had opportunities to make autopsies upon some of them. Then he published a little book containing not much more reading matter than a modern medical journal article of moderate length. This little book absolutely settled the subject of percussion and its value as a diagnostic medium in thoracic disease for all time.

There were two great professors of medicine in Vienna at this time, each of them when writing systems of medicine. One, the famous Van Swieten, published some sixteen volumes on medicine, two of them with regard to thoracic diseases. Van Swieten does not even mention Auenbrugger's work, or the possibility of its having significance, though he does confess that thoracic diseases are the most difficult in diagnosis in the whole range of medicine. The other professor was De Haan, who also wrote extensively on medicine, some eleven volumes altogether, yet made no mention of Auenbrugger's work.

One might have expected that Auenbrugger himself would have thought of putting his ear down to the chest and so have discovered auscultation, but even genius makes but one step into the unknown. Auenbrugger's work did not receive proper credit until it was taken up by the French school under Corvisart, about thirty years later. Corvisart used the method of percussion on Napoleon, who thought it a very practical idea that a physician should try to learn something about his patient by such direct means rather than by looking at his tongue and feeling of his pulse. Accordingly, Corvisart was made professor at the University of Paris, and his protegé, Laennec, became impressed with the importance of Auenbrugger's work.

It was to Laennec that the world was to owe the diagnostic method of auscultation. He, too, began his successful studies on thoracic disease when he was under twenty-five. It took him about twelve years to complete his book on the subject. When he had finished it, the subject of auscultation had sprung as perfect from his brain as Minerva from that of Jove. Nothing further was needed to finish it. Some eighty years have passed since that time. There are three things, it is said by the recent biographer of Laennec with regard to auscultation in pulmonary diseases, that have been added since the original master's time. Their comparative insignificance can be best judged when I mention them. They are the *bruit d'airain* of Trousseau, the prolonged expiration at the end of expiration in the initial stage of pulmonary tuberculosis, and finally the dubiously significant sign, Bacelli's ægophony —only these after nearly a century of medical work to be added to the twelve years observation of one young man. Verily, in the words of Augustine Birrel at the end of his essay on Carlyle, "Fellow mortals, lend me your ears and

let me whisper into their furry depths, don't let us quarrel with genius. We haven't any of it ourselves and the worst of it is we cannot get along without it."

It might have been expected then that Laennec, listening to so many chests, would have discovered the secrets of heart disease. Let me repeat, even genius makes only one step into the unknown. That was left for the Irish school of medicine, for Graves, Stokes, and Corrigan, and that is why I am going to talk this evening about this school.

It must not be thought that it is only in medicine that the history of discovery goes skipping round from country to country in the way that I have just detailed. A typical example of the contrary of any such false impression is easily to be seen in the sketch of the development of electricity at about the same time as these advances in clinical medicine were being made. Our own Franklin made the first step by demonstrating that the lightning and trivial electric phenomena here on earth were due to the same cause, though even in this he is said to have been anticipated by a Bohemian clergyman. The next step came from Galvani in Italy. Volta tried to contradict Galvani and made some great discoveries, but no further good work was done in Italy. The next step came, some 2000 miles away, from Oersted, a Dane, who showed the identity of magnetism and electricity. Then the distinguished French scientist Ampère, making his observations at Paris, developed this idea, while a German mathematical savant, Ohm, worked out the laws of resistance. After this English electrical scientists came in for a series of important observations and demonstrations in the rising science.

The first and most important name in the Irish School of Medicine is that of Dr. Robert Graves, who received his degree of bachelor of medicine at the University of Dublin in 1818. Undoubtedly his genius for original observation of high order was fostered by the fact that after his graduation he spent some time in most of the large cities of the world in which important work in medicine was being done. He was at London, for instance, for several months. He then spent three years on the continent, dividing his time between Berlin, Gottingen, Vienna, and Copenhagen, and eventually getting around to Paris and down to Italy, always noting what was being done in medicine wherever he wandered. Before returning to Dublin, he passed some months at Edinburgh and here was brought in contact with Stokes and Corrigan, who were later to be his colleagues in Dublin. Stokes and he became fast friends and remained such for the rest of their lives.

Like practically all of the great medical men who have proved to be original workers, Graves' interest was not confined alone to medicine. During his sojourn in Italy he became acquainted with Turner, the celebrated English landscape painter, and was his companion in many journeys. Graves himself was possessed of no mean artistic powers, as his friend Stokes tells us, and his sketches are characterized by natural vigor and truth. His thorough appreciation of his companion, however, and the breadth of his sympathy and admiration for the great painter of nature can perhaps best be understood from some candid expressions of his with regard to their work in common. " I used to work away," he said, " for an hour or more and put down as well as I could every object in the scene before me, copying form and color as faithfully as was possible in the time. When our work was done and we compared drawings the difference was strange. I assure you there was not a single stroke in Turner's drawing that I could see like nature, not a line nor an object, and yet my work was worthless in comparison with his. The whole glory of the scene was there."

It is not too much to say that Graves owed not a little of his faculty for observation, for seeing things that others had missed, though readily to be perceived after he had pointed them out, to these educational experiences with the great artist. It is the power to observe more than the store of information that the medical student needs. As Dr. Stokes very well says: " In this large and truly liberal education, which embraced the training of the school, the university, and the world, we can discover in part the foundations of his subsequent eminence. He did not content himself, as is so commonly the case, with commencing—to use his own words —' the life of a practitioner without practice,' but he made himself intimate with the recent discoveries and modes of thinking in every great school of medicine, whether abroad or at home, and formed friendships with the leading physiologists and physicians of Europe, with many of whom he kept up a correspondence during his life."

Graves spent thirty years of fruitful study of medicine after this in Dublin, leaving his mark very prominently on every chapter of medical investigation that he took up—fevers, diseases of the chest, intestinal diseases, nervous diseases, and especially in diagnosis and treatment.

It is with regard to fevers especially that Graves' work will count for all time, because he set their treatment on so practical a basis. The trained nurse is quite a modern institution, yet seventy-five years ago Dr. Graves insisted that the services of a properly-qualified nurse in severe, continued fever are inestimable. He emphasized the necessity for moral management in .fever, and friends and relatives are seldom capable of discharging this office.

" If they chance to discover from the physician's remarks or questions the weak points of the patient's case they generally contrive to let him know them in some way or another. If the patient is restless, for instance, the ill-judged anxiety of his friends will most certainly prevent him from sleeping. If he happens to take an opiate and they are aware of the nature of his medicine they will surely inform him of it in some way or another, though it may be only by a hint, and his anxiety for sleep conjoined with their disturbing inquiries prevents its due operation."

We are apt to think that the modern aphorism, nursing (meaning trained care), is more important than medicine in the treatment of fever, is the result of observations in our own day. Dr. Graves, however, felt very deeply that the most important element in the treatment was the conservation of the patient's strength with the preservation of his *morale,* and this can be best accomplished when the patient is constantly under the care of an experienced nurse, noting every symptom and saving every possible source of worry and every form of exhaustion of energy.

Another interesting anticipation of modern methods was with regard to child feeding in summer diarrhœa. It is often thought that only in recent years with the development of the science of bacteriology the danger of continuing milk feeding when infants are already ill in the summer time has come to be recognized. Milk is now known to be an excellent culture medium for various forms of bacteria, that is, it is a substance on which microbes grow plentifully, and it is often used in the laboratory to raise microbes. Dr. Graves, however, without any knowledge of modern bacteriology, but from clinical observation alone, pointed out that the only way to avoid a summer diarrhœa was to stop all milk feeding.

" Let the infant," he says, " abstain from milk in any shape for twenty-four hours, sometimes for the space of two, or even three, days. It is incredible how small a portion of milk, even in the most diluted state, will keep up this disease, acting like a species of poison on the intestinal mucous surface."

Even more interesting in these modern times, however, than Graves' attitude towards the treatment of fever is the position he took with regard to the habits of life that were best for the consumptive. At that time tuberculosis of the lungs was considered to be an inflammatory disease requiring the patient to be in the house most of the time, carefully protected from cold, and during any rise of temperature kept in warm rooms, and without any special encouragement to take food. Graves and Stokes changed all that, and for the time completely revolutionized the principles of treatment for this serious ailment. Alas, their work, notwithstanding the good results shown in a certain number of cases, failed to attract widespread attention and it was not until our own time that the principles they laid down as the rational basis of successful therapeutics for tuberculosis came to be generally adopted.

Graves insisted that his patients when suffering from beginning tuberculosis should not be confined to the house, but on the contrary should be out of doors most of the time. He emphasized what he called the taking of exercise, but in such a way that he agrees much more than might be thought with modern ideas on this subject. Now it is insisted that tuberculosis patients must not overtire themselves by taking exercise, though they must be out in the open air a large part of the time. Graves explains the exercises that he would like to have them take by saying that they should spend four or five hours every day riding in a carriage, or as he seems to prefer in an open jaunting-car. And that they should spend at least as much time sitting outside in quiet.

Besides this the most important element in treatment he

considers to be the encouragement of the appetite—as might be expected from the man who first fed fevers. His directions in this matter are very explicit, and he suggests various methods by which patients can be tempted to eat more and more food, and emphasizes the use of cereals and of milk and eggs as likely to be of most service in enabling these patients to gain in weight and strength so as to be able to resist the further advance of the disease. This, it may be said in passing, is just the ideal treatment for the consumptive at the present time.

Others of Graves' ideas in regard to tuberculosis are in general surprisingly modern. He insists, for instance, that the main causes of the disease are the overcrowding in towns, the long hours of hard work in factories, and the abuse of alcohol. He considers that the population of country places though fed no better as a rule than in the city do not develop the disease so frequently because of their opportunity for fresh air. He placed very little confidence in the idea that cold had anything to do with tuberculosis, though he disputed Laennec's dictum that bronchitis was never the beginning of tuberculosis. Graves advises his students not to try to protect their throats by means of mufflers, for this will only render them more liable to cold. His advice is rather to harden themselves against cold. For this he suggests the use of water plentifully on the chest and throat, to be employed not too cold during the winter time, unless one is used to it. He also suggests the use of vinegar and alcohol as hardening fluids. They should be applied freely, and in his experience were effective.

It is no wonder that Dr. Graves' work was properly appreciated even by those who were not his countrymen and who did not know him personally. The distinguished French clinician, Trousseau, at that time the leader of thought in European medicine, said of him:

"For many years I have spoken of Graves in my clinical lectures; I recommend the perusal of his work; I entreat those of my pupils who understand English to consider it as their breviary; I say and repeat that, of all the practical works published in our time, I am acquainted with none more useful, more intellectual, and I have always regretted that the clinical lectures of the great Dublin practitioner had not been translated into our language."

A little later in the same lecture he said:

"And, nevertheless, when he inculcated the necessity of giving nourishment in long-continued fevers, the Dublin physician, single-handed, assailed an opinion which appeared to be justified by the practice of all ages; for low diet was then regarded as an indispensable condition in the treatment of fevers. Had he rendered no other service than that of completely reversing the medical practice upon this point, Graves would, by that act alone, have acquired an indefeasible claim to our gratitude."

His tribute closes with the following very striking passage:

"I freely confess that I had some difficulty in accepting,

notwithstanding the imposing authority of Graves, what he states of the influence of certain remedies, such as mercurials, essence of turpentine, spirituous preparations, nitrate of silver, etc.; but the Dublin Professor speaks with so much conviction that I ventured to follow his precepts, and I must say that my early trials very soon encouraged me to adopt unreservedly what at first I accepted only with misgiving. There is not a day that I do not in my practice employ some of the modes of treatment which Graves excels in describing with the minuteness of the true practitioner, and not a day that I do not, from the bottom of my heart, thank the Dublin physician for the information he has given me.

"Graves is, in my acceptation of the term, a perfect clinical teacher. An attentive observer, a profound philosopher, an ingenious artist, an able therapeutist, he commends to our admiration the art whose domain he enlarges, and the practice which he renders more useful and more fertile."

The second of the great leaders of the Irish School of Medicine is William Stokes, the son of the Regius Professor of the Practice of Medicine of Trinity College, a post to which in due course of time he succeeded. As a boy he was not much given to study and, indeed, was somewhat the despair of his parents. He spent much of his time in reading poetry and romance, and the Scottish Border Ballads, which had just then been made so popular by Sir Walter Scott, were his favorite readings. He is said to have spent days in committing them to memory. This was a source of special anxiety to his mother, and one day, having fallen asleep while reading his favorite author, Sir Walter Scott, he was awakened by her tears falling on him as she bent over him. It is said that after this the dreamy indolent boy became the ardent and enthusiastic student. His love, however, for the olden times never left him and he remained a faithful student of Celtic antiquities and, indeed, his daughter is one of the authorities on this subject.

Stokes amply made up for any neglect of study there might have been in his boyhood days as soon as he entered upon the medical course to which he felt called. Here he came to be looked upon as one of the most ardent and painstaking of students.

His preliminary medical studies were begun in Dublin at the Meath Hospital. Chemistry he learned in the laboratory of Trinity College, and anatomy in the Royal College of Surgeons. After spending several years thus he went to Glasgow where for two years more he was occupied mainly at chemistry in the laboratory of Professor Thompson. Like most of the young Irishmen of his time, he next proceeded to Edinburgh in order to complete his education in clinical medicine and if possible obtain his medical degree from that famous institution. It was at Edinburgh, under the magnetic influence of that great teacher, Allison, that Stokes began to develop the rare powers of original observation which at an early age placed him in the front rank of the best medical men of the time.

It is interesting to note that before he left Edinburgh he published his first medical work, a treatise on the use of the stethoscope, which was undoubtedly the means of bringing that instrument—and with it Laennec's fruitful system of physical diagnosis by means of auscultation—to the general notice of the English-speaking medical profession. Even after all that has been written on the subject, it remains a very valuable little book. It was dedicated to the famous Cullen, who had already published a series of cases which had been illustrated by the use of the stethoscope and to whom Stokes probably owed the idea of the need for a formal little treatise on the subject. It is typical of the slow adoption of medical novelties that more than ten years afterwards, old time, though distinguished, physicians not infrequently made fun of Stokes for spending so much time in the study of cases with the stethoscope, since they were apt to consider it as little more than a toy. Stokes, however, intensely practical in his way, realized the value of the instrument, and as the result of his teaching it soon began to be more generally used, thus introducing that exact knowledge of diseases of the chest, which can only be obtained by means of this little instrument and the methods of auscultation which are associated with it.

Perhaps the most interesting phases of Stokes' purely medical work during the first part of his career is his treatment of the subject of consumption. When not quite thirty-three he wrote a treatise on the diagnosis and treatment of diseases of the chest. His familiarity with the work of Graves and of Auenbrugger gave him command of all the modern methods of physical diagnosis, so that he was able to study tuberculosis to the best possible advantage and with the least possible chance of too favorable judgment with regard to its cure. Notwithstanding the accuracy of his knowledge, however, he insisted that the disease was curable and that the important point with regard to it was the recognition of it as early as possible, in order that the patient might be given the best chance for life.

At that time most physicians considered tuberculosis to be an hereditary disease, without any idea of its being possibly contagious, and this idea of heredity seemed to set the stamp of inevitable fatality on the heads of victims of the disease. To announce the curability of tuberculosis then was to run counter to all the medical traditions of the time, and Stokes in doing so must have had in support of his teaching many observations of patients who had been cured notwithstanding the fact that they were assured sufferers from this supposedly fatal disease. We know at the present time that Stokes was surely correct in his judgment in this matter, and realize too that his method of treatment, which included abundant feeding and long hours each day in the outdoor air, constitutes the best elements of the modern treatment of tuberculosis.

Stokes devoted most of his life to the study of diseases of the chest and undoubtedly came to be one of the best diagnosticians in heart disease that the world has ever known.

Down even to the present time his book is an authority on the subject and will remain so unless some new method of physical diagnosis makes revelations hitherto undreamt of in regard to heart affections. It is rather interesting to find then that Stokes, far from insisting on how wonderfully exact in detail cardiac diagnosis has become, rather deprecates the pretension of too exact diagnosis so common among younger heart specialists. As a matter of fact, I know no set of expressions likely to encourage a young man more in his study of heart cases than Stokes' modest disclaimer on his part, of being able to tell many things that are supposed to be clear to the expert, and his insistence that too much is claimed for the possibilities of cardiac diagnosis. He says:

"We read that a murmur with the first sound, under certain circumstances, indicates lesion of the mitral valves. And, again, that a murmur with the second sound has this or that value. All this may be very true, but is it always easy to determine which of the sounds is the first, and which the second? Every candid observer must answer this question in the negative. In certain cases of weakened hearts acting rapidly and irregularly, it is often scarcely possible to determine the point. Again, even where the pulsations of the heart are not much increased in rapidity, it sometimes, when a loud murmur exists, becomes difficult to say with which sound the murmur is associated. The murmur may mask not only the sound with which it is properly synchronous, but also that with which it has no connection, so that in some cases even of regularly acting hearts, with a distinct systolic impulse, and the back stroke with the second sound, nothing is to be heard but one loud murmur.

"So great is the difficulty in some cases, that we cannot resist altering our opinions from day to day as to which is the first and which the second sound. . . .

"To the inexperienced the detailed descriptions of such phenomena as the intensification of the sounds of the pulmonary valves, of constrictive murmurs as distinguished from non-constrictive; of associations of different murmurs at the opposite sides of the heart; of pre-systolic and post-systolic. pre-diastolic and post-diastolic murmurs, act injuriously first, by conveying the idea that the separate existence of these phenomena is certain, and that their diagnostic value is established; and secondly, by diverting attention from the great object, which—it cannot be too often repeated—is to ascertain if the murmur proceeds from an organic cause, and, again, to determine the vital and physical state of the cavities of the heart. . . .

"If the question as to the practicability of the negative diagnosis, with reference to either orifice, be raised, it appears probable that where a mitral murmur is manifest it will be easier to determine the absence of disease of the aortic valves than to declare the integrity of the mitral valves in a case of aortic patency. The experience of each succeeding day devoted to the study of diseases of the heart will make us less and less confident in pronouncing as to the absence of disease in any one orifice, although no physical sign of such a lesion exist, if there be manifest disease in another, or, again, if there be symptoms of an organic affection of the heart."

Both Graves and Stokes insisted very much on the necessity of bedside teaching for medical students. It is surprising to think that considerably more than half a century passed away before anything like an organized effort was made to put into practice generally their counsels in this matter. Every one admitted the necessity, but every one feared the labor involved. Graves particularly railed at the fact that medical students were sent out to practice without ever having written a prescription. Men were taught all sorts of things in their medical course but not the practice of medicine. Thanks to the labors of Professor Osler, at last the opprobrium of absence of bedside teaching is gradually passing away. There is another phase of the subject of teaching on which Stokes had something to say that remains of interest, however, and from his words a precious lesson for the present generation might be gleaned. He makes the application of his words to all teaching, as well as that of medicine, and personally I think that his expressions might well be printed as a motto for every class-room:

" One word as to the duty of teachers, and this applies to those of other sciences as well as medicine. It is not to convey all the facts of a subject to their hearers, but it is, by precept and example, to teach them how to teach and guide themselves. If they succeed in this they have done their duty in the largest sense of the word."

On another occasion Stokes stated more definitely what he considered the duty of the medical teacher. " To teach the individual pupil, to encourage him to learn, to show him how to teach himself, to bring him into the true relation in which he ought to stand with his instructors, to make him familiar with bedside medicine, to show him the value of every new fact and observation in medicine, and to have him know the duties as well as make him face the pleasure of original investigation. These are the duties of the teacher in medicine."

Perhaps the most salient trait in Dr. Stokes' character was his treatment of the poor. He was kindness itself even to the most abject. The smile with which even those who were suffering severely greeted his arrival was the best evidence of this. After this, his great characteristic was his sympathy with his professional brethren. He succeeded in obtaining for the Irish physicians who devoted themselves to the care of the poor for the miserable pittance allowed by government, better conditions than those which had hitherto obtained, by representing very strongly to a Parliamentary committee that the death rate among Irish physicians, owing to the prevalence of virulent fever in Ireland, was nearly twice as high as that among army officers in the field during war times.

One tribute to his goodness of heart from the pen of a personal friend who had known him for many years seems to deserve a place at the close of this short sketch of his career:

" Those who have seen Dr. Stokes at the bedside of the sick know how gentle, how refined, how kindly was his bearing towards the patient. Amid all the ardor of clinical observation and research he never for one moment forgot the sufferer before him—no thoughtles word from his lips, no rough or unkind action ever ruffled the calm confidence reposed in him by those who sought his skill and care. In many eloquent lectures delivered in the Meath Hospital he inculcated those Christian lessons of charity and thoughtfulness; and so by precept and example he strove to teach the duties of a true and God-fearing physician."

The third of the Irish School is Sir Dominic Corrigan, whose name is probably more familiar to the ordinary student of medicine than either of his distinguished colleagues, because of its association with the form of pulse which occurs in aortic heart disease. Corrigan's career should prove a stimulating example to the young physician just taking up that real post-graduate work in medicine which comes after he has received his degree, finished, perhaps, his hospital work, and is beginning his practice. Corrigan was only twenty-seven when he began the series of observations on which was founded his paper on aortic heart disease, which was published when he was about thirty. In this matter of youthful accomplishment, Corrigan is not alone among his distinguished Irish contemporaries. Stokes, it will be remembered, wrote his little book on the stethoscope when he was only twenty-one, and had made some very important observations on diseases of the chest before he reached the age of thirty. Graves had showed very clearly the sound metal of his intelligence before he was twenty-five, and had described the cases of the nervous diseases which have since come to be called after his name, Graves disease, before his third decade had run more than a year or two. In fact, these young men accomplished so much by their careful observation and dependence on their own resources that the medical writer of the modern times is tempted to wonder if perhaps that most precious quality of the human mind in the young adult, its originality, is not obscured by the amount of information that it is expected to digest before it is tempted to do any thinking for itself.

There is another remarkable feature of Corrigan's achievement, in the recognition and description of this form of heart disease. At the time he was the physician to a hospital which had only room for six medical patients. This appointment to the little Jervis Street Hospital in Dublin had been secured only after competition, and Corrigan had to pay for the privilege of being the attending physician. This he could ill afford to do at the time, and so he resolved to make all his opportunities for the study of patients count to the greatest possible extent. He did not visit his hospital merely to see patients, but to study the cases carefully. His success is only another example of the necessity for seeing much, and not many things, if there is to be any real progress. In our day, physicians scarcely consider that they have any hospital experience unless they are the attending physicians to several hospitals, seeing at least one hundred patients a week. The result is that patients do not receive the skilled care they should, and that advance in medicine suffers because of the wasted opportunities for clinical observation while a busy attending physician rushes through a ward and the resident physician has only time for the routine work that enables him to keep just sufficiently in touch with the progress of his cases to satisfy the hurrying chief physican.

Before publishing his classic paper on the permanent patency of the aortic valve, on which his reputation as a wonderful clinical observer in medicine rests, Corrigan had called attention to some mistakes in the classification of heart murmurs made by Laennec in Paris. At this time Laennec was considered to be the best authority in Europe on diseases within the thorax. As regards diseases of the lungs, he well deserved the reputation. It is to him that the medical world owes all that it knows about diseases of the chest as far as these can be detected by means of the ear. His young contemporary in Ireland, however, was able to show that in diseases of the heart some of the ideas acquired in long years of study of the lungs were leading Laennec into false conclusions as regards the significance of murmurs in the heart. Even genius does not often succeed in doing more than one thing well, and while the Frenchman might have been thought just the one to complete the work begun on the heart this duty was to devolve on his Irish contemporaries.

Any one who wishes to realize how well Corrigan did his work should turn to that marvellously concise, complete article from which I select only the author's division of aortic heart affection:

" The morbid affections of the valves and aorta permitting this regurgitation are the following:

" 1st. The valves may be absorbed in patches, and thus become reticulated and present holes, through which the blood flows back into the ventricle.

" 2d. One or more of the valves may be ruptured; the ruptured valves when pressed, flapping back into the ventricle instead of catching and supporting the column of blood in the aorta, the blood then regurgitating through the space left by the broken valves.

" 3d. The valves may be tightened or curled in against the sides of the aorta, so that they cannot spread across its mouth; and an opening is then left between the valves, in the center of the vessel, through which the blood flows freely back into the ventricle.

" 4th. The valves without any proper organic lesion may be rendered inadequate to their function by dilatation of the mouth of the aorta. The aorta affected by aneurism, or dilated, as it frequently is in elderly persons, about its arch, will sometimes have the dilatation extending to the mouth of the vessel, and in such a case the valves become inadequate to their function, not from any disease in themselves, but from the mouth of the aorta dilating to such a diameter as to render the valves unable to meet its center; the blood then, as in the other instances, regurgitates freely into the ventricle."

I doubt if any better classification has been made even after three quarters of a century of additional study.

Another very distinct contribution of Corrigan to the medicine of his time was his insistence on the distinction that existed between typhoid and typhus fever. This is one of the most interesting features of his little book on the " Nature and Treatment of Fever." With our present knowledge, it seems hard to understand that these two fevers should have been so long confounded, but, as a matter of fact, it was not until the middle of the nineteenth century that the distinction between them was recognized even by the most acute observers. In this matter the French and Americans anticipated most of the rest of the world, though Corrigan's teaching in the matter had been correct for many years before others in the British Isles came to the true position.

Within a few years after his essay on aortic heart disease, Corrigan published a paper on chronic pneumonia or, as he called it, cirrhosis of the lungs. Corrigan's successful achievements in medicine depended mainly on the fact that he studied the pathological anatomy of fatal cases with the greatest care. He had detected that in certain cases of chronic pneumonia the process seemed to be quite different from that of tuberculosis. Observations, made post mortem, showed that his clinical observations were justified by the differences observed in the organ. As a result he formulated his opinions on the subject. He called particular attention to the fact that what he found corresponded very closely with the pathological process that had been observed by Laennec in the liver, and to which the French medical pathologist had given the name of cirrhosis. It would seem as though the pathology of the time was so crude that Corrigan must surely fall into serious error in his account of what he saw. Twenty years later, Virchow was to revolutionize pathology by the publication of his " Cellular Pathology." Notwithstanding the progress made since his time, however, Corrigan's description of the condition of the lungs that he noted, and of the pathological process observed, is so true that even to the present day this paper remains of distinct value in medicine and represents the beginning of correct ideas on the subject.

After Corrigan's death in 1880, the London Lancet said: " In the light of recent pathology Corrigan's speculations on cirrhosis of the lungs are more meritorious than ever and continue to be regarded as in the main sound. They anticipated by forty years much of the present pathology." Needless to say it is only a genius of a very high order that is thus capable of rising above the limitations of its environment.

The Irish School of Medicine has in Graves and Stokes and Corrigan a greater group of contemporaries than has been given to any other nation at one time. If we were to eliminate from nineteenth century medicine all of the inspiration derived from their work there would be much of value that would be lacking from the history of medical progress. These men were deeply imbued with the professional side of their work as physicians, and were not, in any sense of the word, money-makers. Another very interesting phase in all their careers is that no one of them occupied himself exclusively with medical studies. All of them had hobbies followed faithfully and successfully together with medicine, and all of them were deeply interested in the uplifting of the medical profession, especially in securing the rights of its members and saving poor sick people from exploitation by quacks and charlatans. All of them gave of their time, their most precious possession, for the political and social interests of their fellow men, and felt in so doing that they were only accomplishing their duty in helping their generation to solve the problems that lay immediately before them.

Undoubtedly the most important lesson of the work of the Irish School of Medicine is that real advances in medical teaching and science are due much more to clinical observation, the actual careful study of patients, than to the application of supposed theoretic principles of science that seem to explain much. Always in the history of medicine there has been an abundance of theory and most of it has been outlived in the course of time. Clinical observation, however, even when for a moment its significance may be mistaken, always retains a permanent value. In our age we are no different from those of former generations, and while we may consider that laboratory work apart from the patient will do much to explain disease, and help medicine, we are likely to find that in this we are as much mistaken as have been our forefathers whenever they abandoned the close study of groups of patients.

There is no doubt that there is as much room for advance in medicine by clinical observation at the present moment as there has been at any time in the history of our science. It is not at all improbable that, for instance, the infectious diseases will prove to be more numerous than they have so far been considered. It took a long time for even acute medical observers, and nowhere is this clearer than in studying the

Irish School of Medicine, to realize that typhoid fever was quite distinct from typhus fever, and our generation has seen the practical acceptance of a third disease in the group, paratyphoid fever, and has come to the threshold of the thought that there are further disease entities in this same series. The scarlatina-measles group has been increased by a third disease, German measles, and probably also by a fourth, the so-called Duke's fourth disease.

There remain other disease groups that need differentiation very sadly. It has been pointed out over and over again that the word rheumatism covers a multitude of diagnostic sins and shortcomings and forms an excuse for lack of thoughtful observation of patients. The uric acid diathesis has been an abomination for half a century and is only now beginning to find its way properly into the limbo of things to be forgotten. The word neurasthenia has been almost as much abused as rheumatism and has proved just as fruitful of evil in preventing proper differentiation of diseased conditions. There seems no doubt that such words as hysteria and functional neurosis of various kinds are being abused in the same way. As a matter of fact, words are constantly serving as cloaks for ignorance and as excuses for negligence. Malaria as a universal refuge has gone out to a great extent, but since the great epidemic of 1890 influenza has come into explain most of the obscure febrile conditions of the winter time.

Our hope must be that the young men, for it is always the man under thirty-five who does original work in medicine of higher order, will not accept these ready-made substitutes for thought and observation, but will set himself to the problem of further developing diagnosis in the practice of medicine. The work of Graves and Stokes and Corrigan, the best elements of which saw the light before they were thirty, is a proof of how much can be accomplished by men who will try to see things for themselves without being prejudiced by the loose indefinite notions of the past, wrapped up though they may be in taking theory.

JOHN HUXHAM OF DEVONSHIRE (1692-1768).[1]

By William J. Vogeler, M. D.

John Huxham, who at the beginning of the 18th century enjoyed more than a local reputation both as a writer and a physician, is stated by some, apparently on insufficient evidence, to have been born the son of a butcher of Haberton. Though the reports of his parentage are at variance, it seems well ascertained that he was actually born at Totness, in the county of Devonshire, England, in or about the year 1692.

By most careful and industrious habits (traits that he handed down to his son), Huxham's father had acquired a small estate in the parish of Staverton, which became the property of this, his eldest son, who disposed of most of it

[1] Read before the Johns Hopkins Historical Club, March 13, 1905.

when he reached the age of 21, to defray the expenses of his medical education. According to Edward Meeres, whose excellent account of Huxham's early life I have carefully followed, as being the most accurate, he was left to the guardianship of a Mr. Thomas Edgeley, a dissenting minister of Totness; but in a short time he was removed to a private academy at Exeter. Selecting medicine for his profession Huxham proceeded to Leyden, and was entered on the Physic line in 1715, being then 23 years of age; how he had been occupied for some years before this is not known.

The University of Leyden was then at the zenith of its reputation and Boerhaave in his prime; his reputation was more than European, and students were flocking from all parts of the civilized world to hear him—in fact, so well known was he that any letter from distant parts of the world addressed to " Boerhaave, Europe," would reach its destination. Huxham, it is said, shared in the general admiration and enthusiasm, and most of his future excellence and success may be traced to his lifelong recollection of the example and exhortation of his celebrated teacher.

Although in later years his practice made him more than a wealthy man, at this time Huxham's pecuniary means were inadequate to complete the usual course of study for a medical degree at Leyden which extended over a period of three years, so after a time he left, going to Rheims, where he took the degree of Doctor of Medicine.

On his return to England, he first settled at Totness, but soon removed to Plymouth to take up his abode with Mr. Colker, one of the most influential of the Plymouth dissenters. He not long afterward married, with the view (Meeres tells us) of securing the additional advantage of family interest.

Huxham neglected no efforts which he thought might conduce to his professional advancement, and believing that the appearance of being extensively sought for and employed was one of the most certain means of actually becoming so, descended to expedients, which his better judgment could not have approved. He would, it is said, go to Chapel, order his servants to call him out in haste, when he was not really wanted, get upon his horse and ride

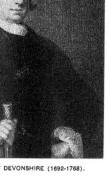

JOHN HUXHAM OF DEVONSHIRE (1692-1768).

furiously out of one gate of the town and in at the other. He affected great gravity, dignity of manner, and peculiarity of dress, and wore as his ordinary costume, a scarlet coat with ruffles at the wrist and a cocked hat—scarlet, I may observe, was sometimes, though rarely, worn by a few physicians of the 17th century, as was common with Mead and a few others. He carried a gold-headed cane, and in hot weather had his man-servant following him, carrying his gloves.

Notwithstanding these efforts, Dr. Huxham's progress for some years was slow, and it was not until the death of Dr. Seymour, who then engrossed the medical practice of Plymouth and vicinity, that Huxham made much advance. This period, however, was not lost; if he did not add greatly to his practical knowledge, he constantly increased his stock of medical learning. How deeply he was read in the great medical authorities of Greece and Rome, his published works testify.

Hippocrates, he regarded with the utmost veneration, and in his " Essay on Fevers " he speaks thus of his estimation of the medical writings of antiquity. " I will not take upon me to say a person cannot be a good physician without consulting that great oracle of physic (meaning Hippocrates) and reading the ancients, but this let me say, he will make a much better physician for so doing, and I believe few, if any, ever made any considerable figure in the profession who had not studied them."

Although, at Plymouth, he had several competitors of character and great respectability, none were able to compete with him in energy and assiduity, none in extent of professional knowledge or in the tact with which he applied it to the recognition and alleviation of disease. His aptitude in seizing on the really important points of a case, and his facility in the selection of means wherewith to meet them, are points in his professional character which, handed down by tradition, are abundantly exemplified in his writings. Though bred a Dissenter, he, after a time. conformed to the Established Church, a change which doubtless tended to his professional advancement.

Huxham was twice married, and in his second volume of " Observations," he gives a pathetic account of the death of his wife, who died in 1742, aged 40 years, of dropsy, after having been twice tapped. He had two daughters and one son, John Corham Huxham, who graduated from Exeter College, Oxford, became F. R. S. and edited several of his father's works. In 1739 Huxham was elected Fellow of the Royal Society, and an honorary fellow of the College of Physicians of Edinburgh in 1735; in that year also the Royal Society awarded him the Copley Medal for his observations upon Antimony. By a long and successful practice he accumulated a considerable fortune, died on August 11, 1768, aged 76, and was buried on the north side of St. Andrew's Church, Plymouth.

II. Writings.

Huxham early distinguished himself as a writer—his first contribution to the " Philosophical Transactions " having appeared in 1723.

I. In 1731 he wrote " Observations on Air and Epidemic Diseases " (Observationes de aere et Morbis epidemicis), of which a second edition appeared in 1752, and a third volume, after his death in 1770. These two volumes contain daily observations on the weather and the prevailing diseases, and the object was to ascertain the relation between atmospheric condition and disease, a subject probably suggested by the writings of Sydenham, who years before had studied along the same line.

II. In 1739 appeared the book on which the author's fame chiefly rests, his "Essay on Fevers" (etc.). In this he describes the course and treatment of simple fevers, nervous fevers (in which the modern typhoid is included, and in which, as Dr. Osler puts it, he had "taken notice of the very great difference there is between the putrid malignant and the slow nervous fever"). In this work also appear small-pox, pleurisy, inflammation of the lungs and bronchitis (then designated peri-pneumonia notha). This essay was received with the greatest applause and gained for him a European reputation. It reappeared in 1750, 1757, and 1764, and reprints of the last edition (4th) in '67, '69 and '82· The work was translated into Latin and into most of the European languages. The accuracy of his descriptions and the practical value of his distinctions have never been seriously questioned. Huxham's French biographer as late as 1822 asserts that it is infinitely superior to any treatise on fever which has been subsequently published in England, not even excepting that of Cullen; whilst the German historian of medicine, Sprengel, admits it to be the best that appeared during the first half of that century.

A high mark of distinction befell Dr. Huxham in consequence of this publication described by Polwhele as follows: "The Queen of Portugal being ill of a fever, and being reduced to the last extremity notwithstanding the efforts of a physician of the country, his majesty hearing of the eminence of a physician of the factory at Lisbon, sent for him and inquired if it were in his power to give any assistance? He replied in the affirmative, the disorder took a favorable turn and in a short time the Queen was restored to perfect health. The doctor being complimented by the King upon his ability and success, said he had no claim to the application, that the merit was due to Dr. Huxham, an eminent physician of Plymouth, whose tract on the management of fevers he had implicitly followed. Upon which the King immediately procured the treatment, had it translated into the Portuguese language and sent it richly bound to Huxham, as an acknowledgment of his debt of gratitude on the recovery of the Queen."

The chapters of the book are full of original observations and are written in a lucid style. The author, in fact, seems to derive most of his information from his own observations, and though he copies none, is clearly a follower of Sydenham, a student of sick men rather than of physician's books, but at the same time eager to recognize and apply remarks drawn from original observations whenever he meets them in the works of the ancients or of modern. He more than once quotes with praise the remarks of Hippocrates, that "whoever knows the nature of the disease knows the method of care," but he is at the same time careful and rational in his use of drugs and general method of treatment, and to show this it

might be well mentioned here that the compound tincture of cinchona bark, at present in the British Pharmacopœia, which also contains bitter orange peel, serpentary root, saffron and cochineal mixed with spirits, was devised by him, and was for some time called Huxham's tincture, the original formula still holding good!

III. In 1747 (30th September) he wrote from Plymouth to the "General Evening Post" on the occasion of the return after a voyage of only thirteen weeks, of Admiral Martin's fleet with 1200 men disabled by scurvy, recommending vegetable food as a preventive and urging a fuller supply of it to the Navy. These remarks with additions were reprinted as a book, entitled "De scurbuto," at Venice in 1776.

IV. In 1752 he published a short book, "De Morbo Colico Domnomiensi" (Devonshire colic). He describes very justly the symptoms of the terrible disease, which was formerly quite a scourge in the west of England, and tries hard to explain them, but without success. He was keen enough to observe that the colic was commonest when the fresh cider came, but it was reserved for Sir George Baker in 1767 (on the authority, however, of Huxham's previous description of the symptoms) to observe that the real cause was the lead used in the apple presses and dissolved by the cider, Devonshire colic being nothing more or less than lead poisoning, "causing obstruction of the bowels, paralysis and death."

V. Medical and chemical observations upon Antimony, originally published in the Phil. Trans by the Royal Society, subsequently appeared in book form, giving a full account of the method of preparing and prescribing antimonial medicines. A preparation of this important medicine was formerly vended under the name "Huxham's Antimonial Wine."

VI. In 1757 appeared a dissertation "On the malignant, ulcerous sore throat," which contains an excellent account of what is now called diphtheria and he deserves the credit of being the first to observe the palsy of the soft palate common to the disease, but failed to distinguish cases of diphtheria from those of scarlatina anginosa.

VII. In addition to the important works just mentioned, Dr. Huxham published several papers in the Philosophical Transactions, which, after his death, were collected into a very small volume by his son. They are:

I. Anomalous, epidemic small-pox.

II. Letter to Dr. Mortimer, Concerning polypi of the heart.

III. Letter to Dr. Mortimer, Case of Hannah Hitchcock.

IV. Letter to Thomas Slack, Venereal case.

V. Letter to Dr. ———, Emphysema.

His works have appeared in numerous editions, and his writings published as late as 1829 in Leipsic, under editorship of Hænel as part of the "Scriptorum classicorum de Praxi Medica nonullorum opera collecta."

CONCLUSION.

In conclusion it might be well to sum up the qualities of the man, good and bad. In spite of the fact that in the early days of his practice he may have descended to expedients which were not all the most lofty, still in his works his main object was simplicity, and he wrote so clearly that everyone could understand him, following the motto of his illustrious teacher, Boerhaave, " Simplex sigillum veri." With industry he combined perseverance and the courage to express his opinions boldly, when founded on what he honestly felt to be the truth, and if not the whole truth, nothing but the truth.

He had a patience that was inexhaustible, a devotion to labor unsurpassed, and a slow but sure and reliant comprehension. He combined with a stolid firmness a rare talent for penetration into hitherto obscure problems, and for casting aside objects which were coincident or accidental.

As Sir Benjamin Richardson has said of Sydenham, so it might be said of Huxham, " He wrote from what he saw in medicine and his sphere was the sick room. He had not many remedies, and what he had he used sparingly but he did his work with precision and therefore with confidence." The faculties of the man were well balanced and so strong that they would have been powerful in any age. It was fortunate for him and for us that they came into operation just at a time when they could be applied with the greatest advantage to their owner and to the world.

Finally what better can be said of any man than that he was a reader of Hippocrates, a scholar of Boerhaave, a follower of Sydenham, and a contemporary of William and John Hunter.

POPULAR MEDICINE IN THE EIGHTEENTH CENTURY.

By EBEN C. HILL.

As is apparent in the many semi-scientific articles which have appeared during late years, the present tendency in medicine is toward small doses frequently administered rather than the large " tablespoonfuls " which in olden times made the visit of the physician so dreaded by the defenseless patient. The heroic doses of Castor oil were not disguised and the ever ready " bitters " were everything that the name signifies. In the present day, however, the fear of injuring the patient by some ill-chosen remedy is so great that the doses are small and the maxim most frequently emphasized in all lectures on therapeutics is " do no harm even if you can do no good."

It is not the purpose of this sketch to elaborate the causes which have produced these marked changes, for they have been most thoroughly discussed, and it is sufficient to say that science now fully appreciates that no drug is specific in its action and that each decoction is a many-edged tool. However, in looking through some old medical books I found a small leather-bound volume written by John Wesley, M. A., during the middle part of the eighteenth century, a few extracts from which will give an interesting survey of the popular materia medica of his time. The work was intended more especially to aid the clergy in meeting the frequent demands of their flock in cases where physicians were not easily accessible. It met with greater popularity than was anticipated by its author, however, and the book passed through twenty or more editions.

The purpose of the work is characteristically set forth in the preface, and although throughout the treatise the good Wesley maintained a scientific attitude, yet it has many quaint touches of theology. I have taken a few extracts from this preface in order to show how logically he justifies himself for presenting the public with remedies to avoid the pain and suffering which he confesses are sent as a punishment for the sins of our forefathers:

When man came first out of the hands of the great Creator clothed in body as well as in soul, with immortality and incorruption, there was no place for physic, or the art of healing. As he knew no sin, so he knew no pain, no sickness, weakness or bodily disorder. The habitation wherein the angelic mind, the

Divinæ particula Auræ abode, though originally formed out of the dust of the earth, was liable to no decay. It had no seeds of corruption or dissolution within itself. And there was nothing without to injure it: Heaven and earth and all the hosts were mild, benign and friendly to human nature. The entire creation was at peace with man, so long as man was at peace with his Creator. So that well might " the morning stars sing together and all the sons of God shout for joy."

But since man rebelled against the Sovereign of the earth and heaven, how entirely is the scene changed! The incorruptible frame hath put on corruption, the immortal hath put on mortality. The seeds of weakness and pain, of sickness and death, are now lodged in our inmost substance; whence a thousand disorders spring without the aid of external violence. And how is the number of these increased by everything round about us! The heavens, the earth and all things contained therein, conspire to punish the rebels against their Creator. The sun and moon shed unwholesome influences from above; the earth exhales poisonous damps from beneath; the beasts of the field, the birds of the air, the fishes of the sea, are in a state of hostility: the air that surrounds us on every side is replete with the shafts of death: yea the food we eat, daily saps the foundation of the life which cannot be sustained without it. So has the Lord of all secured the execution of his decree—" Dust thou art and unto dust thou shalt return." ·

But can there nothing be found to lessen these inconveniences, which cannot be wholly removed? To soften the evils of life, and prevent in part the sickness and pain to which we are continually exposed? Without question there may. One grand preventive of pain and sickness of various kinds, seems intimated by the great Author of nature in the very sentence that entails death upon us: " In the sweat of thy face shalt thou eat bread till thou return to the ground." The power of exercise, both to preserve and restore health, is greater than can be well conceived; especially in those who add temperance thereto; who if they do not confine themselves altogether to eat either " bread or the herb of the field " (which God does not require them to do) yet steadily observe both the kind and measure of food which experience shows to be most friendly to health and strength.

'Tis probable, physic, as well as religion, was in the first ages chiefly traditional: every father delivering down to his sons, what he had himself in like manner received, concerning the manner of healing both outward hurts and the diseases incident to each climate, and the medicines which were of the greatest efficacy for the cure of each disorder. · · ·

* * * * * * * * * * *

As to the manner of using the medicines here set down I should advise: As soon as you know your distemper (which is very easy, unless in a complication of disorders, and then you would do well to apply to a physician that fears God): First. Use the first of the remedies for the disease which occurs in the ensuing collection (unless some other of them be easier to be had, and then it may do just as well). Secondly. After a competent time, if it takes no effect, use the second, the third, and so on. . . . . Third. Observe all the time the greatest exactness in your regimen or manner of living. . . . Drink only water if it agrees with your stomach; if not, good, clear, small beer. Above all, add to the rest (for it is not labor lost), that old unfashionable medicine—prayer.

Then follow some general rules of life, among which we find:

Malt liquors (except clear, small beer, or small ale, of a due age), are exceedingly hurtful to tender persons. Such persons ought constantly to go to bed about nine and rise at four or five. Those who read or write much should learn to do it standing; otherwise it will impair their health.

In the postscript to a more recent edition published in 1755 we find expressions of pleasurable surprise at the popularity of the book, and in mentioning the additions to this new edition there is an interesting apology for the omission of certain "strong drugs." He writes:

It is because they are not safe, but extremely dangerous, that I have omitted together with antimony the four Herculean medicines—opium, the bark, steel, and most of the preparations of quicksilver. Herculean indeed! Far too strong for common men to grapple with. How many fatal effects have these produced, even in the hands of no ordinary physicians? And whereas quicksilver, the fifth, is in its native form as innocent as bread or water: has not the art been discovered so to prepare it as to make it the most deadly of all poisons? . . . But they have not yet taught them how to wound at a distance; and honest men are under no necessity of touching them, or coming within their reach.

In uncommon or complicated diseases, where life is more immediately in danger, I again advise every man, without delay, to apply to a physician that fears God. . . . From one who does not, be his fame ever so great, I should expect a curse rather than a blessing.

After this excellent advice follows the "collection of receipts." Those remedies which the good Wesley from personal experience could recommend were marked with an asterisk. The diseases are arranged alphabetically, and I have selected a few at random. The cold bath and drinking water either sitting or standing seemed to be the most frequently prescribed, though being "electrified" seemed to have produced most satisfactory results. There is no explanation of just how this was to be done, but it was almost a panacea. Most of the remedies could be obtained in the woods, and it was not necessary to go to an apothecary. Indeed, there seemed to be as much dread of this compounder of drugs as of his godless colleague, the physician. For "perhaps he has not the drug prescribed by the physician and so puts in its place what will do as well. Perhaps he has it, but it is stale and perished; yet you would not have him throw it away. Indeed, he cannot afford to." So Wesley prescribes those remedies which are easily obtained, as is exemplified in the following treatments:

For Ague.—Go into a cold bath before the cold fit. Or, make six middling pills of cobwebs, take one a little before the cold fit; two a little before the next fit; the other three if need be a little before the third fit. This seldom fails. Or, eat a small lemon, rind and all.

To Cure Baldness.—Rub the part morning and evening with onions, till it is red, and rub it afterwards with honey.

The Colic.—Drink a pint of cold water. Tried. Or, drink a quart of warm water. Or apply outwardly a bag of hot oats. Parched peas eaten freely have had the most happy effects when all other means have failed.

The delightfully simple way in which consumption is disposed of would indicate that the many tuberculosis conferences held in recent years were useless, for the following simple remedies have cured "many deep consumptives."

One in a deep consumption was advised to drink nothing but water, and to eat nothing but water-gruel, without salt or sugar. In three months time he was perfectly well. Or, take a pint of skimmed milk, with half a pint of small beer. Boil in this whey about twenty ivy leaves, and two or three sprigs of hyssop. Drink over night half, the rest in the morning. Do this if needful for two months daily. This has cured in a desperate case. Tried.

Or, take a cow-heel from the tripe-house ready dressed, two quarts of new milk, two ounces of isinglass, a quarter of a pound of sugar candy, and a trace of ginger. Put all these in a pot, and set them in an oven after the bread is drawn. Let it continue there till the oven is near cold and let the patient live on this. I have known this to cure a deep consumption more than once.

Or, every morning cut up a little turf of fresh earth, and lying down, breath into the hole for a quarter of an hour. Tried. Mr. Masters, of Evesham, was so far gone that he could not stand alone. I advised him to lose six ounces of blood each day for a fortnight, if he lived so long, and then every other day, for the same time. In three months he was well.

Or, take for a quarter of an hour, morning and evening, the steam of white rosin and beeswax, boiling on a hot shovel. This has cured one who was in the third stage of consumption.

These read like the testimonials of some of the patent remedies, and it all goes to prove that people will recover even under the most "heroic" treatment. At the present time it would be considered homicide to prescribe blood letting in a desperate case of tuberculosis, yet we find Wesley vouching for a cure in a patient "far gone." Almost every disease has among the list of remedies cold baths, drinking water lying down or sitting up, or being "electrified." These, or at least all except the last, may not have been so unpleasant, but a large toasted cheese bound to a cut, or onions and honey in the ears, or the juice of rotten apples in the eyes were not so delightful. In cases of extreme madness we are advised to "set the patient under a great water fall, as long as his strength will bear it." Fortunately this treatment seems to have been abandoned, else it would be a most difficult matter to find suitable places for asylums. It certainly is unpleasant to think how nearly we lost Niagara as a pleasure resort, for undoubtedly the argument that the greater the fall the more speedy the cure would have resulted in lining the banks with sanitariums for the demented.

Before concluding the treatise Wesley makes a final plea for cold bathing which, besides curing every known and imaginable malady, "*prevents the growth of hereditary diseases*" such as blindness, deafness, and melancholy.

THE AMERICAN HOOKWORM (NECATOR AMERICANUS) IN GUAM AND CHINA.

BY CH. WARDELL STILES, PH. D.,

Chief of Division of Zoology, Hygienic Laboratory, U. S. Public Health and Marine Hospital Service.

In 1902, I described the common hookworm of this country under the specific name *americanus*, because it was so distinct from the species reported for other parts of the world.

Since then, Looss has shown that earlier observers had specimens of this worm mixed in with their material of *Agchylostoma duodenale*, but that they had failed to recognize that they were dealing with more than one form. He has also found the American species in Africa, while Siccardi has reported the same worm for Italy. I have found the American form in soldiers who had returned from the Philippines, but as it was not excluded that the men had become infected in the United States, it seemed hazardous to conclude that *Necator americanus* should be considered a Philippine worm also. Recently, specimens of hookworms have been received at this laboratory taken by Dr. O. T. Logan, an enthusiastic collector, in Changteh, Hunan, China (U. S. P. H. & M. H. S., No. 9906); specimens (U. S. P. H. & M. H. S., No. 9915) have also been received from Assistant Surgeon O. J. Mink, U. S. Navy, collected from a native child in the Island of Guam. In both of these sendings, the worms seem to agree, both generically and specifically, with *Necator americanus.*

It will thus be seen that the American hookworm has a much more extensive geographic distribution than was at first assumed. This fact has no influence, however, upon the specific name *americanus*, for America still remains the type locality of the species from a nomenclatural point of view, although the interpretation that the species is originally of American origin is naturally weakened by the more recent findings.

SAHLI'S DESMOID REACTION IN GASTRIC DIAGNOSIS.

BY THOMAS R. BOGGS, B. SC., M. D.,

Associate in Medicine. The Johns Hopkins University; Assistant Resident Physician, The Johns Hopkins Hospital.

(From the Clinical Laboratory of the Johns Hopkins Hospital and University.)

In 1905 Sahli (1) published a new method for testing gastric function without using the stomach tube.

This method is based on the assumption that catgut in the raw state is soluble in the peptic secretions of the stomach but entirely indigestible in the pancreatic juices. Ad. Schmidt (2).

To carry out the test one encloses a pill (of methylene blue 0.05 gram or iodoform 0.1 gram or both together with sufficient ext. glycyrrhizæ to make a pill not over 3 or 4 mm. diameter) in a rubber sack made by twisting the pill in the center of a square piece of thin rubber dam and tying the twisted neck with three turns of number 00 raw catgut previously soaked in cold water until soft, care being taken that the knots are both on the same side of the bag. The rubber is then trimmed away carefully so that only a little free edge of about 3 mm. remains beyond the ligature. It is essential to see that the cut edges of the rubber do not cohere, that the complete pill sinks instantly in water and is watertight.

This " desmoid pill " is given with or just after the midday meal, and the urine collected at periods of 5, 7, and 18-20 hours later is examined for methylene blue or iodine or both. The methylene blue is recognized by the greenish-blue color imparted to the urine or in absence of color, the urine is boiled with ⅓ volume of glacial acetic acid when a greenish-blue color appears if the chromogen of methylene blue is present. The chromogen alone is seldom found; most cases without color are due to the fact that the gut has not dissolved.

Iodine is recognized by strongly acidifying the urine with pure nitric or sulphuric acid and shaking out with a little chloroform, when the rose color is readily detected.

It may be tested also in the saliva with starch paper or acid.

If the methylene blue or iodine be found within the 18-20 hours after the ingestion of the pill the test is called positive, otherwise negative. .

The advantages claimed for the test are that it is simple in application, that it causes the patient no distress, and more important yet, that, as it is given with the principal meal, it is subjected to the activities of the gastric functions when they are stimulated to do their utmost.

For, in accordance with Moritz' (3) observation, the pill being relatively heavy will remain in the stomach the maximum length of time and so test fully the activity of the gastric juice.

The desmoid will, therefore, often give a positive result when with the test breakfast we get an absence of free hydrochloric acid. This is, as Sahli pointed out, a matter of considerable diagnostic importance in distinguishing cases with true achylia, carcinoma, or pernicious anæmia from less serious disorders in which the stimulus of the Ewald breakfast is insufficient to cause an excess of hydrochloric acid.

In the recent literature several extended reports have appeared which substantiate to a large extent Sahli's claims for his test. Notably those of Eichler (4), Kuhn (5), and Kaliski (6).

In this clinic, with the kind permission of Dr. Barker, I have examined some 34 cases in which there was impairment of the gastric function, in addition to 12 normal persons. These latter were all positive and are not included in the table. The pathological cases are arranged below in tabular form. In each instance, with two exceptions in which it was impossible to pass the stomach tube, the result of the test was compared with the findings of the Ewald breakfast or Fischer's meal or both.

As will be seen in the table of the carcinoma cases, all but one gave a negative test. This patient was an ignorant negro man who may have bitten the capsule or the tying may have been insecure. It was unfortunately impossible to repeat the test. At operation a large pyloric carcinoma was found involving also the lesser curvature.

With the same uniformity all of the seven cases of pernicious anæmia gave negative tests. Of these two had no gastric analysis, Case XXVIII being too ill and Case XXXII refusing to take the tube. It is interesting to note that this patient, while steadily improving as to blood count, gave constantly a negative desmoid test with persistent achlorhydria. In contrast, Case XXXIII with a secondary anæmia of long duration and of even lower grade (R. B. C. not over 1,500,000 in past three years) gave constantly a positive test.

Cases VIII and XXXIV, general carcinomatosis and carci-

Case Number.	Name.	Age.	Sex.	Race.	Diagnosis.	Free HCl.	Total acidity.	Lactic acid.	Desmoid reaction	Remarks.
I	C. T. T.	64	M.	Bl.	Carcinoma Ventriculi.	0	36	0	Neg.	Fischer meal.
II	M. F.	59	F.	W.	" "	0	2.5	+	Neg.	
III	J. K.	43	M.	W.	" "	0	24	+ +	Neg.	
IV	G. W. E.	66	M.	W.	" "	0	4	0	Neg.	
V	C. W.	48	M.	Bl.	" "	0	4	+	Pos.	
VI	M. M.	47	M.	W.	" "	0	51.	0	Neg.	Fischer meal.
VII	H. C. S.	57	M.	W.	" "	0	2	+	Neg.	
VIII	F. L.	54	M.	W.	General carcinomatosis.	0	5.	+	Neg.	
IX	L. O.	45	M.	W.	Chronic gastritis I. Carcinoma ventric (?) Lues secondaria.	0	38	0	Neg.	Marked alcoholism. Free HCl constantly O. Total acidity, 14-38.
X	M. J.	67	F.	W.	Cholelithiasis I. Carcinoma ventric (?)	6	30	0	Pos.	
XI	M. F.	56	F.	W.	Cholelithiasis I. Achlorhydria.	0	8	0	Neg.	Fischer meal. Desmoid positive after attack. Persistent achlorhydria with Ewald breakfast.
XII	W. M.	46	M.	W.	Chronic gastritis.	.0	4	0	Pos.	Marked alcoholism, much mucus.
XIII	J. B. S.	37	M.	W.	Achylia gastrica (?) Tuberculous peritonitis.	0	5	0	Pos.	
XIV	A. H.	41	M.	W.	Chronic enteritis.	0	25	0	Pos.	
XV	J. A. N.	40	M.	Bl.	Gastric ulcer (?)	11	28	0	Pos.	Fischer meal. Doubtful case; strong possibility of cancer.
XVI	H. T. W.	28	M.	Bl.	Gastric ulcer.	22	43	0	Pos.	
XVII	A. E.	21	F.	Bl.	Gastralgia I. Gastric ulcer (?)	0	33	0	Pos.	Pain. Varying acidity. Blood (?)
XVIII	H. M.	35	F.	W.	Gastric tetany.	0	8	0	Neg.	Persistent achlorhydria with Ewald test breakfast. Typical tetany attacks.
XIX	M. E. G.	34	F.	W.	Benign stricture of pylorus.	0	21	0	Pos.	Operation.
XX	C. L.	35	M.	W.	" " " "	0	21	0	Neg.	Pt. getting no food by mouth. Operation.
XXI	J. M.	48	M.	W.	Primary splenomegaly.	0	8	0	Pos.	Second desmoid Neg. day after severe hemorrhage pt. on low diet.
XXII	W. D.	52	M.	W.	Cirrhosis of liver.	0	8	0	Pos.	Possibility of early carcinoma.
XXIII	A. G.	37	M.	W.	Cirrhosis of liver. Psoriasis.	0	2	0	Pos.	Later tests showed Free HCl 7-21.
XXIV	W. H. F.	44	M.	W.	Myxœdema.	0	16	0	Pos.	Marked azotorrhœa.
XXV	S. vT. C.	36	M.	W.	Neurasthenia I. Achlorhydria.	0	5	0	Neg.	Nervous dyspepsia 10 years. Desmoid positive with administration of HCl.
XXVI	F. I.	43	M.	W.	Pernicious anæmia.	0	10	0	Neg.	
XXVII	H. E. J.	47	F.	W.	" "	0	3	0	Neg.	
XXVIII	H. H.	30	M.	W.	" "	—	—	—	Neg.	No gastric contents obtained. Stomach negative at autopsy.
XXIX	L. B.	57	M.	W.	" "	0	0.2	0	Neg.	
XXX	G. L.	54	M.	W.	" "	0	9.	0	Neg.	
XXXI	C. B.	26	M.	W.	" "	0	1	0	Neg.	
XXXII	W. B. O.	31	M.	W.	" "	—	—	—	Neg.	No analysis possible. Desmoid still negative after 6 weeks.
XXXIII	F. E. C.	28	M.	W.	Hæmoglobinuria secondary anæmia; pulmonary tuberculosis.	15	40	0	Pos.	Long continued intermittent hæmoglobinuria. R.B.C. 824,000. Hb. 17%. Blood count not over 1,500,000 in 3 years.
XXXIV	F. K.	49	M.	W.	Carcinoma of pancreas.	0	20	0	Neg.	Marked azotorrhœa.

NOTE—Free HCl by Dimethylamidoazobenzol. Total acidity by phenolpthalein. Lactic acid by Uffelmann's test on the ether extract. Fischer's meal: Ewald breakfast plus ¼ lb. finely chopped lean beef lightly broiled and seasoned. Removed after three hours.

noma of pancreas, respectively, also gave negative tests, and absence of free hydrochloric acid.

Two cases of inoperable carcinoma of uterus with cachexia and low free hydrochloric acid gave positive tests. They are not included in the table.

Other interesting negative tests were obtained in Case IX, chronic alcoholic gastritis with secondary lues, who was strongly suspected of early carcinoma, but refused exploratory laparotomy. This case contrasted well with XII, who gave a positive test with his initial low acidity and improved under treatment until his free HCl was normal, while Case IX maintained a constant achlorhydria.

Case XI showed persistent achlorhydria with all $_t$e$_{st}$ meals and gave a negative desmoid during the gallstone attack, with a positive test and increased total acidity in the interval.

Case XVIII, gastric tetany with persistent achlorhydria, gave a negative desmoid.

The negative result in Case XX is reasonably attributable to the fact that the patient was being fed per rectum only and there was thus no adequate stimulus to gastric secretion.

Case XXV, neurasthenia with achlorhydria, gave a negative test and later a positive desmoid while taking hydrochloric acid.

The positive outcome in the hepatic cases with low acidity is interesting. Cases XXI to XXIII.

A consideration of the above data seems to bear out Sahli's contention that the desmoid pill does show the ability of the stomach under the best conditions. Particularly is this true with regard to the presence of free HCl. In fact I feel inclined to agree with Eichler and Kuhn that its principal value is as a test for free HCl.

It cannot replace the test meal, but is a useful adjunct to this most essential measure.

Kaliski, I think, goes entirely too far in his deductions as to the nature and severity of the involvement, from the time of appearance and the intensity of the color.

Einhorn's (7) unfavorable opinion is open to legitimate criticism in that his observations were very limited and his glass bead test for the digestibility of gut in the intestinal juices is not proved accurate. Fat splitting ferments in the stomach and mechanical freeing of the gut must be taken into consideration.

I have exposed the well-soaked raw gut in solutions of the most active artificial pancreatic juice for periods of 15 days in the thermostat at 37° C. without the least damage to the gut. While a few hours in ordinary pepsin-HCl digesting fluid will dissolve it completely. Solution begun in pepsin-HCl mixture seems quickly checked in pancreatic fluid.

The pills found in the stools of the negative cases showed no evidence of digestion, yet in most cases the intestinal digestion of foods, including meats, was good. This fact speaks strongly for the specificity of the test for gastric digestion.

LITERATURE.

1. Sahli: Corresp. Bl. f. Schweiz, Aertzte, 1905, S. 241 and 286.

2. Ad. Schmidt: Deutsche Med. Woch., 1899, S. 811.

3. Moritz: Münch. Med. Woch., 1895, XLII, S. 1143.

4. Eichler: Berl. Klin. Woch., 1905, XLII, S. 1493.

5. Kuhn: Münch. Med. Woch., 1905, LII, S. 2412.

6. Kaliski: Deutsche Med. Woch., 1906, S. 185.

7. Einhorn: Journ. Am. Med. Assn., 1906, XLVI, p. 1434.

NOTES ON NEW BOOKS.

Counsels and Ideals from the Writings of William Osler. (*Boston and New York: Houghton, Mifflin & Company, 1905.*)

In this compilation, so judiciously made by Dr. Camac, one is struck by an aptness of quotation, a felicity of statement, a freshness of treatment, an elevation of thought, and a clearness of vision which are stimulating and illuminating. The extent and variety of the author's reading, his charity, his breadth of view, his high ideals, and the eminently human quality of his utterances all commend them to lovers of good literature, whether physicians or laymen. After once testing their exactness, the reader is impelled to go back to the original essays, to follow once more the author's guidance to rich fields of living thought. The extracts are happily chosen and the selection has been made by an appreciative friend.

Liverpool School of Tropical Medicine. Memoir XVI. Trypanosomes, Trypanosomiasis, and Sleeping Sickness: Pathology and Treatment. By H. WOLFERSTAN THOMAS and ANTON BREINL. (*London: Williams & Norgate, Publishers, 1905.*)

In connection with the studies of Dutton and Todd on Sleeping Sickness in the Congo Free State, Thomas and Breinl carried on the laboratory work at Liverpool, and have published a very exhaustive report of endless observations which were carried out on particularly rich animal material.

They first deal with the description of seven cases of sleeping sickness which were sent to England from the Congo Free State. Three of these were "sleeping sickness" and the other four "trypanosome fever." The periodicity of the presence of the parasites in the peripheral blood was very well shown in these cases, though the rises of temperature were not necessarily coincident with the increase of the number of parasites in the peripheral blood. This shows the difficulty in making a diagnosis by the examination of peripheral blood unless the examinations are made daily and for a long time. The second part of their report deals with inoculation experiments with *Trypanosoma Gambiense* upon baboons, monkeys, horses, donkeys, cows, sheep, goats, dogs, cats, rabbits, and guinea-pigs. They found that the *Trypanosoma Gambiense* was identical in animal reaction and morphology with trypanosomes found in the cerebro-spinal fluid in cases of sleeping sickness from Uganda and the Congo Free State as well as with the blood of trypanosome fever cases from the Congo Free State, and in Europeans affected in the Congo. They consider that there is no acquired immunity against infection, nor is there any transmission of the immunity to the offspring. In many experimental animals the infection is of a very mild character, but the blood is still infective a year after the orignal inoculation. They further found that in the case of the horse the parasites are still seen, and the blood is still infective after a lapse of 28 months. They found no attenuation in the passing of a strain from a susceptible to a resisting animal, but that the parasites in an animal had apparently increased at times their virulency. In all their cases both in man and beast the periodicity of the parasite is a very prominent feature, and they found further that there was no change in the morphological characters of the trypanosome after being passed through many hundreds of animals during a period of three years. They further deal with different forms of trypanosome strains especially that in the Gambian horse disease, that of dourine and mal de caderas as well as surra. These authors did not find as good results from the use of gland puncture as did Dutton and Todd, nor were they frequently able to find the blood in the exudate of blisters. They followed Novy and McNeal in attempting to cultivate the trypanosomes, especially the Gambian form and the "Trypanosoma dimorphon" horse disease. They were able to keep the former alive for 68 days, but after the 17th day they found it no longer capable of infecting a · susceptible animal; changing the media in many ways did not bring them any nearer success, although they speak hopefully of their belief in the ultimate success of this procedure. In the tubes they found that Trypanosoma equinum did seem to actually grow.

A very large number of experiments were made with regard to the treatment of trypanosome infection. They found that arsenic was the only drug which seemed to exert any action other than transient. The best results were obtained with the largest amounts of arsenic, and they consider that the treatment ought to be long continued, even after the apparent necessity therefor has disappeared. The so-called "trypaned" was of some use, and they think that the combination of arsenic and trypanred is even better; but the toxicity of arsenic is a drawback to its employment. The authors give very full accounts of post-mortem examinations, with the macroscopic and microscopic changes in four human cases as well as many animals.

Ibid. Gland Puncture, in Trypanosomiasis. By the late J. E. DUTTON and J. L. TODD.

These authors found that puncture of the enlarged glands was by far the most satisfactory method of finding the trypanosomes. The gland is punctured with a needle, the material is diluted to prevent coagulation and centrifugalised, and they conclude that the examination of the fluid of the glands though not infallible is a very efficient method of detecting the parasite.

Liverpool School of Tropical Medicine. Memoir XVII. The Nature of Human Tick-Fever in the Western Part of the Congo Free State. By the late J. E. DUTTON and J. L. TODD. (London: Williams & Norgate, Publishers, 1905.)

Dutton and Todd cabled to Liverpool in November, 1904, that they had discovered that a spirochaete was the pathogenic agent of the human tick-fever, and that they had been able to infect monkeys through the bites of ticks. This was at the very time at which Ross and Milne published their notes on tick-fever in the British Medical Journal, so that the priority really belongs to the latter named, although Dutton and Todd made their discovery independently. About the time of this discovery both observers fell ill with recurrent fever and in February the lamented death of Dr. Dutton occurred. Todd has published the results of their joint work in the Congo. Shortly after entering the Free State they were able to collect ticks, and they had an autopsy upon a fatal case of tick-fever. From transmission experiments they were able to show that tick-fever is a relapsing fever produced by a spirochaete, probably identical with *Spirochaete Obermeieri*,

and that this organism can be transmitted by the bite of the tick. Further, in one experiment they transmitted the spirillum by the bites of young ticks hatched in the laboratory from eggs laid by infected parents. They report on the history of human tick-fever in the Oriental Province of the Congo Free State, and add their clinical observations of a number of cases, including their own. Centrifugalisation of the blood is not very useful in demonstrating the organism and they succeeded best in using thick dehæmoglobinised blood films stained with weak carbol-fuchsin, or a modified Romanowski method. They give a considerable amount of information upon the distribution of the human tick in the Free State and conclude that tick-fever is clinically identical with a relapsing fever and is caused by a spirochaete, probably Obermeieri, and is transmitted from animal to animal by the tick (Ornithodorus). They consider that the transmission is not merely mechanical but that probably a developmental process is carried on in the tick and that a considerable degree of immunity can be acquired to the spirochaete.

Beobachtungen über Riesenzellen. Von DR. VICTOR BABES, University of Bucarest. (*Stuttgart: Verlag von Edwin Nägele, 1905.*)

In this monograph of 128 pages the author considers at length the formation of giant cells in various pathological processes, in particular in chronic productive inflammations, in the infectious granulomata, and in neoplasms, emphasizing the genesis of the cells rather than the finer details of structure. He gives the results of the study of an extensive material and his interpretation of the same with a generous consideration of the literature of the subject. In brief, it may be said that Babes concludes that giant cells may be formed from a great variety of cells; that they are formed not by fusion of cells, but by the process of nuclear division and by budding of cells—processes which are hindered by some injurious agent from their normal completion. In the inflammatory processes, he is unable to convince himself that the mononuclear leucocytes play a part in the formation of the giant cells, but derives them in great part if not entirely from vascular, endothelial, sprouts. A similar origin is attributed to the tubercle giant cell. The cells are not developed for the purpose of phagocytosis, but are somewhat abortive attempts at regeneration. The article is accompanied by some excellent plates and by a good bibliography.

A Text-Book of Clinical Diagnosis by Laboratory Methods. By L. NAPOLEON BOSTON, A. M., M. D. (*Philadelphia: W. B. Saunders & Company, 1904.*)

This text-book covers the clinical examination of the blood, urine, gastric contents, feces, sputum, buccal secretion, nasal secretion, discharges from the ear and eye, secretion of the genital organs, transudates, exudates, cerebro-spinal and synovial fluids, diseases of the skin, and milk. It is illustrated with 320 illustrations, many of them in colors. The directions seem to suppose no previous knowledge of microscopy or chemistry, even the pictures of a glass slide and cover glass are given; the "simple spelling" of technical terms is used. The publishers have done their part fairly well. The illustrations are numerous enough, cover the ground fairly well, but many could be properly dispensed with. The same may be said of the text, for many directions are not complimentary to the intelligence of an ordinary medical student. A little learning is a dangerous thing, and this applies with especial force to the subjects with which this book deals. The student should not be allowed to begin the study of general biology and chemistry with the study of clinical microscopy and clinical chemistry, and if he tries to do so the simplest tests should be taught, not the hard ones. Again, the latter do not admit of "boiling down" for the expert, much less for the beginner. The sufficiently prepared student does not need to be told "to grasp the test-tube between the thumb and index finger." the well trained one would certainly like to discuss certain steps in the methods, realizing that they could not be followed according to any fixed directions, of "one, two, three, etc.," and that even to slightly acidify some solutions isn't nearly as easy as it sounds. The author has condensed methods to the danger point. He does not discuss the steps to render them intelligible. The clinical results are also condensed dry. The author uses the first personal pronoun singular with startling frequency.

Clinical Methods, A Guide to the Practical Study of Medicine. By ROBERT HUTCHISON, M. D., F. R. C. P., and HARRY RAINY, M. A., F. R. C. P. Ed., F. R. S. E. Third edition. *(Chicago, 1905.)*

This book has evidently been popular, since its first and second editions were each reprinted three times. It is not a treatise on medical diagnosis, but a compendium of methods which should be applied in the diagnosis of any given case; methods of physical diagnosis, of clinical microscopy and chemistry, of parasitology, of the diagnosis of nervous disorders, of the diseases of the spinal nerves, of diseases of children, and of clinical bacteriology. And yet the volume is pocket size, of 634 pages. It is quite profusely illustrated. Here we have a vast amount of information well "boiled down " to very small volume. Undoubtedly such books have a very great value, as digests of larger works and handy laboratory guides, but that the student could from these alone get a very valuable knowledge of a subject we very much doubt.

Medical Diagnosis. Special Diagnosis of Internal Medicine. A Handbook for Physicians and Students. By DR. WILHELM V. LEUBE. Authorized translation from the sixth German edition, edited, with annotations, by JULIUS L. SALINGER, M. D. *(D. Appleton & Company, 1904.)*

The translation of this book places at the disposal of those who do not read German readily one of the most important works on the diagnosis of medical diseases. This has long been the standard book in Germany, and an invaluable aid to many American students. Why it should not have been translated some time ago it is difficult to understand.

The translating has evidently been very carefully done, perhaps too carefully, for the long involved English sentences do not read nearly as easily as do the German, of which they are a literal translation. Sentences of eight or more clauses seldom read smoothly and some require study to gain their meaning. The publishers have done their work well. The use of italics for words and long sentences has been carried to an extreme. The figures and cuts are fair.

Indigestion. The Diagnosis and Treatment of the Functional Derangements of the Stomach with an Appendix on the Preparation of Food by Cooking, with Especial Reference to its Use in the Treatment of Affections of the Stomach. By GEORGE HERSCHELL, M. D., Lond. Third Edition, Entirely Rewritten. *(Chicago: W. T. Keener & Co., 90 Wabash Avenue. London: Henry J. Glaisher, 57 Wigmore Street, Cavendish Square, W., 1905.)*

When one recognizes the fact that a very large percentage of patients in private practice seek medical advice for some disorder of digestion, a practical book on this subject such as the present one is invaluable to the practitioner. This, the third edition of the work, is a material improvement on the last one. The subject matter is simply and clearly presented and a successful effort seems to have been made to avoid making a mystery of gastric disorders and gastric chemistry which too often has been the case in works treating on this subject.

The volume opens with a concise account of the normal processes of gastric and intestinal digestion. The causes, symptoms, chemistry, and treatment of the various forms of indigestion due to disturbances of the gastric secretion are then taken up. The author deals more especially with the various types of gastric neurasthenia.

Lack of knowledge of the proper way of cooking food in the domestic household of the present day is one of the most fruitful causes of indigestion. One of the great deficiencies in the teaching in our medical schools of to-day is the almost entire absence of instruction in dietetics and in the manner in which food should be properly cooked. When the student becomes a practitioner he is utterly incapable of instructing his patients as to how their food should be cooked or how some of the more simple articles of diet for the sick-room should be prepared. Consequently, a section by Herschell on the preparation of food with especial reference to its use in the treatment of affections of the stomach will be found most valuable to the practitioner.

Clinical Treatises on the Pathology and Therapy of Disorders of Metabolism and Nutrition. By CARL VON NOORDEN, Physician-in-Chief to the City Hospital, Frankfurt A. M. Authorized American Translation. Edited by BOARDMAN REED, M. D. Translated by FLORENCE BUCHANON, D. SC. and I. WALKER HALL, M. D. Part VII. Diabetes Mellitus. Its Pathological Chemistry and Treatment. Lectures delivered in the University and Bellevue Hospital Medical College. New York Herter Lectureship Foundation. *(New York: E. B. Treat & Co., 1905.)*

As von Noorden's name has been so closely associated with, and he has so long been considered an authority on diabetes mellitus, the profession receives with keen interest any fresh contribution to the subject from this writer. The present series of lectures deals mainly with the disturbances of metabolism in diabetes, and with the therapeutics of the disease based on its pathological chemistry. The subject matter and its general arrangement bear a striking similarity to the author's treatment of the same part of the subject in his article in Volume II, of The Twentieth Century Practice of Medicine. It has been brought more up to date, however, by the inclusion of the results of recent researches by the author himself and by others. Although some of the views held by von Noorden have not received general acceptance, he has the faculty of presenting the most difficult and most important part of the disease—its pathological chemistry—in a manner in which the practitioner can obtain an intelligent grasp of it.

Only a few points can be touched on in this review. Von Noorden states that Cohnheim's recent theory, that the glucose of the blood is normally disposed of by the interaction of ferment-like bodies produced by the muscles and pancreas, is quite erroneous and that the disappearance of the glucose in his experiments was due to the effect of bacterial contamination. This was shown by the work of Embden and Claus carried out in the author's laboratory. Von Noorden has his own theory to account for the appearance of diabetes in certain lesions of the pancreas. He believes that the pancreas supplies to the blood a substance which has something to do either with the building up or with the breaking down of glycogen. This might be a ferment which favors the act of polymerisation in the formation of glycogen, or it might be an antiferment which prevents too rapid destruction of glycogen. In both cases poverty of glycogen in the organs and hyperglycæmia would be the inevitable consequence and the cardinal symptoms of diabetes would naturally follow. The author thinks that, as yet, it is not clearly established that the islands of Langerhans are essentially different from the rest of the pancreatic gland. It is claimed by some that they are only early stages of the ordinary secreting gland acini. He holds that further evidence is necessary to prove that lesions of the glands of Langerhans and diabetes bear the relationship to each other of cause and effect.

Although for many years it was held that the acetone bodies were derived from proteid alone, the view at first cautiously advanced by Geelmuyden, Magnus, Levy, and Schwartz that they are really derived largely from fat is the one now generally accepted and the one supported by the author.

There is a very practical section on the therapeutics of diabetes. It will serve as a good guide-to the practitioner in outlining the treatment in each individual case, rather than blindly following the same routine in all cases of the disease. The volume concludes with a series of food tables and tables of equivalents giving the percentages of proteid, fat, and carbohydrates in the more important articles of diet.

On Carbohydrate Metabolism, with an Appendix on the Assimilation of Carbohydrate into Proteid and Fat, Followed by the Fundamental Principles, and the Treatment of Diabetes Diabetically Discussed. By F. W. PAVY, M. D., L. L. D., F. R. S. (London: J. & A. Churchill, 7 Great Marlborough Street, 1906. Philadelphia: P. Blakiston's Son & Co.)

This volume of 138 pages gives Pavy's latest conception regarding the warehousing of carbohydrates in health and in diabetes. Although nearly all modern physiologists support the theory of the glycogenic function of the liver first advanced by Claude Bernard, Pavy for years has claimed that this theory is untenable. In this view he stands almost alone. As his work on diabetes and carbohydrate metabolism has been of so high a character and has always commanded the attention of the best physiologists and physiological chemists, we are forced to treat his opinions with the greatest respect. The fact that the recent work of Cohnheim, which at the time seemed to clearly solve the method in which the glucose of the system is disposed of, having been met with considerable opposition in certain quarters, together with the very diverse views advanced regarding the physiology of the carbohydrates, is ample evidence that the question is far from being a solved one. There is, therefore, all the more reason why Pavy's views, although differing markedly from those usually held, should be treated with consideration.

According to the glycogenic theory, the carbohydrates of the food are converted through processes of digestion chiefly into glucose, which passes by way of the portal vessels to the liver where it is converted by the liver cells into glycogen. The glycogen remains stored up in the liver until the system requires carbohydrates, when it is reconverted into glucose which is conveyed to the tissues by the general circulation.

Pavy, as stated, refutes the glycogenic theory as generally accepted. He believes that the lymphocytes play a most important part in the assimilation of the carbohydrates. He holds that the glucose, resulting from the alimentary digestion of carbohydrate food, enters into combination with the growing bioplasm of the lymphocytes of the intestinal villi, which contain lymphocytes in enormous numbers. These lymphocytes with their " locked up " glucose then reach the general circulation by way of the lacteals rather than by passing through the walls of the portal capillaries in the villi. Pavy thinks that if glucose reached the general circulation in a free form it would be filtered off by the kidneys at once, and that it is only by being " locked up " in the lymphocytes in the manner stated that this is prevented. After reaching the tissues incorporated in the lymphocytes the glucose is yielded off to them for combustion. The writer admits that when carbohydrates are taken in excess some of the glucose escapes the treatment above noted. This portion of the glucose passes by way of the portal capillaries to the liver where it is transformed into glycogen by the protoplasm of the liver cells and there stored up.

This glycogen is later retransformed into glucose. Pavy holds that the glucose is not transported to the tissues for consumption in the free state; otherwise it would filter through the kidneys and produce glycosuria. He claims that the glucose is taken on as a side chain by a proteid constituent of the blood and transported in this combined form to the tissues, where it is broken up for subjection to utilization.

The writer's theory is an interesting one but is quite contrary to the general teaching at the present day. Whether his view be the correct one or not will be eventually shown by the subsequent work of other competent physiologists and physiological chemists. The sections on the assimilation of carbohydrates into fats and proteids and on the treatment of diabetes contain many points of practical interest.

Uric Acid. The Chemistry, Physiology, and Pathology of Uric Acid and the Physiologically Important Purin Bodies, with a Discussion of Metabolism in Gout. By FRANCIS H. McCRUDDEN. (New York: Paul B. Hoeber, 69 East 59th Street.)

In 1901 McCrudden began a study of the metabolism in certain bone diseases, rheumatoid arthritis, osteo-arthritis, osteitis deformans, etc., under the direction of Doctors Goldthwait, Painter, and Osgood, of Boston, who have added much to our knowledge of these diseases, especially of rheumatoid arthritis, preferably termed arthritis deformans, through their surgical treatment of these affections. It soon became apparent to the author that a thorough appreciation of our present knowledge concerning the chemistry of the purin bodies, uric acid and the so-called xanthin bases, and their relationship to the various joint affections, was indispensable. Accordingly, he reviewed and compiled the enormous mass of literature that has appeared up to August, 1905, on the chemistry of the purins and on the relationship of these bodies to gout. As this material has never been completely brought together and published in English for ready reference, McCrudden decided to issue the present monograph of 318 pages, giving his exhaustive analysis of the literature. The material is systematically arranged and data on any desired point is easily accessible. The volume is invaluable to anyone interested in the metabolism of gout and of allied joint affections.

The chemical investigations of the last few years have added much to our knowledge of the source and mode of formation of uric acid. Following the classification of Burian and Schur, we now speak of uric acid as being either exogenous or endogenous in origin. The exogenous uric acid is that derived from the ingested food, whilst the endogenous uric acid is an acid product of cellular metabolism in the body. So far as we are aware the uric acid in both instances is derived practically entirely from the nucleo-proteids, either of the food or of the body. Burian has recently shown, however, that a large proportion of the endogenous uric acid is derived from the hypoxanthin of the muscles which results from muscular activity. This hypoxanthin undoubtedly is in part derived from the nuclei of the muscle cells. A feature that must be emphasized is that uric acid is derived almost alone from the nucleo-proteids and not from the simple proteids such as egg albumen.

It is only within the last three years that we have learned that specific ferments play a most important part in the transformation of the nucleic acid, which is split off from the nucleo-proteids, into uric acid. This knowledge has been acquired chiefly through the investigations of Burian, Walter Jones, and Schittenhelm. The following quotation from McCrudden gives concisely our present knowledge on this point. " The action of spleen, liver, and other organs in the transformation of purin bases to uric acid has been much studied recently. It will be remembered that in the study of the occurrence of purin bases in the tissues, we saw that different purin bases were obtained in fresh organs from those obtained in organs which had undergone self-digestion. The results of Levene, who studied this subject, show that the amino purins change to the oxypurins in the process of autolysis. According to Jones, there is an enzyme in thymus which can decompose the nucleoproteid and give the free amino purins, and another enzyme which changes the amino purins to the oxypurins. In the pancreas there is an enzyme which changes the guanin to xanthin. In the spleen there is an enzyme which changes adenin to hypoxanthin. According to Jones, "guanase," the ferment which changes guanin in xanthin, is a different body from "adenase," which changes adenin to hypoxanthin, for in the liver the adenin changes to hypoxanthin, but the guanin does not change to xanthin. Schenck agrees with Jones that the guanase and adenase are different ferments, but he differed from Jones in finding an adenase but not guanase in pancreas. The view of Schittenhelm seems more probable. According to this author, there is one ferment which splits the purin bases from nucleic acid; another which changes the amino purins to the oxypurins, and a third which oxidizes hypoxanthin and xanthin to uric acid. These ferments are widely distributed in the various organs, liver, spleen, lungs, and muscle. Schittenhelm isolated both the oxidase and the ferment which splits off the amino group to some extent. These ferments do not act on the nucleic acid. This author believes that the ferment which changes the amino purins to the oxypurins is the "desamidierende" enzyme which Lang has found widely distributed in the organism. Burian likewise has found in organs an enzyme which oxidizes oxypurins to uric acid.

As to the four theories advanced to explain the increased uric acid in the blood in gout—increased formation, retention, decreased destruction, and change in chemical composition—McCrudden fails to express any definite opinion as to which he thinks the most plausible one. He emphasizes an important fact, namely, that physical chemistry has taught us that the acidity and the alkalinity of many complex mixtures of electrolytes such as blood and urine cannot be determined by titration methods. Only recently has an accurate method been offered by which the acidity of the urine and the alkalinity of the blood can be determined. By means of this method Höber has shown that the prevailing views concerning the acidity of the urine and the alkalinity of the blood are far from correct. The work of His and Höber puts an end to many theories concerning uric acid in the blood and urine and to any scientific basis for the alkali therapeutics in gout. McCrudden points out that the work of Burian and Schur, Soetbeer, Ibrahim, and Salkowski shows that uric acid is excreted in great part unchanged by man. He states that this is a final death blow to the old view that uric acid is an antecedent of urea in the destructive metabolism of proteid.

Gall-Stones and Their Surgical Treatment. By B. G. A. MOYNIHAN, M. S. (Lond.), F. R. C. S. Leeds. Fully illustrated with colored and black and white drawings (*Philadelphia: W. B. Saunders & Co., 1905.*)

The appearance of this book by such a well-known author as Moynihan is warmly welcomed. The subject is systematically treated in eleven chapters and the book is well indexed. It is well printed on good thick paper and contains numerous illustrations in color and in black and white.

The first fifty-seven pages are devoted to the anatomy of the gall-bladder and gall-ducts and to a study of the constitution and origin of gall-stones. About fifty pages are devoted to the pathology of gall-stone disease, a hundred to the symptoms and physical signs, and about fifty more to the complications and sequelæ. The remainder of the book is devoted to a description of operative procedures.

Moynihan states that the valves of Heister are not arranged spirally; that in two-thirds of the cases the pancreatic portion of the common duct can only be reached by dividing pancreatic tissue; and he calls attention to the importance of Opie's work in explaining acute pancreatitis.

According to Moynihan the earliest symptom in almost all cases of gall-stone disease is "indigestion." He notes also that jaundice is a rare symptom. He credits Courvoisier with the discovery that, in persistent jaundice due to stones, the gall-bladder is contracted in over eighty per cent of the cases and that persistent jaundice with distention of the gall-bladder, in over nine-tenths of the cases, was caused by a pressure from without the duct, chiefly from carcinoma of the head of the pancreas. He points out that in the case of stone in the common duct there is an ebb and flow in the jaundice, while in cancer the jaundice steadily increases and has more of a greenish hue.

Moynihan considers that chronic pancreatitis is the condition most difficult to differentiate from stone in the common duct. He states that after the stone is passed "the thickening of the head of the pancreas which has been left behind may cause a remarkable mimicry of the symptoms of stone."

In the chapters on operative procedures he gives full directions for the preparation necessary in the case of the surgeon, assistants, patient, etc. He states that only one assistant is necessary or desirable.

For suture material he uses catgut, prepared according to the method of Claudius, and Hagenstecher's celluloid thread. He gives a careful and detailed description of his method of performing the various operations upon the bile passages and describes many illustrative cases.

O. B. P.

Food and Diet in Health and Disease. By ROBERT F. WILLIAMS, M.A., M.D., Professor of the practice of medicine in the Medical College of Virginia. (*Philadelphia and New York: Lea Brothers & Co.; 1906.*)

This little book seems well fitted for its purpose. It contains little or nothing that is new, but as the author states in the preface that he has drawn largely upon literature in its preparation, originality is not to be expected. The most distinctive thing about it is that the author deviates from the time-honored usage which divides foods into animal and vegetable and considers them according to their predominating essential constituents from an alimentary point of view, an arrangement which is certainly more rational.

The choice of material is good and the arrangement is well-suited to the end in view; moreover, the style is interesting and readable, a matter of no small importance in a book of this kind, for in all works upon food the question must arise whether the systematic consideration of food from the point of its nourishing qualities does not destroy our appetite for it. To fix our attention upon what we eat solely, or even mainly, with the idea of benefit to be derived from it must in the end induce a detached state of mind similar to that of the man described by Mr. William Dean Howells "who took his meals in a detached manner as if he were feeding an engine." Such a mental attitude must, we should think, be destructive to all enjoyment, and yet enjoyment physiologists tell us, is a potent factor in digestion and assimilation. The only way out of the difficulty would seem to be that systematic treatises should be read by the few who may then make use of the knowledge thus acquired in the interests of the many.

A Text-Book of Diseases of Women. By BARTON COOKE HIRST, M.D., Professor of Obstetrics in the University of Pennsylvania. With 655 illustrations, many of them in colors. (*Philadelphia and London: W. B. Saunders & Co., 1903.*)

This work seems well adapted for the purpose of a text-book, for it is written in a clear condensed style, which assumes that the acquisition of information, not the discussion of theories, is the reader's object in reading it. The range of subjects is, of course, the same as that contained in all books of the kind and there seems to be little that is original or even distinctive. The author has, we think, done wisely in laying stress on the palliative or restorative side of gynecology, which has received too little attention from gynecological specialists since its surgical aspect came into prominence.

The illustrations are not, perhaps, of the highest order of merit from an artistic point of view, but they are sufficiently good for their purpose, and it is better that they should fall short of the utmost perfection than that the price of the book should be raised to an unreasonable amount in order that they should be carried to the greatest degree of artistic excellence.

One minor matter, we think, deserves a word of comment. It is to be regretted that a man of reputation should lend the sanction of example to the present practice of writing compound words in one. Such words as fibromyomata, bulbocavernosus, pseudohæmaphroditism, etc., in our opinion demand a hyphen between their two component parts, first, because it serves a useful purpose in showing that the word has two sources, and, second, because the length of most compound words makes them a weariness to the eye and the mind in reading. We have reason to congratulate ourselves that our native language is free from the clumsiness which such words induce in the German tongue. Why then should we voluntarily introduce the defect?

Diseases of the Nervous System. A text-book for students and practitioners of medicine. By H. OPPENHEIM, M. D., Professor at the University of Berlin. Translated and edited by EDWARD A. MEYER, M. D., Pittsburg, Pa. Second American edition, revised and enlarged, with 343 illustrations. (*Philadelphia: J. B. Lippincott & Co., 1904.*)

The author of this book has wisely devoted his energies and his well-known acquaintance with the subject to the production of a work adapted exclusively to the needs of students and general practitioners, and has made no effort to render it suitable for specialists in the study of the nervous system. In this decision he has, we think, shown excellent judgment, since an attempt to fulfill both purposes would certainly have failed of success with either. The clinical side of his subject is gone into with the utmost thoroughness and the discussion of its therapeutics is as satisfactory as it is possible that it should be in the present condition of our knowledge concerning it. References to literature have been intentionally avoided as tending to impair the continuity of the text, but it is quite plain that the writer's knowledge with all that has been written on the subject has been thoroughly assimilated and the best of it brought forward in the manner most profitable to the reader. The translator has done his work well, on the whole, although words occasionally occur which do not, to our thinking, render the best equivalent for the original.

Medical and Surgical Reports of the Boston City Hospital. Fifteenth Series. Edited by H. L. BURRELL, M. D., W. T. COUNCILMAN, M. D., and C. F. WITHINGTON, M. D. (*Boston: Published by the Trustees, 1905.*)

The report of the Boston City Hospital for the year 1905 contains some very interesting reading. Sixty cases of extra-uterine pregnancy, reported by P. S. Newell, occurring in five and a half years, seems a much larger number for one hospital than our present knowledge of the condition would have led us to suppose possible. One of the points connected with the condition upon which our minds are now receiving enlightenment, however, is that it is of greater frequency than we have hitherto supposed and the length of this particular record is valuable confirmatory evidence to this effect. A careful study of these cases also brings out sundry other points in which, it would appear, we have been

under a misapprehension. For example, it has been asserted without contradiction that most cases of ectopic gestation give a history of sterility for a number of years before its occurrence, and the inference has, therefore, been that the majority of cases occurred in elderly primaparæ or in multiparæ who had become pregnant after a period of sterility. The series in question shows, on the contrary, that only nine patients were pregnant for the first time and the ages of these varied from twenty to thirty-six; of the remaining fifty-one cases, all but one had been pregnant at a recent date and their ages varied from twenty to forty-two. It would seem, therefore, that ectopic gestation is most frequent in the middle child-bearing period of life and in women who have recently been pregnant. Or rather, as the writer puts it, " the condition may arise in any woman exposed to pregnancy at any time."

A fully reported case of Pott's disease in the monkey, by E. E. Southard, is of considerable interest to comparative pathology. So far as it goes it tends to show that the morbid processes of our poor relation differ but little from our own.

A case of oxyuris vermicularis in the vermiform appendix, reported by S. T. Otron, is one more added to the number, which is still very small. Kelly and Hurdon, as the writer states, report only seven instances of the condition collected from literature.

Five cases of glanders, by Abner Post, are a contribution to a subject which is little discussed. One of these cases occurred in the Boston City Hospital during 1905, and the others were collected from the records since 1864, the date when it first received inmates. They are all given at length for purposes of comparison, and although they are, of course, too few for any definite conclusions to be drawn from them, they indicate, so far as they go, that an initial pneumonic process is more frequent than has been usually supposed.

These are but a few of the interesting articles contained in this report, indeed there is hardly one which does not contain something that specially recommends it, either from the point of view of rarity or from that of careful consideration and tabulation. The editors may be congratulated on having issued a report of unusual interest and originality.

Walter Reed and Yellow Fever. By HOWARD A. KELLY, M. D., Professor of Gynecological Surgery, The Johns Hopkins University. (*New York: McClure, Phillips & Co., 1906.*)

No more stimulating and interesting book of medical biography has appeared since Radot's Life of Pasteur, which it resembles in many respects and its lesson for the medical profession is of equal importance. It is the story of the life and achievements of one who unquestionably has made the most important medical discovery of any American, a discovery which as far as the saving of human life is concerned must be placed beside that of Jenner, a hundred years ago. The tale of Walter Reed's life may be told in a few words: Of English stock originally, the son of a Methodist clergyman, born in Gloucester County, Virginia, in 1851, he received his education principally at the University of Virginia, graduating in medicine in his eighteenth year. He pursued his medical studies subsequently in New York and received a degree also from Bellevue Hospital Medical College. He served thereafter in several hospitals in New York, and recently and finally became a sanitary inspector in Brooklyn. In 1874 he was appointed an assistant surgeon in the U. S. Army, and during the following sixteen years saw service in Arizona, Nebraska, Alabama, and Washington, D. C. In 1890 he came to Baltimore and began the study of bacteriology and pathology under Prof. Welch at the laboratory then just opened by the Johns Hopkins Hospital, prior to the organization of the Johns Hopkins Medical School. In 1893 he became curator of the U. S. Army Medical Museum and professor of pathology and clinical microscopy in the U. S. Army Medical School founded by the zeal and scientific initiative of Surgeon-General Sternberg. Here he did excellent work as a teacher and investigator and laid the foundation of a scientific reputation which, during the Spanish-American War, led to his appointment as a member of a Commission to investigate the epidemic occurrence of typhoid fever among the troops in their camps. In 1899 he with Dr. Carroll demonstrated the incorrectness of Sanarelli's claim that he had discovered the causative agent of yellow fever. In 1900 he was sent to Havana at the head of a commission to investigate the etiology of yellow fever and by a series of brilliant and conclusive experiments demonstrated that yellow fever was transmitted from man to man by the bite of a variety of mosquito, the Stegomyia fasciati. In November, 1902, he died of appendicitis while engaged in his duties at the Army Medical Museum, after a brief illness.

The story of his life has been told simply and attractively by the author of this book, which deserves to be widely read. The letters which Reed wrote while an army surgeon are graphic and full of incident. The chapters which treat of yellow fever in America and the rise and fall of the numerous theories as to its causation are valuable contributions to the literature of the disease. The account of the development of the theory of the causative relation of the mosquito to the spread of the dread disease is well told and the book as a whole is worthy to take its place among the standard biographies of eminent medical men. It is a matter of genuine surprise to those who are familiar with the varied activities of the accomplished author in many fields, that he should have found time to pen this graceful, painstaking and affectionate tribute to the work and worth of Walter Reed.

BOOKS RECEIVED.

Differential Diagnosis and Treatment of Disease. By Augustus Caillé, M. D. With two hundred and twenty-eight illustrations in the text. 1906. 8vo. 867 pages. D. Appleton & Company, New York and London.

A Manual of Materia Medica and Pharmacology. Comprising all Organic and Inorganic Drugs which are or have been Official in the United States Pharmacopœia. By David M. R. Culbreth, Ph. G., M. D. Fourth edition, enlarged and thoroughly revised. With four hundred and eighty-seven illustrations. 1906. 8vo. 976 pages. Lea Brothers & Company, Philadelphia and New York.

A Laboratory Manual of Physiological Chemistry. By Elbert W. Rockwood, M. D., Ph. D. Second edition, revised and enlarged. With one colored plate and three plates of microscopic preparations. 1906. 12mo. 229 pages. F. A. Davis Company, Philadelphia.

Refraction Including Muscle Imbalance and the Adjustment of Glasses. By Royal S. Copeland, A. M., M. D., and Adolph E. Ibershoff, M. D. 1906. 8vo. 144 pages. Boericke & Tafel, Philadelphia.

The Diseases of Infancy and Childhood. Designed for the Use of Students and Practitioners of Medicine. By Henry Koplik, M. D. Second edition, thoroughly revised and enlarged. Illustrated with 184 engravings and 33 plates in color and monochrome. 1906. 8vo. 885 pages. Lea Brothers & Company, New York and Philadelphia.

Lectures on Tropical Diseases. Being the Lane Lectures for 1905. Delivered at Cooper Medical College, San Francisco, U. S. A. August, 1905. By Sir Patrick Manson. 1905. 8vo. 230 pages. W. T. Keener & Company, Chicago.

A Text-Book of Diseases of the Nose and Throat. By D. Braden Kyle, M. D. With 175 illustrations, 24 of them in colors. Third edition, revised and enlarged. 1904. 8vo. 669 pages. W. B. Saunders & Company, Philadelphia, New York, London.

THE JOHNS HOPKINS HOSPITAL REPORTS.

VOLS. XIII AND XIV,

OF ABOUT 600 PAGES EACH, WITH NUMEROUS ILLUSTRATIONS.

(NOW IN PRESS.)

STUDIES IN GENITO-URINARY SURGERY. By HUGH H. YOUNG, M. D., Associate Professor of Genito-Urinary Surgery, The Johns Hopkins University, and Associate in Genito-Urinary Surgery, The Johns Hopkins Hospital, and F. H. BAETJER, M. D., of Baltimore; HENRY A. FOWLER, M. D., of Washington, D. C.; STEPHEN H. WATTS, M. D., of Baltimore; JOHN W. CHURCHMAN, M. D., of Breslau; LOUIS C. LEHR, M. D., of Washington, D. C.; J. T. GERAGHTY, M. D., of Baltimore, and A. R. STEVENS, M. D., of Baltimore.

CONTENTS.

1. The Seven Glass Test. By Hugh H. Young, M. D.
2. The Possibility of Avoiding Confusion by Bacillus Smegmatis (Smegma bacillus) in the Diagnosis of Urinary and Genital Tuberculosis. An Experimental Study. By Hugh H. Young, M. D., and John W. Churchman, M. D.
3. Urethral Diverticula. By Stephen H. Watts, M. D.
4. Case of Urethrorrhagia. By H. A. Fowler, M. D.
5. Paraurethritis. By John W. Churchman, M. D.
6. Use of Ointments in the Urethra. By Hugh H. Young, M. D.
7. Treatment of Stricture of the Urethra. By Hugh H. Young, M. D., and John T. Geraghty, M. D.
8. The Treatment of Impermeable Stricture of the Urethra. By Hugh H. Young, M. D.
9. The Treatment of Bacteriuria by Medication. By John W. Churchman, M. D.
10. Use of the Cystoscope in the Diagnosis of Diseases of the Prostate. By Hugh H. Young, M. D.
11. Chronic Prostatitis. An Analysis of 358 Cases. By Hugh H. Young, M. D., John T. Geraghty, M. D., and A. R. Stevens, M. D.
12. The Treatment of Prostatic Hypertrophy. By Hugh H. Young, M. D.
13. Recto-Urethral Fistulæ. By Hugh H. Young, M. D.
14. Modern Method of Performing Perineal Lithotomy. By Hugh H. Young, M. D.
15. Early Diagnosis and Radical Cure of Carcinoma of the Prostate. By Hugh H. Young, M. D.
16. Operative Treatment of Vesical Diverticula. By Hugh H. Young, M. D.
17. Case of Double Renal Pelvis and Bifid Ureter. By Hugh H. Young, M. D.
18. Pyonephrosis Due to B. Typhosus. By Hugh H. Young, M. D., and Louis C. Lehr, M. D.
19. The Use of the X-ray in the Diagnosis of Renal and Ureteral Calculi. By F. H. Baetjer, M. D.
20. Nephritis and Hematuria. By H. A. Fowler, M. D.
21. Microscopic Study of Urinary Calculi of Oxalate of Lime. By H. A. Fowler, M. D.
22. Cystinuria and the Formation of Calculi. By H. A. Fowler, M. D.
23. Post-Traumatic Atrophy of the Testicle. By John W. Churchman, M. D.

Price per volume in paper, $5.00; in cloth, $5.50.

Orders should be addressed to

THE JOHNS HOPKINS PRESS, BALTIMORE, MD.

THE JOHNS HOPKINS HOSPITAL REPORTS.

VOLUME I. 423 pages, 99 plates.

VOLUME II. 570 pages, with 28 plates and figures.

VOLUME III. 766 pages, with 69 plates and figures.

VOLUME IV. 504 pages, 33 charts and illustrations.

VOLUME V. 480 pages, with 32 charts and illustrations.

CONTENTS:

The Malarial Fevers of Baltimore. By W. S. THAYER, M. D., and J. HEWETSON, M. D.

A Study of some Fatal Cases of Malaria. By LEWELLYS F. BARKER, M. B.

Studies in Typhoid Fever.

By WILLIAM OSLER, M. D., with additional papers by G. BLUMER, M. D., SIMON FLEXNER, M. D., WALTER REED, M. D., and H. C. PARSONS, M. D.

VOLUME VI. 414 pages, with 79 plates and figures.

Report in Neurology.

Studies on the Lesions Produced by the Action of Certain Poisons on the Cortical Nerve Cell (Studies Nos. I to V). By HENRY J. BERKLEY, M. D.

Introductory.—Recent Literature on the Pathology of Diseases of the Brain by the Chromate of Silver Methods; Part I.—Alcohol Poisoning.—Experimental Lesions Produced by Chronic Alcoholic Poisoning (Ethyl Alcohol). 2. Experimental Lesions Produced by Acute Alcoholic Poisoning (Ethyl Alcohol); Part II.—Serum Poisoning.—Experimental Lesions induced by the Action of the Dog's Serum on the Cortical Nerve Cell; Part III.—Ricin Poisoning.—Experimental Lesions induced by Acute Ricin Poisoning. 2. Experimental Lesions induced by Chronic Ricin Poisoning; Part IV.—Hydrophobic Toxæmia.—Lesions of the Cortical Nerve Cell produced by the Toxine of Experimental Rabies; Part V.—Pathological Alterations in the Nuclei and Nucleoli of Nerve Cells from the Effects of Alcohol and Ricin Intoxication; Nerve Fibre Terminal Apparatus; Asthenic Bulbar Paralysis. By HENRY J. BERKLEY, M. D.

Report in Pathology.

Fatal Puerperal Sepsis due to the Introduction of an Elm Tent. By THOMAS S. CULLEN, M. B.

Pregnancy in a Rudimentary Uterine Horn. Rupture, Death, Probable Migration of Ovum and Spermatozoa. By THOMAS S. CULLEN, M. B., and G. L. WILKINS, M. D.

Adeno-Myoma Uteri Diffusum Benignum. By THOMAS S. CULLEN, M. B.

A Bacteriological and Anatomical Study of the Summer Diarrhœas of Infants. By WILLIAM D. BOOKER, M. D.

The Pathology of Toxalbumin Intoxications. By SIMON FLEXNER, M. D.

VOLUME VII. 537 pages with illustrations.

   I. A Critical Review of Seventeen Hundred Cases of Abdominal Section from the standpoint of Intra-peritoneal Drainage. By J. G. LARK, M. D.

   II. The Etiology and Structure of true Vaginal Cysts. By JAMES ERNEST STOKES, M. D.

   III. A Review of the Pathology of Superficial Burns, with a Contribution to our Knowledge of the Pathological Changes in the Organs in cases of rapidly fatal burns. By CHARLES RUSSELL BARDEEN, M. D.

   IV. The Origin, Growth and Fate of the Corpus Luteum. By J. G. CLARK, M. D.

   V. The Results of Operations for the Cure of Inguinal Hernia. By JOSEPH C. BLOODGOOD, M. D.

VOLUME VIII. 552 pages with illustrations.

On the rôle of Insecta, Arachnida, and Myriapods as carriers in the spread of Bacterial and Parasitic Diseases of Man and Animals. By GEORGE H. F. NUTTALL, M. D., PH. D.

Studies in Typhoid Fever.

By WILLIAM OSLER, M. D., with additional papers by J. M. T. FINNEY, M. D., S. FLEXNER, M. D., I. P. LYON, M. D., L. F. HAMBURGER, M. D., H. W. CUSHING, M. D., J. F. MITCHELL, M. D., C. N. B. CAMAC, M. D., N. B. GWYN, M. D., CHARLES P. EMERSON, M. D., H. H. YOUNG, M. D., and W. S. THAYER, M. D.

VOLUME IX. 1060 pages, 66 plates and 210 other illustrations.

Contributions to the Science of Medicine.

Dedicated by his Pupils to WILLIAM HENRY WELCH, on the twenty-fifth anniversary of his Doctorate. This volume contains 38 separate papers.

VOLUME X. 516 pages, 12 plates and 25 charts.

Structure of the Malarial Parasites. Plate I. By JESSE W. LAZEAR, M. D.

The Bacteriology of Cystitis, Pyelitis and Pyelonephritis in Women, with a Consideration of the Accessory Etiological Factors in these Conditions, and of the Various Chemical and Microscopical Questions involved. By THOMAS R. BROWN, M. D.

Cases of Infection with Strongyloides Intestinalis. (First Reported Occurrence in North America.) Plates II and III. By RICHARD P. STRONG, M. D.

On the Pathological Changes in Hodgkin's Disease, with Especial Reference to its Relation to Tuberculosis. Plates IV-VII. By DOROTHY M. REED, M. D.

Diabetes Insipidus, with a Report of Five Cases. By THOMAS B. FUTCHER, M. B. (Tor.).

Observations on the Origin and Occurrence of Cells with Eosinophile Granulations in Normal and Pathological Tissues. Plate VIII. By W. T. HOWARD, M. D., and R. G. PERKINS, M. D.

Placental Transmissions, with Report of a Case during Typhoid Fever. By FRANK W. LYNCH, M. D.

Metabolism in Albuminuria. By CHAS. P. EMERSON, A. B., M. D.

Regenerative Changes in the Liver after Acute Yellow Atrophy. Plates IX-XII. By W. G. MACCALLUM, M. D.

Surgical Features of Typhoid Fever. By THOS. MCCRAE, M. B., M. R. C. P. (Lond.), and JAMES F. MITCHELL, M. D.

The Symptoms, Diagnosis and Surgical Treatment of Ureteral Calculus. By BENJAMIN R. SCHENCK, M. D.

VOLUME XI. 555 pages, with 38 charts and illustrations.

Pneumothorax: A historical, clinical and experimental study. By CHARLES P. EMERSON, M. D.

Clinical Observations on Blood Pressure. By HENRY W. COOK, M. D., and JOHN B. BRIGGS, M. D.

The value of Tuberculin in Surgical Diagnosis. By MARTIN B. TINKER, M. D.

VOLUME XII. 548 pages, 12 plates and other illustrations.

The Connective Tissue of the Salivary Glands and Pancreas with its Development in the Glandula Submaxillaris. Plates I-III. By JOSEPH MARSHALL FLINT, M. D.

A New Instrument for Determining the Minimum and Maximum Blood-Pressures in Man. Plates IV-X. By JOSEPH ERLANGER, M. D.

Metabolism in Pregnancy, Labor, and the Puerperium. By J. MORRIS SLEMONS, M. D.

An Experimental Study of Blood-Pressure and of Pulse-Pressure in Man. Plates XI and XII. By JOSEPH ERLANGER, M. D., and DONALD R. HOOKER, A. B., M. S.

Typhoid Meningitis. By RUFUS I. COLE, M. D.

The Pathological Anatomy of Meningitis due to Bacillus Typhosur. By WILLIAM G. MACCALLUM, M. D.

A Comparative Study of White and Negro Pelves, with a Consideration of the Size of the Child and Its Relation to Presentation and Character of Labor in the Two Races. By THEODORE F. RIGGS, M. D.

Renal Tuberculosis. By GEORGE WALKER, M. D.

VOLUME XIII. (In press).

The Johns Hopkins Hospital Bulletins are issued monthly. They are printed by the FRIEDENWALD CO., Baltimore. Single copies may be procured from NUNN & CO. and the BALTIMORE NEWS CO., Baltimore. Subscriptions, $2.00 a year, may be addressed to the publishers, THE JOHNS HOPKINS PRESS, BALTIMORE; single copies will be sent by mail for twenty-five cents each.

BULLETIN ·

OF

THE JOHNS HOPKINS HOSPITAL

Entered as Second-Class Matter at the Baltimore, Maryland, Postoffice.

Vol. XVII.—No. 187.]   BALTIMORE, OCTOBER, 1906.   [Price, 25 Cents

CONTENTS.

BACTERIOLOGICAL EXAMINATIONS OF THE CONJUNCTIVAL SAC IN TYPHOID FEVER AND IN PNEUMONIA.

BASED UPON AN EXAMINATION OF 100 CASES OF TYPHOID FEVER AND 48 CASES OF LOBAR PNEUMONIA OCCURRING IN THE WARDS OF THE JOHNS HOPKINS HOSPITAL.

By ROBERT L. RANDOLPH, M. D.

The study of the bacterial flora of the conjunctival sac in health and disease has been the subject of many investigations, but it has left still unsolved many problems of interest and importance. The nature of the infection and the mode of not a few conjunctival infections are unsettled. There are several ways by which microorganisms can gain access to the conjunctiva, viz.: (1) From the exterior either through air infection, through dust or droplets, or by direct contact; (2) from the throat and nose by way of the naso-lacrymal duct; (3) by the blood circulation either directly to the conjunctiva or by elimination of microorganisms in the secretion of the lacrymal glands; (4) by the lymphatics, and (5) by direct extension from infection of neighboring parts. In many instances it is often difficult or impossible at present to determine by which of these various paths the infection has been conveyed.

We are also, in some cases, in doubt either as to the nature or the source of the specific organism concerned in the infection. Here a question of much interest relates to the relative frequency of conjunctival infections by the microorganisms causing a primary infection elsewhere or by secondary invaders. For a considerable number of diseases it has been demonstrated that the bacteria of the primary disease may cause also an associated conjunctival infection. This is true of gonorrhœa, cerebrospinal meningitis, pneumonia, diphtheria,

influenza, tuberculosis, erysipelas, pyæmia, septicæmia, bubonic plague, Malta fever and leprosy, but in the case of some, at least, of these affections a complicating conjunctivitis is due more frequently to secondary invaders than to the bacterium causing the primary disease. As regards the inflammations of the mucous membranes including the conjunctiva which so often complicate scarlet fever, small pox, measles, and other exanthematous fevers, our inability to demonstrate satisfactorily the specific parasites of these diseases makes it impossible at present to state positively, in any case, in any degree directly responsible for such inflammations. Without denying the possibility of the direct participation of these unknown microorganisms in the complications in question, the existing evidence favors the view that secondary invaders are the chief excitants of this class of affections, *Streptococcus pyogenes* being most frequently concerned. Other secondary invaders to be reckoned with in these cases of conjunctivitis are the pneumococcus, the pyogenic staphylococcus, influenza, and pseudo-influenza bacilli, xerosis and other pseudo-diphtheria bacilli. It is probable that in most instances these bacteria were not introduced from without, but being already present in the throat, nose or conjunctiva were enabled to multiply and produce their pathogenic effects in consequence of lowered resistance resulting from the primary infection. This latter interpretation of the facts, which is the one generally held, renders of especial interest the examination of the bacterial flora of the normal conjunctival sac.

Several years ago I reported the results of my bacterial examinations of the normal conjunctiva of 100 persons. In 88 per cent M. albus, the ordinary skin coccus, was recovered in culture from the conjunctival sac, and subsequent examinations have convinced me that this organism is a regular inhabitant of the normal conjunctiva. The genuine M. aureus, which has been found frequently by some others in this situation, I have encountered only in a small minority of cases, and I must believe that there has been some error in identification by those who claim that it is frequently present. The frequency with which certain other bacteria are found in the conjunctival sac will doubtless depend upon the technique employed. This is true especially of influenza bacilli, the Koch-Weeks bacillus, the Morax-Axenfeld diplobacillus, certain pseudo-diphtheria bacilli, and in a measure the pneumococcus which grow best upon media of special composition. In opposition to Gasparrini and more in accord with Oertzen, Axenfeld, Lawson, and the majority of investigators, I have found the pneumococcus in only one or two per cent of normal conjunctivæ.

As a small contribution to the solution of certain of the problems indicated I have undertaken the bacteriological examination of the conjunctival sac in a series of cases of typhoid fever and of pneumonia.

The occurrence of the typhoid bacillus in the blood, urine, sputum and fæces of patients with typhoid fever, or, in other words, the wide distribution of this bacillus throughout the body in this disease added to its resisting powers and ready adaptation to its environment suggests the possibility of the occasional appearance of the bacillus also in the conjunctival sac. Conjunctivitis is a recognized complication of typhoid fever, but while the search for the typhoid bacillus is of especial interest in this complication, it might readily be that the bacillus occasionally gained access to the conjunctiva without exercising any injurious effect. Although rare in contrast to otitis media, conjunctivitis is not an uncommon complication of acute pneumonia.

The following method was employed in making the cultures. Through the cotton plug of a test tube containing one cubic centimeter of sterile bouillon ran a glass rod, on which was tightly wrapped some cotton wool, thus making a swab. This rod, with the plug, was removed at the bedside, and both conjunctival sacs above and below were well swabbed, care being taken not to touch the lids and lashes. Then, with a pair of sterile forceps, the lower end of the rod just above the swab was broken off and dropped back into the bouillon at the bottom of the tube. It is hardly necessary to say that before the tube was opened everything within it had been thoroughly sterilized. The plug was then replaced and the tube taken over to the laboratory. The usual quantity of fluid agar for a plate culture was poured into this tube and well shaken up and plate cultures made in the usual manner in Petri dishes and placed in the oven at a temperature of 35 C. - 37 C. The interval of time between the inoculation of the bouillon and

the pouring of the plates never exceeded fifteen minutes, and was usually less. In this manner inoculations were made from 100 cases of typhoid fever and 48 cases of lobar pneumonia. I might say that the inoculations were never made from any but undoubted cases of typhoid fever, that is to say, from individuals with continued fever with "positive Widal" and with other characteristic signs and symptoms of this disease. Cases in any respect doubtful were not utilized. The predominant colony in the plates was almost always Micrococcus albus, and familiarity with its appearance obviated the necessity of making cover slips from each colony in the plate. Frequent examinations, however, were made even from these round white colonies to assure me that my interpretation was correct. Whenever a colony showed the slightest deviation from what I have learned to expect in the appearance of this organism in plate culture cover slips were made, and if necessary the organism was subjected to the proper cultural tests.

In glancing over the findings one must be surprised at the frequency with which M. albus comes to the front. This organism occurred in the typhoid cases 59 times alone; in other words, there was no other organism in the plate. It actually thus occurred oftener, for in one case (Case 24) inoculations were made on nine different occasions and M. albus was found six times, while in the remaining three times it was found six with M. aureus. The same should be said of Case 78, in which it was thought proper to make inoculations every day for three weeks. Inoculations were made from this patient 18 times, and in only four instances did M. albus fail to appear. Not counting these two cases M. albus was found associated with other bacteria in 23 cases, so that out of the 100 cases this organism was found 82 times. In eight cases M. aureus was found alone, while in 13 cases it was found associated with other bacteria, in two out of the 13 with M. albus. Streptococcus pyogenes was found three times, and in two of these cases along with M. albus. The Morax-Axenfeld diplobacillus was found once and was associated with M. albus. The xerosis bacillus was found three times, and in two of these cases was associated with M. albus. B. pyocyaneus occurred once. B. subtilis occurred four times and in three of these along with M. albus. The plates were sterile in two cases, and in two others impurities predominated to such an extent as to make the observation worthless. Out of the 100 cases then the conjunctival sac was found to contain bacteria in 96. What is remarkable is that the typhoid bacillus was absent throughout. There were three cases of conjunctivitis, and inoculations made from the conjunctiva showed in two instances M. albus, and in the other case M. albus and M. aureus.

In the other series 48 cases of lobar pneumonia were examined, and in these cases M. albus was found alone in 24 cases, and along with other bacteria 14 times; in other words, this organism was found in 38 out of 48 cases. The pneumococcus was found twice, once alone and once along with M. albus. B. subtilis was found three times alone and once along with M. albus. M. aureus occurred 10 times, once alone and nine times associated with M. albus. There were three sterile plates in this series. The Morax-Axenfeld diplobacillus was found once and the xerosis bacillus once. In five cases there was conjunctivitis, and inoculations from three of these five cases showed only *M. albus*, one showing *M. aureus* and the remaining one the pneumococcus. In a few instances there appeared an occasional colony of some unidentified bacterium of no apparent significance.

The question naturally arose in the course of these observations, whether the typhoid bacillus might not be found at some particular stage of the disease, and this question was answered by making the inoculations at different stages of the fever. In one case (Case 78) inoculations were made practically every day throughout the course of the disease, and even in convalescence attempts were repeatedly made to recover the organism from the conjunctival sac, but always with negative results. As regards the pneumonia cases the pneumococcus was found twice, and in one of the patients its presence was associated with a conjunctivitis. The conjunctival sac in pneumonia must be regarded then as a very unlikely place in which to find the pneumococcus.

My own investigations into the bacterial flora of the conjunctival sac, not only in healthy individuals, but in those under the influence of a general infection, as, for instance, typhoid fever, have resulted so consistently in the discovery of one organism that I am confirmed in the belief that this organism is an invariable inhabitant of the conjunctival sac, and that among the defensive mechanisms, either by its numerical superiority or by its products, it may aid in rendering this part of the body a soil unfavorable for the growth and multiplication of those bacteria which are regarded as especially pathogenic for the eye and which occasionally find their way into this location oftener, I believe, than is generally thought. The possibility is suggested then that this organism, slightly pathogenic and quite numerous in the conjunctival sac, gives rise to conditions which are antagonistic to such organisms, for instance, as *B. diphtheriæ*, the gonococcus, Koch-Weeks' bacillus and the organism of trachoma, whatever that may be. What a very common disease is gonorrhœa, and yet how comparatively infrequent is gonorrhœal ophthalmia. It can hardly be otherwise that the gonorrhœal virus gains access to the conjunctival sac without setting up inflammation, and it must happen that in cases of highly infectious inflammation of one eye infectious germs are often conveyed to the other eye without resulting injury. It is true, as I have shown elsewhere, that an intact epithelium is a great safeguard

against infection of the conjunctiva, but the frequency with which *M. albus* is found in the conjunctival sac leads me to think that this organism in this location plays the part of an enemy to many invaders. The antagonism which exists between certain organisms or the inhibitory influence which some bacteria exert upon the growth of others is a familiar and well established fact. In this connection I am reminded of the observations of Menge and Krönig,[1] who introduced into the vagina 23 times *B. pyocyaneus*, 30 times *M. aureus*, and 27 times *Streptococcus pyogenes*. The staphylococcus was obtained from a breast abscess, the streptococcus came from the purulent exudate found in the abdominal cavity of a woman who had died of an acute septic peritonitis. *B. pyocyaneus* was obtained from green pus. There was no doubt then that these bacteria possessed virulence and freshness in a high degree. No trace of these organisms could be found in the vaginal tract after 26 hours. The conditions then in the normal vaginal canal for the development of pathogenic bacteria are unfavorable, conditions probably due to a considerable extent to the presence in the canal of *B. vaginalis Doederlein*, which organism, Doederlein holds, is largely responsible for the peculiar reaction of the vaginal secretion, a reaction which helps to keep sterile this part of the genital apparatus, that is to say, sterile so far as its freedom from pathogenic bacteria is concerned. It has been observed in large obstetric wards that fever was more often seen in women in whom the effort was made to disinfect the vaginal canal by means of the so-called chemical disinfectants, than in women in whom no such attempt had been made. Efforts to disinfect the alimentary canal through the same means are equally futile, and when made, are frequently followed by distressing symptoms. Attempts to render the conjunctiva sterile have equally failed.

CONCLUSIONS.

The bacterial flora of the conjunctival sac during typhoid fever and pneumonia shows practically no difference from the conjunctival flora of individuals who are in perfect health.

It does not seem unreasonable to suggest that the exposed mucous surfaces throughout the body are inhabited by bacteria which perform for their resting place functions of a protective character by making the surroundings uncongenial to bacteria of other kinds.

[1] Bakteriologie des weiblichen Genitalkanales, S. 68.

TUBERCULOSIS WORK IN EUROPE.[1]

By Joseph Walsh, M. D.

At the International Congress of Tuberculosis held in Paris last October there were over 3000 delegates from all parts of the world.

Discussion revealed no new method or specific in the treat-

[1] Read before the Lænnec Society, March 21, 1906.

ment of tuberculosis, and it was generally agreed that sufficient rest, sufficient fresh air and sufficient good nourishment were the only elements in the treatment at present known to science.

The official seal, as it were, of the Congress was put on

various efforts towards the cure and prevention of tuberculosis namely, sanatoria for adults and for children, hospitals for advanced cases, supporting dispensaries, park convalescent camps (day camps) and societies for the education of the public. In addition to hearing the discussions as to the work done in the various countries I had the pleasure of investigating, personally, the work done in England, France and Germany.

Sanatoria are found in all the countries of Europe. The greatest number of them are found in Germany where the sanatorium idea originated, the smallest number in France, the natural antagonist to Germany and German ideas.

The first sanatorium in the world was founded by Brehmer at Gœbersdsorf about 1860, and it is within the last forty years that sanatoria have sprung up elsewhere.

It is interesting to note that the first man in our own country to advocate the curability of tuberculosis, namely Benjamin Rush, was ably seconded by the greatest layman of his time, namely, Benjamin Franklin; and again that the foundation of Brehmer's Sanatorium was largely due to the greatest layman of fifty years ago, namely, Alexander von Humboldt. The layman has had his hand in the crusade against tuberculosis from the beginning; his aid is now recognized to be definitely necessary; it ought not to be difficult to obtain.

The Germans believe the purpose of the sanatorium to be threefold. (1) The cure of the patient. (2) The education of the patient in the way of prevention in order to avoid further contagion. (3) The prevention of further contagion on the part of the patient for the time he is in the sanatorium.

The German sanatoria have been built regardless of cost and are magnificently endowed.

England possesses the next largest number of sanatoria and these are surpassed in magnificence only by those in Germany itself. Like in Germany no money has been spared on the building of English sanatoria, but there the funds have stopped, and there is not a sanatorium on the island that does not show a woeful lack of means for maintenance.

On account of the lack of maintenance English sanatoria are very much hampered in their work. Whatever maintenance they have is kept up by means of subscribers. Depending on the amount of the subscription each subscriber has the right to send one or several cases a year to the sanatorium. The sanatoria are, therefore, practically obliged to take cases even when they are unsuitable. Moreover the subscriber demands the admission of his full quota of cases yearly, thereby making the stay of the individual patient short. A common stay is six weeks, and it is uncommon to keep a patient more than three months.

This method of subscription and its *quid pro quo* seems to be pretty thoroughly rooted in England. We all remember in our novels of English life how the landed proprietor of the village, if he built a church, insisted that his family should always retain the right to name the rector.

On account of the unsuitableness of the cases and the shortness of their stay results in individual cases are not very good. Moreover the length of time the patient is kept under control

thereby preventing further infection in the home is insignificant. Consequently in England the purpose of the sanatorium is considered to be merely educational.

France with her natural antagonism to Germany succeeded in bringing arguments against the usefulness of sanatoria until within these last ten years. Among other things, the French schools insisted that contagion practically always took place about the family hearth in childhood and when the disease broke out in the adult, the patient's resistance was exhausted and the likelihood of cure small. Moreover, by this time he had done practically all the damage in the way of contagion that was worth while considering. The French, therefore, directed all their efforts to the prevention of tuberculosis in the child and to the treatment of the child. I think it is safe to say that they have more sanatoria for children throughout France than in all other countries combined. Their marine sanatoria for the cure of tuberculosis in children are the best known in the world.

While, therefore, antagonizing Germany they developed a new and important phase of the crusade against tuberculosis, namely, the care of the children, and by coming eventually around to sanatoria for adults they furnished the best proof of their usefulness and importance.

On account of our geographical position and our mental attitude towards the rest of the world, the United States stands in an especially favorable position for the development of new ideas. We are reasonably quick at taking up new ideas and taking them up without prejudice. It is not strange, therefore, that the sanatorium in the United States developed along more rational lines and that as a consequence the results accomplished are the best in the world. We consider the purpose of the sanatorium twofold, namely, first the cure of the patient, second the education of the patient and his friends.

The objection to the public charity sanatoria in Germany is their extreme elaborateness and the lack of enthusiasm of the men usually in charge of them. In the United States we have not yet gotten beyond the stage where each sanatorium still remains under the control of the enthusiasm that built it. On account of the number of sanatoria in Europe compared with the United States they have better control of the general tuberculosis situation but I believe are behind us in individual results.

The private sanatoria that I visited in Germany were Brehmers and Rompler's at Gœbersdsorf, Hohenhonnef, Falkenstein and Rupertshaim. Brehmer's ideas and his energy in pushing them deserve to put him in the position he occupies in connection with tuberculosis work.

Brehmer's idea was that fresh air was the principal element in the cure and that exercise was a powerful adjunct. It was the dictum of the century before when Sydenham insisted that the outside of a horse was good for the inside of a man. From the time of entrance to the sanatorium, Brehmer put his patients on mountain climbing. The grounds of Brehmer's sanatorium consist of a most beautiful park on a rather steep mountain side traversed by walks among trees and rocks, here cut through a small tunnel, there beautified by a fountain surrounded by nymphs, the whole charming as enthusiasm could make it. Despite the progress in the treatment of tuberculosis Brehmer's ideas continue to be carried out most religiously. Patients are still put on exercise from the moment of entrance practically regardless of the disease condition present.

The next step in the treatment of tuberculosis after fresh air, was introduced by Detweiler, who realized that exercise instead of being an adjunct was in many cases harmful. The indications for and against exercise not being properly understood, Detweiler put all patients on rest and kept them on rest.

Exactly across the street from Brehmer's sanatorium is a sanatorium founded by Rompler, a follower of Detweiler. Rompler, too, is dead but Rompler's ideas still hold sway and in Rompler's sanatorium, though the patients may stay for a year, they practically never get off their steamer chairs. The grounds around Rompler's sanatorium are quite as beautiful and quite as suitable for exercise as those about Brehmer's though they are never used.

Moreover though the idea as to the necessity for unlimited fresh air still remains, the private sanatoria in Germany presented the greatest inducements to remain in-doors. In Falkenstein, in Rompler's and in Brehmer's they have the most beautiful reception rooms, reading rooms, libraries, closed winter gardens, etc., in each of which a certain number of patients can be constantly found.

In the private sanatoria are seen no arrangements for sleeping out-of-doors, on balconies or the like, and whether the windows are left open at night or not depends to a considerable extent on the whim of the patient. In the charity sanatoria throughout Europe arrangements are most complete for sleeping on balconies or sleeping in very open wards, but in the private sanatoria though fresh air is insisted on theoretically it does not seem to be urged practically.

The private sanatoria throughout Germany are handsome massive stone or brick buildings built like the cathedrals in Europe to last forever with landscape gardening about them that any park in the world might envy. They do not, however, begin to compete with the public charity or semi-charity institutions.

To an American the elaborateness and completeness of the charity sanatoria throughout England are astonishing. They are built like the modern European hospital, with all conveniences, and everything in the way of equipment that can be desired or imagined. Some of the older sanatoria in England, like at Bournemouth and Ventnor on the Isle of Wight are just handsome old sanatoria, but the recently built sanatoria in England are models of architecture.

The sanatoria at Northwood, Frimley and Pinewood are splendid examples of this recent style, though the new King's Sanatorium at Midhurst will easily surpass them all. The King's Sanatorium has now been building three years and will be building two years more before ready for the reception of a single patient. It will cost when finished $1,000,000.

Despite the amount of money that is being put into the King's, Northwood, Frimley and Pinewood, which are not far from it, have only half their quota of patients. Northwood has accommodation for 120 and has about 68 with Frimley and Pinewood in the same plight. The reason for this is not that they have not sufficient patients to fill these sanatoria, but they have not sufficient maintenance to run them. Looking at them one cannot help comparing the American and the English way of building sanatoria.

Saranac Lake Sanatorium was begun by one patient in a shack, the buildings increasing as patients and money increased. White Haven Sanatorium began with three or four patients in a barn, and has gradually grown till it accommodates 166 and practically always has a waiting list. In the case of the King's a million dollars is standing idle while the sanatorium is being built and during the same period no patients are being treated.

We find it sufficiently difficult in this country to get maintenance for our hospitals, yet we never dream of building new parts until the old parts are overcrowded. It is rare, therefore, in America to find empty wards. Throughout England it is the common finding. There is scarcely a hospital in London (none that I personally know of) with its quota of patients. In Brompton and the City of London Hospital, whole wards are vacant.

In the United States we bring our donors in and show them wards overcrowded to the last degree as an inducement for further donations. In England they use just the opposite argument, namely, an empty ward completely equipped crying out as it were for patients to fill it.

Throughout England they insist on fresh air to even a greater extent than we do in this country, possibly on account of all the vacant space they have. In the charity sanatoria it is common to find the largest wards containing only three and four beds.

In the public sanatoria in Germany the wards are a little more crowded, though even there they allow a little more space than we usually do in the United States.

In the public sanatoria in England they endeavor to make the patient do a certain amount of work, especially light gardening, etc., but from my talks with the residents I was inclined to believe this work was more in name than in actuality.

Except in Brehmer's the theoretical ideas in regard to work are about the same all over Europe, namely, rest while there is elevation of the temperature or of the pulse and graduated exercise afterwards.

In many of the sanatoria elaborate douche rooms are found. This is especially true of the sanatoria in Germany, all of which whether private or public are furnished with douche rooms.

The douche rooms at Falkenstein, at Hohenhonnef and Rompler's fell into disuse years ago, though the douche room at Brehmer's is still in action. The douche room in Brehmer's is a common room in the basement with an extremely strong douche falling from a distance of about 12 feet above the patient's head. The douche is manipulated from a room absolutely separate and unconnected with the douche room and with the patient's chart before him the physician regulates the strength and duration of the douche.

Despite the fact that the majority of the private sanatoria in Germany have given up douches the recent public sanatoria have installed the most elaborate douche rooms that I have ever seen. The story of these douche rooms is usually similar to that at Belzig.

Belzig is an elaborate half charity sanatorium about 14 miles from Berlin where they charge about five dollars a week. It has three departments, one for males, one for females and one for children. The two former were opened about six years ago; the last about a year ago. Each of the three departments contains its own elaborate marble-tiled douche room, magnificently equipped with every kind of douche known to modern medicine. Everything about the room is beautifully nickel plated and one could only imagine it a room in a very luxurious and well patronized Turkish bath. I asked the resident how much use was made of these rooms and he said though hé had been there three years he had never seen them used once. In other words despite the fact that the first two rooms had never been used they had recently built the same sort of a douché room in the new children's department.

True, in Germany they possess the ideal way of supporting public sanatoria, namely through the insurance companies and krankenkasse. These insurance companies take in all the people in the State especially working people. Every working man and every working woman must be insured, not only against death but also against disability from sickness or other cause, the employer paying the insurance. When a person falls ill, therefore, the insurance company stands behind to support him. Moreover, many of these public sanatoria have been built entirely or in part by the insurance companies, and money was not spared in the building or equipment. This is true of the sanatorium at Beelitz.

The sanatorium at Beelitz is so complete that it is doubtful if any sanatorium will ever be built to surpass it. It has 600 beds; 300 for tuberculosis and 300 for general constitutional diseases like chronic rheumatism, nervous disease, etc. The two departments are quite widely separated from one another and the males and females are also separated in each department.

The absolute completeness of everything at Beelitz is shown by their elaborate wash rooms. There is a wash room at both ends of each floor. These rooms are handsomely tiled and contain the most improved modern marble wash-basins with all their appurtenances. In addition there are a dozen of places (as many as there are wash basins) in the middle of the room for washing the teeth. These places are separated one from another by zinc enamelled partitions and contain a self-washing porcelain basin somewhat similar to our dentist's basin with a spigot eighteen inches above. The arrangement is ideal though undoubtedly very expensive. Our dentist's basin costs forty dollars; it is impossible to imagine what all their elaborate system would come to.

Each of the four departments of Beelitz has its own elaborate douche room more elaborate and more beautifully equipped and according to the statement of the resident as rarely used as those at Belzig. In other words because Brehmer advocated douches forty years ago, they are still installing douche rooms even where they do not believe in them.

The details of the equipment of Beelitz that are out of the common would necessitate more time than can be devoted to them in one evening. Not a few of these elaborate details are superfluous, yet there is an excuse for Beelitz which does not exist for the elaborate sanatoria in other countries especially England. In the first place all the public sanatoria in Germany are magnificently maintained so that there is no feeling that more money should have been put into maintenance; secondly, Beelitz itself was built by the People's Insurance Company (the Landesversicherung) which found itself in the position where a certain amount of money had to be gotten rid of or it would probably go elsewhere.

The Berlin branch of the Landesversicherung had a surplus of something over thirteen million marks when the idea arose that sanatoria should be built by the insurance companies. Since practically every city and state was to have its own sanatorium, the Berlin branch feared that unless all this money was used some of it would go to other places, consequently instead of seeing for how little they could build a sanatorium they were obliged to try to get rid of the thirteen million marks or something over three million dollars. They have put into Beelitz Sanatorium this whole sum.

In all the sanatoria of Europe they insist on good nourishment, though the details of the nourishment differ somewhat. In most places they simply supply six meals a day, three substantial ones, and three lighter ones, the latter usually composed of milk and raw eggs.

There is practically no insistence on altitude or climate. The recent sanatoria over the continent are at all degrees of elevation and the very handsomest and most elaborate are not elevated at all, at least not more than will give them a free sweep of the country more on account of the view than any other reason.

Sea-coast, too, appears to make no difference in their minds. The older English sanatoria like Ventnor and Bournemouth are on the sea-coast, the more recent ones in the country near the large cities.

In France where the adult sanatoria are all recent the great majority are on the sea-coast. In Germany they have taken no pains but to put them near the large cities, the handsomest ones that I saw, namely Buch, Belzig, and Beelitz being built on the level without view of any kind (except their own landscape gardening) just outside of Berlin.

I found no special methods of treatment. As in this country, in some sanatoria they use tuberculin freely, in others not at all. Many of the sanatoria show very handsome and splendidly equipped inhalation rooms. On inquiry in the private sanatoria I found that creosote was the most common medicament inhaled. I asked if they thought they derived any benefit from it and they answered that they did not except whatever mental impression it had on the patient. In the public sanatoria like Beelitz these inhalation rooms are not used at all.

Everywhere throughout Europe the house sputum cup was of china shaped like a shaving mug with a removable depressed cuspidor top, and the outside cup a Detweiler blue glass pocket cup, open at one end by a spring top and at the other by a screw top. The germicide usually used was lysol; in one or two places they still used carbolic acid and in one, Bournemouth, they were still using bichloride of mercury. Only two claimed to have made a study of the best germicide for sputum, namely, Ventnor and Hohenhonnef: in both these places they were using caustic potash. I mention this with a certain amount of pride since at the Phipps Institute in Philadelphia we have always used caustic potash in the form of lye. I would like to add also that I never before came in close contact with the Detweiler pocket sputum cup and I was not impressed by it. Even with the utmost care the top and bottom loosen in a short time allowing the sputum to continually contaminate the pocket and, therefore, also the hands.

Hospitals for advanced cases serve the purpose of the prevention of tuberculosis by removing the case in its most contagious period and so preventing it acting as a further focus of contagion in the home. The cases ordinarily seen in these hospitals are from among the poor. Such cases may live in a helpless condition six months or a year or even longer. During this period the tubercle bacilli appear more virulent and the wage-earner or housekeeper is not only taken from the family but extra work is thrown on the others in the household by the nursing and care of the invalid. Moreover, among the poor it is not uncommon to find a dying case sleeping in the dining room or the living room in order that unnecessary steps may be saved the attendant.

The usefulness of a hospital for advanced cases is, therefore, evident. Special hospitals for advanced cases are found in all the countries of Europe but the best known are in England. Among those I might mention the Royal Hospital for Diseases of the Chest founded in 1814, Brompton Hospital founded in 1841, the City of London Hospital founded in 1848, North London Hospital, etc.

It is a remarkable fact that London, the largest and one of the most crowded cities in the world, has the lowest death rate from tuberculosis, and it appears to me that this can be accounted for only by the fact that London has had for so many years hospitals for advanced cases.

There is another very important purpose served by the hospital for advanced cases, namely, the better instruction of physicians by means of the autopsies. Brompton Hospital, for instance, has 190 autopsies a year and the others in London a corresponding number. In some ways the physician, especially the conservative physician, is lagging behind the layman in the crusade against tuberculosis. The autopsy table of the hospital for advanced cases is, therefore, an urgent need.

The only special hospital for advanced cases of tuberculosis that I saw in Berlin was the Invalidenheim. This is as yet only an experiment, accommodating a small number of cases, but the need for such hospitals is recognized and they expect to proceed further with them. The general hospitals, however, of Berlin and Paris have special wards for consumptives, thereby deriving the benefit of the special hospital. In this country we have driven the advanced consumptive out of the general hospital and except in one or two cities have given him nothing in return.

The most modern machine in the fight against tuberculosis and one that stands in the foremost ranks on account of its power of controlling the tuberculosis situation, is the tuberculosis dispensary. The dispensary of the past saw and treated its case and thought no more about it till it returned; the modern tuberculosis dispensary follows the case to its home and endeavors to control the situation throughout the household.

As Calmette says: " The physician in the tuberculosis dispensary must act very differently to the physician in an ordinary dispensary. In the ordinary dispensary the physician examines the patient and gives him a prescription; he pays little or no attention to the lodgings, resources, the best mode of assistance or the environment of the patient. Such an attitude was all right fifty years ago when the powers of resistance and the care of the patient were not well understood, when it was not known that further spread of the disease could be accomplished, when the disease was thought a dispensation of Providence and could not be prevented by human means; but with the progress of science, with the knowledge of the cause of diseases and how to prevent them, the duty of the physician has been very distinctly broadened. He must not only cure the disease in the patient but he must prevent its extension further. He must not only treat the patient but he must coöperate actively with public charity, he must teach families how to live, advise mothers on the proper raising of their children, decide on the salubrity of lodgings, etc., so that taking all in all his rôle as educator becomes more important than that of examining physician." In ancient mythology Apollo was regarded as the god of medicine and as the announcer of death, the tuberculosis dispensary of to-day would make him also the preventer of disease.

There are two names especially notable in the foundation of the tuberculosis dispensary, namely, Phillips of Edinburgh and Calmette of Lille in France. The tuberculosis dispensary at Lille, or as it is called by Calmette the preventorium, was founded in 1901. According to Calmette's own account the preventorium is not merely to diagnose the case and distribute medicine to the poor but to investigate and draw under control cases affected with tuberculosis; to give these cases sufficiently often or over a sufficiently long time whatever care they need; to properly advise them and their family; to give them when they are obliged to stop work proper nourishment, clothes, bedding, spit cups and germicides; to make their lodging hygienic; to insist on frequent cleansing and disinfection; to procure for them when necessary a more hygienic lodging; to gratuitously wash their linen in order to avoid contagion in their family and elsewhere; to see that private benefaction is properly expended and to obtain succor for the patient in every way.

In the preventorium at Lille when the patient comes in he is sent to a bath room and while he is taking a bath his clothing is disinfected. The patient then comes to the physician for examination. This examination is very complete both as regards the condition of the patient and the details of his ocupation and general environment. If the patient has tuberculosis or the disease is suspected he is given directions how to live in order to recover and in order to prevent infecting other people. He is also given a pocket spit-cup, a house spit-cup and a liter of a 2% solution of lysol with very definite instructions how to use it. A day or two later a nurse is sent to the house to get in touch with the rest of the family, explain to them how the patient ought to live in order to get well, and how they ought to live in order to prevent infection.

If the apartments are not suitable she advises change; if the patient is not in a position to obtain sufficient nourishment she reports it and the dispensary helps him out. The dispensary supplies milk, eggs, meat, coal, and sometimes lodging. In addition it takes care of all the patient's laundry in order to make sure that it is frequently washed and to avoid the possibility of infecting the laundress. It is considered that no matter how careful the patient is it is practically imposible to avoid contamination of his clothes, thus leaving him a menace to himself and others. Printed pamphlets are also given to the patient insisting among other things on moist, not dry, sweeping.

Calmette says: " Such a preventorium should be installed in one of the populous quarters of the town. It is in no way a menace to the neighborhood, in fact it is much less dangerous than the ordinary dispensary or charity organization quarters where diseases of all kinds are seen and where sufficiently vigorous measures are lacking to avoid dissemination of germs of all kinds. Such a preventorium can be created and supported by private benefaction, by beneficial societies, by charitable societies or by cities themselves."

Calmette's statistics on the general cost of such a dispensary is about 30 cents per day per patient. In 1904, 287 families were thus assisted at a cost of $5,400.

Throughout Paris they have opened up three or four dispensaries on the order of the one at Lille. I personally visited only one of these, namely Beaujon Dispensary. This imitates Lille very closely, and probably the only thing worthy of particular mention about it is the fact that its expenses are entirely borne by one enthusiastic young woman of 23 who, though possessing no means herself, collects the money for this dispensary yearly. Practically the only support given in the Beaujon Dispensary at present is in the form of meat, and since ordinary meats are quite expensive in Paris patients are supplied when necessary with 100 g. of horse meat daily. As at Lille, however, the physician follows the patient into the home and insists on proper discipline and proper precautionary measures.

Though practically founded in France the tuberculosis dispensary appears to have had its greatest development in Germany. Berlin has three or four of these preventoriums which prepossess one as most thorough in their work. In Germany they are called Fürsorgestelle.

In my opinion Berlin has the best control of the tuberculosis situation of any city in the world. It has three very handsome and very large sanatoria, four tuberculosis dispensaries, three park convalescent camps and various societies which aid in the prevention of tuberculosis.

Considerable of this magnificent control is due to Prof. Pannewitz. The head of the dispensary system in Berlin is Dr. Puetter who was brought to Berlin from Halle for this purpose on account of his success in Halle. The park convalescent camps are the result of the earnest work of Dr. Becher encouraged and assisted by Prof. Pannewitz.

I was especially prepossessed by the general economy especially of the physician's time in the Berlin Fürsorgestelle. The system was about as follows: There were three connecting rooms; in the first the patient waited his turn, in the second were two or three nurses who took the histories, and in the third the physician made the examination. The nurses took the complete history of the patient not only relative to his occupation and home surroundings but even in relation to his previous diseases, his present symptoms, etc.

In both France and Germany the history sheets are models that might be imitated everywhere. The German one appears to me especially complete.

After the nurse has gotten the complete history the patient again waits his turn and goes into the doctor for examination. The examination was more or less perfunctory and not very detailed. In other words the Fürsorgestelle cater more to the treatment of the patient and the further prevention of the disease than to the study of the individual case. The physician decided only that the patient had tuberculosis, the general stage of advance and the probable prognosis. After the examination the patient was sent home without treatment and a day or two later the nurse visited the house and investigated the home conditions as to destitution, surroundings, etc. If the patient were suitable from the standpoint of destitution the patient and his whole family returned to the dispensary on another day. Each member of the family or of the household was examined and all instructed how to take care of themselves either to cure or prevent the condition. If the house or apartments in which they lived were unsuitable they were not only encouraged to seek other quarters but it was insisted on. A member of the family was at once sent out to seek these quarters and when found the nurse decided on their suitability. If these quarters were more expensive than the old ones and the patient could not afford to pay the extra price the dispensary paid the difference between the old and new lodgings.

If the patient or patients were extremely early cases and could continue their occupation while recovering they were allowed to do so. If the family income was insufficient to procure proper nourishment, proper nourishment was supplied by the dispensary. If the case was more advanced but still curable it was sent to a sanatorium. If the patient was quite advanced but could be handled at home the patient was encouraged to go daily to a day camp and particular attention in the way of prevention was paid to the rest of the family. If the patient was very advanced and the surrounding circumstances were unfavorable to his remaining at home he was sent to the Invalidenheim.

The control of the tuberculosis situation in Berlin is complete on account of all the different institutions working in harmony. It thus happened that if a patient could not be controlled in one way he could be controlled in another. Each part of this magnificent system was controlled by its special men yet all parts worked together so as to control the situation.

In these dispensaries the nurses did very good and very intelligent work. I sat for hours in these dispensaries listening to different nurses extracting histories from patients and it seemed to me that they did it quite as well as a physician. I am remarking this side of it on account of the general economy of this method and the large number of cases that the physician is thereby enabled to see.

The nurse visited the home of the patient once a week, or once every two weeks, in order to see that the instructions were being properly carried out. The patient visits the dispensary, if a curable case, about once a month and, if incurable, even less frequently.

Another very good thing which originated in Berlin is the park convalescent camp (Walderholungsstätte). I visited these in company with their founder, Dr. Becher. The principal one is at the edge of the Grünewald or Green Forest, eight miles from the centre of the city. It consists of a rather pretty Queen Anne cottage one story high with a little distance from it a long rough kiosk, the whole surrounded by about an acre of ground enclosed by a wire fence. The cottage contains quite a large kitchen from which can be fed two hundred people at a time. The dining room is furnished with rather rough benches and tables and seats about sixty.

This camp is intended for patients too advanced for sanatorium treatment but capable of caring for themselves at home, and for patients who are forced to stay at home from work on account of temporary indisposition.

The patient comes here early in the morning, between 8 and 10 o'clock, and remains till between 4 and 6 o'clock in the afternoon. The kiosk is furnished with steamer chairs giving the patient an opportunity to sit out all day in company with others. The camp supplies the mid-day meal at the nominal sum of seven cents and gives the patient free of charge a pint of milk at 10 a. m. and at 3 p. m. This scheme works very much better in Germany than in the United States. In the first place the meals and the milk are supplied by the insurance companies, in the second place the railroads give the patients special rates, for instance, the ordinary charge to Grünewald by train is eight cents, railroad working men and patients for the camp pay only two cents. Moreover, the street cars and omnibuses give special rates of seventy-five cents a month for an unlimited number of rides in both directions.

These camps are undoubtedly good for several reasons: (1) They give the patient what he needs, namely, plenty of fresh air, and they encourage him to take it by the companionship of those about him. (2) They give him the nourishment necessary and teach him what nourishment he should take. (3) They keep him away from his own apartments and, therefore, his family for a considerable part of the twenty-four hours. (4) They encourage methods of prevention by insisting on the practice of those methods at the camp.

These park convalescent camps are managed by a nurse and two or three kitchen women. The camp supplies the necessary blankets and the general comforts. With the city contributing the ground near one of its parks such a camp can be installed for about $1500 to $2000 initial expense, and kept up for probably $60 per month, provided the meals are paid for. Any physician in town is entitled to send his patients to these camps. The patient is not treated at the camp and so remains entirely under the control of his home physician. The patients have the privilege of resting all day or walking about through the woods depending on the directions of their physician.

My principal object in visiting Berlin was to study the convalescent camp with the idea of starting one in Philadelphia. I was not as much prepossessed as I expected to be; yet I thought them a very good adjunct in the crusade. Anything tending to educate the patient or remind him of the care he should constantly take cannot help but be serviceable.

From experience I have learned how soon patients forget their teaching, even when it has been instilled by months of routine in a sanatorium. One day a month spent in a convalescent camp would I believe keep the patients on the *qui vive*, consequently the usefulness of the camps is apparent.

The fifth thing in the crusade against tuberculosis is the tuberculosis society composed of physicians and lay people, the principal object of which is the education of the people in the prevention of the disease. The oldest society in the world with this main object is the Pennsylvania Society for the Prevention of Tuberculosis founded in 1892. Though the United States possesses the oldest society of this kind in the world, the Europeans have developed it in a way that might easily make us blush. In New York and Chicago the Anti-Tuberculosis Society is developing along the lines popularized in Europe, but even they are not yet far advanced. In Europe they have combined with the Anti-Tuberculosis Society every other society, no matter what the general object, which might in any way aid the crusade against tuberculosis. Boards of Health, Charity Organization Societies, Children's Aid Societies, Day Nurseries, Labor Unions, Workingmen's Beneficial Associations, Civic Betterment Societies, Tenement House Societies, City Park Societies, Anti-Dust Societies, Temperance or Total Abstinence Societies, are all brought in to aid the cause.

What was learned from the Congress and the investigation of the tuberculosis work in Europe?

(1) That although the sanatoria in the United States are

probably accomplishing better results in individual cases, we have not a sufficient number of sanatoria. Germany with only two-thirds our population, not one-tenth our area and not one-twentieth our wealth has more sanatoria and is spending three times the amount of money on them.

(2) We are not using all the means that might be employed to build and maintain sanatoria, like insurance companies, beneficial societies, etc.

(3) We are lacking in hospitals for advanced cases, and until we get them, wards in general hospitals should be set aside for the care of the tuberculous. Such wards in addition

to caring for the consumptive will help in the education of the general physician, the residents, the nurses and the patients.

(4) The tuberculosis dispensary as managed in France or in Germany is the most important element in the crusade against tuberculosis and we are woefully lacking in them. A city the size of Philadelphia should have at least half a dozen, and it has one. Baltimore should have three or four and it has one. Such dispensaries might be supported as follows: One by the city (as in New York City), one by charity, and one by a combination of beneficial societies.

MOSES MAIMONIDES.[1]

(*In Memoriam 1205-1905 C. E.*)

By David Israel Macht.

Though the subject of this paper is rather out of the ordinary and the atmosphere into which I wish to introduce you an unfamiliar and foreign one, I think it hardly necessary to beg for gracious indulgence and respectful attention from an audience such as is here assembled.

The most superficial student of Semitic literature and history cannot fail to be impressed by the general ignorance prevailing on these subjects, even among the most cultured, and to this the field of medicine is no exception. To the average western student of medicine the history of his noble art begins with the Greeks, and then, with one vast stride, passes directly to the achievements of the modern English, French, and German physician; all the rest is considered of no importance. The work of other peoples, the contributions of other races are usually overlooked, sometimes ignored, and often, what is worst of all, misrepresented. Anyone who makes at all a study of the subject meets now and again with many and many a false inference, and unwarranted conclusion, a misstatement with regard to some work or personality, based on nothing more substantial than a few paltry quotations and those not in the original, but translated, and drawn by those who condemn what they do not understand.

Of Maimonides, the subject of this paper, the following is the note made by Osaibya, a distinguished Arabic physician and historian.

"He, Abu Amram Musa ben Maimuni, was a man deeply versed in the sciences and philosophy, who both in theoretical and practical medicine held the foremost place among the physicians of his time."

Of the same Maimonides, a modern English authority writes: "At his death, the grief at the loss of the 'Light of the Age,' was universal in East as well as in the West, and he has been recognized universally as one of the noblest and grandest men of all times, gifted with the most powerful and brilliant qualities of mind, possessed of the most varied and astounding knowledge." (Chambers' Encyclopædia.)

[1] Read before the Johns Hopkins Hospital Historical Club, December 11, 1905.

But recently, the seven hundredth anniversary of Maimonides' death was celebrated by Jews the world over: How many in this assembly have even heard of his name? And yet, the field of medicine is supposed to be the most universal, the most cosmopolitan of all the arts and sciences! This fact is perhaps sufficient apology for the following humble sketch.

Moses Maimonides, or as he is more commonly known among the Jews, from the initial consonants of his name (*Rabbi Moses Ben Maimon*) *Rambam*, the greatest Jewish philosopher of modern times, a pre-eminent religious authority, a proficient mathematician, and, according to Arabic historians, one of the most prominent physicians of his time, was born in the city of Cordova, Spain, on the 14th day of the Hebrew month Nissan (30th of March) 1135 C. E. His father, a pupil of the then famous Joseph ibn Migash, was quite a learned man, and could trace his descent from the House of King David. He early took cognizance of his young son's precocity and brightness of intellect, and endeavored to give him that most precious of wealth, which is the ideal of every Jewish parent, a complete and thorough, all-round education. Maimonides imbibed his early knowledge in the cities of Cordova and Lucena. His father himself taught him the Torah (Bible) and Talmud; from the Arabs, who dominated Spain at that time, he learned mathematics, astronomy, philosophy, the natural sciences, and especially the science and art of medicine.

The peaceful life of the Maimuni family was early disturbed by the Almohades, a wild tribe of Arabs from North Africa who captured Cordova in 1148, and offered to both Christians and Jews the choice of either Islam, or death. The Maimuni family preferred to emigrate.

After quite a long period of wandering life in Christian Spain, they at last made their abode in the city of Fez, in 1159. Here, the worthy Caliph Abdelmummen was not so zealous in his religious persecutions. He contented himself with requiring the outward observance of some Moslem customs only; with the private life and practices of his subjects he did not directly interfere. The Maimuni family remained here for some years, the young Maimonides all this time, in spite of their wanderings and tribulations, being deeply engrossed in his studies. It was at this time that he published the first of his great works, the Pirush Ha-mishniyoth, Commentary to the Mishna, the legal portion of Talmud. This work, though primarily a religious one, is of interest to us as containing quite a considerable amount of medical matter especially on anatomy and hygiene.

The precarious life of practicing their religion in secret was not to the taste of the Maimuni family. This and the martyrdom of the revered Rabbi Yehuda Hakohen of Fez prompted them again to grasp the wanderer's staff. They took ship for Acco, Palestine, in 1165 C. E., where after a very stormy and perilous voyage they at length landed. So great was their joy that the date of their landing remained a day of thanksgiving in the family for years to come. Their wanderings, however, were still not over. Lack of sustenance made life even in the Holy Land, an impossibility, and it was only in Egypt in the city of Fostat, or old Cairo, that they at length found a permanent home.

It is in Fostat that Maimonides' greatest work was done and his fame established. His path to glory, however, was not bestrewn with roses. More troubles were at hand. His father died soon after their coming; then two children; and, closely following, his elder brother David, the support of the family and his best friend suffered ship-wreck, lost his whole fortune, and was himself drowned. Rambam's only consolation was in his work and faith. He now rapidly gained renown. As a Jew he became chief Rabbi of Kahira, an eminent position spiritually, though of no value as far as remuneration was concerned. Socially, he made rapid strides in his medical profession, and was soon at the head of his compeers. The poet and kadhi, Alsaid Ibn-Sina Almulk wrote of him:

Galen's art heals only the body,
But Abu Amram's (Maimonides') the body and soul;
With his wisdom he could heal the sickness of ignorance.
If the moon would but submit to his art,
He would deliver her of her spots at the time of full moon,
Cure her of the periodic defects,
And at the time of her conjunction save her from waning.

He gained the favor of the vizier Alfadhel and through him came to the notice of that remarkable romantic figure, standing out so conspicuously in the history of the Middle Ages—The Sultan Saladin Jussuf ben Ajuh, or as he is commonly known, Saladin. Saladin appointed Maimonides his court physican, a position which Rambam retained the rest of his life, under both Saladin and his successor Alfadhel. This assured him his living so that he could devote more time to his studies and works. That his hands were full at this time there can be no doubt. In a letter to one of his pupils, R. Juda Ibn Tibbon—a letter which has become a classic in modern Hebrew literature, and is quoted in almost every Jewish history—he gives us the following glimpse at his life:

" With respect to your wish to come here to me, I cannot but say how greatly your visit would delight me, for I truly long to communicate with you and would anticipate our meeting with even greater joy than you. Yet I must advise you not to expose yourself to the perils of the voyage, for beyond seeing me, and my doing all I could to honor you, you would not derive any advantage from your visit. Do not expect to be able to confer with me on any scientific subject for even one hour either by day or by night; for the following is my daily occupation: I dwell in Mizr (Fostat) and the Sultan resides at Kahiro; those two places are two Sabbath days' journeys (one and a half miles) distant from each other. My duties to the Sultan are very heavy. I am obliged to visit him every day, early in the morning and when he, or any of his children, or any of the inmates of his harem are indisposed, I dare not quit Kahira, but must stay during the greater part of the day in the palace. It also frequently happens that one or two of the officers fall sick and I must attend to their healing. Hence, as a rule, I repair to Kahira very early in the day and even if nothing unusual happens I do not return to Mizr until the afternoon. Then I am almost dying with hunger. I find the antechambers filled with people, both Jews and Gentiles, nobles and common people, judges and bailiffs, friends and foes—a mixed multitude who await the time of my return. I dismount from my animal, wash my hands, go forth to my patients, and entreat them to bear with me while I partake of some light refreshment, the only meal I take in twenty-four hours. Then I go forth to attend to my patients, write prescriptions and directions for their several ailments. Patients go in and out until night-fall, and sometimes even, I solemnly assure you, until two hours and more in the night. I converse with them, and prescribe for them, while lying down from sheer fatigue; and when night falls I am so exhausted that I can scarcely speak. In consequence of this, no Israelite can have any private interview with me, except on Sabbath Day. On that day the whole congregation, or at least, the majority come unto me after the morning service when I instruct them as to their proceedings during the whole week; we stay together a little until noon, when they depart. Some of them return and read with me after the afternoon service until evening prayers. In this manner I spend that day. I have here related to you only a part of what you would see if you were to visit me."

With all this, he found time to write a number of medical works, as we shall see, and published his great religious work, the Mishna Torah, a complete code of Jewish law, and his greatest philosophical treatise—the Moreh Nebuchim or " Guide of the Perplexed,"—a work which has ever since remained famous and was even then admired by the Christian scholars, Thomas Aquinas and Albertus Magnus. Certainly of him we could not quote the lines from Chaucer:

Nowher so bisy a man as he ther was,
And yet he semed bisier than he was.
—Prologue, ll. 321-2.

It was at this time that Maimonides received an invitation from King Richard, the Lion-Hearted, the soul of the Third Crusade, to become his physician in ordinary; but Rambam declined. Those who have read Scott's charming little novel, " The Talisman," will perhaps recollect that author's descrip-

tion of the Arabic physician Al Hakim, whom Saladin is supposed to have sent to cure Richard. It is more than possible
that this character was suggested by Maimonides.

Maimonides lived to the age of sixty-nine. Hard work, sympathy for his brethren, the victims of the inhuman persecutions of the Dark Ages, and personal misfortunes hastened his
death, which took place on the 20th day of the Hebrew month
Teves (Dec. 13) 1204 C. E. A public mourning was pro-
claimed by both Jews and Gentiles; and he was buried with
honors in the city of Tiberias.

The works of Maimonides fall into three categories: (1)
Religious. (2) Philosophical. (3) Medical.

Though it is with his medical works that we are here chiefly
concerned we cannot give a fair estimate of Maimonides as a
physician without a brief reference to some of his other writings; for after all, a great man's work, whether it be in the
domain of speculative philosophy or in the field of inductive
science, is bound to reflect his personality. Maimonides' aim
in life was first and above all to be true unto himself—to be a
perfect, consistent Jew, in the highest and noblest sense of
the word. He early recognized the utter futility of the attempt to eradicate indelible differences by forsaking the Torah
or Sacred Law, in an effort to promote the universal brother-
hood of men, but thought it rather much better to further that
purpose, by each one proving true unto himself, and acting
his part well. And so he remained loyal to his colors; he
staunchly clung to what he regarded as Truth; and he tried
to do his best in the world by living up to the Law. He sa-
credly observed his Sabbath, strictly followed the Jewish dietary laws, scrupulously carried out every religious and moral
injunction of his people, and all his vast store of philosophical
and scientific information went but to strengthen his faith.

It is, therefore, not surprising to find his great religious
work Mishna Torah (or Code of Jewish Law), his most important philosophical treatise the "Moreh Nebuchim" or
"Guide for the Perplexed," and many of his other works—replete with much useful information on physics, mathematics,
astronomy, anatomy and especially hygiene. In his Hilchoth
Deoth, a part of the afore-mentioned Mishnah Torah, Maimonides builds up a system of ethics, and no small part of
that work is devoted to the consideration of one's duties to his
body—the care of health. Far ahead of the monastic and as-
cetic tendencies of his age, which saw a special virtue in destroying flesh by burdening the body with chains of iron, he
boldly asserts that a healthy soul requires a healthy temple to
dwell in, or as he puts it—a perfect body is an essential to the
proper serving of God. Together with the injunctions to love
vur neighbors as ourselves, to curb pride, to love the stranger,
widow, and orphan, and to practice humility and charity, he
admonishes us to take care of our health, avoid excesses, to
regulate our diet and sleep. The Biblical verse, "He that
guardeth his mouth and tongue, keepeth his Soul from distress" (Prov. XXI, 23), he interprets literally as well as spiritually: "He that taketh care of what he eateth and drinketh
will keep his soul from distress." Indeed in his Ethics, Rambam gives us a pretty complete system of practical hygiene,

so modern in tone that it could well compare with the most
recent text-books on the subject. He goes minutely into the
dietary; discusses the relative values of various foods; the effects of the summer and winter seasons; the care of bowels;
the importance of proper sleep and exercise. He dwells on
the subjects of clothing and hydrotherapy. *Lack of exercise,
over-eating, alcohol,* and *sexual excesses,* he summarizes, are
responsible for the cause of most diseases. Any disturbance
in the excretory functions of the body will lead to pathological conditions. He concludes with the assurance that any
one attending to the simple advice given will be pretty sure
of maintaining good health, *unless* his condition has already
been undermined (1) by disease; (2) by some herditary taint
cr defect, or (3) by "Exposure to the scourge of some epidemic."

In Chapter XXIII he mentions the ten réquisites for any
town to be fit to dwell in: (1) a proficient physician, (2) a
proficient surgeon, (3) proper bathing facilities, (4) proper
sewerage, (5) a fresh water supply, (6) a place of worship,
(7) a proper school, (8) a scribe or notary public, (9) a court
of justice, (10) a charity organization.

Of Maimonides' strictly medical works there exists quite a
collection, though many of them are either in Arabic or Hebrew, with a few translations in Latin, Spanish, and German.

The following is a pretty exhaustive list (Cf. Bodleian
Catalogue). I have arranged them under five headings:

I. *Expositions of and Commentaries on older authorities.*
    1. Firké Mosheh (Aphorisms.)
    2. Commentary on Hippocrates.
    3. Compend of Galen.
    4. Translation of Avicenna.
II. *Works on Hygiene.*
    1. De Regimine Sanitatis.
    2. Notes on Dietetics for Saladin.
    3. The Ethics of Maimonides (above mentioned).
    4. Consultation on Various Accidents.
III. *Works of Physiological Character.*
    1. On Foods.
    2. On medicaments.
    3. Sefer Hassamim or Toxicology.
IV. *Works on Special Subjects.*
    1. On Hemorrhoids.
    2. On Gout (Podagra).
    3. On sexual relations.
    4. On asthma.
    5. Sefer Refuoth.
    6. On psychology, etc.
V. *De Causis et Indiciis Morborum.*

The Firké Mosheh is a book of aphorisms from the older
writers Hippocrates, Galen, Al-Razi, the Hebrew physician
Ebn Zohar, or as he is more commonly known Avenzoar, and
others. It consists of 25 sections or chapters, and was originally written in Arabic and later translated into Hebrew and
Latin. The following are the subjects treated of, as far as I
could learn from the Hebrew translation.

To go more minutely into his treatment of the subjects would take too long.

De Regimine Sanitatis is a "Makrobiotic," or Book on Hygiene written by Maimonides at the instigation of Sultan Alafdal, successor of Saladin. The same was a sickly man and asked Maimonides to write him some rules of life. Maimonides promptly responded with wholesome, though perhaps not very flattering and agreeable advice. Quoting from Hippocrates he boldly tells the profligate monarch that we preserve our health in proportion to our abstinence from over-eating and other excesses. "For the preservation of health and length of days," he goes on further, "above all, moral purity and spiritual activity are necessary; whereas a loose life will bring one quickly to his grave. One must, therefore, strive to attain to perfect self-control. But it is only those that draw their moral strength from philosophy and religion, that can attain to such a state." He then gives the Sultan various medical advice, prescribes a dietary and medicine and concludes with the prayer: "May the health and strength of the Sultan be prolonged as it is the wish of his humble servant Moses ben Maimon."

Of the third group of works, the Sefer Hassamin or Maimonides' Work on Poisons is perhaps the best known. A German translation with notes by Steinschneider is found in Virchow's Archiv, Vol. LVII. Maimonides was led to write the book at the request of the Sultan on account of the unusual number of cases of bites by poisonous animals occurring at that time. The book is of considerable interest on account of the large amount of exceedingly practical and useful information it contains.

The first part treats of the bites of poisonous animals, and the treatment in such cases, both general and specific. The second part speaks of "internal poisonings," prophylaxis and antidotes. The advice, as Hæser says, is throughout very appropriate. Maimonides speaks of the prevention of the spread of the poison from an infected wound by prompt ligation of the member, by suction of the wound with lips previously anointed with oil, etc. He mentions various specifics and discusses antidotes and emetics. He then takes up the poisonings by particular animals, such as scorpions, snakes, mad dogs, etc.; the bites of man; and again by various poisonous plants, such as hyoscyamus, mandragora, cantharides, various mushrooms and toadstools, etc. The book was very popular. Originally written in Arabic, it was translated into Hebrew, and later under the title "De Venenis" by Amergau and Blasius into Latin.

In the Sefer Refuoth, Maimonides discusses affections of the stomach, tumor of the brain, affection of the meninges, etc.

Of his work on gout, I do not know much beyond the fact that it was written in Arabic and translated into Spanish by Abu Amam ben Abdallah of Cordova.

In forming a critical estimate of Maimonides' position in the history of medicine, we must class him with the so-called Arabic school, and yet, there are differences between him and other members of that group, which give him a distinct and eminent place by himself.

In the first place he is a rationalist, and is bitterly opposed to astrology and other occult arts in which the Arabs were so fond of dabbling. "The eyes look forward and not backward," he tells us in one of his letters; and so, he would never prescribe a remedy which he did not either test himself or receive from some good authority. The use of amulets and incantations he considered an abomination, though he conceded their possible effect as placebos, in pacifying the spirits of the simple-minded. A quack he calls a murderer. Imbued with a pure faith and clear intellect he spurns superstitions and accepts naught which has no solid foundation. In one of his epistles to the Jews of Marseilles in regard to astrology, he gives his views on the subject:

"Know, my Lords, that man ought to believe only one of three things—firstly, something which he can clearly grasp through pure reason, as, for instance, the science of arithmetic or geometry or astronomy; secondly, something which he can perceive with one of his five senses, as, for instance, when he sees, or tastes, or hears; and thirdly, something which he learns from the prophets and sages of blessed memory.

"And a man that has common sense, ought to sift and classify, both in thinking and reasoning, those things which he regards as true and those which he does not, and he should say unto himself, I believe this to be true because I perceive it through my senses, or I believe this to be true through pure reason; or I believe this to be true because I have been told so by the prophets and sages, but he who believes a thing which does not fall under any of these three classes of him it is said: 'The simple believeth everything.' (Prov. XIV.)

"You should also bear in mind that there are fools who have

composed thousands of books, and that many 'great men'—
great in years, but not in wisdom—have spent their days in
the study of them, and these conceited stupids imagine that
these books contain great wisdom; and so their hearts become
elated, and they think that they are great wise men because
they know that wisdom, and it is just in this wherein most, if
not all, the world is in error, with the exception of the few."

In the second place, Maimonides, unlike his contemporaries
who revelled in vague and mysterious concoctions of multitudinous drugs was, far ahead of his time, a great opponent of
poly-pharmacy, and a warm advocate of the Nature-cure. On
this subject he gives us some definite views:

"Now most physicians are greatly in error," says he, "in
that they think that medicine strengthens the health; it weakens and perverts it; and for this reason hath Aristotle said that
most of the patients who die, do so through the medicine of the
physicians. When the interference of the physician is indicated, his task should be (merely) to sustain the strength of
the patient and to promote Nature in its effort at repair.
Most physicians, however, act wrongly and while they think
they help Nature, they hinder it, and destroy its beneficent activity." On reading this passage, we cannot help recalling Dr.
Treves' latest utterances on the nature of disease.

In the third place, Maimonides, far in advance of his age,
seems to have taken the modern standpoint of looking at disease from the *etiological* or *causal* point of view. It is a great
pity that his most important work, the "Sefer Hassiboth"
or "De Causis et Indiciis Morborum" has never yet been
published, but is in manuscript form in Oxford and Paris;
for, as Dr. Alfred Nossig remarks (Die Socialhygiene der
Juden, 1899) :

"The very manner in which he undertakes his task in this
his greatest work, the very fact that seven hundred years before the medicine of to-day, he already looks upon diseases
from the etiological point of view, his search for the *causes*
of sickness—point to the man's keen intellect, and explain,
why he was regarded as such a great physician and rose to
such fame."

But, as a historian (Grætz) remarks, "It was not only his
wide and deep knowledge and his fame as a physician, but his
character which constituted Maimonides' distinction. He was
a perfect sage, in the most beautiful and venerable sense of
the word." Well-digested knowledge, calm deliberation, mature conviction, and mighty performance, were harmoniously
blended in him. He was possessed of the deepest and most
refined sense of religion, of the most conscientious morality,
of philosophical wisdom and of the keenest scientific insight;
or rather, these various elements, which are generally hostile
to each other, had in him come to a complete reconciliation.
That which he recognized as truth was to him inviolable law;
from it he never lapsed for a moment, but sought to realize it
by his actions throughout his whole life, unconcerned as to
the disadvantages that might accrue. "From the point of
view of learning, he occupied the first place of his time, in religion and morality he was rivaled by but few of his compeers,
but in his strongly marked individuality he surpassed all his

contemporaries. His actions corresponded to his mind. Maimonides was imbued with a most profound earnestness which
considered life not as an opportunity for pleasure or gain, but
as a serious mission to labor nobly and to confirm by deeds the
great truth, that man is an image of God.

"The mean, the false, and the impure were abhorred by
him, and were not permitted to approach him."

Maimonides gave the world the Jewish ideal of a physician!
And we may all profit by his example.

Perhaps I may appropriately conclude this sketch with a
translation of an invocation which he is said to have repeated
daily before turning to his day's work :

And now, I turn unto my calling;
Oh, stand by me, my God, in this truly important task!
Grant me success! For—
Without Thy loving counsel and support,
Man can avail but naught.
Inspire me with true love for this my art
And for Thy crea-tures,
Oh, grant—
That neither greed for gain, nor thirst for fame, nor vain
    ambition,
May interfere with my activity.
For these, I know, are enemies of Truth and Love of men,
And might beguile one in profession,
From furthering the welfare of Thy creatures.
Oh, strengthen me!
Grant energy unto both body and the soul,
That I may e'er unhindered ready be
To mitigate the woes,
Sustain and help,
The rich and poor, the good and bad, the enemy and friend,
Oh, let me e'er behold in the afflicted and the suffering,
Only the human being!

Balto. Kislev 8 (Dec. 6) 5666.

תם ונשלם שבח לאל בורא :עולם

BIBLIOGRAPHY.

1. Chambers' Encyclopedia: Maimonides.
2. Encyclopædia Britaannica: Maimonides.
3. Jewish Encyclopædia: Maimonides.
4. Maimonides: Works.
5. Dr. Richard Landau: Geschichte der Jüdischen Aerzte.
(Berlin, 1895 C. E.).
6. C. Cannoly: Histoire des Médecins Juifs.
7. Grætz: History of the Jews, Vol. III.
8. S. M. Dubnoff: Istoria Yévreieff (Odessa 1901 C. E.).
9. Hæser: Geschichte der Medizin, Vol. II.
10. Yellin and Abrahams: "Maimonides."
11. Dr. J Münz: "Jüdische Aerzte in Mittelalter."
12. Dr. J. Münz: "Maimonides als Medizinische Autori-
tät. (Berlin, 1895 C. E.).
13. Dr. Alferd Nossig: "Die Socialhygiene der Juden,
1899.
14. Virchow's Archiv. Vol. 52 (Toxicologische Schifte der
Araben von M. Steinschweider).
15. Virchow's Archiv. Vol. 57. (Gifte und ihre Heilung
des Maimon. von M. Steinschneider).

16. Rabbinowitz, J. M.: "Traité des Poisons de Maimonides." (Delahaye 1867-8).

17. Macht, David I.: "Iggereth Rambam." Jewish Comment 1903, C. E., Vol. XVII, No. 9.

18. Friedländer: "The Guide of the Perplexed" of Maimonides.

19. Rosin: Die Ethik des Maimonides.

20. Hilchoth Deoth (The Ethics of M.) by R. S. Sofer. New York, 1899.

21. Scott, Sir Walter: "The Talisman."

22. Kaiserling, Dr. M.: Allg. Zeitung des Juden, 1863 (M.'s prayer).

23. Orient: 1898, p. 341.

24. Kerem Chemed III, p. 15.

25. Treves, F.: British Med. Journal, Nov. 11, 1905, C. E.

OBSERVATIONS UPON PAROXYSMAL TACHYCARDIA.

By Arthur D. Hirschfelder, M. D.

(From the Medical Service of the Johns Hopkins Hospital.)

In 1903 August Hofmann (1) called attention to the fact that during an attack of paroxysmal tachycardia the pulse rate was exactly or nearly double that present between attacks. This observation has been confirmed in the articles of D. Gerhardt (2), Lommel (3), Rihl (4), Hofmann's second article (5), and more recently Hewlett (6); and as no exceptions have been reported, it is probable that tachycardia, due to sudden doubling of the pulse rate, may be considered a disease entity as definite as Stokes Adam's disease.

The following theories have been advanced to explain this sudden doubling of the heart rate: 1. The theory originally advanced by August Hofmann (1) that owing to some increase in irritability of the heart or to the sudden occurrence of extra stimuli, each regular systole was followed by an extrasystole which occurred exactly in the middle of the interval between the two regular systoles. This view was adhered to by Gerhardt and Lommel, and tracings were given by them showing the occurrence of occasional small systoles midway between regular systoles during the periods between attacks. It was assumed that these were extrasystoles, probably ventricular in origin—the interpolated ventricular extrasystoles of Hering (7) and Rihl (8); but no venous tracings have furnished any evidence in support of this view.

2. James Mackenzie (9) assumes that the tachycardia is due to a prolonged series of ventricular extrasystoles, replacing the regular rhythm. He states that short series of such extrasystoles are not uncommon and calls attention to the fact that the venous tracing in his cases always shows the ventricular type of venous pulse during the attack. This is further borne out by the tracing obtained by Hofmann during an attack, and also by the tracing in the case to be reported below.

Against this view are the facts that in the tachycardia the rate is always doubled; that in most of these cases there is during the attack other signs of tricuspid insufficiency (dyspnœa, enlargement of liver during the attack, œdema of angles, etc.), which would in itself account for the occurrence of a ventricular type of venous pulse. Further, the absence of proof that such short series of ventricular extrasystoles do occur in these cases. Lastly, the tracings of Rihl, and Hof-

man, and in our own case to be reported below, indicating that in some cases at least the tachycardia has its origin above the ventricle, in either the auricle or the sinus.

3. August Hofmann, in his second paper (5), called attention not only to a sudden doubling of the pulse rate, e. g., from 60 to 120 per minute, but sometimes to a further doubling, e. g. from 120 to 240, both changes occurring suddenly without a transitional increase in rate. Subsidence of the tachycardia also occurred by halving of the pulse rate equally sudden. These sudden changes and the 2 : 1 ratio of the pulse rates caused him to suggest that the heart responded to all the impulses arising at the sinus only during the periods of tachycardia; that between attacks, owing to a diminution in conductivity, which he referred to the sino-auricular region, auricles and ventricles responded to only alternate or sometimes only every fourth impulse from the sinus. The latter condition he thought might be due to depression of conductivity in two places, as suggested by v. Kries (10) to explain such successive responses to gradually diminishing conductivity.

4. J. Rhil (4) has given an excellent venous tracing taken during an attack of paroxysmal tachycardia in which each ventricular contraction was preceded by an auricular contraction, and in which, between attacks, the venous pulse showed that the auricle continued to beat at twice the rate of the ventricle (namely, at about the same rate as during the attack); in other words, that there was a partial heart block at the auriculo-ventricular bundle of His. Hofmann (5) also cites one of his cases as showing a similar condition between attacks.

These two cases are somewhat against the third view (Hofmann's) as to the site of the block, indicating that in them, at least, it is at the auriculo-ventricular junction rather than above it.

However, as yet the number of cases in which venous tracings have been given, and hence in which we have any information regarding the contractions of the auricles, is too small to allow of generalities; and it is largely with a view to adding further material for comparison that our own case is reported. For the privilege of doing so, I wish to express my thanks to Prof. L. F. Barker, in whose wards the case ' occurred.

Patient G. D. R., General No. 53,892, Medical No. 19,360, aged 72, American, proprietor of a hotel in North Carolina. Admitted February 22, 1906, complaining of palpitation of the heart. Family history and past history negative, has always been healthy and has had no infectious diseases whatever, and no other cardiac manifestations.

The first attack of palpitation came on suddenly after ' retiring one evening twenty years ago, causing him great fear but no pain. It lasted six hours and left him weak but otherwise well. Attacks similar in character recurred once every month or so until the last winter (1905-06) since when they have occurred once or twice a week, and have been somewhat more severe than before, sometimes lasting ten hours. During the attacks he passes large amounts of urine. He never notices palpitation between attacks.

P. E. Patient is a large, well nourished man. He does not look especially ill. Color good. Pupils equal and react to light and during accommodation. Thorax barrel-shaped. Angulus Ludovici prominent. Left upper front more prominent than right. Costal angle over 100°. Expansion slight. Chest moves as a whole. Percussion note hyperresonant 'in front, normal behind. Breath sounds distant but clear.

Heart impulse not seen nor felt. Heart sounds best heard in fifth left interspace 11 cm. from midsternal line. Dulness extends 4 cm. beyond this point to nipple line. Relative cardiac dulness begins above the third rib, and cannot be made out to the right of the sternum. Heart sounds at apex distant but apparently clear; second sound louder than right. At base sounds are very distant, no murmur, even when patient sits up. Pulse 64 per minute, regular in force and rhythm; good volume and tension. Vessel wall sclerotic. Blood pressure between attacks. Maximum, 165-190; minimum, 100-115.

Abdomen large and flabby, considerable panniculus. Relative hepatic dulness begins at fifth interspace, absolute hepatic dulness at sixth interspace and reaches to costal margin. Liver and spleen not felt. *Genitalia* appear normal. *Extremities*—shins smooth; knee kicks present; no ankle or patellar clonus. Small venules distended in inner side of left thigh. Large, mottled, brownish areas on inner side of each knee. Plantar response normal.

History while in hospital.—On February 23 and March 1, patient had attacks of tachycardia, the pulse rate suddenly rising from 80-88 to 160 per minute, respiration remaining 20 per minute throughout; no enlargement of liver, no œdema. During the attacks he has a feeling of terror and weakness, but on the whole he thinks himself better than before admission.

On March 15, patient had two attacks, the first beginning suddenly at 7 a. m., just after returning to bed from going to the closet, where he passed a soft, fluid stool without effort. Tracings were made from over the jugular vein and carotid and brachial arteries during this attack (Figs. 1-3), which lasted until 10 a. m., when patient yawned and the attack

suddenly subsided, the pulse rate falling from 152 to 80 or 88 per minute. Venous tracings made during the attacks showed venous pulse of the ventricular type, with no presystolic auricular notch (Figs. 2-3). The blood pressure during attack was maximum 130, minimum 95-100. Tracings made immediately afterward (Figs. 4-5) showed a definite venous pulse of the auricular type identical in rate and form with the tracings obtained at other times between attacks (Fig. 7). There is no sign whatever of a wave midway between the two auricular waves a-a such as might correspond with the persistence of rapid rhythm in the auricles after slowing of the ventricles as found by Hofmann (5) and Rihl (l. c.). On the contrary, although such an auricular contraction would occur before the tricuspid valves have opened (i. e., before the wave v), hence would give a larger wave on the venous pulse than does the normal auricular contraction (c. f. Rihl) (11), the absence of any such wave enables one to be quite certain that no abnormal auricular contraction has taken place. The auricular rate had fallen to half the rate as well as that of the ventricles. This is exactly opposite to what occurred in the cases of Hofmann and Rihl.

At noon patient was shown at the medical clinic, which caused him much annoyance, and he was brought back to the ward about 1 p. m. About 3.10 p. m. a second attack of palpitation began suddenly and lasted till 7.30 p. m., pulse rate (140 to 160) and pulse form being exactly as in the first attack. Pressure on the vagus in front of the sterno cleido mastoid, digitalin 1.5 mg. hypo., spiritus ætheris nitrosi by mouth, pressure on abdomen, and deep breathing were all without effect, as had been the application of an ice-bag to the heart on previous occasions. Yawning which had stopped the first attack was tried (voluntarily), but although one beat was dropped in the arterial pulse on one attempt, and on another a small beat produced between two large ones (Figs. 9-10), no change was otherwise manifest in either the rhythm or the force of the ventricles; and the attack was not (Figs. 9-10) aborted. It ceased spontaneously with sudden halving of the rate at 7.30 p. m., and no irregular beats occurred after cessation of the attack.

On March 21, the patient's pulse was somewhat irregular, as shown on tracings (Figs. 11, 12, 13). Unfortunately the Jacquet chronograph was at this time not available and measurements had to be made in millimeters of the smoked paper, the average pulse rate being 76 per minute. However, the drum, as shown during several months of use, when controlled by the chronograph, moved with great regularity, and these measurements therefore represent time relations almost as accurately as though the chronograph had been used.

It will be noticed on these tracings that many of the pulse intervals cover but 7-8 mm., while next to them are intervals of 12-15 mm., almost exactly double; which would correspond with the theory of Hofmann, that the heart in the long intervals was omitting a response to one stimulus. Here again, however, there is no sign of a wave midway between the auricular waves a, a; and for the reasons given above it may be assumed that the auricular contraction also is omitted.

These interspersed long and short beats with a time relation of 2 : 1 are not the only beats present, numerous others covering 10-12 mm. being also seen, and the relation of these latter to the irregular beats is $7 + 15 = 2 \times 11$ (systole + extrasystole = twice regular pulse interval), indicating that these represent the regular rhythm and the others auricular extrasystoles. On the other hand, this "regular" interval is sufficiently close to the prolonged period to represent extrasystoles arising at the sino-auricular junction (cf. Engelmann (12)).

This form of irregularity, with the appearance of some beats at half the usual interval, seems to be a very common one in cases of paroxysmal tachycardia, as it frequently occurs also in the cases of Hofmann, Gerhardt, Lommel, and Hewlett (l. c.). Unfortunately these authors (except Hofmann) give no venous tracings which alone would show the contractions of the auricles, and furnish a clew to the mechanism of the irregularity. Hewlett's radial tracings also show an occasional 3 : 1 interval; but as this also appears on the brachial tracings from our case, when the venous tracings (Figs. 12-13) show that one ventricular contraction had occurred but had not been forcible enough to force open the aortic valves, it is not unlikely that in his case the apparent 3 : 1 interval is made up of one 2 : 1 + one 1 : 1 interval.

The prevalence of the 2 : 1 relation in all the conditions between attacks, as well as in the ratio between the normal pulse rate and that during the attack, is further evidence in favor of Hofmann's theory that the periods between attacks are due to dropping of alternate auricular impulses. Our own case, in which the auricles did not continue to beat at the tachycardia rate after the ventricular rate had become slow, and in which even during the period of interspersed long and short beats, the auricle still kept the same rhythm as the ventricle gives evidence that such a block could not be at the auriculo-ventricular bundle as in the cases of Hofmann and Rihl, but would have to be at the sino-auricular junction. This is more in accordance with Hofmann's own theory than was his own case, which was really against it.

But in our own case the question of the origin of the beats occurring at intervals of 10-12 mm., i. e., entirely out of the 2 : 1 relation remains to be explained, and it is quite possible that this stage of irregularity bears no relation at all to the tachycardia, although at best it indicates a somewhat increased irritability of the auricle; and favors the view that the auricle would take part in originating or transmitting a series of rapid beats.

As to the experimental evidence bearing upon Hofmann's theory, there are some facts of considerable interest: Bayliss and Starling (13) and later Rihl (l. c.) showed that if induction shocks were thrown into the auricle too rapidly for it to follow, it responded only to alternate beats. As shown by MacWilliam (14) this depends upon the intensity as well as upon the frequency of the stimulus, and in experiments which I have performed I have been able to confirm this observation for rhythmic stimuli as well as for single stimuli.

If the auricle is responding to only alternate induction shocks at a rapid rate, an increase in the intensity of the shocks without change in rate may cause it to respond to all of them. The ventricle may or may not respond to all the contractions of the auricle, the number of dropped beats depending largely upon the degree of asphyxia, as shown by Hering and Rihl (l. c.). I have been able to obtain exactly the same results when the electrodes (fish hooks with all but tips insulated) are applied to the sinus instead of the auricles. If, moreover, the irritability of the auricle be increased as by pouring on hot physiological salt solution, while it is responding only to alternate stimuli, it may suddenly double its rate and respond to every stimulus; or may reach this doubled rate gradually after a series of beats in which some are responses to successive and some to alternate stimuli (Figs. 14-15). When the hot salt solution is discontinued the half rate is resumed either suddenly or gradually after a similar transition.

This represents exactly the condition suggested by Hofmann as underlying the attack of paroxysmal tachycardia, although the block is here a purely functional one. Similar functional blocks have been shown by Bayliss and Starling and also by Rihl to be brought on or removed by nerve influence. For example, if rapid rhythmic shocks are thrown into the auricle, stimulation of the vagus may cause the ventricle to respond to only alternate auricular impulses instead of to all. Similarly when some of the ventricular beats are dropped, stimulation of the accelerators causes the ventricles to respond to all by improving the conductivity. Reid Hunt (15) has shown that a similar dropping of alternate ventricular beats in a large number of mammals occurs during vagus stimulation or during periods of increased vagus tone. In these animals, the period of vagus inhibition corresponds to the periods between attacks in the patient with paroxysmal tachycardia (at least in the patients of Hofmann and Rihl), while the normal animal corresponds to the patient during the attack. Another fact common to them is that the systolic pressure during the periods of vagus tone, as between the attacks, is higher than during the periods of rapid pulse rate.

It is quite probable that just as the vagus may produce a partial block from auricle to ventricle, it may also diminish the conductivity from sinus to auricle, as shown in the frog by Engelmann (l. c.) and Gaskell (16), and in the dog by Knoll (17), although no such 2 : 1 ratio has been produced here experimentally. Nevertheless this is only a question of degree.

Reid Hunt (l. c.) was able to demonstrate that accelerator stimulation could also produce temporary slowing of the ventricles due to the rapid rate of the auricles which the ventricles could not follow at first. This was followed by sudden doubling of the pulse rate due to the improved conductivity, the ventricle then responding to all the auricular contractions.

Naturally, it was of interest to determine in our case whether the doubling of the rate was due to loss of vagus tone, or whether some other influence was necessary. The

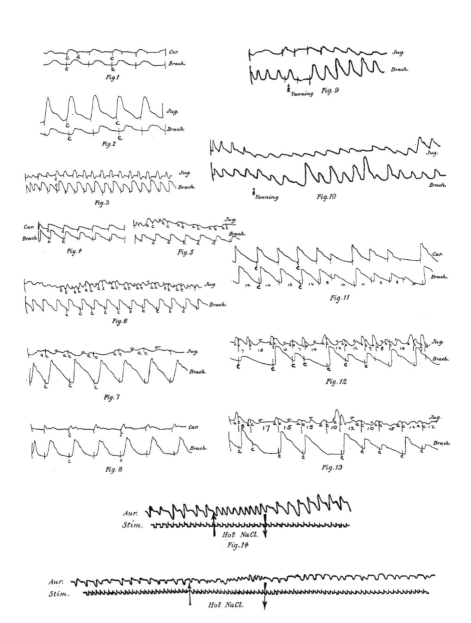

Fig.1

Fig.2

Fig.3

Fig.4

Fig.5

Fig.6

Fig.7

Fig.8

Fig.9

Fig.10

Fig.11

Fig.12

Fig.13

Fig.14

latter is evidently true; for on March 22 and March 23 the patient was given 2 mg. atropin within two hours, and although his mouth was dry and his pupils slightly dilated, and he felt quite weak and giddy, none the less the pulse rate remained at 76 per minute, unchanged by the atropin. On March 23, while under the influence of the atropin, he was made to walk about the ward, which caused him a considerable effort. Nevertheless there was only a momentary and gradual rise of pulse rate to 96, from which it fell to 76 before a record could be made. He was then made to perform vigorous arm exercises while in bed with a similar result. Fig. 7 shows the venous pulse taken immediately after the exercise, the rate having already fallen back to 76. None of the tracings made at this time show any abnormal auricular contractions.

On March 24, patient was made to inhale two pearls of amyl nitrite, and although his systolic pressure fell from 200 mm. to 170 mm., his face flushed and he complained of heat and throbbing, nevertheless the pulse rate remained at 76.

Both the atropin and the amyl nitrite must have removed the vagus from the field of action, and yet no change of pulse rate occurred. Evidently in this patient the normal vagus tone was very slight, which is not surprising in a man 72 years of age. But it is equally evident that the doubling of the heart rate is not due to loss of vagus tone.

Gerhardt (l. c.) has also shown that giving atropin to such a patient does not bring on an attack, although in his case there was a certain degree of vagus tone present, and the pulse rate quickened after atropin. Unfortunately, we have no means of determining clinically whether there is an increased action of the accelerators, nor have we any means of paralyzing the accelerators as we can the vagus. The rate of the accelerators in these cases must therefore remain a matter of conjecture, although the view put forward by Franze (18) that all heart neuroses, and among them paroxysmal tachycardia, are due to disturbed function of the sympathetic nerves, is rather alluring. For the present, this question must remain open.

On the other hand, practically all the means that have been used successfully to suppress the attacks—ice-bag to the heart, deep inspiration, pressure on the abdomen, galvanism to the vagus nerve in the neck, digitalin, pressure upon the vagus—depend for their efficacy upon the direct or reflex stimulation of the vagus. As might be expected from the uncertainty of their stimulating power, the results of these methods have been uncertain and variable. The one drug which exerts the purest and most certain action in stimulating the vagus, namely aconite, so far as I have been able to learn, has not been used.

Our patient had no further attacks from March 15 to his departure from the hospital on March 25, and as no other cases of paroxysmal tachycardia have been available, the use of this drug in small doses (five minims of the 1900 pharmacopœial tincture repeated once or twice at half hour intervals), can therefore only be suggested for the present.

REFERENCES.

1. Hofmann, August: "Ueber Herzjagen." Deutsches Archiv für klinische Medizin, 1903, Vol. 78, p. 39.

2. Gerhardt, D.: "Beitrag zur Lehre von den Extrasystolen." Deutsches Archiv für klinische Medizin, 1905, Vol. 82, p. 509.

3. Lommel, Felix: "Ueber anfallsweise auftretende Verdoppelung der Herzfrequenz." Deutsches Archiv für klinische Medizin, 1905, Vol. 82, p. 495.

4. Rihl, J.: "Analyse von fünf Fällen von Ueberleitungsstörungen." Zeitschrift für experimentelle Pathologic und Therapie (Berlin), 1905, Vol. 2, p. 83.

5. Hofmann, August: "Ueber Verdoppelung des Herzfrequenz." Zeitschrift für klinische Medizin (Berlin), 1904, Vol. 53, p. 206.

6. Hewlett, A. W.: "Doubling of the Cardiac Rhythm and its Relation to Paroxysmal Tachycardia." Journal of the American Medical Association (Chicago), 1906, p. 941.

7. Hering, H. E.: "Ergebnisse experimenteller und klinischer Untersuchungen ueber den Vorhofvenenpuls bei Extrasystolen." Zeitschrift für experimentelle Pathologie und Therapie (Berlin), 1905, Vol. 1, p. 26.

8. Rihl, J.: "Experimentelle Analyse des Venenpulses bei den durch Extrasystolen verursachten Undegelmässigkeiten des Säugetierherzens." Zeitschrift für experimentelle Pathologic und Therapie (Berlin), 1905, Vol. 1, p. 43.

9. Mackenzie, James: "On the Inception of the Rhythm of the Heart by the Ventricles." British Medical Journal (London), 1904, Vol. 1, p. 529; also, "New Methods in the Study of Affections of the Heart." Ibid, 1905, Vol. 1, p. 813.

10. v. Kries, J.: "Ueber eine Art polyrhythmischer Herzthätigkeit." Archiv für Anatomic und Physiologic. Physiologische Abtheilung (Leipzig), 1902, p. 477.

11. Rihl, J. (l. c.).

12. Engelmann, Th. W.: "Ueber den Ursprung der Herzbewegungen." Archiv für die gesammte Physiologic (Bonn), 1897, Vol. 65, p. 109.

13. Bayliss, W. M. and Starling, E. H.: "On Some Points in the Innervation of the Mammalian Heart." Journal of Physiology (Cambridge), 1892, Vol. 13, p. 407.

14. MacWilliam, J. A.: "On the Rhythm of the Mammalian Heart." Journal of Physiology (Cambridge), 1888, Vol. 9, p. 167.

15. Hunt, Reid: "Direct and Reflex Acceleration of the Mammalian Heart." American Journal of Physiology (Boston), 1899, Vol. 2, p. 395; also, "Experiments on the Relation of the Cardio-Inhibitory to the Accelerator Nerves in the Heart." Journal of Experimental Medicine, 1897, Vol. 2, p. 151.

Hunt, Reid and Harrington, D. W.: "Notes on the Physiology of the Cardiac Nerves in the Opossum." Ibid, 1897, Vol. 2, p. 711.

Hunt, Reid and Harrington, D. W.: "Note on the Physiology of the Cardiac Nerves of the Calf." Ibid, 1897, Vol. 2, p. 723.

16. Gaskell: Article on Innervation of the Heart in Schaefer's Physiology (MacMillan & Co., London), 1900.

17. Knoll, Philipp: "Ueber den Einfluss des Herzvagus auf die Zusammenziehungen der Vena Cava Superior beim Sängethier." Archiv für die gesammte Physiologie (Bonn), 1897, Vol. 68, p. 339.

18. Franze, P. C.: "Ueber Herzneurosen." Berliner Klinische Wochenschrift (Berlin), 1905, Vol. 42, p. 1111.

DESCRIPTION OF FIGURES.

Car. = Carotid pulse tracing.
Jug. = Pulsation over the right external jugular vein.
Brach. = Pulse tracing from cuff of Erlanger blood-pressure, apparatus, applied to upper arm at diastolic pressure.
c = Beginning of upstroke upon carotid pulse.
a = Beginning of auricular presystolic wave.
v = Crest of mid-diastolic wave (corresponding to opening of tricuspid valve), *i. e.*, the *vs* wave of Hering and Rihl (*l. c.*).
d = Dicrotic notch upon carotid tracing.
Lettering of figures is uniform throughout.

FIG. 1.—Carotid and brachial pulses taken simultaneously at 8.00 a. m., March 15, during attack. Pulse rate 140 per minute. Drum revolving at highest speed.
FIG. 2.—Jugular and brachial pulses taken simultaneously at 8.15 a. m., March 15, during the attack. Pulse rate 152. Drum at highest speed. Tracing shows jugular pulse exactly synchronous with carotid.

FIG. 3.—Same as Fig. 2, drum at slower speed. Tracing taken at 9.55 a. m., just before end of attack.
FIG. 4.—Carotid and brachial pulses at 10.00 a. m., Pulse rate 88.
FIG. 5.—Jugular and brachial pulses at 10.05 a. m., showing presystolic wave *a-c* not present in Fig. 3. Pulse rate 88.
FIG. 6.—Same at 10.20 a. m., showing the presystolic wave *a-c*. and the diastolic wave *v*. It is to be noted that there is no wave midway between *a* and *a*.
FIG. 7.—Jugular and brachial tracings made on March 23, at 3.00 p. m. Patient had received within two hours two doses of 1 mg. atropin hypo, and had just walked around the ward. The venous pulse is in every way identical with that obtained at other times between attacks.
FIG. 8.—Carotid and brachial pulses taken at same time as Fig. 7.
FIGS. 9 and 10.—Jugular and brachial tracings taken during the afternoon attack (March 15), showing the effect of voluntary yawning.
FIG. 11.—Carotid and brachial tracings, March 21. Figures indicate pulse interval in millimeters on the curve .15 mm. one sec. (approx.).
FIGS. 12 and 13.—Jugular and brachial tracings taken just after Fig. 11. Figures indicate the pulse interval (in millimeters).
FIG. 14.—Tracings from the auricle (Aur.) of a dog. Rhythmic induction shocks applied to the sinus venosus as shown by the electro-magnetic signal below (Stim.). Auricle responding to alternate stimuli. Between the arrow heads ↑ and ↓ hot 0.6 per cent. Na Cl is being poured over the auricle.
FIG. 15.—Same as Fig. 14, from another dog. Showing some beats responding to every stimulus, some only to alternate stimuli.

A SIMPLE METHOD FOR THE QUANTITATIVE DETERMINATION OF PROTEIDS IN MILK.

By THOS. R. BOGGS, M. D.,

Associate in Medicine, The Johns Hopkins University; Assistant Resident Physician, The Johns Hopkins Hospital.

(*From the Clinical Laboratory of the Johns Hopkins Hospital.*)

The increasing interest in the study of metabolism in infants, whether fed artificially or at the breast, has emphasized the need of some means of determining the proteids of milk, which is at the same time applicable by those with a minimal laboratory equipment and technical experience, and yet sufficiently accurate to be a basis for rational deductions.

The gravimetric and Kjeldahl nitrogen methods are out of the question for the busy practitioner, as they demand time and special laboratory facilities. A method was published by Woodward (Philadelphia M. J., 1898, Vol. 1) some time since based on the separation of fat by heat in the thermostat, the subsequent precipitation of the proteids with Esbach's solution and then centrifugalization in graduated tubes. This procedure requires a rather elaborate equipment and very constant conditions as to speed of centrifugalization, length of armature, etc., to secure uniform results, in addition to the fact that picric acid is not an ideal precipitant for milk proteids.

The method in common use is to estimate the total solids from the specific gravity, to determine the fat, and so arrive at the proteids by difference. The sugar is considered a constant factor, as are the salts.

Among other objections may be mentioned that the small lactometers or aerometers used are often very inaccurate. This is especially true in the analysis of human milk since the available material is small in amount.

The idea that Esbach's tube or some similar device might be adapted to this purpose was suggested to me by Dr. Slemons, and a series of experiments was undertaken to determine if this were practicable.

In the attempt to solve the difficulty a number of precipitants were tried and discarded for various reasons. Among others Esbach's solution, which gave a very coarsely flocculent precipitate. This did not settle evenly, often floated, and so rendered the readings valueless.

With mercuric nitrate the precipitate was finer but also tended to float after standing 10 to 14 hours, apparently from the development of tiny gas bubbles throughout the precipitate, which caused the whole to rise *en bloc* to the top of the tube.

Tannic acid gave an excellent, finely divided precipitate, but this contracted laterally as well as vertically, and regularly toppled over so as to render measurements inaccurate.

Finally an apparently ideal precipitant was found in phosphotungstic acid in hydrochloric acid solution. This substance precipitates instantly all the proteids in a finely divided condition. The precipitate contracts evenly in a vertical direction and reaches a constant minimum volume within twenty-four hours. The supernatant fluid is perfectly clear and gives no trace of proteid by any tests. The solution finally settled upon as the optimum is composed as follows:

Phosphotungstic acid, 25 grams; distilled water, 125 cc.

After thorough solution is obtained there is added:

Hydrochloric acid (conc.), 25 cc., diluted with distilled water, 100 cc.

This yields 250 cc. of a 10 per cent solution of phosphotungstic acid in about 3 per cent HCl. The solution is quite stable if kept in a dark bottle, and gives satisfactory results after months of standing. It is desirable that the components be mixed as indicated, i. e., the well diluted HCl added after solution of the phosphotungstic acid, in order to avoid precipitation.

Having found a satisfactory precipitant, a series of observations was made with human and cow's milk and with various artificial compounds of the latter used in infant feeding, in order to determine under what conditions of dilution, temperature, etc.; direct reading in percentage could be obtained. These readings were carefully controlled in every instance by Kjeldahl nitrogen determinations made in duplicate from the same specimens at the same time.

The milk samples were diluted with distilled water, using normal pipettes and flasks to secure the maximum accuracy. The Esbach's tubes of the standard patterns, reading from 1 to 7 grams per litre, were used. Those reading from 1 to 12 were found to be less uniform in calibration and gave unsatisfactory results.

The diluted milk is poured into the tube to the mark U, being careful to read from the bottom of the meniscus. The phosphotungstic acid solution is added to the mark R, the tube corked and slowly inverted 12 times to secure thorough mixing. Care being had to avoid shaking roughly and thus mixing air in the fluid. The tube is then placed in a rack for 24 hours and the percentage read off at the level of the top of the precipitate. Fractions of percent between the graduations are readily judged by the eye. At dilutions of one part in ten, percentage of proteid is read directly from the scale, while if the dilution be one in twenty we multiply the reading by two, if one in five we divide by two.

The optimum dilution for human milk is 1 in 10. That for cow's milk 1 in 20. If the proteid content be found extremely low we may use 1 in 5 for human milk and 1 in 10 for cow's milk.

As temperature has a definite influence on the volume of the precipitate it is desirable that the tubes be not exposed to extremes, although the differences noted in this precipitate were not nearly so great as when Esbach's solution was used.

No considerable variation was found in volume of precipitates, with temperatures ranging between 15°-25° C. (59°-77° F.), while in thermostat at 37° C. all floated, and in the ice-box at 5° C. (41° F.) all read appreciably higher than at room temperatures averaging 20° C. (68° F.).

The minimum volume of the precipitate is reached in twenty-four hours. Readings at thirty and forty-eight hours showed no appreciable variations.

The presence or absence of cream in the milk also seemed unimportant as far as the volume of the precipitate is concerned. Repeated observations on the same specimens of milk before and after separation of the cream yielded results which tallied precisely.

This observation on the natural milk was confirmed by results obtained from the analysis of artificial mixtures where the percentages of fat were very high in proportion to the proteids.

In a series of over 300 precipitations of various milks the results were surprisingly uniform, particularly in human milk when the mean difference from the Kjeldahl percentage was 0.2 per cent with an extreme of 0.5 per cent. With cow's milk, owing to a slightly coarser precipitate the variations were a trifle wider, mean 0.3 per cent, extreme, 0.7 per cent.

In order to secure accurate dilution of the small quantities of human milk available it is necessary to use accurate pipettes and flasks. A convenient outfit consists of a 2 cc. pipette graduated in one-tenths and a small standard flask of 20 cc. These may be obtained from the chemical supply houses at a cost of about fifty cents. With this apparatus in addition to the Esbach's tubes possessed by every practitioner, a satisfactory determination of the proteids may be made with 2 cc. of milk, giving a dilution of 1 in 10. As in any quantitative analysis it is essential that care be exercised in carrying out the details of the method if accurate results are to be obtained, particularly as the process is purely empirical. But five minutes work will suffice to give a good determination to be read off twenty-four hours later.

THE JOHNS HOPKINS UNIVERSITY.
MEDICAL DEPARTMENT.

THE HERTER LECTURES.

The third course of lectures on the Herter Foundation will be delivered by

SIR ALMROTH E. WRIGHT, M. D.,

late Professor of Pathology, Army Medical School, Netley, Pathologist to St. Mary's Hospital, London, on Monday, Tuesday and Wednesday, October 8, 9 and 10, 1906, at 4:30 p. m. in the auditorium of the Physiological Building, Johns Hopkins Medical School, Washington and Monument Streets.

The lectures will relate to the investigations of Sir A. E. Wright upon opsonins and bacterial vaccines.

You are cordially invited to attend these lectures.

IRA REMSEN, President.

NOTES ON NEW BOOKS.

Case Teaching in Medicine. A Series of Graduated Exercises in the Differential Diagnosis, Prognosis, and Treatment of Actual Cases of Disease. By RICHARD C. CABOT, A. B., M. D. 8vo. Cloth. Pp. x-214. *(Boston: D. C. Heath & Co., 1906.)*

The book, as indicated in the title, is a collection of case histories with questions and answers covering various points of diagnosis, prognosis, treatment, etc.

"To aid the teacher in training his pupils to think clearly, cogently, and sensibly about the data gathered by physical examination," is the object of the book, as stated in the preface.

The value of such a work has always seemed rather problematical, especially where actual cases are available for study. There is a strong tendency in such exercises toward too dogmatic and diagrammatic delineation of cases with not a little encouragement to a snap diagnosis. In not a few instances in the book under consideration the details of the case supplied seem very inadequate and hardly warrant the certainty of the diagnosis given.

To those, however, who employ this method of teaching, the book will prove interesting and furnish a number of good cases for discussion.

The Examination of the Function of the Intestines by Means of the Test-Diet. By PROF. DR. ADOLF SCHMIDT. Authorized Translation from the latest German Edition, by CHARLES D. AARON, M. D. With a frontispiece plate in colors. Crown octavo, 91 pages. *(Philadelphia: F. A. Davis Company, Publishers, 1906.)*

This little book is a presentation of the results of the researches of Adoph Schmidt and his pupils into changes of intestinal function as evidenced by the fæces. He properly emphasizes the necessity of a fixed uniform diet for comparable results.

Full details are given for the application of the method, and many useful diagnostic and natural therapeutic points are brought out.

The translation is comprehensive, though it lacks somewhat in smoothness.

International Clinics. A Quarterly of Illustrated Clinical Lectures and Especially Prepared Original Articles on Treatment, Medicine, Surgery, etc. By leading members of the Medical Profession throughout the world. Edited by A. O. J. KELLY, M. D., Philadelphia. Volume I. Sixteenth Series, 1906. *(Philadelphia and London: J. B. Lippincott Company, 1906.)*

The volume before us has sections upon Treatment, Medicine, Surgery, Obstetrics and Gynecology, and Pathology; also summaries of Medicine and Surgery during the year 1905. The summaries although not exhaustive are well done and fairly complete, and the lectures are presented in an interesting form and are valuable contributions to their respective branches of medicine.

Liverpool School of Tropical Medicine. Memoir XIX. Yellow Fever Prophylaxis in New Orleans in 1905. By ROBERT BOYCE, M. B., F. R. S. *(London: Published for the Committee of the Liverpool School of Tropical Medicine by Williams & Norgate, 1¼ Henrietta St., Covent Garden, April, 1906.)*

This memoir is a graphic and clear account of the measures which were taken last year to free New Orleans from yellow fever, written by a representative of the Liverpool School of Tropical Medicine, who had been sent to New Orleans to observe the epidemic. The object of Dr. Boyce is to "show what can

be done by a community without recourse to force in a mixed population and laboring under many other disadvantages," to destroy the *Stegomyia fasciata.* He further says, "The practicability of the systematic extermination of the Stegomyia will also in my opinion pave the way to a far more determined and scientific effort to get rid of the malaria-bearing Anopheles, towards which, unfortunately, a large section of mankind seems to have grown tolerant and apathetic, although it is now known to be the greatest cause of the hindrance to progress in the tropics." The book deserves to be widely read.

An Introduction to the Study of Materia Medica and Pharmacology, Including the Elements of Medical Pharmacy, Prescription Writing, Medical Latin, Toxicology, and Methods of Local Treatment. For the Use of Students of Medicine and Pharmacy. By OLIVER T. OSBORNE, A. M., M. D., Professor of Materia Medica, Therapeutics, and Clinical Medicine in Yale University. *(Philadelphia and New York: Lea Brothers & Co., Publishers, 1906.)*

The name of the author of this little volume serves to stamp it as a book in which one may look for a great deal of practical information. The object of the book is " to introduce the student to the study of Materia Medica and Pharmacology." So well has it been done that even the busy physician will find it somewhat useful to have it close at hand.

The sections on Treatment of Poisoning and Special Treatments contain some very valuable information for easy reference, while the sections on Prescription Writing, Dosage, and Weights and Measures, will be found exceptionally valuable to the students of Medicine and Pharmacy. The method of grouping the Pharmacopœial preparations is excellent, but the usefulness of the book would have been increased by giving a full list of the preparations.

J. L. W.

Progressive Medicine. A Quarterly Digest of Advances, Discoveries, and Improvements in the Medical and Surgical Sciences. Edited by HOBART AMORY HARE, M. D., Professor of Therapeutics and Material Medica in the Jefferson Medical College of Philadelphia, etc., assisted by H. R. M. LANDIS, M. D. Volume I. March, 1906. Surgery of the Head, Neck, and Thorax, Infectious Diseases, Pneumonia and Influenza, Diseases of Children, Rhinology, and Laryngology, Otology. *(Philadelphia and New York: Lea Brothers & Co., 1906.)*

Reference has been made to this valuable digest of medical and surgical advances and discoveries in previous issues of the BULLETIN, and little remains to be said, except to add that the present volume seems fully equal to any of its predecessors. We are interested to notice that Dr. Frazier speaks with commendable plainness upon the passing of the tendency to do craniectomies upon idiot children. The section upon trigiminal neuralgia by the same author is presented clearly and with discrimination. Dr. Preble gives an excellent résumé of the present condition of our knowledge of infectious diseases; Dr. Crandall speaks of infant foods and infant feeding; Dr. Kyle treats of laryngology and Dr. Randall of otology. The letter press and illustrations are good. A few mis-spelled names are noted as McCullom for McCollum, Wimie for Winnie, Le Garde for La Garde.

The Morphology of Normal and Pathological Blood. By GEORGE A. BUCKMASTER, D. M. (Oxon.) University College, London, *(Philadelphia: P. Blakiston's Son & Co., 1906.)*

The subject matter of this volume is divided into a series of lectures which discuss in turn: (1) The various improved methods and results of calculating the blood mass; (2) erythrocytes and their structure; (3) hæmolysis within the body; (4) the origin of the different white cells; (5) the significance of leucocytosis and the various types; (6) blood platelets; (7) the more recent delicate tests for detecting blood; and concludes with a lecture on the morphology of pathological blood. The book is progressive and contains a fairly complete abstract of the various results obtained in the fields discussed. Where the author has not performed original work, a resume of the results of the better known investigators sets forth the latest conclusions. The treatment of pathological blood is too brief to do the subject credit, and in some instances rather radical statements are made which are not always borne out by clinical experience, but the book is stimulating and a distinct contribution to the study of the blood.

BOOKS RECEIVED.

International Clinics. A Quarterly of Illustrated Clinical Lectures and Especially Prepared Original Articles. By Leading Members of the Medical Profession Throughout the World. Edited by A. O. J. Kelly, A. M., M. D., Philadelphia. Volume I. Sixteenth Series, 1906. 8vo. 309 pages. J. B. Lippincott Company, Philadelphia.

Scientific Memoirs. (*New Series.*) *No. 22.* By Officers of the Medical and Sanitary Departments of the Government of India. *Mediterranean Fever in India: Isolation of the Micrococcus Melitensis.* By Captain George Lamb, M. D., I. M. S., and Assistant Surgeon M. Kesara Pai, M. B., C. M. (Madras). 1906. Fol. 22 pages. Office of the Superintendent of Government Printing, India.

On Carbohydrate Metabolism. (A Course of Advanced Lectures in Physiology delivered at the University of London, May, 1905). With an Appendix on the Assimilation of Carbohydrate into Proteid and Fat, Followed by the Fundamental Principles, and the Treatment, of Diabetes Dialectically Discussed. By F. W. Pavy, M. D., LL. D., F. R. S. 1906. 8vo. 138 pages. J. and A. Churchill, London.

Scientific Memoirs. (*New Series.*) *No. 21.* By Officers of the Medical and Sanitary Departments of the Government of India. *On the Standardisation of Anti-Typhoid Vaccine.* By Captain George Lamb, M. D., I. M. S., and Captain W. B. C. Forster, M. B., D. P. H., I. M. S. 1905. Fol. 15 pages. Office of the Superintendent of Government Printing, India.

Infection, Immunity, and Serum Therapy. In Relation to the Infectious Diseases which Attack Man; with Considerations of the Allied Subjects of Agglutination, Precipitation, Hemolysis, etc. By H. T. Ricketts, M. D. 1906. 12mo. 599 pages. American Medical Association Press, Chicago.

Twenty-ninth Annual Report of the Board of Health of the State of New Jersey, 1905, and Annual Report of the Bureau of Vital Statistics. 8vo. 1906. 396 pages. Trenton, New Jersey.

Die Placentation beim Menschen. Von J. Clarence Webster. Ins Deutsche Übersetzt von Dr. Gustav Kolischer, Chicago, Mitt 18 Abbildungen im Text und 27 Tafeln. 1906. Fol. 84 pages. Verlag von Oscar Coblentz, Berlin. W. T. Keener & Co., Chicago.

A Compend of Operative Gynecology. Based on Lectures in the Course of Operative Gynecology on the Cadaver at the New York Post-Graduate Medical School and Hospital. Delivered by William Seaman Bainbridge, M. D. Compiled, with Additional Notes, in Collaboration with Harold D. Meeker, M. D. 1906. 12mo. 66 pages. The Grafton Press, New York.

The Practitioner's Library. The Practice of Pediatrics. In Original Contributions by American and English Authors. Edited by Walter Lester Carr, A. M., M. D. Illustrated with 199 engravings and 32 full-page plates. 1906. 8vo. 1014 pages. Lea Brothers & Co., Philadelphia and New York.

International Clinics. A Quarterly of Illustrated Clinical Lectures and Especially Prepared Articles. By Leading Members of the Medical Profession Throughout the World. Edited by A. O. J. Kelly, A. M., M. D. Volume II. Sixteenth Series. 1906. 8vo. 302 pages. J. B. Lippincott Company, Philadelphia and London.

Surgical Suggestions. Practical Brevities in Diagnosis and Treatment. By Walter M. Brickner, M. D., and Eli Moschcowitz, M. D. 1906. 16mo. 58 pages. Surgery Publishing Company, New York.

The Morphology of Normal and Pathological Blood. By George A. Buckmaster, D. M. (Oxon.) 1906. 8vo. 244 pages. P. Blakiston's Son & Co., Philadelphia.

Physiology of the Nervous System. By J. P. Morat. Authorized English edition translated and edited by H. W. Syers, M. A., M. D. (Canlab.). With 263 illustrations (66 in colours). 1906. 4vo. 680 pages. W. T. Keener & Co., Chicago.

Materia Medica and Therapeutics. An Introduction to the Rational Treatment of Disease. By J. Mitchell Bruce, M. A., LL. D. (Hon.), Aberd., M. D. Lond. New and enlarged edition, revised throughout, and containing the Indian and Colonial Addendum to the British Pharmacopœia. 1906. 16vo. 632 pages. W. T. Keener & Co., Chicago.

A Manual of Medical Treatment or Clinical Therapeutics. By I. Burney Yeo, M. D., F. R. C. P. Fourteenth edition. Two volumes. 1906. 12mo. W. T. Keener & Co., Chicago.

Case Teaching in Medicine. A Series of Graduated Exercises in the Differential Diagnosis, Prognosis, and Treatment of Actual Cases of Disease. By Richard C. Cabot, A. B., M. D. (Harvard). 1906. 8vo. 214 pages. D. C. Heath & Co., Boston.

The Medical Diseases of Infancy and Childhood. With Points on the Anatomy, Physiology, and Hygiene Peculiar to the Developing Period. By Alfred Cleveland Cotton, A. M., M. D. 1906. 8vo. 670 pages. J. B. Lippincott Company, Philadelphia and London.

Transactions of the Medical Society of London. Volume the twenty-eighth. Edited by H. J. Waring, M. S., F. R. C. S., and J. S. Risien Russell, M. D., F. R. C. P. 1905. 8vo. 350 pages. Printed for the Society, London.

Report Relating to the Registration of Births, Marriages, and Deaths in the Province of Ontario. For the year ending 31st of December, 1903. 8vo. 47 + 223 pages. 1905. L. K. Cameron, Toronto.

The Health-Care of the Baby. A Handbook for Mothers and Nurses. By Louis Fischer, M. D. 1906. 12mo. 144 pages. Funk and Wagnalls Company, New York and London.

Walter Reed and Yellow Fever. By Howard A. Kelly, Professor of Gynecological Surgery, Johns Hopkins University. 1906. 12mo. 293 pages. McClure, Phillips & Co., New York.

The Eye and Nervous System. Their Diagnostic Relations. By Various Authors. Edited by William Campbell Posey, A. B., M. D., and William G. Spiller, M. D. Illustrated. 1906. 8vo. 988 pages. J. B. Lippincott Company, Philadelphia and London.

Progressive Medicine. A Quarterly Digest of Advances, Discoveries, and Improvements in the Medical and Surgical Sciences. Edited by Hobart Amory Hare, M. D., assisted by H. R. M. Landis, M. D. Volume 2. June, 1906. 8vo. 368 pages. Lea Brothers & Co., Philadelphia and New York.

The Practice of Gynecology. In Original Contributions. By American Authors. Edited by J. Wesley Bovée, M. D. Illustrated with 382 engravings and 60 full-page plates. 1906. 8vo. 836 pages. Lea Brothers & Co., Philadelphia and New York.

On Leprosy and Fish-Eating. A statement of Facts and Explanations. By Jonathan Hutchinson, F. R. S., and F. R. C. S., LL. D. 1906. 8vo. 420 pages. Archibald Constable & Co., London; W. T. Keener & Co., Chicago.

The Subconscious. By Joseph Jastrow. 1906. 8vo. 549 pages. Houghton, Mifflin and Company, Boston and New York.

Operative Otology. Surgical Pathology and .Treatment of Diseases of the Ear. By Clarence John Blake, M. D., and Henry Ottridge Reik, M. D., 1906. 8vo. 359 pages. D. Appleton and Company, New York and London.

The Operative Treatment of Prolapse and Retroversion of the Uterus. By J. Inglis Parsons, M. D., M. R. C. P., M. R. C. S. 1906. 8vo. 90 pages. John Bale, Sons and Danielsson, London.

Introduction to Materia Medica and Pharmacology. Including the Elements of Medical Pharmacy, Prescription Writing, Medical Latin, Toxicology, and Methods of Local Treatment. By Oliver T. Osborne, M. A., M. D. 1906. 12mo. 167 pages. Lea Brothers & Co., Philadelphia and New York.

Scientific Memoirs. (*New Series.*) *No. 23.* By Officers of the Medical and Sanitary Departments of the Government of India. *The Anatomy and Histology of Ticks.* By Captain S. R. Christophers, M. B., I. M. S. 1906. Fol. 55 pages. Office of the Superintendent of Government Printing, India.

The Examination of the Function of the Intestines by Means of the Test-Diet. Its Application in Medical Practice and its Diagnostic and Therapeutic Value. By Prof. Dr. Adolf Schmidt. Authorized translation from the latest German edition, by Charles D. Aaron, M. D. 1906. 8vo. 91 pages. F. A. Davis Company, Philadelphia.

International Clinics. A Quarterly of Illustrated Clinical Lectures and Especially Prepared Original Articles. By Leading Members of the Medical Profession Throughout the World. Edited by A. O. J. Kelly, A. M., M. D. Philadelphia. Volume IV. Fifteenth Series. 1906. 8vo. 312 pages. J. B. Lippincott Company, Philadelphia and London.

Transactions of the American Surgical Association. Volume the twenty-third. Edited by Richard H. Harte, M. D., Recorder of the Association. 1905. 8vo. 392 pages. Printed for the Association. William J. Dornan, Philadelphia.

Progressive Medicine. A Quarterly Digest of Advances, Discoveries, and Improvements in the Medical and Surgical Sciences. Edited by Hobart Amory Hare, M. D., assisted by H. R. M. Landis, M. D. Volume I. March, 1906. 8vo. 304 pages. Lea Brothers & Co., Philadelphia and New York.

Nursing: Its Principles and Practice. For Hospital and Private Use. By Isabel Hampton Robb. Third edition, revised and enlarged. Illustrated. 1906. 12mo. 565 pages. E. C. Koeckert, Cleveland.

THE JOHNS HOPKINS HOSPITAL REPORTS.

VOLS. XIII AND XIV,

OF ABOUT 600 PAGES EACH, WITH NUMEROUS ILLUSTRATIONS.

(NOW IN PRESS.)

STUDIES IN GENITO-URINARY SURGERY. By Hugh H. Young, M. D., Associate Professor of Genito-Urinary Surgery, The Johns Hopkins University, and Associate in Genito-Urinary Surgery, The Johns Hopkins Hospital, and F. H. Baetjer, M. D., of Baltimore; Henry A. Fowler, M. D., of Washington, D. C.; Stephen H. Watts, M. D., of Baltimore; John W. Churchman, M. D., of Breslau; Louis C. Lehr, M. D., of Washington, D. C.; J. T. Geraghty, M. D., of Baltimore, and A. R. Stevens, M. D., of Baltimore.

CONTENTS.

1. The Seven Glass Test. By Hugh H. Young, M. D.
2. The Possibility of Avoiding Confusion by Bacillus Smegmatis (Smegma bacillus) in the Diagnosis of Urinary and Genital Tuberculosis. An Experimental Study. By Hugh H. Young, M. D., and John W. Churchman, M. D.
3. Urethral Diverticula. By Stephen H. Watts, M. D.
4. Case of Urethrorrhagia. By H. A. Fowler, M. D.
5. Paraurethritis. By John W. Churchman, M. D.
6. Use of Ointments in the Urethra. By Hugh H. Young, M. D.
7. Treatment of Stricture of the Urethra. By Hugh H. Young, M. D., and John T. Geraghty, M. D.
8. The Treatment of Impermeable Stricture of the Urethra. By Hugh H. Young, M. D.
9. The Treatment of Bacteriuria by Medication. By John W. Churchman, M. D.
10. Use of the Cystoscope in the Diagnosis of Diseases of the Prostate. By Hugh H. Young, M. D.
11. Chronic Prostatitis. An Analysis of 358 Cases. By Hugh H. Young, M. D., John T. Geraghty, M. D., and A. R. Stevens, M. D.
12. The Treatment of Prostatic Hypertrophy. By Hugh H. Young, M. D.
13. Recto-Urethral Fistulæ. By Hugh H. Young, M. D.
14. Modern Method of Performing Perineal Lithotomy. By Hugh H. Young, M. D.
15. Early Diagnosis and Radical Cure of Carcinoma of the Prostate. By Hugh H. Young, M. D.
16. Operative Treatment of Vesical Diverticula. By Hugh H. Young, M. D.
17. Case of Double Renal Pelvis and Bifid Ureter. By Hugh H. Young, M. D.
18. Pyonephrosis Due to B. Typhosus. By Hugh H. Young, M. D., and Louis C. Lehr, M. D.
19. The Use of the X-ray in the Diagnosis of Renal and Ureteral Calculi. By F. H. Baetjer, M. D.
20. Nephritis and Hematuria. By H. A. Fowler, M. D.
21. Microscopic Study of Urinary Calculi of Oxalate of Lime. By H. A. Fowler, M. D.
22. Cystinuria and the Formation of Calculi. By H. A. Fowler, M. D.
23. Post-Traumatic Atrophy of the Testicle. By John W. Churchman, M. D.

Price per volume in paper, $5.00; in cloth, $5.50.

Orders should be addressed to

The Johns Hopkins Press, Baltimore, Md.

BULLETIN

OF

THE JOHNS HOPKINS HOSPITAL

Entered as Second-Class Matter at the Baltimore, Maryland, Postoffice.

Vol. XVII.—No. 188.]   BALTIMORE, NOVEMBER, 1906.   [Price, 25 Cents

CONTENTS.

THE FUTURE OF THE MEDICAL PROFESSION.[1]

By Charles W. Eliot, LL. D.,

President of Harvard University.

The future occupations and interests of the medical profession are to be in some respects different from those of the past, and they are to be more various. The ordinary physician has for the last hundred years been almost exclusively a man devoted to the treatment of diseases already developed in human bodies or of injuries already incurred. He made his diagnosis, and then sought remedies and a cure. He was the sympathetic and skillful helper of sick or injured persons. Most of the cases that came under his care were cases considered plain as to symptoms, period and accepted treatment. The minority of cases were obscure, and called for unusual knowledge and skill in discerning the seat of the disorder, or the approximate cause of the bodily disturbance. Hence the special value of the experienced consultant, who was ordinarily a man of some peculiar natural gift of body, mind, or temperament, possessing also in high degree the faculty of keen observation, and the habit of eliminating irrelevant considerations, and ultimately finding his way to the accurate, limited inference from the facts before him. Both the ordinary physician and the consultant have already been much helped by the extraordinary progress made in medical science during the last thirty years, but they have been helped, chiefly, to a surer recognition of diseases established

[1] Address delivered, Sept. 26, 1906, in Sanders Theatre, Cambridge, on the occasion of the dedication of the new buildings of the Harvard Medical School.

in human bodies, and to a better treatment of their patients' diseases when recognized.

The physician or surgeon commonly renders a personal service to an individual, sometimes for a pecuniary recompense, but often without money compensation. He is often a trusted adviser in the most intimate family concerns. Births and deaths alike bring the physician into the home. In rendering these services he must be tender, sympathetic, considerate, pure-minded and judicious. There will always be need, crying need, of the physician and surgeon in this sense and for these functions; and whatever else the regular education of the physician provides in the future, it must provide all the elements of the best training for the practising physician who is to treat diseased or crippled human bodies, and give advice about the sudden and the chronic ills which afflict humanity. So much will continue to be demanded of all good medical schools; but much more they must do.

The progress of what we call civilization exposes human beings more and more to the ravages of disease. When savages come in contact with men called civilized, they invariably suffer from diseases new to them. When a rural population crowds into cities, it falls a victim to diseases from which in the country it had been exempt. When hundreds of thousands of people huddle into small areas and create there smoke, dust and noise, they suffer not only from new diseases, but from the exacerbation of diseases not wholly unknown to them in the rural condition. Under such favorable conditions of residence and labor the human body degenerates in many respects, and, losing vigor, becomes in some respects less able to resist the attacks of disease.

Against these bodily evils which result from civilization the physician has thus far struggled chiefly by treating more or less successfully the numerous individuals who are attacked by disease. Doubtless, the treatment of sick and injured persons has substantially improved, but, nevertheless, the death-rate in our cities diminishes slowly, and the heavy economic losses which result from disease and premature death continue. Moreover, the improvement of treatment in hospitals and private practice has been accompanied by a great increase in the cost of treatment, so that the charges upon the community resulting from sickness and injuries have, within the last thirty years, rapidly mounted, and these heavy charges are, after all, incurred for the palliation of evils already suffered, and not for the prevention of such evils. Again, in different parts of the habitable globe, mankind has been exposed for centuries to dangers more or less localized,—in one region to the attacks of venomous reptiles; in another of fierce carnivora; in another to the ravages of flights of insects which devour every green thing; in another to the constant presence of formidable diseases.

For the most part, the human race has learned how to exterminate the offending creatures, or at least, to limit their ravages; and where grave infectious diseases are always present, in greater or smaller degree, or frequently recur, a considerable proportion of the population becomes in some degree immune to them. Mankind is now in face of enemies which are not localized, but which, on the contrary, are carried all over the habitable globe on the ubiquitous routes of travel and commerce. The worst of the new enemies are minute, multitudinous and mysterious, in that their relations and connections are unknown; they infest many of the animals with which man is associated, or pass into man from the animals and plants of which he makes use. Untrammeled dissemination of noxious things has taken the place of centuries-long localization, a localization which sometimes secured checks, antidotes, or immunities. Since then, modern society cannot help incurring new risks; it should seek new defenses. These defenses it may reasonably expect medical education to plan, and public and private expenditure to provide.

If civilized society is to endure under its new exposures and dangers, it is clear that the medical profession must take up with new ardor the work of preventing approaching disease in addition to the work of treating disease arrived. The profession must recognize that health is eminently a social product, just as the psychologists have recognized that the mind of a civilized man is a social product.

When we consider what has already been learned about the production, transmission and prevention of smallpox, cholera, yellow fever, the black death, typhoid fever, diphtheria, anthrax, rabies and tetanus, we cannot resist the conclusion that in the future medical science must include the study of causes and sequences which will carry the student through a large

portion of the animal and vegetable kingdoms, and particularly into the habits and habitats of their minute parasitic forms. Systematic medical education must therefore produce a considerable number of men capable of studying in this region the causes of disease, and the ways of interrupting the means of communication, or breaking the chain of sequences, through which at last the germs of disease get a chance to produce their malignant effects within the human body. Considering the great obscurity of the physiological processes which go on within the body and the dense ignorance of mankind concerning the microscopic animal kingdom, it is a great wonder that medical science in its imperfect state has constructed so many effective defenses capable of studying disease within the last thirty years. Indeed, we are now using some efficient defensive methods, the real nature of which we but imperfectly understood, as, for instance, the vaccinations against smallpox and hydrophobia. Although we are not yet able absolutely to prevent disease, we are able in many cases to restrict the communication of diseases and to modify their course in the individuals attacked.

The medicine of the future has, therefore, to deal much more extensively than in the past with preventive medicine, or, in other words, with the causes of disease as it attacks society, the community, or the state, rather than the individual. The object in view will be not only to arrest or modify a malady which has appeared in the body of a patient, but, as in the recent case of yellow fever, to learn how the disease is communicated and how to prevent that communication. The study of mitigations, remedies and cures is to continue; but the study of the causes of disease and the means of prevention is to be greatly developed. The function of the nineteenth century physician will continue, and, indeed, will become more effective through a better knowledge of the forces which may be made to act upon his patient, both from within and from without; but another sort of physician will be at work in the twentieth century, preventing the access of epidemics, limiting them when they arrive, defending society against bad food and drink, and reducing to lowest terms the manifold evils which result from the congestion of population.

The explorers and pioneers in the field of medicine must be encouraged to press on their patient work of analyzing all the processes which accompany disease, in order that they may learn their actual sequences. Only through the knowledge of these sequences can real control over disease be certainly gained. And this work will be endless; for civilization involves constant changes in the environment of the human race; and it is on medical science that the race must depend for protecting it from the new dangers which accompany each novel environment. The medical scientists being provided and furthered, medical education must also train large bodies of men to clear and cultivate the regions through which the pioneers have made trails, or, in plainer words, to apply to millions of men and women in all sorts of climate and environment the discoveries of the scientists. Thus thousands of physicians all over our southern states must for years be teaching the people how to protect themselves from yellow

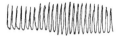

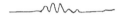

TRACING No. 1.—From a clinical case of Cheyne-Stokes respiration in association with increased intracranial tension. The upper curve represents the pulse tracing obtained from the brachial artery by means of the Erlanger sphygmomanometer. The instrument was permanently set at a point midway between systolic and diastolic blood pressures. An increase in size of the pulse waves represents a rise in blood pressure, a decrease a fall in blood pressure. The middle curve represents the respirations recorded by means of a Marey double tambour, the upstroke representing inspiration. The lowermost line records the time in one second intervals. The record is to be read from left to right.

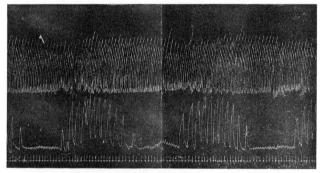

TRACING No. 2.—A similar record obtained from a case of Cheyne-Stokes respiration occurring clinically in association with cardiac insufficiency. The curves are to be interpreted as in Tracing No. 1.

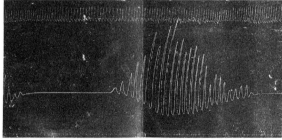

TRACING No. 3.—Record of experiment in which a normal individual endeavored to simulate Cheyne-Stokes respiration. The tracing is to be interpreted as records 1 and 2.

ERRATUM.
These curves should have accompanied Dr. Eyster's "Blood Pressure Changes in Cheyne-Stokes Respiration," p. 296, September BULLETIN.

fever. Major Walter Reed and his colleagues proved how yellow fever is communicated, and—what was equally important—how it is not communicated; but thousands of medical men must see to it that intelligent application is made of that precious knowledge.

Recent events have brought into strong light a new function of the medical profession which is sure to be amplified and made more effective in the near future. I mean the function of teaching the whole population how diseases are caused and communicated, and what are the corresponding means of prevention. The recent campaign against tuberculosis is a good illustration of this new function of the profession. To discharge it well requires, in medical men, the power of interesting exposition, with telling illustration and moving exhortation. Obviously, the function calls for disinterestedness and public spirit on the part of the profession; but to this call it is certain that the profession will respond. It also calls for some new adjustments and new functions in medical schools, which should hereafter be careful to provide means of popular exposition concerning water supplies, foods, drinks, drugs, the parasitic causes or consequences of disease in men, plants and animals, and the modes of communication of all communicable diseases.

Medical museums should be arranged, in part, for the instruction of the public, and, with some suitable reservations, should be statedly open to the public. The medical schools should also habitually provide popular lectures on medical subjects, and these lectures should be given without charge on days and at hours when working people can attend. In other words, selected physicians should become public preachers, as well as private practitioners. America has much to learn from Europe in regard to this public-spirited service on the part of the profession.

In another respect the teaching of medicine must be broadened in the century we have now entered on. Medical study has been, in time past, far too exclusively the study for man's body by itself. Hereafter, the study of medicine must be largely comparative, or, in other words, must include man's relations to the animal and vegetable kingdoms. The Harvard Medical School enters into possession of its new buildings with three professorships of comparative medicine already established,—the professorships of comparative anatomy, comparative physiology and comparative pathology. This tendency to comparative study has been already well developed in other subjects, as, for example, in comparative psychology, legislation and religion. Wherever this study by comparison wins adequate place, it makes the study of the subject broader and more liberalizing, and the results obtained more comprehensive and just.

Medical students should, therefore, have studied zoölogy and botany before beginning the study of medicine, and should have acquired some skill in the use of the scalpel and microscope. It is absurd that anybody should begin with the human body the practice of dissection or of surgery; and, furthermore, it is wholly irrational that any young man who means to be a physician should not have mastered the elements of biology, chemistry and physics years before he enters a medical school. The mental constitution of the physician is essentially that of the naturalist; and the tastes and capacities of the naturalist reveal themselves, and, indeed, demand satisfaction long before twenty-one years of age, which is a good age for entering a medical school. The Harvard Medical School has derived great advantages from its requirement of a previous degree for admission; but in view of the fact that many young men procure a bachelor's degree without ever having studied any science, the school needs an additional and more specific requirement, namely, a previous knowledge of biology, physics and organic chemistry, and an acquaintance with laboratory methods in all three subjects.

As at the preliminary stages of the medical career, so at its climax there is an increasing need of men who have a working knowledge of several sciences which were formerly treated as distinct, and whose best representatives in medical schools labored apart, each in his own field. The most promising medical research of our day makes use of biological, chemical and physical science combined. Physiology advances by making applications of the principles, the methods, and the implements of all three sciences. The physiologist listens to the normal or abnormal sounds in the bodies of man and animals with a modified telephone, and may record by electricity almost all the phenomena he studies. Bacteriology and biological chemistry go hand in hand in serving pathology and the public health.

A great number of new chemical substances, coming from organic sources, and yet as definite and uniform in composition as salt or alum, prove serviceable in pharmacology and in physiological and pathological research, although they were neither discovered nor manufactured with any such purpose in view. The stainings of bacteriological technique, and the quantitative color tests for characteristic ingredients in the various secretions of the body, ingredients which fluctuate in amount in health or in disease, illustrate the present dependence of medical research on chemistry and physics.

For the effective study of the toxins and antitoxins, within and without the body, the bacteriologist and the biological chemist must co-operate. Many of the effects produced by the toxins in the living body are definite chemical changes, such, for instance, as may be produced by the activation of certain ferments, and the antagonism of toxin and antitoxin is probably a chemical reaction. Many of the great discoveries of the future will come through the cooperation of sympathetic groups of medical scientists representing different modes of attacking the same problem. There will be a like necessity for cooperation between the clinician, the pathological anatomist, the physiological chemist and the bacteriologist.

The world has observed and will not forget that some of the greatest contributors to the progress of medicine and surgery during the past thirty years have been, not physicians, but naturalists and chemists. Pasteur was a chemist; Cohn, the teacher of Koch, a botanist, and Metschnikoff, a zoölogist. Students of disease must, therefore, be competent to utilize in their great task every aid which natural science can furnish. How vastly is the range of medical science and medical education broadened by this plain necessity! The dignity and serviceableness of the medical profession are heightened by every new demand on the intelligence and devotion of its members.

The recent liberal endowment of the Harvard Medical School by private persons is an indication that the more intelligent and public-spirited portion of the American people is beginning to understand that most diseases would be preventable if only mankind had acquired the knowledge needed to prevent them. The urgent duty of society to-day is to spend the money needed to get that knowledge. How to spend it we have learned; witness the admirable work of the Massachusetts Board of Health for thirty years past, aggressive work, both defensive and offensive; witness also the remarkable results of the medical institutes, both in this country and in Europe.

The medical profession of the future will have the satisfaction not only of ameliorating the condition or prolonging the life of the suffering individual, but also of exterminating or closely limiting the preventable diseases.

THE UNITY OF THE MEDICAL SCIENCES.[1]

By WILLIAM H. WELCH, M. D.

The dedication of the new buildings of the Harvard Medical School is an occasion for rejoicing not to Harvard University alone but to all in this country and elsewhere interested in the progress of medical education and of medical science, and in behalf of all such I beg to offer to this University hearty congratulations upon this magnificent addition to its resources for medical teaching and study. Medicine everywhere and especially in America has reason to be profoundly grateful to the generous and public-spirited donors who have made possible the construction of this group of buildings, unsurpassed in the imposing beauty and the harmony of their architectural design and in their ample, internal arrangements. This design is adapted from the Greek, and it is peculiarly fitting that the medical sciences should be housed in a style which suggests the spirit of ancient Greece, where first flowed the springs of medical science and art—living springs even to this day. In the singular harmony of the architecture of the group of buildings devoted to the various medical sciences are typified the unity of purpose of these sciences and their combination into the one great science of medicine. What I shall have to say on this occasion is suggested in part by this thought of the " Unity of the Medical Sciences."

The good fortune of the Harvard Medical School in coming into possession of the splendid laboratories now formally dedicated is well merited by the leading position which this institution has held in this country since its foundation, by its union with Harvard University, and by the assurance that the greatly enlarged opportunities will here be used to the highest advantage. Since the appointment in 1782 of its first professors, John Warren and Benjamin Waterhouse, of enduring fame, this school has had a long line of honored names upon its roll of teachers, lustrous not only for such single stars as Channing and Ware and Holmes and Ellis and Cheever, but especially for its clustered stars, the Warrens, the Jacksons, the Bigelows, the Shattucks, the Wymans, the Bowditches, the Minots; and it will not be deemed invidious on this occasion to mention of the latter group the names of two members of the present distinguished faculty to whose services this school is so largely indebted for securing the funds for the new buildings, Professor Henry P. Bowditch, the eminent leader of American physiologists, and Professor John Collins Warren, who, as surgeon, writer and teacher, has so worthily maintained and enhanced the ancestral fame.

The Harvard Medical School has been a pioneer in this country in many improvements of medical education; it has stood successfully in an historic city and commonwealth for high standards of professional attainment and honor, and for just recognition of the dignity and usefulness of the profession; it has made valuable contributions to the advancement of medical knowledge and practice, and above all there issued from this school and the Massachusetts General Hospital through John Collins Warren, the elder, and Samuel G. Morton medicine's supreme gift to suffering humanity of surgical anæsthesia.

This school, however, has no possession so valuable or which gives such assurance of its stability and growth for untold generations to come and of the worthy bestowal of the great gifts which were dedicated yesterday as its union with Harvard University, and it is befitting that the significance of this university relationship should be emphasized by including among the dedicatory ceremonies this academic function in the halls of this great university.

The severance of the historical union of medical school and university, leading to the establishment of a multitude of independent medical schools without responsible control, and usurping the right to confer the doctor's degree and the license to practise, is accountable in large measure for the low position to which medical education in this country sank during the larger part of the last century, and from which it has now risen in our better schools to a height which we can contemplate with increasing satisfaction. Nor would it be difficult to show, if this were the suitable occasion, that

[1] An address delivered September 26, 1906, at Harvard University, at the dedication of the new buildings of the Harvard Medical School.

our universities on their side have suffered from the loss of a member which has brought renown to many foreign universities and that many of the embarrassing anomalies of our collegiate system of education are due to lack of personal contact on the part of colleges and universities with the needs of professional, especially medical, training. There is, of course, no saving grace in a merely nominal connection of medical school and university; the union to be of mutual benefit must be a real and vital one; ideals of the university must inspire the whole life and activities of the medical department.

To have recognized fully, from the beginning of his administration, the importance of this vitalizing union of the medical school with the university, to have striven patiently with full grasp of the problems and with intelligent sympathy with the needs of medicine for the uplifting of the standards of medical education, and, with the aid of his medical colleagues, to have planted these standards where they now are in the Harvard Medical School, is not the least of the many enduring services which President Eliot has rendered to American education, and, in behalf of our profession, I wish to make to you, sir, on this occasion, grateful acknowledgment of this great and beneficent work.

The opening of the new laboratories of the Harvard Medical School marks the culmination, up to the present time, of an educational and scientific movement which has been the most distinctive characteristic of the development of medicine during the past fifty years, and which has transformed the face of modern medicine. To have some idea of the extent and the direction of this development, consider how inconceivable would have been the mere existence of such laboratories a century ago, and how impossible it would have been for even a Bichat or a Laënnec to have put them to any use or to have imagined their use. The only scientific laboratory which existed at that time was the anatomical, and this had been in existence for at least two hundred and fifty years, although not in a form which meets our present ideas of such a laboratory.

The modern scientific laboratory was born in Germany in 1824 when Purkinje established the first physiological laboratory, thus antedating by one year the foundation of Liebig's chemical laboratory, which had a much greater influence upon the subsequent development of laboratories. As might naturally be expected, anatomical and physiological laboratories had attained a considerable development before the first pathological laboratory was founded in Berlin by Virchow. The opening and activities of this laboratory, which has recently celebrated its fiftieth anniversary, mark an era in the progress of medicine. With the exception of the modest beginning of a pharmacological laboratory by Buchheim about 1850, all of the other medical laboratories—those of physiological chemistry, of hygiene, of bacteriology, of clinical medicine—originated at a much later date.

This remarkable growth of laboratories for the cultivation of the various medical sciences has been at once the cause and the result of the rapid progress of medicine in recent years. By teaching and exemplifying the only fruitful method of advancing natural knowledge, laboratories have overthrown the dominance of authority and dogma and speculation and have turned medicine irrevocably into the paths of science, establishing the medical sciences as important departments of biology; by demonstrating that the only abiding, living knowledge, powerful for right action, comes from intimate, personal contact with the objects of study, they have revolutionized the methods of medical teaching; by discovery they have widened the boundaries of old domains and opened to exploration entirely new fields of knowledge, by the application of which man's power over disease has been greatly increased.

Medicine, as a science, is occupied with the systematic study of the structures and functions of the human and animal body in health, of their changes by disease and injury, and of the agencies by which such morbid changes may be prevented, alleviated or removed. Its ultimate aim, which indicates also its method, is that of all science, the deduction of general concepts and laws from the comparison of the relationships and sequences of ascertained facts, and the application of these laws to the promotion of human welfare. This goal, to-day far from realization, is most nearly approached where the principles of physics and of chemistry can be applied, but there remains a large biological field awaiting reclamation for the application of these principles. The subject-matter of medical study, as thus indicated, is of supreme import to mankind, but complex and difficult far beyond that of any other natural or physical science.

The places where such study may be most advantageously carried on are laboratories and hospitals supplied with the material for study, with the necessary instruments, appliances and books, and with trained workers. By growth of medical knowledge the field to be covered has become so vast as to require much subdivision of labor, nor is it to be supposed that the end of this subdivision has been even approximately reached.

From human anatomy, the mother of medical as well as of many other natural sciences, there branched off in the eighteenth century physiology, and, still later, pathological anatomy. As if to replace these losses anatomy gave birth to comparative anatomy, embryology and microscopic anatomy as more or less separate branches. During the past century physiological chemistry and pharmacology have separated from physiology, and comparative pathology and experimental pathological physiology are asserting their independence from pathological anatomy. Hygiene and bacteriology are of recent and more independent growth. The latter, lusty stripling, with the rise of medical zoology, especially protozoology, is seeking a more comprehensive and appropriate designation. The latest and perhaps the most significant development is the clinical laboratory in its various forms.

Specialization in scientific work should not be decried; it is demanded by the necessities of the case and has been the great instrument of progress, but the further division of labor is carried, the more necessary does it become to emphasize essential unity of purpose and to secure coordination and cordial cooperation of allied sciences. Especially urgent is full recognition of the unity and cooperation of the clinic and the laboratory.

During the last two decades we have witnessed in this country the extraordinary rise of practical laboratory instruction from the weakest to the strongest and best organized part of the medical curriculum of our better schools. Our laboratory courses are, I believe, in several instances, more elaborate and occupy more time than corresponding ones in most foreign universities.

It is, however, as was emphasized by Dr. Dwight and Dr. Shattuck in their remarks yesterday, an error to suppose that from the point of view of science any fundamental distinction exists between the clinical and the so-called laboratory subjects other than that based upon differences in the subject-matter of study. The problems of the living patient are just as capable of study by scientific methods and in the scientific spirit, and they pertain to independent branches of medical science, just as truly as those of anatomy, physiology or the other so-called laboratory subjects. All of the medical sciences are interdependent, but each has its own problems and methods, and each is most fruitfully cultivated for its own sake by those specially trained for the work.

There is a highly significant and hopeful scientific movement in internal medicine and surgery to-day characterized by the establishment of laboratories for clinical research, by the application of refined physical, chemical and biological methods to the problems of diagnosis and therapy, and by the scientific investigation along broad lines of the special problems furnished by the living patient. The most urgent need in medical education at the present time in this country I believe to be the organization of our clinics both for teaching and for research in the spirit of this modern movement and with provision for as intimate, prolonged, personal contact of the student with the subject of study as he finds in the laboratory.

In addition to undergraduate instruction our laboratories at present furnish better opportunities for the prolonged, advanced training of those intending to make their careers in anatomy, physiology, pathology and other sciences, than are afforded by most of our hospitals to those who aim at the higher careers in medicine and surgery. A further clinical disadvantage is that while the former class after good scientific work may reasonably look forward to desirable positions as teachers and directors of laboratories, the latter, however high their attainments, in consequence of the separation of the medical school from any control over the appointments to the hospital staff, cannot anticipate with any degree of assurance similar promotion in their chosen lines of work, and consequently the medical faculty has not so wide a field of choice in filling the clinical chairs as in filling those of the auxiliary sciences.

The removal of these deficiencies on the clinical side of medical education in America requires some reorganization of its staff on the part of the hospital and the control by the medical school of its hospital, or, at least, its voice in appointments to the hospital staff. So far as our resources permit, we have, I think, accomplished this reform at the Johns Hopkins Medical School and Hospital.

The welfare of the patient is the first obligation of the trustees of hospitals and of physicians in attendance, but nothing is more certain than that cordial cooperation between medical school and hospital best subserves the promotion of this welfare. Fortunate the hospital and fortunate the patients brought into such relations with the Harvard Medical School.

As is strikingly illustrated by the new buildings of this school, the educational machinery of medicine to-day is vastly complicated and costly compared with the simplicity of the days when a lecture room, a dissecting room, a simple chemical laboratory, and a clinical amphitheatre were all that was needed. The purpose of medical education, however, remains to-day what it has always been and will continue to be— the training of the student for the future practice of his profession, and to this end in an harmonious scheme of education the various medical sciences all work together. Right action requires abundant knowledge, nowhere more so than in medical practice, and the all-sufficient justification for the position held by the various sciences in the preliminary and the professional education of the physician is that they furnish knowledge and discipline of mind needed in the preparation for his future work. The social position of the medical man and his influence in the community depend to a considerable extent upon his preliminary education and general culture. For this reason, as well as for his intellectual pleasure in his profession and as a sound foundation for his future studies, the student should enter the medical school with a liberal education, which should include training in the sciences fundamental to medicine.

The unity of the various medical sciences is manifested not only in their historical development and in their co-operation in the scheme of medical education, but especially in their contributions to the upbuilding and progress of medicine as a whole.

There is no branch of medicine or even of physical science which has not played an important part in the evolution of our present medical knowledge and beliefs. The great lesson taught by the history of this development of medicine through the centuries has been the unconditional reverence for facts revealed by observation, experiment, and just inference, as contrasted with the sterility of mere speculation and reliance upon transmitted authority. The great epochs of this history have been characterized by some great discovery, by the introduction of some new method, or by the appearance of some man of genius to push investigation and scientific inference to limits not attainable by ordinary minds. The history of medicine has a greater unity and continuity, and extends over a longer period of time, than that of any other science.

The first clear note, which has rung down the ages, was sounded by Hippocrates when he taught the value of the inductive method by simple, objective study of the symptoms of disease, and the cry "Back to Hippocrates!" has more than once recalled medicine from dogmas and systems into sane and rational paths. Medicine, however, was handed on from the Greeks and Romans in bondage to a system of doctrine, constructed by Galen, so completely satisfying to the mediæval mind that this system remained practically untouched for over a thousand years.

With the liberation of intellect through the renaissance came the great emancipators, in the sixteenth century Vesalius, and in the seventeenth, Harvey, the former placing human anatomy upon a firm foundation and bringing medicine into touch with the most solid basis of fact in its domain, the latter bringing to light in the demonstration of the circulation of the blood the central fact of physiology and applying for the first time in a large and fruitful way to medicine the most powerful lever of scientific advance, the method of experiment.

In the century of Galileo, Harvey and Newton instruments of precision, as the chronometer, the thermometer, the balance, the microscope, were first applied to the investigation of medical problems, and physics began to render those services to medicine which, continued from Galileo to Röntgen, have been of simply incalculable value. The debt of medicine to chemistry began even with the rise of alchemy, received an immense increment from the researches of Lavoisier, the founder of modern chemistry, concerning the function of respiration and the sources of animal heat, and has grown unceasingly and to enormous proportions up to these days of physical chemistry, which has found such important applications in physiology and pathology.

How disastrous may be to medicine the loss of the sense of unity in all its branches has been very clearly and admirably shown by Professor Allbutt in depicting the effects which, for centuries, followed the casting off from medicine of surgery as a subject unworthy the attention of the medical faculty. Thereby internal medicine lost touch with reality and the inductive method, and remained sterile and fantastic until the days of Harvey, Sydenham and Boerhaave. The services of surgery to medicine as a whole, so brilliantly exemplified in the experimental work of John Hunter in the eighteenth century, have become a distinguishing feature of the medicine of the present day.

The great awakening of clinical medicine came in the early part of the nineteenth century from the introduction of the new methods of physical diagnosis by Laënnec and from pathological anatomy. The subsequent development of scientific and practical medicine has far exceeded that of all the preceding centuries. It has kept pace with the progress during the same wonderful century of all the sciences of nature and has contributed even more to the promotion of human happiness.

In anatomy with embryology and histology, in physiology, pathology, physiological chemistry, pharmacology, hygiene, bacteriology—sciences which are ancillary to medicine and at the same time important branches of biological science—there have been marvelous activity and expansion. For physiology and the understanding of disease, the establishment of the cell doctrine by the aid of botany, embryology, and pathology has been the greatest achievement. By the combined aid of physiology, physiological chemistry, experimental pathology, improved methods of diagnosis and clinical study, medicine has gained new and higher points of view in passing from too exclusive emphasis upon the final stages of disease revealed by morbid anatomy to clearer conceptions of the beginning and progress of morbid processes as indicated by disturbances of function, and above all has penetrated to the knowledge of the causation of an important class of diseases, the infectious. As a result of this rapid growth of knowledge in many directions has come a great increase of the physician's power to do good by the relief of suffering and the prevention and cure of disease.

In this connection I wish especially to emphasize the mutual helpfulness of the various medical sciences in the development of medical knowledge and practice. Attention is generally so concentrated upon the final achievement that there is danger of losing sight of the manifold sources which have contributed to the result. Let my medical hearers consider, for example, the indispensable share of embryology, of anatomy, gross and microscopic, of physiology, of pathological anatomy, of clinical study in the evolution of our knowledge of the latest contribution to diseases of the circulatory system —that disturbance of the cardiac rhythm called "heart-block." Similar illustrations of the unity of the medical sciences and of the cooperation of the laboratory and the clinic might be multiplied indefinitely from all classes of disease.

The same phenomenon is exhibited in medicine as in all science, that the search for knowledge with exclusive reference to its practical application is generally unrewarded. The student of nature must find his satisfaction in search for the truth, and in the consciousness that he has contributed something to the fund of knowledge on which reposes man's dominion over reluctant matter and inexorable forces.

How readily better action attends upon increased knowledge is shown by the part which the art of medicine is playing and is destined to play even more prominently in the world's progress. The value of this work of modern medicine is to be measured in part, but only in part, by the standard applied by the average man, namely, improvement, which, indeed, has been great, in the treatment of disease and injury. It is, however, its increasing power to check the incalculable waste of life, of energy, of money from preventable disease that places medicine to-day in the front rank of forces for the advancement of civilization and the improvement of human society. Economists and other students of social conditions have begun to realize this, but governments and the people are not half awake, and medicine, shaking off all mystery and with a sense of high public duty, has before it a great campaign of popular education.

The knowledge which has placed preventive medicine upon a sound basis and has given it the power to restrain and in some instances even to exterminate such diseases as cholera, plague, yellow fever, malaria, typhoid fever, tuberculosis and other infections, has come from exploration of the fields opened by Pasteur and by Koch. This power and the certainty of increasing it has given great strength to appeals for the endowment of medical research and the construction of laboratories. What is all the money ever expended for medical education and medical science compared with the one gift to humanity of Walter Reed and his colleagues of the Army Commission—the power to rid the world of yellow fever?

Great as has been the advance of medicine in the past half century, it is small indeed in comparison with what remains to be accomplished. Only a corner of the veil has been lifted. On every hand there are still unsolved problems of disease of overshadowing importance. The ultimate problems relate to the nature and fundamental properties of living matter, and the power to modify these properties in desired directions. Here our levers are far from the satisfactory fulcrum. But knowledge breeds new knowledge, and we cannot doubt that research will be even more productive in the future than it has been in the past. It would be hazardous in the extreme to attempt to predict the particular direction of future discovery. How unpredictable even to the most far-sighted of a past generation would have been such discoveries as the principles of antiseptic surgery, antitoxins, bacterial vaccines, opsonins, the extermination of yellow fever or malaria by destruction of a particular species of mosquito, and many other recent contributions to medical knowledge!

The activities within the new buildings of the Harvard Medical School begin at a period of medical development full of present interest and full of hope for the future, and it may be confidently predicted that they will have an important share in the onward movement, educational and scientific, of medicine.

One side of these activities will be devoted, under conditions most admirable as regards teachers, methods and opportunities, to the training of medical students and to advanced instruction. Supplemented by similar opportunities for undergraduate and advanced training in the hospital wards and dispensary, these conditions will be ideal.

The inspection of these noble new buildings, however, shows clearly that those who have planned them with such care, foresight and sagacity, while recognizing fully their important educational uses, have had also another and a main thought in their arrangements, namely, their adaptation to the purposes of original research. It is this dual function of imparting and of advancing knowledge which justifies the expenditure of money and which insures a return of the capital invested in buildings, equipment, and operation with a high rate of interest in the form of benefits to mankind.

The most ample and freely available facilities are an important condition for productive research, but on this creative side of university work men count for more than stately edifice and all the pride and pomp of outward life. Research is not to be bought in the market-place, nor does it follow the commercial law of supply and demand. The multitude can acquire knowledge; many there are who can impart it skillfully; smaller, but still considerable, is the number of those who can add new facts to the store of knowledge, but rare indeed are the thinkers, born with the genius for discovery and with the gift of the scientific imagination to interpret in broad generalizations and laws the phenomena of nature. These last are the glory of a university. Search for them far and wide beyond college gate and city wall, and when found cherish them as a possession beyond all price.

By the possession of investigators such as these, by the character and work of teachers and taught, by the advancement of knowledge and improvement of practice, may this new home of the Harvard Medical School be a centre for the diffusion of truth in medicine, the abode of productive research, a fortress in the warfare against disease, and thereby dedicated to the service of humanity!

REMARKS UPON THE INTERNATIONAL CONGRESS OF TUBERCU-LOSIS, PARIS, 1905.[1]

By HENRY BARTON JACOBS, M. D.

The International Congress of Tuberculosis held in Paris October, 1905, was attended by three or four thousand people interested in the work of the Congress. To realize why such a large number of people should have been brought together, consider for a moment the importance of the work; tuberculosis is by far the greatest scourge of the human race. Wars, smallpox, yellow fever, plague, railway disaster, these cause momentary outbursts of great excitement and fear, even heavy mortality, but this mortality is small as compared to this silent, ever-present foe, tuberculosis, which so stealthily and yet so unceasingly lies in wait for its victims.

The statistics of our own city may be taken as a fairly accurate expression of the statistics of the whole civilized world; notice them week by week, always the same thing; deaths from tuberculosis leading the list, except perhaps now and then in the winter months when pneumonia may run ahead, but season in and season out it is tuberculosis which is killing the greater number of the people. This fact alone would seem sufficient to incite men and women to an interest in its study, but when we consider that it has been completely demonstrated that this disease is dependent upon an agency which can be *destroyed* and can be *avoided* so that the disease need not exist, then we realize more fully the interest called forth

[1] Read at a meeting of the Laennec Society, March 19, 1906.

the world over in all efforts to comprehend the nature of the disease and the best methods of suppressing it.

The three thousand or more enthusiasts in Paris were by no means disappointed in the results of this last meeting; they came from the nations encircling the globe; all brought some tribute to the cause, not the least of which was an eagerness to see and know what others were doing, thus to receive stimulation for better work at home. Such inspiration is not necessarily to be gathered wholly from papers read; it comes from intermingling and conversing, with even looking upon the great leaders in the cause and so breathing in enthusiasm by the mere contemplation of the life and work of such men. It is also to be derived from exhibitions, not only of the practical results of labor but also of the scientific attainments recorded from many sources, and again from actual visits to the institutions where work is being done, noting conditions, how far they agree, how better and how far inferior to those at home. So it is that the Congress in Paris may be said to have been interesting, instructive and stimulating by the papers presented, the exhibits of many things relative to the subject, the entertainments in which the members met together, learned to know each other and informally derived new ideas and enthusiasm; and excursions to existing institutions where methods and plans were seen and discussed.

At three o'clock on the afternoon of October 2, 1905, the opening session was held under the direct auspices of the President of the Republic and the officers of Government with such military and other formal surroundings as accompany full state functions. The ambassadors of various countries in official dress, and delegates in full uniform all tended to give picturesqueness and dignity to the first meeting and to emphasize the importance of the movement which the Congress represented. At this session there was little but formal words of welcome and salutations of respect for France and her President. The United States was represented by Dr. Beyer, of the Navy, who in full uniform as Surgeon and Commandant, in a few well chosen words spoken in French brought greetings from America.

The real scientific work of the Congress began the next day, papers being read simultaneously in four sections:

Section 1 being devoted to the medical aspects of tuberculosis;

Section 2 to its surgical aspects;

Section 3 to the protection and aid of children;

And Section 4 to the protection and aid of adults, including social hygiene in its broadest aspects.

To the papers and discussions of these sections I will refer briefly, especially to those representing at this time thoughts which are uppermost in the minds of those working for the prevention and relief of tuberculosis.

Each Congress marks, as it were, a stage of progress in the work. We have the period in which Bremer, Detweiler and others demonstrated the efficacy of the open air treatment of early tuberculosis in specially constructed sanatoria. Then the period following Koch's discovery of the specific cause of

the disease. At another Congress Koch advocated tuberculin as a curative agent, and in the period following, this substance was the all absorbing subject of investigation and discussion.

In 1901 Koch made the assertion that the tuberculosis of cattle was to be considered of little or no importance as a factor in the production of the disease in the human race. In the period since, this question largely has occupied the minds of investigators.

In all these periods progress has been making in many correlative branches, and at the various Congresses there has been a form of "rounding up," and a "taking of stock," so to say, of our knowledge as to the whole range of subjects embraced in the study of the disease, its physical and bacteriological nature, its sources and means of transmission, prevention and cure.

That this last Congress will take its place with those preceding it in marking a similar distinct epoch in the work I have no doubt. There are old questions which seem to have been settled and laid aside and others have been brought forward which are new and will need the test of time and much investigation to ascertain their truthfulness and value.

It seems safe to say that one of the most far reaching conclusions arrived at in Paris is that it must be assumed that tuberculosis in cattle may be a source of tuberculosis in man.

We, therefore, start in this new period following this last International Congress with the conviction that the fullest attention must be paid to our milk supply, especially if fed to young children, lest it become a source of infection. Renewed activity should be exercised by our State veterinarians and State boards of health to see to it that the farmers are selling only milk from cows free from tuberculosis. So convinced of this was the medical section that it voted almost unanimously [two dissenting voices], that it was not only indispensable to prevent contagion from man to man, but also necessary to protect the human race against the tuberculosis of cattle by statutes and municipal laws.

In reference to the transmission of the disease directly from man to man there was one paper by Dr. Mongour of Bordeaux which should tend to allay the great fear many have of contracting the disease directly from the affected one. Dr. Mongour studied 440 cases where in the family either the husband or the wife was ill with consumption or had died of this disease. In these 440 instances he found only 16 cases where the partner in marriage was also afflicted; i. e., less than 4 per cent. His conclusion is that consumption is contagious, but that with proper restraints it is so feebly so that parents and friends should be much more calm and courageous. Again, the idea of the inheritance of tuberculosis has received in the Paris Congress many hard blows, and it must be believed that the disease in descendants is mainly dependent upon the greater opportunity of infection and not on the direct transmission of the disease, though it is admitted that a soil favorable to tuberculosis may be inherited.

Additional stress was laid upon early diagnosis, and some new features leading to this desirable end were suggested, with the view of discovering the cases of consumption even before the individual himself realizes he is ill, for the earlier the disease is discovered the greater the chance of recovery. In this connection it may be said the French lay great stress upon the importance of giving attention to a class which they define as the "pre-tuberculous," meaning by that term those who from one cause or another are so built or so reduced in vitality that they seem likely subjects for infection with tuberculosis. They insist these individuals should be treated much as if they were already tuberculous in order to prevent them from becoming such. If this is done many may be saved from acquiring the disease; young, pale, delicate individuals, or those with greatly reduced chest capacity, particularly children, may readily be classed as "pre-tuberculous," and by judicious care or treatment may be saved the disease.

On the subject of feeding consumptives there seems to have been pretty general agreement that *correct feeding* is much better than *over feeding*, a sin of commission into which one is so likely to fall when the treatment is reduced to the *cure d'air, cure de repos, et cure d'alimentation*, the "therapeutic triad" of sanatorium physicians. In some of the French clinics great faith is placed upon feeding with raw meat and its advocates maintain that they find quicker and surer improvement with its use than with any other food. It is administered either as the pulp of raw meat, or as the juice of the pulp.

Landouzy and other French observers have called attention to the fact that dogs and cats occasionally are subjects of tuberculosis, and they point out that perhaps more frequently than may have been supposed the lap dogs and cats are the source of infection in man.

Particularly interesting were the papers and discussion in the section devoted to childhood. France leads the world in its efforts in this direction, largely through the energy of Professor Grancher, who presided over the section. In a few words I can perhaps sum up the main features which are worthy of attention. As Professor Grancher sees it, tuberculosis is a contagious malady and nearly always contracted by the small child in a contaminated or infected home; that the tuberculosis of adults is most often a tuberculosis of childhood which has remained latent, that in consequence the preservation and protection of the child is the most effective means of combating the disease. Therefore to preserve the child it is necessary,

1. To make the home clean and hygienic.
2. To sterilize the milk the child consumes.
3. If the home is infected, to remove the child as early as possible.
4. To employ such measures as will tend to strengthen the child's constitution.

In order to remove children still well from infected homes, Professor Grancher has established a society which has for its object the care in the country near Paris of poor children taken from such homes. This society assumes that the children it takes are likely from their surroundings to become tuberculous and so by their removal are saved, and in their new environment become strong, healthy individuals. This represents the latest feature in the development of the prevention of tuberculosis and is akin to the treatment of the "pre-tuberculous" to which I have already referred. It is the new idea and one which will be particularly identified with this last Congress. Other measures in use in France for the upbuilding of weakly children are the maintenance at public expense of the so-called *cantines scolaires*, or free lunches, for those who need more food; and the *vacation colonies* by means of which delicate poor children are sent to the country at public expense for three or four weeks each summer.

By the fuller development of these salutary measures much is to be looked for in saving the coming generation. For children already afflicted no country has made such large provision as France. Something like four thousand beds are at the disposal of children either at the seaside or in the hills, and great encouragement is to be found in studying the results of treatment, particularly in cases of surgical tuberculosis, such as hip disease, scrofula, etc. In this country we have but scarcely made a beginning in this work, Dr. Halsted being the first to send such patients to the Adirondacks and Dr. Brannan in New York, having established a small seaside sanatorium at Coney Island. The Floating Hospital in Boston Harbor is also a development in the same direction. I am glad to say, too, Dr. Lowman in Cleveland has taken up Professor Grancher's idea and is advocating the necessity of removing children from infected homes, sending them to the country and indemnifying the parents if the child has been a source of support.

Great stress was laid upon the importance of school hygiene, out-of-door exercises for the child, and *special instruction* in practical hygiene during school life, so that pupils should not have merely some mental pictures of what is necessary, but rather from daily practical experience and teaching should acquire *automatic habits* of the essential features. In this respect we may look to great improvements in our public schools so that they may become to children what sanatoria are to adults, namely, really schools giving instruction in the simple principles of correct living.

This thought brings me to speak of the important discussion held in Section 4 upon the place of the sanatorium and the dispensary in the fight against tuberculosis. It was a most important discussion participated in by the best men of many countries, and the conclusion reached may seem somewhat disappointing to those whose feelings are centered upon the individual sick patient, rather than upon the greater question of stamping out the disease altogether. This conclusion was that whereas many may be improved and cured, the really great value of the sanatorium and dispensary lies in teaching measures by which tuberculosis can be avoided, *i. e.*, in teaching prophylaxis. The real suppression of tuberculosis, therefore, becomes a social problem in which better housing, less crowding, increased wages, better food, wider streets, more parks, higher intelligence and greater knowledge are the real factors.

The Tuberculosis Exposition held in connection with the Congress was in a larger way an amplification of the Exposition held here in McCoy Hall two years ago. Most European countries contributed, the United States alone omitting to do so, from the fact that no one undertook the task of being responsible for it. Models of sanatoria, charts, maps, reports, tables of statistics, photographs of all sorts, model beds, chairs, rooms, etc., composed the greater part of the exposition, but among the most interesting of all exhibits were the two made by the Pasteur Institute and the Veterinary School at Alfort. In the first were cultures of the tubercle bacillus from every possible source, and in the latter a demonstration of how universally our domestic animals and birds are occasionally afflicted with the disease.

The entertainments and excursions were very enjoyable and instructive. The President of the Congress, Professor Hérard, held a large reception at the Continental Hotel, and the President of the Republic gave a dinner and a large reception at the Elysée Palace. A noteworthy feature of the Congress and one particularly to be approved was the interest taken in the work by the large daily papers—the *Matin* entertaining every one at a theatre performance at which among other things was given Molière's comedy, "Le médicin malgré lui," *The Figaro* giving a reception, and the *Journal* sending a special train to the Riviéra.

At two or three of the previous Congresses there has been one communication which has stood out pre-eminently above all others in interest; in this respect this last Congress did not differ from the preceding. The sensation in Paris was found in Professor von Behring's communication expressing the conviction that he had discovered a substance or a principle which can be used "to protect men threatened with phthisis against the dangerous consequences of tuberculous infection." As yet he is not ready to speak freely of this new substance, for he wishes to make farther researches with it. He names the curative principle T. C. This is what plays the essential rôle in the immunizing action of the bovo-vaccine by means of which he has rendered calves immune to tuberculosis. When this T. C. is introduced into the body it forms in the cells of the body something which he terms T. X., and it is this T. X. which gives the immunity or resistance to the disease, probably a cellular immunity. The T. C. is obtained from the tubercle bacilli and, therefore, it must be assumed that these germs which are in themselves to be considered as *damaging* do contain a substance which is *curative*. It is not a living substance nor self reproducing, but nevertheless "it can be made far superior to the living bacillus in regard to its protective and curative action." In a paper on von Behring's communication Klebs of Chicago concludes with these words, "Considering once more Behring's announcement in the light of his own and other experimental studies, we are allowed to conclude that he has entered on a new line of work and that his further reports will merit great attention. On the whole, it seems that his method is based on principles, elaborated before him by others, especially Metschnikoff and E. Klebs. How much, ultimately, suffering mankind is to profit cannot be predicted, nor can Behring's expressed, though carefully and ambiguously worded expectations, mean anything but a plausible hypothesis, yet unproved by him, of a curative principle, applicable in human tuberculosis."

At the last session of the Congress American representatives presented the invitation of our National Association coupled with Mr. Roosevelt's personal invitation for the next International Congress to be held in Washington. Great enthusiasm greeted these invitations, and it was unanimously voted to go to Washington in 1908.

GOVERNOR JOHN WINTHROP, JR., OF CONNECTICUT, AS A PHYSICIAN.

SECOND PAPER.

By WALTER R. STEINER, A. M., M. D.,

Formerly House Medical Officer, The Johns Hopkins Hospital.

Since writing my first paper on John Winthrop, Jr., as a Physician,[1] I have seen twenty-nine additional Winthrop letters, which all bear on medical topics and show still further the high esteem in which the people held him for his medical knowledge. All of the letters, save three, were addressed to him by those who wanted advice as to treatment for themselves, their families or friends. Two of the remaining three were written by those unknown to Winthrop to some of his acquaintances, asking them for aid in gaining Winthrop's medical advice, while the third letter was written by Winthrop in reply to one included in this list. This collection of medical letters was presented to the Boston Medical Library in 1879 by Hon. R. C. Winthrop, and I am greatly indebted to the late Dr. James R. Chadwick, the former librarian, for his courtesy in allowing me to copy and publish them.

Eighteen of the letters were sent to Winthrop at Pequot (New London), two were addressed to him at Hartford, and eight show no indication as to their final destination. Two were written in 1651, fifteen in 1652, two in 1653, one in 1656, and four in 1663. Windsor, Wethersfield, Saybrook, Hartford,

[1] Steiner, "Governor John Winthrop, Jr., of Connecticut, as a Physician." Johns Hopkins Hospital Bull., 1903, XIV, pp. 294-302.

New Haven and Branford in Connecticut; Springfield, Hadley, Ipswich, Watertown and Rehoboth, in Massachusetts, and Easthampton, Southampton and Southold in Long Island, were the towns in which the writers dwelt. These letters show in eight instances a desire to satisfy Winthrop for his services. Daniel Clark writes: " I wil satisfy his worship for the same, in silver or otherwise, according to his demand," while George Ward, benefited by Winthrop's visit, declares: " If you pleas to show me wherein I may answer your charge and travell I shall be desirous to attend you." Again, Robert Fuller, showing by his letter that he was somewhat illiterate and also poor in this world's goods, declares he will be freely willing in some measure to satisfy Winthrop. William Andrews and his family appear to have been gratuitous patients, as he characterizes Winthrop's services as " a labor of love for us." I have previously given extracts from a number of Goodwin's letters, and some, subsequently written, in this collection, show that Winthrop probably received compensation for his medical labors. In one of them Goodwin wants more medicine for his wife, and adds: " I shall sattisfy for all."

Robert Bond of Easthampton, magistrate of the town as well as gospel minister, sought Winthrop's advice before he removed to Barbadoes on account of an offense, which public sentiment would not condone. For he had previously preached a sermon, not composed by himself, which on its discovery was considered " highly disreputable." He requests aid on a neighbor's behalf, whose children were " destempered with some disease on their heads. It appears to have been a whitish scabb—dry for the most part only uppon their takeinge coullde it have run exceedingly." The duration of the affection was two years and a half and " on the first risinge of it it came in spots like the forme allmost of A ring worme." The scabs gradually increased in thickness and sometimes could be removed by the application of " butter and beare." A violent itching in their heads also troubled the children, most commonly about bed time. Robert Fuller, also anxious about a similar scalp affection, writes a line from Rehoboth. He states his " children's heads, which Winthrop saw, groweth worse, the hair cometh off." His sister, Wheaten, was troubled with small worms and he desired Winthrop to " direct us or her about it."

James Fitch, of Norwich, pastor of the church there, with a tender solicitation for one of his flock, asks Winthrop's help for her " whom its conceaved hath a dropsy which swells her leggs, thighes and bodie up towards the stomacke. Sometimes it does abate and then uppon a catching of cold it increaseth agayne." Her husband, Richard Towslande, had previously received some medicine for her, but as no directions accompanied it he wishes to know how to use it. Fitch also writes about his own stomach trouble. He complained " sometymes with burning heate, sometymes loaded with fleame and much distempered in my heade with fumes of a corrupt stomacke." And Richard Smyth, full of concern about " my son's wife lidia," writes from Wethersfield on February 21, 1652, that she " was full of pain from her navill

to ye crowne of her head when the sickness first tooke her. After three restless weeks she felt something to role within her, and her breath was redie to be stopd. after yt she roused and raised corruption and now alate she vomits up bladders about ye bignes of a walnut and some like to a bullet of cleare water and raiseth corruption wᵗʰ them: She coufs and raiseth filthi stufe." He entreats Winthrop to send her advice and remedies. Sarah Rood, " troubled with ye falling out of ye wome these three years and more after her first child was borne," also besought Winthrop's council and help, and John Clark writes that his wife had taken the portions of medicine which was sent her, but though they were effectual in causing two attacks of vomiting and three movements of the bowels, " yet she voided no worms at all." As " she thinketh that something bobeles up in hear throt still that makes hear think it must be Chest wormes."

Other women patients than these also demand his attention. Andrew Haniford beseeches " Winthrop's favor to consider the case and condition of his wife, craving his council and advise for what to do." She had been troubled with cold feet for a year and a half. Presently her " whole body became likewise affected and suddenly it turned to a flushing heate and extrem paine and weaknes in her back and a great stoping at her stomocke and when she cannot Raise anything is exceeding sicke and when she doth Raise there cometh up blood with it." She had had a child some months before and about thirty days after childbirth " these could and hote fitts tooke her again and so it continueth with extrem weakness and stoping at her stomocke." " Mrs Whitne's trubble in her head " necessitated her husband to write to Winthrop for medical assistance. " The trubble " was described as " not a payne but a swiming as it wear which as wee conceve is ocashioned from a cloging at her stomake and sum times she is overrun with a sudden flashing heat and she is much overrun with malancolly."

Many male patients, too, pour forth their complaints to Winthrop. John Sherman, minister of the gospel at Watertown, informs our worthy governor on June 30, 1663, that " the hernia I have formerly bin troubled with doth still continue with and grow uppon me: noe meanes hitherto used have availed to doe me any good. The tumor is even without any unequall unshapen excrescence in any part and hath not (to feeling) ye hardnes of a scirhus. It is hardest upwards towards my body, and more soft downward, but doth not pitt or retaine any impression: without inflammation or paine. Mr. Clark (after sight and feeling) hath expressed that he conceiveth it to be mostly wind and water and that a seton might doe me good." Joseph Howard, not gaining benefit from the " fiseke " Winthrop had given him, and being much troubled with his water again desires that some remedies be sent him. He writes: " My watter is verie burning to me and my watter is verie thike and att the last there is some blood and I am very costiff in my bodie. I would entreate you to send me a verie stronge purge and some of that water which I had beffore." In a postscript he adds that the bearer of the letter " hath a wife who hath a verie greatte swelling in her brest and would desire you to deirect him about it." William Andrews, poor and afflicted with a " distemper, a flucke and loossness one year and 7 months for the most part," writes from New Haven, giving particulars about this distemper, which the " french doctor could only stay for two weeks when it brock out agayne." He wished his case considered and something sent him by " this bearer." If necessary, he is willing to come to Pequot for treatment. Daniel Hovey, from Ipswich, almost a confirmed dyspeptic, states that the remedies Winthrop had sent caused much relief. At present, he adds : " I find much Confluens of wind in my bowels working up and down my stomack thoe not wth such a Juncter of fiem and mellancolly as formerly I have therw^th bin exsersised . . . . . I find an incapacity to digest and such obstruction of wind allongst wth ye us of food y^t oft tims I have thout best to fast away my ilnes and thout it ye only menes for my cur and I think I have oft thuse escaped but herby my body hath bin brought verie low . . . . . . At times I am troubled with hart burning ye only remedy against wch I find ye us of Curnell of 2 or 3 peach stones Curs. I find y^t after a tedious fit y^t going out I oft find it accompanied with a tedious stitch on my brest somtims on my hart and sometims to sid and chest and about my brest it may be 2 or 3 days wch provoks to a kind of sigs and then it be tedioussome soe to doe." Nathaniel Bliss, likewise numbered among Winthrop's patients, desires further attention as the " powders " would not work.

Besides these the Wards, father and son, have their afflictions to lay before Winthrop. The father appears to have had some difficulty in micturition, due to an enlarged prostate. He had also suffered from a " bastard pleurisy " the previous spring. While the son's " trubel " is this : " At sometims when I am in my sleep I am for the space of half an houer insensibel of any thing somtims shaking in this.tim with my body somtims lying still as on dead, after this in extream pain in my bake : also colde : a pain at my stumake : afterwards in my head : but as the wind doth go from my stumake I have eas again : I hav had 4 of theis fits sinc January last which is all to this tim."

Winthrop was also much sought after to treat many children. William Andrewes, from Hartford, in 1653, desires his daughter, who was staying at Pequot for Winthrop's treatment, to be returned to them by " some Master of the Pinness wch cometh from Pequet to hartford." On May 9 of that year we hear " she returned faint and weak when shee came to us and troubled with a cough." The medicine Winthrop had prescribed had been taken, but the cough had increased. She had also " a payn in her backe and left side" and Andrew feared she was too weak to go again to Pequot, so wished something sent up to her. Summer diarrhoea of infauts affecting the little daughter of John Pynchon of Springfield, aged " about or neere one yeare and three quarters old," caused him anxiously to write to Winthrop in 1663. " She hath not bin very well," he says, " these 3 or 4 days,

but especially yesterday morning was taken wth a greate looseness and vomiting wch doth continue much and excedingly weakens her. She is very restless and unquiet, and sleepes little and is exceding dry craving for drink." Nine years earlier Daniel Clark from Windsor asks Hugh Caukins " to procure me the help of y^t worthy instrument (Winthrop) whom I heare is to be highly prized for his great skill." Clark needed Winthrop's aid as his son, aged four years, as well as his daughter, aged about a year and a quarter, were having much trouble from the rapid decay of their teeth. Abigail Montague, too, required Winthrop's medical services, as her child had some eye trouble.

The most interesting letters in this collection refer to the children of Samuel Stone and Richard Odell. The former was assistant to Thomas Hooker, first pastor of the First Church of Christ, in Hartford. Stone[2] was very much worried over his child's illness. He states " the child is 23 weeks old, hath been somewhat ill 3 or 4 weeks, unquiet his eyes looking yellow, having a cough especially when he takes his victuals. Wee thought he might have been breeding teeth : but about a week past we peceived y^t he hat the yellow Jaundise. By Mrs Hooker her advise we gave him Barbarie barke boyled in beer, with saffron, twice in a day, for two dayes together : and one time saffron alone. Also lice[3] 2 or 3 times, and Tumerick twice. we hoped y^t the Jaundise had been cured : because he was sometimes more chearefull and had a better appetite, but the last Saterdaie at night he was very unquiet, heavie and could not sleep and upon the Sabbath seemed to looke somewhat swart in the face. In the afternoone we gave him about 3 quarters of a grain of your purging powder,[4] which we had of Mrs Haynes which caused him to vomit twice or three and to purge downwards thrice—he slept well the night after and in the morning was somewhat unquiet again as before, wringing and winding back, his cough seemes to increase, as if he had much fleagme. he seems to be sick at times but without any convulsion or starting fits. when he began to be ill he was costive in his bodie but now is in good temper. he doth not burne often, but a little sometimes. I pray Sir send me word whether he may not take some more

[2] I have elsewhere (see " Some Early Autopsies in the United States." Johns Hopkins Hosp. Bull., 1903, XIV, pp. 201-203) spoken of the autopsy on Rev. Mr. Stone, which was probably performed by Dr. Bryan Rossiter, of Guilford, Conn. I there quote from Mathers Magnalia: " As for Mr. Stone, if it were *metaphorically* true (what they *proverbially* said) of Beza, that ' he had no gall,' the physicians that opened him after his death found it *literally* true of this worthy man."

[3] " In 1708 Lady Otway gives two receipes for curing jaundice made up mostly of yellow substances. In one she put lemon, tumeric, and saffron ; the other consisted of 20 head-lice mixed with nutmeg and sugar and powder of tumerick " (Eggleston. " The Transit of Civilization." New York, 1901. See chapter on " Concerning Medical Notions.")

[4] I take this to be a reference to Winthrop's " sovereigne remedy," Rubila. In another letter, in this collection, John Sherman craves Winthrop's kindness in supplying him with a little of ye red powder, which probably refers also to Rubila.

of that pouder and what quantity. If you thinke it convenient to prescribe anything I pray speake to Mr Blinman. I know he will ᵖᶜᵘʳᵉ some Indian to bring your note and I will please him for his journey."

Richard Odell's daughter was troubled with an "ichey humer all over her body." Finally the "humer stoped by degrees but before it was quit stoped shee began to be very plesent and joccund and spoke very plesently the same moment that shee was stricken about the 20 day of October last about 11 or 12 as shee was sitting by the fier shee rise up hastily to fetch som victells shee fell downe upon ou side been set up againe she was neither able to stand nor speak and she hath continued till this Instant haveing lost the use of the right side from the head to the foot she hath gained lately som strength on her lieg she can stand wᵗʰ a littell helpe and is able to sit upright wᵗʰ her body wᵗʰout support— but cannot speak a word she is sensable of feeling through out her lame part it is somthing swelled and very sore in the flesh and hath an exceeding payne in Her other part as in her leg and arme I meane that wᶜʰ shee hath use of. She hath also a stopage in her throat or below the swallow when she drinks that she can scarsely induer to drink or take any liquid mater."

To this Winthrop replied in the following letter, which I quote in full:

PEQUOT, Nov. 27. 1652

SIR.—I received your letter about 2 daies since wherin you desire directions concerning your child, wch indeed is very uncertaine to doe in the absence of the pty. it being difficult to find out the true cause & seat of the originall of such disease by the most diligent & curious observations, where the patient is dayly present: for though by your description I judge it to be a palsy, yet the cause of that disease is often very differing for in some it is through too much drinesse in some too much moisture in some the cause is in the Nerves of the third coniugation of the braine sometymes in other nerves, in others it hath its originall in ye marrow of the back bone: this seemes to be that kind wch we call Hemiplegia where one halfe of the spinall marrow is affected, or [wch is often in others, and makes me doubt it may be so in this child; by reason of the suddainnesse wherewth she was stroken] it may come fro a light apoplexye [a stronger Apoplexye is comoly present in death] this lighter kind of Apoplexy strikes suddainly & leaves comonly one side wthout sence or motion, and after continueth it wholy paraliticall: it may also come fro some thick flegms stopping the influence and distribution of ye vitall spiritts in the nerves, wch may also cause that suddaine apoplecticall stupor. The cure depends upon the knowledge of the right cause, and not only that but the constant and due aplication of such things as may conduce thereto wch is difficult to doe at a distance. I am not provided of things alwaies ready for such cures yt are usuall to be had ready made in other places at the Apothecaries, and am forced to prepare things myselfe in such case where any neighbours doe want helpe and therefore am not able to send you many things that might be usefull, and I suppose it would be as uselesse to prescribe you such receipt as phisitians comend in those cases, wch I know it is not probable any of them to be had wth you. if the child were were me I might doe mine indeavour to provide such things as I could heare make myselfe and see to the due administration therough, otherwise I accont it an hopelesse to direct for the cure of so dangerous a

disease wherin the best meanes often faile of help: some generall things that may be helpfull In all kinds of those diseases I shall mention. there is a Coldnesse comonly accompanes this disease, whatever ther cause be, therfore warmth by aplication of hares or ffox ffure [wch is also specificall to paralitical disteprs] or in want therof Racoones or lamb or swanes or such as can be had: also artificiall meanes of heat by hott clothes, hott trenchers or brickes wraped up in cloths aplied to the place most benumned also oyntments of hott chimicall oyles as of rosmary tyme Origanū also oyle of castor mixed wth a greater quantity of oyle of wormes & fox grease, or for want of these wth fox grease alone: or wch is counted very efficatious the Balsam of Guido if you have any [it is an ordinary knowne oyntment] though at present I have none of it but have sent you another oyntment instead thereof with wch or wth any of the other if they be to be had anoynt the whole backe bone as hott as can be endured & that side that is affected twice a day covering it presently wth hott clothes, also the aplying of cupping glasses to the heads of the muskles, they might be such glasses as have very narrow mouths and must be aplied without scarification, & wth a great & quick flame but must not continue as long as in other cases, but be often reiterated and a plaister of Colophony frankincense & rosin wth the pouder of Bayberries, these mixed wth as much melisett plaister all melted together & made into a plaister, and aplied to the places after the cupping glasses, also some bathes wherin the decoction of Betony Rosmary sage in a quanty of sweete sacke or muskadell but better the spiritts of those herbes & other hott herbes mixed with it: but speciall care must be in the using of a bath least it overcome the patient or too much relax the nerves by being too long in it or too hott aplied: I use in such cases a bath of minerall spiritts wch I find both safe & effectuall in many cases coming neere the virtue of the naturall bathes wch must be used immediately after it is prepared, therefore I never prepare it but as it is used, nor cannot contrive a way to supply you wth it so farre of; I commend also to be used inwardly a decoction of Gualcū & Sassaparilla also some drops of the spirit of rosmary in bere if it may be had, or in want of it Rosemary boyled in broth & so taken, a vomitt in some kind of such disease is usefull but not in every kind, an Issue on the contrary arme or legge as the nature of the disease apeares if most upward in the legge if most downward in the arm may be usefull: but if she be of a very spare bode it will not be good: this is what I cā for the present advise. so with loving salutations to yourselfe & wife wth Mr. Howell & thous I rest   Your loving friend,

J. WINTHROP.

This letter with an ointment and electuary were received by Odell and by the use of the remedies his daughter improved. Odell later writes she can "both walk and talke," though "she speaks imperfectly and walks lamely." Although her strength had much recovered, yet her arm was almost useless. "She can lift it up to her mouth and can grip with it, but she cannot open it when she would . . . . She is as sencable on that part as in the other I doe conceive that the disease lis mostly in her braine and nerves. She hath her apprehension as well as ever. her memory failes exceedingly that shee cannot express herself as she could. we have use the best meens that the plac can afford. we have wrap her in fox furs and anoynted her with fox grease and have keep her very warme." He was unable to send her down to Winthrop, as his wife could not accompany her and it would "kill her" to go alone.

THE ADVANTAGES OF LOCAL SANATORIA IN THE TREATMENT OF PULMONARY TUBERCULOSIS.

By David R. Lyman, M. D.,

Medical Superintendent Gaylord Farm Sanatorium; Clinical Lecturer in Medicine, Yale Medical School.

In discussing the subject of local sanatoria it will be my purpose to deal with them chiefly in relation to those sufferers from tuberculosis who have not the advantage of independent means, and for whom, as well as for the community in which they live, the problem of their treatment, restoration to health, and return to the ranks of the wage earners is infinitely difficult.

There is no question as to the salutary effect of that old and trusted prescription, " a change of climate " in most cases of tuberculosis; nor that rejuvenation of the whole system, with restoration of the normal powers of resistance which is the chief means through which the sanatorium treatment of tuberculosis reaches its desired goal, can be more quickly attained under those climatic conditions which best fulfill the needs of each individual case. Sanatoria for private patients are now to be found in every country, and in localities of climatic conditions so diverse that the man of means has but to decide which will prove best suited to his needs to avail himself of the advantages it offers.

But for the patient whose means are limited the institutions at which he will be received are few; principally situated at a great distance from his home, and of such relatively limited capacity as to admit of their receiving only a small portion of those who seek their aid. By far the larger majority of consumptives who seek health in the leading resorts spend their time while there in boarding houses, and under conditions which of necessity preclude them from obtaining the great advantage of constant medical supervision and careful schooling in their general habits of life which sanatorium treatment affords.

Before taking up the possibilities and advantages of local sanatoria for the reception of this class of cases, it is necessary to answer one question which is still uppermost in the minds of many of the medical profession and most of the general public; and that is as to their efficiency from a medical standpoint. Can tuberculosis be cured under such conditions? Can it be cured anywhere, except in a few justly noted localities, whose fatal influence on the viability of the tubercle bacillus is so firmly believed in as to cause both physicians and friends frequently to overlook the fatal effects of the journey on the patient?

To find the answer to these questions one has but to consider the location of the many institutions now established for the open air treatment of tuberculosis and compare their results. Contrast for example the Adirondack Cottage Sanitarium with that at Fort Bayard, N. M.; or the Agnes Memorial at Denver with Dr. Millet's Sanatorium at East Bridgewater, on the Massachusetts coast; or again the sanatoria in the Swiss Alps and the Black Forest with those on the

banks of the Rhine or with Dr. Phillip's noted institution in the suburbs of Edinburgh. You have localities whose atmospheric conditions and the character of whose soils are wholly dissimilar. Compare their results, and while some will show a greater degree of efficiency than others, yet for similar classes of cases and length of treatment a singular conformity obtains. Surely one must be convinced that for this striking uniformity of their results these institutions do not depend upon the widely different localities in which they are situated, but rather upon some factor common to them all. Further examination proves this to be a fact. We find perhaps each one laying particular stress on some especial feature of the treatment, but all employ the same general routine; rest in the open air, regulated exercise, wholesome food and constant medical supervision whose chief aim is to thoroughly school the patient in the new and rational mode of life so essential to his ultimate recovery.

To those who ask if tuberculosis can be successfully treated under local conditions we can say unhesitatingly, " Yes "; provided that the treatment be carried out under the régime of a modern sanatorium whose situation is such as to combine an atmosphere free from dust and smoke, with ample sun light and good drainage of the soil; and surely such a site is readily accessible to every community.

Having established the feasibility of the successful treatment of tuberculosis wherever the above requirements can be provided, we now come to the consideration of those factors which render the local treatment of its tuberculous members more desirable, not only from the standpoint of the patient, but from that of the community itself.

We must at the outset divide these patients into two distinct classes according to the medical condition they present; the favorable and the far advanced cases; whose distinctive needs demand that they be cared for in absolutely separate institutions. A very brief connection with any sanatorium for incipient tuberculosis will suffice to convince one of the necessity for more adequate provisions for the advanced cases. Institutions for incipient tuberculosis refuse admission each year to as many applicants as they receive, if not more.

Influence of all kinds is brought to bear on those in charge in order to secure admission for these advanced cases, and we are often openly charged with too great a regard for our statistics. And yet, the donors to any charitable work make one universal requirement; evidence that their money is accomplishing definite results. And in this case these results are measured solely by the percentage of cured or arrested cases that these institutions send back to take care of their share of the world's work. Did they fill their beds with the incurable cases that besiege their doors, they would soon have to close those doors for a lack of financial support.

Beyond all such considerations there are, however, sound medical and economic reasons why the two classes should be cared for separately. They require very different treatment. The early cases need but little nursing, but rather medical supervision combined with a careful training for the needs of their future years. The advanced cases, on the other hand, chiefly require careful and constant nursing and treatment, entailing an entirely different equipment from that required in institutions for the care of incipients. Nor is it right or just to the curable cases to take in the incurable among them. Tuberculosis differs from almost every other disease in that its treatment to be successful must extend over many months under conditions of restraint that grow irksome at times to the most stoical; and it is imperative that the patient's environment be made as cheerful and agreeable as possible. It is impossible for a man who has a given disease, no matter in how slight a degree, to be thrown in daily contact with another, hopelessly sick with the same disease, and watch him sinking nearer and nearer to his end without questioning as to the possibility of his own case eventually reaching the same state; and so in simple justice to the curable cases we must refuse admission to the far-advanced. Almost the greatest medical need of any of the larger towns and cities of this country to-day is that of institutions where far-advanced cases of tuberculosis can be given proper care. The general hospitals cannot receive them unless they be given proper facilities for the purpose. Dispensaries for tuberculosis with their staff of visiting physicians and nurses to care for and instruct the patients in their homes, do great good, but can only reach the few. The only way in which these cases can be adequately cared for is in institutions erected and equipped for that sole purpose.

From a humanitarian standpoint no one who has ever seen an advanced case of tuberculosis struggling for life or for bare comfort in the midst of unfavorable home conditions can ever question their usefulness. But what of the economic side of the question, will it pay in dollars and cents for any corporate community to provide accommodations for these cases? I think that a careful consideration of this question will convince anyone that it will, and pay well.

We can even omit all consideration of loss of earning capacity of the member of the family who must act as nurse; and also the well-known economy of caring for many patients together instead of each one separately. All we need ask consideration of is the enormous saving through placing these cases where they will not constantly imperil the lives of all around them. We have all seen whole families wiped out of existence by the ravages of this disease. And while we know that tuberculosis is preventable, we also know that amongst the poorer classes we find neither the knowledge nor the facilities for its cure or prevention. Any large city that provides adequate means for the care of these cases would, purely from a financial standpoint, be amply repaid in the saving of life

and of earning capacity amongst the remaining members of their household.

I look upon hospitals for far-advanced cases of tuberculosis as pre-requisite to the control of the disease.

Let us now consider the question of local sanatoria for the early or curable cases, and see what if any are the advantages they offer over those in distant resorts. What have they to offset the benefit often derived from a marked change of climate?

Their advantages are all derived from the simple fact of their accessibility. It is easier to persuade a patient to go there for treatment. Tuberculosis is often an insidious disease, and its symptoms and physical signs may be apparent to the physician at the time when the patient himself can hardly believe there is anything serious the matter with him. And while he may be persuaded to give up work for a time, yet the expenses and discomfort of a long journey and the separation from his family seem to him hardly necessary. He can be much sooner persuaded to go to a place but a few miles distant and from which he can readily return whenever his health admits; and a difference of a week or two in the commencement of treatment may mean a month or two in the time needed for the arrest of the disease.

Often we find a case that is willing and anxious to go, but who is entirely dependent upon his own scant means. We find him doing extra work at a time when he should be doing none in order to raise the money for railway fares, hotel bills, etc. A local institution saves him not alone the time that he devotes to earning this extra money, but also the sorely needed strength he expends in this extra work, sometimes forever losing his chance of renewed health. More than this, the cost of these travelling expenses would in most cases easily cover the cost of a month or more in a sanatorium, and the permanency of the results of treatment bears a direct ratio to its length.

We find therefore that a patient will be willing to come sooner, and will be able to remain longer in the case of the local institutions.

Another advantage of the local sanatoria is that the patient is not deprived of the comfort of seeing his family and friends. All influences that tend to keep him cheerful and contented have a distinct value for him and must be given due weight. We see cases sent far away from home in whom the element of homesickness or the anxiety concerning home affairs is so strong as to seriously impair the benefits they would otherwise receive, and to these the frequent visits of the family are of great benefit.

The principal value of local treatment from the standpoint of the patient is to be found in this very fact that his friends and relatives can and do visit him. One of the chief dangers to a patient after his return from a distant sanatorium is that those at home have no conception whatever of the life he should lead, or the extreme importance of its routine being closely observed. His letters have been calculated to surprise rather than to instruct. They have told of sitting and sleeping out of doors in all sorts of weather, and have magnified each circumstance until those at home often feel that his recovery is in spite of and not on account of the life he has led. And when he returns he has to contend against the old established opinions as to night air, etc.—a serious drawback.

Often, too, the family themselves are responsible for the patient's relapse from attempting to resume work too soon. The first fact that impresses a visitor to a sanatorium for tuberculosis is that all the patients there look astonishingly healthy; often more so than the visitor himself. Only the physician can realize how far the improvement in the general health outstrips that in the condition of the disease process, and that the real danger-point in tuberculosis is, as expressed by Babcock, the time when the patient first commences to look and feel perfectly well. Let such a patient return to his home where the burden of his care entails expense, self-denial, and often hardship on the other members of his family, and it is but natural that they should expect and often insist upon one who to their minds seems well, doing the work of a healthy man. Many a relapse in a case of arrested tuberculosis can be traced to just this source. Indeed we find that close proximity to the family can become a serious drawback on this account, for sometimes it is necessary to use every possible argument to induce those most concerned in the patient's recovery to allow him to remain under treatment sufficiently long.

As a rule, however, these visits of the family are of inestimable benefit. They see in actual operation the details of a life in a sanatorium, and how simple, sane and practical it all is. They regard it not so much with curiosity as with interest, for the possibility and advantage of their intelligent co-operation are manifest to them. They are no longer dependent upon the meagre details of the patient's letters, but can discuss the régime of the treatment with the physicians and nurses in person. They come to realize that the eventual cure of the patient entails something more than sitting on a porch for two or three months, and that they themselves have an important part to perform after the patient returns home.

In thus securing for the discharged patient the intelligent co-operation of his family local sanatoria have an advantage over distant institutions that can hardly be over-estimated.

To remain in constant touch with affairs at home is a distinct benefit to the patient in yet another way. Almost without exception when he leaves the sanatorium it is to face the problem of his own support. The average patient arriving at one of the noted resorts brings a letter asking if employment cannot be found by means of which he can pay for his treatment, or when that is ended maintain himself in that climate long enough to perfect his cure. But for every suitable position that offers there are a score of applicants, who only ask that the wages be sufficient to enable them to make both ends meet. Only one can obtain the place. The remaining nineteen must turn their faces homeward where in their prolonged absence the interest of their friends and acquaintances may have become inert. When the friends can visit the patient and watch his improvement from month to month this interest is not only kept alive but stimulated, and we find

them interesting their friends in turn, and keeping close watch for all suitable positions that may offer.

Also an occasional visit in person to a former employer results in a patient's old position (if at all suitable) being kept open for him much longer than when his condition and prospects are but indefinitely known.

The ready accessibility of the local institutions is of great benefit to the visitors themselves, and through them to the whole community. They are enabled to appreciate the fact that fresh air and sunlight were not intended solely for the cure of tuberculosis; but that the main principles of sanatorium treatment can be carried out at home to the benefit of the whole household, and as a result we find fresh air and sunshine in homes where they were previously unknown. More than this, the adequate simplicity of the sanitary precautions for the prevention of the disease is impressed upon their minds, and a lively interest in the anti-tuberculosis crusade awakened, thus creating an ever-widening basis of public interest on which to rely for the enactment and enforcement of measures tending to the betterment of the public health.

There is one more important consideration that must not be omitted. It is becoming more and more generally realized that it is not possible to effect a permanent cure of a case of tuberculosis within the few months' term of a sanatorium treatment. The Nomenclature Committee of the National Society recommended the following definition of a "cured" case: "All constitutional symptoms and expectorations with bacilli absent for two years under ordinary conditions of life." This means that the influences which have to bear upon the patient's life and health after his discharge from a sanatorium are of greatest importance, and that whatever tends to lower a patient's general condition, thus rendering him liable to relapse, should be avoided. It is well known that the indefinite influence of a distinct change of climate calls for a readjustment of the whole organism to its requirements; and when we bring a patient back from a totally different climate to resume his work, he has in addition to the increased calls upon his physical strength, to bear the strain of this readjustment. The patient discharged from a local sanatorium has not to contend with this.

There are many to whom these local institutions would be of the greatest benefit whom the distant ones cannot reach at all, and in whose care and control the community is most vitally interested. I refer to the ambulant, curable cases, who, while they would gladly avail themselves of the opportunity to obtain proper treatment, cannot afford to remain in the sanatorium for more than a few weeks. The expense of a long journey would leave no funds to meet their bills and they are forced to remain at home and at work, in utter ignorance of the care they owe to themselves or of the sanitary precautions they owe to their fellow-men. These are the ones whose expectoration upon the side-walks, in the cars, and in public places generally is such a menace to the public health; and in whose care and teaching the community is, therefore, as I have said, so vitally concerned. With railways and hotels no longer to be provided for, these cases gladly come for the limited term their means will allow; and the benefit to all concerned is very great. Often there is an arrest or an abatement of the activity of the disease; always the patient returns home not only with some definite conception as to the mode . of life necessary for his recovery; but with full knowledge as to the simplicity and the importance of the few sanitary precautions so essential to the prevention of the disease. The fact that they reach this class of cases is an advantage of local sanatoria which I would especially emphasize.

I do not wish to be misunderstood as to my opinion of the beneficial effects of climate in the treatment of tuberculosis. I regard it as a distinct benefit to all, and as an essential to some. But for the average patient I hold that treatment in local institutions possesses advantages that more than offset those derived from a change of climate, and that their chief advantages are to the community in or near which they are located. To this they afford a practical demonstration of the value of good hygiene and proper sanitary precautions in the cure and control of tuberculosis; and constantly stimulate an active public interest in all measures tending towards the eradication of the disease.

NOTES ON NEW BOOKS.

Multiple Personality. An Experimental Investigation into the Nature of Human Individuality. By Boris Sidis, M. A., Ph. D., and S. P. Goodhard, Ph. B., M. D. (*New York: D. Apple- ton & Co., 1905.*)

This volume is of value mainly because of the interesting collection of cases of dual or multiple personality which has been made. Some of these cases, notably that of Hanna, have been detailed at great length and form very interesting subject matter for thought and speculation as to the relations of the different personalities to each other. The authors do not believe that these conditions are necessarily associated with epilepsy and regard them rather as the result of a neuropathic disposition or constitution with consequent instability of the mental life. " The higher constellations and clusters of neurons with their concomitant mental systems are not firmly organized in the principal constellations correlative with the synthetic moment of self-consciousness. Thus the very cerebral organization has an inherent tendency to segmentation or even disintegration, under conditions that would in no way affect more stable organizations. A strong stimulus, or even one of medium intensity, may set up a process of disorganization. . . . . The hurtful stimulus may not be of a violent character, acting suddenly, but of a mild nature, acting for a long time on the neural constellations and finally inducing the phenomena of dissociation and disintegration." Such disorders are common in confirmed alcoholism or in epilepsy. The remedy, according to the authors, is through the employment of a species of hypnotism which they denominate the " hypnoleptic state," by which the intervals between the different personalities are made constantly shorter in duration until finally the different stages merge into each other and the dissociation is over.

The book is interesting and suggestive, but as it is confessedly based upon the single case of Hanna it is not wholly conclusive. It deserves careful reading and thoughtful consideration. The whole subject is still *in nubibus* and the solution of the many problems which it presents must come from an unprejudiced study of further similar cases. In the present volume the pathology and treatment of the condition are sought to be explained by an unproved working hypothesis as to the relations of neurons to each other. Something beyond this is unquestionably needed.

A Non-Surgical Treatise on Diseases of the Prostate Gland and Adnexa. By George Whitfield Overall, A. B., M. D. (*Chicago: Rowe Publishing Company, 1906.*)

A notice of the first edition of this book appeared in Vol. XV, p. 145. The present edition, we are told in the preface, has been revised carefully so that it may portray the author's present methods of practice, including new remedies and new instruments. The intention of the book seems unexceptionable; its apparent defect, however, is its absolute reliance upon non-surgical treatment for the relief of diseases of the prostate and adnexa. Granting that the results of the author's methods of treatment are good, the fact still remains that his methods are not applicable to all diseases of the prostate and adnexa. There are many diseases of the prostate which must have surgical treatment and it is to be regretted that the limitations of non-surgical treatment have not been clearly given.

The Subconscious. By Joseph Jastrow, Professor of Psychology in the University of Wisconsin. (*Boston and New York: Houghton, Mifflin & Co. The Riverside Press, Cambridge, 1906.*)

The author of that entertaining book, " Fact and Fable in Psychology," has now given us a volume on " The Subconscious." So much, either mysterious or nonsensical, has been written about the rare and unusual phenomena associated by the laity with this word that it is pleasing to have before us a discussion of the subject by a psychologist of reputation. Professor Jastrow tells us that subconscious functioning plays a very large part in the normal life of everyone; all degrees of transition, he believes, may be traced from experiences with which everyone is familiar to those remarkable phenomena occasionally observable in abnormal persons, namely, the dissociated consciousness and the altered personality.

The book is divided into three parts: I, Normal; II, Abnormal; and III, Theoretical.

In Part I the author tries to make clear the normal relations of the " subconscious " to our fully " conscious " processes; his task is here " the more precise comprehension of those manifestations of consciousness, and of those varieties of its activities, that take place below the threshold of our fully waking minds." This necessitates a description of the function of consciousness in which he finds the principle of utility effective, a discussion of the relation of consciousness to the nervous system, a chapter on consciousness and volition, and another on the distribution of attention. The mechanism of consciousness is next taken up, after which the author passes at once to the subconscious in mental procedure, deals with the subconscious maturing of thought, describes the lapses of consciousness which occur in normal individuals, and concludes this part of the book with a chapter on self-consciousness.

In Part II the " method of the abnormal " is applied to the

study of the subconscious and the phenomena observable when there is mentally a "quiescence of what is normally active" and a "prominence of what is normally subsidiary" are discussed. The author describes "dream-consciousness," and its variants (hypnagogic hallucinations, delirium and drug-intoxication), then passes on to a consideration of the "dissociated consciousness" (including somnambulism, hypnosis and the hysterical consciousness) and finally takes up the genesis of "altered personality" and the nature of "disintegrating lapses of personality." Among the interesting cases cited, Dr. Morton Prince's "multiple Miss B." occupies a prominent place.

The theoretical interpretation of the phenomena of the subconscious, normal and abnormal, is reserved for Part III. The treatment, though too complex to permit of brief analysis here is interesting and worthy of careful reading by all concerned with normal and morbid psychology. Jastrow asserts that "to secure acceptance, an interpretation of the varieties of subconscious activity must readily find place in a system of mental evolution." The subconscious is, he believes, intimately related to the whole mental economy and participates in even the more developed mental concerns. But it, like all other evolved faculties, is liable to arrest and decay, deformity and enfeeblement. The paths of dissolution are manifold and intricate, often puzzlingly divergent. The author's opinion differs entirely from the theory ordinarily spoken of as that of the "subliminal self," which emphasizes the schism of conflicting personalities as fundamental and regards all such phenomena as exceptional in nature, assuming, to explain them, the existence in the mental constitution from its outset of an entirely separate factor, an influence which becomes articulate only in exceptional circumstances when released from the thrall of ordinary consciousness. For Jastrow, the subconscious is "a natural function with the most intimate relations to consciousness, subject with it to like influences, both parts of a common synthesis, though of unlike service therein."

International Clinics. A Quarterly of Illustrated Clinical Lectures and Especially Prepared Original Articles on Treatment, Medicine, Surgery, Neurology, etc. By leading members of the medical profession throughout the world. Edited by A. O. J. Kelly, A. M., M. D., Philadelphia, U. S. A., with the collaboration of many others. Vol. II. Sixteenth Series, 1906. (*Philadelphia and London: J. B. Lippincott Company, 1906.*)

Reference has often been made in previous issues to the International Clinics which are issued twice each year with commendable regularity. The present volume is fully equal to any one of its predecessors and contains many valuable articles. Among them may be especially mentioned "The Prophylaxis of Nervous Disease, with special reference to educational influences in the growing child," by Dr. Zenner of Cincinnati. "The True Significance of Uric Acid," by Dr. Porter of New York, and "Experimental Researches bearing on Surgical Intervention in Nephritis," by Dr. Rovighi, of Bologna.

The Health-Care of the Baby. A Handbook for Mothers and Nurses. By Louis Fischer, M. D., Attending Physician to the Willard Parker and Riverside Hospitals. (*New York and London: Funk & Wagnalls Company, 1906.*)

This book is written for the use of mothers and nurses, but the subjects are treated in so brief a way that one must have considerable knowledge of the care of infants to be able to make use of the author's advice. However, on the whole, the information given is good, but the book would be improved if some of the themes were discussed more fully.

Medical and Surgical Report of the Presbyterian Hospital in the City of New York. Vol. VII. March, 1896. Edited by John S. Thacher, M. D., and George Woolsey, M. D., (*New York: Trow Directory Printing and Bookbinding Company.*)

The papers contained in this volume are of varying interest, but all do credit to the staff of the Presbyterian Hospital and indicate much activity on the part of its members. While it would be invidious to discriminate between them it is proper to mention several of special value. The "Open-air Treatment of Children in Fever and Convalescence," by Dr. Northrup, treats of a therapeutic measure of growing importance in the successful management of acute diseases. The discussion seems rather general in character and the reader cannot help wishing that more specific information had been given and the limitations of the application of the measure to acute diseases had been more fully considered. The procedure in fact seems dealt with in a popular rather than a scientific manner. It is to be feared that the enthusiasm of the author may lead some less experienced physician to attempt the open-air treatment in cases to which it is not well-suited. The paper on "Sporadic Trichinosis," by Dr. Bovaird, Jr., is an example of careful and painstaking study. It is gratifying to note that the writer gives full credit to the observation of Dr. T. R. Brown as to the diagnostic value of an increased eosinophilia in these cases. Dr. George Woolsey's paper on "Typhoid Perforation" is also worthy of note.

In "Suggested Analgesia," by Dr. Kingsbury, the interesting fact is brought out that however great the value of suggestion may be theoretically, practically the analgesic effects of hypnotism are only manifested in about 10 per cent of those cases which are susceptible to hypnotic influence. As the percentage of persons who can be hypnotized is relatively small, it seems very unlikely that hypnotic suggestion will ever play a very important rôle as a substitute for the use of anæsthetics in surgical operations. The volume contains 234 pages and is attractively printed.

Surgical Suggestions. Practical Brevities in Surgical Diagnosis and Treatment. By Walter M. Brickner, M. D., Chief of Surgical Department Mt. Sinai Hospital Dispensary and Eli Mascheowitz, M. D,. Assistant Physician, Mt. Sinai Hospital Dispensary, New York. (*New York Surgery Publishing Company, 1906.*)

These suggestions are terse, often epigrammatic, and constitute interesting reading, however much one may entertain doubts as to the practical utility of concentrated knowledge.

The Medical Diseases of Infancy and Childhood, with points on the Anatomy, Physiology, and Hygiene peculiar to the Developing Period. By Alfred Cleveland Cotton, A. M., M. D. (*Philadelphia and London: J. B. Lippincott Company, 1906.*)

The author has recognized the fact that an understanding of the anatomy, physiology and hygiene peculiar to the developing period is essential to the rational management of children and he presents most of the salient points in a clear and concise manner. We heartily subscribe to his opinion, that infant feeding is a problem of physiology and physiological chemistry and that the knowledge obtained along these lines must be taken into consideration. The importance of such an understanding of the scientific principles which form the basis of the modern conceptions of nutrition prompts us to review this part of the author's work more in detail.

In Part I, Chapter IV, headed "Physiology of the First Year," the statement occurs that a portion of the ingested water is directly absorbed from the surface of the stomach into the blood. This statement is not in accordance with the generally accepted teachings of physiology. The ferments of the small intestines proper seem to be entirely disregarded in the chapter, and thus the peculiar proteolytic enzyme, erepsin, escapes mention. This enzyme may prove of special interest since casein is one of the two native proteids so far known, which is subject to its action. The author copies freely from a paper by Southworth in regard to the chemical behavior of casein in the presence of acids, rennet and pepsin. We must remember that the results of the experiments of Slyke and Hart on which this paper is based do not necessarily apply to the problem of the digestion of human or cow's milk *by the infant.* In the infant, experiments are still to be conducted in regard to the action of human rennin on human milk, etc., since there seems to exist a certain specificity of the different ferments and there certainly exists a difference in the material to be acted upon. We have only to call attention to the inhibiting action of human milk on the coagulation of cow's milk by means of calf's rennin. The statement that young animals do not secrete any acid at first does not hold good for the human species if we can rely on the old data given by Zweifel and which have since been confirmed. The bacterial flora of the intestinal canal and of the feces, and its significance and the conditions under which this flora changes has received little or no attention. The main bacteria found in the feces of the normal breast-fed infant are, according to the author, *B. lactis ærogenes* and *B. coli communis,* the most abundant *B. bifidus, Tissier* is not mentioned.

With the fifth chapter we enter on the hygiene of the first year. The protection of the infant, the nursery, sleep, clothing, baths and exercise are ably considered. The closing sentence is, " an infant during the first year should neither be amusing nor amused." Sins against this rule are frequent!

Chapter VI is devoted to the natural feeding. The author emphasizes the necessity of intelligent control in regard to the act of suckling. Nevertheless, although " woman's instinct may have become perverted or deranged to a certain extent" in regard to the nursing, the instinct of the baby may frequently be relied upon, and if the mothers could be taught to refrain from inducing and encouraging their infants to nurse, when they have dropped the nipple with the apparent desire to go to sleep, much difficulty would be avoided. A fixed rule is given that the infant should be put to the breast every two hours during the day and once at night during the first six weeks. The actual number of meals under this regime is not stated. The fact that the stomach is found empty one and one-half to two hours after a meal certainly speaks against any more frequent nursing. But it does not indicate any necessity of a two-hour rule. Another reason, not expressedly stated by the author, may be advanced for the two-hour rule, and that is, that the single meal should not exceed the capacity of the stomach. Clinical observations, as well as experiments, in regard to the emptying of the stomach after ingestion of fluids, teach us not to lay too much stress on this latter point, and there does not seem to exist any reason whatever, why we should always adhere to the arbitrary two-hour rule laid down by many writers of text books. While the rule, that the time occupied in nursing and the quantity ingested should be controlled by the mother, is perhaps in most of the cases superfluous, in many instances it may be followed with advantage. The author recommends strongly and justly to give the baby water systematically and freely. When giving the constituents of breast milk a little lapse occurs on the part of the author in classifying lactalbumen and lactoglobulin as whey proteids. While these proteids are found in whey, the term whey-proteid (Molkeneiweiss) was introduced by Hammarsten to designate a certain proteid which supposedly is produced by the action of rennin on casein. The statement, that an infant at the breast digesting well and gaining in weight and strength, is ingesting normal milk, regardless of what the analysis may show, should

be taken to heart. The author does not seem to be quite clear in speaking about the reaction of human milk and later of cow's milk. In stating the reaction of milk the indicator must always be given. Thus both milks are alkaline towards lacmoid and acid towards Phenolphtalein. The biological properties of milk have received practically no attention.

In Chapter VII the hygiene of lactation is considered. In this chapter much more stress ought to be laid on the stimulus of suckling to excite the flow of a sufficient milk supply and the dangers of milk stasis are too important not to receive any consideration. Furthermore, it might be well to mention the drugs which are eliminated through the mammary glands.

Chapter VIII treats of milk analysis. The methods of fat determination of Holt, Freser, and Marchand are obsolete and should be discarded. The exact methods for the determination of proteids, ash and sugar should be mentioned, even if briefly. In a chapter on the analysis of breast milk it is just as important to point out how the milk for the analysis should be obtained as to give the methods of analysis. The value of many milk analyses, among others, the widely quoted ones of the Adriances, has been diminished since the publication of Rheyer has called attention to the cautions which have to be observed in collecting the milk.

In Chapter IX supplemental feeding is discussed, also weaning and the contra-indications of weaning. The removal from the breast on account of acute infectious diseases seems to be recommended more on the basis of sentiment than of observation.

Chapters X, XI and XII are devoted to the discussion of artificial feeding. While the author lays much stress on the composition of the food, he strangely omits to give any rules in regard to the total amount of food to be given in 24 hours, or to the amount to be given at a single meal. The author claims to demonstrate the difference between the acid coagula of human and cow's milk by dropping the milk into dilute acetic acid. He is in error on this point in regard to human milk, which gives no coagulum under these conditions.

In talking about the laboratory modification, the methods of which, we may say, have been elaborated by Mr. Gordon, the importance of slight variations in the food is pointed out. If these slight variations are so very important the control analyses of Wentworth make us believe that the accuracy of the method leaves much to be desired. The author is a well-known champion of the use of milk decalcified by means of sodium citrate. But from his exposition of the subject it is evident that he has not a clear conception of the mechanism of the rennin reaction, which has been elucidated by the work of Loevenhart. In other respects the subject of artificial feeding is treated much in the same manner as in other American textbooks. As the author stated previously, scientific infant feeding is a physiological problem, and to obtain the best results we have to take into consideration the data furnished so far by physiology and physiological chemistry. It becomes evident that this problem has to be studied according to the methods in vogue in studying any problem of nutrition, and the peculiarities which belong to the growing organism are to be pointed out. For instance, in adults a very important point is the nitrogen equilibrium, in order to determine the minimal amounts of nitrogenous food necessary. In the growing organism this problem is beset with great difficulties, as a nitrogen equilibrium solely is not sufficient to determine this minimal amount of nitrogenous intake since here the growth demands a nitrogen retention, and the physiological degree of this retention can at present only be fixed arbitrarily. The laboratory modification, as well as the home modifications simply considers how to obtain certain food mixtures, and the relative composition of the food certainly is of importance. But the rules which govern the changes of the formulas are not based on scientific principles, but on clinical observation and therefore they do not offer anything new. The modern efforts to obtain a more scientific basis for the feeding of infants are neglected by the author. Some of the differences, which exist between human and cow's milk, are also disregarded, as are the differences, which exist between the breast-fed and artificially fed infant. I only need to call attention to the work of Heubner and Rubner and Schlossmann in regard to the energy value of the food and its significance, to the conceptions of Schlossmann, Moro, Hamburger and Wassermann in regard to the biological properties of the milk and their significance; to the work of Moro concerning the difference in the alexins contained in the serum of breast-fed and artificially fed infants, etc., none of which are mentioned. The toxic effect of even small amounts of cow's milk on the young infant in some cases has not received any attention, nor has the importance of the knowledge of the decomposition products of the proteids been pointed out. Unfortunately, the importance of these subjects has been lost sight of in the expressions of mutual admiration so common among American writers and instead of marching in the vanguard of scientific infant feeding, as the author supposes, we, as American physicians, can hardly hold our own in this field of investigation.

In Chapter XIII on the hygiene of later infancy the necessity of the often neglected care of the mouth, nose and nasopharynx is duly emphasized.

In Chapter XIV the physiology and hygiene of childhood are discussed, and the warning of the author in regard to the dangers of overexertion sometimes incurred in the kindergarten courses deserves our fullest attention.

Chapter XV treats of the care of the premature infant, and after a short and concise presentation of the congenital malformations in Chapter XVI, we enter on the second part of the book, "The Diseases of Children."

The chapter on the disorders of nutrition is rather short. Just here the influence of a faulty diet with its consequences should find its place. It may perhaps be of advantage to reserve the term "marasmus" for those atrophic conditions of the infant, the etiology of which has not been elucidated, while the secondary forms of this state may be better considered from an etiological point of view. In an otherwise well-written chapter on rhachitis, the early manifestations of this disease with the prominence of the craniotabes are somewhat neglected. The author cites the sterilization of the milk as a factor in the etiology of scurvy. Since recent research has robbed this factor of its preeminence we note with satisfaction that he does not give it the usual prominence. The author is of the opinion that a multitude of clinical facts lend their support to the idea that more or less severe disturbances may be due to difficult dentition. Since the work of Jacobi, Kassowitz and others, it becomes necessary to base such an opinion on a number of carefully observed cases fully reported in literature. Otherwise we cannot acknowledge this multitude of clinical facts. The disturbances caused by adenoid vegetations have received the prominent notice they deserve. The possible etiological factors of summer diarrhœa are shortly though ably discussed. The author arrives at the following conclusion: "Whatever the future may reveal, for the present, at least, the etiology of summer diarrhœa, in its protean forms and lesions, must be regarded as multiplex and more or less obscure as to the relationship of its several factors." This statement voices the conviction of many pediatrists.

In the treatment of laryngismus stridulus we miss the phosphorus medication which has proven beneficial in a great number of cases. The space allotted to the description of tuberculous meningitis—24 lines—is hardly sufficient to illuminate a disease of so many aspects. The therapeutic value of the lumbar puncture in cases of meningitis is not discussed.

The chapter on syphilis seems to have been written before the era of the spirochæta pallida. The bone-lesions as well as the skin eruptions of hereditary syphilis receive rather short treatment.

In regard to the dissemination of tuberculosis the author adheres to the views of Cornet according to whom the infection is mostly carried through dried and pulverized sputum. Flügge's "Tröpfchen" infection is not considered. The author expresses himself very guardedly in regard to the mode of infection in early life. He regards the tuberculin test as of doubtful propriety. Two forms of peritoneal tuberculosis are given, namely, the wet and dry form, or the ascitic and the plastic. As a rule, a third form is accepted, characterized by ulceration and caseation.

The author is rather sanguine in the expression of a hope that diabetes mellitus may perhaps be avoided by controlling the child's development through attention to hygiene.

An appendix is added to the book, in which the author gives directions as to sick-room hygiene, therapeutic suggestions and recipes for the preparation of certain foods, ending up by giving a few formulas for prescriptions.

In this review the main stress is laid on the scientific principles of infant feeding. In justice to the author it must be stated that his presentation of this part of the subject does not differ materially from what we are accustomed to find in most of our text-books. Therefore, the criticism is not so much directed against the author's efforts as against the more or less general disregard of the scientific principles involved in infant feeding so common in works of this kind. It is apparent throughout the book that the author draws on an extensive clinical experience. Although some of his opinions may be debatable, his conclusions are given in a clear and conservative manner, and his book may be perused with advantage. SAMUEL AMBERG.

SEPARATE MONOGRAPHS REPRINTED FROM THE JOHNS HOPKINS HOSPITAL REPORTS.

Studies in Dermatology. By T. C. GILCHRIST, M. D., and EMMET RIXFORD, M. D. 1 volume of 164 pages and 41 full-page plates. Price, bound in paper, $3.00.

The Malarial Fevers of Baltimore. By W. S. THAYER, M. D., and J. HEWETSON, M. D. And A Study of some Fatal Cases of Malaria. By LEWELLYS F. BARKER, M. B. 1 volume of 280 pages. Price, bound in paper, $2.75.

Pathology of Toxalbumin Intoxications. By SIMON FLEXNER, M. D. 1 volume of 150 pages with 4 full-page lithographs. Price, in paper, $2.00.

Pneumothorax. A Historical, Clinical, and Experimental Study. By CHARLES P. EMERSON, M. D. Price, in paper, $4.00.

Operations of 459 Cases of Hernia, in the Johns Hopkins Hospital, from June, 1889, to January, 1899. By Jos. C. BLOODGOOD, M. D. Price, in paper, $3.00.

Orders should be addressed to

The Johns Hopkins Press, Baltimore, Md.

INDEX TO VOLUMES 1-16 OF BULLETIN.

A subject and author index of the first sixteen volumes of the Johns Hopkins Hospital Bulletin is now ready. As the edition will be limited, it is desirable that orders be sent in as promptly as possible.

Price bound in cloth is fifty cents.

Orders should be addressed to the Johns Hopkins Press, Baltimore, Md.

THE JOHNS HOPKINS HOSPITAL REPORTS.

VOLUME I. 423 pages, 99 plates.

VOLUME II. 570 pages, with 28 plates and figures.

VOLUME III. 766 pages, with 69 plates and figures.

VOLUME IV. 504 pages, 33 charts and illustrations.

VOLUME V. 480 pages, with 32 charts and illustrations.

CONTENTS:

The Malarial Fevers of Baltimore. By W. S. THAYER, M. D., and J. HEWETSON, M. D.

A Study of some Fatal Cases of Malaria. By LEWELLYS F. BARKER, M. B.

Studies in Typhoid Fever.

By WILLIAM OSLER, M. D., with additional papers by G. BLUMER, M. D., SIMON FLEXNER, M. D., WALTER REED, M. D., and H. C. PARSONS, M. D.

VOLUME VI. 414 pages, with 79 plates and figures.

Report in Neurology.

Studies on the Lesions Produced by the Action of Certain Poisons on the Cortical Nerve Cell (Studies Nos. I to V). By HENRY J. BERKLEY, M. D.

Introductory.—Recent Literature on the Pathology of Diseases of the Brain by the Chromate of Silver Methods; Part I.—Alcohol Poisoning.—Experimental Lesions Produced by Chronic Alcoholic Poisoning (Ethyl Alcohol). 2. Experimental Lesions produced by Acute Alcoholic Poisoning (Ethyl Alcohol); Part II.—Serum Poisoning.—Experimental Lesions induced by the Action of the Dog's Serum on the Cortical Nerve Cell; Part III.—Ricin Poisoning.—Experimental Lesions induced by Acute Ricin Poisoning. 2. Experimental Lesions induced by Chronic Ricin Poisoning; Part IV.—Hydrophobic Toxæmia.—Lesions of the Cortical Nerve Cell produced by the Toxine of Experimental Rabies; Part V.—Pathological Alterations in the Nuclei and Nucleoli of Nerve Cells from the Effects of Alcohol and Ricin Intoxication; Nerve Fibre Terminal Apparatus; Asthenic Bulbar Paralysis. By HENRY J. BERKLEY, M. D.

Report in Pathology.

Fatal Puerperal Sepsis due to the Introduction of an Elm Tent. By THOMAS S. CULLEN, M. B.

Pregnancy in a Rudimentary Uterine Horn. Rupture, Death, Probable Migration of Ovum and Spermatozoa. By THOMAS S. CULLEN, M. B., and G. L. WILKINS, M. D.

Adeno-Myoma Uteri Diffusum Benignum. By THOMAS S. CULLEN, M. B.

A Bacteriological and Anatomical Study of the Summer Diarrhœas of Infants. By WILLIAM D. BOOKER, M. D.

The Pathology of Toxalbumin Intoxications. By SIMON FLEXNER, M. D.

VOLUME VII. 537 pages with illustrations.

I. A Critical Review of Seventeen Hundred Cases of Abdominal Section from the standpoint of Intra-peritoneal Drainage. By J. G. CLARK, M. D.

II. The Etiology and Structure of true Vaginal Cysts. By JAMES ERNEST STOKES, M. D.

III. A Review of the Pathology of Superficial Burns, with a Contribution to our Knowledge of the Pathological Changes in the Organs in cases of rapidly fatal burns. By CHARLES RUSSELL BARDEEN, M. D.

IV. The Origin, Growth and Fate of the Corpus Luteum. By J. G. CLARK, M. D.

V. The Results of Operations for the Cure of Inguinal Hernia. By JOSEPH C. BLOODGOOD, M. D.

VOLUME VIII. 552 pages with illustrations.

On the role of Insects, Arachnids, and Myriapods as carriers in the spread of Bacterial and Parasitic Diseases of Man and Animals. By GEORGE H. F. NUTTALL, M. D., PH. D.

Studies in Typhoid Fever.

By WILLIAM OSLER, M. D., with additional papers by J. M. T. FINNEY, M. D., S. FLEXNER, M. D., I. P. LYON, M. D., L. F. HAMBURGER, M. D., H. W. CUSHING, M. D., J. F. MITCHELL, M. D., C. N. B. CAMAC, M. D., N. B. GWYN, M. D., CHARLES P. EMERSON, M. D., H. H. YOUNG, M. D., and W. S. THAYER, M. D.

VOLUME IX. 1060 pages, 66 plates and 210 other illustrations.

Contributions to the Science of Medicine.

Dedicated by his Pupils to WILLIAM HENRY WELCH, on the twenty-fifth anniversary of his Doctorate. This volume contains 38 separate papers.

VOLUME X. 516 pages, 12 plates and 25 charts.

Structure of the Malarial Parasites. Plate I. By JESSE W. LAZEAR, M. D.

The Bacteriology of Cystitis, Pyelitis and Pyelonephritis in Women, with a Consideration of the Accessory Etiological Factors in these Conditions, and of the Various Chemical and Microscopical Questions Involved. By THOMAS R. BROWN, M. D.

Cases of Infection with Strongyloides Intestinalis. (First Reported Occurrence in North America.) Plates II and III. By RICHARD P. STRONG, M. D.

On the Pathological Changes in Hodgkin's Disease, with Especial Reference to its Relation to Tuberculosis. Plates IV-VII. By DOROTHY M. REED, M. D.

Diabetes Insipidus, with a Report of Five Cases. By THOMAS B. FUTCHER, M. B. (Tor.).

Observations on the Origin and Occurrence of Cells with Eosinophile Granulations in Normal and Pathological Tissues. Plate VIII. By W. T. HOWARD, M. D., and R. G. PERKINS, M. D.

Placental Transmissions, with Report of a Case during Typhoid Fever. By FRANK W. LYNCH, M. D.

Metabolism in Albuminuria. By CHAS. P. EMERSON, A. B., M. D.

Regenerative Changes in the Liver after Acute Yellow Atrophy. Plates IX-XII. By W. G. MACCALLUM, M. D.

Surgical Features of Typhoid Fever. By THOS. McCRAE, M. B., M. R. C. P. (Lond.), and JAMES F. MITCHELL, M. D.

The Symptoms, Diagnosis and Surgical Treatment of Ureteral Calculus. By BENJAMIN R. SCHENCK, M. D.

VOLUME XI. 555 pages, with 38 charts and illustrations.

Pneumothorax: A historical, clinical and experimental study. By CHARLES P. EMERSON, M. D.

Clinical Observations on Blood Pressure. By HENRY W. COOK, M. D., and JOHN B. BRIGGS, M. D.

The value of Tuberculin in Surgical Diagnosis. By MARTIN B. TINKER, M. D.

VOLUME XII. 548 pages, 12 plates and other illustrations.

The Connective Tissue of the Salivary Glands and Pancreas with its Development in the Glandula Submaxillaris. Plates I-III. By JOSEPH MARSHALL FLINT, M. D.

A New Instrument for Determining the Minimum and Maximum Blood-Pressures in Man. Plates IV-X. By JOSEPH ERLANGER, M. D.

Metabolism in Pregnancy, Labor, and the Puerperium. By J. MORRIS SLEMONS, M. D.

An Experimental Study of Blood-Pressure and of Pulse-Pressure in Man. Plates XI and XII. By JOSEPH ERLANGER, M. D., and DONALD R. HOOKER, A. B., M. S.

Typhoid Meningitis. By RUFUS I. COLE, M. D.

The Pathological Anatomy of Meningitis due to Bacillus Typhosur By WILLIAM G. MACCALLUM, M. D.

A Comparative Study of White and Negro Pelves, with a Consideration of the Size of the Child and its Relation to Presentation and Character of Labor in the Two Races. By THEODORE F. RIGGS, M. D.

Renal Tuberculosis: By GEORGE WALKER, M. D.

VOLUME XIII. (In press.)

Studies in Genito-Urinary Surgery.

VOLUME XIV. (In press.)

Studies in Genito-Urinary Surgery.

The Johns Hopkins Hospital Bulletin are issued monthly. They are printed by the FRIEDENWALD CO., Baltimore. Single copies may be procured from NUNN & CO. and the BALTIMORE NEWS CO., Baltimore. Subscriptions, $2.00 a year, may be addressed to the publishers, THE JOHNS HOPKINS PRESS, BALTIMORE; single copies will be sent by mail for twenty-five cents each.

BULLETIN

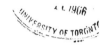

OF

THE JOHNS HOPKINS HOSPITAL

Entered as Second-Class Matter at the Baltimore, Maryland, Postoffice.

Vol. XVII.—No. 189.]   BALTIMORE, DECEMBER, 1906.   [Price, 25 Cents

CONTENTS.

COMPARATIVE SURGERY

SECOND SERIES OF REPORTS.

By F. W. Bancroft and E. S. Cross; G. R. Henry; W. D. Gatch; J. G. Hopkins; A. R. Dochez; W. Von Gerber; and G. J. Heuer.

(From the Hunterian Laboratory of Experimental Medicine.)

Under the above title a series of papers by C. M. Faris, H. C. Thacher, J. F. Ortschild, and F. C. Beall were published in the Johns Hopkins Hospital Bulletin for May, 1905, and in an introductory note mention was made of a building which, through the generosity of the University Trustees, was then being erected in part for the furtherance of the work. This laboratory building and the way in which it is used for the teaching of operative surgery have been fully described in a recent article.[1] It remains only to comment upon the purpose of the building as a hospital, since the portion of our work which is strictly veterinary in character has naturally grown with our improved facilities for the study and care of privately-owned animals.

We have had under treatment during the past year a number of animals suffering from maladies of considerable interest, not only from a surgical but from a general pathological point of view. There have been numerous types of neoplasm, the more common ones being growths affecting the abdominal

mammæ, and of the mixed tissue variety described by Dr. Ortschild a year ago. There have been in addition an epithelioma of the jaw, an osteosarcoma of the humerus (both in the dog and cat), a primary tumor of the spleen, a large papilloma of the bladder wall. The description of a tumor arising in an undescended testicle is included in the present series of papers.

A slight epidemic of distemper has given us an opportunity of making some preliminary bacteriological studies on this etiologically obscure malady. We have seen also some of the peculiar disturbances which not infrequently are a sequel of distemper, as epilepsy and certain forms of (tic spasmodique). One animal, a fox-terrier with a persistent monoplegic tic of the right fore leg, was operated upon, and the contralateral motor cortex, including the entire area for the fore leg, was removed. The spasm continued unabated, showing that this form of tic need not be of cortical origin, as it is generally supposed to be.

Possibly owing to our new and clean quarters, we have not been troubled, as we were a year ago, with a form of hæmorrhagic enteritis, which attacked many of our animals after operation, and the cause of which in many cases may possibly have been an infection with the Coccidium bigeminum, which

[1] Instruction in Operative Medicine, with the description of a course given in the Hunterian Laboratory of Experimental Medicine. The J. H. H. Bulletin, 1906, Vol. XVII, p. 123. The reports appearing in this month's Bulletin are numbered consecutively to those of the first series.

Drs. Cross and Bancroft describe. Few of the stray dogs in this locality fail to have numerous intestinal parasites, and they deserve careful tabulation and study. They offer an unusual opportunity for investigations in parasitology.

Instances of infection with filaria we have observed this year for the first time, and, as Mr. Hopkins has brought out, the presence of the worms in considerable number in the right heart has seemingly proved, in some instances, a fatal complication in the administration of an anæsthetic.

We have seen and treated a number of more or less serious fractures: one small fox-terrier with a fracture of both humeri was successfully put up in a bilateral ambulatory splint so that he could actively hobble about.

We have encountered at autopsy a number of cases of chronic endocarditis in the dog; and evidences of old valvular lesions are not infrequently met with. We have also seen many pathologically interesting lesions of other organs; for example, one of the most advanced cases imaginable of interstitial hepatitis was found to have been the cause of death in a cat whose body was sent to us for examination.

With Dr. James Bordley's aid some ophthalmological work in a small way has been undertaken. Cataract of various forms is especially common in the dog, and is amenable to the same surgical treatment given to the corresponding conditions in man.

In the routine operative courses for graduates and undergraduates more than 120 major operations have been performed with a very low percentage of fatalities. Most of the deaths have been due to unusual causes, such as are met with from time to time after similar operations in man. After abdominal operations we have seen two or three instances of post-operative intussusception, one of them proving fatal. An acute post-operative dilatation of the stomach was the cause of death in another animal. This rare complication we have never before seen after a laparotomy upon animals. It ran a clinical course similar to the rapidly fatal cases of like nature occasionally met with after simple abdominal operations on man. The stomach was enormously distended and almost filled the entire abdominal cavity. No gross or microscopic lesion was found to account for the process. The finding of such post-operative complications as the above; a death from hæmorrhage due to a loosely-placed mass ligature; the needless opening of the abdomen for a supposed tumor which proved to be a fæcal impaction; all such experiences are of the greatest value to beginners in surgery.

The reports which follow, like those made a year ago, are not only interesting in themselves, but they will serve, it is hoped, to encourage others to make similar comparative studies, not only of the surgical but of the pathological aspects of some of the diseases common particularly among our canine population.

HARVEY CUSHING,
P. K. GILMAN.

V. NOTE ON THE FINDING OF COCCIDIUM BIGEMINUM.

By F. W. BANCROFT and E. S. CROSS.

So far as we know the Coccidium bigeminum has been observed only once before in this country, and then by Charles Wardell Stiles. Having encountered it again in its typical form, we considered it to be of sufficient interest to warrant the publication of this note.

The organisms were found during the routine examination of sections from the organs of a dog which had died eleven days after an operation for excision of the cæcum with lateral intestinal anastomosis during the course of operative surgery in the Johns Hopkins Medical School.

The dog was a well-nourished, apparently normal fox-terrier of the ordinary kind, presenting no marked peculiarities. The operation was performed under ether anæsthesia and was successfully carried through. Two days after the operation the wound was noted to be clean and in good condition; the dog seemed well and was taking milk. In a day or two, however, the dog was noticeably losing; he refused to eat and staggered when attempting to walk. Bloody diarrhœa with mucus-containing stools appeared. Weakness increased and the animal died on the eleventh day following the operation.

The autopsy showed the body of an emaciated dog. The heart and lungs were normal. The peritoneal cavity contained about 20 cc. of a dark-brownish fluid; there were fairly firm adhesions around the operative wound; the mesentery was intensely injected. The parts of the intestines that were not bound down by adhesions were covered with smooth and glistening peritoneum.

Stomach.—Contained some fluid; mucosa appeared normal.

Duodenum.—Near the upper part of the duodenum the mucosa appeared normal, but near the lower part it became slightly thickened, red, and covered with a thick layer of mucus.

Jejunum and Ileum.—Throughout the entire length the surface was covered with a thick layer of mucus. In places the mucosa was red and swollen; in others it seemed to be eroded and the sub-mucosa swollen and infiltrated as if the superficial vessels were engorged with blood.

Colon.—The mucosa here had a greyish coloration. The hæmorrhagic appearance was lost and the superficial vessels did not seem to be engorged. Over this entire surface, too, there was a heavy layer of mucus.

Microscopical examination of stained specimens of the intestines showed the following:

Peritoneum, muscular layer, and muscularis mucosæ appeared normal. Mucosa: in the glands of Lieberkühn the epithelium appeared normal, as did the submucosa. Villi: the tips of the villi seemed thickened and club-shaped. The superficial vessels were dilated and there was slight increase in the amount of connective tissue. No polymorphonuclear leucocytes were seen, though there was some increase in lymphoid cells observed. On the surface of the villi the epithelial layer had almost entirely disappeared, but the epithelial covering of the glands seemed normal.

Scattered through the ends of the villi were seen small round and oval structures consisting of a clear sac or shell containing several apparently solid bodies of a round or elongated shape, staining deeply with hæmatoxylin, but not occupying more than half the size of the shell. They were nearly always near the surface of the villi, sometimes immediately beneath areas from which the epithelial layer had disappeared. They were never found deeply imbedded in the sub-mucosa.

It was suggested by Dr. McCallum that these structures might be coccidia. Investigation was immediately made among the dogs in that part of the kennels from which the case had come, and several were found which showed a somewhat similar condition, viz., emaciation, weakness, and diarrhœa. The stools were carefully examined for bodies similar to those observed in the sections, but none were found even in those cases in which there occurred bloody mucous discharges such as our first dog showed.

The viscera of the infected dog had been kept on ice, and scrapings from the intestinal mucous membrane showed the organisms more clearly and distinctly than did the sections. Apparently the hardening and staining of the tissues had obscured the real structures. In fact we did not succeed in staining the coccidia at all by methylene blue, carbol fuchsin, or in fresh smears.

The organism as we first saw it consisted of a clear cyst closed in by a membrane of double contour, apparently of some stiffness, as we never saw any indentations or irregularities in it. Contained in the cyst were several, usually four elongated, greenish, somewhat refractile, falciform bodies (sporoblasts), rather irregularly piled upon one another, but always with their long axes parallel to that of the cyst. On a lateral view the cyst was uniformly of an oval shape. We

FIG. 1. FIG. 2. FIG. 3.

FIG. 1.—Typical form, showing thin capsule. Each cyst or twin contains sporoblasts and a protoplasmic rest.

FIG. 2.—Single forms are frequently seen, perhaps freed from capsule by some traumatism.

FIG. 3.—Single form, evidently before division into the twin forms.

did not make accurate measurements, but Stiles says these cysts average about .013 by .009 mm. In addition the cysts contained several round, greenish, refractile bodies, rather irregularly arranged and probably representing the portion of protoplasm remaining after the division of the cell contents into the sporoblasts. This was the usual appearance on a lateral view. End views were also obtained, and here the cyst showed a circular form, having the same double-contoured membrane, but on this view the sporoblasts were represented by circular masses of greenish, refractile substance. The protoplasmic rests were practically the same in appearance as in the lateral view. It was the rule for two of these cysts, enclosed by a thin and delicate membrane, to lie side by side with their long axes parallel.

A third form was noted, viz., a single cell about the size of the double cyst, showing the same double-contoured membrane, tending to be rather more nearly circular in shape, and containing fairly large masses of circular, greenish, refractile granules, not unlike the protoplasmic rests of the double and single cysts. According to Stiles, this represents the undivided coccidium. The single cysts probably represent merely half of one of the organisms, the membrane of which has ruptured, perhaps from some external force; or it may be that only one cyst matured, the other one aborting.

Portions of the intestine of the infected dog were then fed to a supposedly normal dog, to see if a similar condition could be produced artificially. A week passed during which the animal showed no diarrhœa or signs of emaciation, when it was accidentally killed and no autopsy was obtained. This experiment, then, showed only that the infection was not of a very virulent or rapid nature.

The attempt was made to see if any light could be thrown upon the life cycle of the organism by the production of other forms when the infected mucosa was incubated in a thermostat at 37° C. in the presence of a weak solution of boric acid. The latter was to lessen if possible the putrefaction without injuring the organisms. The forms originally described were seen in preparations from these cultures, but no new ones.

The viscera of several other dogs were now examined, in which an interesting variety of parasites was discovered. In five of the number uncinariasis was disclosed. Such intestines were lined with a thick layer of mucus, and scrapings showed the typical eggs of uncinaria, while adult worms in large numbers were macroscopically visible. Tæniæ were found in two dogs, one of which harbored three of these parasites. In one dog Coccidium bigeminum was again found.

Concerning this last dog a note of March 27, 1905, reads as follows: "Supposedly normal dog etherized to-day; it came from another part of the dog-house than that in which the infection was supposed to exist. The intestines were not hæmorrhagic, but the epithelial surface was covered with mucus to a marked degree. Three tape-worms were present and very numerous uncinaria worms. Scrapings from the mucosa showed the Coccidium bigeminum in twin form, and disclosed more clearly than ever that in this condition the two are inclosed in a thin, transparent capsule. Not all were in this form, however, some being single as before." The large round cells with the mass of granules in the center were also present.

On looking up the literature upon this subject we found that Döflein in "Die Protozen" gave a very brief mention of the Coccidium bigeminum, crediting the form to Stiles. He says it always consists of two spore-holding cysts originating from the oöcyst which divides into two equal parts, and each of these again gives rise to four spores. He notes their occurrence in various mammals, dogs, cats, and rarely man, in the intestinal villi under the epithelial layer, and concludes that the group needs further investigation.

Charles Wardell Stiles, in the Journal of Comparative Medicine and Veterinary Archives, September, 1892, says: "In the literature on the sporozoa we find frequent mention of a parasitic protozoön in the intestinal tract of domestic

dogs.[1] R. Virchow described a case where the intestinal lining was fairly packed with coccidia. Several authors mention the presence in the dog of Coccidium perforans, the intestinal Coccidium of rabbits. Rivolta described a Cystospermium villosum intestinalis canis which Railliet and Lucet consider identical with a parasite they found in the intestinal villosities of Parisian dogs. They recognized that it was a true coccidium, and also that it generally occurs in pairs, a fact they were inclined to explain by assuming a division of the original cell."

Railliet and Lucet have published a second note in which they state that this parasite was originally found in the villosities of cats by Finck in 1854, who gave a very good description of it. He, however, did not understand the true nature of it, as he called the parasites "corpuscles geminés," and doubting their parasitic nature thought they stood in some relation to the mechanism of fat absorption.

VI. CHRONIC ENDOCARDITIS WITH BLOODY ASCITES.

By GLADYS R. HENRY.

CASE REPORT.—A mongrel black and white curly-haired dog of Newfoundland type was admitted to the hospital on November 28, 1905, because of a rapidly increasing abdominal enlargement.

According to his master, he had always been a healthy animal of amiable disposition until two weeks before admission, when he had become irritable and snapped at his friends. Coincident with this change in disposition, abdominal swelling and shortness of breath were noted. During the two weeks preceding admission the abdomen had progressively increased in size, and the hind legs had become swollen (Fig. 4).

The note made on November 29, the day after admission, describes the patient as a large, well-nourished dog, suffering from dyspnœa even when at rest. He had marked ascites with extensive anasarca in the tissues of the hinder part of the body and legs, and possibly a slight swelling of the left fore leg. He is barely able to stand and take a few steps. His pulse was irregular both in force and rhythm, averaging 100 beats per minute. The heart sounds were irregular in rhythm and in tensity, and were accompanied by an indistinct murmur. Ophthalmoscopic examination was negative.

By paracentesis on the same day four thousand cubic centimeters of a blood-stained serous fluid were withdrawn from the abdomen, the first of it being under considerable tension. An equal amount must have been left behind, but owing to the weakness and rapidity of the heart action after the removal of this amount of fluid it was deemed wise to leave the remainder. This fluid contained no gross particles. Its reaction towards litmus was slightly alkaline, and its specific gravity was 1010. It contained thirteen grams of albumin to the litre, and gave reduction by Trommer's test. The sediment obtained by centrifuging a portion consisted chiefly of red blood cells, a few large and small mononuclear and polymorphonuclear leucocytes with occasional clumps of apparently normal peritoneal cells.

After the paracentesis, two tumor masses were felt on palpa-

tion through the somewhat relaxed abdominal wall. One of them was a stony-hard, elongated, nodular, quite freely movable mass, which lay in the left side of the cavity. In the right

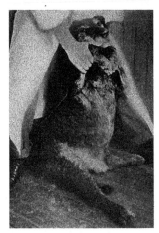

FIG. 4.—Case of general anasarca with bloody ascites from cardiac insufficiency after valvular disease.

upper quadrant there was a firm, smooth mass reaching 8 to 10 cm. below the costal margin. An edge could not be made out,

---

[1] R. Virchow, Rivolta, R. Leuckart, Railliet, etc.

though it was presumed to be the liver. The inguinal glands were not palpable.

.The existence of tumor masses in the abdomen, together with a bloody ascitic fluid, led to the tentative diagnosis of a malignant growth, and two days later an exploratory laparotomy was performed.

Operation.—December 2, 1905. The abdominal cavity, when opened, was found to contain about two litres of fluid similar to that removed by paracentesis. The peritoneal surfaces were smooth, and the mass which had been palpated in the right upper quadrant was found to be an enlarged liver of purplish hue, which showed a honeycomb tracing on its surface. A small piece from the edge of the organ was excised for examination. The freshly cut surface was yellowish and greasy in appearance.

The cylindrical tumor on the left proved to be the descending colon packed with hard fæcal matter. After the fæcal impaction had been broken up by intra-abdominal manipulation and passed along so that it could be removed in part per anum, the excess of peritoneal fluid was sponged out and the abdominal wound closed without drainage.

On his recovery from the anæsthetic a turpentine enema was administered, and this led to the further evacuation of a considerable amount of stony-hard fæcal material. Though the removal of the ascites seemed to leave the patient more comfortable for a day or two after the operation, the fluid rapidly reaccumulated; and with it a return of the dyspnœa. By the fourth day the swelling and the shortness of breath became very pronounced and the animal succumbed.

The autopsy report reads as follows: "The body is that of a large animal with a shaggy coat. There is a recent laparotomy wound which has been healing without reaction. There is marked œdema of the hind legs and probably some of the fore legs also. The abdomen is uniformly distended. On median incision the panniculus adiposus is well preserved and the peritoneal surfaces are smooth and glistening, except for occasional flakes of pink fibrin coagula. The abdominal cavity contains about 4000 cc. of a clear, reddish, serous fluid similar to that removed at the operation.

The liver is greatly enlarged and of a purplish color. Its surface is smooth and shows a honeycomb marking. The lobulation is distinct. The central vein of each lobule is dilated and dark red, and the periphery is a yellowish gray. The omentum is adherent to the liver, where it was stitched during the operation to cover the raw surface left by the removal of a portion of the liver for examination.

Microscopically the capillaries at the center of the lobule are widely dilated and congested. There is atrophy of the parenchymatous cells in the central zone, and fatty degeneration of those at the periphery, with a slight increase of stroma about the hepatic veins.

The left kidney is readily stripped of its capsule, and shows a smooth, dark red surface with a few grayish, translucent, depressed areas. The organ is firm, and the edges of its cut surface are sharp. The cortex is not narrowed, except beneath the depressed areas noted on the surface. The glomeruli are prominent and the vessels of the medulla are injected. The right kidney is similar to the left.

The spleen and pancreas show little more than the evidences of passive congestion present in all the abdominal organs. The capsule of the spleen is thickened and the Malpighian corpuscles and trabeculæ stand out distinctly.

The stomach is distended, and the vessels of its serous surface are injected, as are those of the mesentery and peritoneal covering of the intestine. The mucosa of the stomach is dark red and shows areas of submucous hæmorrhage. Microscopically the vessels of the mucosa are widened and congested. There

are minute hæmorrhages just beneath the surface epithelium. There is marked cellular proliferation and slight fibrous increase in the stroma in certain areas over which the mucosa appears thinner than normal. A few of the glands are dilated and show the presence of many goblet cells in their lining membrane, with a few polymorphonuclear leucocytes and desquamated cells in their lumen.

There are minute hæmorrhages in the mucosa of the duodenum, jejunum, and the upper part of the ileum. The large bowel is partially filled with small masses of fæcal material.

The inner surface of the bladder is reddened by dilated vessels.

There is no fluid in the pleural cavities. The lungs are mottled, red, air containing throughout, and covered with smooth, shining pleura. On section both lungs are of a yellowish red color and somewhat moist. The bronchi are clear. Sections show that the alveoli are free from exudate, except for occasional desquamated epithelial cells, some of which contain rounded refractile yellowish granules of pigment. Others contain angular masses of coal pigment. The capillaries are dilated. The smooth muscle bundles about the orifices of the atria are hypertrophied.

The heart as it lies in the thorax appears much enlarged. The pericardial surfaces are smooth, and the sac contains no excess of fluid. On removing the heart from the thorax, it is found considerably hpertrophied. The right auricle contains a post-mortem clot that extends into the right ventricle. The latter is greatly dilated. The dilatation is most marked in the conus arteriosus. The wall of the right ventricle is markedly thickened. The right auriculo-ventricular ring is stretched so that the tricuspid valve cannot reach across it. The septal leaflet of the tricuspid valve is somewhat thickened and there is a patch of sclerosis at its base. The right leaflet is slightly thickened. The pulmonary valves are normal in appearance. The left auricle and ventricle are dilated, and their walls are thickened. The mitral valve shows shortening of both leaflets and of their chordæ tendineæ. The posterior leaflet is particularly affected, and it is so shortened and thickened that there is marked insufficiency at the mitral orifice. The endocardium of the ventricles presents a mottled appearance, and section of the heart wall shows yellow streaks in the myocardium. There are also translucent, whitish areas to be seen. The aortic valves are free and delicate.

Anatomical diagnosis.—Chronic endocarditis; mitral insufficiency; cardiac hypertrophy; chronic fibrous myocarditis and fatty degeneration of the heart muscle; dilatation of the heart; relative tricuspid insufficiency; chronic passive congestion of the lungs, liver, spleen, kidneys, gastric and intestinal mucosa; bloody ascites and anasarca; chronic gastritis of mild grade."

DISCUSSION.

We were at first led to believe, by the extensive general anasarca and the ascites, that this patient was suffering from some chronic cardiac or renal lesion, but we were thrown off the track by finding, upon paracentesis, that the peritoneal fluid was bloody. Unaware that the passive congestion from a leaking tricuspid valve could lead to such a form of ascites, and finding the hard, movable, nodular mass in the abdomen, a tentative diagnosis of malignant disease was made and a laparotomy performed. The experience of opening the abdomen in the expectation of finding a malignant tumor which has turned out to be a fæcal impaction, has come to many surgeons—an error which once made is not likely to be repeated.

A digital examination of the rectum should be a routine procedure, especially in all obscure abdominal diseases, and the true condition might have been revealed before the operation, had this been done; this, however, is doubtful, since the hard masses were in the descending colon and their lower end high above the brim of the pelvis.

In the course of the post-mortem examinations held during the past winter we have seen a number of hearts which have given evidence of old valvular disease and it does not seem to be a particularly uncommon lesion. In none of these cases, however, was there any valvular insufficiency, and in none of them ascites.

With the primary object of reproducing this condition of bloody ascites, due to simple passive congestion, we have made a series of experimental vascular lesions, in order to study their late effects. Dr. W. G. MacCallum had been successful in reproducing experimentally most of the valvular lesions (insufficiency, by means of a cutting hook which he has devised and stenosis, by ligature) the acute physiological effects of which he has been studying. The idea occurred to us that we might produce these same lesions and secure surgical recover-ies. This has been done by a thoracotomy, either carried out through the pectoral region by means of a muscle-splitting operation and the excision of a rib, or else by splitting the sternum in the mid line and springing the chest open by retraction. Artificial respiration in the meantime has been carried out through an external tracheotomy. The wounds in the throat and thorax have always been immediately closed after the production of the lesion, and primary union has been invariably secured in the neck, and with only one or two exceptions, in the thoracic wounds. The pericardium and pleura are very unresistent to infection, and a number of animals have subsequently died from empyema in spite of all precautions.

We have limited ourselves chiefly to the production of mitral and tricuspid lesions, and the deltails of the operative methods followed and the results obtained will be published in another communication. Of the recovered cases, none of them have shown lesions which have not allowed of early compensation and as yet we have had no instance of œdema or ascites such as was found in the patient whose history is recorded above.

VII. THE RADICAL CURE OF PROLAPSUS VAGINÆ.

By W. D. Gatch.

This paper has a three-fold object: first, to supplement H. C. Thacher's report of a year ago; second, to give the somewhat meager literature on vaginal prolapsus in the dog; third, to suggest an operative treatment for this condition in dogs and other animals. Dr. Thacher[1] reported in full two cases of utero-vaginal prolapse, and in a note referred to a third case which had been successfully operated upon. The prolapse in one of these animals had occurred as an acute sequel of parturition; in the others it was associated with the period of œstrum.

During the present year we have seen three additional instances of the form of prolapse which recurs during the period of heat, the protrusion finally assuming such proportions that it becomes irreducible in the interval. The origin of the trobule seems to bear no relation to pregnancy, nor to the traumatism of coition or parturition; and these animals, aside from the unsightly tumor, were in perfect physicial condition. The protrusion may possibly result from an unduly relaxed state of the tissues subjacent to the vaginal wall, which favors their eversion when the mucous membranes are highly vascularized during heat. When once the protrusion has occurred, venous stasis and œdema finally lead to a thickening of the tissues, just as in cases of extensive prolapse in the human, so that reduction becomes more and more difficult.

Two of these animals were members of the same family, and there may be an hereditary tendency to the lesion. Our experience would lead us to believe that it occurs more frequently in highly-bred than in mongrel animals, though this impression may be due to the fact that the former are more likely to be brought to us for treatment. The condition is progressive, more and more of the vaginal wall becoming everted at each successive period of heat, until the prolapsed mass finally may contain the peritoneal reflection from the pelvic wall to the uterus, and thus hold not only the pelvic organs, but also loops of intestine. Disturbances of micturition naturally follow, and the consequent straining favors the increasing growth of the hernia.

Other ill effects of such prolapse are the unsightly appearance of the tumor, the discomfort which the animal suffers, and the difficulty or impossibility of using her for breeding purposes. However, unless the condition is extreme, impregnation and an uncomplicated pregnancy may take place, even after development of a prolapse of considerable proportions, as will be related in the first of these histories.

Case I.—The patient, a valuable and highly-bred Boston terrier bitch, was admitted to the clinic November 29, 1905. Her age was a little over three years. When about a year old she was in heat for the first time, and a considerable prolapse of the vagina occurred, which prevented her from being successfully covered. The protrusion subsequently disappeared, but the same experience was repeated during her second period. When in heat for the third time, though the protrusion was greater than on the previous occasions, it was reduced by a

[1] The J. H. H. Bull., 1905, Vol. XVI, p. 184.

veterinarian, and she was impregnated. After this act there was no return of the prolapse and she went through a normal pregnancy and labor, giving birth to four healthy pups in April, 1904.

She remained well until September, 1904, when occurred the first period subsequent to her pregnancy, and with it an enormous protrusion of the vagina. The tumor became so large that it trailed upon the ground when she walked. When her period had passed the protrusion did not subside as it had done before, but remained out until, with a second period, it

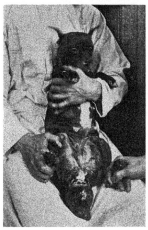

FIG. 5.—Case I. Large vaginal prolapse.

further increased in size and the patient was brought to the clinic for treatment.

Physical Examination.—Proves negative other than for the local lesion. Protruding through the vulva there is an enormous pear-shaped mass covered by brightly injected, distended and œdematous vaginal mucous membrane (Fig. 5). The mass is constricted at the proximal end, bulges out, and then tapers off to a point where there is an orifice, just within which the external os of the uterus can be palpated. The mucous membrane covering the mass is inflamed, and in one area in its ventral surface covered by a superficial ulceration. The urethral orifice is visible on the ventral surface of the tumor 2 cm. from the vulvar margin and urine dribbles constantly over the surface. The animal makes frequent straining efforts, as though suffering from retention, but on catheterizing the bladder only two or three ounces of urine are found. There is some difficulty in catheterization, for the urethra is found to be kinked, and the glass catheter passes first for about 2 cm. toward the tip of the protrusion and then must be turned in the opposite direction before it enters the bladder. It is possible to palpate the tip of the catheter through the abdominal parietes above the pubes, so that the bladder does not form a part of the tumor, as was feared. The urethra alone seems to be drawn down with the vaginal wall into the prolapse. The protrusion, however, is so great that it seems probable that it must contain not

only the uterus and tubes, but also bowel as well. The enclosing tissues are too densely œdematous to enable one to determine the nature of the contained organs.

Operation.—December 1, 1905. Morphia: ether anæsthesia. After thoroughly shaving and cleaning the surrounding area and putting the animal in the perineal position, a catheter was once more re-inserted into the bladder in order to insure the straightening of the urethra and its withdrawal away from the tumor mass to be removed. Then a circular incision was made through the œdematous vaginal wall near the vulvar margin and just behind the urethral opening. This circular incision was gradually carried down to the central core of the tumor; namely, the inverted uterus. It was hoped that by stripping back the tissues by blunt dissection, as in Whitehead's operation for rectal prolapse, it would be possible to approach the central lumen of the inverted tube without opening the peritoneum. We were, however, disappointed in this, for the peritoneal reflection was drawn by the prolapse far out beyond the vulva, and it was necessary to enter the cavity. It was thus found that not only were there loops of bowel in the prolapse, but the uterine tubes and their loose and fatty broad ligaments as well.

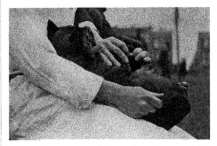

FIG. 6.—Case II. Offspring of Case I, with small vaginal prolapse.

These structures were reduced and held in place by gauze packing, while the uterus was amputated near its bifurcation. The circular opening into the peritoneal cavity was then closed about the stump, and finally the raw vulvar margins were united to those of the amputated uterus. This necessitated the closure of the tissue in a raquet shape, as the vulvar opening was much the larger of the two circles. When the union had been completed the body of the uterus, which meanwhile had been held down by traction, was freed. It withdrew into the pelvis, carrying the circular line of union with it, so that the line of union was well within the vulvar orifice. The latter, however, was so large and flaccid, owing to the pre-existing condition of things, that it seemed best to gather in the tissues on the dorsal part of the opening. This was done by a simple perineorrhaphy after denudation of the surface.

Post-operative.—The animal recovered from the operation without complication. The wound healed perfectly, and she was returned to her home ten days later. Since then there has been no evidence of recurrence of the trouble, and she is reported to be in perfect health.

CASE II.—The patient, a Boston terrier, a daughter of Case I, eleven months of age, was brought to the clinic March 8, 1906. She has always been perfectly sound and well until her first period of heat six weeks before her admission. At that time a protrusion of the vagina occurred just as has been related in the preceding story. Though the swelling has subsided somewhat, it has not completely gone, and the owner, fearing a sequence of events like those related above, is desirous of having an earlier operation performed. An effort has already been made in this direction by a veterinarian, who after reduction of the prolapse closed the vulvar orifice in the usual method by sewing the labia together. The sutures finally cut through and the protrusion recurred.

Physical examination.—The dog is a young, active and well-nourished animal of highly bred terrier type. Protruding from the vulva is a round, œdematous mass of prolapsed mucous membrane, moist, bright red in color and about the size of a hen's egg. Fig. 6.

The prolapse can be reduced, but it immediately recurs on any movement of the animal. The perineum is greatly relaxed and the vaginal outlet large. There is a perforation about 1 cm. in diameter through each of the labia, with cicatricial margins, as the result of the operation above mentioned. The prolapse in its present condition is made up mostly of the anterior vaginal wall. The mucous membrane is thickened and there are a few patches of superficial ulceration. The orifice of the urethra is pulled down on to the ventral surface of the protrusion. The vaginal wall is greatly relaxed, and through its canal two fingers may be easily introduced far enough to be palpated over the pubes.

Operation.—March 10, 1906. Morphia: ether anæsthesia. The prolapsed vagina was withdrawn so as to form a symmetrical double walled cylinder, and a catheter was introduced into the urethra. Close to the junction of skin and mucous membrane an incision was then made encircling the protrusion just distal to the urethral orifice. The incision was then carried down through the œdematous tissue to the lumen of the prolapsed tissue; namely, to the as yet uneverted part of the vaginal canal. Largely by blunt dissection the tissue to be amputated was then dissected back from the vagina, as the latter was drawn down into view, just as is done in the radical cure of prolapse of the rectal mucous membrane by Whitehead's method. The tissues were carefully stripped away from the bladder and rectum, and the peritoneum was not opened in this case. The cylinder of vagina thus exposed, with its inner lining of mucous membrane and outer raw surface, including the prolapsed portion, was amputated a short distance below the cervix uteri, and the circular margin was sutured to the edge of the original circular incision made near the external attachment of the prolapse. When the traction upon the vagina was released, the line of sutures withdrew back out of sight. Finding that the vaginal outlet remained relaxed and large, and in order to insure against the risk of any future protrusion, the outlet was narrowed on the perineal side by the usual splitting operation of perineorrhaphy, as performed for simple cases of relaxed vaginal outlet in the human. After a semilunar incision at the muco-cutaneous junction, a triangle of mucous membrane was dissected up and the denuded area closed by sutures placed from side to side.

The time required for the operation was only thirty-five minutes. Ether was well taken. The animal made a good recovery, the perineal wound healing per primam and leaving a normally small vaginal outlet. She was discharged March 20, and has remained well. There has been no recurrence of the trouble.

DISCUSSION.

The literature on vaginal prolapse in the dog is scant. A careful search at the Surgeon-General's Library and at the Bureau of Animal Industry brought to light only three books or articles giving anything more than a mere mention of the condition. The best descriptions were found in the works of Müller (1), Hobday (2), and Hill (3). Hill states that the causes of vaginal prolapse are " frequent pregnancies, relaxed and debilitated conditions of the system, and violent separations at coitus." All three authors advocate the same general treatment; namely, replacement of the prolapse and its retention in place by a pessary of some sort, and, in case this fails, by surgical treatment. The latter has so far been the ligation of the mass, as a whole or in part, close to the vulva, followed by amputation of the tissues distal to the ligature, either by the knife, the cautery, or by the process of sloughing. Crude though such an operation is, the animals usually get well; but they are liable to have incontinence of urine because of the inclusion of the urethra by the ligature. Stitches through the lips of the vulva to hold the prolapse in place, are also advocated; but, as we have observed in one of our cases thus treated, the method is inefficient. The former methods in a severe case of total prolapse (*e. g.*, Case I) would certainly result in the animal's death.

The treatment of vaginal prolapse in the domestic animals is a matter of considerable commercial importance, as is shown by the large literature on the condition, especially as occurring in the horse and cow. Prolapse occurs also in sheep and goats. The bad effects and the causes are about the same for other animals as for the dog, though for the heavier animals great stress is laid upon too great a backward slope of the stall as a factor in the production. The operative treatment usually followed in case replacement has failed, consists, as with the dog, in ligating or crushing off the mass. But from the very few cases reported—and those of very doubtful success—it is apparent that the operation leaves much to be desired.

I see no reason why the methods which we have employed in the treatment of these cases cannot be used on all animals. These consist, (*a*) in the excision of the prolapsed vaginal mucosa by a method similar to Whitehead's operation for prolapsed rectal mucosa, and (*b*) if necessary, in contracting the relaxed vaginal outlet, as described, by a perineorrhaphy.

These operations, judging from our six successful cases, insure a cure of the condition, and should not interfere with the future use of the animal for breeding purposes. As methods of anæsthetizing larger animals are now in use, these operations can even be performed on horses and cows when the value of the animal would justify the expense of an operation.

LITERATURE CONSULTED.

1. Die Krankheiten des Hundes und ihre Behandlung. Georg Müller, Berlin, 1892. Verlag von Paul Parry.

2. Surgical Diseases of the Dog and Cat. F. T. G. Hobday, London, 1906. Baillière, Tindall and Co.

3. Management and Diseases of the Dog. Hill, New York, 1900. The Macmillan Company.

4. Fleming's Veterinary Obstetrics. Fleming, New York. 1892.

5. The Sheep. Rushworth, Buffalo, 1899.

6. Special Report on Diseases of Cattle. Bureau of Animal Industry, 1904.

7. Special Report on Diseases of the Horse. Bureau of Animal Industry, 1903.

8. Pregnancy and Parturition in the Cow. Crichton, The Veterinary Review, London, Vol. VI, 1902.

9. Veterinary Medicine. Courtenay, edited by Hobday, London, 1902.

VIII. SIX CASES OF INFECTION WITH FILARIA IMMITIS.

By J. G. Hopkins.

During the past winter infection with Filaria immitis has been observed in six dogs in the course of post-mortem examinations held in the laboratory. Three of these animals died quite suddenly on the operating table soon after beginning the administration of ether; in the other three, the worms had no apparent causal relation whatever to the death of the animals.

Case I.—January 5, 1906. The animal was a healthy fox-terrier dog, and nothing abnormal was noted in his condition before the operation. A few minutes after the first administration of ether he suddenly ceased breathing, and artificial

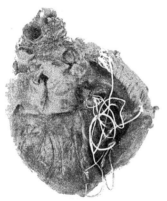

Fig. 7.—Filaria immitis in the right ventricle.

respiration failed to revive him. An autopsy was held, and on opening the right auricle numerous coils of worms were seen protruding from the tricuspid orifice. They were white and wax-like and about 1 mm. in diameter. On pulling them out of the ventricle they proved to be about 20 cm. in length. The right ventricle, when opened, presented a very striking picture. It was slightly dilated and closely packed with intertwined worms, twelve or more in number. Two or three of the bodies

extended up through the pulmonic orifice. The accompanying illustration (Fig. 7) is from a photograph of this heart after a number of the worms had been removed. Smears taken from the blood showed numerous nematode embryos about 3 mm. in length. No other lesions were found.

Case II.—On January 5, 1906, a splenectomy was performed on a mongrel terrier. The animal took ether well and made an uneventful operative recovery. The patient died suddenly on January 17. The autopsy findings were negative, except that in the right heart was a large, dark red clot, adherent to the tricuspid valve, which contained numerous filariæ.

Case III.—An operation for the removal of the cæcal region with anastomosis between ileum and ascending colon was performed on a mongrel terrier January 13, 1906. The animal succumbed on the following day. The autopsy showed acute dilatation of the stomach. In the heart were found two worms, one male and one female. Blood smears from the femoral vein, spleen and liver showed numerous embryos.

Case IV.—March 30, 1906. A large dog of the Newfoundland type died under anæsthesia before the operation could be begun. About ten worms were found in the right ventricle and pulmonary artery, some extending a little way beyond the hilum of the lung. Numerous actively motile embryos were found in the blood.

Case V.—April 9, 1906. This dog also died under anæsthesia. The only abnormality noticed at autopsy was one male filaria in the pulmonary artery. No embryos could be found in the blood.

Case VI.—On May 19, 1906, a small terrier dog who had been ill was found dead in one of the laboratories. The alimentary tract showed the lesions of an acute corrosive poisoning. On opening the heart one female filaria about 27 cm. in length was found coiled in the first part of the pulmonary artery. The wall of the artery for a distance of 2 cm. above the valve was found studded with fine granules which on section proved to be subendothelial fibrous nodules. Examination of the blood was negative.

It is impossible to say how long the heart worms of dogs have been known. In 1856, Leidy (1) reported two cases and named the parasite Filaria immitis. The other names under which the same worms have been described are, Filaria canis cordis (Leidy, 1850) and Filaria papillosa hematica canis domestici (Gruby and Delafond, 1852).

Braun (2) describes the parasite as follows: "The body is thin and filiform; the posterior extremity is pointed and the anterior end rounded off; the mouth is terminal, and behind it are six small papillæ; the anus opens near the posterior extremity; the male measures 12-18 cm. in length, 0.7-0.9 mm. in breadth; the tail is slender and twisted like a cork-screw; it has a fold of skin at either side and four pairs of large pre-anal, and some smaller post-anal papillæ, the surface of which exhibit a smooth appearance. The female measures 25-30 cm. in length and 1.0-1.3 mm. in breadth; the vulva is about 7 mm. distant from the anterior extremity; vivaparous; the larvæ measure 0.285-0.295 mm. in length and .005 mm. in breadth; the posterior extremity terminates in a very thin point."

The adult worms are found usually in the right of the heart and frequently in the pulmonary artery and venæ cavæ. They have also been found in the other large systemic veins. I found three cases reported in which they occurred in the left heart. In one, a coiled mass of worms extended from the right auricle through an opening in the interauricular septum into the left heart (3); in another case, worms were also found in many of the systemic arteries (4); in the third there were forty worms in the left auricle and ventricle, and the right pulmonary artery was likewise filled with them (5). They have also been found in the pleural cavity, in the bronchi, and in the œsophagus. They number from one to fifty or more. It is not known how long they may live in the host. The embryos, which are actively motile, are found in the blood at all times of day, but are most numerous in the peripheral circulation at night. They are also found in the urine.

Filariasis is a common disease of dogs in many countries. According to Janson (4) about one-half the dogs in Japan are affected and in China about two-thirds. The disease also occurs in Australia, Italy, and Southern France. All the cases which I have seen described from England and Germany were imported from the Orient. From time to time cases have been reported as curiosities from various parts of this country. A number of cases, however, have been found in the past in the laboratories here, which have never been published, and apparently the disease is much more common than the reports would indicate. It might be noted that at least two of the dogs in this series came from the same locality, which suggests that the infection may be more prevalent in certain districts than in others.

Various symptoms in dogs have been ascribed to filariasis (convulsions, emaciation, etc.), but the causal relation is doubtful. In many cases certainly the infection has no manifest effect on the animal. No symptoms were observed in any of the dogs in this series.

The most extensive observations seem to be those of Janson. In three-quarters of his cases no disturbance was noted which could be attributed to the worms. He regards the effects as purely mechanical, due usually to interference with the heart valves by the adults. As long as the worms remain in the ventricle they produce no symptoms, he thinks, but

if they wander out through the orifices they may produce insufficiency by holding the valves back, or stenosis by blocking the passage of blood. He found five cases of complete blocking of the pulmonary artery. He also observed anæmia and atalectasis of the lung and chronic passive congestion of the liver, ascites, hydrothorax, contracted kidney, and gastro-intestinal catarrh. He also thinks that the embryos may cause disturbances by blocking capillaries, e. g., in the brain, or by stimulating connective-tissue growth. Deffke (6) reports a case of nephritis in which the embryos were found in the interstitial kidney tissue as well as in the blood. Seven of Janson's cases had an aneurism of the pulmonary artery. In this connection the endarteritis observed in Case VI might be noted. Some of Janson's dogs had periodical attacks of complete collapse lasting only a few minutes, from which the dog would recover and seem perfectly well. Hæmaturia was observed in some cases. Van Meter (3) reports in his case a continuous cardiac murmur with a palpable thrill. The susceptibility of these dogs to ether, in three cases out of five anæsthetized, could hardly have been a coincidence. It would seem that the mechanical effect of the worms in the heart, either in diminishing the capacity of the ventricles, or in preventing the closure of the valves, might explain this. Although Case II with a number of worms took ether well, whereas Case V with only one succumbed, it may be that in the latter case the worm extended past the pulmonary orifice during life, and so embarrassed the valve action more than would several worms entirely within the ventricle.

The intermediate host of Filaria immitis is the mosquito, as has been shown by the work of Grassi and Noè (7), and of T. L. Bancroft (8). Grassi first succeeded in transmitting the disease through Anopheles maculipennis. Bancroft used Culex fatigans in his experiments. Both these species are thought to act as intermediate host for F. bancrofti also. Earlier attempts to transmit the worms, using another species of mosquito, Culex vigilax, were negative. Experiments were also made with fleas, lice, ticks, horse-flies, and intestinal worms. It was found that while these parasites sucked in the embryos with the blood, the latter failed to develop.

When sucked into the stomach of their intermediate host, the embryos make their way to the Malpighian tubes. Here they undergo a metamorphosis similar to that of F. bancrofti in the thoracic muscles. Leaving behind their old cuticle, they pass into the labium, where they lie in what seems to be a continuation of the body cavity. According to Bancroft, when the mosquito bites, the worms escape through a hole in the labellæ, which embrace the stylets at the point where they enter the wound, and make their way into the puncture. This agrees with Lebredo's subsequent observations on F. bancrofti (9), but has not yet been confirmed by other observers for F. immitis. Eighteen to twenty days are required for the filariæ to complete their development in the mosquito.

After a dog is infected it is nine months before embryos

appear in the blood. Adult worms were found in the heart in one case seven months after inoculation, but the uteri of the females contained no embryos. In autopsies made shortly after infection no trace of the worms is found as a rule, and it is not known where they develop before they appear in the heart. In one instance Grassi found fragments of a small worm in the connective tissue near the genitals. Bancroft has observed small worms in the lungs of dogs with fully-developed heart worms, and thinks that development may take place in the branches of the pulmonary artery.

Janson reports a case of transmission through the placenta. There are no well-established cases of infection of man by this parasite. Three possible cases are mentioned. Braun (2) examined some worms which were obtained from the veins of a Russian at Dorpat. He recognized them as filariæ, but did not identify the species. In 1889 Bowlby (10) reported in the Lancet two cases of Bilharzia infection. A review of his article by Kurth (11) is entitled "Two Cases of Filaria Immitis in Man." As a result of this error these cases have been frequently referred to as instances of the infection in man. If it were possible for man to be infected it would seem that the disease would be common in the Orient, where it is so prevalent among dogs.

The only known heart worm of man is F. magalhaesi. This was discovered at Rio de Janeiro by Magalhaes in the left ventricle of the heart of a child, the cause of whose death was unknown (12). It is a distinct species.

The other filariæ reported for the dog are:

F. recondita (Grassi) (13). The embryos of this worm also appear in the blood. The adults are 3 cm. in length and have been found only in the areolar tissue. A flea and a tick act as intermediate hosts.

F. sanguinolenta (Schneider) (14), also called Spiroptera sanguinolenta. This worm is found in the walls of the œsophagus, where it forms a small tumor the size of a bean. Less frequently it occurs in the stomach or the aorta. The adult female is three to four inches in length, the male a little over one inch (15). The worm is oviparous. Grassi thinks that the embryos described by Manson in the blood were embryos of F. recondita.

F. trispinulosa (Diesing) (16) was reported once. It was found in the eye.

Besides Filaria immitis, Eustrongylas gigas and Strongylas vasorum are reported to have been found in the dog's heart (15).

The articles on F. immitis are very numerous and some of them inaccessible, so no attempt has been made in this report to make a complete review of them. The best article on the pathology, etc., is Janson's (4); and Bancroft's articles give the most complete account of the life cycle.

References.

1. Leidy: Proc. Acad. Nat. Sci., Phila., 1856, Vol. V, p. 118.

2. Braun: Animal Parasites of Man, trans. Falcke, ed. 1906, p. 285.

3. Van Meter: Trans. Col. State Med. Soc., 1892, Vol. XXII, p. 288.

4. Janson: Deutsche Gesells. f. Natur. u. Völkerk. Ostasiens, Vol. V, p. 349.

5. W. E. French: American Veterinary Review, Vol. XXIII, 1899-1900.

6. Deffke (Rev. by Braun): Centr. f. Bakt. u. Parasitenk., 1890, Vol. VII, p. 515.

7. Grassi and Noè: Centr. f. Bakt. u. Parasitenk., 1900, Vol. XXVIII, p. 652.

8. T. L. Bancroft: Proc. Roy. Soc., New South Wales. 1901, Vol. XXXV, p. 41; and Proc. Roy. Soc., New South Wales, 1903, Vol. XXXVII, p. 254.

9. Lebredo: Jour. Infec. Diseases, May, 1905, Supplement No. 1, p. 332.

10. Bowlby: Lancet, 1889, Vol. I, p. 786.

11. Kurth: Centr. f. Bakt. u. Parasitenk., 1889, Vol. VI, p. 190.

12. Magalhaes: Rev. des Cursos theor. e. prat. d. Fac. d. Med. d. Rio di Janeiro, 1886, Anno III, No. 3.

13. Grassi: Centr. f. Bakt. u. Parasitenk., 1888, Vol. IV, p. 609; and Centr. f. Bakt. u. Parasitenk., 1890, Vol. VII, p. 18.

14. Schneider: Mono de Nematod, p. 100.

15. A. J. P. Silva Aranjo: Lyon Med., 1878, Vol. XXIX, pp. 319, 363.

16. Diesing: Syst. Helm., Vol. II, p. 274.

IX. A FURTHER REPORT ON HERNIA IN DOGS.

By A. R. DOCHEZ.

CASE I.—*Large irreducible right inguinal hernia.*

The patient, a black and white fox-terrier bitch, 8 years old, was brought to the clinic December 1. 1905. The history of her first two years is not obtainable. She is thought never to have been pregnant. Six years ago when she came into the possession of her present master, she had a swelling in the right inguinal region about the size of an English walnut. This swelling has gradually increased up to its present large dimensions. It has apparently not led to any disturbance other than the inconvenience occasioned by its large size and position.

Examination shows a rather old, inactive, well-nourished

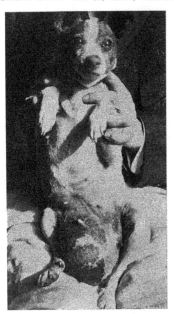

FIG. 8.—Case 1. Right inguinal hernia containing the intestine, the uterus and its appendages.

animal, with no apparent abnormality except for the enormous tumor, which hung from the lower right quadrant of the abdomen. Its size is best shown by the accompanying photograph (Fig. 8). The tumor is rather tense, firm, and on manipulation cannot be reduced. The skin over it appears somewhat stretched and the superficial veins are greatly dilated. Palpation fails to reveal the presence of viscera in the tumor, nor is there any evidence of fluid or gas. No peristalsis is observed.

Operation.—December 3, 1905. Morphia: ether. *Herniotomy.* All attempts to reduce the hernia, after the animal was relaxed under anæsthesia, proved unavailing. An incision was made over the sac and its neck was exposed at the external ring and the aponeurosis of the external oblique divided. The sac was then opened. Its contents were found to consist of the tubes, the cornua and body of the uterus, and the entire small intestine. A portion of the right cornu of the uterus was firmly adherent to the posterior wall of the sac. The left tube and cornu showed cystic changes just above their junction with the body of the uterus. Considerable difficulty was experienced in replacing the intestine, owing to the contracted condition of the abdominal wall from the long duration of the hernia, but this was finally accomplished. The uterus, the fatty broad ligaments and the tubes, it was thought best to remove; consequently a total hysterectomy was performed. The wound in the abdominal wall was closed as described in the cases reported by Dr. Beall (1) in the Bulletin a year ago,

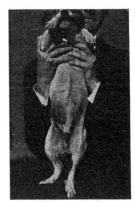

FIG. 9.—Case 1. Late operative result.

the operation resembling very closely the ordinary method of cure for inguinal hernia in women. The animal made an uneventful recovery and the wound healed per primam.

Pathological note.—The tissues removed consisted of the body of the uterus, together with its appendages. The uterus and the right cornu were normal. The left tube showed a double cystic condition. The cysts were thin walled, the size of hickory nuts, and were found to contain a thick, brown, grumous, fluid material, and to communicate with one another by a small opening 2 mm. in diameter. The lumen of the tube elsewhere was apparently occluded.

CASE II.—*Double inguinal hernia.*

Fanny, a medium-sized, brindled bull bitch, of uncertain age, a great favorite from her reputation as a ratter, was admitted on February 23, 1906. The following meagre history was obtained. A small mass was first noticed in the left groin three years ago, following pregnancy. The mass slowly increased in size until six months ago, since when it has grown more rapidly. From its size, it has caused the animal great inconvenience in locomotion, and gives her a peculiarly awkward gait. She has not been pregnant since the tumor appeared.

Examination shows a healthy, well-nourished animal, who walks with a marked limp. The left femur is distinctly bowed and the left leg turned outward in walking or running, apparently in the effort to avoid striking against the large pendulous mass which hangs in the left inguinal region. The dimensions of this mass are shown in the photograph (Fig. 10). It extends well forward on to the abdomen and hangs below the level of the patient's heel. The tumor is divided into two distinct portions by a marked constriction, an anterior large mass and a posterior small one, as shown in the photograph. The smaller mass extends backward almost to the vulva. The skin over the large tumor is thin, stretched, and has carried with it on to the surface of the tumor, the left

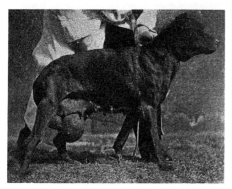

FIG. 10.—Case 2. Large double inguinal hernia.

inguinal nipple. The superficial veins are large and well defined. The skin is freely movable over the underlying structures. Palpation reveals coils of intestine, though no visible peristalsis is observed. The mass can be traced back to a pedicle at the left inguinal ring, which measures 5 or 6 cm. in diameter. It is impossible to reduce the tumor.

In the right inguinal region, on the other hand, is an easily reducible small tumor mass, which even disappears on a change in posture. When this mass is reduced it is found that the ring easily admits one or two fingers.

Operation.—February 23, 1906. Morphia: ether. *Radical cure left inguinal hernia.*

By the method we have heretofore described, the large left hernia was operated upon. When the sac had been freed and its neck opened, it was found to contain omentum and what seemed to be the entire small intestine. The uterus and tubes were not found within the sac. The intestines were reduced without great difficulty. The abdominal wall was closed in layers by overlapping, and the wound closed. The animal made an uneventful recovery and the wound healed per primam.

The bowed condition of the left leg has, of course, not been affected by the operation, and the animal walks with a peculiar

gait. She is expected to return for operation upon the other hernia.

CASE III.—*Double inguinal hernia.*

A nervous skye-terrier bitch, six years of age, a household

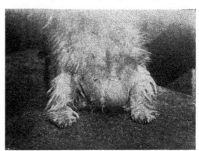

FIG. 11.—Case 3. Small double inguinal hernia.

pet, well cared for and in excellent condition, was brought to the clinic March 2, 1906. The owner does not believe that she has ever been pregnant. Three years ago a small swelling was noticed in left groin. This has increased gradually in size until it is now as large as a lemon (Fig. 11). Three months ago a similar swelling appeared in the right groin, which has gradually increased in size. There is no known cause for the appearance of these tumors. They seem to have affected the dog considerably, as she is easily exhausted and suffers from marked constipation.

Examination.—The patient is a small, well-nourished and

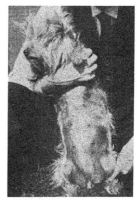

FIG. 12.—Case 3. Late operative result.

healthy looking animal, with clean, glossy skin. Aside from the bilateral swellings in the inguinal regions, examination is negative. The nipples are long and suggest a previous pregnancy. When the animal barks or struggles, the inguinal swellings become larger. The swelling on the right is not especially prominent. It is soft, easily reducible, but the character of its contents not apparent. In the left inguinal region, which is occupied by the larger mass, there is a firm, elastic swelling, which cannot be entirely reduced. It cannot be told by palpation whether or not the sac contains intestine. No peristalsis is visible.

Operation.—March 3, 1906. Morphia: ether. *Radical cure of hernia; hysterectomy.*

When the sac was opened in this case, it was found to contain the broad ligaments and uterus. There were many adhesions rendering reduction difficult and it was thought best to do a hysterectomy, for it was hoped that removal of the uterus and appendages would lessen the likelihood of a recurrence and might, at the same time, obviate the necessity of a subsequent operation on the right side. The neck of the sac was ligated off and the wound closed by overlapping in layers. Healing occurred by primary union. The result is shown in Fig. 12.

Discussion.

The literature on the subject of hernia in dogs is not very extensive. Dr. Beall (1) was able to report a series of three cases of inguinal hernia with operation, in females, and gave references to 14 other cases, one of which was a scrotal hernia. Apparently cases of scrotal hernia are rare. In the new edition of his Operative Surgery, Hobday gives pictures of one or two cases which had been under his care, and he also comments upon the not infrequent form of perineal hernia, instances of which we have never seen.

In a perusal of the literature, we have been able to find 26 other cases of hernia which have been operated upon. From a study of all the cases of which we have cognizance, it would seem that the viscera most commonly found in the hernial sac, in the order of their frequency, are: the pregnant uterus in five cases; the non-pregnant uterus and tubes in five cases; the small intestine alone in four cases, in one of which it was strangulated; the small intestine and omentum in four cases; the intestine, uterus, and cornua in three cases; and practically all of the abdominal viscera in two cases. In six of the reports, the contents of the sac were either not determined or were not mentioned.

It will be seen from the above that the uterus and appendages alone or in association with other viscera were found in 15 out of 23 cases. This is interesting from a comparative standpoint, in the light of a recent paper by F. T. Andrews (2) on hernia of the female pelvic organs in woman. In this paper he has collected 366 cases, of which 46 cases of hernia containing the tube without the ovary; 80 the tube with the ovary; 267 the ovary without the tube; 46 the non-gravid uterus, and 30 the pregnant uterus. In the dog, of course, it is more to be expected that the hernial sac would contain tube than ovary, owing to the high position and degree of fixation of the latter. In the human, the anatomical conditions are just reversed.

Owing to the small number of reported cases in the dog of scrotal hernia and of hernia of the pregnant uterus, it is thought to be of sufficient interest to record these cases here.

Scrotal hernia.—Colin (3) reports a scrotal hernia which was noted three weeks after birth. It attained the size of a hen's egg. At nine weeks of age the pup became very ill, the mass became hard, resistant, tender to pressure, and irreducible. Operation. The sac contained a strangulated, somewhat gangrenous loop of bowel. The bowel containing a mass of hard straw was resected. Recovery.

Hobday (4). A toy Manchester terrier, 6 weeks old, had a large scrotal hernia. Operation. Death from collapse.

Cases with pregnant uterus.—1. Veterinary Review (5). A mongrel bitch, 7 years old, had a litter of puppies and subsequently developed an inguinal hernia. Became pregnant again the following year. One normal puppy was born and lived four days. Meanwhile the mass in the inguinal region had increased greatly and was regarded as a tumor. It subsequently ulcerated and discharged a dead fœtus. The mother died from infection. At post-mortem, a horn of the uterus, containing the remains of a second fœtus was found in the hernial sac.

2. Sutton (6). A small, toy, bull-bitch had vomited frequently the night before admission. She was pregnant and there was a bloody discharge from the vagina. There was a tumor in the right groin, which was diagnosed hernia of the pregnant uterus. Palpation disclosed a fœtus, and digital examination per vaginam revealed a paw. It was impossible to effect delivery, owing to the diminutive pelvis. Laparotomy was performed. The hernia was reduced by taxis, combined by compression upon the fœtal head. After reduction of the herniated uterus, it was impossible, owing to the small pelvis, to effect delivery even with forceps. A Porro-Cæsarean operation was done, with recovery.

3. Hobday (7). A meager history of a herniated uterus containing a dead fœtus, with laparotomy; removal of fœtus and recovery.

4. Hobday (4). A fox-terrier bitch, 5 years of age, had an irreducible, left inguinal hernia. On operation the sac was found to contain the left horn of the uterus, in which were two fœtuses four or five weeks old. Hysterectomy was performed and death from peritonitis resulted.

5. Hobday (8). A mongrel fox-terrier bitch, 2 years old and pregnant, had a left inguinal hernia. At operation the sac was found to contain the horn of the uterus with a single fœtus and omentum. The left horn of the uterus with the fœtus was removed. The dog recovered from the operation and 17 days later gave birth to a normal puppy.

One of the most remarkable cases of hernia is reported by Hobday (4), in which most of the abdominal viscera had prolapsed into the sac. A Manchester terrier bitch, 8 years of age, had a double hernia; on the left side, the size of a duck egg; on the right, the size of a child's head. At operation the sac on the right side was found to contain the small intestine, omentum, pancreas, uterus, cæcum, rectum, and bladder. The organs were replaced and the right horn of the uterus removed. Death occurred 36 hours after the operation from peritonitis.

LITERATURE.

1. Beall: Hernia in Dogs. Johns Hopkins Hospital Bulletin, 1905, Vol. XVI.

2. Andrews, Frank T.: Hernia of the Tube without the Ovary. Jour. Amer. Med. Assn., Nov. 25, 1905, p. 1625.

3. Colin: Hernie étranglée chez un chien avec pelote stercorale dans l'ansed'hernie. Rec. de Med. Vét., 1901, 8me.

4. Hobday: Jour. of Comp. Pathology and Therapeutics, 1897, Vol. X.

5. ——— Hernia of uterus in slut. American Veterinary Review, 1878, Vol. II.

6. Sutton: Pregnant Herniated Uterus. Reduction by Taxis, Followed by Porro's Operation in Bitch. Veterinary Record, Nov. 26, 1904, Vol. XVII.

7. Hobday: Journal of Comp. Pathology and Therapeutics, 1895, Vol. VIII.

8. Hobday: Surgical Diseases of the Dog and Cat, 1906, 2d edition, Ballière, Tyndall and Cox, London.

X. SARCOMA OF AN UNDESCENDED TESTIS.

By W. Von Gerber.

CASE —.—*Small round celled sarcoma of the left undescended testis.*

The patient, a well-bred Irish terrier, said to be about eight years of age. was admitted to the clinic November 23, 1905. Six years ago its owner first noticed a tumor about the size of a pigeon's egg in the left inguinal region. This has gradually increased in size until at the present time it forms a mass the size of a closed fist. The dog had always been well.

Examination.—The animal is a small, shaggy dog, seemingly

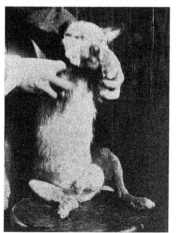

FIG. 13.—Tumor of retained testis.

in excellent physical condition despite the evidences of age. Aside from the tumor no abnormalities are found.

In the left inguinal region is a large ovoid growth measuring 10 x 7 x 6 cm. On palpation it is found to be firm in consistency and unelastic. The surface is everywhere smooth, and the

tumor is apparently encapsulated. The overlying skin is not adherent, and the mass itself can be moved somewhat freely from side to side over the underlying tissues. It lies in a superficial position just above Poupart's ligament (Fig. 13). There is but one testis, the right, in the scrotum; it is apparently normal. The left half of the scrotum is atrophied.

Operation.—November 24, 1905. Morphia: ether. A double incision was made through the skin in the long diameter of the tumor, the two incisions meeting at either end like a spindle. The skin was retracted on each side, exposing a growth covered by a smooth, tense capsule. There was very little adherent tissue, except at the inferior pole of the tumor. The mass was shelled out, the anterior portion with ease, the posterior portion with more difficulty, owing to numerous vascular attachments there. These latter were ligated and the wound kept as bloodless as possible throughout the operation. The upper pole of the tumor was attached to a pedicle containing many blood vessels, the spermatic cord and an open process of peritoneum. This pedicle was drawn down, perforated, ligated en masse, and divided between two ligatures about 3 cm. above the tumor. The stump was allowed to retract behind the abdominal wall through the external abdominal ring. After the wound had been sponged and made ready for closure there was a sudden gush of blood through the external ring. This was immediately opened by splitting the external oblique, and the tissues at the site of the hæmmorhage were clamped quickly and again ligated—securely, it was supposed. The opening in the abdominal parietes, the subcutaneous fasciæ and the skin were then sutured as quickly as possible. The animal's condition was not good, as ether had been badly taken from the first. He was given strychnine hypodermically and wrapped up warmly. Though he rallied somewhat for a time, in the course of an hour his pulse again became rapid and feeble, and he died before fully coming out of the anæsthetic.

Autopsy.—On opening the thorax, the lungs did not collapse completely. Section showed a uniformly dark red surface from which thick fluid exuded. The heart was normal in size. The edges of the mitral valves were slightly thickened. The abdominal cavity contained a large amount of fluid blood. Under the internal abdominal ring there was a large, fresh blood clot. The abdominal viscera, aside from their pallor, were normal in appearance.

The severed cord was exposed and found to be only partially secured by the ligatures. Hæmorrhage had evidently taken place directly into the abdominal cavity through the patent processus vaginalis, which had been cut but had slipped out of the ligature together with some of the larger vessels.

Anatomical diagnosis.—Recent operative wound; engorgement of the lungs; slight thickening of the edges of the mitral valves; hæmorrhage from the severed spermatic cord into the peritoneal cavity.

On fresh longitudinal section of the tumor (Fig. 14) it presents a fairly homogeneous, moist, greyish surface from which cellular elements are not easily scraped. It is broken up into several lobules by bands of connective tissue which radiate from a central point to the dense capsule underlying the tunica vaginalis. This trabecular structure somewhat resembles that of the normal gland in its distribution. No normal glandular tissue is to

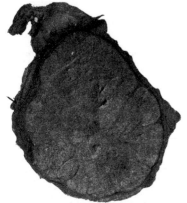

Fig. 14.—Photograph of median section of hardened tumor.

be made out by the naked eye; and only a small margin crowded toward the mediastinum testis was detected subsequently by the microscope. Though its visceral and parietal layers are somewhat adherent, the two surfaces of the tunica vaginalis can be easily peeled away from one another, showing the growth to be everywhere encapsulated by the tunica vaginalis. The tunica vaginalis passes up along the cord, the processus peritonei being unobliterated. The blood vessels of the cord are enlarged and numerous, and the section of the tumor shows it to be a vascular growth, the openings of many large vessels being visible in the cut surface.

Histologically the tumor is found to be made up of a single type of small round cells which are massed together with little intercellular structure in the spaces between the intersecting fibrous trabeculæ.

Histological diagnosis.—Small round celled sarcoma.

DISCUSSION.

This operation, through its technical error and the fatality which resulted therefrom, served to emphasize to the operator and the assistants the need of extreme care in the placing of ligatures about a pedicle of any size, especially when they are tied with the pedicle under some tension. Post-operative

hæmorrhage from the slipping of a mass ligature, or from a rise in arterial pressure, or an increased venous stasis which forces blood through a ligature which seemed to serve its purpose at the time of the operation, is an experience which is not uncommon. The lesson once learned is not likely to be forgotten. Separation and individual ligation of the vessels, double ligation on the proximal side of the proposed site of division, or ligation of the tissues thinned out by crushing with heavy, smooth-bladed clamps before the ligature is tied, are precautions to be taken in order to prevent such an accident.

This is the first instance of a testicular tumor among the laboratory records of surgical lesions in the dog. The condition is interesting from the standpoint of the growth itself, as well as from its appearance in an organ incompletely descended.

Retention of the testicle is mentioned in the medical writings of the ancients, but little was known of the conditions underlying the malady until the description by John Hunter in his earliest published work of the normal descent of the gland during fœtal life and the variations which this descent may undergo. During the past fifty years there have been a number of papers dealing with the subject of cryptorchidism in general, as well as with its complications and treatment. Curling's book on Diseases of the Testicle (London, 1866), the Hunterian Lectures on "The Imperfectly Descended Testicle" (The Lancet, 1902), delivered by Eccles, and the excellent monograph by Odiorne and Simmons in the Annals of Surgery for 1904, may be consulted for full details of the subject.

It has been found that in many of the lower vertebrates the testicle never descends to the scrotum. In the frog and pigeon, for example, it remains in its original position in the abdomen; in the hedge-hog it is close to the inguinal canal, while in the hare it is contained within the canal. In apes the testicle makes a complete descent, but the processus vaginalis remains patent, and this, so far as our experience goes, is invariably the case in the dog. These differences in position which exist normally in some animals, correspond more or less closely to the different degrees of non-descent that may occur pathologically. The testicle develops as an abdominal organ situated in front of the lower pole of the kidney, and in most mammals it migrates downwards towards the internal abdominal ring and through the inguinal canal, reaching the bottom of the scrotum shortly before birth. Abnormalities, either in the path of its descent, or in the structure of the gland itself, may cause retention. Among these abnormalities the most important are connected with the mesorchium, which may be too long or may be adherent; with the testis itself or the length of the spermatic cord and vessels; with the gubernaculum, which is often partially deficient or misplaced or may fail to contract; or with an ill-developed inguinal canal or abdominal ring.

Retention may be of various degrees. If the testicle remains in its original position in the abdomen it is said to be complete. In iliac retention it lies on the psoas muscle close to the internal abdominal ring. Inguinal retention, possibly the most common form, is frequently associated with hernia of the congenital type. Besides these there is a cruro-scrotal retention, in which the testicle lies just outside of the external abdominal ring, as was the case in our patient. According to Marshall's statistics, there is some grade of retention in one out of every nine hundred recruits. As a result of imperfect descent there may be atrophy, an incompletely descended testicle being usually functionless; and non-development of both testes is frequently associated with poor general development. Generally there is abnormal mobility of the retained organ, nearly 50 per cent of the cases of torsion being in retained testicles, and reports of strangulation from a twisted pedicle are not uncommon. Hernia is a frequent complication in man, and may possibly be due to his erect posture rather than to the patency of the peritoneal process; for this normally fails to close in a large number of animal species in whom hernia is almost unknown.

Another important complication, both in man and animals,

is the susceptibility to malignant disease of the illy-developed and abnormally-placed testicle. Tumor of the testicle is relatively far less common in the normally descended gland, and for this reason its retention is regarded by many writers as a distinct menace. Odiorne and Simmons found that out of 54 cases of testicular tumors in the Massachusetts General Hospital, six, or eleven per cent, were associated with arrested descent,—a large proportion, considering the relative infrequency of the latter condition. Carcinomata and sarcomata are the usual forms, the latter occurring more frequently. The sarcomata are as a rule either small round-celled or spindle-celled tumors. In man the disease is almost always fatal; the growth either advances along the cord or desseminates itself by metastases. Early castration offers the only hope of cure.

In this particular case there were no post-mortem macroscopical evidences of spread of the disease beyond the confines of the glandular capsule, and it is possible, had the operation terminated favorably, there would have been no recurrence.

XI. OBSERVATIONS ON DISTEMPER.

By G. J. Heuer.

Etiology.

Considerable work has been done on the etiology of the disease. Its contagiousness was recognized by Edward Jenner (18) in 1809, at which time he stated that it is as easily transmitted among dogs as the small-pox, measles, or scarlet fever is among the human species; and that the contagious miasmata, like those arising from the diseases just mentioned, retain their infectious properties a long time after separation from the distempered animal. He noted that young hounds brought in a state of health into a kennel where others have gone through the distemper seldom escape it. · He endeavored to destroy the contagion by ordering every part of the kennel to be carefully washed with water and then whitewashed, and finally to be repeatedly fumigated with the vapors of acid. He, however, obtained no good results by these methods.

Hill (14) in 1877 also recognized the contagiousness of the disease, and states: " It is highly contagious but oftimes is undoubtedly self-generated." He noted that age is no preventative, yet it is a disease more particularly of youth and is more frequent and fatal among high-bred and pampered animals. He states that one attack does not render a dog secure from a second. He suggests a possible identity between typhoid and distemper.

Millais (25) in 1890 published a paper on the pathogenic microbe of distemper in dogs, wherein he states that it is a specific infectious disease, one attack conferring immunity. From the nasal secretion of dogs sick with the distemper he obtained in gelatine tubes three organisms, a micrococcus and two bacilli. · By isolating these and performing inoculation

experiments on young pups he came to the conclusion that one of the bacilli, designated Bacillus B., is the cause of the disease, while the micrococcus is a potent factor in producing the pneumonia which so frequently follows distemper. With the above organism he was able to reproduce the disease, and young pups placed with a dog infected by experimental inoculation also acquired the affection. A complete description of these organisms is not given in his paper. According to the picture, Bacillus B. is a medium-sized bacillus occurring singly or in short chains. It liquefies gelatine, descending as a flaky mass in almost clear fluid, which is covered by a whitish scum. The micrococcus also produces a clear liquefaction.

Wadams (43) (1895) upheld the infectious nature of the disease, but stated that one attack does not confer immunity against a second. The incubation period he places between ten days and two weeks.

Martinet (22) (1895) states that the disease is always an infection and never occurs spontaneously. It is peculiar in the number of its complications and sequelæ and resembles measles in man.

Galli Valerio (12) (1896) isolated from dogs sick with the distemper an oval bacillus which was present in the lungs, brain, spinal marrow, and the pus in the frontal sinuses. It presented the following characteristics:

Morphology.—An oval bacillus, 2.5 x .31 μ in size. In the body of the dog it is not observed as an oval bacillus but as a coccus; hence the organism may change its morphological characters. It is *motile* in all cultures and takes the *Gram stain.*

Gelatine.—Along the stab, gas bubbles appear. The stab culture shows small white points of growth; no liquefaction in several months. Stained preparations show oval bacilli, in pairs, with polar staining.

Agar.—Small white colonies.

Horse Serum.—Cloudy growth along the streak in coagulated serum. In fluid serum a flocculent precipitate appears at the bottom of the tube.

Bouillon.—Cloudy. After several days a sediment appears at the bottom of the tube.

Potato.—24 hours. A white transparent growth.

Milk.—Good growth. The milk is not coagulated.

Peptone bouillon.—Growth, but no gas.

Milk sugar.—Growth, but no gas.

Indol reaction.—Negative.

Lignieres (20) (1903) isolated and described an organism which was also worked upon by Phisalix (29). These observers obtained from the blood of the heart and internal organs an organism in the form of a long bacillus which, after passage through a guinea-pig or on cultures, soon changed into a short cocco-bacillus. To this organism was given the name Pasteurella canis. In general character it simulates the organisms belonging to the fowl-cholera group, which includes fowl cholera, swine plague, pneumo-enteritis of cattle, sheep, goats, and buffalo; equine influenza, guinea-pig distemper, and so forth. With this organism Phisalix was able to reproduce the disease in the dog and cat. Inoculation of a culture into the veins gave the characteristic symptoms of the disease, and these were found to vary with the strength of the culture, amount injected, etc. He found that the organisms were attenuated by growth and successive transfer on media, and both he and Lignieres were able to determine the various clinical manifestations of distemper, such as meningoencephalitis, chorea, paralysis, vesicular pustules, opalescent and ulcerative keratitis, gastroenteritis, lung complications, arthritis, and catarrhal symptoms. According to Phisalix, the Pasteurella canis forms a soluble poison in artificial cultures which, when injected, acts principally on the nervous system and gives rise to disturbances of nutrition, lowers resistance, and offers a favorable soil for secondary infection. The morphology and cultural characteristics are as follows:

The organism is a cocco-bacillus; non-motile; does not take the Gram stain. It is very polymorphous and shows many involution forms. It is chiefly aerobic, but may also be anaerobic. Its virulence is variable, but is generally great.

Gelatine.—Shows growth, but no liquefaction.

Milk.—No acid formation; no coagulation. The reaction remains normal.

Potato.—No visible culture on natural acid potato.

Gelose of Würtz.—Not reddened.

No *indol* in pancreatic bouillon.

In his paper, Gray (9) states that Monckton Copeman claims to have found a microbe 15 years before Lignieres' discovery, when working with Millais. He described a small

cocco-bacillus, staining with ordinary analine dyes but decolorized by Gram's; *gelatine* in time tends to become liquefied; grown with difficulty on *potato*. He isolated the germ from the lungs, tracheal mucosa, and nasal secretion, not from the heart, liver, kidney, or spleen.

It will be seen that there is considerable difference in the morphological and cultural characteristics of the various organisms above described. The differences between the Mallais-Copeman organism and the Lignieres and Phisalix organism have been pointed out by Gray. The *former* is (*a*) larger and grows in chains; (*b*) it has a tendency to liquefy gelatine; (*c*) it grows slightly on potato, forming a pale buff color, and (*d*) it is found not in the blood of the heart or organs but in the nasal, bronchial, and pulmonary mucous. The *latter* is (*a*) a very small cocco-bacillus which does not form chains; (*b*) it does not liquefy gelatine; (*c*) it does not grow on potato; (*d*) it has not been isolated from the nasal, tracheal, or pulmonary mucous, but is found in the blood of the heart and organs during the early stages of distemper, and (*e*) it causes the various clinical forms of distemper, such as meningoencephalitis, chorea, etc. The organism of Galli Valerio is also described as (*a*) a small cocco-bacillus; (*b*) it does not liquefy gelatine; (*c*) it does not change milk. In these respects it resembles the organism of Legnieres and Phisalix. On the other hand it is described as a motile organism, which stains by Gram and shows a visible growth on potato. Again it was isolated from the lungs, brain, spinal marrow, and pus in the frontal sinuses. In these respects it differs quite markedly.

All of the organisms are said to produce symptoms characteristic of the disease, so we must conclude either, that several organisms can produce the disease, or that the same organism is capable of considerable morphological and cultural variation.

VACCINATION EXPERIMENTS.

Millais, quoted above, did some experiments in attenuation and protection. In all cases in which he was able to produce distemper by inoculation he states that he obtained but a mild form of the disease. Hence he thought that by inoculating dogs with attenuated cultures of Bacillus B. he could render them immune. He first inoculated two valuable dogs with such cultures and got a mild distemper in each case, the temperature never rising above 102.5°. In a second experiment he inoculated 2 pups with a diluted culture heated at 60° for 10 minutes. No ill effects resulted; after a week, to allow the effects of the virus to take place, he inoculated the same pups with a pure culture of Bacillus B. and to make the experiment more striking, placed them in a kennel previously inhabited by dogs with distemper. No disease followed. He repeated these experiments, and of 12 pups so treated, 5 did not develop distemper. In the remaining 7 the disease developed, complicated with pneumonia. One dog died. Again he inoculated 2 out of 17, St. Bernard dogs, infected with the distemper. Of the 17 dogs 15 died, the only 2 living being those inoculated.

The most extensive vaccination experiments have been those of Phisalix. With the organism worked out by Lignieres and himself as a basis he prepared a serum and worked out a careful method for vaccinating dogs.[1] His results are as follows: Of 1250 vaccinations performed between May 15, 1901, and May 15, 1902, *65*, or 5.2 per cent, were infected with the disease; *36*, or 2.88 per cent, died, and *29*, or 2.4 per cent, had only a benign attack. Of 1035 dogs vaccinated between May 15, 1902, and May 15, 1903, *47*, or 4.4 per cent, gave symptoms of the disease; *18*, or 1.75 per cent, died, and *29*, or 2.84 per cent, had only a benign attack. In the hands of other workers equally good results have not been obtained. Thus Lignieres worked with the virus of Phisalix and obtained very unsatisfactory results. In his first attempt he inoculated 2 young dogs three times; they both died. Again in another series the dogs showed no trace of a reaction. In a third experiment he inoculated 4 young dogs with vaccine prepared by Phisalix and according to his directions; 2 dogs with virulent virus and 2 with weak. All died. In a second paper the same author reports further experiments. In two-thirds of his cases the dogs showed signs of the disease and his mortality was practically 100 per cent. In the other one-third of his cases many died from the disease, while others had a grave infection. Therefore, Lignieres maintains that the results of vaccination are as yet not at all conclusive.

Gray agrees with the results of Phisalix, while Parker (*47*) records a series of 60 inoculations upon healthy pups, in which he found a higher mortality in the vaccinated pups than in the same number unvaccinated. Of those 60 vaccinated, 42 contracted distemper afterward; 14 were unaffected. Of the 42 which contracted the disease later, 8 recovered, 22 died, and 19 were killed because of the disease.

The *morbid anatomy, symptoms, course,* and *treatment* of the disease are well given in the various papers quoted in the literature and in the various text-books on veterinary pathology. A good account is that in Friedberger and Fröhner's Veterinary Pathology. It is not within the scope of this paper to review them.

The cases which are reported in the following pages were all seen among the patients in the Hunterian Laboratory between November, 1905, and May, 1906. It is to be regretted that the malady, in each instance, was not observed at an earlier stage. Among those who have worked upon the disease it seems the general opinion that the infective agent is active early in the disease and that secondary invaders are already present when the more prominent symptoms call attention to the disease. In Case I the disease was well advanced, for one of the most frequent complications which follow the distemper, namely, pneumonia, was undoubtedly present when the animal was first seen. Case II seemed most favorable for study, since here the progress of the disease was followed almost from the beginning. The infection was evi-

[1] Method in Vet. Record, Aug. 30, 1902.

dently a severe one and the animal died before any of the common complications had set in. Case III resembled Case I, in that it presented the severe symptoms of distemper coupled with a pneumonia. In Case IV an extensive pneumonia was the most distinctive lesion, and we cannot feel positive, although it is highly probable, that it was preceded by the distemper.

CASE I.—*Dog 10 37.*

When first observed, the disease was evidently well advanced. The caretaker was not certain when the dog first became sick, but believed that it had been ill for a week or two. When seen the dog was lying in a corner, his head out-stretched upon the floor between his paws, a thick, creamy, greenish-yellow discharge issuing from his nose and eyes. The dog was hot and feverish, the respirations rapid and noisy, and every now and then he would make an effort to expell the purulent material from his respiratory passages. He remained in this condition for two days, taking no food and being aroused only with great difficulty. It was decided to kill the animal and this was done by over anæsthetization.

Necropsy.—The body is that of a medium-sized, emaciated male dog, 65 cm. in length. Both eyes are partially stuck together by a thick purulent exudate. There is an abundant white, creamy discharge from both nostrils. Over the lower portion of the abdomen are several ulcerated areas, the largest measuring 1.5 cm. in diameter, the smallest .8 cm. These ulcers are shallow, with a hyperæmic base and a sharply marked, fairly regular margin. On the inner surface of each thigh are similar areas of ulceration.

Head.—The skull-cap was removed by a circular incision around the top of the cranium. The dura is shiny and glistening and apparently normal. The arachnoid space contains a small quantity of clear fluid. On removing the brain its surface is found to be normal in appearance throughout. There is no marked congestion of the cerebral vessels. (Cultures made from the cerebrospinal fluid).

Frontal sinuses.—Both frontal sinuses are completely filled with a thick, creamy purulent exudate (cultures). The mucous membranes lining the sinuses are rather pale in appearance. On continuing the opening downward all the nasal passages are found to contain a quantity of this purulent material. The trachea, lungs and heart were removed en masse.

LUNGS.—*Left Lung.* The outer surface of the *upper lobe* is covered with a rather dry, white, purulent-looking exudate. With a forceps, small pieces of this exudate can be readily stripped off. The lobe is grayish-pink in color, voluminous and is found to be completely consolidated. On section a quantity of creamy, purulent material gushes out of the smaller bronchi. The cut surface is uniformly pale, grayish-pink in color and slightly granular in appearance. The *lower lobe* is air containing throughout and on section presents a normal appearance. No areas of consolidation are made out.

Right Lung.—The upper lobes are free from adhesions and their surfaces are smooth and glistening. They appear rather pale. No areas of consolidation are made out and the tissue is everywhere air containing. On section the cut surface is normal in appearance. The lower lobe presents a smooth and shiny surface. In palpation two or three small nodular masses are made out which are quite hard and firm. The largest measures about .5 cm. in diameter. Otherwise the lobe is air-containing and crepitant throughout. On section these nodules are fairly circumscribed, firm and smooth and the cut surface projects slightly above the surrounding tissue. The surface is deep red in color and appears hæmorrhagic.

Trachea and bronchi.—The trachea is found to contain a considerable quantity of a white purulent exudate mixed with mucus. The mucous membrane is quite uniformly pale. Both the larger and smaller *bronchi* contain an exudate similar to that found in the trachea but it is thicker and in greater amount. On the left side, especially in the consolidated lobe the smaller bronchi are completely filled with purulent exudate. The mucous membrane is pale throughout.

Heart.—The pericardial cavity contains a small quantity of clear fluid. The epicardium is everywhere smooth and glistening. The heart does not appear enlarged. (Cultures from the auricle). On section the cavities of the heart do not appear dilated. The mitral, tri-cuspid, aortic and pulmonary valves are thin and delicate and apparently competent. The myocardium is rather pale in appearance and perhaps of softer consistence than normal.

Abdomen.—The peritoneal cavity contains no excess of fluid. The peritoneal surfaces are everywhere smooth and glistening.

Spleen.—Is of normal size. The capsule is slightly wrinkled but otherwise the surface is smooth. The organ is dark red in color; rather firm on palpation. The cut surface is smooth and the edge quite sharp. The malpighian bodies are plainly visible but not especially enlarged. The trabeculæ are well marked. There is no increase in the red spleen pulp.

Kidneys.—The kidneys present no distinct lesions. The cortex is perhaps thickened and shows a slight degree of cloudy swelling.

Liver.—The liver is not enlarged. The surface is everywhere smooth and shiny. The color is reddish-brown. On section the cut surface is smooth and of a brownish color. The lobulation is fairly well marked, the central veins of the lobules being distinctly seen. Several areas are found in which the central vein is surrounded by a paler, more opaque cortex, apparently areas of degeneration. The *gall-bladder* is distended with a greenish-brown, rather viscid bile.

Stomach.—The stomach is distended with fluid. (Old operation). On section, the mucosa is thrown into numerous folds which are uniformly pale, but otherwise normal in appearance.

Intestines.—The mucosa is uniformly pale except for two areas in the duodenum which are red and congested. The mucosa here is somewhat thickened and more folded than usual. No macroscopic lesions are demonstrable.

Lymph glands.—The mesenteric lymph glands appear enlarged and are firm and hard. On section they present a uniformly grayish-white appearance.

CASE II.—*History.* A family of four cats, all of which were suffering from snuffles or distemper, was seen on Monday, February 12, 1906. The owner, who spent a great part of her time with her pets, was very positive as to the course of events and the following history was obtained: On Friday, February 9, owner noticed that one of her black cats, an animal three years old, was not well and the first thing observed was a watery discharge from the nose and eyes. Later in the day there was difficulty in breathing and the animal's neck, the owner says, was distinctly swollen. The next day the discharge from the nose and eyes was thick and purulent and streaked with blood. There was noisy respiration and difficulty in swallowing. The animal coughed a good deal. Late Saturday afternoon a great amount of purulent material came from the nose and mouth and after this occurrence the cat was evidently much relieved. It has taken no food for three days. It had no movement of the bowels until to-day (four days). It slept a great deal; when aroused it seemed stiff and couldn't walk well. When seen on February 12 the animal was much better. There was still some purulent discharge from the eyes, nose and mouth. Respiration labored (but not rapid) and noisy as if the respiratory passages were filled with purulent exudate. It coughs a good deal, but cough is looser than previously. It has taken some food and its bowels moved to-day.

The second cat to be attacked was an animal two years old. This cat, the owner said, had had a cold for some time. Saturday morning, however, a day after the above cat was affected, she noticed a watery discharge from its nose and eyes. This became purulent Sunday. This animal presented exactly the same symptoms as the previous one, but they were not so severe and when seen on Monday there was but a slight purulent discharge from the nose and eyes and the animal seemed fairly lively. It had a cough and sneezed frequently and there was some difficulty in respiration.

A third cat, an animal one year old, had but a very slight attack of the disease. The symptoms first appeared on Saturday, there being a watery discharge from the eyes and nose. The discharge became purulent Sunday, but was small in amount and the cat did not seem very ill at any time. When seen February 12 there was some discharge from the nose and eyes, but the cat was lively and seemed in good condition.

The fourth of the group, an old cat ten years of age, was the most seriously affected. Symptoms first appeared February 9 with a watery discharge from the nose and eyes. This discharge rapidly became purulent and so great in amount that there was great difficulty in respiration. It became dull and apathetic, crouched upon the floor wherever placed, and could not be roused sufficiently to take food. On February 11 it gave birth, prematurely, to two dead fœtuses about 9 cm. in length. When seen February 12 there was an abundant thick purulent discharge from the eyes, nose and mouth. The respiration was noisy, a long-labored, snoring respiration being followed by a shorter forcible expiration. There was difficulty in swallowing. Rectal temperature, 102.6. Pulse, very rapid. Over both sides of the chest respiration and expiration were prolonged, although there was no distinct tubular breathing. Expiration was accompanied by moist and sonorous râles. Heart rapid but sounds clear at apex and base.

Subsequent history.—February 13, 1906. Cats seen in the afternoon. The three younger animals better and evidently the worst part of the attack has passed. There is still some discharge from the eyes and nose and they sneeze and cough a good deal. They eat well, however, and seem livelier than when last seen. The old cat is about the same as when last seen. There is a thick purulent discharge from the eyes and nose. It crouches in the corner with head on the floor and can scarcely be aroused at all. Has taken no food and bowels haven't moved since onset of attack. Was given calomel gr. ¾ in a little milk. Boric acid advised for eyes.

February 14, 1906.—Cats seen in evening. The three younger animals better. The old cat also seems much better. There was an abundant discharge from its nose last evening and owner thinks that relieved it a great deal. It takes notice of things and has walked about the room. It has eaten nothing. Owner does not know whether or not its bowels have moved.

February 15, 1906.—Cats seen in the evening. The younger animals are doing well. There is still some discharge from the nose and eyes. The old cat is not so well as on yesterday. Its eyes are much better, but there is an abundant discharge from the nose. It crouches in the corner and takes no notice of things about. Does not eat. Sleeps a great deal. Its bowels have not moved. Given calomel gr. i in a little milk. Eyes treated as before.

February 18, 1906.—Cats seen in the morning. The three younger animals are practically entirely well. The old cat died at 2.30 a. m. this morning. A necropsy was permitted.

CASE II.—*Cat.*—*Necropsy.* The body is that of a well-nourished maltese cat. Rigor mortis is well marked. Both eyes are glued together by a purulent discharge which has formed crusts upon the eyelids. There is a purulent discharge mixed with *blood* from the nose and mouth. The mucous membranes of the mouth show areas of ulceration along the gums and on the inside of the cheeks. There are no skin lesions upon the body.

Head.—The skull-cap was removed by a circular incision. The meninges are not thickened and are glistening in appearance. There is no excess of fluid. The surface of the brain shows no lesions. The cerebral vessels are not especially congested.

The *frontal sinuses* are filled with a greenish-yellow purulent exudate. The mucous membranes of the sinuses are pale in appearance.

Chest.—The *left lung* presents a smooth and glistening surface. There are no adhesions. The color is rather pale. The lobulation is plainly marked by an abundance of pigment. On palpation the lung is crepitant and air-containing throughout. No areas of consolidation can be found. On section the cut surface is uniformly grayish-pink in color and rather dry. The bronchi are free from exudate and the mucous membranes are pale.

The *right lung* presents an appearance very similar to the left. The lung is air-containing throughout and shows no demonstrable lesions. The bronchi are clear.

Trachea.—In the upper portion of the trachea there is a small amount of frothy purulent exudate. The lower part of the trachea is clear. The mucous membrane is uniformly pale.

Heart.—The pericardial cavity contains a very small quantity of clear fluid. There are no adhesions. The epicardium is smooth and shiny. On section the cavities of the heart do not appear dilated. The valves are delicate and apparently competent. (Cultures from auricle).

Abdomen.—The peritoneal cavity contains no excess of fluid. The surfaces are smooth and glistening.

Spleen.—The surface is smooth and the capsule not thickened or wrinkled. The spleen is pale in color and rather soft on palpation. On section the cut edge is not sharply marked and the tissue bulges. The malpighian bodies are plainly visible but not greatly enlarged. The trabeculæ are distinctly made out. The red spleen pulp appears slightly increased in amount.

Kidneys.—The *right kidney* is of a pale red color. The capsule strips readily leaving a smooth surface. On section the cortex appears thickened, is very pale and granular in appearance. The straight vessels are well marked and the glomeruli are visible as minute red points. The whole cortex is opaque and cloudy and definitely shows cloudy swelling. The medulla is red and the straight vessels are plainly marked and filled with blood. The *left kidney* is similar in appearance to the right.

Stomach.—The stomach is not distended. It contains a small quantity of dark fluid. The mucosa is pale except for a few slightly congested areas.

Liver.—The liver appears rather large. Its surface is smooth and shiny and presents a mottled coloring, red areas alternating with yellowish-white. On section the cut surface is very friable and soft. The cortex looks opaque and cloudy. There is the same mottled appearance seen on the surface. In the yellowish-white areas the central veins of the lobules are seen as red dots surrounded by a zone of opaque yellowish white cortex. These are areas of degeneration. The cut surface also shows other irregular, not very sharply marked areas in which the liver substance is of a dirty brown color and very soft so that it can almost be wiped away with the finger; evidently areas of focal necrosis.

Uterus.—The right cornua of the uterus contains a dead fœtus 9 cm. in length.

Bladder.—The bladder contains a small quantity of rather highly colored ammoniacal urine. The mucosa is pale and shows no lesions.

Intestines.—The lower portion of the intestine contains a quantity of fecal matter. The mucosa is pale throughout and shows no lesions.

Lymph glands.—The lymph glands are not enlarged.

CASE III.—A small black dog, first seen on February 15, 1906. He presented the typical picture of distemper. Was very much emaciated and lay in a corner with his head outstretched on the floor, a purulent discharge running from his nose. He could be aroused, but only with difficulty. He took no food. No history was obtainable other than that the dog had been sick for a few days. When seen on Saturday, February 16, 1906, the purulent discharge from the nose was streaked with blood and there was an abundant discharge from the eyes. The respiration was rapid. He was aroused with great difficulty and on auscultation over the thorax there were tubular breath sounds on either side, most marked on the left. The dog died on Sunday, February 17, 1906.

Necropsy. February 18, 1906, p. m.—The body is that of a very much emaciated small black male dog. Rigor mortis well marked. The eyes are stuck together by crusts of purulent material. There is scarcely any discharge from the nose.

Mouth.—The mucous membranes of the mouth show discrete patches of ulceration, the largest being 2.5 x 1.5 cm. in diameter situated in the upper left cheek. Teeth in good condition.

There are no ulcers over the body.

Head.—Skull opened by a circular incision. The meninges and brain are clear throughout.

The *frontal sinuses* contain a very small amount of muco-purulent exudate (cultures). The mucous membranes are pale.

CHEST.—*Right lung.* Is large and voluminous. There are no adhesions between the parietal and visceral pleuræ. The upper lobe is pink in color and air-containing throughout. The lower lobe is crepitant along the borders; its center is occupied by a dark red mottled area which projects above the surrounding lung surface and which has a definite outline. This area is hard, firm and non-air-containing. On section a quantity of muco purulent material with some serous fluid issues from the cut surface (cultures). The cut surface is of a rather uniform grayish-pink color and is marked by white dots of pus which apparently fills the smaller bronchi.

Left Lung.—The left lung is large and voluminous. There are no adhesions between the parietal and visceral pleuræ. The middle lobe is voluminous, dark red in color and completely consolidated. From the cut surface there issues a muco-purulent material similar to right lung. The lower half of the upper lobe and the middle third of the lower lobe are likewise consolidated and present an appearance similar to the middle lobe.

Heart.—(Cultures). There are no adhesions between the pleuræ and pericardium. The pericardial cavity contains a small quantity of clear straw-colored fluid. The heart appears of normal size. The right auricle and ventricle are distended by a postmortem clot. The tri-cuspid valve is apparently competent and normal except for a dark colored, almost black vesicle about 2 mm. in diameter which projects upward from the base of the posterior flap. On pricking with a knife the contents of the vesicle are bloody in nature.

Abdomen.—The peritoneal cavity contains no excess of fluid. The peritoneal surfaces are everywhere smooth and glistening.

Left Kidney.—The capsule strips readily, leaving a smooth dark red surface. On section the cortex appears opaque and has a boiled appearance (cloudy swelling). The glomeruli are made out with difficulty. The straight vessels of the medulla are well marked and filled with blood.

Right Kidney.—Similar to left in appearance.

Spleen.—Is of a dark red color. The surface is smooth and the capsule does not appear thickened. It is rather firm in consistence. On section, the cut surface is dark red. The trabeculæ are plainly marked as fibrous bands. The malpighian bodies are visible. There is no apparent increase in red spleen pulp.

Stomach, intestines and *pancreas* are normal in appearance.

Liver.—Is large. Its surface is smooth and mottled in appearance, dark red areas alternating with others almost white. On section the cut surface is cloudy and opaque. It is mottled as on the surface, the pale areas surrounding the central veins of the lobules and appearing as areas of degeneration. The *gall bladder* is distended with a greenish thick bile. The ducts are patent.

Mesenteric lymph glands.—Are not especially enlarged. They are dark gray in color and much pigmented.

CASE IV.—This animal, a rather large, long-haired white and brown dog, was first seen about the hospital on February 20, 1906. No definite history could be obtained. The caretaker said that the dog when brought in was thin and emaciated. When seen he was lying in a corner of the room, listless, with his head on the floor. His eyes were heavy and around the lids there was a sticky purulent discharge. There was no discharge from the nose. His nose was hot and his respiration rapid and labored. On auscultation tubular breathing was present on both sides and pneumonia was strongly suspected. The dog was very irritable and could not be approached. He died two days later.

Necropsy.—The body is that of an emaciated, long-haired, brown and white dog. Rigor mortis is well marked. The eyes are stuck together with a purulent, yellowish-green exudate. There is no discharge from the nose. The oral mucous membranes show several patches of ulceration. The teeth are in good condition. There are no ulcers on the skin.

Head.—The *meninges* and *brain* show no macroscopical lesions. The *frontal sinuses* and nasal passages are free from exudate and no signs of inflammation are apparent.

Lungs.—The *left lung* is voluminous. There are no adhesions between it and the chest wall. It presents a mottled appearance, patches of grayish-pink alternating with areas of deeper red. The surface is smooth and shiny. On examination the *two upper lobes* are found to be completely consolidated and airless. On section a quantity of purulent material issues from the lung substance. The cut surface is uniformly grayish-pink in color, firm, granular and much like the liver in consistence. The *lower lobe* is air-containing throughout and on section is normal in appearance. The *right lung* is also voluminous. There are no adhesions present between it and the chest wall. In color it resembles the left lung. Its surface is smooth and glistening. The upper lobe is completely consolidated and airless. On section a muco-purulent material escapes from the lung substance. The cut surface is similar in all respects to that found in the two upper lobes of the left lung. The remainder of this lung is air-containing throughout and the bronchi are clear.

Heart.—There are no adhesions between the pericardium and pleuræ. The pericardial cavity contains a small amount of clear fluid. The epicardium is everywhere smooth and glistening. The heart does not appear enlarged. On section the cavities of the heart appear normal in size. The heart valves are all delicate and apparently competent.

Abdomen.—The peritoneal cavity contains no excess of fluid. The surfaces are smooth and glistening.

The *spleen* is dark red in color. The capsule appears slightly thickened and roughened. The organ is less firm than normal. On section the malpighian bodies are plainly visible, although not apparently enlarged. The trabeculæ stand out plainly. The red spleen pulp is perhaps slightly increased in amount.

Kidneys.—The *left kidney* is about of normal size. The capsule strips readily leaving a smooth dark red surface. On section the cortex is grayish-red in color, of normal thickness, and appears slightly cloudy. The malpighian corpuscles are visible as red dots. The straight vessels are distinctly marked and appear filled with blood. The *right kidney* is similar to the left in appearance.

Liver.—The liver is large and reaches well below the costal margin. It is dark red, but mottled so that the lobulation appears plainly marked on its surface. On section the cut surface is dark reddish-brown in color. The lobulation is plainly seen. Each central vein appears as a red dot surrounded by a wide yellowish zone of parenchyma, this in turn being encircled by a narrow zone of red. The appearance is that of a central degeneration.

The *stomach* and *intestines* are normal in appearance.

BACTERIOLOGICAL REPORT.—In Case I, smears were made from the eye, frontal sinuses, nose, and small bronchi. That from the eye, stained with gentian-violet, showed numerous pus cells and many microorganisms, the predominant form being that of a medium-sized coccus which was quite uniformly scattered, singly or in clumps. A few large bacilli were seen. The smear from the frontal sinus stained by Gram's showed a similar picture. The cocci took the Gram stain. Those from the nose and bronchi, stained with gentian-violet and methylene-blue, respectively, also presented the same picture. In the smear taken from the nose bacilli were more numerous.

Cultures were taken from the meninges, the frontal sinuses, the nose, the smaller bronchi, the lungs, and the blood (right auricle). All the cultures were plated and the various organisms separated in pure culture. They were transferred upon the various media and followed through in the usual way. It will be unnecessary to give all the cultural reactions. The cocci were obtained almost in pure culture from the frontal sinuses, nose, eyes, bronchi, and pus from the lungs, and gave the reactions of the pyogenic staphylococci, the staphylococcus albus being most frequently found although the staphylococcus aureus was often present. The few bacilli seen in the smears from the nose and eye proved to be B. subtilis. From the blood an organism was isolated which morphologically and culturally corresponds closely to the Pasteurella Canis or cocco bacillus of Lignieres. Its morphological characters and cultural reactions are as follows:

Forty-eight-hour agar plates show small circular colonies from pin-point size to 1 mm. in diameter. White by reflected light; slightly translucent by transmitted light. Under the microscope the edges are fairly regular and well defined. The colonies are granular with flocculent masses. Rather brownish in color.

A hanging drop preparation shows a small, very short bacillus, seen singly or occasionally in pairs. There is an active dancing movement but no definite movement from place to place. (The preparation was made after several transfers were made so that it represented an organism several generations old.)

A preparation made from the first transfer and stained with gentian-violet showed a longer bacillus than was seen in later generations so that the organism is polymorphous and on media tends to become shorter. The organism stains freely with methylene-blue. It does not take the Gram stain. A preparation from a milk culture stained with methylene-blue shows polar bodies.

Agar.—At 21 hours there is a fine white growth which is translucent when held to the light. The edges are irregular and marked by small discrete circular colonies. The growth at 45 hours and up to 3 weeks showed no change.

Bouillon.—At 21 hours the bouillon is slightly cloudy, a finely granular sediment is present with stringy masses at the bottom of the tube. Excepting that the sediment increased there was no change in 3 weeks.

Potato.—At 21 hours there is no perceptible growth; at 45 hours it was thought that the growth was just visible; at 69 hours and thereafter up to 3 weeks there was no visible growth.

Milk.—At 21 hours there is no acid reaction; no curd nor digestion. The medium remained unchanged until the third day when there was a very slight change to an acid reaction. There was no curd nor digestion. The milk culture remained thus without change until the third week. Stained preparations showed the bacillus present in fairly large numbers having a tendency to polar staining.

Gelatin.—At 21 hours there is a white growth along the stab. No liquefaction. There was no liquefaction up to the third week.

Glucose fermentation tube.—Showed a good growth but no gas formation.

Glucose litmus agar.—Good growth. Acid reaction. No gas.

Lactose litmus agar.—Good growth. Acid reaction in 48 hours. At 1 week color almost entirely gone except for a faint pink ring at the surface of the media. No gas formation.

Mannite litmus agar.—Good growth. No acid reaction. No gas.

Saccharose litmus agar.—An abundant growth on the surface of the media which shows a bluish coloration. The surface of the agar is blue while below, by transmitted light, it is red. No gas formation.

The cultures from the meninges showed no growth.

In Case II cultures were made from the meninges, frontal sinuses, eyes, nose, and blood (right auricle). They were plated as in Case I. Due to some fault in technique the plates were quickly overgrown with B. vulgaris and therefore we cannot feel certain that some organism did not escape us. The colonies on the plates were all similar in appearance and a large number were transferred to agar slopes. For the most part the colonies were formed of cocci which gave the cultural and staining reactions of the pyogenic staphylococci, and of these the staphylococcus albus was alone present, there being no development of color on the media and no digestion of gelatin. An organism which differed from the above was isolated from the frontal sinuses. It was a coccus giving a white growth on agar, but there was no acid formation in litmus milk which gave a normal reaction throughout. There was but a faint white growth on gelatin which appeared only after 5 days. No liquefaction occurred.

The cultures from the meninges showed no growth.

In Case III cultures were taken from the meninges, frontal sinuses, eyes, lungs, and blood (auricle). They were plated

on agar and gelatin plates. The colonies were all small and circular or oval, ranging from pin-point to 1 mm. in diameter. The same organisms were found as in Case II. A coccus, corresponding to the one described above, giving no acid reaction in milk and a slow growth with no digestion on gelatin, was isolated both from the frontal sinuses and heart's blood. It did not give a very definite Gram's stain. The short bacillus isolated from the blood of Case I was carefully searched for but not found.

In Case IV no cultures were obtained.

INOCULATION EXPERIMENTS.—A few animal inoculations were made. They are not many enough to warrant any conclusions. No experiments, furthermore, were made with the organisms most frequently found and which were thought to belong definitely to the pyogenic staphylococci. The experiments were confined to the short bacillus isolated from the blood in Case I and the coccus isolated from the frontal sinuses and blood of Cases II and III.

Experiment I.—About 3 cc. of a bouillon suspension of a 36-hour agar culture of the bacillus from blood of Case I was injected into the subcutaneous tissue of a very young puppy which was known not to have had the distemper. The pup was carefully watched for 10 days. It developed no symptoms. There was a slight exudate about the point of puncture on the third day but no distinct reaction. The pup became emaciated, but this was thought to be due to the fact that its mother did not feed it properly. It died 16 days later. At the necropsy the peritoneal cavity contained an excess of clear fluid. No other lesions were found. No organisms were recovered.

Experiment II.—About 2 cc. of a bouillon suspension of a 24-hour agar culture of the same organism as in Experiment I were injected into the mucous membranes of the nose and into the subcutaneous tissue of the abdomen. On the following day there was a slight discharge from the nose but no distinct reaction. No symptoms developed in 2 weeks and the organism was not recovered. The animal was an adult dog of uncertain age and it was not known whether or not it had had the distemper.

Experiment III.—A similar injection as in Experiment II was made on a puppy which was known not to have had distemper. No symptoms developed.

Experiment IV.—About 3 cc. of a bouillon suspension of a 24-hour agar culture of the same organism was injected into the saphenus vein of a young kitten. It was watched for over 2 weeks. No symptoms developed.

Similar experiments were performed with the coccus with similar results. It also produced no symptoms referable to the disease.

CONCLUSIONS.

It is apparent from a perusal of the literature on the subject, that the etiological factor in distemper has not been definitely established.

A number of organisms have been described by various authors, all of which differ morphologically and culturally, as well as in their staining properties. They all are said to produce, when inoculated artifically, symptoms characteristic of the disease. The symptoms which they produce have not been described in sufficient detail. They are described as mild symptoms, but it could not be determined what was to be inferred from that term.

The organism most fully described and accepted as the etiological factor by the greatest number of authors is the Pasteurella canis, described by Lignieres and Phisalix. This organism in their hands produced, when injected artificially, symptoms of the disease. Phisalix made a virus from it and performed over 2000 vaccinations, which he considered very successful. Yet in the hands of others, as we have seen, neither the virus nor the method of vaccination were at all successful.

An organism identical (the only difference was a very slight possible acid reaction in milk) with the Pasteurella canis, morphologically, culturally, and in staining properties, was isolated from the blood in Case I. When inoculated into animals (*Felis* and *Canis*), which could not have been rendered immune by a previous attack of the disease, it produced no symptoms. However, the inoculation experiments were very few in number and perhaps incomplete. Also the organism has been described as of varying pathogenicity, some strains being but very slightly pathogenic; and in the hands of previous observers the organism had passed through several generations before being used for animal inoculations.

LITERATURE ON DISTEMPER.

1. Ainslie: Canine Distemper. Proc. of Vet. Med. Assoc., January, 1838.

2. Bull, W. A.: Notes on Canine Distemper Vaccine. Vet. Record, London, 1902-3, XV, 732.

3. Cadéac: Ency. de Path. Interne. Art.-Maladie des Chiens, Vol. VI, 1897.

4. Carré, H.: Sur la Maladie des Chiens. Bull. Soc. Centr. de Méd. Vét., Paris, 1905, LXXX, 313.

5. Delabere (P. Blanc): Diseases of Dogs; with an Appendix on Diseases of the Cat and also Canine Pathology. 4th edition, 1841.

6. Eloire, Aug.: La Vaccination Contre la Maladie des Chiens. Aviculteur, Paris, 1902, XXII, 224-226.

7. Friedberger and Fröhner. Vet. Path. Transl. by Capt. Hayes.

8. Gray, H.: Dr. Copeman's Vaccine and Mr. Sewell's Experiments. Vet. Record, London, 1902-3, XV, 374.

9. ——— On the Etiology and some of the Phases of Canine Distemper. Vet. Record, 1903-4, XVI, 381-386.

10. ——— Bilious form of Canine Distemper, or Epizoötic Jaundice in the Dog. Vet. Record, London, 1905-6, XVIII, 235.

11. ——— Recurrence of Canine Distemper. Vet. Record, London, 1905-6, XVIII, 89.

12. Galli Valerio: Le Microbe de la Maladie des Jeunes

Chiens. Trans. in Centralbl. f. Bak., 1 abth., Jena, 1896, XIX, 694-698.

13. Hertwig, C. H.: Krankheiten der Hunden. 2d edit., 1880.

14. Hill, J. W.: Canine Distemper. Vet. J. and Ann. Comp. Path., London, 1877, V, 260-272.

15. Hodge: Action of Alcohol on Dogs as Regards non-Viability and Malformation of Young and Severity of Attack in an Epidemic of Distemper. J. Boston Soc. M. Sc., 1897-98, II, No. 4, 35-38.

16. Hofer: Der Abd. Typhus der Hunde. Rep. der Thierheilkunde, Vol. XIII, 1852.

17. Howatson: Canine Distemper; Preventative Inoculation of the Flint and Denbigh Fox Hounds with Dr. Phisalix's Vaccine. Vet. Journal, London, N. S. VII, 270-272; also Vet. Record, London, 1902-3, XV, 698.

18. Jenner, E.: Observations on Distemper in Dogs. Med. Chir. Tr., 3d ed., London, 1815, I, 265-270.

19. Lepinay: La Maladie des Jeunes Chiens. Argus Méd., Paris, 1901, III, Nos. 12 and 13, 1-5.

20. Lignieres: Le vaccination de la Maladie des Chiens; Critique des Statistiques de M. Phisalix. Comp. Rend. Soc. de Biol., Paris, 1903, LV, 1087..

21. ——— Sur la Vaccination Contre la Maladie des Chiens. Bull. Soc. Centr. de Méd. Vét., Paris, 1903, N. S. XXI, 40; also [Abstr.] Comp. Rend. Soc. de Biol., Paris, 1903, LV, 919-921.

22. Martinet, W. H.: Canine Distemper. J. of Comp. Med. and Vet. Arch., Vol, XVI, 1895, p. 292.

23. Mayhew: On the Dog, 1854, and Veterinarian, 1854.

24. Meguin: Le Chien, 3d Edit., Vols. I and II, 1893-94.

25. Millais, E.: The Pathogenic Microbe of Distemper in Dogs and its use for Protective Inoculation. Vet. J. and Ann. Comp. Path., London, 1890, XXX, 313-321; also Brit. M. J., London, 1890, I, 856-859.

26. ——— Distemper in the Dog and Experiments Therein in St. Thomas's Hospital. Vet. J. and Ann. Comp. Path., London, 1891, XXXII, 313-328.

27. Müller: Diseases of the Dog. Trans. by Alex. Glass, 1897.

28. Nocard and Leclainche: Les Maladies Microbiennes des Animeaux. 3d Edition, 1903.

29. Phisalix, C.: Maladie des Jeunes Chiens; Statistiques des vaccination pratiques du 15 Mai, 1901, au 15 Mai, 1902. Compt. Rend. Acad. d. Sc., Paris, 1902, CXXXIV, 1252; [Repr.] Progrès Méd., Paris, 1902, 3 S., XIV, 385-389.

30. ——— Maladie des Jeunes Chiens; Statistiques des vaccination practiques depuis le 15 Mai, 1902, Jusqu, au 11 Juillet, 1903. Compt. Rend. Soc. de Biol., Paris, 1903, LV, 980-982.

31. ——— Apropos du Microbe et de la Vaccination de la Maladie des Jeunes Chiens. Ibid., 1085.

32. ——— Recherches Sur la Maladie des Chiens; vaccination du chien contre l'infection experimentale par le bacilli

specifique. Compt. Rend. Soc de Biol., Paris, 1901, LIII, 601-604.

33. Phisalix and Rabieaux: Sur la Vaccination Contre la Maladie des Chiens. Bull. Soc. Centr. de Méd. Vét., Paris, 1903, N. S. XXI.

34. Renault: Veterinarian, 1844.

35. Schantyr: Unters. uber Mikro örgan. der Hundesstaupe. Deut. Zeit. für Thier. Med., Vol. XVIII, 1892.

36. Sewell, A. J.: Phisalix Antidistemper Vaccine. Vet. Record, London, 1902-3, XV, 375.

37. Toplin, Wm.: Practical Observations on Thorn Wounds, Punctured Tendons, and Ligamentary Lameness in Horses, etc.; and an appendix on Distemper in Dogs. About 1790.

38. Taussig, S.: Die Hundskrankheit, Endemischer Magenkatarrh in der Herzegowina. Wien. Klin. Wchnschr., 1905, XVIII, 129-163.

39. Trasbot: Rec. de Méd. Vét., 1868. Arch. Vét., p. 161.

40. —— Dict. de Méd. Vét. de Bouley, Vol. XVIII, 1890.

41. Viborg, E.: Veterinar Skriften, 3 Copenhagen, 1795.

42. Viborg and Greve: Erfahrungen über Krankh. der Hausthiere, Oldenburg, 1818.

43. Wadams, E.: Canine Distemper; its Causes, Symptoms, Sequels, and Treatment. J. Comp. Med. and Vet. Arch., Phila., 1895, XVI, 92-99.

44. Williams: Principles and Practice of Vet. Med., 8th Edition, 1897.

45. Youatt, Wm.: On the Dog, 1845; Distemper in the Dog. Veterinarian, 1830.

46. Zundel: Dict. de Méd. Vét. de Hurtrel D'arboval. Article, Maladie des Chiens. Vol. III, 612-630, Paris, 1857.

TUBERCULOSIS, A SOCIAL DISEASE.[1]

By S. A. KNOPF, M. D., New York.

Associate Director of the Clinic for Pulmonary Diseases of the Health Department of New York City.

Tuberculosis, a social disease, is the subject assigned for my address this evening. The desire to attack this disease from its social side seems to have come into more than usual prominence at the present time. A few months ago I returned from the International Tuberculosis Congress in Paris, where I had the good fortune to meet your distinguished president, Professor Henry Barton Jacobs, who will bear me out when I tell you that this gathering was the largest of its kind which has ever taken place. There distinguished laymen and medical men united to learn from each other how to treat, cure and prevent tuberculosis, considered not only as a medical, but also as a social disease. While in Paris I received an invitation by cable to speak before the Massachusetts State Federation of Charities on November 9, on "The Social Aspect of Tuberculosis." The People's Forum of Yonkers begged for the same lecture for their meeting on the following Sunday, and to-day I am here to treat the same subject before this selected audience of students of tuberculosis.

For the honor of again appearing before you I am indebted to no less a person than our great and beloved teacher, Professor Osler. It must please you to think that he planned this symposium on the social aspect of tuberculosis on the eve of his departure. Knowing that he could not be with us in person he wrote me, "I shall be with you in spirit." The forethought in arranging a discussion on this subject shows the love and deep interest he has in the society which owes its existence to his genius.

Your society is the first which consecrated itself to the exclusive study of tuberculosis. You have advanced so far in your studies, that I fear I shall not be able to tell you anything new, yet the name of him under whom your society is called, the immortal Laennec, and the large gathering here of you, his earnest followers, should be an inspiration to me. I am, however, only

a physician, and if I fall short in my sociological reasoning, I pray you to ascribe it to lack of understanding and not to lack of heart or good will to do the best I can.

Were our great Osler in my place, he would probably in his own inimitable way treat the subject as if it were a clinical case. He would begin with the etiology, then describe the symptoms, then the prevention and the curative measures, and lastly, the prognosis—the outlook. I will endeavor to carry out this idea as well as I can in my present address, also beginning at the bottom of the social ladder with the children.

Tuberculosis in infancy is indirectly due, on the one hand, to either an hereditary or acquired predisposition, and directly, on the other hand, to a postnatal infection. Direct hereditary transmission of the tuberculous germ from parent to child is of exceedingly rare occurrence. When the father or mother is tuberculous the child may inherit a predisposition, which I like to describe as a physiological poverty, giving the child less resisting power to the invasion of tuberculous diseases. The same condition may be produced when the child, instead of being raised at the breast of a healthy mother or wetnurse, is fed from a bottle. Such a child, unless the greatest care is bestowed on the artificial feeding, will almost invariably remain below par in health. The earliest postnatal infection takes place if a tuberculous mother or tuberculous wetnurse is allowed to give the breast to the child, or if she carelessly coughs over the child, kisses it on the mouth, or if, when feeding it, she puts the nipple of the milk bottle or the spoon alternately into her mouth and then into the baby's in order to test temperature or sweetness. Furthermore, we must not forget the very probable source of infection through milk from tuberculous cows used as food for the infant. Lastly, there is another source of infant infection, threaten-

---

[1] Address delivered by invitation before the Laennec Society for the study of Tuberculosis of Johns Hopkins Hospital, Baltimore, Md., Nov. 23, 1905. Revised for publication in The Johns Hopkins Hospital Bulletin, May 1, 1906.

ing particularly infant foundlings or deserted little ones who have at first been inmates of foundling asylums or infant hospitals, and because of their not having done very well, have been given to the care of families residing in the country. In institution life there is, of course, always some danger of infection from a tuberculous infant to a healthy one; secondly, from tuberculous milk supply; and, thirdly, though more rarely, from tuberculous attendants. To my mind, the danger to the little ones given out to families living in the country, is far greater than in an institution. Do you know that the majority of families who make boarding babies a business confide them to the care of the invalid of the family, who, perhaps nine times out of ten, is a consumptive? The danger which arises to these little ones from such a consumptive attendant is obvious, particularly when we consider the usually inferior hygiene in such homes and the ignorance of the inmates of the nature and prevention of tuberculosis.

Before going any further let us see what we may be able to suggest in order to combat these various sources of tuberculous predisposition and actual infection. The prophylaxis regarding the transmission of a predisposition of tuberculosis lies, of course, in preventing tuberculous individuals from marrying and procreating a predisposed race. It is not always easy to prevent the marriage of tuberculous individuals, for some marry without knowing that they are tuberculous, and some who even know that they are so marry nevertheless, no matter what the doctor says, and there is no law to prevent them from doing so. In such instances, unfortunate as they are, the physician has a duty to perform in preserving the life of the tuberculous mother, which is always endangered by pregnancy, and preventing the transmission of a tuberculous diathesis to an innocent child. I feel very strongly on this subject, and though I know that there are many worthy men and women, inside and outside of the medical profession, who differ with me, I am willing to take the responsibility before the law and God for each time I have taught a consumptive husband and wife not to procreate a tuberculous race.

Certain authors have made the statement that tuberculous parents confer on their children an immunity against the contraction of the disease. In twenty years of labor, exclusively devoted to tuberculous patients, I have not found the slightest evidence for this deduction; on the contrary, I have found children of tuberculous parents, owing to their inherited physiological poverty, anything but immune.

What can we do to have more breastfed and vigorous babies and thus a more vigorous race, a healthier type of American men and women, strong enough to resist a tuberculous invasion, or, for that matter, any other infectious disease to which a weakened organism easily falls prey. With all due respect to our beloved President, let me say that as a physician with a somewhat large experience among the poor and poorest of the poor, the middle classes and also among the well-to-do, and as a student of sociology as well as of preventive medicine, I am not for quantity but for quality.

I know I am in the presence of earnest students who, by careful study of the social as well as the medical aspect of tuberculosis, are anxious to better the condition of their fellowmen. For this reason I speak plainly and am willing to give you the result of some interesting observations from my own practice which, I think, justify me in taking this position. It is invariably my custom when examining a patient to take down the family history, and one of the questions asked is, "How many children were in your family?" and, "Were you born the first, second, or third?" etc. In the majority of cases, when there is a large family, it is the 5th, 6th, 7th, 8th or 9th born who has contracted tuberculosis. This is to be explained, on the one hand, by physiological reasons, the parents being in advanced life and less vigorous; on the other, by economic reasons: the later born children cannot, because of increased expense, receive that particular care and that good and ample nourishment which was the privilege of the first ones to receive when the family was still small. No amount of wealth, no family prestige or social connection can give the child that inheritance which it receives when born of vigorous parents, nursed by its own mother, and tenderly cared for until able to care for itself.

Let the mothers who, for the sake of pleasure and convenience, abandon the divine privilege of nursing their own children, change this unnatural practice. I feel certain that if they but knew the difference in the physical and intellectual make-up of their sons and daughters if tenderly nursed by themselves, or when handed over to strangers to become bottle-fed babies, they surely would do differently. I know it will be said that not every mother can nurse her infant. This is true in some instances; but to the women, the future mothers of mothers, I like to say that it has been statistically demonstrated that if one generation of mothers fails to give their infants, and particularly female infants, food from the source which nature has designed, the next generation of mothers will have great difficulty in the natural feeding of their infants. The reverse has also been demonstrated, and it has even been shown that when mothers, not fully able to supply the infant with food, have supplemented the artificial feeding as best they could with their own breast, their daughters have been able to fulfill the divine duty of nursing their infants, if not always entirely, at least to a much larger degree than the preceding generation.

Let us draw a lesson from this scientific fact, which is corroborated by nature's own laws. This lesson once learned, the coming generation of American men and women may yet surpass all other nations in physical beauty, intellectual attainments, and moral strength.

Against post-natal infection, arising as aforesaid from a careless mother, father, or attendant, there is but one remedy, and that is education—education of the prospective mother, education in all that appertains to the prevention of tuberculosis and other infectious and preventable diseases, in school, colleges, etc. Against the contraction of tuberculosis from infected milk our sanitary authorities should protect us. Regular tuberculin tests of all milch cows, inspection of stables, milk transportation and milk depots, should be practiced in all well regulated communities. But we ourselves can protect our babies from infected milk by boiling or sterilizing the milk whenever we are not certain of its absolute purity. In this connection I cannot help paying a tribute to Mr. Nathan Straus of New York, who has done such grand and life-saving work by presenting to several communities large plants for sterilizing milk to be distributed to the poor at cost.

In institutions for infants, isolation of tuberculous children should be practiced as far as possible. No tuberculous individual should be employed in a hospital to take care of infants, and no child should be given into the care of a family unless the hospital authorities are absolutely certain that the infant will not be attended by a consumptive.

We come now to tuberculosis in childhood, which may likewise be contracted from either tuberculous parents, tuberculous relatives, friends or boarders. A tuberculous individual living in such a home, particularly if it is small and unhygienic, need only be careless with his expectoration, and the little child, crawling on the floor, is sure to come in contact with it, touching everything with its fingers which are often put into its mouth afterwards, or scratching its delicate skin with the infected nails. If the tuberculous sputum has had a chance to dry and become pulverized the bacilli-laden atmosphere, always heavier in the lower strata of the air, is sure to be inhaled by the little one. You have thus a source of infection which may cause a tuberculous from ingestion, from inhalation, and from inoculation; in other words, the child has a chance of having its intestines, its lungs and its skin tuberculously infected at the same time.

The remedy for this again lies in education—education of the tuberculous and education of those living with them.

There is one more source of infection arising in children of which I must speak and which is often overlooked by our hygienists and social workers. I refer to the life of little ones in day nurseries. These institutions should be most carefully watched and supervised; in fact, I firmly believe that not only tuberculosis, but diphtheria, measles, and other children's diseases would be greatly diminished if our sanitary authorities would insist upon a daily medical inspection of the children in these nurseries. The isolation and particular watching of tuberculous children could then be easily accomplished.

Before taking up the third phase, "Tuberculosis during the School Age," I would like to say one word more in regard to the management of the predisposed child when it no longer receives the healthy mother's or foster mother's breast. In the eyes of the utilitarian or materialist, or, perhaps, also in the eyes of a certain class of sociologists, the question, how to raise a child predisposed to tuberculosis, might seem a paradox. In defense of our views in this respect, let me repeat that while in my humble opinion it belongs to the highest

mission of the physician to prevent the procreation of a tuberculous race, when, in spite of his warnings and teachings, a child is born of tuberculous parents, it is his most sacred duty to do all in his power to save the child's life and, if at all possible, make it strong, healthy and vigorous; and we physicians should use the clinical experience of the best authorities to guide us in this respect.

Predisposed children are almost all born bad eaters. They will have a disinclination to many kinds of food and be often unwilling to eat when they should. Only by beginning at the earliest possible period with a firm discipline can these children be made to eat as other healthy children. The old practice of folding our hands, resigning ourselves to fate, and saying that because the father or mother had tuberculosis the child must also be doomed, with our present knowledge of phthisiology is thoroughly reprehensible. Sensible parents, even if tuberculous, can often be very helpful in combating a hereditary predisposition in their children if able to give them proper physical and intellectual care and training, combined with good food, much outdoor life and sensible dress.

In the homes of the poor such an ideal training of the child is not always easy. French phthisiotherapeutists and philanthropists have realized the importance of caring for offsprings of tuberculous parents who would have to live in a *milieu tuberculeux*, and have a special organization called "Oeuvre de Prevention de l'Enfance contre la Tuberculose." This work was started by my esteemed master and teacher, the great children's physician, Professor Grancher of Paris, in November, 1903, by a large personal gift from Mrs. Grancher and himself. It consists in the main in removing the children of poor tuberculous parents from the center of infection, either to good sanitary private homes in the country or to seaside or inland sanatoria. There is no time limit; the children may stay away until, in the opinion of the supervising physician, they are strong enough to resist a tuberculous invasion. The removal of these children is, of course, always done with the consent of the parents. The first complete report of the work of this society was given out at the recent Tuberculosis Congress at Paris and showed most gratifying results.

What are the predisposing causes of tuberculosis during the school age? Badly ventilated school rooms, overtaxing of the child's brain to the detriment of its physical development, unhygienic dress, particularly of the school girl, and among the poor, underfeeding, insufficient clothing, and bad housing, often combined with child labor in workshops, factory and even at home.

What are the direct causes of tuberculous infection during school life? Close association with tuberculous fellow pupils; very much more rarely the carelessness of a tuberculous teacher.

To describe the various sources of infection during school life, I believe I cannot do better than to repeat here the little list of rules which I like to see school teachers give to their pupils, which might serve as an alphabet in the prevention of tuberculosis.[2]

1. Every child or adult can help to fight consumption. School children can be helpful by complying with the following rules:

2. Do not spit except in a spittoon, or a piece of cloth, or a handkerchief used for that purpose alone. On your return home have the cloth burned by your mother, or the handkerchief put in water until ready for the wash.

3. Never spit on a slate, floor, sidewalk, or playground.

4. Do not put your fingers in your mouth.

5. Do not pick your nose or wipe it on your hand or sleeve.

6. Do not wet your finger in your mouth when turning the leaves of books.

7. Do not put pencils in your mouth or wet them with your lips.

8. Do not hold money in your mouth.

9. Do not put pins in your mouth.

10. Do not put anything in your mouth except food and drink.

11. Do not swap apple cores, candy, chewing gum, half-eaten food, whistles, bean blowers, or anything that is put in the mouth.

12. Peel or wash your fruit before eating it.

13. Never cough or sneeze in a person's face. Turn your face to one side or hold a handkerchief before your mouth.

14. Keep your face and hands and finger-nails clean; wash your hands with soap and water before each meal.

15. Do not kiss anyone on the mouth, nor allow anyone to do so to you.

16. When you don't feel well, have cut yourself, or have been hurt by others, do not be afraid to report to the teacher.

17. Be just as careful and cleanly about your person at home as in school.

18. Clean your teeth with toothbrush and water, if possible, after each meal, but at least on getting up in the morning and on going to bed at night.

19. Learn to love fresh air, learn to breathe deeply, and do it often.

Another good method of teaching school children the prevention of tuberculosis has been inaugurated in France in a most ingenious way. My distinguished teacher, Professor Letulle, suggested to the Minister of Education of France that the coverings of the books used by school children might serve as a means of instructing the pupils concerning the prevention of tuberculosis. He himself wrote two pages of instruction for the purpose. The outside cover represents the exterior of a sanatorium, and the text is illustrated by a number of

pictures. Permit me to give you here the translation of the subjects, which are treated in a most concise and comprehensible way on these two pages:

" The air we breathe and the respiratory organs."

" Tuberculosis decimates humanity."

" Tuberculosis is contagious."

" Tuberculosis and its microbe."

" Robert Koch, the discoverer of the microbe of tuberculosis (consumption)."

"Tuberculous infection from man to animal and from animal to man."

" Tuberculosis can be prevented."

" Sure way to prevent consumption."

" Never use strong drinks."

" Tuberculosis can be cured."

" Tuberculosis is a social disease."

To remove all possible causes which might render a child susceptible to the invasion of tuberculosis during school life, we must appeal to school boards, superintendents, teachers and school physicians to do all in their power. Permit me to quote here what I said on this subject in an address delivered last year before the American Academy of Medicine. The School Board, or board of education, as it is called in some localities, should, in choosing a site for a school, bear in mind that, whenever possible, a somewhat elevated region, where the streets are wide and the surrounding houses not too high and not too close together, and where the traffic is not too heavy, should be selected in building a public school. About the construction of a modern and model school house much could be said. The essentials of such construction are well known to all sanitarians and up-to-date architects. In relation to the prevention of tuberculosis I would suggest only a few points. Where the site or locality does not permit of having a large playground, a roof garden which can be covered in winter is absolutely necessary. Instead of our American windows, which can only be opened to one-half of their extent, I should wish to see French windows in every school house, or windows sliding in the wall, or those that turn on a pivot, all of which permit twice the amount of foul air to go out and of good air to come in that our ordinary windows do. Heating and general ventilation of school rooms should, of course, be of the most improved kind. The walls and wood-work of school rooms should be plain to make the accumulation of dust virtually impossible and the cleansing easy. All corners should be rounded off, and the walls painted. The interior equipment—that is to say, the school furniture, benches and desks—should be so arranged that they can be easily moved or folded together, so that a thorough cleaning of the floors is made possible after each daily session. It goes without saying that the drinking cup should be replaced by the hygienic drinking fountain, which makes the use of a cup unnecessary, and thus eliminates one method of transmission of microbic diseases.

Every public school should have a well equipped gymnasium and a swimming tank with constantly running fresh and salt

[2] My inspiration to compile this set of rules I received from a little leaflet which I found during my visit to Providence. I have since learned that they were written by Prof. Theobald Smith of Harvard, who wrote them at the suggestion of Dr. Chapin of Providence, R. I., and I am anxious to give these gentlemen credit for their work. I have ventured to make some additions and some changes in order to cover the entire ground of first principles in the prevention of tuberculosis.

water, warmed to a suitable temperature in winter. Each pupil should be given the opportunity to bathe several times during the week. To learn to swim should be made obligatory and every class should be supervised by a competent swimming master. Leaving aside the great hygiene gain to be derived from such an installation, especially when the pupils are recruited from homes where bath rooms are rare and where regular bathing is considered superfluous, the swimming lessons will be of value to every boy and girl, and in case of such disaster as the recent Slocum tragedy there will be a much smaller loss of life. There is hardly a college in existence in America where the gymnasium and the swimming tank do not form an important part of the equipments, and a college without them would surely suffer in prestige. The public school where the children of the masses receive their education should not be behind the private college in its equipments.

I am convinced not only that the public school which has a well-equipped swimming establishment and which makes regular bathing and instruction in swimming obligatory for every pupil, will have fewer cases of infectious and contagious diseases, particularly scrofula and tuberculosis, but that the intellectual and moral status of its pupils will also be higher.

The duties of the superintendent of a public school in the prevention of tuberculosis are manifold. In arranging the curriculum he should bear in mind never to push the intellectual training to the detriment of the bodily development or physical welfare of the children in his school. There has been, and is yet, altogether too much overtaxing of the brain and the nervous system of our boys and girls in public and also in private schools. Our gynecologists and nerve specialists have given us enough illustrations of the detrimental effects of the overtaxing and overstraining of the mind and the nervous system of the young girls at the age of their development into womanhood. Many of our college pupils, male and female, do not get enough rest; they are overworked and sleep too little. Those of us who have given to tuberculosis a somewhat closer study also know that it is often at the period of entering puberty that the predisposed individual becomes most susceptible to the invasion of the bacillus, particularly when additional strain is put upon the physical or mental system. This holds good of both sexes. A judiciously divided curriculum, combined with gymnastics, swimming and as much outdoor instruction as possible, would seem to me a most important factor in the prevention, not only of tuberculosis, but of all indoor diseases and nervous troubles.

By outdoor instruction I mean not only botanizing tours and geological excursions, but also outdoor singing and outdoor recitation. In my textbook on tuberculosis[2] as well as in my article on the subject in the Twentieth Century Practice of Medicine,[3] I quoted Barth, of Köslin, who had made a

[2] "Pulmonary Tuberculosis, Its Modern Prophylaxis and the Treatment in Special Institutions and at Home," P. Blakiston's Son & Co., Philadelphia.

[3] Twentieth Century Practice of Medicine, Vol. XX, p. 230.

careful study of the effects of singing on the action of the lungs, the pulmonary circulation, diseases of the heart, the blood, the vocal apparatus, the upper air passages, the ear, the general health, the development of the chest, and the activity of the digestive organs. As a result of his studies he came to the conclusion that singing should be considered one of the exercises most conducive to health. I am willing to go even further and say that outdoor singing and outdoor recitation, when the weather is neither too windy nor too cold, is a most excellent means of preventing the development of pulmonary diseases. You have all heard of the numerous cases of open-air speakers, such as political campaigners, evangelists, etc., having developed their respiratory capacities and strengthened their lungs as a result of their peculiar profession. Some even profess to have been cured of consumption as a result of their outdoor speaking. The German military authorities, who have the reputation of instituting all exercises which tend to prevent disease and invigorate the soldiers, have of late much encouraged singing during the marching of the troops.

To every class in the public school opportunity should be given in fairly good weather to have recitation and singing at least once a day in the playground, adjoining garden, or roof garden. Breathing exercises should, of course, be instituted for at least a few minutes at a time during recess for all classes. This should be done either in the open air or when the windows are wide open, and a number of times each day. The simple breathing exercises which I recommended as a prevention of pulmonary diseases, I have published and illustrated in my books, as well as in various articles, and also in my popular essay on tuberculosis[4] and I don't feel that it will be necessary to describe them here again. The selection of rational textbooks on physiology and general hygiene must be left to the good judgment of the board of education and the superintendent.

The duties of the superintendent and those of the school teacher are, of course, interdependent. The former makes out and supervises the curriculum; the latter carries it out. The lessons in physiology and hygiene must be adapted to the age and understanding of the pupils. The school teacher should, of course, be familiar with all the practical and feasible methods in vogue in regard to the prevention of tuberculosis as an infectious and communicable disease.

Let me finally mention a place where tubercle bacilli abound and where you find at certain hours more children than even at school. I refer you to our menageries. To visit the ape-house in the zoological gardens and to remain there as long as possible is the delight of children; and yet, perhaps next to cattle, there are no animals so subjected to tuberculosis as apes, nearly 90 per cent being afflicted with the disease. Add to this the commotion, dust, and impure air in the average ape-house at the usual time of the children's visits, and one cannot help thinking of an absolute danger. There seems no reason,

[4] "Tuberculosis as a Disease of the Masses and How to Combat It." Fred. Flori, 514 East 82nd St., New York, Publisher.

why an ape-house, containing numerous consumptive animals, should not be as much a source of infection as a tenement house, where ignorant and careless tuberculous individuals have expectorated indiscriminately.

Before closing the paragraph on the prevention of tuberculosis during school age, I must call your attention to the term scrofulosis, which really means tuberculosis in a milder form, and which is particularly frequent among school children in the districts of the poor and is the result of bad housing and particularly of underfeeding. To prevent scrofulosis—the milder form of tuberculosis—I must revert once more to the duties of the school board, for what can the teacher or superintendent do with the underfed children of the poor attending our public schools? Breathing exercises will not supplement their lack of food, but, if anything, they will increase the appetite of the pupil, and an apple and a cracker are not enough for a growing boy or girl and altogether too little to make their cheeks red. I would therefore suggest to the board of education a philanthropic enterprise in which the generous and good-hearted people of every city would most gladly join. It may thus become possible to provide these half-starved little ones with a luncheon of a few meat sandwiches and one or two glasses of good milk, and I am convinced that fewer will develop tuberculosis and scrofulosis, and they will do better work at school and at home. To avoid a pauperizing tendency a few cents may be charged for these lunches. If I have been well informed, I believe this practice is in vogue in Boston, Milwaukee, and in a few other cities. I do not know whether statistics have been kept regarding the results, but I know that in some European cities the persistent administration of a nutritious luncheon resulted in the physical and intellectual improvement of the children and in a considerable gain in weight.

The problem of the underfed school child is a much more serious one, than is usually believed. Let me quote in this connection from Mr. John Spargo's recent book, "The Bitter Cry of the Children." "When it was suggested that 60,000 or 70,000 children go to school in our greatest city in an underfed condition, and when Dr. W. H. Maxwell, Superintendent of the Board of Education of New York City, declares, in a public address, that there are hundreds of thousands of children in the public schools of the nation unable to study or learn because of their hunger, something of a sensation was caused from one end of the land to the other." Underfeeding predisposes to tuberculosis and thus you see that in school children tuberculosis has a very decided social aspect

One more word on the duties of the school physician, and of course every school should have one or several. These duties should consist in the constant supervision of the sanitary condition of the school buildings; regular visits to the gymnasium and the swimming school, and lastly, the most important function of all, the monthly weighing of the pupils and the periodical examination of the chests of all pupils, teachers and employes of the school. The weeding out of all such individuals as might constitute a source of infection, or those whose treatment becomes an imperative necessity, and

the advice to be given to parents of a tuberculous child, will make the school physician a most important factor in the solution of the tuberculosis problem.

It goes without saying that the school physician, who must devote so much time to this duty in order to do it faithfully, should receive ample remuneration for his service.

I do not wish to have it understood that our public schools and kindergartens are the only institutions which need sanitary supervisions. Boarding schools, parochial schools, seminaries, etc., often need the watchful eye and frequent visits of a trained sanitarian just as much, if not more, in order to prevent the spread of tuberculosis and other infectious diseases.

Before leaving the subject of tuberculosis in schools, it is but right that we should devote a few earnest words to the subject of "What to do with the tuberculous school child and naries, etc., need often the watchful eye and frequent visits of the tuberculous school teacher." Permit me to quote here from a recent address which I delivered before the teachers of the Public Schools of New York at the occasion of the American Tuberculosis Exhibition held under the auspices of our National and our New York Anti-Tuberculosis Associations. A number of states have taken very radical measures in this respect. My interest in the subject was first aroused by a letter received last February from my friend, Dr. Herbert Maxon King, the physician-in-chief of the Loomis Sanatorium at Liberty. He sent me a clipping announcing the decision of the Board of Education of Jersey City, that no teacher having consumption would hereafter be allowed to teach in a public school. In commenting on this decision, Dr. King said: "It occurs to me that if such action shall be taken on the part of the various Boards of Education throughout the country, much injustice is going to be done." Since then, according to the *Medical Record* of November 25, 1905, the State of Iowa, and, according to the *Medical News* of December 30, the State of Illinois, have joined the list of those that exclude tuberculosis from the public schools, and these boards have issued an order notifying the superintendents of schools throughout the State to exclude all teachers, pupils, and employes suffering from the malady. They exclude the teacher, and they exclude the child and I approve of this decision, but I must ask: "Have those states which exclude the tuberculous teacher, who nine times out of ten has contracted this disease in the performance of his or her duty, provided a pension for her, so that she can devote a year, perhaps more, to doing nothing but getting well?" Or, "Has she been able to accumulate enough means to live the rest of her life without care in case she shall not be cured entirely and not be readmitted to the school?" I doubt if this will be the case in many instances.

A French Commission was recently appointed to look into this matter and they recommended that all tuberculous school teachers employed in the Republic of France, should receive for at least three years a sum sufficiently large to provide for proper sanatorium treatment at home, and this without losing the right to be pensioned later on.

And what is done in our American schools for the children who are tuberculous? How many seaside—or inland—sanatoria for tuberculous children have we where the child may be cured of its disease and concomitant with its physical improvements receive an education? We in the great city of New York have just one seaside sanatorium for tuberculous children which fulfills this mission, but its capacity is limited to 54 beds, and we have in New York about six thousand tuberculous children needing sanatorium treatment.

I approve of weeding out both tuberculous child and tuberculous teacher from our public schools, but I also believe that it is our most sacred duty to provide for these tuberculous teachers and tuberculous children. Let us multiply our sanatoria for children and employ in them as many teachers as we can from the unfortunate ones who have contracted tuberculosis.

Now, what are we to do with the rest, who cannot find employment in these institutions? One of our most beloved, large-hearted and generous philanthropists and distinguished fellow townsmen, Mr. Andrew Carnegie, recently created a fund to pension teachers in academic schools who are beyond a certain age and no longer able to earn their livelihood. Mr. Carnegie very justly recognized that our college professors are, as a rule, too poorly paid to accumulate a sufficient fortune to live in comfort during their declining years. This is a grand and beautiful philanthropy, and I sincerely hope that the example of Mr. Carnegie may be emulated by other philanthropists; but I hope and pray that in the future gifts for pensioning educators, our ordinary school teachers will not be forgotten. They must have served at least twenty years before they are entitled to any pension, and then it is but small. Then they, too, have often very little chance to accumulate enough to enable them to live in comfort during old age; and I am certain that when misfortune strikes one in the prime of life, when the school teacher contracts tuberculosis and must leave the school, nine times out of ten she will have saved very little or no money. Yet is costs money to provide for at least a year in which to cure a tuberculous patient, and it requires even more to make her comfortable when she is not curable but is forced to live in idleness for two years or more. Let the municipality which excludes the tuberculous teacher and the tuberculous child provide school sanatoria for the children, and, whenever possible, employ therein the tuberculous teachers in the earlier stages of the disease. Let our good and generous fellow-citizens who love to devote part of their wealth to the relief of the suffering and misery of their fellowmen, remember in their benefaction the school teacher who has had the misfortune to contract consumption. Whether such a benefaction be in the shape of a special sanatorium for tuberculous school teachers or a special fund whereby these school teachers can be sent to existing sanatoria, or be treated at home, is immaterial.

What need have I, before an audience of this kind, to speak of the baneful influence of child labor? A few states of the Union have endeavored to do their best in enacting and enforcing laws against this shameful practice. But there is yet much to be done. Let all American legislatures understand that nothing predisposes a child's delicate and growing organism to tuberculosis more than the great physical strain produced by hours, and often long hours, of indoor labor, which time the child should spend in outdoor play. Child labor makes physical and nervous wrecks of normal children and because of its influence on the nervous system of the growing boy and girl, I hold child labor responsible for a good deal of alcoholism among our young people.

President Roosevelt, in his recent message at the opening of the last session of Congress, recommended in strong terms a model child labor law, in order that Congress might set a worthy example to the States in which it has no power to legislate on this subject, by wise and discriminating legislation for the District of Columbia, over which it has the necessary power.

Permit me to read to you a few suggestions from an appeal issued recently by the National Child Labor Committee,[*] which, I think, speak for themselves:

" We request the friends of the twenty-nine million children under 16 years of age in the United States, for whose industrial guardianship and for the protection of whose rights to healthy physical development, education, and leisure the National Committee is organized, to co-operate in recommending this bill to the favorable attention of their members in Congress. It will mean much for our cause in every State to have at the National Capital a reasonably strong and fair law on the subject of child labor. Members and friends of local child labor committees, of educational, charitable, and philanthropic societies, of women's clubs, and all other organizations interested in this movement, are earnestly requested to write at once to their respective senators and members of Congress, sending them, if possible, the enclosed copy of the bill to be presented, and urging the passage of this bill."

There is, of course, also a kind of child labor at home for which school superintendents, teachers or parents are alone responsible. When the child is given too many lessons to study at home so that it must rise very early or can only retire at a late hour, the result on its nervous and general system is the same as child labor performed in a factory or shop. Like the overworked college student above referred to, those children do not sleep enough. They are habitually in want of sleep. Children up in the age of 16 should have nine hours sleep in summer and nine to ten in winter. This certainly offers a field for reform in arranging the curricula of our public schools.

One of the saddest forms of child labor is the one imposed upon the child of thoughtless parents who, in addition to the school lessons at home, expect their children to devote nearly all their time, which should be spent in play or recreation, to helping in the household.

---

[*] This appeal was accompanied by a copy of a most excellent bill proposed to regulate the employment of child labor in the District of Columbia.

I have seen so-called "little mothers" in our New York tenement homes who were veritable heroines and who sacrificed their little lives on the altar of devotion to their little brothers and sisters and in obedience to their thoughtless and often cruel parents. I have seen a widow leaving a 10-year-old daughter to take care of three smaller children, one a babe, and expecting her to do the cooking besides. Is it a wonder that such a child cannot resist the invasion of the tubercle bacilli so prevalent in the crowded tenement districts of our large cities?

To treat the children of the poor when they are afflicted with tuberculous and scrofulous diseases, the seaside sanatorium, as has been said, is the ideal place, but inland-sanatoria will also answer the purpose if the coast is at too great a distance. It goes without saying, a school should be attached to every sanatorium for children so that the intellectual training keeps pace with the physical improvement of the sanatorium inmate. The results obtained in these children's sanatoria are surprisingly good; they vary from 50 to 75 per cent of cures.

The great social and economic advantage resulting to a community which takes care of the tuberculous and scrofulous children of the poor must be obvious. Such a sanatorium not only spares the community the expense of taking care of more consumptive adults, because of the cures accomplished among the children, but it lessens the number of crippled, deformed, and helpless individuals. Every case of Pott's disease cured, means a hunchback less in the world; every case of tuberculous hip or knee joint cured means a well person and a bread-winner, instead of a cripple who is likely to become a pauper.

The dangers of contracting tuberculosis during the age of adolescence in college or high school are about the same as those during the school age. I have already referred to the detrimental effects of overtaxing and overstraining the mind and nervous system of young girls. The young man choosing a college career should bear in mind that while a reasonable amount of athletics are conducive to health, physical overtaxing is a strong predisposing factor to tuberculosis, and, strange as it may seem, when the overtrained athlete contracts tuberculosis, the disease more frequently takes an unfavorable turn than in other instances. I have examined a number of men, recently from college, who had distinguished themselves as athletes, and as a rule I had the painful experience of finding them in worse condition to battle with the disease than individuals who had never practiced athletics. The remedy for all this lies, of course, with the college authorities, who should regulate the sports so that they may become a benefit and not a detriment to the students.

The young man or woman who is obliged to go to work in a shop, factory, office, or store, in order to make a living, has the same risk of contracting tuberculosis as the adult. However, even the close contact with a tuberculous individual is not dangerous if the latter is trained to take care of his tuberculous sputum and is careful to hold his hand or handkerchief before his mouth when coughing, even when he does not expectorate, so as to prevent the droplets or the possibly infectious spray from doing any harm. Right here, I wish to state distinctly that the conscientious consumptive is as safe an individual to associate with as any healthy person. To treat the conscientious consumptive as an outcast is a cruelty and most inhumane, and phthisiophobia, that is to say, the exaggerated fear of the presence of the consumptive is a condition which all social workers and physicians must combat. Let us teach the masses and the individual consumptive the effective and yet so simple means of preventing the dissemination of consumption through carelessness. Teach them never to expectorate except into a proper receptacle, never to cough unless it is really necessary, and then always to hold a handkerchief or the hand before the mouth. Let our sanitary authorities, our railway and street car companies see to it that in every public place where people congregate a sufficient number of well-kept spittoons are provided. Let them furthermore change the working of the formula "Don't spit," which, as we know only too well, is frequently disobeyed, to the formula "Spit here."

Our factories, workshops, the notorious sweatshops, our offices and department stores, and smaller ones also, our railroad stations and trains should receive the visits of sanitary inspectors so that it may be assured that the men and women employed or congregating in them are reasonably protected from the diseases arising through bad ventilation and other unsanitary conditions.

To improve the hygiene in the homes of the poor and prevent as far as possible the propagation of tuberculosis through dust, I beg leave to reproduce here some rules which, upon the suggestion of our distinguished co-worker, Professor T. Mitchel Prudden, were issued by our New York Committee on the Prevention of Tuberculosis.

SWEEPING AND DUSTING.

"When you sweep a room raise as little dust as possible, because this dust when breathed irritates the nose and throat and may set up catarrh. Some of the dust breathed in dusty air reaches the lungs, making parts of them black and hard and useless."

"If the dust in the air you breathe contains germs of consumption—tubercle bacilli—which have come from consumptives spitting on the floors, you run the risk of getting consumption yourself. If consumptives use proper spit cups and are careful in coughing or sneezing to hold the hand or handkerchief over the nose and mouth so as not to scatter spittle about in the air, the risk of getting the disease by living in the same room is mostly removed."

"To prevent making a great dust in sweeping, use moist sawdust on bare floors. When the room is carpeted, moisten a newspaper and tear it into small scraps and scatter these over the carpet when you begin sweeping. As you sweep brush the paper along by the broom and they will catch most of the dust and hold it fast, just as the sawdust does on bare floors. Do not have either the paper or the sawdust dripping wet, only moist."

"In dusting a room, do not use a feather duster, because

this does not remove the dust from the room, but only brushes it into the air so that you breathe it in; or it settles down and then you have to do the work over again."

"Use soft, dry cloths to dust with and shake them frequently out of the window; or use slightly moistened cloths and rinse them out in water when you have finished. In this way you get the dust out of the room."

"In cleaning rooms you should remember that dust settles upon the floors as well as on the furniture, and is stirred into the air we breathe by walking over them. You can easily remove all this dust in rooms which have bare floors, in houses, stores, shops, schoolrooms, etc., after the dust has settled, by passing over the floor a mop which has been wrung out so as to be only moist, but not dripping wet."

One of the strong predisposing factors to an acquired tuberculosis in adult life is always the fearful scourge, alcoholism. How to combat this is in itself a problem. I confess, that to my mind the only rational way is to follow the example of Norway and some of the cantons of Switzerland, by making the manufacture and the sale of alcohol a government affair. Experience in those countries has shown that through such means alone have they been able to reduce alcoholism and its consequent evils—disease, crime, poverty, misery, and want.

Educational propaganda regarding alcoholism will also be helpful. Concerning tuberculosis it should be impressed upon the masses that alcohol, in whatever form it may have been administered, has never been either a prevention nor a cure for consumption. Since we have not yet any laws prohibiting the sale of patent preparations and proprietary medicines, containing a large percentage of alcohol and other deleterious substances under the guise of medicine, we must educate the people to the true state of affairs.

Such work as Mr. Bock's, Professor Osborne's, Mr. Adam's, Dr. Grinnell's, Mrs. Allen's, etc., should be printed and reprinted and receive the largest possible circulation among all intellectual classes, our statesmen and our ecclesiastics. These latter will perhaps then refrain from endorsing patent medicines, of the composition and effect of which they have not the slightest idea. There happened recently an incident which came to my notice and which is well worth telling. I will reproduce the story here textually, as it appeared in the *Journal of the American Medical Association* of August 5, 1905, under the title "A Family Tragedy."

"The following is a true tale of a receat happening in an American city. It is a good story to relate to patients and legislators in the campaign against nostrums and against adulterated foods and drugs. A respected clergyman fell ill and the family physician was called. After examining the patient carefully, the doctor asked for a private interview with the patient's adult son.

"'Harry,' said the doctor, 'do you know what is the matter with your father?'

"'No. We sent for you to tell us that.'

"'Well,' the physician said, 'I am sorry to tell you that your father undoubtedly is suffering from chronic alcoholism.'

"'Chronic alcoholism; why, that's ridiculous; father never

drank a drop of liquor in his life, and we know all there is to know about his habits.'

"'Well, my boy, it's chronic alcoholism nevertheless, and at this moment your father is drunk. How has his health been recently? Has he been taking any medicine?'

"'Why, for some time, six months I should say, father has often complained of feeling unusually tired. A few months ago a friend of his recommended "Peruna" to him, assuring him that it would build him up. Since then he has taken many bottles of it, and I am quite sure that he has taken nothing else.'"

In this connection it might be added that a very prominent anti-saloon worker, a clergyman, lately said that in shame he was compelled to admit that he had run across indubitable proof that there are ministers of the gospel who receive pecuniary commissions from the makers of alcoholic nostrums whose wares they recommend; than this there can be no worse form of graft. The time is here for the organized profession to join hands with all other workers and organizations, whether anti-saloon leagues, temperance unions, or courageous anti-nostrum publications, to set a definite limit to the progress of "respectable and innocent" intemperance.

For the benefit of the statesman, legislator, and the clergyman who recommend the public press which lends its columns to advertise, and the people who consume patent medicines, I would like to make a few more quotations from important authorities on the subject:

Mr. Adams, in his second article on "The Great American Fraud" in *Collier's Weekly* of October 28, 1905, entitled "Peruna and the Bracers," has this to say on the manufacture of Peruna:

"Any one wishing to make Peruna for home consumption may do so by mixing half a pint of cologne spirits, 90 proof, with a pint and a half of water, adding thereto a little cubebs for flavor and a little burned sugar for color. It will cost, in small quantities, perhaps seven or eight cents per quart. Manufactured in bulk, so a former Peruna agent estimates, its cost, including bottle and wrapper, is about eight and one-half cents. Its price is $1.00. Because of this handsome margin of profit, and by way of making hay in the stolen sunshine of Peruna advertising, many imitations have sprung up to harass the proprietors of the alcohol-and-water product. Pe-ru-vi-na, P-ru-na, Purina, Anurep (an obvious inversion); these, bottled and labeled to resemble Peruna, are self-confessed imitations. From what the Peruna people tell me, I gather that they are dangerous and damnable frauds, and that they cure nothing.

"What does Peruna cure? Catarrh. That is the modest claim for it; nothing but catarrh. To be sure, a careful study of its literature will suggest its value as a tonic, and a preventive of lassitude. But its reputation rests upon catarrh. What is catarrh? Whatever ails you. No matter what you've got, you will be not only enabled, but compelled, after reading Dr. Hartman's Peruna book, "The Ills of Life," to diagnose your illness as catarrh, and to realize that Peruna alone will save you. Pneumonia is catarrh of the lungs; so is consumption. Dyspepsia is catarrh of the stomach. Enteritis is catarrh of the intestines. Appendicitis—surgeons, please note before operating—is catarrh of the appendix. Bright's disease is catarrh of the kidneys. Heart disease is catarrh of the heart. Canker sores are catarrh of the mouth. Measles is, perhaps, catarrh of the skin, since "a teaspoonful of Peruna thrice daily or oftener is an effectual cure."

Professor A. Jacobi of New York City, my venerable friend and the teacher of thousands of American physicians for the past fifty years, has come to the conclusion, from a careful estimate, that the American people spend an average of $200,-000,000 a year for patent medicines.

Professor Oliver T. Osborne of Yale, in his address on "The Scourge of Nostrums," etc.,[1] expresses himself regarding the public press and patent medicines as follows: "Were it not for the daily papers and periodicals this enormous sale of patent medicines could not take place. This autosuggestion of disease and disease symptoms and then the positive promise of cure causes frail human nature to give the stuff a trial, and, as is expected, the narcotic and the alcohol give a taste for more."

According to a statement published in connection with Mr. Adams' article, Dr. Ashbel P. Grinnell of New York City, who has made a statistical study of patent medicines, asserts as a provable fact that " more alcohol is consumed in this country in patent medicines than is dispensed in a legal way by licensed liquor venders, barring the sale of ale and beer."

Next to alcoholism, unsanitary tenements and lack of air and light are the strongest predisposing factors to tuberculosis. The building of model tenement houses where the honest laborer may have a cheerful home at a reasonable rate, the creating of tenement house commissions in large and smaller cities to compel greedy contractors to remodel unsanitary tenement houses and build only sanitary ones, is one way of combating this evil. Not enough praise can be bestowed upon men like Mr. Phipps and others who devote their wealth to the building of sanitary homes for laborers. These are certainly more needed than monuments, libraries, general hospitals, and even churches. To me, the man who builds such homes, which render thousands of American laborers and their families happy, serves his creator better than the builder of cathedrals and churches, for the former serves God by serving his fellowmen, and if we are to believe the beautiful story told us of Abu ben Adhem —

> Midst those whom love of God has blessed
> The lover of his kind leads all the rest.

I have always maintained that if we can give the honest laborer a cheerful home and a wife who knows how to cook a good, plain, but appetizing meal, the saloon with its bright lights will have less attraction to him and alcoholism will be indirectly combated. When duty calls me into the houses of the poor, and I see the dingy, untidy rooms of the laborers and the woman unskilled in the plainest household duties, get-

ting the meals from the nearest delicatessen store instead of preparing them herself, I do not blame the laborer when, instead of returning directly home from his occupation, he enters the saloon to take a drink, thinking it will cheer him up. The laborer's wife who, after leaving school, had to enter the workshop or store, and thus never had a chance to learn to cook or learn the first principles of housekeeping, is not to blame for her ignorance, but society is, and we should seek to remedy such conditions by not allowing our girls to leave the public school without having learned to be housekeepers and cooks.

It would furthermore pay economically and socially if our philanthropists and communities would establish places of amusement where a man might go with his family to spend his leisure time, partake of non-alcoholic drinks and enjoy good music, or other healthful amusement. All this will help to strengthen family ties, prevent alcoholism, and indirectly prevent tuberculosis and other diseases.

In most of our cities we need more parks, large and small, more playgrounds, more recreation piers and public roof gardens. These places represent the lungs of a great city; without them a city cannot be in a healthy condition. Sanitary houses, public baths and healthful places for amusement are, however, not only necessary for our city population, but are equally important for people living in the country. Home sanitation, love for fresh air, general and personal hygiene, must be taught to the country people as well. They have the good air of the country, but how often do they shut themselves up in badly ventilated rooms, being more afraid of fresh air than even city people, fearing the little draught—the only way of purifying foul air—as if it was disease producing. The lack of healthful amusement in the country is the cause of so many young people migrating to the cities. Here is a new field of philanthropy. The man who, by creating a system of healthful amusements for country people, can stop the ever-increasing migration to the cities, or perhaps even induce laboring families to migrate from our crowded cities to the country, will bestow a lasting benefit on present and future generations.

If we wish to diminish tuberculosis among the masses, we must pay our laborers in city and country reasonable wages so that they can live decently, eat sufficient good and nourishing food, and provide food and shelter for themselves and families for a time when work is lacking. Labor bureaus should be established everywhere by states, cities, and smaller communities. There should be constant interchange between all of them so as to regulate the demand and supply as far as practicable. Then, the abnormality that one section of the country suffers from the want of laborers while another has an army of "the unemployed" will be a thing of the past. Some man or woman having been cured of pulmonary tuberculosis may find outdoor employment through such an exchange which will ensure his or her recovery and guard against a relapse which so often follows from a return to unsanitary environments. Our federal government could materially help these labor ex-

---

[1] "The Scourge of Nostrums and Irregular Practitioners." Journal of the American Medical Association, July 2, 1904.

changes in their grand work·by arranging for cheap transportation whenever it seems expedient to do so.

In relation to employment, travel and transportation, there comes to my mind another means of contagion which I consider dangerous, and that is dust. We are in the habit of calling tuberculosis a house disease, and well it deserves this name, but it might also be called a dust disease, and we shall not be able to eradicate tuberculosis if we do not find means to lessen the amount of dust we breathe. Even so-called noninfectious dust is apt to irritate the pulmonary surfaces and thus make the respiratory system more receptive to the invasion of the bacillus. The dust uselessly raised in our factories and workshops could be materially lessened by automatic dust-collectors. The cleaning of such establishments, and also department stores, churches, theaters, concert halls, offices, schools, railway stations and railroad and street cars, should not be done in the old-fashioned way, with a broom, but by the modern electric exhaustion process now in use in some establishments, which is certainly far superior and thoroughly hygienic. The same process of cleaning should be employed for carpets in preference to beating them in the back yards, in closely settled communities. Sweeping a street in its dry state should be considered a municipal crime, and the same holds good of the collecting of ashes in uncovered carts.

What to do to prevent the dust raised by speeding electric street cars and automobiles is indeed a difficult problem. Our fellow-citizens on the Pacific coast have used an oily substance to allay the dust. I submit this problem to the street-cleaning commissioners and city engineers of our great Eastern cities in the hope that their ingenuity may find a solution.

The dust in a railway car should be greatly minimized by proper ventilation and the more simple construction and equipment of sleepers and passenger coaches. But in addition to this a regulation should be enforced which will make it punishable by dismissal for any colored porter to brush a passenger about to leave the car, in the presence of the others. To my mind, it is an unpardonable offense on the part of any company not to prevent this practice on the part of their employees, who, as we all know, resort to it in order to solicit a gratuity. I have been told that the wages of colored porters on Pullman and parlor cars are so small that they must rely on an additional source of income from "tips." I do not know whether this is so or not, or whether the companies, the porters or the passengers are to blame, but tipping the colored porter has become habit with the American public and would probably be difficult to stop. However, I think a rule that brushing garments should only be allowed in the vestibule of the cars, should be enforced.

Dust collectors should be an obligatory equipment in the workshops of our prisons. In a recent investigation of some of our penal institutions I found a deplorable state of affairs in regard to this, besides the many other unhygienic conditions tending to propagate tuberculosis, which I had occasion to observe.[a]

[a] "The Tuberculosis Situation in Penal Institutions," Medical Record, May 13, 1905.

No matter how serious a crime the individual may have committed, society has no right to add to years of imprisonment additional punishment by giving the individual tuberculosis through unhygienic prisons and workshops.

In speaking of the social aspect of tuberculosis, we cannot overlook the tuberculosis situation in prisons and reformatories. Isolation and treatment of tuberculous prisoners in special wards or agricultural colonies are some of the means which must be resorted to to diminish consumption among this class of people. Some prisoners return to their families. This cannot be desirable if they have become tuberculous during prison life. They should have been treated and cured of their disease before discharge. The practice of discharging prisoners in the last stage of tuberculosis, often virtually dying, without previous investigation to see that the freed individual will find a home where he will not constitute a source of infection and receive proper medical care, is thoroughly reprehensible.

What is the social duty, the duty of a community, in regard to an average individual afflicted with tuberculosis? The rich consumptive will be able to take care of himself; he can be cured at home, in health resorts, or private sanatoria; but for the comparatively poor, or middle classes, there should be institutions where, for a moderate price, equally good chances for cure can be offered. No community has a right to pauperize its citizens; many are willing to pay, and he who can pay but will not should be made to pay. We have in this country a number of high-priced institutions, and a number of purely charitable institutions, while for the middle classes and for the more advanced cases of consumption we have virtually nothing. There should be a sufficient number of city and county sanatoria to take in the moderately and absolutely poor consumptives in all stages of the disease. That it is cheaper to take care of a consumptive at the right time and in the right place until he is well, instead of taking care of him at the wrong time (in the advanced stage) and at the wrong place (general hospital) until he is dead, has been often enough demonstrated to not need any further proof.[b]

But how are we to discover a patient at the right time? By educating the public in the early signs of tuberculosis, by establishing special tuberculosis dispensaries, by having periodical examinations of the chests of all public employes, pupils of public and private schools, colleges, etc., by urging the well-to-do to employ a family physician, not only to take care of them when they are ill, but to watch over them while well and examine every member of the family from time to time so as to discover an early tuberculosis if such is developing. The special tuberculosis dispensary will serve the poor for the purpose of seeking early advice, although I hope that at not too distant a time communities will realize that it will pay them to pay physicians, each one to be assigned to a number of poor families as a healer and a teacher—that is to say, to cure and to prevent disease.

[b] John H. Pryor, M. D., "What Shall the State Do for the Consumptive?" Medical News, October, 1900.

Will it pay a community to treat its consumptive poor at the right time and in the right place? Most assuredly and by doing so the State and municipality will be the moral and financial gainers in the end. We will take the State of New York, which is the State having the largest population, for example. It is estimated that there are in this State about 50,000 tuberculous invalids. Of these probably one-fifth belong to that class of patients which sooner or later become a burden to the community. These 10,000 consumptives, absolutely poor, will sooner or later have to be taken care of by the public general hospitals. While they may not stay in one hospital twelve months continuously, they will certainly occupy a bed in one of the public institutions for that length of time before they die. According to a recent report of the public charity hospitals of New York City the average cost per patient per day in the general hospitals was $1.16. Thus the cost to the Commonwealth will be $4,234,000 per year for caring for the 10,000 consumptives.

What would be the expense if they were taken care of in a sanatorium? Experience in this country has demonstrated that the maintenance of incipient cases in well-conducted sanatoria can well be carried out for $1.00 per day. If these 10,000 would be sent to a sanatorium in time, at least 6,000 of them could be lastingly cured after a maximum sojourn of 250 days, at an average expense of $250 per capita. Thus for $1,500,000 6,000 would be made again breadwinners and useful citizens. If the remaining 4,000 invalids were kept in the sanatorium one year before they died, it would cost $1,460,000. Thus taking away from the tenement districts 10,000 consumptives, curing more than half of them and caring for the other half, and destroying 10,000 foci of infection will cost $2,960,000. Not taking care of them in the earlier stages of this disease they will probably all die, since this 10,000 represents the absolutely poor who now live under most unhygienic conditions; they will have infected a perhaps equally large or larger number of individuals living with them but before dying they will have cost the community $4,234,000.

If we could imitate the German State Invalidity Insurance Companies, I think we would make a good step forward toward the betterment of the lot of our working population and make a wonderful stride toward the solution of the tuberculosis problem. Every laborer and employe in the German empire, earning less than 800 marks, must be insured against accident, old age, and disease, including tuberculosis. The German insurance companies, under state supervision, soon realized that the earlier they took care of the policyholders who happened to become tuberculous, the greater was the chance of their cure and the smaller the expense to the company. They urge their policyholders, at the slightest indication of pulmonary trouble, to go to the physician paid by the company, for examination, and tuberculosis is thus discovered very often in the most incipient and consequently the most curable stage. The patient is then sent to a sanatorium, very often built and maintained by the insurance company, near large centers of population and independent of climatic conditions. Nevertheless, the absolute and lasting

cures often amount to 75 and 85 per cent. In the meantime, the family of the consumptive laborer is looked after, so that it may not be in want.

What is the social aspect, the social advantage of such an institution, which the Germans very justly call a " Volksheil-anstalt "—a people's healing institution, or sanatorium? Time does not permit me to dwell at length on all that is accomplished by the sanatorium in regard to the social aspect of the disease under consideration. I had the honor, a few months ago, to address the Tuberculosis Congress in Paris on the subject of the Sanatorium for Tuberculous Patients and Its Medical and Social Mission. Let me recapitulate rapidly the essential points of the latter, that is to say, the social mission, which I enumerated in that address.

By the admission of a patient to a sanatorium a frequently dangerous center of infection is made inoffensive and the patient is given the greatest possible chance of cure. If he is in the advanced stage he is made as comfortable as lies in the power of human skill with all the modern therapeutic means at command. The statistics of sanatoria show that the careful and trained consumptive is no danger to his immediate surroundings, and the sanatorium no danger to the neighborhood. The contraction of tuberculosis by physicians, nurses and employes in sanatoria is of the rarest occurrence. The tuberculosis mortality in villages surrounding well-conducted sanatoria decreases because of the imitation by the inhabitants of the example in cleanly habits set before them by the inmates of the sanatorium.[10] The sanatorium cures the consumptive whenever he is curable, and thus demonstrates the curability of the disease independent of climatic conditions. This is important when we consider that the majority of patients must be treated and cured in the same, or nearly the same, climate where they will have to live and labor after their restoration to health. This cure is not established by quacks, patent medicines, faith cure, or other mysterious means, but simply by the judicious use of God's fresh air, sunshine, good food, pure water, and sometimes a little medicine, and all under the careful guidance of a competent physician. The sanatorium makes the patient a hygienic factor when he returns to his former environments and thus demonstrates the preventability of tuberculous diseases. The patient has been taught the love of fresh air by day and by night, taught to shun vitiated atmosphere and the air of the saloon and of crowded meeting places. He has learned the value of simple, pure and good food, and how much more advantageous it is for him and his family to spend his money for food instead of for intoxicating liquors.

In the private as well as in the people's sanatorium there is much opportunity for cultivating compassion, benevolence and true democracy. It was my good fortune, ten years ago, when serving as assistant to my immortal teacher, Professor Dettweiler, at Falkenstein, to see the birth of the first sanatorium for the consumptive poor. The wealthy and aristocratic pa-

---

[10] This is shown by statistics of Goerbersdorf and Falkenstein in Germany, and Rutland, Mass., in this country.

tients at Falkenstein, being so much benefited by their sojourn there, manifested a deep feeling for the sufferings of the consumptive poor, deprived of the care and comfort of institutional treatment. They collected a large fund, which became the nucleus of the largest people's institution in Germany, now located at Ruppertshain.

Many of these people's sanatoria give their patients educational advantages through lectures and regular classes of instruction. Some of our American sanatoria, I am happy to say, have imitated this good practice.[11] The young medical man, entering the sanatorium as assistant, is given an opportunity to become a trained diagnostician of incipient tuberculosis. The addition of such a doctor to a community means a great step toward the solution of the tuberculosis problem.

[11] In the Muskoka Sanatorium, a Canadian institution, Dr. Elliott takes his patients on botanizing tours and geological excursions. A botany club has recently been formed at the Adirondack Cottage Sanatorium with a view to entertaining and instructing the tuberculous invalids of that institution.

Do not consider me too sanguine if I say the sanatorium teaches true democracy, compassion and benevolence to the aristocratic, the rich and the indifferent. It teaches the intemperate to become temperate, the disorderly to become orderly. It offers opportunity for education to the uneducated, and by teaching its inmates personal and general cleanliness and hygiene and love for fresh air, it not only indirectly prevents tuberculosis but also many other diseases whose origin must be traced to lack of fresh air, to filth, bad food, unsanitary habitation, and bad habits.

Let me conclude this altogether too lengthy paper by saying that to my mind the solution of the tuberculosis problem means the solution of the social problem. Whatever prevents the development of tuberculosis will prevent social misery; whatever cures it will help to cure the social ills. Inasmuch as we diminish tuberculosis among the masses we will diminish suffering, misery, and social discontent, and when the problem of tuberculosis will have been solved, we will be nearer the millennium than we have ever been before.

ON THE INFLUENCE OF AGGRESSINES UPON THE OCCURRENCE OF GENERAL INFECTION FOLLOWING THE INTRODUCTION OF PATHOGENIC BACTERIA INTO THE UNINJURED GENITAL TRACT OF ANIMALS

By Caroline B. Towles, M. D.

(From the Bacteriological Laboratory of the Medical Clinic of Prof. Von Jaksch, Prag.)

The following series of experiments was undertaken to determine whether a general or a local reaction could be produced by the introduction of pathogenic micro-organisms into the upper part of the vagina or uterus of animals, no lesion of the epithelial wall having been produced. While examination of the normal vaginal flora has given diverse results, there has been usually the same outcome from the introduction of bacteria into the vaginæ both of human beings and animals. A few experiments of this character are quoted showing this negative result.

Doederlein[1] introduced staphylococci into the vagina of a girl and in a few days was unable to demonstrate them.

Bumm[2] did the same experiment with the same result in two women.

Menge[3] introduced B. pyocyaneus twenty-three times, staphylococcus thirty times, streptococcus twenty-seven times into the vagina of women and found that it rapidly cleared itself of the organisms.

Krönig[4] used B. pyocyaneus with the same result.

Stroganoff[5] introduced staphylococcus seventeen times, and streptococcus four times into the vagina of rabbits and found that the organisms had disappeared when he examined the vaginal secretion a few days later.

Cahanescu[6] introduced streptococcus and staphylococcus into the vagina of dogs, rabbits, hares and guinea-pigs without general or local reaction and found that the cocci disappeared in a short time.

Caselli[7] introduced tampons saturated with a culture of streptococcus into the vagina of three rabbits by means of a glass sound avoiding injury to the wall. The animals remained well, except that one had a streptococcus infection following the birth of her young a month later.

Heinricius[8] infected a number of rabbits by introducing streptococcus cultures into the uterus by means of a catheter. Most of these animals died after a considerable time, but with no demonstrable infection. Some died in a very short time, but as laparotomy was done in each case in order to guide the catheter, and as in many rabbits the vaginal opening is extremely minute their vitality must have been lowered considerably and there was also a chance of local injury in spite of the greatest care.

The organisms used in these experiments were either laboratory cultures or obtained from abscesses, and in almost all cases cultured at least once, and accordingly must have been of a light degree of virulence—as Professor Bumm[9] says:

Wir erkennen die verschiedenen Grade der Virulenz der Streptokokken aus der Verschiedenheit ihrer Wirkung beim Thier-Experiment; wir sehen die Virulenz bei der künstlichen Züchtung der Streptokokken im Kulturglas gewöhnlich rasch abnehmen, können sie im Kulturglas aber nicht künstlich vermehren, und wissen nicht warum und wodurch die Keime bei ihrem Wachsthum im Thierkörper eine höhere Virulenz gewinnen.

Professor Bail[16] has classified micro-organisms in regard to their virulence as follows:

CLASS A. *True Parasites.*—Included under this head are such organisms as produce illness or death of an animal if one or at least very few of the group be present in its tissues. Examples of this are: anthrax for rabbits, chicken cholera for chickens, and possibly plague for human beings.

CLASS B. *One-half Parasites.*—Included under this head are most of the bacteria pathogenic for man—typhoid, cholera, streptococcus. It is conceivable that members of this class may under favorable conditions attain sufficient pathogenic power to be included under class A.

CLASS C. *Saprophytes.*—Includes such micro-organisms as are never pathogenic to man in the ordinary sense of the term. It must, however, be remembered that an organism generally harmless may under certain conditions become pathogenic. For example, *B. subtilis* is a saprophyte for the body generally, but becomes pathogenic when introduced into the eye; since the adjustment of this organ is so delicate that the ordinary mild inflammatory reaction produced is sufficient to cause its impairment (Ullrich.)

Since cultures in nutrient media soon fall from class B to class C, or at least nearer to it, it was decided in these experiments to use only such organisms as had been brought as near as possible to the degree of virulence included under class A.

The striking results obtained by Prof. Bail and his pupils with aggressines led to its being employed in the hope that here, too, it would supplement the power of otherwise ineffective organisms. Prof. Bail's work with cholera and typhoid showed that the body fluids, œdema, ascites, or pleural exudate, produced by the infection of a sensitive animal, contained a property antagonistic to the protective power of the animal body against the organism employed. The idea that this might be the case was suggested some time ago by Prof. Kruse,[17] and the active principle was called by him lysine. It was, however, first elaborated in a series of experiments by Prof. Bail.

Working with cholera and typhoid organisms the latter found that the exudate, produced by the infection of an animal, after being sterilized, was capable of producing severe lesions or death, when used in association with a number of micro-organisms which, when injected alone, produced only a mild reaction in animals of the same weight. This effect was apparently due to the very rapid multiplication of the bacteria injected. The sterile fluid seeming to possess some property which enabled it to neutralize the opposition of the animal body and to produce conditions favorable for the growth and reproduction of the bacteria. A name for this property was necessary, and, in the place of the term

lysine which had come to have another significance, Prof. Bail called it aggressine at the suggestion of Prof. Kruse.

It is necessary to differentiate between aggressivity and virulence. The latter term always means the pathogenic power of an organism, while aggressivity refers only to its power of multiplication.

Of course in most instances if a micro-organism can multiply unchecked in the animal body it has pathogenic properties. That this is not always the case, however, is shown by the action of trypanosoma in rats, the organism reproducing enormously without detriment to the host. On the other hand the pathogenic power may depend but little upon the number of bacteria present, as in the case of diphtheria.

The term aggressivity, then, does not necessarily include pathogenic power, but only in those cases in which that power is intimately connected with the number of organisms present. (For further details see article of Kikuchi.[18])

The method employed in my experiments consisted in bringing the micro-organisms used as near to class A as possible, and then introducing them into the vagina of animals without producing any lesion of the epithelium. Pairs of animals of equal weight were treated in this way, one being injected subcutaneously with aggressine and the other with a neutral fluid, such as normal serum of the same species or aseptic exudate produced by aleuronal (Buchner). Streptococcus was taken first and large quantities of an ordinary laboratory culture were injected into a rabbit. This animal died the next day, and after the exudate was shown to contain streptococcus in pure culture it was injected into a second rabbit. This process was repeated a number of times until only a few loopfuls of the exudate were necessary to produce a lethal effect. A large rabbit then received an intrapleural injection of this exudate and died in about nine hours; after which the pleural exudate was drawn off without any attempt to keep separate that obtained from the two sides. This exudate was shown to contain streptococcus in pure culture.

The aggressine of streptococcus had not been prepared before, Dr. Weil[19] being then at work upon his article which is now in press. It was prepared in the same way as by Bail with anthrax, cholera, typhoid and tubercle, by Hoke,[20] with staphylococcus and diplococcus, by Weil with hen cholera, Kikuchi with dysentery and by Salus[21] with colon. The turbid blood-tinged pleural exudate was drawn off into a sterile pipette into test tubes and centrifugalized for several hours. The supernatant fluid was then poured off and rendered sterile with toluol, which was afterward removed by evaporation. One cubic centimeter of this fluid was put in serum bouillon and kept in the thermostat for forty-eight hours. If no growth resulted, the aggressine was considered sterile and ready for use; if not, toluol was added again and the process repeated from that point. The fluid which was used in the control animal was subjected to the same process in order that exactly similar conditions might be present.

The organisms for vaginal infection were all obtained in the same way. The day before the experiment was to be made an animal received an intra-pleural or abdominal injection of the sediment obtained after centrifugalizing the exudate for the aggressine, and the fluid so obtained was used fresh from the body of the animal.

Rabbits were tried first, but much difficulty was encountered on account of their anatomical structure; there being a common outlet for the bladder and sexual organs so that the vagina does not possess a separate lumen until the upper part of the symphysis is reached. Guinea-pigs were therefore substituted as better adapted to my purposes since they have a separate outlet for bladder, sexual organs and rectum.

EXPERIMENT FIRST.

October 6. A full grown guinea-pig weighing 620 grms. received 3 cc. of aggressine fluid in its abdominal cavity and a piece of cotton saturated with fresh exudate containing a pure culture of streptococcus was introduced into the vagina. This was effected by laying the cotton upon the vulva and gently pushing it in as far as possible with a glass sound. October 7 the weight was 510 grms., the temperature 104.2° F., and the animal seemed very sick. It died in the night between 3 and 7 a. m. of October 8.

On section the guinea-pig presented a normal appearance; there was no peritonitis, no enlargement of the spleen nor injection of the uterus or vagina. The pledgets of cotton were not found in the vagina. Cultures from the uterus and heart's blood in bouillon gave a growth of streptococcus.

October 6. The control guinea-pig weighed 580 grms; it received 3 cc. of rabbit's serum, treated in the same way as the aggressine, and the same amount of cotton in the vagina saturated with the same exudate used for the first animal. October 7 the weight was 600 grms., the temperature 102° F. and the animal appeared ill. The temperature varied, but became steady on the fourth day at 97.2°. Since that time the guinea-pig has been well and of its usual weight.

EXPERIMENT SECOND.

October 15. By means of a hypodermic syringe without its canula, an Angora guinea-pig weighing 750 grms. received ½ cc. of fresh exudate containing a pure culture of streptococcus in the vagina, and a pledget of cotton saturated in the same fluid was introduced as before. 4 cc. of aggressine fluid were injected subcutaneously as before. October 16 it weighed 720 grms., had a temperature of 102.6°, and died late the next afternoon.

On section, which was done immediately after death, a well-marked subcutaneous oedema was found. The abdominal cavity was normal, showing no peritonitis nor fluid. Spleen was not enlarged. Uterus was pregnant in both horns, the embryos being about 1 cm. long. The foetal membranes were transparent and the amniotic fluid clear. The membranes were opened between two pairs of forceps and a loopful of the fluid placed in serum bouillon. Next morning there was a profuse growth of streptococcus in pure culture. Smears taken from the maternal side of the placenta and the maternal

heart's blood showed streptococcus in pure culture. A specimen from one horn of the uterus above the embryonic distension showed masses of cocci in the muscularis and a few cocci in the endometrium, but there was no infiltration with small cells.

October 15. Control guinea-pig weighed 850 grms. It received the same treatment as the above, except that instead of the aggressine fluid 4 cc. of aseptic exudate, produced by the injection of aleuronal, which had been treated in the same way as the aggressine fluid, were injected subcutaneously. Just as this was completed the guinea-pig met with an accident, having a fall of about five feet and striking violently against a stone jar. It was badly stunned but partially recovered. On October 16 it had chills and at a temperature of 101.2°, weighed 790 grms. On the evening of the 16th a marked increase in the size of the abdomen was noted. On the 17th it was very sick in the morning, was dying at noon, so it was killed at 12.30 p. m.

On section there was marked oedema of the subcutaneous tissues. Abdomen was free from fluid and of normal appearance. The uterus showed one horn very large, containing three dead half-grown embryos. The membranes were close around each foetus and no amniotic fluid was present. Free in the uterine cavity outside the embryonic sacs was a large amount of blood-stained fluid, which showed masses of cocci and a few leucocytes. The heart's blood, spleen and uterine epithelium all showed numbers of cocci.

A number of attempts were made to obtain a similar result in an animal that was pregnant and treated with exudate from aleuronal and cotton in the vagina. Animals were taken in all stages of pregnancy but in no other instance was any result obtained. The guinea-pig in each case simply appeared sick on the following day and then recovered completely. This being the case, the above mentioned result was considered as due to the accident.

October 16. A guinea-pig weighing 700 grms, received 4 cc. of aggressine fluid subcutaneously. October 17 it had a temperature of 100.8°, seemed a little sick, and lost a few grams in weight. On the 18th it was quite well and has remained so since.

In view of the likelihood of an adult animal being pregnant the other experiments were done on half-grown guinea-pigs.

THIRD EXPERIMENT.

October 18. A guinea-pig weighing 340 grms. received cotton in the vagina prepared as before and 3 cc. of aggressine fluid subcutaneously. It died on October 19 at 1 p. m. On section it appeared normal in all organs, but smears from the heart's blood, spleen, and tissue fluid showed large numbers of cocci.

The control guinea-pig which weighed 370 grms. received cotton in the vagina as above and 3 cc. of normal serum. It was killed at 4 p. m. on the afternoon of the 20th as it was dying. On section it appeared normal except that the uterus was enlarged and injected in both horns. On opening the horns the inner surface seemed to be covered with a necrotic mass and the cavity filled with a muco-purulent material. The smear showed cocci in this and also in the heart's blood.

FOURTH EXPERIMENT.

October 26. Young guinea-pig weighing 250 grms. received cotton in the vagina as usual and 3 cc. of aggressine subcutaneously. Died in the night of the 27th. Smear showed cocci in uterus and heart's blood.

The control guinea-pig which weighed 225 grms. received cotton as usual in vagina and 3 cc. of bouillon subcutaneously. It died in the early morning of the 29th. On section it showed the same picture as the other animal, all organs appearing normal. Smears showed cocci in the uterus, heart's blood, and spleen.

FIFTH EXPERIMENT:

November 13. A guinea-pig late in pregnancy weighing 990 grms. received cotton as before in the vagina and 3 cc. of aggressine fluid subcutaneously. It died at 10 a. m. on the 17th of November. No peritonitis. One horn contained three almost fully developed dead embryos. This horn was removed as a whole, being clamped at each end, burned in a flame and laid upon a sterile cloth. The uterus was laid open without injury to the embryonic sacs and found to contain necrotic material and a muco-purulent fluid. The amniotic fluid was turbid but not purulent. Serum bouillon cultures made from the amniotic fluid, the mother's heart's blood, and the placental tissue, showed a luxurious growth of streptococcus. But cultures taken from the umbilical vessels and fœtal heart's blood were sterile.

November 1. One of the guinea-pigs that had received infected cotton in the vagina and normal serum subcutaneously, as a repetition of the control which had been hurt on the 16th of October, was delivered of two young, both unusually large. The mother had been perfectly well for the ten days which had elapsed since the cotton was introduced. The two young seemed well and nursed several times. Both died in the night and on section showed in the smears taken from the tissue fluid, heart's blood, and spleen great numbers of streptococci in pure culture. The mother died on November 4. Both uterine horns were large and showed the placental sites; there was no necrotic material or exudate; the surface seemed healthy. No peritonitis; spleen not enlarged. A great increase in the pericardial fluid was found and adhesions between the auricles and the base of the pericardium. No pleural exudates. Smears showed a few cocci in uterus and heart's blood and many in the pericardial fluid.

Briefly, the results of the five experiments were as follows: *Three of the* experiments were done upon adult guinea-pigs, two pairs of which were pregnant. In the non-pregnant pair, the animal which received aggressine in addition to the infected cotton died in less than two days, showing a general streptococcus infection, while the other, after a slight reaction, remained alive and well. An old animal, which was treated with aggressine alone, has also remained alive and well.

In the two experiments upon pregnant guinea-pigs, the animal receiving the aggressine fluid in addition to the infected cotton died undelivered, showing a general infection with streptococcus; while those not receiving the aggressine remained alive and well until delivered, except in one case in which the guinea-pig sustained a severe injury. Several control experiments also gave negative results.

Two of the experiments were done on half-grown guinea-pigs. All four of these animals died, but those which had received the aggressine died twenty-four and thirty hours earlier than the control animals. From these results it seems permissible to conclude:

1st. That animals can, under special conditions, i. e., with a very virulent organism, in very young animals or after the addition of aggressine, receive general infection from streptococci introduced into the uninjured vagina and uterus.

2d. That in adult guinea-pigs, whether pregnant or not, a general infection cannot be produced by the mere presence of streptococcus, however virulent in the uninjured vagina or uterus; on the other hand, the subcutaneous injection of aggressine fluid, associated with the introduction of bacteria, promptly results in general infection and death, no matter whether the animal be pregnant or not.

3d. That a young guinea-pig may contract a general infection, and die from the mere presence of streptococcus in the vagina and uterus, but that death occurs much more rapidly if in addition aggressine fluid be injected subcutaneously.

It is a pleasure to take this opportunity to thank Prof. von Jaksch for the kindness that has made this work possible.

BIBLIOGRAPHY.

1. Doederlein: Das Sheidensekret u. s. Bedeutung f. d. puer. Fieber; Leipzig, 1892.

2. Bumm: Die Micro-Organismen der gonor. Schleimhaut-Erkrank., II. Aufl., Wiesbaden. (Quoted from Menge & Krönig.)

Menge: Bacteriologie d. weiblichen genital Kanales, Teil I, S. 68, 1897 Leip.

4. Krönig: The same, Teil II, S. 18-19.

5. Stroganoff: Monatsschr. Geb. u. Gyn., 1895, Bd. II, Heft 5 and 6.

6. Cahanescu: Annales de L'Institut Pasteur 1901, S. 842.

7. Caselli: Centralblatt f. Bacteriol., 1899, XXV, S. 5.

8. Heinricius: Archiv. f. Gyn., LXXIV, S. 292.

9. Bumm: Centralblatt f. Gyn., 1893, S. 975.

10. Bail: Archiv. f. Hygiene, 1905, Bd. LII, S. 272.

11. Ullrich: Græfe's Archiv. f. Ophthalmol., 1904, LVIII, S. 243.

12. Kruse: Ziegler's Beiträge, 1893, Bd. XII, S. 333.

13. Kikuchi: Archiv. f. Hygiene, 1905, Bd. LII, S. 378.

14. Weil: Archiv. f. Hygiene (In press).

15. Hoke: Zeitschr. f. Hygiene, 1905, Bd. L, S. 541.

—— Wiener klin. Wochen., 1905, 1906, XVIII, Nr. 14, XIX, Nr. 2.

16. Salus: Wiener klin. Wochenschr., 1905, Nr. 25.

NOTES ON NEW BOOKS.

Operative Gynecology. By HOWARD A. KELLY, Professor of Gynecological Surgery in the Johns Hopkins University and Gynecologist-in-Chief of the Johns Hopkins Hospital. Illustrations for the most part by MAX BROEDEL, Associate Professor of Art Applied to Medicine in the Johns Hopkins University. Two volumes, pp. 680, 656. (*New York and London: D. Appleton & Co., 1906.*)

The appearance of Kelly's Operative Gynecology marked a new era in Gynecology. Coming with the excellent illustrations by Broedel and Becker, at the time when pelvic surgery had just made great strides, it became the standard work on the subject and to-day is to be found in all parts of the world. Since the appearance of this work, nine years have elapsed, and in the interim much progress has been made.

In the second edition we find many changes. Much old matter has been eliminated and still more new inserted. There is a total net increase of over two-hundred pages of text.

The general appearance of the work is not as pleasing as was that of the first edition. Many of the illustrations are hazy, and do not come out clearly. The printing on one side of the page occasionally shows through on the other side and the margins on the page have been cut down to the limit. All these failings can be readily overcome in the next printing, and we would strongly advise the publishers to use much less ink, more paper, and to pay the necessary attention to the careful underlaying of the illustrations. Even with such poor printing the illustrations are much better than those usually found in medical books. No firm in America has done more exquisite medical book work than did D. Appleton & Co., in Kelly's first edition, and in Cullen's Cancer of the Uterus, and we are anxious to see them maintain the high standard they have set publishers in this country. The binding is much more satisfactory in the new edition.

A short and practical chapter on local and pathological treatment has been added.

The chapter dealing with menstruation and its anomalies is most instructive and well merits a thorough perusal as does also the section dealing with pessaries. In later years we have been inclined to discard pessaries entirely. Their indications are certainly limited, but in some individuals the introduction of a suitable pessary completely relieves the annoying train of nervous phenomena.

The chapter on anæsthesia is well up to date, but the pages of this edition went to press before the simple drop method of administration of ether had been adopted in the clinic. In this method the ether is given in a manner similar to chloroform. There is no asphyxia and little nausea is encountered afterward.

The chapters on vaginal cysts and on Bartholin's glands have been re-written and are well illustrated.

The author has fundamentally changed his method of operating on complete perineal tears. The first and essential point is to dissect out clearly the sphincter ends and to approximate them. This method of treatment has been most satisfactory and the illustrations clearly depict the various steps in the operation.

When Operative Gynecology was published the so-called "scratch mark" method of diagnosing renal or ureteral calculi was still in the experimental stage. A perusal of the second edition will thoroughly convince the reader that this method is a most valuable one, and that it has stood the severest test.

A chapter on the use of the X-ray in detecting calculi has been added. This is unusually interesting and should be read by all physicians and surgeons.

In the chapter dealing with suspension of the uterus, the author gives the after results in a great many of his cases, and frankly discusses the merits and drawbacks in the operation. This chapter should be carefully read by all who deal with retro-displacement of the uterus.

In the chapter on pelvic abscess, we would suggest leaving out Figure 423, showing a sharp pointed scissors piercing the vaginal vault to enter the abscess. It seems preferable to make a transverse incision through the vaginal mucosa just posterior to the cervix and then peal it back toward the abscess as far as possible with a gloved finger. A uterine dilator or a long pair of artery forceps will then readily puncture the abscess, but can in no way injure a loop of gut that may perchance get in the way. This blunt method has been frequently used in Dr. Kelly's clinic for over ten years.

Bisection of the uterus in myoma cases is clearly described, and its use in densely adherent cases also fully dealt with.

The chapter on cancer of the uterus has been thoroughly revised and brought up to date. It gives not only a clear idea of the operative treatment, but also the essential pathological findings. To the chapter on extra-uterine pregnancy much of interest has been added.

The value of this work lies in the fact that it represents the crystalized ideas obtained by careful handling of a vast amount of clinical material coming under the observation of the author and his associates.

The writer has to a great extent developed the technique of hysterectomy for myomata; has by his splitting operation rendered it possible for us to remove the densely adherent pelvis structures that heretofore defied operation; has step after step explored the urinary passages in the female until the diagnosis of renal diseases has become relatively easy; and has finally given us the best instruments for the exploration of the rectum. No other man in America has done as much to advance abdominal surgery as the accomplished author of these volumes.

The first edition of Operative Gynecology was enthusiastically received by the profession at home and abroad. This new edition with its careful revision and its new chapters dealing with subjects met with so frequently by general practitioners will have an even wider sphere of usefulness.

A Compend of Operative Gynecology. By WILLIAM S. BAINBRIDGE, M. D., and HAROLD D. MEEKER, M. D. (*New York: The Grafton Press, Publishers, 1906.*)

This little compend appears to be just what its authors, in the preface, claim it to be, " A brief and necessarily incomplete aid to students taking the course in operative gynecology on the cadaver." It gives, in a very few words, the salient points in the technic, and after treatment of nearly all gynecological operations. There is also brief mention made of several general surgical principals, such as the proper use of instruments, placing of sutures, and control of hemorrhage.

As a guide for the beginner in operative work on the cadaver the book is of value.

Physical Diagnosis. By RICHARD C. CABOT. Third Revised Edition. (*New York: Wm. Wood & Co., 1905.*)

This book is designed for the practitioner. It differs, however, from most books in that it is not filled with technical data and methods beyond the ordinary medical man. It takes up and emphasizes such methods as should be commonly employed.

The author endeavors to break down the distinction between clinical and laboratory diagnosis. The important methods of investigation are grouped together irrespective of clinical or laboratory procedure. As one studies the book one feels that he is getting the personal experiences and opinions of the author and not merely a collection of facts. We are given what he believes to be the most general and useful methods.

The classification of the various subjects is upon an anatomical basis The author first treats of the diseases of the head and then in turn takes up each portion of the body.

The book is a valuable one and especially so to the general practitioner.

A Text-Book of Genito-Urinary Diseases, Including Functional Sexual Disorders in Man. By Dr. Leopold Casper. Translated and Edited with Additions by Charles W. Bonney, B. L., M. D. *(Philadelphia: P. Blakiston's Son & Co., 1906.)*

Several years of service have proven the usefulness of Casper's text-book and there is no doubt about the wisdom of extending this usefulness by making the book available for English speaking students. The particular need of a good text-book of genito-urinary diseases is apparent to any one working in this field, who is sure to have had cause to lament that it is supplied in this respect, rather well than wisely. No one could, however, claim that Casper has written an ideal text-book. It labors, .for one thing, under the handicap due to the rather anomalous position in which genito-urinary surgery finds itself; and it must certainly appeal to custom or arbitrary selection, rather than to logic to explain why a text-book of genito-urinary diseases, which treats of syphilis of the prostate, of the testicle, of the urethra, and of the kidney should have no word to say of the primary venereal sore itself; or why chancroid should be treated in detail and chancre not at all. The author has consciously, though hardly logically, eleminated this from the field; one is thankful, at any rate, that he has not produced a verbose discussion of the venereal diseases such as is to be found in the text-book of White and Martin. The book is concise and should be very useful for students. One notices slight defects here and there (for instance the scant consideration given to the work of Metz and Bartrina in explaining urinary infiltration of the perineum); but the excellences far outweigh them.

The translation is fairly satisfactory. It is not, however, always smooth; in some cases it is exceedingly careless; and the text is marred by wretched proof-reading. "But yet," it is hardly an elegant rendering of "aber"; and "composition" (p. 1905) can hardly be said to give the meaning of "Zersetzung." Nor are words like these particularly pleasing to the eye: shpincter, Musie Guyon, tuberculousis, tensemus, displococcus, anterio-sclerotic. "Qui vide" may suggest the sense of "Siehe diese," but is hardly Latin that one could call classic. These, and numerous other small mistakes, should be corrected in the second edition of this book, which will doubtless be called for. The attention of the American editor is drawn to the following sentence on page 208, which demands correction in a future edition: "A large number of drugs, among which may be mentioned salicylic, benzoic, camphoric, carbolic and boric acid, potassium chlorate, and nitrate, the balsamics, arbutin (the active principle of uva ursa), salol, urotropin, and helmitol."

The additions which Dr. Bonney has made to the German edition have distinctly increased the value of the book.

Infection, Immunity, and Serum Therapy. By H. T. Ricketts, M. D., Instructor in Pathology, University of Chicago. *(Chicago: Journal of the American Medical Association, 1906.)*

Only good words should be spoken of this excellent short treatise on the etiology and nature of the infectious diseases. The material has been selected with excellent critical judgment, and the important points of this rather complicated and somewhat confusing subject are presented with great clear-

ness and lucidity. It is the one work of which we know, dealing with the question of infection and immunity in this way, except the very large comprehensive work of Kolle and Wassermann, *"Handbuch der pathogenen Mikroorganismen,"* which is too extensive except for the specialist, and is accessible only to readers of German. While the size of Dr. Rickett's book prevents a very comprehensive treatment, this book will prove very satisfactory to any one desiring a short survey of the subject, but in which the latest ideas are presented. The author has very wisely refrained from attempting to give an extensive bibliography. An inspection of the book, however, reveals the wide reading of the author, and shows his thorough knowledge of the whole subject.

We feel that the first or general portion of the book is more valuable than the second or special one, as it is manifestly very difficult to discuss the nature of infection, immunity, etc., of each disease in the few pages devoted to it. Bacteriology as often taught in the medical schools deals too much with the cultural characteristics of the various bacteria, and the student feels sometimes that the last word has been said in regard to the specific infections when the etiological agent has been described and its cultural characteristics ascertained; he forgets that this is but the initial step, and that the discovery of the process by which the organism produces the infection, the way in which the symptoms are produced and the manner in which immunity is brought about is of still greater importance in extending our real knowledge of the disease. Much work has been done along these lines and more is being accomplished, and this book will be of great value in bringing this aspect of the subject and these problems to the attention of students and practitioners.

Some criticism might be made of the effort to classify the infectious diseases on the basis of the nature of the immunity, since in so many of these our knowledge on this point is still obscure. The author fully recognizes, however, that this classification is "provisional and imperfect."

The work first appeared as a series of articles published in the Journal of the American Medical Association, and forms one of the excellent series of articles published by this journal upon medical topics of paramount interest. This mode of publication and the fact that the plates were not recast made necessary the wide page margins, and so renders the book much more bulky than it would otherwise be, and detracts from its otherwise typographical excellence. This is not a serious fault, however, and to some may add to the book's attractiveness.

Both the author and the publishers are to be congratulated upon the production of such an excellent and valuable presentation of this important subject.

Operative Otology. Surgical Pathology and Treatment of Diseases of the Ear. By Clarence John Blake, M. D., and Henry Ottridge Reik, M. D. *(New York and London: D. Appleton & Co., 1906.)*

This book fills a place long vacant in the literature of otology and is sure to find favor at the hands of otologists. Some of the chapters are not excelled by any work of the same scope in otology. Take as an instance the chapter entitled, "Middle-Ear Operations,' which is the clearest and best treatise we have yet seen. The chapter on "Aseptic. Technique" is also well written. All in all the book is a very creditable piece of work.

While we are willing to grant that there must be some overlapping of certain specialties, we cannot help taking exception to the very broad statement of the authors as to the relations of the otologist to brain surgery. It seems hardly proper to censure the general surgeon for entering the mastoid and at the same time advise the otologist to enter the brain. If it is a sin for the general surgeon to perform operations for the relief of mastoiditis, it is equally a sin for the otologist to explore the brain

In searching for the evil consequences of ear diseases. The most serious criticism, however, of the book is that it is incomplete. While this in no manner lessens its value as a reference book, it would materially restrict its usefulness as a text-book for students and general practitioners.

Operative Treatment of Prolapse and Retroversion of the Uterus. By J. INGLIS PARSONS, M. D., M. R. C. P., M. R. C. S. (*London: John Bale, Sons & Danielsson, Ltd., 1906.*)

In this monograph the author gives the results of his experience during twenty years at a special hospital for women. The anatomy of the pelvis in relation to prolapse and the relative value of the general anatomical elements in keeping the uterus in its normal position, are briefly considered in the first chapters. The etiology, the various stages of these displacements and the non-operative as well as operative treatment are discussed.

The author's views are, in general, those commonly accepted by conservative surgeons. His method of treating prolapse by injecting some irritating substance into the base of the broad ligament, however, appeals to a surgeon only as a make-shift; but his results are excellent and compare well with those obtained by other means. In non-operative cases the injection should certainly be given a trial.

Suspension of a prolapsed and painful ovary to the uterine cornu, if no disease is present, is to be preferred to removal, as advocated by the author.

There is as yet no unanimity of opinion as to the best operation for retroversion of the uterus. The author discusses the merits of three procedures—ventrosuspension, intraperitoneal shortening of the round ligaments, Alexander's operation—giving the preference to ventrosuspension.

The Surgery of the Diseases of the Appendix Vermiformis and their Complications. By WILLIAM HENRY BATTLE and ELDRED M. CORNER. 8vo. 203 pp. (*Chicago: W. T. Keener & Co.*)

This small book of two hundred pages by two St. Thomas Hospital surgeons is chiefly interesting to American surgeons, because it represents an English view of the treatment of this common disease. It covers the subject in a concise way from the history of appendicitis to its relations with life insurance. It is well written and printed, but rather poorly illustrated.

A few extracts will be of interest: "It has been and is the custom to treat cases of appendicitis with milk, beef tea, etc., as food, rest in bed, fomentations to the abdomen, doses of opium, etc. With regard to the opium the least possible amount should be given."

"If the case is seen shortly after the onset and the vomiting allows of it, a purgative is a good thing." "Whilst we do not urge immediate and therefore clinically indiscriminate operations, as the diagnosis will be in some cases most uncertain, we do urge that the decision for surgical procedure should be formed, whenever possible, within forty-eight hours of the onset. . . . . Of course this is difficult and implies that the case will have been seen, perhaps, more than once within forty-eight hours of the onset."

"Far be it from us to recommend anything like indiscriminate operations as then doubtless many cases of other abdominal diseases, or even pneumonia, would be subjected to a needless appendicectomy, but in some cases it is better to advise early operation than to risk waiting."

In removing the appendix, they advise crushing of the base of the appendix with a special clamp, which divides the mucous membrane and muscular coats, leaving the "peritoneal" surfaces in apposition for about one-third of an inch. The stump is tied off with fine silk and inverted.

They advise entering the abdomen through the Battle incision, which is described in detail, and recommend the early opening of abscesses. If the appendix is not removed at the time of operation in abscess cases, a later operation for the removal of the appendix is urged. In general peritonitis, they clean the abdominal cavity by irrigation.

OMAR PANCOAST.

A Manual of Otology. By GORHAM BACON, A. B., M. D., Professor of Otology in the College of Physicians and Surgeons, Columbia University, New York; Aural Surgeon, New York Eye and Ear Infirmary. Fourth edition, revised and enlarged. (*New York and Philadelphia: Lea Brothers & Co., 1906.*)

The previous editions of this book have been favorably mentioned in these columns, and we congratulate the author upon a degree of success, which has demanded four editions within eight years. The work is concise, well illustrated, and prepared in a way to appeal especially to the undergraduate student. This last edition contains a number of improvements. Nearly all of the new pictures are helpful; we would take exception only to one plate, that which purports to give the appearances of the tympanic membrane under varying circumstances; our objection to it is that the colors are not true to life.

Among the new topics introduced into this volume are Osteomyelitis, Primary Jugular Bulb Thrombosis, and Suppurative Labyrinthitis, all of which are treated of briefly, yet with perhaps sufficient fullness to impress their importance upon the student. The only feature of the book which we would criticise is the appendix dealing with the examination of pathologic aural secretions; this is so incomplete as to be practically useless.

The intimate relationship between affections of the ear and nasopharyngeal disease leads the author, wisely, to include a chapter on this subject and his treatment of it is in the main unquestionably correct. There is one point in it, however, which it seems to us is open to criticism. When speaking of the treatment of Hypertrophied Tonsils, it is stated that, "It is advisable to try to reduce the size of the tonsils by internal medication and by local treatment whenever possible." And again, under the head of treatment of Adenoids, "Much may be accomplished by the administration of tonics and alteratives, especially if the general health is impaired." We hope Dr. Bacon will alter this chapter before the next edition of his book for it is utterly unreasonable to expect internal medication or local medicinal applications to reduce hypertrophied tonsils or remove adenoids.

H. O. R.

A Monograph on the Anopheles Mosquitoes of India. By S. P. JAMES, M. B., Q. M. S., and W. GLEN LISTON, M. D., Q. M. S. (*Calcutta: Thacker, Spink & Co., 1904.*)

This monograph by James and Liston gives a good description of the species of anopheles found in India, where the mosquito, in its relation to disease, has been thoroughly studied.

The most complete work on mosquitoes, entomologically, is the monograph of Theobald, of England, in four volumes. Theobald has classified the sub-family anophelina, basing his generic and specific differences upon minute variations in the scales of the adult insect. James and Liston, however, say that generic classification should be based not only on adult, but also upon larval differences and this view is more and more the accepted one among entomologists.

The authors give good descriptions of the various species found in India, and make a classification of their own which includes about 80 species, but only a very few of them have been shown to be concerned in the transmission of malaria. When one tries to identify species of foreign countries with those of his own, difficulties are encountered from the fact that the nomenclature of species is by no means uniform.

Coquillet, of the Department of Agriculture, has recently published "A Classification of the Mosquitoes of North and Middle America," in which he gives five genera of anophelina, comprising 13 species, only one or two of which have been shown to transmit malaria in this country.

The work of James and Liston contains some excellent plates in colors of the species common in India.

T. H. COFFIN, M. D

A System of Physiologic Therapeutics. Vol. XI. Serum Therapy; Organotherapy; Radium, Thorium, and Radioactivity; Counterirritation, External Applications, Bloodletting; An Outline of the Principles of Therapeutics with Especial Reference to Physiologic Therapeutics; Addendum on X-Ray Therapy; An Index-Digest of the Complete System of Eleven Volumes. Edited by SOLOMON SOLIS COHEN, A. M., M. D. (*Philadelphia: P. Blakiston's Son & Co., 1905.*)

In this, the concluding volume of the system, perhaps the most interesting article is that by the editor, Dr. Cohen, on "The Principles of Therapeutics with Especial Reference to Physiologic Therapeutics." In this he discusses the general principles which most govern all treatment. The views here expressed are those which should guide us in the methods of treating patients and diseases. Unfortunately, many of the profession never realize them and there are too many who having known them, forget to carry them into practice. We are all too apt to associate special remedies with particular diseases and lose sight of the general principles by which all treatment should be directed. To read such a section as Dr. Cohen has written, serves to impress this, and it would be an excellent thing if the profession could have such an article brought to its attention frequently.

Of the articles in this volume, Joseph McFarland contributes that on "Serum Therapy" and Oliver T. Osborne on "Organotherapy;" they are both well worthy of study. The subject of "Radium, Thorium, and Radioactivity," is dealt with by Samuel G. Tracy, and in addition there is an addendum on "X-Ray Therapy," which discusses much of the newer work.

The section on "Counterirritation, External Applications, and Bloodletting" was written by the late Frederick A. Packard. He discusses clearly the various methods, many of which might well be more used at the present day. There is a complete index-digest to the volumes of the system occupying somewhat over a hundred pages, which adds greatly to the value of the work.

There is one matter to be mentioned, namely, the weight of the book. It seems unfortunate that it has not been possible to have used lighter paper. However, this is a detail that may depend largely on one's individual preference, and there may be readers who prefer the heavy volume.

International Clinics. Edited by A. J. O. KELLY, M. D., Vol. III. 16th Series. (*Philadelphia: J. B. Lippincott Co., 1906.*)

In this volume of clinical lectures which maintains the high level of excellence of its predecessors are to be found several articles of exceptional interest. To those who have read Fournier's classical works on lues, the article by Dr. Saingery on "Professor Fournier's Recent Modification of His Treatment of Syphilis" will specially appeal. Dr. Fournier recommends to-day a more interrupted course of treatment than heretofore; formerly his advice was to continue the administration of mercury and iodide for three successive years after the primary infection with short intermissions. He now advises that after the first two years an interval of two years be allowed to pass without any medication when it is again actively resumed for a year; and after a pause of one or two years more, the same treatment as earlier be resumed again for a year. In this manner he believes that paresis is more surely escaped as a late manifestation.

Another admirable lecture, the value of which is much enhanced by good illustrations is by Dr. C. H. Bradford on "The Hyperæmia Treatment of Swollen Joints"; in which he demonstrates the real benefit that may be obtained in some cases of stiff joints from the use of very hot dry air.

"Life in the Antarctic from a Medical Point of View," by Dr. J. H. Harvey Pirie, will interest a broad circle of readers, lay as well as medical. In these times when numerous expeditions are setting forth for one or the other pole, we cannot have too much information on all matters relating to the preservation of the health and care of the men, who risk their lives in these ventures.

The last paper in the volume by Dr. G. Banti on "Leukæmia and Sarcomatosis," will doubtless surprise many in its conclusion. The author says: "From these facts I hope you are convinced that the leukæmias are not hyperplasias of normal tissues, but diseases of a neoplastic nature, belonging to the vast and proteiform class of sarcomas. I am not able to explain their etiology, tho' I am convinced that they are infectious sarcomatoses, but heretofore all my researches to discover the specific agent have had a negative result." This quotation should lead all who have devoted themselves to the study of the blood in leukæmia and allied diseases, to carefully read the entire article, written as it is by an authority on the subject, and one who has gained for himself the distinction if not honor of having a disease spoken of by his name, the so-called "Banti's Disease."

This volume contains articles of equal merit, and interest for specialists in other branches than those touched upon by the reviewer, who cannot however be expected to treat in detail the two dozen or more lectures therein contained.

R. N.

INDEX TO VOLUME XVII OF THE JOHNS HOPKINS HOSPITAL BULLETIN.

ILLUSTRATIONS.

THE JOHNS HOPKINS HOSPITAL REPORTS.

VOLUME I.　423 pages, 99 plates.

VOLUME II.　570 pages, with 28 plates and figures.

VOLUME III.　766 pages, with 69 plates and figures.

VOLUME IV.　504 pages, 33 charts and illustrations.

VOLUME V.　480 pages, with 32 charts and illustrations.

CONTENTS:

The Malarial Fevers of Baltimore. By W. S. THAYER, M. D., and J. HEWETSON, M. D.

A Study of some Fatal Cases of Malaria. By LEWELLYS F. BARKER, M. B.

Studies in Typhoid Fever.

By WILLIAM OSLER, M. D., with additional papers by G. BLUMER, M. D., SIMON FLEXNER, M. D., WALTER REED, M. D., and H. C. PARSONS, M. D.

VOLUME VI.　414 pages, with 79 plates and figures.

Report in Neurology.

Studies on the Lesions Produced by the Action of Certain Poisons on the Cortical Nerve Cell (Studies Nos. I to V). By HENRY J. BERKLEY, M. D.

Introductory.—Recent Literature on the Pathology of Diseases of the Brain by the Chromate of Silver Methods; Part I.—Alcohol Poisoning.—Experimental Lesions produced by Chronic Alcoholic Poisoning (Ethyl Alcohol). 2. Experimental Lesions produced by Acute Alcoholic Poisoning (Ethyl Alcohol); Part II.—Serum Poisoning.—Experimental Lesions induced by the Action of the Dog's Serum on the Cortical Nerve Cell; Part III.—Ricin Poisoning.—Experimental Lesions induced by Acute Ricin Poisoning. 2. Experimental Lesions induced by Chronic Ricin Poisoning; Part IV.—Hydrophobic Toxæmia.—Lesions of the Cortical Nerve Cell produced by the Toxine of Experimental Rabies; Part V.—Pathological Alterations in the Nuclei and Nucleoli of Nerve Cells from the Effects of Alcohol and Ricin Intoxication; Nerve Fibre Terminal Apparatus; Asthenic Bulbar Paralysis. By HENRY J. BERKLEY, M. D.

Report in Pathology.

Fatal Puerperal Sepsis due to the Introduction of an Elm Tent. By THOMAS S. CULLEN, M.B.

Pregnancy in a Rudimentary Uterine Horn. Rupture, Death, Probable Migration of Ovum and Spermatozoa. By THOMAS S. CULLEN, M. B., and G. L. WILKINS, M. D.

Adeno-Myoma Uteri Diffusum Benignum. By THOMAS S. CULLEN, M. B.

A Bacteriological and Anatomical Study of the Summer Diarrhœas of Infants. By WILLIAM D. BOOKER, M. D.

The Pathology of Toxalbumin Intoxications. By SIMON FLEXNER, M. D.

VOLUME VII.　537 pages with illustrations.

I. A Critical Review of Seventeen Hundred Cases of Abdominal Section from the standpoint of Intra-peritoneal Drainage. By J. G. CLARK, M. D.

II. The Etiology and Structure of true Vaginal Cysts. By JAMES ERNEST STOKES, M. D.

III. A Review of the Pathology of Superficial Burns, with a Contribution to our Knowledge of the Pathological Changes in the Organs in cases of rapidly fatal burns. By CHARLES RUSSELL BARDEEN, M. D.

IV. The Origin, Growth and Fate of the Corpus Luteum. By J. G. CLARK, M. D.

V. The Results of Operations for the Cure of Inguinal Hernia. By JOSEPH C. BLOODGOOD, M. D.

VOLUME VIII.　552 pages with illustrations.

On the role of Insects, Arachnids, and Myriapods as carriers in the spread of Bacterial and Parasitic Diseases of Man and Animals. By GEORGE H. F. NUTTALL, M. D., PH. D.

Studies in Typhoid Fever.

By WILLIAM OSLER, M. D., with additional papers by J. M. T. FINNEY, M. D., S. FLEXNER, M. D., I. P. LYON, M. D., L. P. HAMBURGER, M. D., H. W. CUSHING, M. D., J. F. MITCHELL, M. D., C. N. B. CAMAC, M. D., N. B. GWYN, M. D., CHARLES P. EMERSON, M. D., H. H. YOUNG, M. D., and W. S. THAYER, M. D.

VOLUME IX.　1060 pages, 66 plates and 210 other illustrations.

Contributions to the Science of Medicine.

Dedicated by his Pupils to WILLIAM HENRY WELCH, on the twenty-fifth anniversary of his Doctorate. This volume contains 38 separate papers.

VOLUME X.　516 pages, 12 plates and 25 charts.

Structure of the Malarial Parasites, Plate I. By JESSE W. LAZEAR, M. D.

The Bacteriology of Cystitis, Pyelitis and Pyelonephritis in Women, with a Consideration of the Accessory Etiological Factors in these Conditions, and of the Various Chemical and Microscopical Questions involved. By THOMAS R. BROWN, M. D.

Cases of Infection with Strongyloides Intestinalis. (First Reported Occurrence in North America.) Plates II and III. By RICHARD P. STRONG, M. D.

On the Pathological Changes in Hodgkin's Disease, with Especial Reference to its Relation to Tuberculosis. Plates IV-VII. By DOROTHY M. REED, M. D.

Diabetes Insipidus, with a Report of Five Cases. By THOMAS B. FUTCHER, M. B. (Tor.).

Observations on the Origin and Occurrence of Cells with Eosinophile Granulations in Normal and Pathological Tissues. Plate VIII. By W. T. HOWARD, M. D., and R. G. PERKINS, M. D.

Placental Transmissions, with Report of a Case during Typhoid Fever. By FRANK W. LYNCH, M. D.

Metabolism in Albuminuria. By CHAS. P. EMERSON, A. B., M. D.

Regenerative Changes in the Liver after Acute Yellow Atrophy. Plates IX-XII. By W. G. MACCALLUM, M. D.

Surgical Features of Typhoid Fever. By THOS. McCRAE, M. B., M. R. C. P. (Lond.), and JAMES F. MITCHELL, M. D.

The Symptoms, Diagnosis and Surgical Treatment of Ureteral Calculus. By BENJAMIN R. SCHENCK, M. D.

VOLUME XI.　555 pages, with 38 charts and illustrations.

Pneumothorax: A historical, clinical and experimental study. By CHARLES P. EMERSON, M. D.

Clinical Observations on Blood Pressure. By HENRY W. COOK, M. D., and JOHN B. BRIGGS, M. D.

The value of Tuberculin in Surgical Diagnosis. By MARTIN B. TINKER, M. D.

VOLUME XII.　548 pages, 12 plates and other illustrations.

The Connective Tissue of the Salivary Glands and Pancreas with its Development in the Glandula Submaxillaris. By JOSEPH MARSHALL FLINT, M. D.

A New Instrument for Determining the Minimum and Maximum Blood-Pressures in Man. Plates IV-X. By JOSEPH ERLANGER, M. D.

Metabolism in Pregnancy, Labor and the Puerperium. By J. MORRIS SLEMONS, M. D.

An Experimental Study of Blood-Pressure and of Pulse-Pressure in Man. Plates XI and XII. By JOSEPH ERLANGER, M. D., and DONALD R. HOOKER, A. B., M. S.

Typhoid Meningitis. By RUFUS I. COLE, M. D.

The Pathological Anatomy of Meningitis due to Bacillus Typhosus. By WILLIAM G. MACCALLUM, M. D.

A Comparative Study of White and Negro Pelves, with a Consideration of the Size of the Child and Its Relation to Presentation and Character of Labor in the Two Races. By THEODORE F. RIGGS, M. D.

Renal Tuberculosis. By GEORGE WALKER, M. D.

The set of twelve volumes will be sold for $65 net. Volume II will not be sold separately. Volumes I, III, IV, V, VI, VII, VIII, X, XI and XII will be sold for $5 in paper and $5.50 cloth, net, each. Volume IX will be sold for $10 net.

VOLUME XIII.　(In press.) About 584 pages, with 201 figures in the text, 2 plates, and 1 colored chart.

Studies in Genito-Urinary Surgery.

VOLUME XIV.　(In press.) About 632 pages, with 97 figures in the text.

Studies in Genito-Urinary Surgery.

Orders should be addressed to The Johns Hopkins Press, Baltimore, Md.

The Johns Hopkins Hospital Bulletins are issued monthly. They are printed by the FRIEDENWALD CO., Baltimore. Single copies may be procured from NUNN & CO. and the BALTIMORE NEWS CO., Baltimore. Subscriptions, $2.00 a year (foreign postage 50 cents), may be addressed to the publishers, THE JOHNS HOPKINS PRESS, BALTIMORE; single copies will be sent by mail for twenty-five cents each.

Lightning Source UK Ltd.
Milton Keynes UK
UKHW011204240219
337912UK00010B/550/P

9 781397 313195